VOLUME FOUR

CAMPBELL'S
OPERATIVE ORTHOPAEDICS

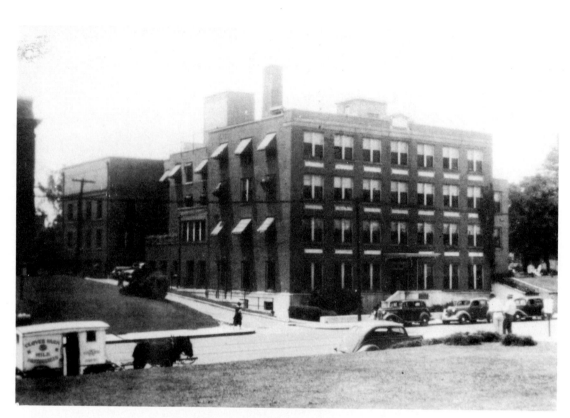

The Campbell Clinic circa 1938

VOLUME FOUR

Seventh Edition

CAMPBELL'S OPERATIVE ORTHOPAEDICS

Edited by
A.H. CRENSHAW

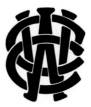

with 6917 illustrations and 8 color plates

The C. V. Mosby Company

ST. LOUIS • WASHINGTON, D.C. • TORONTO   1987

A TRADITION OF PUBLISHING EXCELLENCE

Acquisition editor: Eugenia A. Klein
Developmental editor: Kathryn H. Falk
Project editor: Teri Merchant
Editing and production: Robert A. Kelly,
    Mary G. Stueck, Suzanne C. Glazer
Design: John Rokusek

SEVENTH EDITION

The C.V. Mosby Company
11830 Westline Industrial Drive, St. Louis, Missouri 63146

Library of Congress Cataloging-in-Publication Data

Campbell, Willis C. (Willis Cohoon), 1880-1941.
  Campbell's operative orthopaedics.

  Includes bibliographies and index.
  1. Orthopedic surgery. I. Crenshaw, A. H. (Andrew
Hoyt), 1920-   . II. Title. III. Title: Operative
orthopaedics.   [DNLM: 1. Orthopedics.   WE 168 C192o]
RD731.C28   1987   617′.3   86-23562
ISBN 0-8016-1065-6

C/VH/VH 9 8 7 6 5 4 3 2 1   02/A/210

Contributors

JAMES H. BEATY, M.D.

Chapters 61, 62, and 63

Clinical Assistant Professor of Orthopaedic Surgery, University of Tennessee, Memphis, Tenn.; Chief, Tennessee Crippled Children's Service; Active Staff, Campbell Clinic, Baptist Memorial Hospital, LeBonheur Children's Medical Center, Regional Medical Center at Memphis, University of Tennessee Medical Center/William F. Bowld Hospital; Consultant Staff, Veterans Administration Medical Center, Arlington Developmental Center.

ROCCO A. CALANDRUCCIO, M.D.

Chapter 41

Professor of Orthopaedic Surgery and Chairman of Department of Orthopaedic Surgery, University of Tennessee, Memphis, Tenn.; Chief of Staff Emeritus, Campbell Clinic; Active Staff, Baptist Memorial Hospital, Regional Medical Center at Memphis; Consultant Staff, University of Tennessee Medical Center/William F. Bowld Hospital.

S. TERRY CANALE, M.D.

Chapters 36, 47, and 55

Clinical Associate Professor of Orthopaedic Surgery, University of Tennessee, Memphis, Tenn.; Chief of Pediatric Orthopaedics, LaBonheur Children's Medical Center; Active Staff, Campbell Clinic, Baptist Memorial Hospital, and Regional Medical Center at Memphis.

PETER G. CARNESALE, M.D.

Chapters 26 through 34

Clinical Associate Professor of Orthopaedic Surgery, University of Tennessee, Memphis, Tenn.; Active Staff, Campbell Clinic, Baptist Memorial Hospital, and Regional Medical Center at Memphis; Consultant Staff, St. Joseph Hospital, LeBonheur Children's Medical Center, St. Jude Children's Research Hospital, and Veteran's Administration Medical Center; Courtesy Staff, Methodist Hospital.

A.H. CRENSHAW, M.D.

Chapters 1, 2, and 49

Clinical Professor of Orthopaedic Surgery, University of Tennessee, Memphis, Tenn.; Active Staff, Campbell Clinic, Baptist Memorial Hospital and Regional Medical Center at Memphis; Consultant Staff, Methodist Hospital; Associate Staff, LeBonheur Children's Medical Center.

ALLEN S. EDMONSON, M.D.

Chapters 68, 70, 71, and 72

Clinical Professor of Orthopaedic Surgery, University of Tennessee, Memphis, Tenn.; Active Staff, Campbell Clinic, Baptist Memorial Hospital, Regional Medical Center at Memphis and LeBonheur Children's Medical Center.

BARNEY L. FREEMAN III, M.D.

Chapters 50, 51, 52, and 69

Clinical Assistant Professor of Orthopaedic Surgery, University of Tennessee, Memphis, Tenn.; Active Staff, Campbell Clinic, Baptist Memorial Hospital, Regional Medical Center at Memphis; Consultant Staff, LeBonheur Children's Medical Center, and Veterans Administration Medical Center.

ALVIN J. INGRAM, M.D.

Chapter 66

Professor and Chairman Emeritus, Department of Orthopaedic Surgery, University of Tennessee, Memphis, Tenn.; Chief of Staff Emeritus, Campbell Clinic; Orthopaedic Consultant, Richards Medical Company; Emeritus Staff, Baptist Memorial Hospital and LeBonheur Children's Medical Center.

E. JEFF JUSTIS, JR., M.D.

Chapters 53 and 54

Clinical Associate Professor of Orthopaedic Surgery, University of Tennessee, Memphis, Tenn.; Active Staff, Campbell Clinic, Baptist Memorial Hospital, Regional Medical Center at Memphis; Consultant Staff, Arlington Developmental Center, LeBonheur Children's Medical Center, Veterans Administration Medical Center; Courtesy Staff, Methodist Hospital; Consultant to the Surgeon-General, United States Air Force; Consultant in Hand Surgery, Mississippi and Tennessee Crippled Children's Services.

DAVID G. LAVELLE, M.D.

Chapter 41 (Section on Deep Venous Thrombosis and Pulmonary Embolism)

Clinical Instructor of Orthopaedic Surgery, University of Tennessee, Memphis, Tenn.; Active Staff, Campbell Clinic, Baptist Memorial Hospital, Regional Medical Center at Memphis, University of Tennessee Medical Center/William F. Bowld Hospital; Consultant Staff, LeBonheur Children's Medical Center and Veterans Administration Medical Center.

LEE MILFORD, M.D.

Chapters 3 through 20

Clinical Professor of Orthopaedic Surgery, University of Tennessee, Memphis, Tenn., Chief of Staff, Campbell Clinic; Active Staff, Baptist Memorial Hospital and Regional Medical Center at Memphis; Consultant Staff, University of Tennessee Medical Center/William F. Bowld Hospital.

E. GREER RICHARDSON, M.D.

Chapters 35, 37, and 44 (section on Foot and Ankle)

Clinical Associate Professor of Orthopaedic Surgery, University of Tennessee, Memphis, Tenn.; Active Staff, Campbell Clinic, Baptist Memorial Hospital, University of Tennessee Hospital, and Regional Medical Center at Memphis; Consultant Staff, Veterans Administration Medical Center and University of Tennessee Medical Center/William F. Bowld Hospital; Courtesy Staff, LeBonheur Children's Medical Center.

THOMAS A. RUSSELL, M.D.

Chapters 38, 39, and 48

Clinical Instructor of Orthopaedic Surgery, University of Tennessee, Memphis, Tenn.; Chief of Orthopaedic Service, Presley Trauma Center; Active Staff, Campbell Clinic, Baptist Memorial Hospital, Regional Medical Center at Memphis, University of Tennessee Medical Center/ William F. Bowld Hospital, Consultant Staff, Veterans Administration Medical Center.

FRED P. SAGE, M.D.

Chapters 65 and 67

Clinical Professor of Orthopaedic Surgery, University of Tennessee, Memphis, Tenn.; Active Staff, Campbell Clinic, Baptist Memorial Hospital, and Regional Medical Center at Memphis; Chief of Staff, Crippled Children's Hospital; Consultant Staff, LeBonheur Children's Medical Center and Methodist Hospital.

T. DAVID SISK, M.D.

Chapters 42, 43, 44, 45, 46, 56, 58, 59, and 60

Clinical Professor of Orthopaedic Surgery, University of Tennessee, Memphis, Tenn.; Active Staff, Campbell Clinic, Baptist Memorial Hospital, LeBonheur Children's Medical Center, and Regional Medical Center at Memphis.

ROBERT E. TOOMS, M.D.

Chapters 22, 23, 24, 25, and 40

Professor of Orthopaedic Surgery, University of Tennessee, Memphis, Tenn.; Active Staff, Campbell Clinic, Baptist Memorial Hospital; Consultant Staff, LeBonheur Children's Medical Center and Regional Medical Center at Memphis; Medical Director, University of Tennessee Rehabilitation Engineering Center; Medical Director, Regional Spinal Cord Injury Center; Chief, Child Amputee Clinic and St. Jude Amputee Clinic.

GEORGE W. WOOD II, M.D.

Chapters 70, 73, 74, and 75

Clinical Associate Professor of Orthopaedic Surgery, University of Tennessee, Memphis, Tenn.; Active Staff, Campbell Clinic, Baptist Memorial Hospital, Regional Medical Center at Memphis; Consultant Staff, LeBonheur Children's Medical Center, Veterans Administration Medical Center, University of Tennessee Medical Center/William F. Bowld Hospital.

PHILLIP E. WRIGHT, M.D.

Chapters 21, 42, 57, and 64

Clinical Associate Professor of Orthopaedic Surgery, University of Tennessee, Memphis, Tenn.; Chief, Hand Surgery Service, Regional Medical Center at Memphis; Active Staff, Campbell Clinic, Baptist Memorial Hospital, and Regional Medical Center at Memphis; Consultant Staff, LeBonheur Children's Medical Center, Veterans Administration Medical Center, and Active Staff University of Tennessee Medical Center/William F. Bowld Hospital.

TO
HUGH SMITH

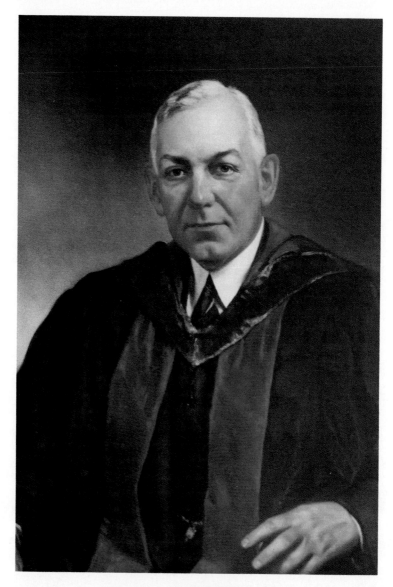

WILLIS C. CAMPBELL, M.D.

1880–1941

Preface to seventh edition

The format for this edition has been changed completely from that of previous editions. The material has been reorganized into 75 chapters divided into 17 parts for better presentation. Some chapters as such have been deleted and new ones on microsurgery, fractures in children, osteonecrosis, foot in adolescents and adults, low back pain and disorders of intervertebral discs, arthroscopy, paralytic disorders, and inheritable progressive neuromuscular diseases have been added. All retained chapters have been rewritten or revised extensively. For the first time since the First Edition all contributors are members of the staff of the Campbell Clinic.

For ease in handling, the material is divided among four volumes instead of two. Of approximately 6900 illustrations, 3000 are new. Included are eight four-color plates.

We have continued to use almost entirely the method of measuring joint motion that has been advocated by the American Academy of Orthopaedic Surgeons. The neutral

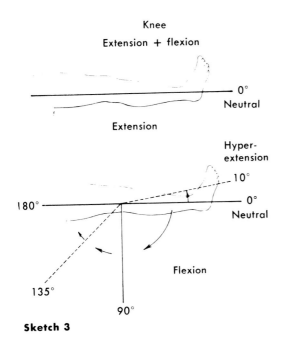

Sketch 1

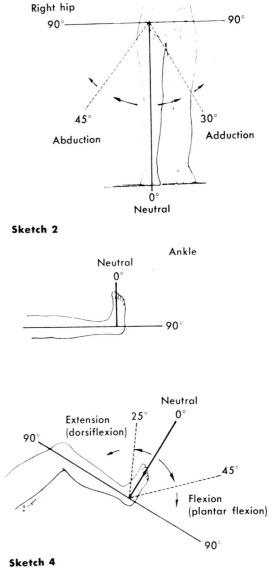

Sketch 2

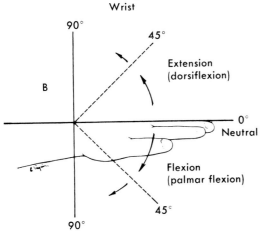

Sketch 3

Sketch 4

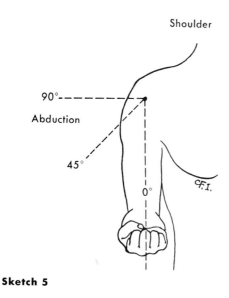

Sketch 5

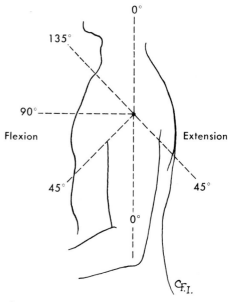

Sketch 6

position is 0 degrees instead of 180 degrees as in the first three editions (see sketches 1 through 4*). For the shoulder, however, the method of the Academy seems too complicated for adoption here. Although the neutral position is 0 degrees as for other joints, the direction of movement in adduction, abduction, flexion, and extension is the same as that used in previous editions (see sketches 5 and 6).

The editor and other members of the staff of the clinic

*Reproduced by courtesy of the American Academy of Orthopaedic Surgeons.

wish to thank Lee Danley, Richard Fritzler, Sarah C. McQueen, Rick Mendius, and Rivers Wilkinson for their artwork for this edition.

I wish especially to express my appreciation to Kay Daugherty, our librarian and medical editor, for her skillful help with the manuscript and references, and to Eugenia Klein, senior editor, Kathy Falk, developmental editor, and Teri Merchant, Bob Kelly, Mary Stueck, and Suzanne Glazer at C.V. Mosby for their expert help.

A.H. Crenshaw, M.D.

Preface to first edition

The title of this book, *Operative Orthopedics,* is not intended to convey the impression that the chief or most important method of treatment of orthopedic affections is open surgery. Although many orthopedic affections are best treated by operative measures alone, the majority are successfully treated by more conservative means. Further, such measures are often essential adjuncts either before or after operation.

This volume has been written to meet the current need for a comprehensive work on operative orthopedics, not only for the specialist, but also for many industrial and general surgeons who are doing excellent work in some branches of orthopedic surgery, and are making valuable contributions to this field.

The evolution of orthopedic surgery has been exceedingly slow as compared to that of surgery in general. Not until aseptic technic had been materially refined was surgery of the bones and joints feasible. The statement is often made that the World War afforded the experience which made possible the rapid development of orthopedic surgery during the past two decades. The surgery of the war, however, was chiefly the surgery of sepsis; there was little of the refined asepsis which is required in reconstruction surgery. Undoubtedly, the demonstration during the war of the necessity and importance of this field led many able men to specialize in orthopedics, and to them considerable credit is due for its subsequent progress.

No classification of orthopedic affections is entirely satisfactory; consequently, any arrangement of operative procedures is subject to similar criticism. With the exception of the chapters on Arthroplasty and Arthrodesis, operations described in this text are grouped together according to their applicability to a given affection. This involves less repetition as to generalities of etiology, pathology, and treatment than would be necessary in a classification according to anatomic location. Operative procedures appropriate to two or more affections are described in the discussion of the one wherein they are most commonly employed.

To overcome the too widespread conception of orthopedic surgery as a purely mechanical equation, an effort is made in the first chapter of this book to correlate the mechanical, surgical, and physiologic principles of orthopedic practice, and throughout the book to emphasize the practical application of these physiologic principles. A special chapter has been written on surgical technic, for the purpose of stressing certain details in preparation and aftertreatment which vary to some extent from those described in works on general surgery. A thorough knowledge of these phases of treatment is a requisite to success.

To avoid constant repetition, chapters have been included on apparatus and on surgical approaches; repeated reference is made to these chapters. The aftertreatment is given in detail for practically all operative technics. This is a most essential, yet too often neglected, factor in the success of any surgical treatment.

In giving the position or range of motion of a joint, only one system has been followed: with the exception of the ankle and wrist, the joint is in neutral position when parallel with the long axis of the body in the anteroposterior and lateral planes. As the joint proceeds from the neutral position in any direction, the number of degrees in which such movement is recorded decreases progressively from 180 to 170, 160, and so on, to the anatomic limit of motion in that particular direction. To illustrate, complete extension of the knee is 180 degrees; when the joint is flexed 30 degrees, the position is recorded as the angle formed between the component parts of the joint, i.e., the leg and thigh, or 150 degrees. Flexion to a right angle is 90 degrees, and full flexion 30 degrees. In the wrist, the joint is at 180 degrees, or in the neutral position, when midway between supination and pronation, and flexion and extension. In the ankle joint, motion is recorded as follows: the extreme of dorsiflexion, 75 degrees; right angle, 90 degrees; and the extreme of plantar flexion, 140 degrees.

In some instances, the exact end results have been given, to the best of our knowledge. So many factors are involved in any one condition, that a survey of end results can be of only questionable value unless the minute details of each case are considered. Following arthroplasty of the knee, for example, one must consider the etiology, pathology, position of the ankylosed joint, the structure of the bones comprising the joint, the distribution of the ankylosis, and the age of the patient, in estimating the end result in each case. Further, a true survey should include the results of *all* patients treated over a period of *many* years, and should be made by the surgeon himself, rather than by a group of assistants, or by correspondence.

In our private clinic and the hospitals with which we are associated, a sufficient amount of material on every phase of orthopedic surgery has been accumulated during the past twenty years or more to justify an evaluation of the various procedures. From this personal experience, we also feel that definite conclusions may be drawn in regard to the indications, contraindications, complications, and other considerations entering into orthopedic treatment. In all surgical cases, mature judgment is required for the selection of the most appropriate procedure. With this in mind, the technics which have proved most efficient in the author's experience have been given preference in the text.

In addition, after a comprehensive search of the literature, operative measures have been selected which in the judgment of the author are most practicable.

Although no attempt has been made to produce an atlas of orthopedic surgery, an effort has been made to describe those procedures which conform to mechanical and physiologic principles and will meet all individual requirements. In any work of this nature, there are sins of omission; also, many surgeons in the same field may arrive independently at the same conclusions and devise identical procedures. We have endeavored, however, to give credit where credit was due. If there are errors, correction will gladly be made. In some of the chapters we have drawn heavily from authoritative articles on special subjects; the author gratefully acknowledges his indebtedness for this material. He also wishes to thank those authors who have so graciously granted permission for the reproduction of original drawings.

In conclusion, I cannot too deeply express my sincere appreciation and gratitude to my associate, Dr. Hugh Smith, who has untiringly and most efficiently devoted practically all of his time during the past two years to collaboration with me in the compilation and preparation of material, which alone has made this work possible. I also desire to express appreciation to Dr. J. S. Speed for his collaboration on the sections on Spastic Cerebral Paralysis and Peripheral Nerve Injuries; to Dr. Harold Boyd for anatomic dissections verifying all surgical approaches described, and for his assistance in preparing the chapter on this subject; to Dr. Don Slocum for his aid in the preparation of the chapter on Physiology and Pathology; to Mrs. Allene Jefferson for her efficient editorial services, and to Mr. Ivan Summers and Mr. Charles Ingram for their excellent illustrations.

Willis C. Campbell

1939

Contents

Color Plates

PART XIV

Arthroscopy

CHAPTER 58

General principles of arthroscopy

T. David Sisk

Progress in arthroscopy, especially in arthroscopic surgery, has been particularly rapid during the past several years. The arthroscope has dramatically changed the way in which orthopaedic surgeons approach the diagnosis and treatment of a variety of joint ailments, especially those about the knee. A thorough history and physical examination supplemented by careful viewing of the joint permit a high degree of diagnostic accuracy; it is a medical dictum that the efficiency of treatment improves with the accuracy of the diagnosis. A high degree of accuracy is clearly possible once a surgeon gains experience in arthroscopic techniques. The low morbidity associated with arthroscopy makes the procedure justifiable in a variety of joint disorders as a possible adjunct to diagnosis, to determine prognosis, and as a treatment. It should be emphasized that arthroscopic procedures should serve as adjuncts to and not as replacements for thorough clinical evaluation; arthroscopy is not a substitute for clinical skills.

Recent improvements in the lens systems of arthroscopes and fiberoptic systems, in miniaturization, and in the accessory operative instruments have made therapeutic or operative arthroscopy the logical extension of diagnostic arthroscopy. Nevertheless, neither diagnostic nor operative arthroscopy is new.

HISTORY OF ARTHROSCOPY

Although crude instruments thought to have been used for viewing body cavities can be traced to ancient civili-

zations, it was not until 1805 that Philip Bozzini of Frankfurt-am-Main devised his ''Lichtleiter,'' or light conductor. Bozzini used this bifid tubular instrument primarily for viewing the vagina and rectum; it consisted of one chamber illuminated with a candle and another chamber that served as a viewing tube, the desired field for examination being illuminated by the reflected light from the candle. (Fig. 58-1).

Instruments of many types have followed the Lichtleiter. Desormaux introduced a cystoscope in 1853 (Fig. 58-2) that consisted of a series of tubes attached to a gastrogen lamp. The light source was produced by burning a mixture of turpentie and alcohol and the observer looked through a perforated concave mirror that reflected the light into the bladder and the urethra. Andrews developed a better light source in 1867 that used a magnesium filament, and Bruck, a dentist, was the first to introduce a light source using a platinum filament, which he inserted into the rectum. This device had serious disadvantages because of the heat produced by the light source. Before the discovery of electricity, reflected light provided the only means of illumination. In 1876 Nitze, a German physician, devised an instrument using a platinum loop that could be inserted into the bladder (Fig. 58-3). The platinum loop had to be cooled by water flowing around it and the instrument had a crude lens system. Light sources continued to improve at the beginning of the twentieth century with Edison's invention of the incandescent lamp, with small electric bulbs being used in cystoscopes. About 1890 Nitze was the first to photograph the interior of the bladder using a cystoscope, and by the beginning of the twentieth century, cystoscopy had become an important urologic tool.

About 1918 Professor Takagi of Tokyo became the first to examine the interior of the knee joint of a cadaver with a cystoscope. This first viewing was made with a 7.3 mm instrument, which was impractical for routine use. Over the next several years, refinements in these instruments, primarily reductions in size, increased the practicality of their use and increased the curiosity of orthopaedic surgeons. In 1921 Bircher published the results of several arthroscopic examinations of the knee using a Jacobaeus laparoscope. In 1925 Kreuscher became the first American to report on the use of the arthroscope for diagnosis of knee disorders. While working independently in 1931, Finkelstein and Mayer and Burman reported experiences with viewing the interior of the knee joint and punch biopsy procedures. Burman not only reported his experience with arthroscopy of the knee, but also included descriptions of

arthroscopic procedures of the hip, ankle, shoulder, elbow, and wrist. This was the first publication describing the arthroscopic appearance of joints other than the knee, and it remains a classic on the fundamental principles of the procedures. In 1934 Burman, Finkelstein, and Mayer reported on their findings in 30 knees and discussed the value of arthroscopy in the diagnosis of knee disorders. Although they advised further development of instruments and techniques, interest in the use of the arthroscope as an aid in the examination and diagnosis of pathologic changes in the knee joint was short lived because the optical instruments had many technical imperfections. In Germany, Sommer in 1937, Vaubel in 1938, and Hurter in 1955 reported their continued interest and experience in arthroscopy. Continued difficulties and imperfections in instrumentation prevented acceptance of the technique for widespread use. These imperfections were recognized by Professors Takagi and Watanabe, who continued to improve the arthroscopic instrument. In 1957 Watanabe published his *Atlas of Arthroscopy,* which was revised in 1969.

It was not until the late 1960s that much enthusiasm for the technique developed in North America. In 1971 Casscells published the first analytical paper in the United States, and in 1972 Jackson and Abe of Toronto reported

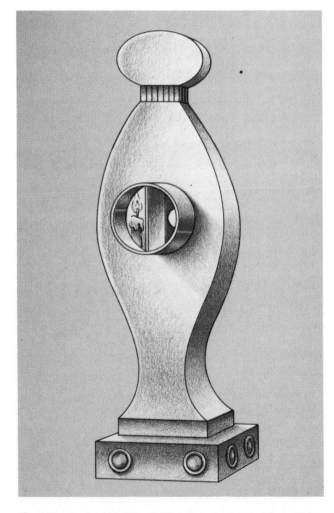

Fig. 58-1. Bozzini Lichtleiter (1805). (From Joyce, J.J., III, In O'Connor, R.L. (ed.): Arthroscopy, Kalamazoo, Mich., 1977, The Upjohn Co.)

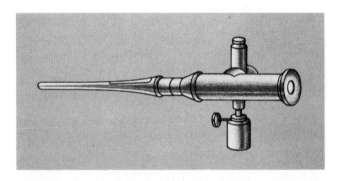

Fig. 58-2. Desormaux's gastrogen endoscope. (From Joyce, J.J., III, In O'Connor, R.L. (ed.): Arthroscopy, Kalamazoo, Mich., 1977, The Upjohn Co.)

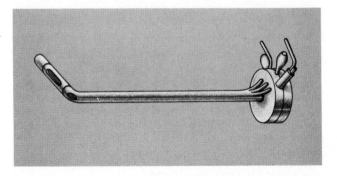

Fig. 58-3. Early model of Nitze cystocope. (From Joyce, J.J., III, In O'Connor, R.L. (ed.): Arthroscopy, Kalamazoo, Mich. 1977, The Upjohn Co.)

on 200 arthroscopic examinations in a carefully documented study. These authors were using the Watanabe No. 21 arthroscope. These reports generated marked enthusiasm in North America, and in 1974 O'Connor of Los Angeles described his extensive experiences with both diagnostic arthroscopy and intraarticular arthroscopic surgery. During the 1970s, numerous reports by Johnson, De-Haven, O'Connor, and Ikeuchi and others increased the enthusiasm for this technique. This enthusiasm resulted in increased interest by the instrument manufacturers, and a quantum leap occurred in the refinement of arthroscopes and related instruments during the next decade. Numerous reports in the 1970s and 1980s by McGinty and Matza, Metcalf, Gillquist et al., and others established the value of arthroscopy in the diagnosis and treatment of a variety of knee disorders.

INSTRUMENTS AND EQUIPMENT
Arthroscope

An arthroscope is an optical instrument. Three basic optical systems are used in rigid arthroscopes: (1) the classic thin-lens system, (2) the rod-lens system designed by Hop-

kins, and (3) the graded index (GRIN) lens system (Fig. 58-4). In the classic thin-lens system, the lenses are thin in comparison with their diameters and air spaces separate the conventional lenses. The light and images are transmitted through the relay lens system to an ocular lens, which then transmits the image to the observer's eye. In the rod-lens system designed by Professor Hopkins of Redding, England, the lenses are thick compared with their diameter and the air space between successive lenses is relatively small. This system provides a number of advantages in construction and performance, and most modern arthroscopes use this optical system. In the graded index lens system, the entire instrument consists of a slender rod of glass. The *Watanabe* No. 24 arthroscope (1.7 mm diameter) and *Dyonics* needle scope use this type of basic optical lens system.

The so-called fiberoptic arthroscopes generally consist of a rod-lens system surrounded by multiple light-conducting glass fibrils. These two systems are enclosed in a specially treated rigid metal sheath (Fig. 58-5).

Certain features determine the optical characteristics of an endoscope. Most important are the direction of view

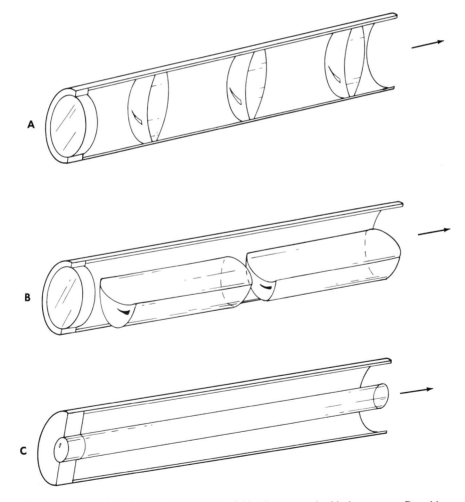

Fig. 58-4. Three basic optical systems used in rigid arthroscopes: **A,** thin lens system, **B,** rod-lens system designed by Hopkins, and **C,** graded index (GRIN) lens system. (From Johnson, L.L.: Arthroscopic surgery, St. Louis, 1986, The C.V. Mosby Co.)

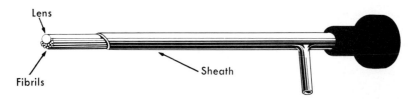

Fig. 58-5. Fiberoptic arthroscope. Note light-conducting fibrils surrounding Hopkins rod-lens system. (From Jackson, R.W.: In American Academy of Orthopaedic Surgeons: Symposium on arthroscopy and arthrography, St. Louis, 1978, The C.V. Mosby Co.)

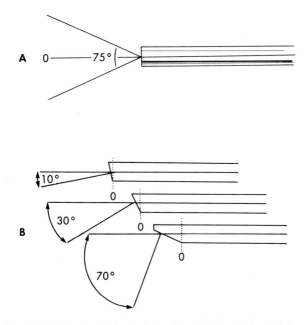

Fig. 58-6. Direction of view and viewing angle. **A,** Angle of vision of an arthroscope (75 degrees) and direction of view (0 degrees). **B,** Comparison of angle of inclination in three arthroscopes: in 10-degree offset arthroscope, line bisecting the angle of vision deviates 10 degrees from axis of scope; in 30-degree offset arthroscope, angle is 30 degrees; and in 70-degree offset arthroscope, angle is 70 degrees. (From Shahriaree, H.: O'Connor's textbook of arthroscopic surgery, Philadelphia, 1984, J.B. Lippincott Co.)

and the viewing angle. The direction of view of an arthroscope is normally the angle between the axis of the endoscope and a line connecting the tip of the endoscope and the center of its field of view. In arthroscopy, this is most frequently 0 degrees, 10 degrees, 30 degrees, and 70 degrees (Fig. 58-6, A and B); the forward viewing (0-degree) and the forward oblique viewing (30-degree) are most often used. Rotation of the forward viewing arthroscope around its longitudinal axis does not increase the field of view (Fig. 58-7), whereas rotation of the forward oblique viewing (30-degree) instrument allows a much larger area of the joint to be observed (Fig. 58-8). The 70-degree and 90-degree arthroscopes are useful in seeing around corners, but have the disadvantage of making orientation by the observer quite difficult (Fig. 58-9).

The viewing angle refers to the field encompassed by the lens (Fig. 58-6, A). The visible area varies according

to the design of the optical system. Wider viewing angles make orientation by the observer much easier.

Arthroscopes consist of an optical lens system, light-conducting fiberoptics, and surrounding sheaths; they vary in diameter from approximately 2 to 6 mm. The 5 and 6 mm arthroscopes are the workhorses of most diagnostic and operative arthroscopic procedures, whereas the smaller 2 mm arthroscope is used for diagnostic and operative arthroscopy involving smaller joints, such as the elbow, wrist, and ankle.

Two arthroscopic instrument designs are available, one for viewing and one for operating. The viewing arthroscope is used for most diagnostic and intraarticular operative procedures using triangulation techniques, which are discussed on p. 2541. Operating arthroscopes allow items such as scissors, biopsy forceps, knives, and grasping instruments to pass through the sheath containing the lens and fiberoptic lighting systems (Fig. 58-10). The advantage of this arrangement is that the tip of the instrument is directly in the field of vision. Operating arthroscopes are usually used in special circumstances during the course of intraarticular surgery or when triangulation techniques prove difficult. It is the surgeon's own preference as to whether he selects the viewing arthroscope and accessory surgical instruments or the operating arthroscope for these intraarticular surgical tasks.

Fiberoptic light sources

The development of fiberoptic lighting eliminated many problems associated with older methods. The fiberoptic cable consists of a bundle of specially prepared glass fibers encased in a protective sheath. One end of the bundle or cable is attached to a light source that is remote from the operative field. The other end is attached to the arthroscope, which is surrounded by fiberoptic fibrils. It is important to note that these strands of glass fiber are quite fragile and will not take significant abuse. Bending the cables, coiling them tightly, or placing heavy instruments on them tends to break the fibers and reduce the intensity and quality of light transmission. For routine general diagnostic inspection and surgery in a joint, a 150-watt tungsten bulb is usually sufficient. If photography and video viewing or recording are desired, more intense power sources, such as the higher-intensity tungsten and xenon systems, are preferable.

Accessory instruments

The following instruments are used in performing all routine arthroscopic surgical procedures. Additional instru-

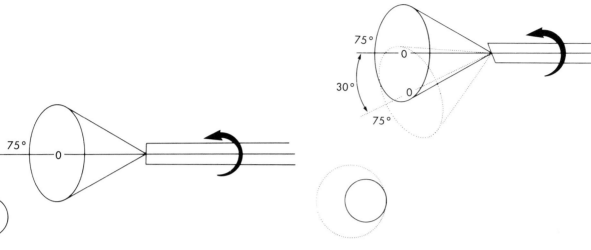

Fig. 58-7. Field of view of straight-ahead arthroscope. *Small circle* indicates field of view covered by rotation of arthroscope. (From Shahriaree, H.: O'Connor's textbook of arthroscopic surgery, Philadelphia, 1984, J.B. Lippincott Co.)

Fig. 58-8. Rotation of arthroscope with 30-degree angle of inclination, which causes scanning effect that increases field of view by about three times. *Dotted circle* shows field of view and is compared at lower left with *small circle* that shows field of view of 0-degree arthroscope. (From Shahriaree, H.: O'Connor's textbook of arthroscopic surgery, Philadelphia, 1984, J.B. Lippincott Co.)

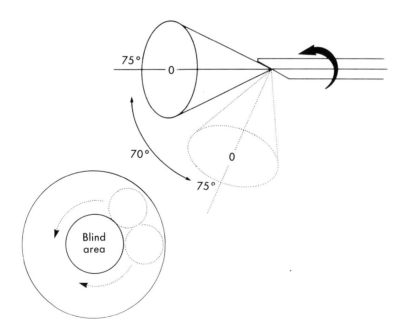

Fig. 58-9. Rotation of arthroscope with 70-degree angle of inclination. This scans large circle but creates blind area directly ahead of it in which nothing can be seen. (From Shahriaree, H.: O'Connor's textbook of arthroscopic surgery, Philadelphia, 1984, J.B. Lippincott Co.)

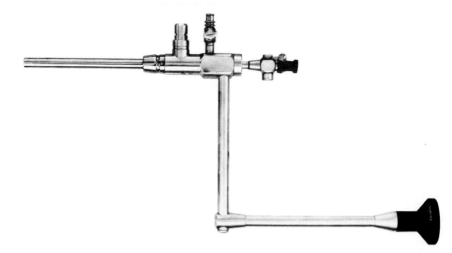

Fig. 58-10. O'Connor operating scope with instrument channel to accommodate 3.4 mm surgical instruments. (From Shahriaree, H.: O'Connor's textbook of arthroscopic surgery, Philadelphia, 1984, J.B. Lippincott Co.)

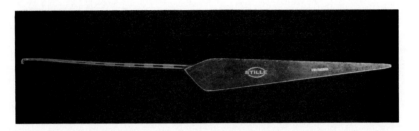

Fig. 58-11. Arthroscopic probe used in exploring intraarticular structures during arthroscopic triangulation techniques.

ments are available and are occasionally used in special circumstances. Each surgeon will have personal preferences in the type, design, and manufacturer of each instrument. All instruments should be approximately the same length as the arthroscope. This makes triangulation easier because the length of the instruments can be compared with that of the arthroscope to judge placement of the tip of the instrument within the joint. The basic instrument kit consists of the following:

Arthroscopes, 0- and 30-degree
Probe
Scissors
Basket forceps
Grasping clamps
Knife with variety of disposable blades
Kerrison rongeur
Motorized meniscus cutter and shaver
Miscellaneous equipment

PROBE

The probe is perhaps the most important diagnostic instrument apart from the arthroscope itself (Fig. 58-11). The probe has become known over the years as "the extension of the arthroscopist's finger." It is used in both diagnostic and operative arthroscopy and is the safest instrument that one can use in learning triangulation techniques. The probe is an essential instrument for palpating intraarticular structures and in planning the approach to a surgical procedure. A tactile sensation soon develops as to what is normal and what is abnormal. It is better to "see and feel" rather than to just "see" alone. It can be used to feel the consistency of a structure, such as the articular cartilage; to determine the depth of chondromalacic areas; to retract loose structures within the joint, such as tears of the menisci; to maneuver loose bodies into more accessible grasping positions; to move the anterior cruciate ligament and determine the tension in the ligamentous and synovial structures within the joint; to retract structures within the joint for exposure; to elevate a meniscus so its undersurface can be viewed; and to probe the fossae and recesses such as the popliteal hiatus within the joint. The known size of the hook of the probe can also be used to measure the size of lesions. Care should be taken when using the tip of the probe, and much of the palpating and maneuvering of the probe within the joint are actually done with the elbow of the probe rather than the tip or toe of the instrument.

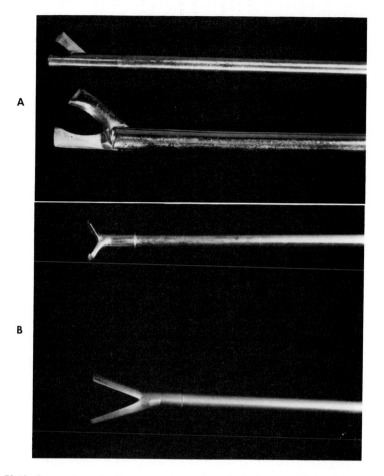

Fig. 58-12. Commonly used arthroscopic scissors: **A,** hooked scissors, and **B,** angled rotary scissors.

SCISSORS

The arthroscopic scissors should be 3 to 4 mm in diameter and may be of the straight or hooked scissors variety (Fig. 58-12). The hooked scissors, as *end-biting* meniscal scissors, are preferred over the straight scissors, which tend to push the material away from the jaws. The configuration of the jaws of the hook scissors tends to hook the tissue and pull it between the cutting edges of the scissors. Optional accessory scissors designs include the right and left curved scissors and the angled cutting scissors. The difference between these two designs is that the shank of the curved scissors is gently curved to accommodate right and left positioning, whereas the angled scissors, usually with a rotating type of jaw mechanism, actually cut at an angle to the shaft of the scissors. These accessory designs may be useful in detaching difficult to reach meniscal fragments.

BASKET FORCEPS

The basket, or punch biopsy, forceps is one of the most commonly used operative arthroscopic instruments (Fig. 58-13, *A*). Removal of the base of the basket forceps permits each punch or bite of tissue to drop free within the joint and does not require removing the instrument from the joint with each bite. Small fragments of tissue that

drop free within the joint through the open-floor punch or basket forceps can be irrigated out or subsequently removed from the joint by suction. This instrument is available in 3 to 5 mm sizes with a straight or curved shaft. It is useful in trimming the peripheral rim of the meniscus or it can be used instead of scissors to cut across meniscal or other tissue. The configuration of the jaws of the basket forceps may be straight or hooked; the hooked configuration is preferred because the hooked jaws tend to grasp the meniscus, pull it, and bite it. As with other arthroscopic instruments, the proper technique is to make small bites to avoid excessive pressure on the joints and pins of the instrument and prevent frequent breakage. The Acuflex rotary biting 90-degree basket forceps are especially useful for trimming the anterior portions of the rim of a resected meniscus.

GRASPING FORCEPS

Many designs of grasping forceps are available, varying from the common operating room pituitary ronguer to the small standard Kocher clamp (Fig. 58-14). Grasping forceps are necessary to place meniscal flaps and other tissues under tension to make the use of a second cutting instrument easier in removing a fragment. Most grasping forceps have some type of ratchet closure on the handle to secure

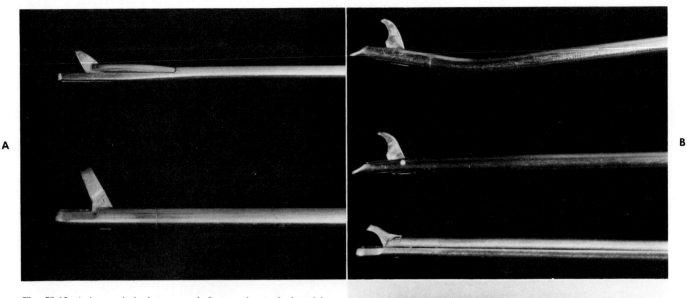

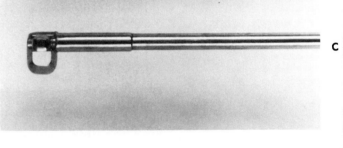

Fig. 58-13. Arthroscopic basket or punch forceps: **A,** standard straight jaw forceps, **B,** hooked jaw forceps, and **C,** Acuflex rotary punch forceps.

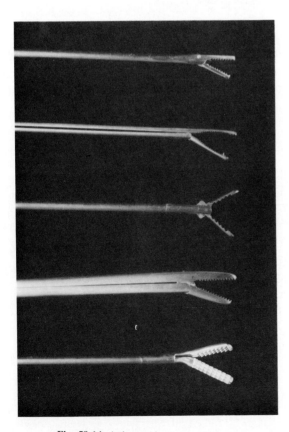

Fig. 58-14. Arthroscopic grasping forceps.

the tissue within its jaws. The jaws of the grasping forceps may be of single action or double action design and may have regular serrated interdigitating teeth, or one or two sharp teeth to better secure the grasped tissue. The double-action grasping forceps, both jaws of which open, are especially preferred for securing an osteocartilaginous loose body because the single-action types frequently allow it to slip from between the jaws.

KNIFE BLADES

Disposable knife blades are generally preferred over those that can be sharpened (Fig. 58-15) even though they have the disadvantage of an increased chance of breaking or slipping free and becoming lost within the joint. However, they are always sharp and many can be bent and contoured to make the cutting in specific instances easier. A variety of disposable blade designs are currently available: hooked or retrograde blades; regular downcutting blades, both straight and curved; and Smillie-type end-cutting blades. The handles holding the disposable blades should be inserted through cannula sheaths or be encased within retractable sheath mechanisms so that the cutting portion of the blade is exposed, not as it enters through the entry portal, but only when it enters the field of arthroscopic vision.

The principle disadvantage of the nondisposable cutting knife blades is that they become dulled quite quickly with use and with sterilization, and although they can be sharp-

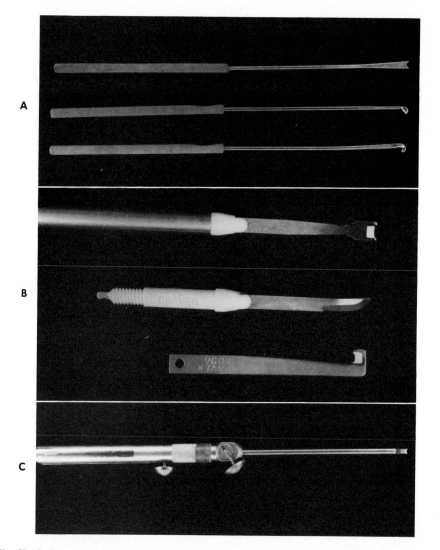

Fig. 58-15. Common arthroscopic knives: **A,** Nondisposable knives, **B,** disposable blades, **C,** blade that can be retracted into protective sheath.

ened, keeping optimally sharp edges is difficult. Therefore the surgeon is often working with dull blades.

KERRISON RONGEUR

The downbiting Kerrison rongeur is an important instrument in meniscal surgery, being used mainly for trimming and excising the anterior horns of the menisci, areas that are quite inaccessible to the standard basket forceps (Fig. 58-16). The disadvantage of the Kerrison rongeur is that the tissue remains within its jaws after each bite, and therefore it must be removed from the joint, cleansed, and reinserted after each bite. The rotary Acuflex basket forceps can be used in place of the downbiting Kerrison rongeur for this task.

MOTORIZED MENISCUS CUTTER AND SHAVER

A motorized meniscus cutter and shaver is useful for debriding soft tissues within the joint and vacuuming the joint to remove loose debris (Fig. 58-17). It is especially useful for shaving or trimming fibrillated or fragmented articular cartilage or removing hypertrophied synovium and small irregularities of the retained rim of a partially resected meniscus. These instruments are most efficient in cutting fibrillated soft tissue; they have difficulty in cutting firm meniscal tissue, which is better cut with the basket forceps, knives, and scissors. The motorized meniscus cutter is then used to trim up imperfections after using these other instruments and to remove debris created by morcellized tissue. All of the motorized meniscal cutters and shavers are basically alike, consisting of a hollow, fenestrated cylinder containing a rotating, two-edged, cylindrical blade that spins within the hollow tube, the blade being driven by a motor. Suction through the cylinder brings the fragments of soft tissue into the window, and as the blade rotates they are amputated, sucked to the outside, and collected in a suction trap. The diameter of the cutting tip is usually 3 to 4 mm, with two cutting tip designs commonly available: one has a window on the side and is useful for

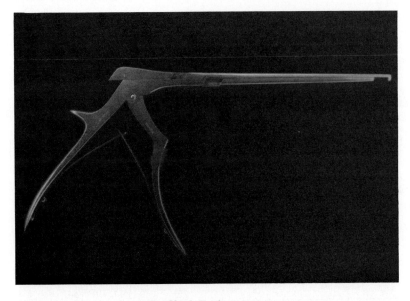

Fig. 58-16. Kerrison rongeur.

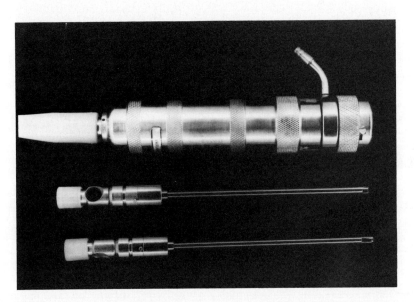

Fig. 58-17. Motorized cutter and trimmer.

shaving smooth articular surfaces and resecting synovium; the other has a corner cutting mechanism, which is more aggressive and more commonly used to trim meniscal tissue. The motorized cutters have forward and reverse controls for the cutting blade, so that the lumen of the shaver does not become occluded with debris. Reversing the rotation of the cutting blade from time to time during the cutting procedure often improves its cutting efficiency. To keep a clear view of the field in which one is shaving, a careful balance between the inflow and outflow of the irrigating solution is essential. If the outflow exceeds the inflow, distention is lost, and turbulence from the suction creates bubbles. If this happens, close the window of the cutting instrument, allow the inflow to again distend the

joint, and then proceed with a clear view of the area. Care should be taken not to activate the rotary cutter without the instrument being within the visual field, and the position of the window should be located before the rotary motion of the blade is activated. Always turn off the fluid egress cannula, to prevent inadvertent suction of potentially contaminated irrigating fluids back through the joint.

Motorized cutters have been found to be useful for shaving areas of chondromalacia on the articular surfaces of the patella and the femoral and tibial condyles; for removing any hypertrophic fat pad and synovium blocking clear arthroscopic vision; for excising synovial plicae and adhesions, and partial synovectomies; for removing stumps or fragments of previously torn anterior cruciate ligaments; for partial meniscectomy and trimming of subtotal meniscal rims; for removing small loose bodies within the joint; and for vacuuming articular debris created by other arthroscopic instruments.

MISCELLANEOUS EQUIPMENT

A variety of sheaths and trocars are required for arthroscopic surgery, and they must accommodate the arthroscope and accessory equipment being used. Sharp instruments should, when possible, be placed through sheaths to protect the soft tissues of the skin portals. The motorized shaver and cutter requires entry through portals using the appropriate sheaths. Both sharp and blunt trocars are required for accurate positioning of the sheaths. The initial perforation through the capsular and synovial tissue requires the use of a sharp trocar passed through the appropriate instrument sheath. Pituitary rongeurs, small currets, small Kocher clamps, small osteotomes, Kirschner wires, and drills may be required for specific arthroscopic procedures. These latter instruments are not used routinely, but in specific instances they are essential.

Care and sterilization of instruments

Because most fiberoptic scopes and cables will not tolerate steam autoclaving, the best method of sterilizing them is by gas (ethylene oxide). However, keeping on hand a suffcient number of steam or gas-sterilized arthroscopes and arthroscopic equipment is not possible in the usual operating room, so most arthroscopists used activated glutaraldehyde (Cidex) for cold disinfection of equipment between successive procedures during the course of a day. Experience with thousands of diagnostic and operative arthroscopic procedures has proven that this is effective and safe. Instruments such as knives, graspers, basket forceps, and suction and irrigation adapters should be sterilized by gas autoclaving after each procedure, but the light cables, power shaving and cutting equipment, and fiberoptic scopes should be soaked for 15 minutes in a glutaraldehyde solution after each procedure.

Irrigation systems

Irrigation and distention of the joint are essential to all arthroscopic procedures (Fig. 58-18). Synovial folds that block the view are usually the result of lack of distention. Joint distention is maintained by normal saline or Ringer's lactate solution during arthroscopy. The inflow may pass directly through the arthroscopic sheath or through a separate portal by means of a needle or a cannula. Either continuous flow or intermittent distention may be used, as preferred. Ringer's lactate solution is now used routinely, because it is more physiologic, especially if continuous flow and prolonged arthroscopic surgery are undertaken. Fewer synovial and articualr surface changes develop with the use of Ringer's lactate solution than with normal saline. If intraarticular electrocoagulation is required, then one must use a nonelectrolytic solution, evacuate the knee of the saline or Ringer's lactate, and use either a carbon dioxide gas medium or water for distention and irrigation.

We prefer continuous irrigation by means of a large bore cannula inserted in the suprapatellar bursa. Continuous ir-

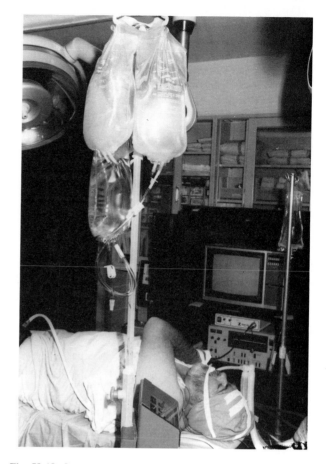

Fig. 58-18. One or more 3 liter irrigating solution bags, used for distention and irrigation of joint during arthroscopy. These are elevated 1 to 2 meters above level of patient.

rigation keeps the fluid clear for optimal viewing, and the ingress of fluids through a large cannula and egress through the smaller outflow of the arthroscope sheath maintains optimal hydrostatic pressure within the joint and therefore maintains joint distention. The one disadvantage of this irrigation system is that any cloudiness within the fluid medium tends to accumulate at the tip of the scope where the outflow egress is located. The inflow and outflow may be changed alternately to improve viewing and distention.

Usually, one or more 3 liter plastic bags of Ringer's lactate solution are suspended at least 2 meters above the level of the patient. The joint is lavaged until the fluid is clear, and the inflow cannula is connected. The two factors that determine the hydrostatic pressure within the joint are the height of the fluid bag and diameter of the tubing. To increase joint distention, one elevates the irrigant container and uses a large-diameter tubing. We have not found the use of pumps to be of any advantage in increasing or maintaining joint distention, and they may potentially increase extravasation of fluid within the soft tissues. Therefore they are not advised for routine use.

As mentioned previously, the outflow stopcock should be closed when suctioning or using motorized cutting instruments with suction to prevent the retrograde suction of potentially contaminated fluid into the joint through the normal outflow cannula.

If electrocoagulation is used, as in lateral retinacular releases or for coagulation of visible open blood vessels, then the joint should be evacuated of the normal saline or Ringer's lactate solution, and water should be instilled for clarity and distention.

It is essential that the inflow cannula not be located in a subsynovial position; otherwise large amounts of the irrigating solution may be injected beneath the synovium, which may totally obliterate the viewing area of the joint. Moving the cannula about freely in the joint or directly viewing its location with the arthroscope ensures that its tip is not beneath the synovium and is a safeguard against subsynovial installation of large amounts of irrigating fluid.

Distention is an important aid in the arthroscopic viewing of any joint, expanding its internal capacity to allow a greater area through which the scope can be maneuvered, and pushing folds of synovium and other soft tissues out of the way in the viewing area. It may also be important in defining proper portal entry points into many joints. Distention is especially critical in making posteromedial and posterolateral entries into the knee for comprehensive examination of these joint compartments. The joint should be maximally distended, with the knee in 60 to 90 degrees of flexion. This permits the posterior capsule to balloon out both medially and laterally, presenting a distended "bubble" for insertion of the sheath and sharp trocar. Attempts to enter the posteromedial and posterolateral compartments of the knee without maximum joint distention are usually difficult or unsuccessful.

Tourniquet

In arthroscopic procedures of the knee, ankle, elbow, and other distal joints, a tourniquet is always applied and is inflated as needed. Normally it is inflated unless there is some specific contraindication, such as a history of thrombophlebitis. The disadvantage of routine tourniquet use is that exsanguination of the limb and tourniquet inflation result in blanching of the synovium, making it difficult to differentiate and diagnose various synovial disorders. One may choose not to inflate the tourniquet routinely unless bleeding develops that cannot be controlled by intermittent irrigation. Many of the commercial leg holders used in knee arthroscopy require the tourniquet to be placed within it. These holders may function quite satisfactorily whether the tourniquet is inflated or not.

Leg holders

The biggest advantage of a leg holder is that it permits application of stress primarily to open the posteromedial compartment for better viewing, manipulation of the meniscus, and posterior horn meniscal surgery (Fig. 58-19). A surgical assistant may provide similar stresses but is subject to such factors as inconsistency and fatigue. A leg holder is especially useful in tight knees, in which the pathology is in the medial and posteromedial compartments. Significant valgus stress applied to the knee firmly gripped in a leg holder may allow significant distraction of the medial compartment to easily permit most operative procedures within this compartment. A leg holder has disadvantages, especially for operations in the lateral compartment or in the patellofemoral joint. It obstructs the placement of the arthroscope and other instruments in the superomedial and superolateral portals, and makes it more difficult to flex the joint without dropping the end of the table or placing the leg in the figure-four position for work in the lateral compartment. Since the thigh is firmly held by the leg holder, the number of different positions in which the leg can be placed is somewhat limited. An alternative to using an encompassing leg holder is to use a lateral post attached

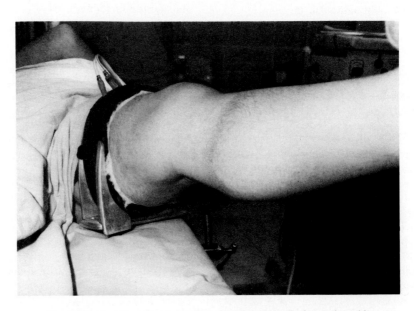

Fig. 58-19. Commercial leg holder that clamps to side rail of operating table.

to the siderail of the operating table, against which the distal thigh can be levered for opening of the posteromedial compartment. The lateral stress post does not confine or prevent the knee from being positioned in an almost unlimited number of positions, does not prevent knee flexion, and does not prevent positioning the knee in the figure four position; therefore it has advantages over many of the expensive commercial leg holding devices.

Furthermore, the routine use of a leg holder, especially one that incorporates a tourniquet within the confines of the holder, may present other difficulties. In such an arrangement wide fluctuations in the tourniquet pressures may occur when stress is applied to the leg; however, we have had no specific complications related to this. Also, the leg-holding device may fix the distal femur so securely that the applied stress can result in fractures about the knee or tearing of the ligamentous structures; such occurrences have been reported.

Thus if the clinical evaluation leads one to suspect medial compartment meniscal pathology, then a leg holder can be of significant assistance. On the other hand, if one anticipates a patellofemoral joint or a lateral compartment problem, then one may elect not to use an encompassing leg holder and resort to a valgus stress post to make viewing of the patellofemoral joint or lateral compartment easier.

ANESTHESIA

Diagnostic arthroscopy can be performed with the patient under local, regional, or general anesthesia. Some intraarticular operative procedures can be performed using regional and local anesthetics.

Local anesthesia can be used for routine diagnostic arthroscopy in a cooperative patient. The choice of local anesthesia to some degree depends on the experience and skill of the arthroscopist, the nature of the knee problem, the patient's tolerance level, and, if a correctable surgical condition is encountered, whether the patient wants to proceed or to come back on another day to have a general anesthetic for a significant intraarticular procedure. The simple removal of loose bodies or small flap tears of the meniscus and other uncomplicated intraarticular procedures may be carried out, under optimum circumstances, with local anesthetics.

General anesthesia is more often used or indicated in the acutely injured knee, where pain is an important factor, when significant intraarticular surgery is anticipated, or when the patient is not cooperative or is especially apprehensive. Allergy to local anesthetics, of course, dictates that a general anesthestic be administered. Arthroscopic surgeons who are less experienced and who are unfamiliar with all of the techniques probably are best advised to select a general anesthetic. If one anticipates proceeding with an intraarticular surgical procedure, then the choice of general anesthesia may be wise, especially if a prolonged procedure, such as complicated meniscal resection or multiple intraoperative procedures, is required. If one anticipates the need for a tourniquet to control bleeding, as in partial or complete synovectomies or excision of adhesions, then general anesthesia permitting the use of a tourniquet is required. Most arthroscopic procedures performed at this clinic are for anticapated operative procedures, and when given the option of having a local anesthetic for diagnostic purposes and coming back on a separate occasion to have the more complicated procedure performed, the patient usually volunteers to have a general anesthetic.

A tourniquet and a leg holder are not used if a local anesthetic is administered. The extraarticular tissues—that is, the skin, subcutaneous tissue, and capsule—are infiltrated with 25 to 30 ml of Xylocaine (lidocaine, 0.5%), mixed with 25 to 30 ml of Marcaine (bupivacaine, 0.5%) with epinephrine. These extraarticular tissues are the major source of pain fibers about the knee. The intraarticular structures, such as the articular surfaces and the menisci, are without sensitive nerve endings. The synovium is sensitive to distention and stretching, but not to cutting. Therefore, the local anesthetic for arthroscopic procedures is concentrated in the skin, subcutaneous tissues, and capsular structures. The addition of a small amount of epinephrine to the Xylocaine/Marcaine mixture helps maintain hemostasis and increases the duration of action of the short-acting Xylocaine. The effect of the Marcaine lasts for several hours, and makes the postarthroscopic period much less uncomfortable. A small amount of Xylocaine may be added to the initial intraarticular distention bolus for those nerve endings within the synovium.

A spinal or regional block anesthetic may be selected for patients who have specific contraindications to general or local anesthetic administration. We rarely use this method of anesthesia, because the disadvantages usually outweigh the advantages. Despite adequate spinal anesthesia for prolonged intraarticular lower extremity surgery, the patient frequently complains of significant discomfort if the tourniquet is inflated, and therefore it has very little advantage over a general anesthetic. Thus, most intraarticular arthroscopic procedures are performed with a general anesthetic that permits long procedures and the safe and comfortable use of a tourniquet.

DOCUMENTATION

The documentation of arthroscopic findings and surgical procedures can be carried out in the following three manners:

1. Carefully constructed drawings can be made to depict the pathology and the operative procedure carried out. These are perhaps the most practical and can be attached to the patient's record for easy reference.
2. A 35 mm reflex camera can be used to photograph the inside of the joint and to document the pathology and operative procedure.
3. Video recordings can be made of the actual pathology and the surgical procedure as it is carried out. The videotapes serve as excellent teaching guides for patients, students, residents in training, and practitioners wishing to learn arthroscopic techniques (Fig. 58-20).

Any 35 mm reflex camera with a lens adapter between the camera and the arthroscope can produce clear, beautiful pictures of intraarticular findings. A focal length of 100 mm will usually provide the best overall image size and

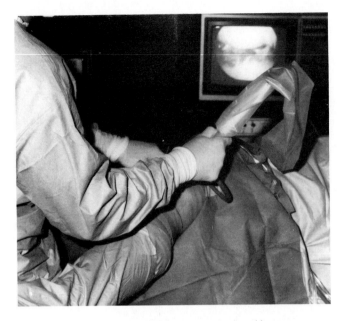

Fig. 58-20. Documentation of findings using videotape.

clarity. The normal ground-glass viewing screen is removed from the camera and replaced with a clear glass viewing screen to focus through the viewfinder. To make high-quality 35 mm slides, a high intensity light source should be available. Although film with higher ASA numbers offers some advantage, generally the higher the ASA reading, the grainier the slide picture. The surgeon interested in documenting arthroscopic findings with 35 mm slides should use his own light source and experiment with a variety of Kodachrome and Ektachrome films of various speeds to see which film and camera setting produce the best slides for his particular light source.

Although recording intraarticular findings and intraoperative procedures on videotape can produce dynamic views of the structures within the joint, it can be quite expensive and time consuming to edit and store. The current commercial tube cameras or solid state cameras all produce excellent video pictures and videotape recordings. If one is especially interested in using dynamic arthroscopic findings for teaching purposes, then video recordings, even with their disadvantages, may be the best means.

ADVANTAGES

The advantages of arthroscopic procedures far outweigh the disadvantages. Among the advantages when compared with arthrotomy are as follows:

1. *Reduced postoperative morbidity.* The patient can return to sedentary work almost immediately and to more vigorous work activities within 1 to 2 weeks after most arthroscopic procedures.
2. *Smaller incisions.* Diagnostic arthroscopic and therapeutic procedures can be carried out through multiple small incisons about the joint (Plate 5, *A*). This is less likely to produce a disfiguring scar.
3. *Less intense inflammatory response.* The small incisions through the capsule and synovium result in a much less intense inflammatory response than does

the standard arthrotomy. This results in less postoperative pain, faster rehabilitation, and faster return to work.

4. *Improved thoroughness of diagnosis.* The diagnosis made on clinical grounds may encompass the most striking symptoms and findings, but often additional less dramatic disorders may be found by thorough arthroscopic examination. Most investigators report that diagnoses based purely on clinical grounds are incomplete in a significant percentage of patients.
5. *Absence of secondary effects.* The secondary effects of arthrotomy about the joints, such as neuroma formation, painful disfiguring scars, and potential functional imbalance (for example, of the extensor mechanism of the knee), are eliminated by arthroscopic techniques.
6. *Reduced hospital cost.* Many arthroscopic procedures can be performed on an outpatient basis. If hospitalization is required, 1 or 2 days is generally the maximum compared with several days required for arthrotomy procedures.
7. *Reduced complication rate.* Only infrequent complications of arthroscopic procedures have been reported.
8. *Improved follow-up evaluation.* The minimal morbidity associated with arthroscopy allows the effects of a previous operative procedure such as synovectomy and partial meniscectomy to be evaluated. These are often referred to as "re-look" procedures.
9. *Possibility of performing surgical procedures that are difficult or impossible to perform through open arthrotomy.* A number of surgical procedures are more easily performed with arthroscopic techniques than through open arthrotomy incisions. For example, partial meniscectomy is usually possible using arthroscopic techniques, whereas trimming and contouring of the inner posterior edge of a meniscus by open means is extremely difficult. With arthrotomy, the entire meniscus is often removed, but the retention of a portion of the meniscus may reduce the degenerative changes that are common after open total meniscectomy.

DISADVANTAGES

The disadvantages of arthroscopy are few, but they may be significant to the individual arthroscopic surgeon. Not every surgeon has the temperament to perform arthroscopic surgery because it requires working through small portals with delicate and fragile instruments. Especially in one's early experience, the procedures can be extremely time consuming. Extensive and expensive specialized equipment is required. The need to maneuver the instruments within the tight confines of the intraarticular space may produce significant scuffing and scoring of the articular surfaces, especially by an inexperienced surgeon.

Although these disadvantages can be quite significant, the advantages to the patients generally far outweigh them.

INDICATIONS AND CONTRAINDICATIONS

Although the original indication for arthroscopy was the so-called problem case, it is now obvious that arthroscopy is useful for a large variety of joint problems, including

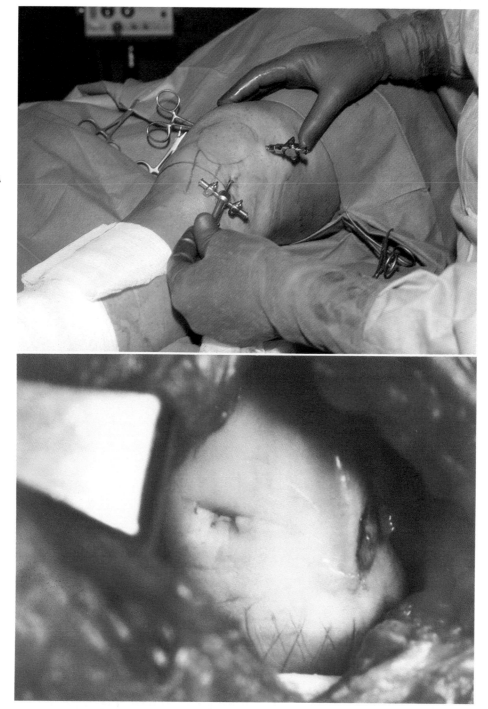

Plate 5. A, Incision for standard anterolateral arthroscopic portal; inflow cannula is superolateral. **B,** Arthroscopic photograph of severe articular scuffing secondary to arthroscopic procedure.

trauma and other disorders. No absolute indications for arthroscopic procedures can be given and the contraindications are few. Diagnostic arthroscopy is indicated for preoperative evaluation and confirmation of the clinical diagnosis before an arthroscopic or open surgical procedure. It may also be indicated for the documentation of specific lesions when medicolegal concerns, workmen's compensation insurance, or other secondary gains may be a factor. Arthroscopy provides an important method of evaluating and studying the pathophysiology of certain diseases.

The contraindications are few. Arthroscopy should not be used in a minimally deranged joint that will respond to the usual conservative methods of treatment. Furthermore, the surgeon should not consider arthroscopy before a careful history, physical examination, and standard noninvasive diagnostic procedures have been carried out. Arthroscopy is contraindicated when the risk of joint sepsis from a local skin condition is present or when a remote infection may be seeded in the operative site. Partial or complete ankylosis that makes maneuverability of the arthroscope and instruments about the joint difficult is also a contraindication. Major collateral ligamentous and capsular disruptions of the joint that will permit excessive extravasation of irrigating solutions into the soft tissues are relative contraindications to arthroscopy.

BASIC ARTHROSCOPIC TECHNIQUES

To learn arthroscopic techniques requires a great deal of patience and persistence. They are mostly self-taught and require mastering a type of surgical skill different from other orthopaedic surgical techniques. The instruments are small and delicate and must be maneuvered in tight, confining compartments. Everything is magnified and, because the arthroscope is monocular and two dimensional, depth perception is a matter of experience rather than observation.

The technique can be difficult and frustrating to learn and probably will not appeal to every orthopaedic surgeon. Traditional open knee operations are still valuable and should not be abandoned. Especially in one's early experience with arthroscopic techniques, it may often be wise to abort a procedure and return to an open method that has given good results in the past.

An absolute prerequisite for arthroscopic surgery is proficiency in diagnostic arthroscopy. Patients' expectations from the use of arthroscopic techniques have placed tremendous demands on practicing orthopaedic surgeons. A surgeon should not be persuaded by these pressures to perform a difficult arthroscopic procedure for which he has yet to develop sufficient skills. A skillful meniscectomy performed through an open arthrotomy is preferable to a poorly performed arthroscopic meniscectomy. Metcalf suggests the following arthroscopic operations on the knee in order of increasing difficulty:
1. Resection of synovial plica
2. Removal of suprapatellar loose body
3. Patellar debridement with motorized shaver
4. Excision of flap tear of medial meniscus
5. Excision of bucket handle tear of either meniscus
6. Lateral retinacular release
7. Excision of flap tear of lateral meniscus

8. Removal of loose body from posteromedial compartment
9. Abrasion or drilling of chondral defect
10. Excision of posterior horn tear of medial meniscus
11. Synovectomy
12. Excision of horizontal tear of posterior horn of lateral meniscus
13. Total meniscectomy
14. Treatment of osteochondritis dissecans
15. Meniscus repair
16. Arthroscopic replacement or reconstruction of anterior cruciate ligament

It is easy to use excessive time in arthroscopic surgery, so it is a good idea to set rigid time limits and adhere to them. If a procedure is not progressing toward a satisfactory conclusion within 45 to 60 minutes, it is better to stop, reprepare and drape the patient, and proceed with an arthrotomy. If unexpected additional pathology is encountered (for example, a complex tear of both menisci instead of a simple tear in either), then the potential time constraints on safe tourniquet and anesthetic use should be observed and an open arthrotomy should be performed instead of risking an overly long arthroscopic procedure.

The learning process for arthroscopic surgery is often a slow and tedious one. Although artificial models and amputation specimens may initially be used for practice, rarely is the realism sufficient or the specimens plentiful enough to develop proficiency. The surgeon who desires to learn arthroscopic techniques should do so by diagnostic arthroscopy of every knee for which open arthrotomy is planned. Depending on the length of time needed for the arthrotomy procedure, 20 to 30 minutes are set aside for arthroscopic practice. Doing this again and again will refine diagnostic arthroscopy skills. Once one can view most of the intraarticular structures, and can insert a probe through an accessory portal and use it to lift, depress, retract, and palpate the structures viewed, one has begun learning the triangulation principles for arthroscopic surgery.

Triangulation technique

Triangulation involves the use of one or more instruments inserted through separate portals and brought into the optical field of the arthroscope, the tip of the instrument and the arthroscope forming the apex of a triangle. Although it is sometimes useful to pass cutting instruments through the central channel in the arthroscope, triangulation techniques are sufficient for handling most of the disorders suitable for arthroscopic surgery. There are several advantages of triangulation over using an operative arthroscope. Viewing is improved because diagnostic telescopes are larger than operating arthroscopes and the optical angle of the telescope can be varied. The triangulated surgical instrument is at an angle to the optical channel in the telescope rather than in line with it, which aids in depth perception. Larger surgical instruments can be used, and one is not restricted to the smaller instruments that will fit along the instrument channel of the operating arthroscope. Perhaps the most significant advantage, however, is that triangulation permits independent movement of the telescope and the surgical instrument, which is not possible with an operating arthroscope.

The only disadvantage of triangulation is the necessity of mastering the psychomotor skills to bring two or more objects together in a confined space while using monocular vision (which eliminates the convergence that provides depth perception with binocular vison). Becoming familiar and skillful with the use of the probe in diagnostic arthroscopy is the critical learning maneuver.

Once diagnostic proficiency in simple triangulation with a probe is mastered, additional skills may be developed. Triangulation of more than one instrument into the optical field of the arthroscope is frequently required in arthroscopic surgery. A straight ahead lens (0-degree) arthroscope makes the learning of triangulation techniques easier. The more angled the fore lens of the arthroscope, the more difficult are the orientation and triangulation procedures.

Thorough recognition of the intraarticular anatomy (for example, recognizing the intercondylar notch and the anterior cruciate ligament, or dividing the menisci into thirds and directing the instruments toward that known structure) increases triangulation skills. If the surgeon becomes disoriented and has difficulty in triangulation, bringing the accessory instrument into the joint, touching or feeling the sheath of the arthroscope with it, and sliding it down the sheath to the arthroscope tip and into the field of vision may be successful. With practice, a surgeon develops a stereoscopic sense that allows him to place the instrument into the field of view immediately.

After this stereoscopic sense develops, the ability to change from one portal to another to locate optimum accessory portals and switch arthroscopes and accessory instruments enables the surgeon to not only explore but to also operate in all areas of the joint. The first prerequisite for triangulation and successful arthroscopic surgical technique is clear vision. Maximum distention of the joint, a clear fluid medium, and a mechanism to apply stress to the joint and open the compartment are basic. If bleeding occurs and clouds the viewing medium, inflation of the tourniquet or thorough lavage generally solves the problem. If the fat pad or synovium obliterates the view, then further distention, retraction with an accessory instrument, or resection of a portion of the fat pad or synovium can be performed. The ability to solve viewing problems of this sort improves with experience.

COMPLICATIONS

Complications during or following diagnostic surgical arthroscopy are infrequent and fortunately are usually minor. Most are preventable with good preoperative and intraoperative planning and attention to the details of basic techniques.

Damage to intraarticular structures

Damage to intraarticular structures is probably the most important complication. Although any structure within the joint may be damaged, the most frequently damaged are the articular cartilage surfaces. In the knee the anterior horn of the menisci, the anterior cruciate ligament, and the fat pad are especially vulnerable. Scuffing and scoring of the articular cartilage surfaces by the tip of the arthroscope or an accessory instrument occur most often when the arthroscopist is inexperienced, in the very tight joint, or

when the procedure is long and particularly difficult. When initially learning arthroscopic techniques, the inexperienced surgeon frequently has difficulty placing the arthroscope, probe, or accessory tools into the desired field of vision during triangulation efforts. The more the instruments are maneuvered within the joint, the more likely it is that the articular surfaces will be scuffed. Forcing the arthroscope or other instruments between the femoral and tibial condyles into the posterior compartment of the knee or between the humeral head and glenoid cavity in the shoulder may severely score their articular surfaces and lead to progressive chondromalacic changes and degenerative arthritis. Using a leg holder or a leverage post during knee arthroscopy or distraction during shoulder arthroscopy will help open up the joint space to permit safer passage of the instruments into their posterior parts. A poorly placed portal frequently makes instrument passage and maneuvering more difficult. It is better to change the portal site or make an accessory portal than to scuff the articular surface severely by forcing the instrument (Plate 5, *B*). Minor superficial scuffs are inevitable and heal with no residual joint problem.

Damage to menisci

In knee arthroscopy, the anterior horn of either meniscus may be damaged by incision or penetration if the anterior portal is located too inferior. The anterior portal location should be carefully marked with a marking pen before the joint is distended and care should be exercised when the incision is made. Anterior portals should be located approximately 1 to 1.5 cm above the joint line and a comparable distance from the edge of the patellar tendon. The cutting edge of the No. 11 knife blade should be oriented superiorly as it penetrates the capsule and synovium and should generally incise upward rather than downward toward the meniscus. Additional portals needed during the diagnostic or operative procedure should be made under direct arthroscopic intraarticular viewing. For example, if the arthroscope is in an anterolateral portal and an anteromedial portal is needed for another instrument, then the fore lens of the arthroscope is directed anteriorly and a spinal needle is passed through the skin and capsule at the desired portal site. One can view the needle as it penetrates the capsule and synovium above the superior surface of the meniscus. Once the needle is optimally positioned, the portal can be safely made without danger of lacerating the anterior horn of the meniscus. Other accessory portals should be made using similar techniques. Transverse laceration of the anterior horn of a meniscus may go undetected and cause subsequent problems or require meniscectomy if this technique is handled poorly.

Damage to fat pad

Improper portal location and improper direction of instrument insertion during knee arthroscopy may damage the fat pad, resulting in hemorrhage, hypertrophy, or fibrosis. Making the anterior portals 1.0 to 1.5 cm lateral or medial to the edge of the patellar tendon helps to avoid this problem. If the arthroscope or instrument passage through the anterior portal is too horizontally oriented, it may pass repeatedly through the fat pad rather than posterior to it. The scope or instrument should be directed di-

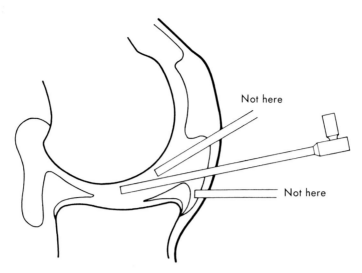

Fig. 58-21. Ideal placement of cannula. If positioned too high, angle of obliquity is such that posterior horn cannot be seen; if too low, it can go through meniscus and limit viewing or mobility. Ideal placement is directly in slot between femur and tibia. (From Johnson, L.L.: Diagnostic and surgical arthroscopy, St. Louis, 1981, The C.V. Mosby Co.)

agonally to the contralateral compartment to avoid the fat pad (Fig. 58-21).

Damage to cruciate ligaments

In knee arthroscopy, either cruciate ligament may be damaged during meniscus excision when an intercondylar attachment is cut. The anterior cruciate ligament is especially vulnerable if the cutting knife, basket forceps, or scissors are misdirected. The suction from the motorized cutter and shaver may result in soft tissue, including synovium and ligaments, being sucked into the cutting aperature of the instrument when one is working near the intercondylar notch. This can be avoided by always keeping the structure being cut in view and carefully controlling the cutting instrument to avoid "plunging" into the intercondylar notch.

Damage to extraarticular structures

BLOOD VESSELS

Damage to the blood vessels about the joint may be the most serious and devastating injury caused by arthroscopic procedures. This may result from either direct penetration or laceration or from pressure caused by excessive fluid extravasation. Major superficial veins may be lacerated when portal site selection is improper. In the knee the saphenous vein may be penetrated by poor posteromedial portal location; in the shoulder the cephalic vein may be penetrated by poor anterior portal site selection. The anterior tibial artery is vulnerable in anterior approaches for ankle arthroscopy, especially the anterior central approach. Posteromedial portals should not be attempted in ankle arthroscopy because of the proximity of the posterior tibial artery to that portal site. The brachial artery coursing over the anterior aspect of the elbow may be injured if accessory portals for extraction of such things as loose bodies from the anterior joint are placed too far anteriorly. These accessory portals should be placed well medial or lateral to the midline of the antecubital fossa. The axillary artery

in shoulder arthroscopy may be injured by arthroscopic instruments plunging through the axillary pouch. More often axillary vessel occlusion is caused by fluid extravasation rather than direct penetration or laceration. Injuries to the popliteal vessels may be devastating. These vessels can be penetrated or lacerated from improper techniques of detaching the intercondylar attachments of the menisci, from improper posteromedial and posterolateral portals, and from improper techniques of passing instruments or arthroscopes through the intercondylar notch to view or examine structures in the posteromedial compartment. During arthroscopic meniscal suture, great care must be exercised when passing the needles to avoid injuring the popliteal vessels when the sutures are placed or passed posteriorly. Direct exposure of the posterior capsule through an appropriate incision and the placement of a suitable protector retractor can minimize dangers to the popliteal vessels.

NERVES

Sensory and motor nerves near the joint may also be damaged. Most commonly injured about the knee are the infrapatellar branches or sartorial branches of the femoral nerve. The location of each of these numerous cutaneous branches is not consistent, and therefore occasional injury to one may be unavoidable if multiple portal techniques are used. If this occurs, in most instances the hypesthesia produced is of minor consequence and causes no problem. Occasionally a painful neuroma may require subsequent resection. Injuries to the common peroneal nerve have been experienced during arthroscopic suture of the posterior horn of the lateral meniscus. Again, these can be avoided by making an open incision down to the capsular structures and passing the meniscal sutures through the capsule under direct vision. In shoulder arthroscopy the branches of the axillary nerve that course along the deep surface of the deltoid and supply it may be injured if either anterior or posterior portal sites are too far inferior. This may result in significant denervation of a portion of the deltoid muscle and subsequent significant functional deficit. Traction neuropraxia of the musculocutaneous nerve, as well as other components of the brachial plexus, has been reported in shoulder arthroscopy when strong traction and distraction of the shoulder have been used. Only the amount of traction needed to distract the joint sufficiently for viewing and maneuvering of instruments should be used. The sural nerve may be injured in the posterolateral approach to the ankle. In elbow arthroscopy the location of the radial nerve must be kept in mind in anterolateral approaches, and the ulnar nerve location must be kept in mind in anteromedial approaches.

LIGAMENTS AND TENDONS

The tibial collateral ligament may be injured by accessory medial portals in diagnostic and operative procedures about the knee, or it may be torn by severe valgus stress in an attempt to open up the medial compartment. This is a real possibility if a rigid leg holder is used and a strong valgus stress is applied. Superior portals through the lateral parts of the rotator cuff in the shoulder for accessory instrument passage or inflow should be avoided. Portals through these parts of the rotator cuff may result in sufficient fraying and rupture of the supraspinatus or infraspinatus tendons or produce sufficient scarring to result in significant impingement and subacromial problems following the arthroscopic procedure. Careful portal placement about the anterior aspect of the ankle after marking the location of the tendons of the tibialis anterior, peroneals, and extensor digitorum longus will avoid significant damage to structures near these portal sites. The patellar tendon can be injured by rough and repeated passages of instruments using the Gilquist technique in knee arthroscopy. If this technique is used, the incision in the tendon should be made vertically; if it is properly placed, injury to the tendon is infrequent and insignificant.

Extravasation of irrigating solutions into the soft tissues about the joint is common; it rarely causes any serious problems but it should be recognized for its potential for serious complications. As already mentioned, this is especially true about the shoulder, where extravasation of fluids through portals or through a connecting bursa may put significant pressures on the neurovascular elements within the axilla. This may result in vascular compromise within the extremity or a significant neuropraxia. Noyes and Spievack have shown that significant extravasation of fluids is possible during arthroscopy of the knee. They have found that rupture of the suprapatellar pouch is not infrequent and that localization of the fluids about the superficial femoral artery can easily dissect all the way to the femoral triangle. They also noted that extravasation by way of a rupture of a semimembranosus bursa was not uncommon, with dissection of fluids into the soft tissues and compartments of the calf. They pointed out that the extravasation of fluids in knee arthroscopy may very well be subtle and significant in prolonged arthroscopic procedures. They recommended that tense distention of the knee be avoided if a flexion position is required and great caution be taken if an inflow system exerts pressure to distend the joint is used.

Improper placement of an inflow cannula in the suprapatellar pouch may result in significant subsynovial instal-lation of large amounts of irrigating solution. The subsynovial location may obliterate the actual viewing of the joint. Careful movement of the inflow cannula in the suprapatellar pouch before the joint is distended will assure that it is not impaled in a subsynovial location and will avoid this potentially troublesome complication. Leakage of irrigating solution into the prepatellar bursa may be marked, but this does not produce any significant problems other than making the procedure technically more difficult.

Hemarthrosis

Hemarthrosis is the most common postoperative complication, most frequently following lateral retinacular releases and total lateral meniscectomies. The superior lateral geniculate vessels are usually cut in lateral retinacular releases. Postoperative hematomas can be minimized by electrocoagulation of these vessels following the release or by the use of a pressure pad over the area for several days following the arthroscopic procedure. If the entire lateral meniscus requires removal, the inferolateral geniculate artery may be lacerated just anterior to the popliteal hiatus. If this is recognized, the vessel should be electrocoagulated.

Thrombophlebitis

Thrombophlebitis is potentially the most dangerous postoperative complication; fortunately it is not common following routine arthroscopic procedures. Some reports suggest that the use of a tourniquet reduces the incidence of thrombophlebitis, whereas others suggest that the incidence is increased by the use of a tourniquet and a leg holder.

Infection

Despite the early fears of infection, the actual number of reported infections has remained extremely low. Watanabe et al. reported no infections in over 2000 cases; Johnson et al. reported a rate of 0.04%, or 5 cases in over 12,500 arthroscopies; and Mulhollen reported only 7 cases of sepsis in over 9000 patients. This low incidence is undoubtedly the result of several factors, including limited incisions, young and healthy patients, short operating time, and irrigation and dilutional effects of the irrigating solutions. Even so, the surgeon should still prepare and drape the joint with the same care as for a major surgical procedure, with the unsterile fields sealed from the sterile area by waterproof drapes. The eyepiece of the arthroscope must be recognized as being unsterile, because it is touched either by the surgeon's eye or the photographic or video couplings, and the stopcock on the outflow cannula should be always closed before using suction or the power cutting equipment. Failure to close the stopcock may pull potentially contaminated solutions in the outflow connection container back into the joint. Gross violation of any of these basic procedures may result in serious pyarthrosis.

Tourniquet paresis

Temporary paresis in the extremity has been observed after tourniquet use to control bleeding in diagnostic or operative arthroscopy, usually following prolonged procedures. If a tourniquet is required, it should be deflated after 90 minutes. Careful monitoring of the tourniquet pressure and testing the accuracy of the tourniquet gauges will minimize these problems. Fortunately, tourniquet paresis is usually mild and resolves within a few days.

Synovial herniation and fistulae

Small globules of fat and synovial tissue may herniate through any of the arthroscope's portals. Usually the larger the portal, the greater the chance of this complication. A large fluid-filled cystic herniation may rarely occur. These fat and synovial herniations are usually small, become asymptomatic over several weeks, and do not require any specific treatment. If a herniation persists and remains symptomatic, then excision of the herniated part with careful closure of the capsule may occasionally be required.

Synovial fistulae are rare, but they have occurred following suture reactions or stitch abscesses. They usually do not produce significant intraarticular infections, but the patient should probably receive antibiotics and the knee should be immobilized for 7 to 10 days to allow the fistula to close spontaneously. Surgical closure is rarely required.

Instrument breakage

Arthroscopic instruments may occasionally break within the joint. The increased use and success of modern arthroscopy parallel the improvement and miniaturization of the arthroscopes and accessory instruments. Delicate cutting and grasping instruments 2 or 3 mm in diameter may be broken unless manipulation within the joint is gentle. These delicate instruments should never be forced into a tight or unusual position where they might bend or break. Cutting instruments with disposable blades, especially knives, not only may break but may become detached from the handle and dropped free within the joint. Adequate locking mechanisms are not currently present on most of the blades and handles to prevent this. If the surgeon notes any loosening of the blade on the handle, he should immediately withdraw the instrument, tighten it, and lock it in place. Although disposable knife blades are popular because they are always sharp and are sufficiently malleable to be contoured, they are more likely to break than one-piece knives and, as already mentioned, may become detached from their handles. However, with sufficient gentleness and care these disposable instruments can be used safely. The basket forceps is another instrument frequently broken, usually by attempting to bite too large a fragment of meniscus or other tissue. The rotational pin holding the biting jaw may break or become dislodged, allowing the jaw to fall free within the joint. A similar breakage may occur with the scissors when too large a bite is attempted. In a survey of over 9000 cases, Mulhollen reported a 0.03% incidence of broken instruments with 0.01% requiring arthrotomy for removal of the broken part. If an instrument breaks, the surgeon should immediately close the outflow cannula, but the inflow should be left open to keep the joint distended. If the broken instrument is within the visual field, total attention to keeping it in view and removing it is essential. Stopping the outflow reduces turbulence and holding the joint still helps prevent it from falling out of sight into another part of the joint. Broken instruments tend to gravitate into the medial or lateral gutters, to hide beneath the menisci, or to drop by gravity into the posterior or most dependent part of the joint. If the broken instrument passes out of the visual field, it may be extremely difficult to locate and retrieve. In the knee, if one cannot locate the piece by searching the medial and lateral gutters, the suprapatellar pouch, and the intercondylar notch, and by carefully probing beneath the menisci, then viewing through posteromedial and posterolateral portals should be considered. If the fragment is still not located, a roentgenogram of the knee should be made. If the broken piece is located, a suction magnet introduced through an accessory portal may stabilize the small broken fragment until a grasping instrument can be inserted through a third portal to secure and extract the piece.

REFERENCES

Bircher, E.: Die arthroendoskopie, Zentralbl. Chir. **48:**1460, 1921.

Burman, M.S.: Arthroscopy or the direct visualization of joints: an experimental cadaver study, J. Bone Joint Surg. **8:**669, 1931.

Burman, M.S., Finkelstein, H., and Mayer, L.: Arthroscopy of the knee joint, J. Bone Joint Surg. **16:**255, 1934.

Casscells, S.W.: Arthroscopy of the knee joint, J. Bone Joint Surg. **53-A:**287, 1971.

Casscells, S.W.: The technique of arthroscopy, Orthopedics **6:**1498, 1983.

DeHaven, K.E.: Principles of triangulation for arthroscopic surgery, Orthop. Clin. North Am. **13**(2):329, 1982.

DeHaven, K.E., and Collins, H.R.: Diagnosis of internal derangement of the knee: the role of arthroscopy, J. Bone Joint Surg. **57-A:**802, 1975.

Eriksson, E.: Problems in recording arthroscopy, Orthop. Clin. North Am. **10:**735, 1979.

Fahmy, N.R., and Patel, D.G.: Hemostatic changes and postoperative deep vein thrombosis associated with use of a pneumatic tourniquet, J. Bone Joint Surg. **63-A:**461, 1981.

Finkelstein, H., and Mayer, L.: The arthroscope: a new method of examining joints, J. Bone Joint Surg. **13:**583, 1931.

Gambardella, R.A., and Tibone, J.E.: Knife blade in the knee joint: a complication of arthroscopic surgery: a case report, Am. J. Sports Med. **11:**267, 1983.

Gillquist, J., and Hagberg, G.: A new modification of the technique of arthroscopy of the knee joint, Acta Chir. Scand. **142:**123, 1976.

Gillquist, J., Hagberg, G., and Oretorp, N.: Therapeutic arthroscopy of the knee, Injury **10:**128, 1978.

Gillquist, J., Hagberg, G., and Oretorp, N.: Arthroscopic examination of the posteromedial compartment of the knee joint, Internat. Orthop. (SICOT) **3:**13, 1979.

Gillquist, J., Hagberg, G., and Oretorp, N.: Arthroscopic visualization of the posteromedial compartment of the knee joint, Orthop. Clin. North Am. **10:**545, 1979.

Hurter, E.: L'arthroscopie, nouvelle methode d'exploration du genou, Rev. Chir. Orthop. **41:**763, 1955.

Ikeuchi, H.: Total meniscectomy of the complete discoid meniscus under arthroscopic control: a case report, J. Jpn. Orthop. Assoc. **44:**374, 1970.

Ikeuchi, H.: Surgery under arthroscopic control, Rheumatology **33:**57, 1976.

Jackson, R.W., and Abe, I.: The role of arthroscopy in the management of disorders of the knee: an analysis of 200 consecutive cases, J. Bone Joint Surg. **54-B:**310, 1972.

Jackson, R.W., and Dandy, D.J.: Arthroscopy of the knee, New York, 1976, Grune & Stratton.

Jackson, D.W., and Strizak, A.M.: Present status of videoarthroscopy, Contemp. Orthop. **2:**521, 1980.

Johnson, L.L.: Diagnostic arthroscopy of the knee. In Ingwersen, O.S. (ed.): The knee joint: proceedings of the International Congress, Rotterdam, September, 1973, Amsterdam, 1974, Excepta Medica.

Johnson, L.L.: Comprehensive arthroscopic examination of the knee, St. Louis, 1977, The C.V. Mosby Co.

Johnson, L.L.: Diagnostic and surgical arthroscopy, St. Louis, 1981, The C.V. Mosby Co.

Johnson, L.L.: Arthroscopic surgery: principles and practice, ed. 3, St. Louis, 1986, The C.V. Mosby Co.

Johnson, L.L., Schneider, D., Goodwin, F.G., and Bullock, J.M.: A sterilization method for arthroscopes using activated dialdehyde, Orthop. Rev. **9:**75, 1977.

Johnson, L.L., et al.: Two per cent glutaraldehyde: a disinfectant in arthroscopy and arthroscopic surgery, J. Bone Joint Surg. **64-A:**237, 1982.

Joyce, J.J., III: Arthroscopic anatomy, Orthopedics **6:**1115, 1983.

Kreuscher, P.H.: Semilunar cartilage disease: a plea for early recognition by means of the arthroscope and early treatment of this condition, Ill. Med. J. **47:**290, 1925.

McGinty, J.B., and Matza, R.A.: Arthroscopy of the knee: evaluation of an out-patient procedure under local anesthesia, J. Bone Joint Surg. **60-A:**787, 1978.

Metcalf, R.W.: Instructional manual of arthroscopic surgery, Salt Lake City, 1980, Press Publishing Ltd.

Metcalf, R.W.: Operative arthroscopy of the knee. In American Academy of Orthopaedic Surgeons: Instructional course lectures, vol. 30, St. Louis, 1981, The C.V. Mosby Co.

Mulhollan, J.S.: Complications of arthroscopic surgery. Presented at the International Arthroscopy Association meeting, Philadelphia, October 4, 1980.

Noyes, F.R., and Spievack, E.S.: Extraarticular fluid dissection in tissues during arthroscopy: a report of clinical cases and a study of intraarticular and thigh pressures in cadavers, Am. J. Sports Med. **10:**346, 1982.

O'Connor, R.L.: Arthroscopy in the diagnosis and treatment of acute ligament injuries of the knee, J. Bone Joint Surg. **56-A:**333, 1974.

O'Connor, R.L.: Arthroscopy, Philadelphia, 1977, J.B. Lippincott Co.

Patel, D., and Guhl, J.F.: The use of bovine knees in operative arthroscopy, Orthopedics **6:**1119, 1983.

Price, A.J., et al: Do tourniquets prevent deep vein thrombosis? J. Bone Joint Surg. **55-A:**106, 1973.

Reagan, B.F., McInerny, V.K., Treadwell, B.V., Zarins, B., and Mankin, H.J.: Irrigating solutions for arthroscopy: a metabolic study, J. Bone Joint Surg. **65-A:**629, 1983.

Schonholtz, G.J.: The use of closed circuit television in arthroscopy, Orthopedics **7:**342, 1984.

Shahriaree, H.: O'Connor's textbook of arthroscopic surgery, Philadelphia, 1984, J.B. Lippincott Co.

Shoji, H., Gutierrez, M.M., and Aldridge, K.E.: The use of 2% glutaraldehyde as a disinfectant for arthroscopes used in septic joints, Orthopedics **7:**241, 1984.

Sommer, R.: Die Endoskopie des Kniegelenkes, Zentralbl. Chir. **64:**1692, 1937.

Takagi, K.: The classic: Arthroscope, Kenji Takagi, J. Jap. Orthop. Assoc., 1939, Clin. Orthop. **167:**6, 1982.

Vaubel, E.: Die Arthroskopie (Endoskopie des Kniegelenkes) ein Beitrag zue Diagnostic der Gelenkkrankheiten. In Jurgens, R. (ed.): Der Rheumatismus, Dresden and Leipzig, 1938, Theodore Steinkopf.

Watanabe, M., and Takeda, S.: The number 21 arthroscope, J. Jpn. Orthop. Assn. **34:**1041, 1960.

Watanabe, M., Takeda, S., and Ikeuchi, H.: Atlas of arthroscopy, Tokyo, 1969, Igaku Shoin Ltd.

Wredmark, T., and Ludh, R.: Arthroscopy under local anesthesia using controlled pressure-irrigation with prilocaine, J. Bone Joint Surg. **64-B:**583, 1982.

CHAPTER 59

Arthroscopy of knee and ankle

T. David Sisk

Arthroscopy of Knee

The knee is the joint in which arthroscopy has its greatest diagnostic and intraarticular surgical application. Considering all the advancements in knee surgery over the past decade, Cassells in 1980 stated that arthroscopy with its diagnostic and surgical potentials stands out as probably the greatest achievement. The increasing popularity of arthroscopic techniques has permitted documentation of the usefulness of the techniques in diagnosis, and it has also been speculated that long-term results of endoscopic meniscectomies may be more satisfactory than those of conventional open meniscectomies because the procedure permits varied and conservative approaches to meniscal lesions.

Arthroscopy has allowed examination of the effectiveness of clinical evaluation, laboratory tests, roentgenograms, arthrographic studies, and other diagnostic tools in knee problems. Johnson (1981) compared clinical impressions with postoperative diagnoses and found a significant amount of additional diagnoses, including diagnoses completely different from the clinical impression in a large percentage of patients. In a study of 229 patients presumed to have a torn medial meniscus, arthroscopy confirmed an isolated diagnosis in surprisingly only 21%, an additional diagnosis in 23%, and a completely different diagnosis in 56%. An unsuspected lateral meniscus tear was noted in 5% of the knees diagnosed as having a torn medial meniscus. Only 10% of Johnson's patients with a torn anterior cruciate ligament had no other identifiable lesion. In 70% of all anterior cruciate ligament tears an accompanying tear of a meniscus was found. Other studies have also confirmed the value of diagnostic arthroscopy compared with clinical impressions, arthrography, and other diagnostic tests.

Curran and Woodward (1980) studied 396 knee arthroscopies and found that the total clinical accuracy rate was only 71%. Diagnostic arthroscopy increased their accuracy to 97%. Of course, statistics will vary from one surgeon to another, depending on his clinical diagnostic acumen and his experience and proficiency with diagnostic arthroscopy.

Noyes et al. (1980) reported some degree of anterior cruciate ligament disruption in 72% of knees undergoing arthroscopy for acute, traumatic hemarthrosis, many knees with negative or equivocal stress tests. DeHaven (1980) and Gillquist and Hagberg (1978) have also documented the high incidence of torn anterior cruciate ligaments and other internal derangements in patients with acute traumatic hemarthrosis when arthroscopy is carried out early in the evaluation process.

Arthroscopy should be considered a diagnostic aid used in conjunction with a good history, complete physical examination, and appropriate roentgenograms. It should serve as an adjunct to, not as a replacement for, a thorough clinical evaluation.

One must become proficient in diagnostic arthroscopy before proceeding to operative arthroscopy. To do so one must become comfortable with the arthroscope and completely familiar with and competent in using multiple portals interchangeably. The ability to make the transition from a high degree of diagnostic accuracy to the simpler intraarticular operative technique will vary from one surgeon to another. Suffice to say if one's orthopaedic practice does not include a large number of patients with knee problems, it is difficult to develop the skills in arthroscopy of the knee. However, no set number of cases must be done to become an arthroscopic surgeon. It is learning to triangulate a second and third instrument into the visual field within the joint that is essential to the transition from diagnostic to operative skills. The use of the probe during diagnostic arthroscopy is the first step in learning this skill.

The general principles, instrumentation, indications, contraindications, and complications of arthroscopy are discussed in Chapter 58.

BASIC DIAGNOSTIC TECHNIQUES
General principles

Arthroscopy of the knee may be carried out as a purely diagnostic procedure, as the essential initial step before proceeding to operative arthroscopy, or before an open arthrotomy. Anesthesia may be local, spinal, or general. If the procedure is for diagnostic evaluation only, it may be carried out using local anesthesia in cooperative patients, especially if the surgeon is experienced in arthroscopy. Diagnostic arthroscopy before arthrotomy or intraarticular surgery is generally best carried out with the patient under general anesthesia, unless this type of anesthesia is contraindicated. If spinal anesthesia is selected because the procedure is long (over 1 hour) and a tourniquet is required, discomfort from the tourniquet may be a problem. Therefore, especially early in one's experience, general anesthesia probably is best unless specifically contraindicated.

The procedure is performed in the operating room under strict sterile conditions. The seriousness of this surgical procedure must not be minimized. While complications such as infection are infrequent, carelessness in surgical scrubbing, preparation, or draping, or careless handling of the irrigating solutions, arthroscopes, and instruments can result in intraarticular infections just as devastating as those following arthrotomy.

A tourniquet is placed about the thigh, but is not inflated in diagnostic arthroscopy, unless troublesome bleeding occurs. Inflation of the tourniquet blanches the synovium and other vascularized tissue and makes diagnostic evaluation of these structures more difficult. The tourniquet usually is inflated after exsanguination of the limb in acute traumatic disorders or if the surgeon anticipates other than the simplest intraarticular surgical procedure.

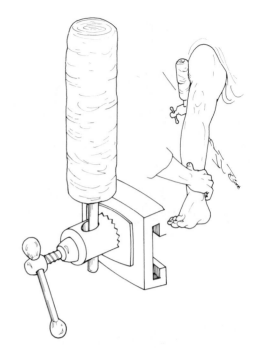

Fig. 59-1. Simple and inexpensive way to apply countertraction to thigh while applying valgus external rotation force to leg allows access to posterior half of medial compartment. Padded metal bar 10 to 12 inches long is secured to operating table and standard stirrup holder. Positioned approximately at midthigh, bar can be moved easily during operative procedure if no longer needed. (From Zarins, B.: Contemp. Orthop. **6**:63, 1977.)

Stressing the knee to open up the various compartments is necessary for either diagnostic or operative procedures. This may be accomplished by using an assistant, a padded lateral post (Fig. 59-1), or a commercial leg-holding device (Fig. 59-2). The use of an assistant to stress the joint is probably the least efficient because of fatigue and the inconsistent amounts of stress that result, among other factors. The use of a padded lateral post attached to the edge of the operating table can be effective for valgus stressing in or near full extension, but does not control rotation. The commercial thigh holders are most effective, but some of their potential dangers must be kept in mind. Also, they are quite expensive. While the use of a leg-holding device makes stressing and opening especially of the posterior compartments easier, these devices do get in the way to some extent when working through the superior portals in the patellofemoral joint. Also, the potential tourniquet effect of the leg-holding devices must be appreciated. We have had no known problems with the commercial leg holder and believe that the advantages of being able to control and stress the joint far outweigh the potential disadvantages.

Surgical draping

Once the patient is anesthetized, the tourniquet and leg holder are applied if desired and the limb from the ankle to the tourniquet is thoroughly scrubbed and surgically prepared, just as for an open arthrotomy. It is essential to

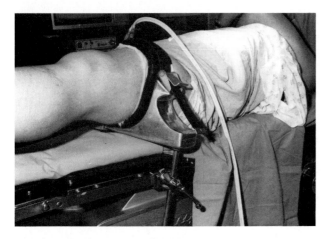

Fig. 59-2. Commercial leg holder that mounts to side rail of standard operating room table. With this particular commercial leg holder, pneumatic tourniquet is placed inside leg holding device.

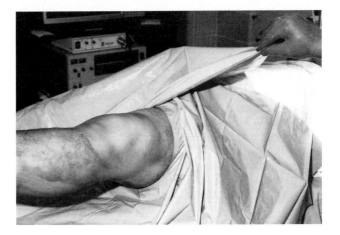

Fig. 59-3. Commercial plastic waterproof underdrape with adhesive strip seals proximal thigh, leg holder, and tourniquet from sterile field.

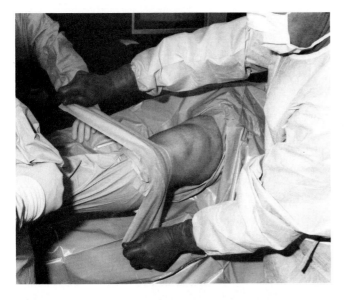

Fig. 59-4. Waterproof stockinette sealed about its proximal end with adhesive strips assures operative field sterility from unsterile foot and leg.

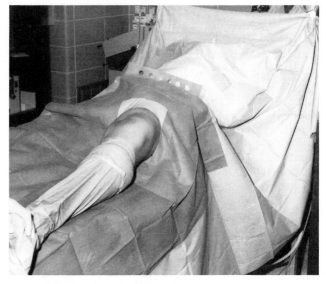

Fig. 59-5. Waterproof outer drape with central rubberized opening seals unsterile proximal thigh from operative field.

seal off the unprepared foot, and the unsterile tourniquet and leg holder, from the sterile field. An adhesive, waterproof, plastic drape is useful here. We prefer to use a special commercial arthroscope draping package for this. A long, adhesive plastic, U underdrape is placed under the leg with the adhesive tails of its proximal end wrapped snugly around the distal thigh just below the tourniquet and above the suprapatellar pouch (Fig. 59-3). This effectively seals off the tourniquet and leg holder. The foot and lower leg are placed in a stockinette with a waterproof covering that is sealed about the upper leg just below the knee (Fig. 59-4). Failure to seal the stockinette below the knee allows leakage from the arthroscope portal and the potential accumulation of large amounts of irrigating so-

lution inside the stockinette. A large table outer drape, with a round, central, rubberized opening is then pulled over the limb, further sealing the distal thigh (Fig. 59-5). This completes the draping—the tourniquet and leg holder sealed by the adhesive U underdrape and the waterproof overdrape, the foot sealed with a waterproof stockinette and adhesive about the proximal leg, and then the distal thigh further sealed with the waterproof overdrape. Thus the leg is draped free for easy maneuvering and stressing. Many of the commercial drapes have tabs for anchoring the suction, inflow, and outflow tubing, and the fiberoptic light cables. These tabs prevent the tubes and cables from sliding off the drape and becoming contaminated.

The surgeon and assistant likewise should wear water-resistant gowns or waterproof aprons to prevent potential contamination.

The prepared and draped limb may be kept lateral to the table or the end of the table may be dropped so both limbs dangle at 90 degrees, depending on the surgeon's preference (Fig. 59-6). If the end of the table is dropped, careful padding and positioning of the opposite leg are essential to avoid potential pressure disorders.

The scrub nurse uses a large back table for instruments. This is positioned for her convenience, usually at the side opposite the knee having surgery. A Mayo stand is placed over the operating table at the level of the upper part of the thighs, and the more commonly used instruments are placed on it. Power cords and light cables are attached to the appropriate sources and are placed on a side table. Irrigation bags are suspended from an intravenous stand at the head of the table and are raised approximately 4 to 5 feet above the level of the patient. The surgeon either stands or sits at the foot of the table, as he desires. The assistant stands to the side of the distal thigh, just below the leg holder, facing the operating surgeon. The assistant can be used to hold various instruments, to stress the leg against the leg-holding device, or if no leg-holding device is used, to hold the leg. If a leg-holding device is in place and the surgeon prefers to stand, he may stand inside the abducted leg, place his outside foot on a small platform, position his hip at approximately 90 degrees, and rest the patient's ankle on his hip and iliac crest area (Fig. 59-7). This frees both the surgeon's hands, and the surgeon can stress the leg into valgus by simply leaning against the leg in the leg holder. One may achieve more consistent stress when needed without fatigue using this technique.

Entry portals

Among the cardinal keys to success in arthroscopy are adequate light, distention of the joint, and *precise* localization of the portals of entry for the scope and accessory instruments. Without adequate illumination, clear vision is

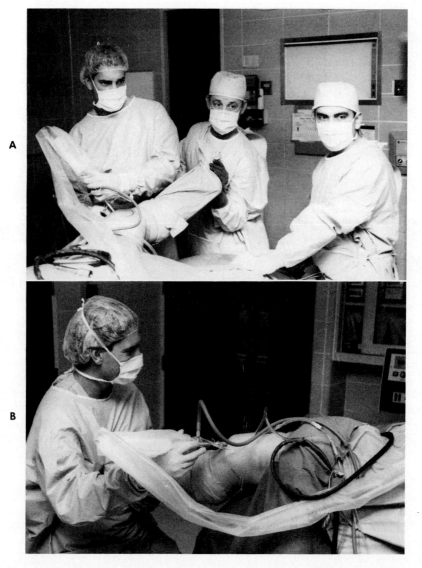

Fig. 59-6. A, Technique of "table flat" position. Surgeon and assistant stand at side of table. **B,** Technique of "table fixed" position. Surgeon sits with sterile draped foot and leg in lap.

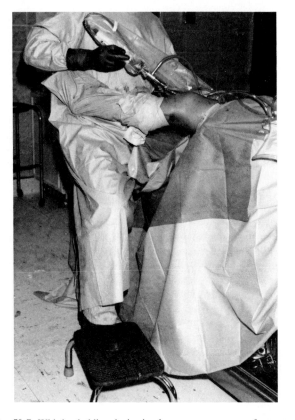

Fig. 59-7. With leg-holding device in place, surgeon may prefer to stand inside patient's abducted leg with outside foot on small platform, hip flexed about 90 degrees, and patient's ankle resting on surgeon's hip and iliac crest area.

impossible; without adequate distention of the joint, the fat pad, synovium, and other soft tissue obstructions obliterate the view; and without precise location of the portals of entry, one will not be able to adequately see all parts of the joint. Then attempts to force the poorly placed arthroscope or instruments will result in articular scuffing, damage to instruments, and other problems. Adequate illumination is assured by proper care of the arthroscope and fiberoptic light cables, changing the light source bulbs when required, cleansing the scope lenses of film from frequent disinfectant soakings, and maintaining a clear irrigation medium. Distention is assured by proper inflow cannula placement, elevating the irrigation fluid bag 4 to 5 feet above the patient, and regulating the stopcock on the outflow tube. Occasionally, in the presence of a florid synovitis, the use of carbon dioxide to distend the joint will force the synovial fronds to "lie down" for better viewing. Precise entry portal location can best be assured by carefully drawing the joint lines and soft tissue and bony landmarks with a skin marking pen before joint distention. All standard and optional portals are marked. Typically, the outlines of the patella and patellar tendon are drawn, the medial and lateral joint lines are palpated with the fingertip and drawn; and the posterior contours of the medial and lateral femoral condyles are marked. The anterior edges of the tibial collateral ligament medially and the fibular collateral ligament laterally are identified and marked. A line across the midpatellar area is drawn to locate the optional midpatellar lateral and midpatellar medial portals (Fig. 59-8).

Once these anatomic landmarks and portals are carefully

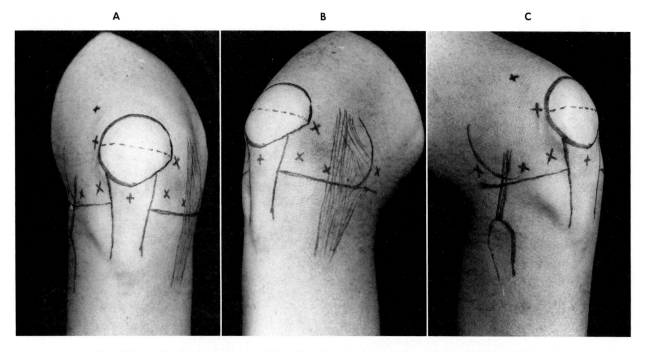

A   B   C

Fig. 59-8. Landmarks drawn on knee before distention. **A,** Anterior view of knee showing standard and optional portal sites and landmarks. Standard portals—anteromedial, anterolateral, and superolateral. Optional portals—transpatellar tendon (central) and midpatellar medial and lateral. **B,** Medial view of knee showing medial skin portal sites and landmarks. **C,** Lateral view of knee showing lateral portal sites and landmarks.

marked, an inflow cannula is inserted, usually into the superomedial suprapatellar pouch. With some arthroscopic systems, the inflow cannula is interchangeable with the sheath for the arthroscope and other instruments. Other systems, or the surgeons' preference, may bring the irrigating solutions through irrigating needles inserted into the suprapatellar pouch, or via the irrigation channels through the arthroscope sheath. Regardless of the system chosen, any blood or effusion within the joint should be removed and observed or submitted for evaluation. If blood is found within the joint, the presence of fat globules may denote an unsuspected fracture; if the fluid is turbid, a sample should be submitted for culture, sensitivity, and synovial fluid analysis. The joint is now thoroughly lavaged and distended.

STANDARD PORTALS

The standard portals for diagnostic arthroscopy are the anterolateral (AL), anteromedial (AM), posteromedial (PM), and superolateral (SL).

Anterolateral portal. If one were allowed only one approach for a diagnostic arthroscopy of the knee joint, the anterolateral portal would be chosen by most arthroscopic surgeons. Using a 30-degree oblique fore lens arthroscope through this anterolateral portal, almost all of the structures within the knee joint can be seen. Through this portal the posterior cruciate ligament, the anterior portion of the lateral meniscus, and in tight knees, the periphery of the posterior horn of the medial meniscus may not be adequately viewed. This portal is located approximately 1 cm above the lateral joint line (previously drawn with a marking pencil) and approximately 1.0 cm lateral to the margin of the patellar tendon. If the portal is placed too near the joint line the anterior horn of the lateral meniscus may be lacerated or otherwise damaged. Also the arthroscope may

be inserted through such a portal either through or beneath the anterior horn of the lateral meniscus. This results in damage to the anterior horn or difficulty in maneuvering the arthroscope within the joint because it is bound down by the overlying meniscus. A portal placement too superior to the joint line does not permit the arthroscope to enter the space between the femoral and tibial condyles, and therefore access for viewing the posterior horns of the menisci and other posterior structures is not possible (Fig. 59-9). Placement of the scope immediately adjacent to the edge of the patellar tendon results in the possible penetration of the fat pad, causing difficulty in viewing and maneuvering the arthroscope within the joint.

Anteromedial portal. In diagnostic arthroscopy the anteromedial portal is most commonly used for viewing the entire lateral compartment and for inserting the probe for palpation of the medial compartment structures. This portal is located in a manner similar to the anterolateral portal, that is, 1 cm above the medial joint line and 1 cm medial to the edge of the patellar tendon.

Posteromedial portal. The posteromedial portal is located in a small, triangular soft spot formed by the posteromedial edge of the femoral condyle and the posteromedial edge of the tibia. Before distention of the joint this small triangle can be palpated easily with the knee flexed to 90 degrees. The landmarks shown in Fig. 59-8, *B* should be drawn on the skin before beginning the diagnostic arthroscopy. The posteromedial compartment is small, but any arthroscope can be inserted into it with proper care and technique. A 30-degree angled scope is necessary for best viewing of all of the structures in this posteromedial compartment. Three guidelines, properly observed, are essential in predictably making this portal easy and routine: (1) the knee must be maximally distended with irrigating solution, so the posteromedial compartment balloons out like

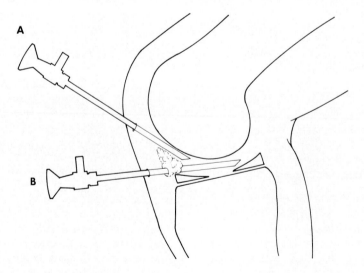

Fig. 59-9. Placement of anterolateral portal. **A,** Arthroscope introduced through portal placed too high above joint line has advantage of avoiding fat pad and being easy to manipulate. However, it is difficult to reach posterior aspect of the joint where most meniscal pathology is located. **B,** With low portal, posterior access is easier since femoral condyle does not get in way, but instrumentation through fat pad is more difficult. Compromise should be made depending on location of intraarticular pathology and tightness of joint. (From Zarins, B.: Contemp. Orthop. **6:**19, 1983.)

a bubble when the knee is flexed to 90 degrees, (2) the knee must be flexed to accomplish this, and (3) the bony landmarks must be drawn before the joint is distended. The location of the portal should be about 1 cm above the posteromedial joint line and precisely at the posteromedial margin of the femoral condyle. The use of the angled lens allows the surgeon to look down on the posterior horn of the medial meniscus and across into the posterior intercondylar notch to view the posterior cruciate ligament. It is usually easy to pierce the distended posteromedial capsule of the flexed knee with the sharp obturator tip, aiming the obturator and sheath parallel or slightly anterior and inferior to the posterior edge of the medial femoral condyle.

Removal of the sharp obturator from the sheath results in escape of the irrigating solution under pressure through the sheath, confirming proper placement within the posteromedial compartment. The meniscocapsular junction of the posterior third of the medial meniscus can be viewed. The posterior periphery of the medial meniscus and the posterior cruciate ligament can be investigated via a probe inserted through the anterolateral portal and passed through the intercondylar notch and into the posterior compartment, or via a probe triangulated from a separate posteromedial portal.

Superolateral portal. The superolateral portal is most useful diagnostically for viewing the dynamics of the patellofemoral articulation. This portal is located just lateral to the quadriceps tendon about 2.5 cm superior to the superolateral corner of the patella. With the arthroscope in this portal, the patellofemoral joint can be viewed and the tracking of the patella can be observed as the knee is carried from extension into varying degrees of flexion, observing its congruity, its lateral overhang, and other characteristics.

OPTIONAL PORTALS

Posterolateral portal. The knee should be flexed 90 degrees and the joint maximally distended. The landmark for the posterolateral portal is at a point where a line drawn along the posterior margin of the femoral shaft intersects a line drawn along the posterior aspect of the fibula. This is about 2 cm above the posterolateral joint line at the posterior edge of the iliotibial band and the anterior edge of the biceps femoris tendon. A 2 to 3 mm skin incision is made, and the distended posterior capsule is penetrated using the arthroscope sheath and sharp trocar. The posterior edge of the femoral condyle is palpated with a trocar, slipping off the posterior condyle parallel to it. Directed slightly inferiorly, the sheath will enter the posterolateral compartment. Care must be taken not to damage the articular surface of the posterior femoral condyle with this maneuver. Also, plunging in with a sharp trocar through the capsule into the popliteal space must be avoided for fear of damaging neurovascular structures. The outflow of irrigation solution on removal of the sharp trocar confirms entry into the joint.

Proximal midpatellar medial and lateral portals. The optional midpatellar portal designations should not be confused with the central transpatellar tendon or Swedish portal, to be described later. These optional portals were described by Patel (1981) to improve the viewing of the anterior compartment structures, the lateral meniscocapsular structures, and the popliteus tunnel and to minimize accessory instrument crowding with the arthroscope during procedures requiring triangulation of several instruments into these compartments. Views of the posterior horns of the menisci are difficult through these portals.

These portals are located just off the medial and lateral edges of the midpatella at the broadest portion of the bone. The selection of the site is critical. A site that is too far superiorly or inferiorly can jeopardize proper viewing. A 30-degree oblique arthroscope is ideal here.

Accessory "far" medial and lateral portals. These inferior optional portals are often used for triangulation of accessory instruments into the knee during operative arthroscopic procedures. They are located approximately 2.5 cm medial or lateral to the standard anteromedial and anterolateral portals. Medially, these portals are near the anterior edge of the tibial collateral ligament; laterally, they should be well anterior to the fibular collateral ligament and popliteus tendon. An excellent technique is to insert a spinal needle through the skin and capsule into the compartment under direct vision with the arthroscope. The needle should enter the joint above the superior surface of the meniscus, which will allow passage to its desired location. After directing the needle to the desired location within the joint, the accessory instrument is also passed to this location with ease. If the needle cannot pass to the desired location, its point of entry is carefully adjusted before making the portal incision. The margin for error is less through these accessory medial and lateral portals; the meniscus or the collateral ligament may be lacerated or the articular margin of the femoral condyle may be damaged.

Central transpatellar tendon, or Swedish portal. The central transpatellar tendon portal is located approximately 1 cm inferior to the lower pole of the patella in the midline of the joint through the patellar tendon. With the patella in higher or lower locations or if the patellar tendon is located entirely lateral to the midline of the joint, adjustments in portal location must be made.

With the knee flexed 90 degrees, a 1 cm incision is made through the skin and subcutaneous tissue, but not through the anterior fibers of the patellar tendon. The tendon is split with the sharp trocar of the arthroscope. Penetration of the tendon is made without the sheath, since the offset of the sheath might rupture tendon fibers. The sharp obturator should pass only into the fat pad. An up and down motion of the sharp obturator splits the tendon vertically. This enlarges the split in the patellar tendon fibers enough to allow atraumatic insertion of the arthroscope sheath and blunt obturator. These are then pushed into the joint with the knee flexed about 45 degrees, aiming the sheath and obturator toward the superomedial compartment. This guarantees passage of the arthroscope above the fat pad. The arthroscope should not pass through the fat pad, because that structure tends to be carried into the joint with the sheath and can obliterate the viewing.

Advocates of this portal cite the following advantages. With the arthroscope in this central position, the standard anteromedial and anterolateral portals are available for bimanual instrument manipulation within the anterior part of the joint. Additionally, this midline location permits movement of the arthroscope through the intercondylar notch into the posterior compartments, allowing a direct view of the posterior joint structures. Probing the posterior structures is then possible through accessory anterior or posterior portals. The use of this midline portal for direct viewing of the posterior structures via the intercondylar notch requires the use of a 70-degree oblique arthroscope, and considerable practice is necessary to master the technique. Further details concerning the use of this portal for meniscectomy will be described later in the section on arthroscopic surgical techniques.

Insertion of scope

If the tourniquet is not to be inflated unless troublesome bleeding occurs, the portal sites should be infiltrated with 4 to 5 ml of a local anesthetic agent mixed with epinephrine. This will reduce bleeding and postoperative pain. More than 4 to 5 ml is not advised, since a larger bolus, especially in the anterolateral and anteromedial portals, may distend the fat pad sufficiently to make viewing difficult. If inflation of the tourniquet is planned the portals are usually not infiltrated.

The anterolateral portal is selected for initial insertion of the arthroscope. This portal site, marked before joint distention, is located 1.0 cm (approximately one fingerbreadth) above the lateral joint line, and approximately 1.0 cm lateral to the edge of the patellar tendon. The knee is flexed approximately 30 degrees, and a 3 to 4 mm incision is made through the skin and subcutaneous tissues using a No. 15 knife blade. Then the cutting edge of the blade is rotated superiorly, and the incision is extended through the capsule. Having the cutting edge of the blade oriented superiorly minimizes the risk of cutting the anterior horn of the lateral meniscus. Care must be taken to avoid overpenetration with the blade to prevent cutting or scuffing of the articular surface of the femoral condyle. With the joint distended with irrigating solution, egress of solution warns of penetration of the synovium, and the blade should be withdrawn. However, it is safer to penetrate the synovium with the arthroscope sheath and a sharp trocar. With the knee flexed to 30 degrees, the arthroscope sheath with its sharp trocar is inserted through the incision in the skin, subcutaneous tissue, and capsule directed at an angle about 45 degrees medially and superiorly to the plane of the leg. This is in the direction of the intercondylar notch. With a gentle push, the synovium is penetrated. When resistance is no longer felt, the sharp trocar is removed from the sheath. The escape of solution through the sheath confirms positioning of the sheath inside the joint. The blunt trocar is inserted through the sheath and the assembly is pushed gently into the anterior intercondylar notch region. With experience, the outline of the intercondylar notch can be

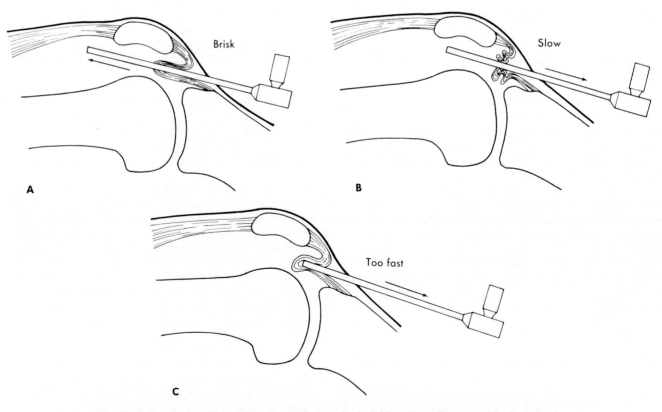

Fig. 59-10. Introduction of scope into suprapatellar pouch. **A,** Brisk motion will penetrate the fat pad and suprapatellar pouch, hanging fat pad and synovium on shank of cannula. **B,** Slow retraction of cannula and endoscope will prevent fat pad from slipping over end of scope. **C,** Fast retraction will pull endoscope into fat pad and obscure viewing. (From Johnson, L.C.: Arthroscopic Surgery, ed. 3, St. Louis, 1986, The C.V. Mosby Co.)

sensed by palpation using the tip of the blunt obturator. As an assistant slowly extends the knee, the tip of the obturator is retracted slightly. As the knee comes into extension, the obturator and sheath are pushed beneath the patella, through the patellofemoral joint, and into the suprapatellar bursa. Once this maneuver is learned, it should be done briskly to allow the synovium to hang up on the sheath; slow withdrawal then pulls the synovium back out of the viewing field (Fig. 59-10). Care must be taken not to rupture the suprapatellar bursa with this maneuver, or distention of the joint during the procedure cannot be maintained.

The blunt obturator is removed and the arthroscope is inserted through the sheath. A 30-degree oblique fore lens arthroscope is used for most diagnostic and operative procedures. The fiberoptic light cable and tubings are connected to the sheath assembly. Some surgeons prefer irrigating solution inflow through the arthroscope sheath channel, others through a separate cannula. Using the sheath channel for inflow assures a clear visual field immediately at the end of the arthroscope. Also, suction can be applied if needed. However, distention of the joint may be lessened, since the volume of solution through this small sheath channel is considerably less than through a larger inflow cannula. Overall, the use of tubings connected to the arthroscope sheath for inflow, suction, or outflow, is determined by the preference of the surgeon. The obliquity of the arthroscope's fore lens relative to the direction of the light cable attachment to the arthroscope should be noted, that is, does it face the cable or away from it? This frequently varies from one commercial brand of arthroscope to the next. This permits easy orientation to the direction of the visual field.

At all times during arthroscopy, the ulnar border of the hand should rest on the leg to give better depth control and avoid fatigue. This position is similar to that used in holding a pencil in writing. If the hand that controls the arthroscope remains in contact with the leg at all times, the arthroscope will not pull out too far or lose position as the knee is manipulated during the examination. Holding the assembly in this manner also keeps the hands away from the unsterile eyepiece of the arthroscope.

It is advisable for the beginning arthroscopist to view directly through the arthroscope, learning to maneuver the scope through the joint, interchanging portals, using the advantages afforded by the arthroscope's angled fore lens, and beginning simple triangulation techniques, rather than using the video camera attached to the arthroscope. Attaching even a miniature video camera to the arthroscope makes maneuverability within the joint and orientation more difficult for the inexperienced arthroscopist.

ARTHROSCOPIC EXAMINATION OF KNEE

The key to successful, accurate, and complete diagnosis of lesions within the knee joint is a systematic approach to viewing. One should develop a methodical sequence of examination, progressing from one compartment to another and systematically carrying out this sequence in every knee. The exact sequence is not critical, but it is important to develop a habit of following it every time. Failure to do so will compromise diagnostic accuracy and completeness (Plate 6).

The knee should be divided routinely into the following compartments for arthroscopic examination:
1. Suprapatellar pouch and patellofemoral joint
2. Medial compartment
3. Intercondylar notch
4. Lateral compartment
5. Posteromedial compartment

In addition, the medial and lateral gutters should be examined. The posterolateral compartment can usually be examined adequately from an anterior portal, but if this compartment is incompletely viewed, a direct posterolateral portal should be chosen.

Suprapatellar pouch and patellofemoral joint

With the arthroscope in the distended suprapatellar pouch and the knee in extension, the surgeon systematically examines the synovium, patella, trochlear notch of the femur, synovial plicae, adhesions, and quadriceps tendon. With the oblique fore lens of the arthroscope directed superiorly, the undersurface of the quadriceps tendon can be inspected. The synovium is usually quite thin in this area.

By rotating the arthroscopic lens alternately to the right and left, the synovium, suprapatellar plicae, adhesions, and other structures within the superior part of the pouch can be seen. One observes the character of the synovial villi, their vascularity, the signs of inflammation, crystalline deposition, and so forth. Suprapatellar plicae and mild adhesions are rarely of pathologic importance. Sweeping the arthroscope from side to side, pistoning it inward and outward, one may carefully focus on the individual structures.

By slowly withdrawing the arthroscope with the fore lens looking upward, one sees the undersurface of the patella (Plate 6, A). With the suprapatellar pouch maximally distended and the knee in full extension, the arthroscope can easily sweep across the patellofemoral joint. The central ridge and medial and lateral facets of the patella are carefully inspected. Manipulation of the patella by the surgeon's free hand, which depresses or tilts each edge, allows inspection of its entire articular surface, the condition of which should be noted.

Rotating the lens so it is looking inferiorly allows similar inspection of the surface of the trochlear notch of the femur. The congruity of the patella in the patellofemoral joint and its dynamics in flexion and extension are best viewed from a superolateral portal. The arthroscope is rotated to point toward the medial peripatellar region. In about 40% of knees, a medial synovial plica can be identified running slightly medial and distal to the patella (Plate 6, B). This synovial and fibrous band usually originates medially from the side wall of the suprapatellar bursa and inserts into the fat pad distally. It may be responsible for anterior knee pain, popping, and chondromalacic changes on the medial femoral condyle when it is thickened and fibrotic from trauma or chronic synovitis. Occasionally a large medial plica will impede the sweep of the arthroscope inferiorly toward the medial compartment. If this occurs, the arthroscope must be partially withdrawn, disengaging it from the plica. With the arthroscope lens looking downward and the horizon of the medial femoral condyle in view, the arthroscope is swept along the medial femoral condyle and down into the anteromedial compartment until the meniscosynovial junction is seen. The knee is then flexed to 30 degrees, a valgus stress is applied, and the arthroscope is moved into the anteromedial compartment.

Medial compartment

Once the arthroscope has been brought into the anteromedial compartment, the free edge of the medial meniscus orients the viewer. The knee is positioned in 10 to 30 degrees of flexion, a valgus stress is applied, and the tibia is externally rotated. For a systematic examination of the medial meniscus, the surgeon divides the meniscus into regions—the posterior, middle, and anterior thirds. By gently wedging the arthroscope, it can usually be slipped between the medial femoral condyle and the medial tibial plateau articular surfaces, assuming the knee is properly positioned and stressed. The arthroscope should not be forced between the condyles, or severe scuffing will result. With the lens directed posteriorly, the inner free edge of the posterior third of the medial meniscus can be viewed from its intercondylar tibial attachment to the posteromedial corner of the knee (Plate 6, *C*). Only in the lax knee can the posterior meniscosynovial and capsular attachments be viewed from this anterolateral portal. Examination of the meniscus is made easier by inserting a probe through an anteromedial portal. The probe is used to lift, to depress, or to gently retract the meniscus. Frequently, tears through the surface of the meniscus, not noted by simple visual inspection, can be demonstrated by probing. Examination of the meniscus is never complete until the entire meniscus is probed. The instrument should be used gently for this. The meniscus can actually be torn by too vigorous probing, especially when the tip of the probe is used. The posterior horn of the meniscus should be viewed with the knee flexed (10 to 30 degrees) and externally rotated and by internally and externally rotating the tibia on the femur.

If a small rim of the medial meniscus is seen instead of a meniscus of normal size, the knee may either have had a prior medial meniscectomy, or a displaced bucket handle tear of the medial meniscus exists, with the major portion of the meniscus displaced into the intercondylar notch. A torn, displaced meniscus in the intercondylar notch can obstruct the arthroscope and make viewing difficult.

Peripheral detachments of the medial meniscus, although not directly viewed, may be suspected when there are abnormal meniscal movements, wrinkling, and so forth. Viewing of the peripheral portion of the meniscus and its attachments can usually best be accomplished through a posteromedial portal or with a 70-degree angled arthroscope passed through the intercondylar notch into the posteromedial compartment (see p. 2557.)

The arthroscope should be withdrawn slightly and the lens rotated directly medially to view the middle third of the medial meniscus. Again, the superior and inferior surfaces and the stability of the meniscus should be observed under probing. The meniscosynovial reflection at the periphery, the synovial covering, and the midmedial capsular and posterior oblique portions of the tibial collateral ligament complex should be evaluated. The peripheral attach-

ment of the middle third of the medial meniscus can be clearly seen.

The surgeon can sweep the arthroscope back into the anteromedial compartment and further rotate the lens anteriorly to examine the anterior horn of the meniscus (Plate 6, *D*). The fat pad may obliterate the view of its most anterior portion. Further distention of the knee by closing the irrigation outflow may push the fat pad away a few millimeters so this area can be viewed. If viewing is still not possible, redirecting the arthroscope, inserting a probe through an anteromedial portal to retract the fat pad, resecting a portion of the fat pad, or moving the arthroscope to a midpatellar portal may allow viewing of this area.

The articular surfaces of the femoral and tibial condyles should be systematically examined for defects indicating chondromalacia or other abnormalities. Flexing the knee will bring greater areas of the femoral condyle into view. With the arthroscope lens directed superiorly and laterally, the surgeon can follow the horizon of the medial femoral condyle into the intercondylar notch.

Intercondylar notch

The anatomic structures to be examined in the intercondylar notch are the anterior cruciate ligament, the ligamentum mucosum, the fat pad, and occasionally the posterior cruciate ligament. As the arthroscope follows the horizon of the medial femoral condyle into the intercondylar notch and superiorly to the top of the intercondylar notch, the femoral origin of the ligamentum mucosum is seen. The ligamentum mucosum runs from the superior intercondylar notch down to the fat pad. It may be a thin, narrow band of synovium or a complete septum dividing the medial and lateral compartments. Difficulty in passing the arthroscope from the lateral to the medial compartment and vice versa may result from an enlarged ligamentum mucosum or a complete septum. More commonly, it is a narrow synovial membrane superior and anterior to the anterior cruciate ligament.

The fat pad may be especially troublesome to the beginning arthroscopist and can make viewing difficult. Dealing with the fat pad is described above.

The cruciate ligaments within the intercondylar notch are best viewed with the knee flexed 45 to 90 degrees. The femoral insertion of the posterior cruciate ligament should be inspected; it is usually covered by synovial tissue. Occasionally the fibers of the posterior cruciate ligament can be viewed and probed; hemorrhage or tearing of this synovial covering can be observed in posterior cruciate ligament avulsions.

The anterior cruciate ligament is the most imposing structure in the intercondylar notch (Plate 6, *E*). The tibial insertion and most of the ligament can be viewed adequately from this anterolateral portal. Viewing and exploration of the femoral attachment of the anterior cruciate ligament may best be carried out with the arthroscope through an anteromedial portal.

The appearance of the anterior cruciate ligament will vary from patient to patient, depending on its anatomy, the presence or absence of injury, and the synovial covering. Occasionally the various anatomic bands of the anterior cruciate ligament will appear as distinct bundles. In the

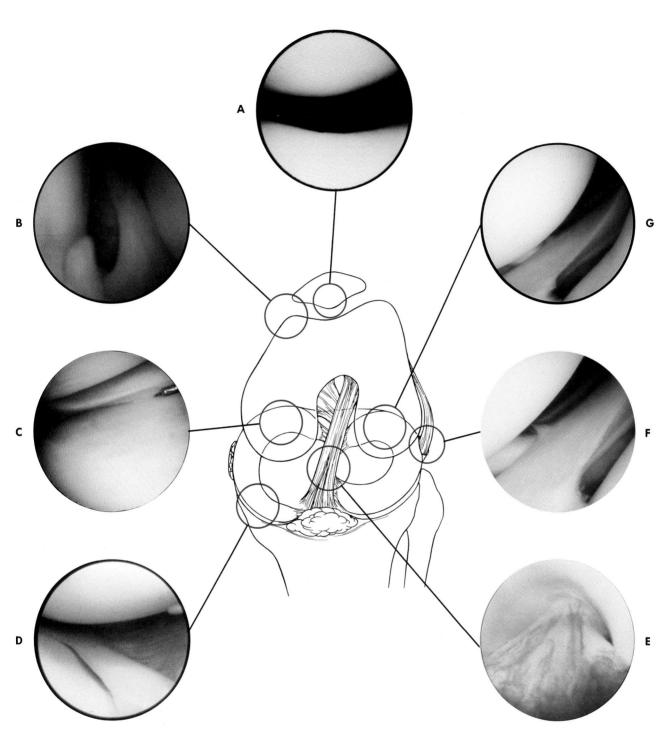

Plate 6. Typical views of normal knee. **A,** Tangential view of patellofemoral articulation; **B,** medial patellar plica; **C,** posterior horn, medial meniscus; **D,** anterior region, medial meniscus; **E,** anterior cruciate ligament; **F,** popliteus tendon; **G,** posterior horn, lateral meniscus.

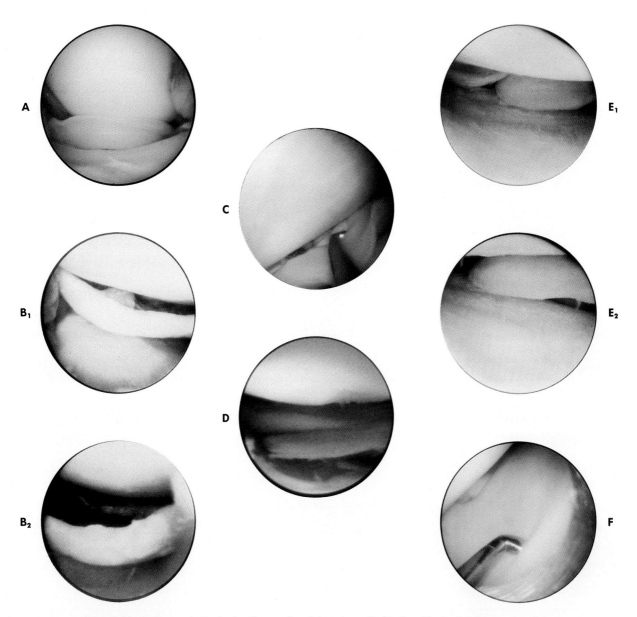

Plate 7. Meniscal tears. **A,** Bucket handle tear of medial meniscus. **B,** Displaced bucket handle tear of medial meniscus. **C,** Undisplaced longitudinal peripheral tear of medial meniscus. **D,** Anterior oblique tear of medial meniscus. **E,** Radial tear of lateral meniscus. **F,** Intact discoid of lateral meniscus.

normal anterior cruciate ligament, the synovial covering is usually thin, with small capillaries coursing on the surface that are obvious with close examination. If considerable synovitis is present, retraction of the ligamentum mucosum and other synovial tissues may be required to observe the underlying anterior cruciate ligament. With complete rupture of the anterior cruciate ligament, considerable hemorrhage within the synovial tissues is first evident. If the synovial covering has also been ruptured, the collagen bundles of the anterior cruciate ligament are apparent as white "mop end" structures. In other instances, the synovial covering may be intact but hemorrhagic. Careful probing and opening of the synovial sheath often demonstrate disrupted anterior cruciate ligament bundles not evident during initial inspection. Thus probing of the anterior cruciate ligament, opening its synovial sheath, and checking its tension with the probe are just as important as probing the menisci. The normal anterior cruciate ligament feels taut or "hard" when hooked with a probing instrument. The torn anterior cruciate ligament feels mushy, without tension. A drawer or a Lachman test may be performed by the assistant while the anterior cruciate ligament is directly viewed. If torn, the ligament can be seen to provide no functional stability to anteroposterior translation of the tibia on the femur.

Lateral compartment

While the lateral compartment of the knee can be viewed with the arthroscope through the anterolateral portal, it is best examined by moving the arthroscope to an anteromedial portal and using a probe through the anterolateral portal. The knee is placed in a figure-four position by flexing and abducting the hip, flexing the knee, and resting the heel and foot on the opposite leg. If a leg holder that encircles the thigh is in place, it makes achieving this figure-four position more difficult, but usually the thigh and hip will externally rotate enough to achieve this position. Downward pressure by the assistant on the thigh just above the knee will result in a varus and internal rotational opening of the lateral compartment. If a constricting leg holder is being used, the alternative to the figure-four position is placing stress on the slightly flexed knee to achieve a varus position with internal rotation of the tibia.

Usually the entire lateral compartment and lateral meniscus can be examined with the arthroscope in the anteromedial portal. As the arthroscope is passed posterior to the fat pad and beneath the ligamentum mucosum, one occasionally encounters difficulty entering the lateral compartment from this anteromedial portal because of the presence of the intercondylar attachment of the anterior horn of the lateral meniscus. Because the lateral meniscus has a more circular orientation than the medial meniscus, the anterior horn comes well posterior into the intercondylar notch, and the arthroscope directed from an anteromedial portal must pass over this portion of the anterior third of the meniscus before it actually enters the lateral compartment. A displaced bucket handle tear of the lateral meniscus incarcerated within the intercondylar notch may also be responsible for difficulty in allowing the scope entry into the anterolateral compartment. With the obliquely angled fore lens directed posteriorly, the posterior third of the lateral meniscus is examined first (Plate 6, *G*). Again, dividing the lateral meniscus into regions or thirds and systematically examining each third assures complete examination. In the figure-four position the entire posterior third of the lateral meniscus can usually be viewed. The lateral meniscus tends to ride up off the lateral tibial condylar surface, and the inferior surface as well as the superior surface of the meniscus can be viewed and probed. The intercondylar attachment of the posterior horn of the lateral meniscus is located much further anteriorly than its medial meniscal counterpart. The meniscosynovial attachment of the posterior horn of the lateral meniscus should be carefully probed to detect any posterior peripheral tears.

At the posterolateral corner of the lateral compartment, the obliquely coursing popliteus tendon can be easily seen (Plate 6, *F*). This usually comes into view when the angled fore lens is slightly rotated to a more lateral position. The popliteus tendon usually appears as a brighter whitish color than the meniscus, which is a more whitish yellow color. The hiatus in the coronary ligament attachment between the edge of the meniscus and capsule should not be confused with a peripheral tear in the meniscus. Careful probing of the anterior and posterior limits of this hiatal opening will show a smooth synovial reflection, which, on close inspection, can be differentiated from the more ragged tear in the coronary ligament attachment of the lateral meniscus. This opening for the popliteus tendon frequently hides small loose bodies.

As the surgeon rotates the lens of the arthroscope to look laterally and slowly retracts the arthroscope, the middle third of the meniscus can be viewed and probed. Further rotation of the obliquely angled fore lens to view anteriorly will result in a good view of the anterior horn of the meniscus with the scope in this anteromedial portal. The anterior horn of the lateral meniscus may be difficult to view with clarity if the arthroscope is in the anterolateral portal, however. Occasionally a hypertrophic, edematous fat pad may block the view of the most anteromedial attachment of the anterior horn of the lateral meniscus, and it may be managed using the techniques described in the discussion of the anteromedial compartment. The articular surfaces of the femoral and tibial condyles should be carefully examined for chondromalacia and other changes.

Posteromedial compartment

The posteromedial compartment may be viewed either through a posteromedial portal, as described above, or with a 70-degree oblique arthroscope passed through the intercondylar notch from a central or transpatellar tendon portal. Use of a 30-degree oblique arthroscope is optimal if viewing is done through a posteromedial portal. Structures examined from these approaches are the peripheral attachment of the posterior horn of the medial meniscus, the posterior meniscosynovial reflection, the distal half of the posterior cruciate ligament (Plate 6, *C*), the posterior femoral condyle, and the confines of the posteromedial capsular and synovial compartment, a compartment to which free loose bodies and meniscal fragments tend to gravitate. When this compartment is viewed by way of a central portal through the intercondylar notch, the posterior cruciate ligament and posterior horn of the medial meniscus can be probed by inserting the probing instrument through a posteromedial accessory portal. Again, the surgeon can use a spinal needle inserted under direct vision to accurately locate the optimal portal site. The posterior attachment of a bucket handle tear of the medial meniscus can be accurately cut by the accessory cutting instrument inserted through a posteromedial portal and the 70-degree scope exposing the posterior horn via a central portal through the intercondylar notch.

Probing the posterior cruciate ligament and viewing the most posterior attachment of the medial meniscus with the 30-degree scope may be accomplished through a posteromedial portal. The probe can be inserted through the anterolateral portal and then passed medial to the anterior cruciate ligament into the posterior intercondylar notch region. The probe comes into view anterior to the posterior cruciate ligament. The most posterior central attachment of the medial meniscus may be probed by this route.

Posterolateral compartment

Structures viewed in the posterolateral compartment are the posterior horn of the lateral meniscus, the meniscosynovial capsular reflection, the popliteus tendon, the posterior limits of the popliteal hiatus, the confines of the posterolateral synovial and capsular compartments, and the posterior articular surface of the lateral femoral condyle.

The horizon for orientation in the posterolateral compartment is the posterior edge of the lateral femoral condyle. Once it is clearly viewed, this horizon is kept in view and followed inferiorly to the capsular and synovial attachments of the posterior horn of the lateral meniscus. As the surgeon looks inferiorly and anteriorly with the oblique lens of the arthroscope, the posterior limits of the popliteal hiatus and the posterior aspects of the popliteus tendon coursing through the hiatus can be examined. Frequently the posterolateral compartment and the popliteal hiatus are areas where loose bodies not seen from the standard anterior portals may be located.

ARTHROSCOPIC SURGERY OF MENISCUS

Classification of the types of meniscal tears encountered during a diagnostic arthroscopy of the knee is essential in planning the subsequent arthroscopic resection or repair. While numerous classifications of meniscal tears exist, the following, proposed by O'Connor, has proven useful. O'Connor classifies the patterns of meniscal tears into the following categories: (1) longitudinal tears; (2) horizontal tears; (3) oblique tears; (4) radial tears; and (5) variations, which include flap tears, complex tears, and degenerative meniscal tears (Fig. 59-11).

Longitudinal tears most commonly occur as a result of trauma to a reasonably normal meniscus. The tear is usually vertically oriented and may extend completely through the thickness of the meniscus, or may extend only partially or incompletely through it (Fig. 59-12). The tear is oriented parallel to the edge of the meniscus, and, if the tear is complete, a displaceable inner fragment is frequently produced. When the inner fragment displaces over into the intercondylar notch, it is commonly referred to as a bucket handle tear (Fig. 59-13). If the tear is near the meniscocapsular attachment of the meniscus, it is commonly re-

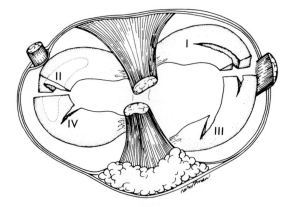

Fig. 59-11. Four basic patterns of meniscal tears: I, longitudinal; II, horizontal; III, oblique; and IV, radial. (From Shahriaree, H.: O'Connor's textbook of arthroscopic surgery, Philadelphia, 1984, J.B. Lippincott Co.)

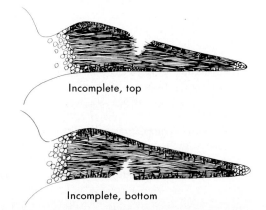

Incomplete, top

Incomplete, bottom

Fig. 59-12. Incomplete superior and inferior longitudinal tears. (From Shahriaree, H.: O'Connor's textbook of arthroscopic surgery, Philadelphia, 1984, J.B. Lippincott Co.)

ferred to as a peripheral tear (Fig. 59-14). If the longitudinal tear is located within the peripheral 25% of the meniscus and the remainder of the meniscus is intact, it may be suitable for suturing with a high expectation of healing, rather than requiring excision.

Horizontal tears tend to be more common in older patients, with the horizontal cleavage plane occurring from shear, which divides the superior and inferior surfaces of the meniscus. These are more commonly seen in the posterior half of the medial meniscus or the midsegment of the lateral meniscus. Many flap tears and complex tears begin initially with a horizontal cleavage component.

Oblique tears are full-thickness tears running obliquely from the inner edge of the meniscus out into the body of the meniscus. If the base of the tear is posterior, it is referred to as a posterior oblique tear; the base of an anterior oblique tear is in the anterior horn of the meniscus (Fig. 59-15).

Radial tears, like oblique tears, are vertically oriented, extending from the inner edge of the meniscus toward its periphery, and may be either complete or incomplete, depending on the extent of involvement. These are probably similar in pathogenesis to oblique tears (Fig. 59-16).

The possible *variations* include flap tears, complex tears, and degenerative meniscal tears.

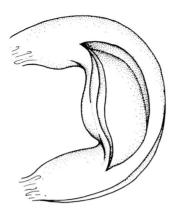

Fig. 59-13. Bucket handle tear, displaced centrally. (From Shahriaree, H.: O'Connor's textbook of arthroscopic surgery, Philadelphia, 1984, J.B. Lippincott Co.)

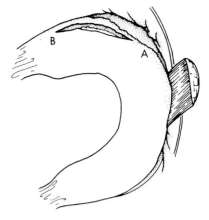

Fig. 59-14. Peripheral tear. *A*, Meniscocapsular tear, and *B*, peripheral longitudinal tear. (From Shahriaree, H.: O'Connor's textbook of arthroscopic surgery, Philadelphia, 1984, J.B. Lippincott Co.)

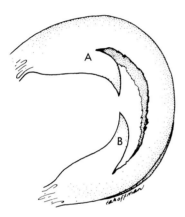

Fig. 59-15. *A*, Posterior oblique tear, and *B*, anterior oblique tear. (From Shahriaree, H.: O'Connor's textbook of arthroscopic surgery, Philadelphia, 1984, J.B. Lippincott Co.)

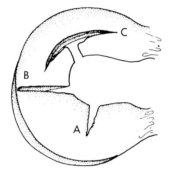

Fig. 59-16. Radial tears. *A*, Incomplete radial tear involves part of width of meniscus. *B*, Complete radial tear extends to periphery. *C*, Incomplete tear extending posteriorly or anteriorly is called "parrot beak" tear. (From Shahriaree, H.: O'Connor's textbook of arthroscopic surgery, Philadelphia, 1984, J.B. Lippincott Co.)

Flap tears are similar to the oblique tears, but usually have a horizontal cleavage element rather than being purely vertical in orientation. Those containing a horizontal element are often referred to as superior or inferior flap tears, depending on where the flap is based on the surface of the meniscus.

Complex tears may contain elements of all of the above types of tears and are more common in chronic meniscal lesions or in older degenerative menisci. These are generally caused by chronic, longstanding, altered mechanics of the meniscus, and the initial tear occurring in the meniscus may not be identifiable once several different planes of tearing have resulted.

The term *degenerative tears* often refers to complex tears. These present with marked irregularity and complex tearing within the meniscus. Again these are most often seen in older patients.

Types of meniscal excisions

O'Connor separated meniscal excisions into three categories depending on the amount of meniscal tissue to be removed (Fig. 59-17).

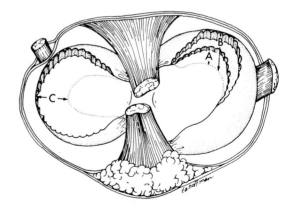

Fig. 59-17. Types of meniscal excision. *A*, Partial meniscectomy. *B*, Subtotal meniscectomy. *C*, Total meniscectomy. (From Shahriaree, H.: O'Connor's textbook of arthroscopic surgery, Philadelphia, 1984, J.B. Lippincott Co.)

Partial meniscectomy. In this type of meniscal excision, only the loose, unstable meniscal fragments are excised, such as the displaceable inner edge in bucket handle tears, the flaps in flap tears, or the flaps in oblique tears. In partial meniscectomies, a stable and balanced peripheral rim of healthy meniscal tissue is preserved.

Subtotal meniscectomy. In this type of meniscectomy, the type and extent of the tear require excision of a portion of the peripheral rim of the meniscus. This is most commonly required in complex or degenerative tears of the posterior horn of either meniscus. Resection of the involved portion by necessity extends out to and includes the peripheral rim of the meniscus. It is termed subtotal, since usually most of the anterior horn and a portion of the middle third of the meniscus is not resected.

Total meniscectomy. Total removal of the meniscus is required when it is detached from its peripheral meniscosynovial attachment and intrameniscal damage and tears are also present. If the body of the peripherally detached meniscus is undamaged, total meniscectomy is not warranted and meniscal suture should be considered.

General principles

Partial meniscectomy is always preferable to subtotal or total meniscectomy. Leaving an intact, balanced, peripheral rim of meniscus aids in the stability of the joint and protects the articular surfaces by its load-bearing functions. Total meniscectomy removes all of the actual load-bearing protection and reduces stability of the joint, especially if a concomitant ligamentous relaxation already exists. Partial meniscectomy, although desirable, is not always possible if the tear extends to the periphery of the meniscus. In such cases, subtotal excision is preferable to complete excision, even though the contoured anterior meniscal tissue left may be subject to subsequent tears or degeneration.

To determine accurately the type of meniscectomy required, one must carefully probe and classify the type of meniscal lesion present and avoid rushing to the task of removing tissue. Failure to accurately and thoroughly classify, probe, and explore the extent and various planes of the tear before proceeding with the meniscus resection often results in needlessly sacrificing healthy meniscal tissue.

Once the meniscal tear has been probed and classified, the surgeon should mentally formulate the methods and steps required to excise the necessary portion of the meniscus. He should be able to visualize the tissues to be removed and the subsequent contour of the peripheral meniscal rim. The objective is to remove the torn, mobile meniscal fragment and contour the peripheral rim, leaving a balanced, stable rim of meniscal tissue.

Excision of the pathologic tissue can be carried out either with en bloc resection of the mobile fragment or by morcellation of the fragments and subsequent removal. It is usually preferable to sharply excise major mobile fragments if possible, rather than proceeding with morcellation, to minimize the potential debris within the joint. Once the tear has been removed, the remaining peripheral rim must be carefully probed to assure that there are no additional tears and that the rim is balanced and stable. Once the surgeon is satisfied that a contoured, balanced, stable peripheral rim is present, the joint should be thor-

oughly lavaged and suctioned to remove any small meniscal fragments or debris that may have dropped into the joint as a result of the resection.

Surgery for specific disorders
TEARS OF MEDIAL MENISCUS

Tears of the medial meniscus may be (1) longitudinal, either intrameniscal or peripheral, complete or incomplete, displaced (bucket handle) or nondisplaced; (2) horizontal; (3) oblique; (4) radial (rarely); (5) flap; (6) complex; or (7) degenerative. While no standard technique must be used in every case, the following techniques are useful in dealing with each of these types of tears via the anteroinferior portals. Examples using the proximal portals or the central or Swedish approach for some tears will also be presented.

LONGITUDINAL DISPLACED COMPLETE INTRAMENISCAL TEARS (BUCKET HANDLE)

TECHNIQUE. After completely examining the knee for ligamentous stability, carry out a complete diagnostic arthroscopic examination. With the arthroscope in the anterolateral portal, view the medial compartment. A large displaced bucket handle tear of the medial meniscus may make passage of the arthroscope into the medial compartment difficult. If you encounter difficulty, direct the arthroscope into the suprapatellar pouch and then sweep it down over the medial femoral condyle, keeping the horizon of the condyle in view, into the anteromedial compartment. This sweeping maneuver usually assures that the scope will pass over the top of a displaced bucket handle tear of the medial meniscus into the anteromedial compartment so that viewing of the medial meniscus is possible. If you note an especially narrow or thin rim of the meniscus, or if its free inner border is ragged, consider the possibility of a displaced bucket handle tear (Plate 7, *A* and *B*). Rotate the 30-degree oblique arthroscope lens to view the intercondylar notch area, and you will see the displaced bucket handle fragment. Make an anteromedial portal, insert a probe, and carefully define the anterior and posterior limits of the displaced fragment (Fig. 59-18, *A*). If it has been displaced into the intercondylar notch for a long time, the longitudinal tear in the meniscus may extend well anteriorly near the fat pad and viewing may be difficult. In such instances, the intercondylar eminence may block viewing of the posterior attachment of the bucket handle fragment if it extends far centrally. You may resect a portion of or retract the fat pad, or move the viewing arthroscope to a midpatellar lateral portal to look down on the anterior horn.

Once the anterior and posterior limits of the bucket handle fragment have been carefully identified by probing, it is usually easier to detach the anterior horn using triangulation techniques. With the probe in the anteromedial portal and the arthroscope in the anterolateral portal, attempt to place the probe tip in the anterior axilla of the anterior horn tear. If this can be accomplished, then insert a small pair of hooked scissors through the anteromedial portal, advance them to the anterior axilla of the tear, and release the anterior horn attachment of the fragment (Fig. 59-18, *B*).

If you cannot advance the scissors into the anterior axilla of the tear, an alternative method is to reduce the displaced bucket handle fragment out of the intercondylar notch and see if this produces a better view (Fig. 59-18, *C*). Reducing the displaced fragment occasionally will bring it far enough away from the fat pad to improve viewing and cutting of the anterior horn attachment. Sometimes blocking off the irrigation fluid outflow will result in sufficient distention to push a fat pad further out of the way. If the anterior axilla of the tear is clearly viewed but the

scissors, knife, or basket forceps cannot be precisely positioned through this anteromedial portal, move the portal further medially to an accessory or far medial portal. Before making such a portal, insert an 18-gauge spinal needle through the portal site selected to see if it can be directed precisely to the anterior axilla of the tear. If so, make the portal, insert the scissors, advance them to the anterior attachment of the bucket handle fragment, and release it. The release of the anterior attachment should be flush

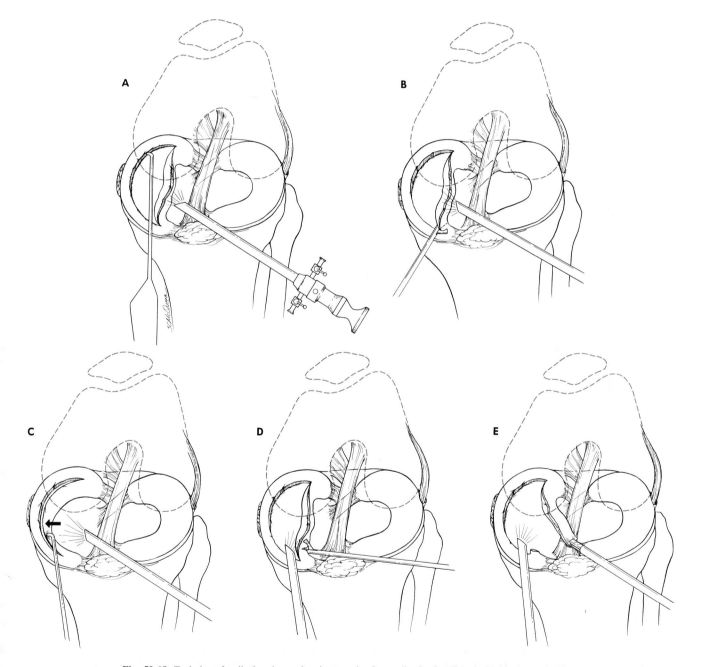

Fig. 59-18. Technique for displaced complete intrameniscal tears (bucket handle). **A,** Probing posterior limits of displaced bucket handle tear of medial meniscus. Probe for additional peripheral tears in meniscal rim. **B,** Hooked scissors through anteromedial portal releases anterior horn attachment. **C,** If anterior attachment of displaced bucket handle tear cannot be released, reduce fragment with probe. **D,** Anterior horn of displaced bucket handle fragment released with scissors through anterolateral portal. **E,** Grasper clamps anterior end of detached fragment and pulls it into intercondylar notch.

Continued.

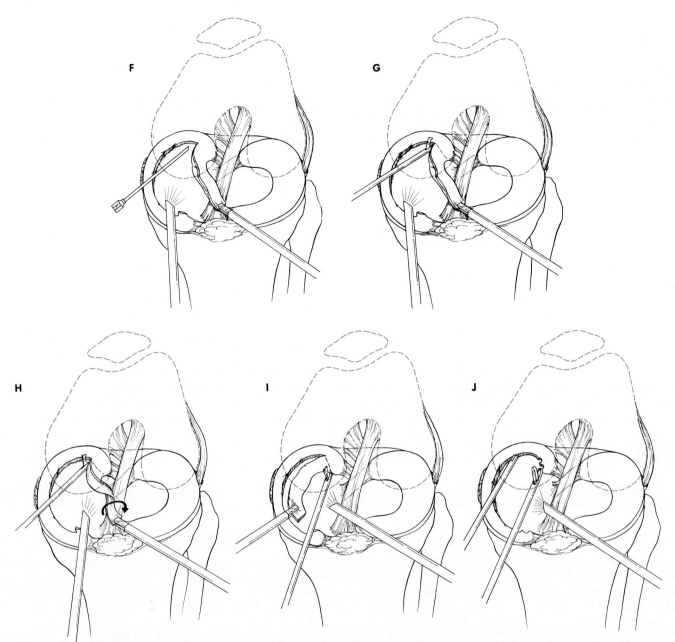

Fig. 59-18, cont'd. F, Accessory medial portal site determined by using spinal needle directed to posterior horn attachment. **G,** Scissors through accessory medial portal detaches posterior horn attachment. **H,** Twisting displaced bucket handle tear may present better edge to cut posterior attachment. **I,** Fragment grasped through accessory medial portal, cut with scissors through anteromedial portal. **J,** Remaining peripheral rim smoothed and contoured with basket forceps or motorized trimmer.

with the intact anterior rim, so no stump or dog-ear will remain.

If the spinal needle cannot be directed to the anterior axilla of the tear, remove the arthroscope from the anterolateral portal and insert it in the anteromedial portal. When the anterior attachment is viewed, bring a probe, then subsequently scissors or a cutting instrument, through the anterolateral portal and release the anterior attachment of the bucket handle fragment (Fig. 59-18, D).

Once this is completed, insert a grasping instrument such as a small Kocher clamp through the anterolateral portal and securely grab the detached anterior tip of the bucket handle fragment. Displace the entire fragment into the intercondylar notch (Fig. 59-18, E).

With the arthroscope in the anteromedial portal, rotate the lens to view the posterior attachment. Alternate gentle pulls on the grasping instrument while viewing the posterior attachment to clearly define where the posterior attachment should be cut. If needed, change the viewing arthroscope at this point for an operative arthroscope to release the posterior attachment by passing the scissors through the arthroscope's instrument channel; most often the posterior attachment is released using triangulation techniques.

With the grasping instrument in the anterolateral portal and the viewing arthroscope in the anteromedial portal, use the spinal needle to locate precisely an accessory medial portal, usually 1.5 to 2.5 cm medial to the anteromedial portal near the anterior edge of the tibial collateral ligament. Pass the needle through the skin, subcutaneous tissues, and capsule under direct vision through the scope, being careful to pass over the intact meniscal rim. By carefully redirecting the passage of the needle, advance its tip precisely to the posterior attachment to be released (Fig. 59-18, *F*).

Once you achieve this portal site and direction with the spinal needle, note its direction, make a 1 cm portal, and pass the scissors or cutting instrument carefully into the medial compartment. If you select a meniscectomy knife or exposed sharp cutting instrument to cut the posterior attachment, pass it through an appropriately sized protective sheath and into view in the medial compartment. Failure to do so may result in laceration of the periphery of the medial meniscus, damage to the articular cartilage, or breakage of the instrument.

Advance the cutting instrument to the posterior attachment and cut it (Fig. 59-18, *G*). Keeping the displaced bucket handle fragment under tension by gentle traction on the grasping instrument will make cutting of the posterior attachment easier. If this posterior attachment is not cleanly incised, twist the fragment by means of the grasping instrument, then use gentle traction maneuvers to expose the portion of the attachment not previously released (Fig. 59-18, *H*).

Complete release of the posterior attachment is achieved when the gentle traction on the grasping instrument indicates it is loose. Then extract the detached fragment from the joint with gentle traction and a to-and-fro twisting motion on the grasping instrument. Slightly enlarging the exit portal if necessary is preferable to having the detached fragment pull from the grasper and become lost as a free fragment within the joint, the subcutaneous tissue, or the edge of the fat pad.

Exercise extreme care in releasing the posterior attachment. The cutting instrument and the tissues being cut must be in view at all times; vascular structures may be injured as a result of blind cutting in the posterior intercondylar notch area, and damage to the cruciate ligaments may result from misdirected aimless cutting. These catastrophes can be avoided if you always view the cutting instrument and what it is cutting.

In longitudinal bucket handle tears of the medial meniscus, when the posterior limit of the tear stops short of the posterior horn attachment, detaching the posterior attachment of the fragment may be difficult with an instrument directed from an anteromedial or an accessory medial portal. In these instances, the direction of a cutting instrument may produce a straight-ahead cut, carrying it into an intact posterior mensical rim. If an angled cutting instrument can be maneuvered into position, release the posterior fragment from the posterior axilla side of the tear. If this angle carries the cutting instrument toward the intact posterior rim, it is best to move to an alternative approach. Move

the viewing arthroscope from the anteromedial back to the anterolateral portal, reduce the bucket handle fragment by way of a probe through the anteromedial portal, and grasp the anterior tip of the bucket handle fragment through an accessory medial portal. With the fragment under tension, by traction on the grasping instrument, insert a thin Smillie meniscus knife or scissors with the appropriate sheath through the anteromedial portal and incise the posterior attachment of the fragment from its free thin inner border, across the fragment to meet the longitudinal intrameniscal tear (Fig. 59-18, *I*). This method is safer than repeatedly attempting to detach the posterior attachment if the instrument cannot be directed at the proper angle. Often a posterior horn tag will be left centrally, which can be easily removed through morcellation with basket forceps through the anteromedial portal.

Once the detached bucket handle fragment has been extracted from the joint, move the viewing arthroscope back to the anterolateral portal and insert the probe through the anteromedial portal. It is essential that the remaining peripheral rim of the meniscus be intact, stable, and balanced. If careful probing of the remaining meniscal rim reveals no further pathology, trim small tags and irregularities along the inner border of the remaining rim using basket forceps or the motorized meniscal cutter (Fig. 59-18, *J*). Thoroughly lavage the joint and remove any articular scuffs or small meniscal fragments remaining within the joint with suction lavage.

LONGITUDINAL UNDISPLACED COMPLETE INTRAMENISCAL TEARS

These tears commonly involve the posterior horn of the medial meniscus (Plate 7, *C*). The shorter the tear, the more difficult it is to diagnose. They are often not displaceable into the joint even with probing. These are longitudinal, full-thickness tears, which if untreated may extend and become displaceable bucket handle tears. Strong valgus and external rotational stress applied to the knee improves viewing if the tear is small and located posteriorly. Partial meniscectomy is usually possible in treating such lesions.

TECHNIQUE. With the viewing arthroscope in the anterolateral portal, view the medial compartment and inner border of the medial meniscus. Insert a probe by way of an anteromedial portal, and probe the posterior horn of the medial meniscus as valgus and external rotational stress is applied. The inner border of the meniscus may not have its normal contour or may be folded on itself, offering a clue to a possible intrameniscal tear. If you carefully probe on both the superior and the inferior surfaces of the posterior horn, the probe tip may fall into such a tear, and with gentle traction of the probe, you may be able to displace the longitudinal vertical tear enough to be noticeable (Fig. 59-19, *A*). Note and carefully probe the anterior and posterior limits of the longitudinal tear.

Next using a thin meniscus knife, small scissors, or basket forceps introduced through the anteromedial portal, incise the free inner edge of the posterior meniscus transversely toward the posterior limit of the longitudinal tear. This incision should stop just short of entering the longitudinal tear (Fig. 59-19, *B*). Now direct attention to the anterior limit of the longitudinal tear. The objective is to

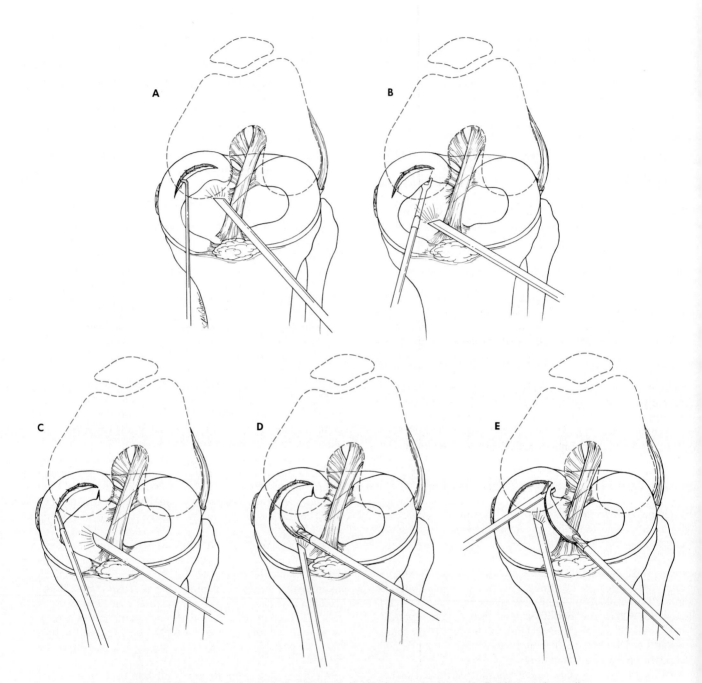

Fig. 59-19. Technique for longitudinal undisplaced complete intrameniscal tears. **A,** Probing complete undisplaced intrameniscal tear, medial meniscus. **B,** Incomplete release, posterior fragment, knife through anteromedial portal. **C,** Release of anterior limit of tear with hooked retrograde cutting knife through anteromedial portal. **D,** Move scope to anteromedial portal, grasper through anterolateral portal. Fragment pulled into intercondylar notch. **E,** Posterior horn attachment release completed with scissors through accessory medial portal.

extend the anterior limit of the tear further anteriorly and obliquely toward the free inner edge of the meniscus. This may be accomplished in several ways. You may insert a retrograde cutting or hook knife with its appropriate sheath through the anteromedial portal. Carefully hook the blade in the anterior axilla of the longitudinal tear, and extend the cut anteriorly and obliquely toward the free inner edge of the meniscus (Fig. 59-19, C). If you are using such a blade, take care not to incise the articular cartilage of the tibial plateau beneath the cut. Once this cut is completed, remove the knife and move the viewing arthroscope to the anteromedial portal. Insert a grasping instrument through the anterolateral portal, grasp the anterior tip of the now posteriorly-based flap, and pull it toward the intercondylar notch (Fig. 59-19, D).

Make an accessory medial portal, first locating precisely its best position by directing a spinal needle through the skin and capsule to the posterior attachment. Complete the posterior detachment with scissors, knife, or basket forceps (Fig. 59-19, E. Contour any irregularities with basket forceps to produce a smooth transition to normal meniscus at the anterior and posterior limits of the resected fragment. Trim small frayed areas with the motorized meniscus cutter, again carefully probing and thoroughly lavaging and suctioning the joint.

LONGITUDINAL INCOMPLETE INTRAMENISCAL TEARS

Longitudinal incomplete intrameniscal tears may extend from the superior surface into the body of the meniscus or may enter from the inferior surface. These are often extremely difficult to view and treat. This type of tear is commonly located in the posterior horn of the medial meniscus and may be only a few millimeters long. By the time such a tear extends more than 1 to 2 cm, it usually becomes complete and often displaceable. Usually severe valgus and external rotational stress of the knee is required to view small tears. One's first suspicion of such a tear may be a wrinkled or buckled inner meniscal border. If the incomplete tear begins from the superior surface, the probe tip will pass into it but not through to the inferior surface. Inferior incomplete tears are even more difficult to view and explore, especially in a tight knee. Again, the tip of the probe passes into the inferior tear but not through to the superior surface of the meniscus. One should avoid vigorously trying to hook the probe into an unseen inferior tear for danger of extending the tear. If such a tear exists, gentle probing may make the inner border of the meniscus buckle and evert. If the clinical diagnosis is reasonably certain and the tear cannot be demonstrated, viewing the undersurface of the posterior horn with a small diameter arthroscope may be helpful. Also, moving the arthroscope to a posteromedial portal or a central portal may allow a view of a superior surface incomplete tear. Excision of these tears may be just as difficult as viewing them.

TECHNIQUE. After you examine the knee for instability, do a complete diagnostic arthroscopy. To carry out arthroscopic excision of longitudinal intrameniscal incomplete tears of the medial meniscus, use triangulation techniques. Insert a 30-degree oblique viewing arthroscope through an anterolateral portal into the anteromedial compartment. Insert a probe through an anteromedial portal. Carry out careful probing as previously described (Fig. 59-20, A). Often the longitudinal limits of an inferior incomplete tear are difficult to determine. The objective is to perform a partial meniscectomy, removing no more meniscus than required to excise the tear and balance and contour the rim. If you could be sure where the tear limits extended, you could sharply incise from the inner edge of

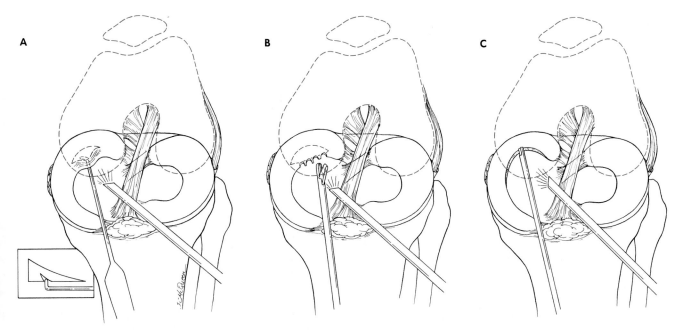

Fig. 59-20. Technique for longitudinal incomplete intrameniscal tears. **A,** Probing longitudinal intrameniscal incomplete inferior surface tear. **B,** Fragment removed bit by bit with basket forceps. **C,** Rim smoothed and contoured with motorized trimmer.

the meniscus at either end of the tear, with removal of the fragment as described for complete tears. Since the limits of the tear, especially in the inferior incomplete tear, cannot always be judged, it is best to remove this fragment by morcellation with basket forceps. Introduce a hook basket forceps through the anteromedial portal and cut the inner edge of the meniscus at the estimated midpoint of the longitudinal tear. Extend this cut into the meniscus bit by bit until the longitudinal tear is encountered (Fig. 59-20, B). Once this is done, careful probing may better delineate the limits of the tear. Continue nibbling along the longitudinal tear until you determine the limits of the tear anteriorly and posteriorly and encounter normal meniscal tissue. Complete the contouring and balancing of the meniscal rim with basket forceps or the motorized trimmer (Fig. 59-20, C). Hook basket forceps with the neck of the instrument angled upward 10 or 15 degrees makes trimming the posterior horn easier. Once you complete the rim contouring, carefully probe the rim to ensure the absence of additional abnormalities, and thoroughly lavage and suction the joint for any loose fragments produced by the morcellation.

LONGITUDINAL PERIPHERAL TEARS

Longitudinal peripheral tears of the medial meniscus may be reparable or nonreparable. Reparable tears are those within the vascularized peripheral 25% of the meniscus (2 to 3 mm) without associated damage to the remaining body of the meniscus. Sufficient evidence now exists that healing is predictable even in chronic tears so that every attempt should be made to repair such lesions. The critical importance of the meniscus for stabilization and for protection of the articular surface from late degenerative arthritis dictates that salvage of the meniscus should always be attempted in such lesions. Few recurrent tears after repair have been reported in stable knees. Repair by suture has most often been accomplished by standard arthrotomy through a posteromedial incision as described in Chapter 56.

Instrumentation is now available for meniscal repair arthroscopically, but few reports have yet appeared comparing open versus arthroscopic techniques of repair. An arthroscopic method of repair is described on p. 2587.

Nonreparable peripheral tears of the medial meniscus are those accompanied by damage to the body of the meniscus, such as multiple tears or cleavage components. These usually require subtotal or complete meniscal excision, depending on the extent of the tears and how far into the anterior meniscus they extend.

TECHNIQUE OF SUBTOTAL MENISCECTOMY. The technique for subtotal meniscal excision is similar to that described for intrameniscal complete vertical tears. After you examine the knee for stability, carry out a complete, systematic diagnostic arthroscopy. With the 30-degree viewing arthroscope in the anterolateral portal, probe the tear through an anteromedial portal as you apply valgus and external rotational stress to the knee. If such probing reveals additional damage to the body of the meniscus, such as flaps, multiple tears, or cleavage components, and repair is not possible, carefully define the anterior and posterior limits of the peripheral tear (Fig. 59-21, A). With the thin Smillie

knife through the anterolateral portal, incise the inner edge of the posterior horn, carrying the incision across the meniscus posteriorly to approach but not enter the peripheral tear (Fig. 59-21, B). Completely releasing this posterior horn tends to make release of the anterior portion more difficult. Then direct attention to the anterior limits of the peripheral tear and its axilla, carefully probing its axilla through the anteromedial portal. You may release the anterior attachment with any cutting instrument such as scissors, basket forceps, or a knife. A retrograde cutting or hook knife works well if some posterior attachment remains to provide fixation of the fragment to cut against. Place the knife blade in the anterior axilla of the tear and pull forward, incising obliquely across the meniscus toward its inner edge (Fig. 59-21, C). Take care not to damage the articular surface of the tibia beneath the meniscus. This anterior cut may be made with scissors or basket forceps through the anteromedial portal if preferred. Using these cutting tools, begin the cut at the inner border of the meniscus anterior to the limits of the peripheral tear, and proceed obliquely across the meniscus to approach and enter the peripheral tear (Fig. 59-21, D).

Once the anterior detachment is completed, move the viewing arthroscope to the anteromedial portal, insert a grasping instrument through the anterolateral portal, firmly grasp the anterior tip of the fragment, and displace the fragment toward the intercondylar notch. Locate an optimal accessory medial portal using the spinal needle directed to the attached posterior fragment. Once the needle can be directed precisely to the area to be detached, make the portal, insert a cutting instrument, and complete the posterior detachment (Fig. 59-29, E). Twisting and tugging intermittently on the grasping instrument better identify the remaining attachment so that it can be incised. Then extract the fragment from the joint. Insert a rotary 90 degree basket forceps (Acuflex) through the anterolateral portal and contour the middle and anterior meniscus to produce a smooth, gradual transition (Fig. 52-21, F).

If the anterior limit of the tear extends into the anterior third of the meniscus, detachment of the anterior portion may be easier if the viewing arthroscope is moved to the anteromedial portal and a cutting instrument is introduced from the anterolateral portal. This usually brings the cutting instrument in toward the meniscal tear at a better angle to release these anteriorly located tears.

TECHNIQUE OF TOTAL MENISCECTOMY. Total meniscectomy should be restricted to cases in which no rim of sound meniscal tissue can be left. In all other cases, subtotal or partial meniscectomy or meniscal repair is indicated. Total meniscectomy is one of the most difficult arthroscopic surgical procedures, taxing the skills of even the experienced surgeon. Unless the surgeon is experienced, total meniscectomy probably should be done through conventional open arthrotomy techniques.

If total meniscectomy is required following a complete diagnostic arthroscopy, move the 30-degree viewing arthroscope to a midpatellar lateral portal and rotate the lens to look down onto the anterior horn of the medial meniscus. Insert a probe through the anterolateral portal, and trace a trial or simulated cut with the probe along the anterior peripheral attachment of the meniscus. If you cannot simulate with the probe the subsequent cut with the knife, adjust the position and direction of the probe. Most often, this requires moving the anterolateral portal slightly more superiorly. Be sure before beginning that nothing prevents the subsequent cutting instrument from following the correct route along the peripheral attachment of the meniscus. If the view of the periphery of the anterior horn is difficult because of the presence of the fat pad, have an assistant

insert a fat pad retractor through the anteromedial portal to expose this area. Once the simulated cut can be traced with the probe, remove the probe and insert the knife through the proper anterolateral portal. The Oretorp special arthroscopy knife with retractable blades works well for this anterior cut. If this knife is used, bring the sheathed knife through the anterolateral portal, position it at the anterior horn, unsheathe the knife blade, and make a cut along the

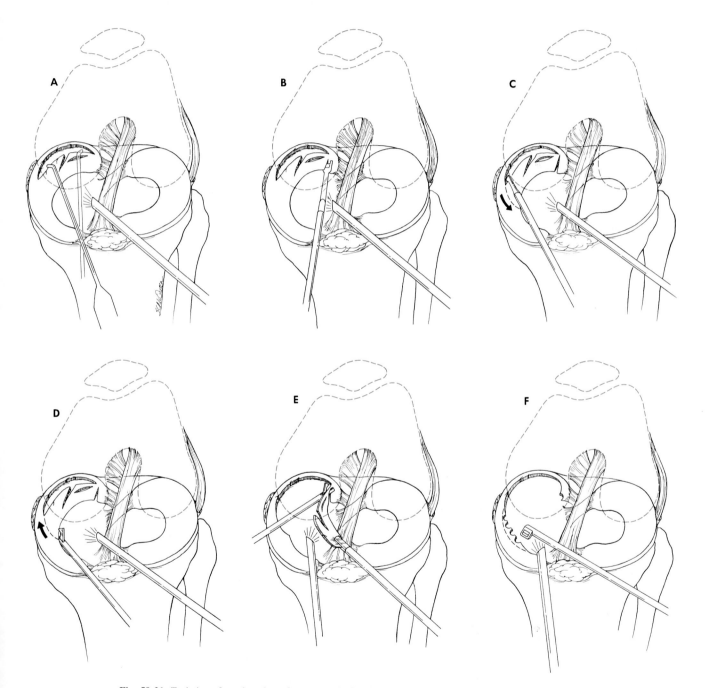

Fig. 59-21. Technique for subtotal meniscectomy. **A,** Probing irreparable longitudinal tear, medial meniscus. **B,** Posterior attachment partially released. **C,** Anterior limit of tear released with retrograde cutting knife. **D,** Anterior limit of tear released with scissors. **E,** Scope moved to anteromedial portal, grasper through anterolateral portal pulls fragment into intercondylar notch. Posterior attachment release completed with scissors through accessory medial portal. **F,** Anterior horn contoured and smoothed with 90 degree rotary basket forceps.

peripheral attachment of the anterior horn (Fig. 59-22, *A*). You may prefer to use the disposable Beaver blades on their long handle to make these cuts. If you choose these, insert them through the appropriate sheath or cannula with the blade not exposed until it is brought clearly into the viewing field. One advantage in using these blades is that they can be gently contoured or bent, allowing the blade to follow around the periphery of the meniscus more easily than a straight blade.

Once the anterior horn is released, remove the knife from the anterolateral portal and introduce it through the anteromedial portal. Identify the medial limit of the previous cut along the periphery of the meniscus, insert the Smillie knife, directing it along the midportion of the meniscus, and incise the periphery of the midsegment of the meniscus (Fig. 59-22, *B*). Again, gently contouring the disposable Smillie Beaver blade makes it easier to follow the rim of the meniscus. Extend the cut to the posterome-

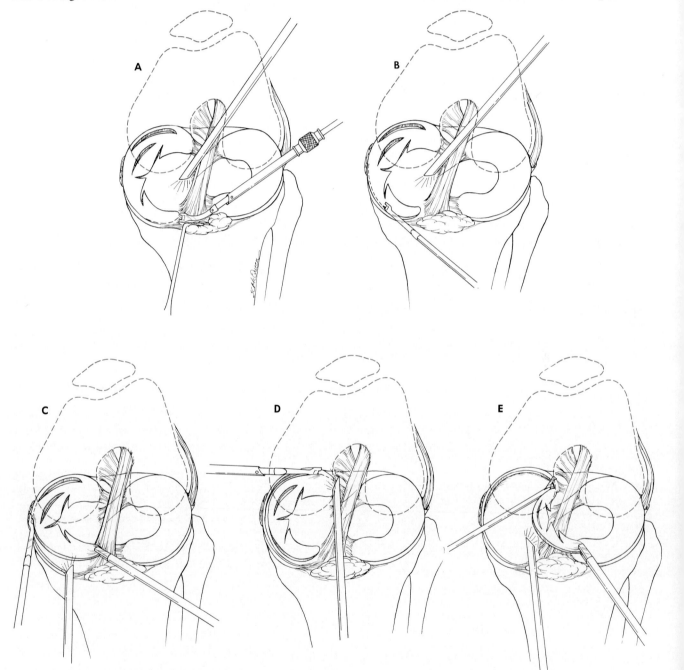

Fig. 59-22. Technique for total meniscectomy. **A,** Release of anterior horn central attachment. Scope is in midpatellar lateral portal, contoured Beaver knife in anterolateral portal. Note fat pad retractor. **B,** Further release of anterior horn and midportion of peripheral attachment. **C,** Middle one third of periphery released through accessory medial portal. **D,** Posterior central attachment released with retrograde cutting knife through posteromedial portal. Seventy degree scope is through intercondylar notch. **E,** Final posterior release, scissors through accessory medial portal.

dial corner behind the tibial collateral ligament. Make all cuts with the cutting edge of the knife clearly in view. Do not push the knife around the posteromedial corner and out of the viewing field. Once the cut is extended to the posteromedial corner behind the tibial collateral ligament, remove the knife from the anteromedial portal. Now move the viewing arthroscope from the midpatellar lateral portal to the anteromedial portal, insert a grasping instrument through the anterolateral portal, and securely grasp the anterior tip of the detached anterior horn. Then pull the detached anterior and middle thirds of the meniscus toward the intercondylar notch with the grasping instrument. Make an accessory medial portal using a spinal needle inserted through the skin and capsule and directed to the posterior limits of the previous peripheral cut. Once the needle is properly positioned and directed, make an accessory medial portal, insert a blunt sheath and trocar to the area where the peripheral cut is to be continued, and insert the knife through the protective sheath. Firm traction on the grasping instrument, pulling the detached anterior two thirds of the meniscus toward the intercondylar notch, usually exposes another 1 to 1.5 cm of periphery that can be safely detached (Fig. 59-22, *C*). Again, gently contouring the cutting blade to conform to the arc of the cut makes this posteromedial release easier. Again, do not push the cutting blade beyond the field of viewing. Remove the knife from the accessory medial portal and the 30-degree viewing arthroscope from the anteromedial portal.

Before inserting the 70-degree arthroscope through the central transpatellar tendon portal into the posteromedial compartment, remove the grasper from the anterolateral portal and reduce the meniscus from the intercondylar notch by means of a pull through the anteromedial portal.

Introduce a 70-degree arthroscope through a central or transpatellar tendon approach directed posteriorly through the intercondylar notch into the posteromedial compartment. Rotate the tip of the arthroscope medially so that the posteromedial corner can be seen. The previous peripheral cut at the posteromedial corner can now be viewed. Make a posteromedial portal, and introduce the cutting knife with its protective sheath into the posteromedial compartment. The knee should be flexed to 90 degrees at this point. Guided by the view through the 70-degree arthroscope, unsheathe the cutting blade and make a cut through the posterior horn close to the synovial junction (Fig. 59-22, *D*). It is safer to change the type of cutting blade from the end cutting Smillie blade used to detach the anterior two thirds to a regular cutting blade for the posterior detachment. It is safer to cut the posterior periphery of the meniscus starting close to the posterior central attachment of the meniscus and cutting toward the posteromedial portal. This cut will join the previous one at the posteromedial corner. To continue the previous anterior cut around the posterior rim toward the popliteal area and the posterior cruciate ligament is riskier for those structures than if the cut begins close to the posterior central attachment of the meniscus and is brought around the posterior periphery to meet the cut at the posteromedial corner.

Once this is completed, the only remaining attachment is the posterior central attachment. Withdraw the 70-degree arthroscope and insert the 30-degree viewing arthroscope through the anteromedial portal. Insert the grasper

again through the anterolateral portal, firmly grasping the anterior tip of the meniscus, and displace the meniscus again into the intercondylar notch. Then release the posterior central attachment using a thin Smillie knife or scissors introduced through the accessory medial portal (Fig. 59-22, *E*). Extract the complete meniscus from the joint with a firm, twisting action on the grasping instrument, and deliver it through the anterolateral portal.

Now check the remaining rim for irregularities and trim it with basket forceps or a motorized trimmer if necessary. Thoroughly lavage and suction the joint to remove any debris.

HORIZONTAL TEARS

Horizontal tears occur most commonly in older patients in the posterior horn of the medial meniscus or in the midportion of the lateral meniscus. The cleavage divides the meniscus into superior and inferior leaves resembling a fishmouth. A simple horizontal cleavage may with time become torn in additional planes and develop into a superior or inferior flap tear or a more complex tear if subjected to repeated injury.

TECHNIQUE. Following a thorough diagnostic arthroscopy, insert the 30-degree oblique viewing arthroscope through the anterolateral portal and advance it into the medial compartment. Insert a probe through an anteromedial portal. Probe the horizontal cleavage split to judge the anterior, posterior, and peripheral limits of the tear (Fig. 59-23, *A*). In this type of tear, it is usually preferable to remove the inner edge of the superior and inferior leaves of the tear with basket forceps. Bit by bit, trim the inner edge toward the peripheral limits of the tear (Fig. 59-23, *B*). When this is accomplished, trim and contour the remaining rim with basket forceps to produce a stable, balanced rim. Careful probing of the rim is necessary to avoid removal of excessive meniscal tissue. Because of the horizontal arrangement of the fibers within the meniscus its cut edge may appear to have small additional cleavage elements in it, and you must judge whether these are portions of the original cleavage component. The subsequent blunted or squared-off edges of the remaining meniscal rim (Fig. 59-23, *C*), with the passage of time and weight bearing, will retriangulate to a significant degree to become a more normal, thin inner meniscal edge. Only with experience can you determine precisely when sufficient meniscal tissue in these older menisci has been removed. Once the tear has been completely excised, thoroughly lavage and suction the joint to remove any remaining bits of meniscus produced by the morcellation.

OBLIQUE TEARS

Oblique tears occur when the thin inner edge of the meniscus is suddenly elongated. This mechanism produces a full-thickness vertical tear extending from the inner edge obliquely into the body of the meniscus. The direction of the base of this oblique tear determines whether it is classified as a posterior oblique or anterior oblique tear (Plate 7, *D*). There is usually no horizontal component.

TECHNIQUE. The technique used for removal of oblique tears is determined by the size, type, and location of the tear. Small, posteriorly based, oblique tears are usually removed by morcellation of the flaps with basket forceps or

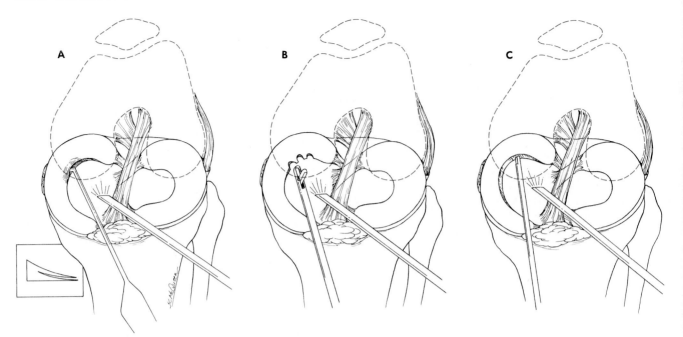

Fig. 59-23. Technique for horizontal tears. **A,** Probe explores horizontal tear, medial meniscus. **B,** Inner edge of meniscus removed bit by bit with basket forceps to limit of tear. **C,** Peripheral rim smoothed and contoured with motorized trimmer.

motorized cutter-trimmer instruments. Insert the 30-degree viewing arthroscope through an anterolateral portal, and examine the limits of the oblique tear with a probe through the anteromedial portal. Insert a hook basket forceps through an anteromedial portal, and bit by bit remove the small tear (Fig. 59-24, *A* and *B*). Then trim and contour the rim. Perform final trimming of the rim with the motorized cutter and probe for additional pathologic conditions (Fig. 59-24, *C*). Lavage and suction the joint.

Large posterior oblique tears may be removed intact if this is preferred. Again, with the 30-degree viewing arthroscope in the anterolateral portal, determine the extent of the tear by probing through an anteromedial portal. Make an accessory medial portal, insert a small grasping instrument, grasp the tip of the posterior oblique tear, and apply tension. Insert a thin Smillie meniscus knife through the anteromedial portal via a protective sheath or cannula, and advance it to the base of the oblique tear. Begin a cut at the inner edge of the meniscus and pass it across the base of the flap to the oblique tear (Fig. 59-24, *D*). Remove this fragment from the joint with the grasping instrument. Trim and contour the intact rim with basket forceps and probe to be certain no additional pathologic condition is present. Lavage and suction the joint to remove any debris.

Anterior oblique tears are also removed using triangulation techniques. If the anterior oblique tear is in the posterior or middle third of the medial meniscus, it is usually excised as a single large fragment. Following a thorough diagnostic arthroscopy, insert the 30-degree viewing arthroscope in the anterolateral portal, and define the anterior oblique tear by probing through the anteromedial portal. View the anterior limit of the oblique tear, remove the

probe, and insert a retrograde or hook knife through a cannula through the anteromedial portal. Advance the knife to the anterior limit of the oblique tear, and hook the tip of the retrograde cutting blade into the axilla of the tear. Incise the meniscus, beginning at the anterior axilla of the tear and proceeding anteriorly and obliquely toward the free inner edge of the meniscus (Fig. 59-24, *E*). It is preferable to complete this cut as a single precise incision through the full thickness of the meniscus, taking care not to incise the articular surface on the tibia beneath the meniscus. Then remove the knife, insert a grasper through the anteromedial portal, and remove the fragment (Fig. 59-24, *F*). If the fragment is completely released by this technique, exercise extreme care to avoid letting the free fragment float out of view before the grasper can be inserted. Turning off the inflow and outflow of irrigation fluids will reduce this risk.

Alternatively, begin the anterior incision through the meniscus at its inner edge just anterior to the oblique tear, so the fragment remains tenuously attached to the intact rim (Fig. 59-24, *G*). Then move the arthroscope to the anteromedial portal and insert a grasping instrument through the anterolateral portal to grab the anterior tip of the fragment. Release the remaining attachment through an accessory medial portal with a knife, scissors, or basket forceps (Fig. 59-24, *H*).

Anterior oblique tears involving the anterior horn of the meniscus are usually removed piecemeal by basket forceps or a down-biting Kerrison rongeur. With the 30-degree viewing arthroscope in the anterolateral portal, probe the anterior oblique tear by way of the anteromedial portal. If the tear and flap of meniscus to be excised are in the anterior third of the meniscus, the instrument through the

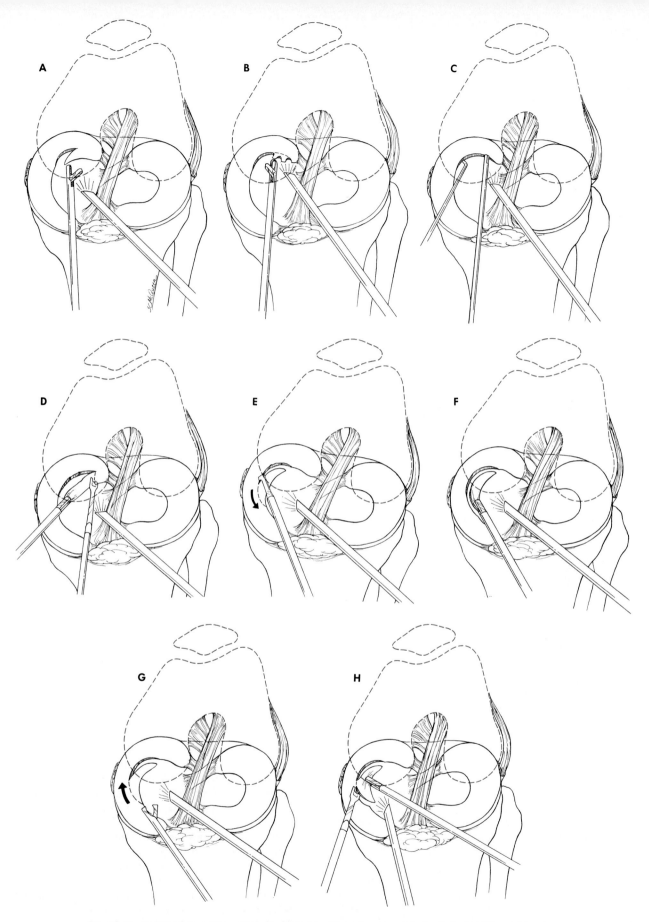

Fig. 59-24. Technique for oblique tears. **A,** Posterior oblique tear approached with basket forceps through anteromedial portal. **B,** Morcellation of fragment with basket forceps. **C,** Peripheral rim smoothed with motorized trimmer. Remaining rim carefully probed for additional tears. **D,** Large posterior oblique tear removed en bloc. **E,** Anterior oblique tear released with retrograde knife. **F,** Anterior oblique tear removed from joint with grasper. **G,** Anterior oblique tear released with scissors. **H,** Anterior oblique tear released with knife—three-portal technique.

anteromedial portal tends to be right on top of the fragment to be excised. For this reason, a down-biting Kerrison rongeur occasionally works well in this location. If accurate resection cannot be accomplished by this means, move the viewing arthroscope to the anteromedial portal, and insert the basket forceps through the anterolateral portal. The 90-degree rotary Acuflex basket forceps is especially useful in removing anterior oblique and flap tears.

Trim or contour the anterior rim to remove the anterior fragment. If it is difficult to see the tear with the arthroscope in the anteromedial portal, switch to a midpatellar lateral location; this gives an excellent view of the anterior horn area. Then resect the fragment produced by the anterior oblique tear with the down-biting Kerrison rongeur through the anteromedial portal, or with the Acuflex basket forceps through an anterolateral portal.

FLAP TEARS

Flap tears most commonly begin as horizontal cleavage tears, in the degenerative tissue of an older patient. They are classified as superior or inferior flaps, depending on the location of the base of the flap. Superior flap tears are usually apparent when the meniscus is viewed, the exception being those that flip up vertically to hide behind the femoral condyle. Those located on the inferior surface of the meniscus may be difficult to see without extensive probing, the inferior flap being tucked underneath the meniscus. With probing and rotation of the tibia, it may be teased or pulled out into the compartment for better viewing. Most flap tears of the medial meniscus involve either the posterior or middle third of the meniscus.

TECHNIQUE. Following a preliminary systematic diagnostic arthroscopic examination, insert the 30-degree viewing arthroscope through an anterolateral portal into the anteromedial compartment. Insert a probe through the anteromedial portal, and thoroughly probe and examine the flap tear (Fig. 59-25, A). It is critical to define precisely the base of the flap. Once this is viewed and a large, superior-based flap tear is seen to be present, remove the probe, insert hooked scissors or basket forceps through the anteromedial portal, and cut the base of the flap, leaving a minimum attachment to the underlying meniscus (Fig. 59-25, B). Remove the scissors or basket forceps, insert a grasper or small pituitary rongeur through the anteromedial portal, grasp the flap, and avulse its remaining tenuous attachment (Fig. 59-25, C). If the base of the flap is initially completely severed, the flap may float away and become lost within the joint during this two-portal technique. You may remove small superiorly based flap tears by morcellation of the flap with basket forceps or the motorized meniscus trimmer.

If a large superior flap tear is present, an alternate technique involves the use of a three-portal approach. With the 30-degree viewing arthroscope in the anterolateral portal, make an accessory far medial portal, using a spinal needle to precisely locate the optimal site. Insert a small grasper through this accessory medial portal, and secure the tip of the flap. Insert a cutting instrument (knife, scissors, or basket forceps) through the anteromedial portal, and sever the base of the flap, maintaining tension on the flap by the grasping instrument. Then extract the flap through the accessory medial portal (Fig. 59-25, D).

Once this superiorly based flap is removed, insert a basket forceps through the anteromedial portal, and trim and contour the rim of the meniscus (Fig. 59-25, E). You may perform final contouring using the motorized meniscal cutter. Many of these tears have a horizontal cleavage element, and judgment must be exercised as to how much of this element of the tear complex should be removed. Flap tears usually occur in older, degenerative menisci, and small cleavage elements may be trimmed all the way to the capsule if you become engrossed in removing every small cleavage. This is where judgment must be exercised. It is permissible to leave small cleavage elements unresected, as long as the peripheral rim is stable, balanced, and contoured. This is preferable to subtotal resection of the peripheral rim.

Excision of inferior flap tears of the medial meniscus is usually best accomplished using basket forceps. With the 30-degree viewing arthroscope through the anterolateral portal, carefully probe the inferior flap through the anteromedial portal. The base of these inferior flaps cannot be as precisely viewed as in superior flap tears, since it is hidden underneath the meniscus. Thus it is usually easier to carefully remove the flap bit by bit with the basket forceps through the anteromedial portal (Fig. 59-25, F). From time to time, lift the meniscus edge with a probe to expose the base for further trimming. Trim and contour the overlying inner meniscal edge with the basket forceps, as described earlier. Carry out final trimming and contouring of the peripheral rim using the motorized meniscal cutter. Thoroughly lavage and suction the joint to remove any remaining debris.

PROXIMAL PORTALS FOR ARTHROSCOPIC MENISCECTOMY (PATEL)

In 1981 Patel described proximal portals for arthroscopic surgery of the knee. Patel believed that insertion of the arthroscope through a more superior portal presented distinct advantages over the standard routine inferior portals, citing better viewing of the anterior horns of the menisci and other anterior compartment structures, less crowding and collision of accessory operating instruments, and less distortion and magnification. Midpatellar medial and lateral portals were advocated by Patel for arthroscope insertion, using a 30-degree oblique viewing arthroscope. Through portals fashioned at the medial or lateral border of the patella at the greatest transverse diameter of the bone, the arthroscope is positioned in a superior location out of the way of accessory instruments introduced through the anteroinferior portals. The principal disadvantages of Patel's portals are that the tibial attachment of the posterior cruciate ligament cannot be seen through them and that experience and practice are required for proper orientation.

While these proximal portals may be used for a variety of intraarticular arthroscopic surgical procedures, the technique for excision of a bucket handle tear of the medial meniscus will be described.

TECHNIQUE. Following a systematic and complete diagnostic arthroscopy, make a 1 cm incision at the lateral edge of the patella at the midpatellar level. The selection of the site is critical. Make the incision at the broadest portion of the patella. Too superior or too inferior an incision can jeopardize proper viewing. A 30-degree oblique viewing arthroscope has been found to be ideal. Flex the knee 15 to 20 degrees, and direct the arthroscope through a midpatellar lateral portal into the anteromedial compartment posterior to the infrapatellar fat pad and ligamentum mucosum. This allows viewing of the anteromedial compartment, consisting of the medial tibial plateau, medial femoral condyle, coronary ligaments, anterior horn of the

medial meniscus, and transverse ligament. Rotating the arthroscope, inspect the tibial attachment and remaining portions of the anterior cruciate ligament and intercondylar notch. Then rotate the arthroscope as necessary to improve the field of vision. External rotation, valgus stress, and an anterior drawer sign test with the knee flexed 15 to 20 degrees help reveal the remaining portion of the medial meniscus, including the posterior horn. Then rotate the arthroscope lens so the anterior third of the medial meniscus and anterior capsule can be seen. Under direct vision, in-

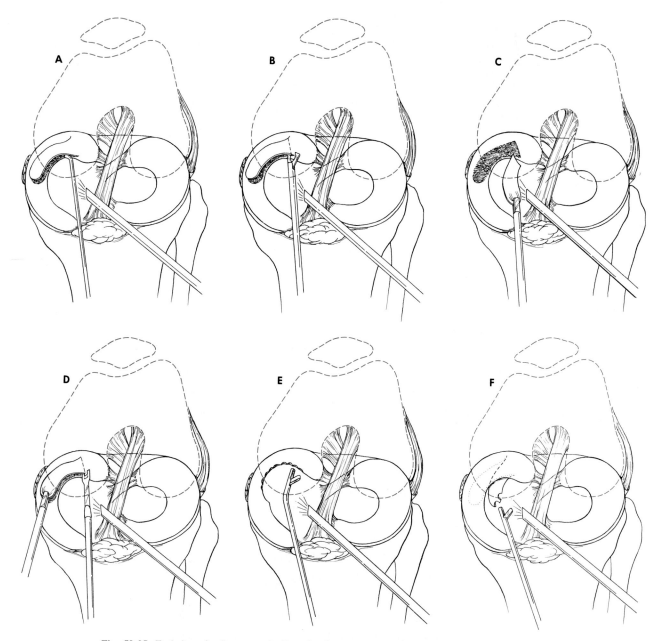

Fig. 59-25. Technique for flap tears. **A,** Posterior flap tear probed. **B,** Base of posterior flap tear released with scissors. **C,** Released posterior flap tear removed with grasper. **D,** Posterior flap tear base released using three-portal technique. **E,** Posterior rim contoured with basket forceps. **F,** Morcellation of posteroinferior flap tear with basket forceps.

troduce an 18-gauge spinal needle inferomedially to select proper placement of the anteromedial portal. If a bucket handle tear of the medial meniscus has been diagnosed, place the needle near the axilla of the bucket handle tear as seen from the midpatellar lateral approach. This anteromedial portal is usually approximately 3.5 to 5 cm medial to the patellar tendon, often referred to as the accessory or far medial portal. Insert a probe through this portal, and carefully probe and identify the extent of the longitudinal tear of the medial meniscus. Divide the anterior horn of the bucket handle tear using scissors or a serrated knife inserted through the accessory medial portal (Fig. 59-26, A). Take specific precautions to make this division flush with the remaining rim to avoid leaving a stub of anterior horn. If the bucket handle fragment of the meniscus is quite mobile, introduce a grasping forceps using a separate anteromedial or anterolateral portal. Grasp the displaced fragment and place it under tension while cutting the anterior horn at its axilla.

Once the anterior attachment of the bucket handle fragment has been released, insert a grasper through an anterolateral portal, and securely grasp the anterior tip of the fragment. Pull the fragment into the intercondylar notch and apply gentle tension. Then insert a probe either through the anteromedial or the accessory medial portal, and direct it toward the posterior attachment of the bucket handle fragment. The selection of which medial portal is best depends on where the probe can be directed most efficiently and properly directed to sever the posterior attachment. Simulating with the probe the subsequent cutting instrument passage to the desired location initially will minimize articular scuffing and potential intraarticular damage. Most often, the accessory medial or far medial

portal presents the best direction for release of the posterior attachment. Insert a small hooked scissors or an end-cutting Smillie meniscus knife with a protective cannula through the accessory medial portal, direct it to the posterior attachment of the bucket handle fragment, and cut the posterior attachment under direct vision (Fig. 59-26, B). Keeping gentle tension on the grasping instrument as the cut is made makes its release easier. Always carry this out under direct vision. Twisting the meniscus with the grasper often allows viewing of portions of the posterior attachment that still remain and facilitates direct viewing for better, more precise cuts. Once the posterior attachment is free, extract the loose bucket handle fragment from the joint with a gentle twisting mechanism as you extract the grasper from the joint. Then carefully probe the peripheral rim of the meniscus for additional tears. If none are present, contour and smooth the remaining peripheral rim using a basket forceps or a motorized meniscal cutter-trimmer introduced through the anteromedial or accessory medial portals. Then thoroughly lavage and suction the joint to remove any remaining debris.

SWEDISH OR CENTRAL APPROACH

Gillquist and associates of Linkoping, Sweden, developed a central approach or portal for arthroscopy with the viewing arthroscope inserted through the patellar tendon, thus the term *central approach*. This is usually combined with two standard inferior portals, anteromedial and anterolateral, for accessory instrument insertion. The position of the arthroscope in the midline is never changed. The arthroscope can be advanced through the intercondylar notch, and with a 70-degree oblique viewing telescope, the posterior horns of the menisci and their meniscosynovial

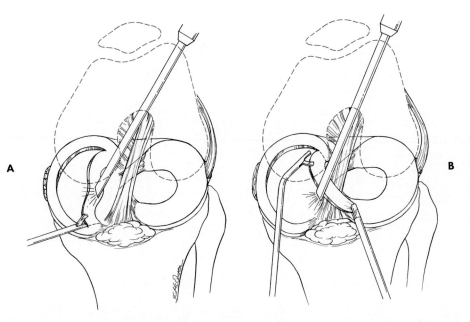

Fig. 59-26. Patel technique for medial meniscectomy. **A,** Anterior horn of bucket handle tear of medial meniscus released with scissors through anteromedial portal. Scope is through midpatellar lateral portal. **B,** Fragment pulled into intercondylar notch by grasper through anterolateral portal. Posterior release with scissors through accessory medial portal.

attachments, as well as the posterior cruciate ligament, can be directly viewed.

TECHNIQUE. Accurate location of these portal sites is one of the most important steps in this system, as with other arthroscopic techniques. The anteromedial and anterolateral portals are approximately one fingerbreadth above the tibial plateau just under the femoral condyle. The central portal is ideally 1 cm inferior to the lower pole of the patella in the midline of the joint (Fig. 59-27).

Make a transverse skin incision, 1 cm below the inferior pole of the patella that extends only through the skin into the subcutaneous tissue and not through the anterior fibers of the patellar tendon. With the knee flexed 90 degrees split the tendon with the sharp trocar of the arthroscope. Then penetrate the tendon without the cannula, since the offset of the cannula edge will rupture some of the tendon fibers. The sharp obturator should pass only into the fat pad. With an up-and-down motion of the sharp obturator, split the tendon vertically. This allows room to insert the blunt obturator and cannula, which are pushed into the joint. Extend the knee as the blunt obturator and cannula are pushed into the joint, aiming toward the superomedial compartment. This guarantees passage of the arthroscope above the fat pad. Once the 30-degree viewing arthroscope is in the joint, bring it down into the intercondylar notch to view the space between the anterior cruciate ligament and the medial femoral condyle. Push the arthroscope directly into this interval with the knee flexed about 70 to 80 degrees, dangling off the end of the operating table (Fig. 59-28). Usually the scope will pass easily and enter the posteromedial compartment. If it does not, slightly increase the amount of knee flexion. Internal rotation of the tibia displaces the posterior cruciate ligament laterally and also eases insertion. If the scope does not pass, substitute the blunt obturator for the arthroscope and cannula. Gentle pressure on the blunt obturator, combined with varying the degrees of knee flexion and tibial rotation, almost always permits entry into the posteromedial compartment. Then remove the obturator or the 30-degree arthroscope, and insert the 70-degree angled arthroscope through the same cannula. Increase knee flexion and internal rotation of the tibia to uncover the posterior aspect of the medial meniscus. Rotate the scope 180 degrees and slightly retract it to reveal the base of the posterior cruciate ligament. Further rotation of the arthroscope follows the cruciate ligament to its origin proximally. The technique for getting both the arthroscope and accessory instruments into the posterior compartments of the knee joint from the front takes practice, but can easily be mastered from these anterior portals.

Instrumentation of the posterolateral compartment is

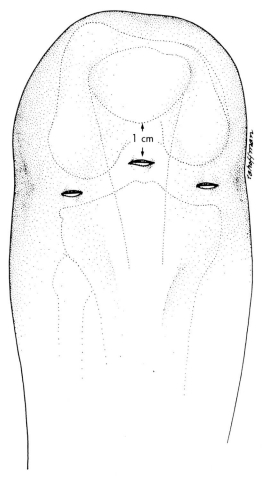

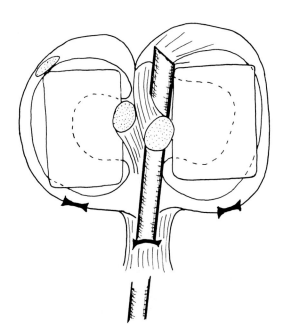

Fig. 59-27. Drawing showing central approach. Anterolateral and anteromedial portals can be used for insertion of other instruments. (From Shahriaree, H.: O'Connor's textbook on arthroscopic surgery, Philadelphia, 1984, J.B. Lippincott Co.)

Fig. 59-28. Arthroscope is passed through central transpatellar tendon portal and through intercondylar notch between medial femoral condyle and posterior cruciate ligament. (From Mulhollan, J.S.: Orthop. Clin. North Am. **13:**349, 1982.)

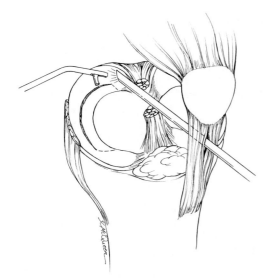

Fig. 59-29. Release of posterior horn attachment of complete longitudinal tear of medial meniscus, using Swedish approach: 70-degree scope is through intercondylar notch, scissors are through posteromedial portal.

performed similarly, but generally with greater ease.

Accessory instruments can be passed into either the posteromedial or posterolateral compartments for probing and for surgical procedures, through the appropriate anteromedial or anterolateral accessory portals.

Carry out meniscal surgery and other operative procedures using the Swedish or central approach much like the conventional triangulation techniques previously prescribed, only with the viewing arthroscope inserted through the central portal and accessory instruments through additional portals. Advocates of this technique cite as the principal advantages the ability to directly view posterior pathologic conditions and to make more precise posterior cuts when excising meniscal fragments. If a displaced bucket handle tear of the meniscus is present, however, reduce it by probing before the arthroscope is passed through the intercondylar notch and into the posterior compartment. Unless the fragment is reduced, passage of the scope posteriorly is impossible. Once the fragment is reduced, pass the arthroscope into the posterior compartment, and directly view the posterior limits of the tear or multiple tears. Then insert a probe through the appropriate anteromedial or anterolateral accessory portal into the posterior compartment, and once the direction and orientation are determined with the probe, insert a retrograde cutting hook knife with its protective cannula along the same line traversed by the probe. Place the hook knife directly in the most peripheral portion of the meniscal tear in the posterior horn and pull it forward, completing the posterior cut. This will often eliminate the dog-ear or nubbin of meniscus that is sometimes left to be trimmed once the principal fragment is removed by conventional triangulation techniques. This is often a clean, fast, and easily accomplished procedure, but practice is required.

Occasionally in tight knees or when the anterior tibial spine is prominent, this posterior meniscal cut may not be possible using an instrument through an anterior portal. In such instances, make an accessory posteromedial portal. Insert an 18-gauge spinal needle into the posteromedial compartment and view it directly with the 70-degree viewing arthroscope as it enters the compartment. Once the optimal position and direction of the spinal needle are determined, bring its tip to the desired location to simulate release of the posterior tear. Then make the portal and select the cutting instrument. This may be hooked scissors or a sheathed knife with an end cutting or Smillie type of blade. Do not use a knife without an appropriate protective cannula through this posteromedial portal. Then directly view the posterior peripheral limit of the meniscal tear and incise the fragment cleanly (Fig. 59-29).

Excise and release the anterior limits of posterior horn tears by triangulation techniques, as described in the previous section, but with the arthroscope located in the appropriate anteromedial or anterolateral compartment of the joint and the operating instrument extending through the appropriate anteromedial or anterolateral accessory portal.

TEARS OF LATERAL MENISCUS

As with tears of the medial meniscus, tears of the lateral meniscus are classified as complete or incomplete, peripheral or intrameniscal, longitudinal or horizontal, and oblique or radial. As a whole, tears of the lateral meniscus are less common than those of the medial meniscus. The radial tear configuration is almost unique to the lateral meniscus, occurring very infrequently in the medial meniscus. Also, the occasional discoid meniscus is rarely encountered in the medial compartment.

Most arthroscopic surgeons find procedures more difficult to perform on the lateral meniscus. The central attachment of the anterior and posterior horns of this meniscus results in a circular configuration of the meniscus. That is, the anterior and posterior horn attachments almost meet in the intercondylar notch, whereas the medial meniscus is more C-shaped. Operating around the tight inner edge of the lateral meniscus is more confining than in the relatively open C shape. Maneuvering the arthroscope and instruments over the intercondylar attachment of the anterior horn of the lateral meniscus from the anteromedial portal is also more difficult for the inexperienced arthroscopic surgeon.

Most lateral meniscus excisions or repairs are carried out with the knee in the so-called figure-four position (Fig. 59-30), that is, with the hip slightly flexed, abducted, and externally rotated, the knee flexed 30 to 90 degrees, and the tibia internally rotated. This position is usually achieved with the table flat, the hip and knee flexed, and the ankle placed on the table surface or on the opposite lower leg. In this position, the hip falls into external rotation, and a varus stress can be applied by pushing downward on the flexed knee. This position may be more difficult if an encircling leg holder is used.

This figure-four position may also reduce overall joint distention by collapsing the suprapatellar pouch, making viewing and the use of the suction motorized cutters and trimmers in the lateral compartment more difficult.

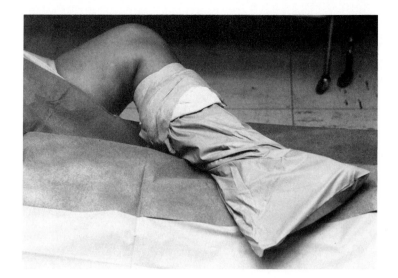

Fig. 59-30. Figure-four position, used to apply varus force to flexed knee to widen lateral compartment.

The principles of excision of tears of the lateral meniscus are quite similar to those described previously for medial meniscus tears, as follows:

1. Partial meniscectomy is always preferred over subtotal meniscus excision, and total meniscectomy is least desired.
2. Triangulation techniques are most commonly used, although the operative arthroscope may be useful in selected circumstances.
3. A balanced, stable, contoured meniscal rim is the usual objective.
4. Articular scuffing should be minimal.

INCOMPLETE INTRAMENISCAL TEARS

Incomplete tears of the lateral meniscus practically always involve the posterior third. Most often, the incomplete tear is a fissure along the superior surface of the posterior horn of the meniscus. By definition, the fissure will not admit a probe through to the undersurface of the posterior horn. The extent may vary from only a few millimeters in length and depth to 1 to 2 cm, extending from the posterior horn attachment to just opposite the popliteus tendon. The inner segment of the tear cannot be displaced into the lateral compartment by the probe.

The surgeon must use judgment when such a tear is encountered. Small tears only a few millimeters in length can be ignored. Longer tears, extending into the depths of the posterior horn a considerable distance, probably are destined to become complete longitudinal tears at some future time and should be removed.

TECHNIQUE. Following thorough examination of the knee for stability and a systematic diagnostic arthroscopy, place the limb in the figure-four position, and move the 30-degree viewing arthroscope to the anteromedial portal. Through this portal, pass the viewing arthroscope obliquely into the anterolateral compartment as varus stress is applied to the knee. Insert a probe through the anterolateral portal, and thoroughly evaluate the extent and depth of the incomplete posterior horn tear (Fig. 59-31, *A*). If

the decision is made to remove this incomplete tear, it is usually best accomplished by basket forceps. Remove the probe, and insert basket forceps through the anterolateral portal. Beginning at the inner edge of the posterior horn of the meniscus opposite the midportion of the incomplete tear, trim and contour the inner border of the meniscus bit by bit, extending peripherally into the meniscus until the incomplete vertical tear is encountered (Fig. 59-31, *B*). Once it is encountered, contour the remaining peripheral rim so a balanced, stable, and smoothly contoured rim is present. Insert a probe through the anterolateral portal, and carefully probe the meniscal rim to rule out additional tears and to be sure that the peripheral rim is stable. In contouring the peripheral rim to be left in place, it is important not to enter the popliteal hiatus; otherwise, a subtotal meniscectomy with removal of the entire posterior horn will be necessary rather than the more desirable partial meniscectomy (Fig. 59-31, *C*). Finally, contour and smooth the peripheral rim using the motorized meniscus cutter (Fig. 59-31, *D*). Then thoroughly lavage and suction the joint to remove all remaining debris.

COMPLETE INTRAMENISCAL TEARS

Complete intrameniscal tears of the lateral meniscus most often involve the posterior horn. Excision of small complete intrameniscal tears may be carried out using basket forceps, as previously described for incomplete tears. Larger complete intrameniscal tears are usually removed by en bloc excision.

TECHNIQUE. Following a complete and systematic diagnostic arthroscopic examination, place the limb in a figure-four position, and insert the 30-degree viewing arthroscope into the anterolateral compartment through the anteromedial portal. Insert a probe through the anterolateral portal, and carefully delineate the extent and limits of the complete intrameniscal tear of the posterior horn. If the tear is determined to be large and en bloc removal is chosen, use either a two-portal or a three-portal technique. If a two-portal approach is chosen, remove the probe, and insert

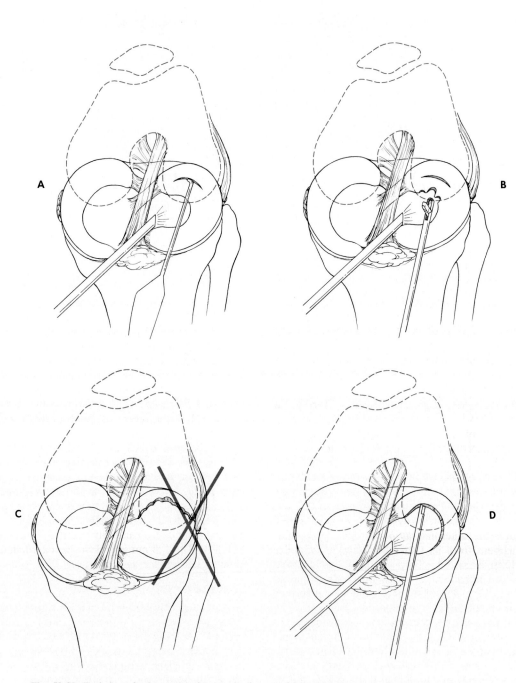

Fig. 59-31. Technique for incomplete intrameniscal tears of lateral meniscus. **A,** Probing incomplete tear, lateral meniscus. **B,** Incomplete tear removed bit by bit with basket forceps. **C,** Popliteus hiatus must not be entered when contouring posterolateral rim. If so, entire posterior rim must be removed. **D,** Peripheral rim is smoothed and contoured with motorized trimmer.

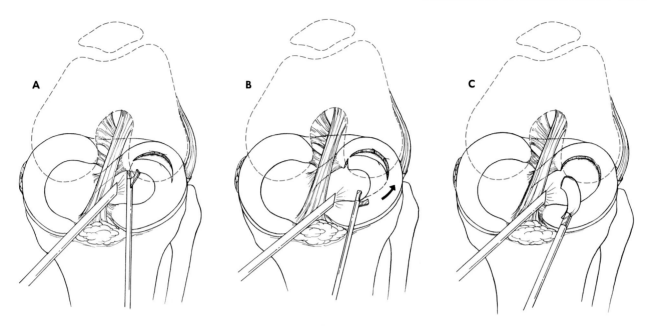

Fig. 59-32. Technique for complete intrameniscal tears of lateral meniscus. **A,** Partial detachment of posterior attachment, complete longitudinal tear, lateral meniscus. **B,** Release of anterior limits of tear with scissors. **C,** Avulsion of remaining posterior attachment with grasper.

hooked scissors or basket forceps through the anterolateral portal. Make a cut opposite the most posterior limits of the tear, proceeding from the inner edge of the posterior horn to approach the posterior limits of the tear (Fig. 59-32, *A*). It is preferable, in making this cut, not to extend completely into the tear, but to leave a small strand of meniscal tissue between the transverse meniscal cut and the horizontal tear. Then position the scissors or hooked basket forceps through the anterolateral portal opposite the most anterior limits of the tear. Beginning on the inner border of the meniscus, make a transverse incision through the meniscus to join the longitudinal tear; complete this cut into the tear (Fig. 59-32, *B*). Remove the scissors or basket forceps, insert a grasping instrument or a small pituitary rongeur through the anterolateral portal, and grasp and avulse the fragment from its tenuous remaining posterior attachment. Then extract the fragment from the joint by the grasping instrument through the anterolateral portal (Fig. 59-32, *C*). Trim the inner rim of the anterior and posterior limits of the en bloc resection, using basket forceps through the anterolateral portal, so that a balanced, smoothly contoured peripheral rim remains. Insert a probe through the anterolateral portal, and carefully probe the remaining peripheral rim of the meniscus for additional pathology. Again in doing this en bloc excision exercise care to avoid entering the popliteal hiatus or a complete excision of the posterior horn will be required, since a balanced stable peripheral rim would not then be possible.

An alternate technique for en bloc excision of large, complete intrameniscal tears of the posterior horn of the lateral meniscus involves the use of three portals. With the 30-degree viewing arthroscope positioned through the anteromedial portal, again carefully examine and determine the limits of the longitudinal intrameniscal tear. Through the anterolateral portal, introduce a scissors or a retrograde

knife to release first the anterior limit of the fragment by making an oblique cut extending from the inner edge of the meniscus out to the anterior limits of the peripheral tear. If the retrograde knife is selected, position the hook of the knife in the anterior axilla of the tear, and carefully incise in an anterior and inward direction (Fig. 59-33, *A*). Bring this cut anteriorly until it meets the inner edge of the meniscus to facilitate grasping the fragment during the next step. Remove the knife or scissors from the anterolateral portal, and move the viewing arthroscope from the anteromedial to the anterolateral portal. Insert a small grasping clamp through the anteromedial portal. Grasp the anterior tip of the detached fragment, and displace it toward the intercondylar notch. Then fashion an accessory far lateral portal by initially inserting an 18-gauge spinal needle 1.5 to 2.5 cm lateral to the anterolateral portal and above the superior surface of the lateral meniscus. Then direct the needle toward the posterior horn of the lateral meniscus to ensure that the instrument through this portal can be directed properly. Once the spinal needle has been properly positioned and directed, make the accessory lateral portal. Insert a knife or scissors through this portal, and as tension is maintained on the displaced fragment, sever the posterior horn attachment (Fig. 59-33, *B*). Use a protective sheath over the knife. If release of the posterior horn attachment of the displaced fragment cannot be completed with the cutting instrument in the accessory lateral portal, push the fragment back into the reduced position with the grasper, remove the grasper, and move the viewing arthroscope back to the anteromedial portal. Then insert the grasper through the accessory lateral portal, grasp the anterior tip of the fragment, and apply gentle traction. Insert a thin-ended cutting knife through a protective cannula through the anterolateral portal to the inner edge, make a cut across the posterior attachment toward the lon-

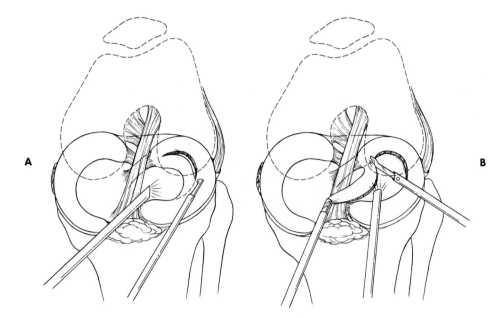

Fig. 59-33. Three-portal technique for complete intrameniscal tears of lateral meniscus. **A,** Release of anterior limits, longitudinal tear, lateral meniscus. **B,** Posterior attachment released using three-portal technique.

gitudinal tear. Release of the posterior attachment requires great care. Do not use the knife or scissors blindly. The tissue edge as well as the cutting instrument must be in the field of vision at all times. To cut blindly may result in cutting the intact posterior meniscal rim or neurovascular damage in the popliteal area.

Once this has been completed, the fragment is free and is extracted from the joint in the jaws of the grasper. Probe the peripheral rim to rule out additional tears. Contour and smooth the rim using basket forceps or a motorized trimmer. As already mentioned it is critical not to cut through the peripheral rim into the popliteal hiatus or else the remainder of the posterior rim will require removal, since rim continuity will be lost and a stable rim will not be possible.

PERIPHERAL TEARS

Peripheral tears of the lateral meniscus, like those medially, may be reparable if they are within the outer vascularized 25% of the meniscus and no additional tears are present within the meniscus. If the peripheral tear is accompanied by multiple other tears, it is best to excise it, usually by a subtotal meniscectomy, with the posterior horn being excised and the middle one third of the meniscus being contoured anterior to the popliteal hiatus.

Repairs of the lateral meniscus may be accomplished either by open suturing (p. 2319) or by arthroscopic techniques described later in this chapter (p. 2594). If the peripheral tear is not reparable and excision is required, it is carried out using the same technique described for en bloc excision of complete intrameniscal tears.

BUCKET HANDLE TEARS

Displaced bucket handle tears usually originate as longitudinal intrameniscal tears. If the anterior limit of the tear extends anteriorly to or beyond the popliteal hiatus, it

may become displaced into the joint and produce locking. Most bucket handle tears of the lateral meniscus are more easily removed if the displaced fragment is first reduced.

TECHNIQUE. After a systematic and complete diagnostic arthroscopy, place the limb in the figure-four position, move the 30-degree viewing arthroscope to the anteromedial portal, and pass it into the lateral compartment. If the bucket-handle tear of the lateral meniscus is displaced into the intercondylar notch, it may block easy passage of the viewing arthroscope into the lateral compartment. If blockage is encountered and viewing the lateral compartment is difficult, pass the scope into the patellofemoral joint and then sweep it down over the lateral femoral condyle into the lateral compartment. This brings the arthroscope down over the top of the displaced fragment, rather than directly into it, as occurs if you attempt to direct the arthroscope through the anteromedial portal directly into the lateral compartment. Insert a probe through the anterolateral portal, and if the bucket handle fragment is displaced into the intercondylar notch, reduce it with the probe (Fig. 59-34, A). This often allows a better view of the compartment and definition of the anterior and posterior axillae of the tear. You can excise the bucket handle fragment using a two-portal technique, that is, anteromedial and anterolateral portals, or, more commonly, a three-portal technique, that is, anterolateral, anteromedial, and accessory lateral portals.

If you choose the two-portal method, retain the arthroscope in the anteromedial portal. Pass a probe through the anterolateral portal and define the anterior and posterior limits of the tear. Remove the probe, and insert a thin end cutting knife, hooked scissors, or basket forceps through the anterolateral portal. Begin cutting across the posterior horn of the meniscus from the inner edge, and direct it toward the posterior limit of the tear. Release this posterior bucket-handle attachment except for a few remaining fibers

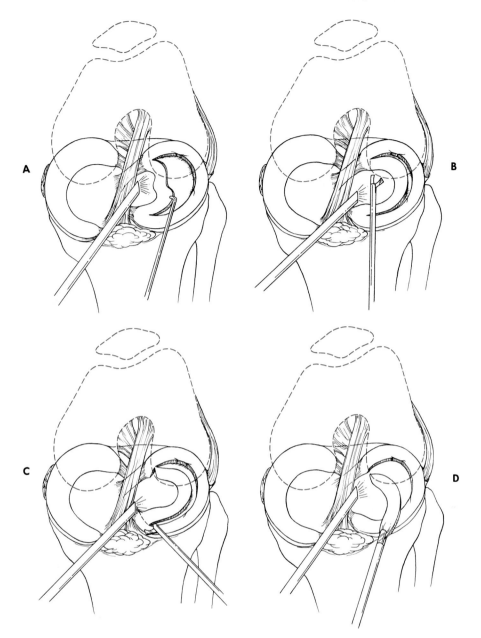

Fig. 59-34. Two-portal technique for bucket-handle tears of lateral meniscus. **A,** Displaced bucket-handle tear of lateral meniscus probed. **B,** Following reduction of displaced bucket handle tear, scissors partially release posterior attachment. **C,** Scissors release anterior attachment. **D,** Tenuous remaining posterior attachment avulsed with grasper and extracted.

(Fig. 59-34, *B*). Then bring the knife, scissors, or basket forceps anteriorly to cut the anterior attachment of the bucket-handle fragment. If the anterior axilla of the tear is far anteriorly, so that the cutting instruments cannot be properly directed to release the attachment, you may elect to move the arthroscope to the anterolateral portal and bring the cutting instrument across to the anterior attachment through the anteromedial portal. The anterior attachment of the bucket handle fragment must be released as near the axilla of the tear as possible to avoid leaving a large anteriorly based flap of remaining meniscus (Fig. 59-34, *C*). Once the anterior attachment is completely re-

leased, insert a grasper and avulse the tenuous attachment remaining posteriorly. Extract the entire bucket handle fragment in a slow twisting motion with the grasper (Fig. 59-34, *D*). Slightly enlarging the exit portal to permit passage of the fragment is preferable to having it pulled from the jaws of the grasper. Then probe the peripheral rim to assess any additional tears, and trim and contour it to produce a smooth, balanced, and stable rim.

More often a three-portal technique is used for bucket handle tears of the lateral meniscus. With the knee in the figure-four position, insert the 30-degree viewing arthroscope through an anteromedial portal into the lateral compartment. If the bucket handle fragment is displaced into the intercondylar notch, reduce it with a probe through the anterolateral portal. Carefully probe the anterior and posterior limits of the tear. If the anterior limit of the tear extends well into the anterior horn, it is usually preferable to move the viewing arthroscope to the anterolateral portal. With the arthroscope now in the anterolateral portal, again carefully probe the anterior axilla of the tear through the anteromedial portal. Once it is clearly defined release the anterior horn with a pair of hooked scissors inserted through this anteromedial portal (Fig. 59-35, *A*). Then remove the scissors and insert a grasping instrument through the anteromedial portal. Firmly grasp the anterior horn of

the bucket-handle fragment and pull the fragment toward the intercondylar notch (Fig. 59-35, *B*). With the fragment now displaced into the intercondylar notch, rotate the arthroscope lens so the posterior attachment of the fragment can be viewed. Gently tugging alternately on the grasper usually allows clear delineation of this attachment. Choose an accessory or far lateral portal by first inserting an 18-gauge spinal needle between the lateral femoral and tibial condyles above the superior surface of the lateral meniscus. The point of entry of the needle can be varied to permit the precise direction to the posterior attachment of the meniscal fragment, but is usually 1.5 to 2.5 cm lateral to the anterolateral portal. Finally adjust the location and di-

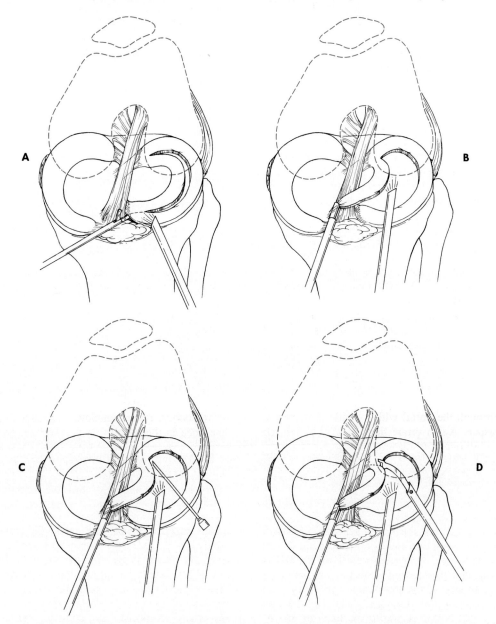

Fig. 59-35. Three-portal technique for bucket handle tear of lateral meniscus. **A,** Anterior horn of bucket handle tear released with scissors. **B,** Released anterior horn pulled into intercondylar notch. **C,** Accessory lateral portal site determined by inserting spinal needle. **D,** Posterior attachment released with contoured knife through accessory lateral portal.

rection of the needle to permit its passage directly to the posterior attachment of the bucket handle fragment so that a cutting instrument passed along the same course can easily reach the attachment (Fig. 59-35, C).

Once this portal site is located, make an incision, carefully protecting the lateral meniscus, for the far lateral accessory portal. Then a thin, end-cutting meniscal knife or curved scissors can be inserted through the accessory lateral portal, directed to the posterior attachment of the displaced bucket handle tear, and used to cut the posterior attachment (Fig. 59-35, D). If the direction of the cutting instrument does not allow complete severance of the posterior attachment, push the bucket handle fragment back into reduced position with the grasper, release the grasper and move to the accessory lateral portal. After reducing the displaced fragment, insert the grasper through the accessory lateral portal, grasp the anterior tip of the fragment, and direct the scissors or knife through the anteromedial portal to release the posterior attachment.

Occasionally, if the posterior limit of the tear extends to the most posterior horn attachment, releasing the posterior horn is difficult. In this instance move the viewing arthroscope back to the anteromedial portal, insert the cutting instrument through the anterolateral portal, and apply gentle traction to the fragment using the grasper in the accessory lateral portal. Alternatively, move the viewing arthroscope from the anteromedial to the anterolateral portal and use the alternate portal for the cutting instrument. This should be employed when difficulty is encountered in releasing the posterior horn attachment. It is imperative that you maintain in your visual field the tip of the cutting instrument and *precisely* those fibers involved in the posterior attachment; do not cut blindly. Often rotating or twisting the meniscal fragment will bring into view fibers of the meniscus that remain attached, permitting more precise cutting. It not only is poor technique but also may result in serious damage to the cruciate ligament and neurovascular structures not to make the effort to view directly the posterior attachment and instead to simply cut blindly.

Once the posterior horn attachment is released, extract the fragment through the portal with a gentle twisting motion of the grasper. Again probe the rim of the meniscus to search for additional pathologic conditions. Using the basket forceps or motorized trimmer, smooth and contour the remaining rim. Thoroughly lavage the joint and suction out any remaining debris.

If a significant anterior flap remains, most often the result of cutting across the anterior attachment of the bucket handle fragment short of the axilla, this is best removed by positioning the viewing arthroscope in the anterolateral portal and introducing the Acuflex rotary basket instrument from the anteromedial portal. The 90-degree cutting action of this instrument allows the inner edge of the anterior horn of the meniscus to be trimmed. An alternative is to position the viewing arthroscope in the anteromedial portal and to use a down-biting Kerrison rongeur inserted through the anterolateral portal. The down-biting mechanism of this rongeur allows irregularities of the anterior horn to be trimmed.

OBLIQUE TEARS

Oblique tears of the lateral meniscus are classified, like their medial counterparts, into anterior and posterior varieties, depending on the direction of the tear and the location of its base. These are much less common in the lateral meniscus than in the medial meniscus. A force that tends to straighten the inner edge of the lateral meniscus because of its shorter inner margin and configuration is more likely to produce a radial than an oblique tear. The converse has been noted medially.

The technique for excision of oblique tears of the lateral meniscus is similar to that described for oblique tears of the medial meniscus, with the arthroscope portals and instrument portals generally reversed. Morcellation of small oblique tears is done with basket forceps; larger oblique tears may be excised either by morcellation or by en bloc excision using principles described in previous sections.

RADIAL TEARS

Radial tears are common in the lateral meniscus (Plate 7, E). Forces that straighten or lengthen the inner edge of the meniscus frequently result in a radially oriented tear extending from the inner edge in varying degrees into the substance of the meniscus. The middle third of the meniscus is most commonly involved. Three varieties of radial tears are encountered: (1) incomplete, (2) complete, and (3) parrot beak. In the incomplete type a vertical, radially oriented tear extends from the inner edge of the meniscus out toward the periphery. No horizontal or flap component exists in this type of tear. This incomplete radial tear is usually the precursor of the complete radial and parrot beak varieties. In the complete radial type, the tear extends all the way from the inner edge to the meniscosynovial rim, in essence dividing the lateral meniscus into anterior and posterior fragments. Again, there is no horizontal or longitudinal element initially, and the middle third of the lateral meniscus is the most frequent site. The parrot beak variety occurs when longitudinal or oblique tears are added to the incomplete or complete radial tears. These anterior or posterior tears extending from the original radial tear may produce mobile flaps or parrot beak extensions.

TECHNIQUE. After complete diagnostic arthroscopy, place the knee in the figure-four position and insert the viewing arthroscope through the anteromedial portal into the lateral compartment. Insert a probe through the anterolateral portal, and carefully examine the peripheral extent of the incomplete radial tear. The objective is to saucerize the inner edge of the meniscus out to the peripheral extent of the incomplete tear (Fig. 59-36, A). Introduce the basket forceps through the anterolateral portal, and excise the posterior leaf of the tear. This is done by fragmentary, bit by bit excision of the inner edge of the meniscus beginning at the transverse tear and gradually tapering and contouring toward the inner edge along the posterior horn of the meniscus (Fig. 59-36, B). It is usually not possible to remove the anterior leaf of the radial tear with the basket forceps in the anterolateral portal, since the cutting edge of the basket generally is parallel rather than perpendicular to the edge to be excised. Remove the basket forceps from the anterolateral portal, and switch the viewing arthroscope

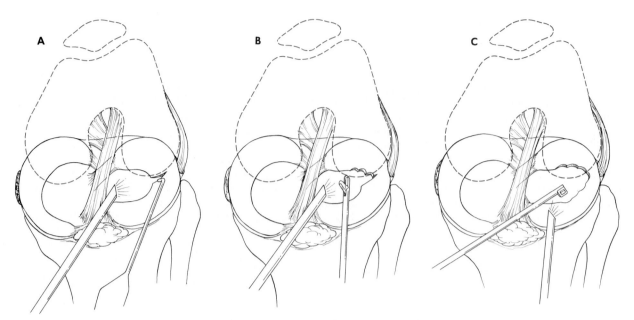

Fig. 59-36. Technique for radial tear of lateral meniscus. **A,** Incomplete radial tear probed. **B,** Basket forceps saucerizes posterior fragment. **C,** 90-degree rotary forceps saucerizes anterior fragment.

from the anteromedial portal to the anterolateral. Introduce the basket forceps through the anteromedial portal and into the lateral compartment, and remove the anterior leaf of the incomplete radial tear bit by bit, contouring the cut edge gradually into the anterior horn of the meniscus. The rotary 90-degree (Acuflex) basket forceps works well (Fig. 59-36, *C*). Bringing the basket forceps in from the antero- medial compartment turns them more perpendicularly to the meniscal edge to be excised. Remove the basket for- ceps and perform final smoothing and contouring of the middle third of the lateral meniscus with the motorized meniscus cutter. Probe the rim of the meniscus and thor- oughly lavage and suction the joint to remove any remain- ing debris.

Excision of parrot beak tears of the lateral meniscus may be performed in a manner similar to that described for in- complete radial tears, using basket forceps to saucerize and contour the meniscus until the lateral limits of the tear have been removed. If the anteriorly or posteriorly based flaps are sufficiently large to be excised en bloc, place the 30-degree viewing arthroscope into the anteromedial portal and introduce a cutting instrument through the anterolateral portal. In such instances hook scissors introduced through the anterolateral portal may cut across the base of the large posterior parrot beak flap extending toward the posterior limit of the horizontal component of the tear. It is wise to stop a few fibers short of entering the longitudinal element of the tear (Fig. 59-37, *A*). Then insert a grasper through the anterolateral portal and avulse the tenuous base of the posterior parrot beak flap (Fig. 59-37, *B*). Smooth and contour the posterior rim of the lateral meniscus by means of basket forceps introduced through the anterolateral por- tal. The midlateral and anterior horn components of the tear may be removed with a down-biting Kerrison rongeur, inserted through the anterolateral portal. With the arthro-

scope in the anterolateral portal, contour the inner edge of the middle and anterior thirds of the lateral meniscus using basket forceps introduced through the anteromedial portal. Straight-hooked basket forceps are satisfactory for con- touring the middle third of the lateral meniscus; however, they are not properly angled to contour the anterior third of the lateral meniscus. The Acuflex rotary basket forceps, which cut 90 degrees to the axis of the instrument, are excellent for balancing and contouring the anterior horn of the lateral meniscus (Fig. 59-37, *C*). Final contouring and trimming are done with the motorized trimmer to fashion a symmetric balance between the anterior, middle, and posterior thirds of the meniscus (Fig. 59-37, *D*).

Excision of complete radial tears of the lateral meniscus is performed in a manner similar to the technique de- scribed for parrot beak tears, only more of the meniscus must be removed. If the radial tear extends all the way to the meniscosynovial junction, a nearly total meniscectomy may be necessary.

With a 30-degree viewing arthroscope in the anterome- dial compartment and the knee in the figure-four position, probe the lateral extent of the tear through the anterolateral portal. If it extends to near the meniscosynovial junction and most of the lateral meniscus requires excision, it is usually easier to remove the anterior half initially, then proceed to the posterior half. Insert a retrograde or hook knife through the anterolateral portal, positioning the hook of the blade near the lateral extent of the radial tear near the meniscosynovial junction. Incise the anterior meniscus from the radial tear to near the anterolateral portal (Fig. 59-38, *A*). Further extension of the anterior cut requires changing the viewing arthroscope to the anterolateral por- tal or to a midpatellar medial portal. Then insert the hook knife through a protective cannula in the anteromedial por- tal across to the anterior horn of the lateral meniscus. Place

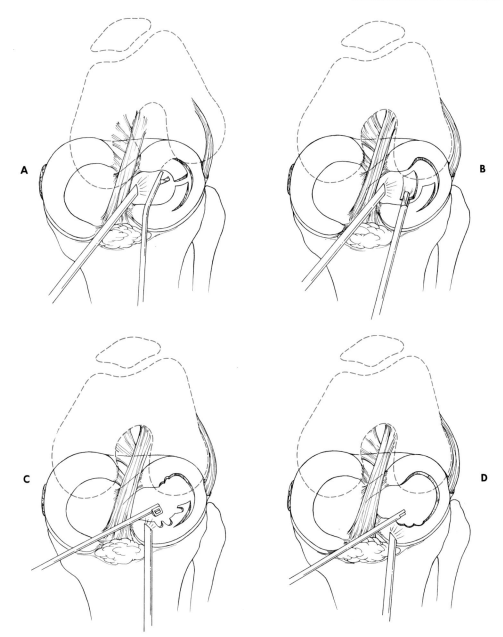

Fig. 59-37. Technique for ''parrot beak'' tears of lateral meniscus. **A,** Base of posterior ''parrot beak'' flap released with scissors. **B,** Fragment avulsed and extracted with grasper. **C,** Morcellation of anterior fragment of parrot beak tear with 90-degree rotary basket forceps. **D,** Final contouring with motorized trimmer.

the hook of the knife into the previous incision in the meniscus and extend the cut as far anteriorly as possible (Fig. 59-38, *B*). This anterior fragment may then be amputated by hook scissors through the anteromedial or anterolateral portal or with a down-biting Kerrison rongeur through the anterolateral portal (Fig. 59-38, *C*). Contour and trim the anterior half with a motorized meniscus cutter through the anteromedial portal. Remove the posterior half of the meniscus bit by bit with basket forceps introduced through the lateral portal with the viewing arthroscope in the anteromedial portal. The entire meniscus may be tediously removed in this manner (Fig. 59-38, *D*). Final trimming is

then completed with the motorized cutter-trimmer (Fig. 59-38, *E*). Thoroughly lavage and suction the joint to remove remaining debris.

DISCOID LATERAL MENISCUS

Most discoid menisci are lateral; compared with other meniscal pathology, the incidence of discoid lateral menisci is exceedingly rare (Plate 7, *F*). A discoid lateral meniscus may be discovered during a systematic examination of the knee in which another pathologic condition may be producing symptoms. The pathologic condition accounting for the symptoms should be appropriately corrected, and

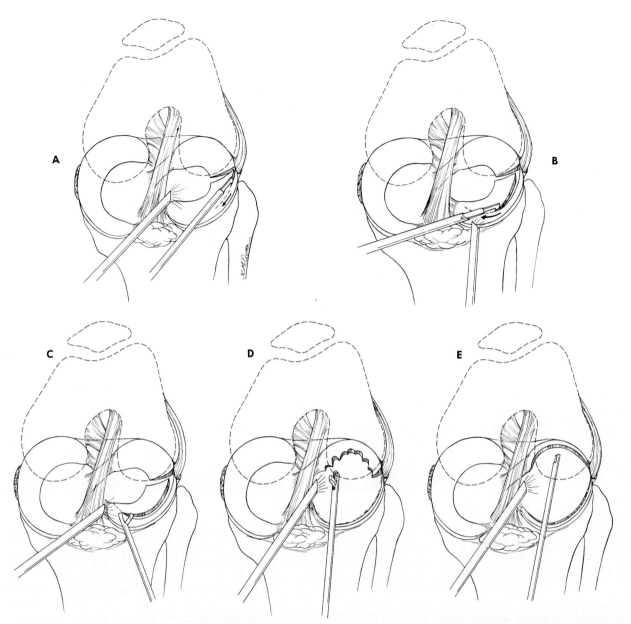

Fig. 59-38. Technique for complete radial tear of lateral meniscus. **A,** Release of middle third of lateral meniscus in complete radial tear. **B,** Release of anterior third attachment. **C,** Release of anterior fragment with scissors. **D,** Morcellation of posterior fragment and of peripheral rim with basket forceps. **E,** Final smoothing, peripheral rim, with motorized trimmer.

unless torn or degenerative, the discoid lateral meniscus probably should be left intact. To excise a torn or degenerative discoid lateral meniscus it is probably best to use conventional arthrotomy except for the most experienced arthroscopic surgeons. A well-performed open arthrotomy and excision of the abnormal meniscus is preferable to a poor arthroscopic excision. Excision of a discoid meniscus is among the most technically demanding arthroscopic procedures.

TECHNIQUE. If arthroscopic excision is attempted, the objective generally is to remove the central portion, leaving a balanced rim of meniscus about the width of the normal lateral meniscus. The width, however, is dictated by the

location and extent of the tear within the meniscus. If the free inner edge of the meniscus is not noted in the systematic diagnostic arthroscopy of the lateral compartment, a discoid lateral meniscus may be responsible. The tibial plateau may be completely covered by the meniscus, and therefore the lateral compartment may appear to be devoid of a lateral meniscus; alternatively, varying portions may be covered. If a discoid meniscus is suspected, carefully explore more centrally in the lateral compartment or over near the intercondylar eminence for a meniscal edge.

If the discoid meniscus is torn and arthroscopic partial excision is attempted, remove and contour the meniscus

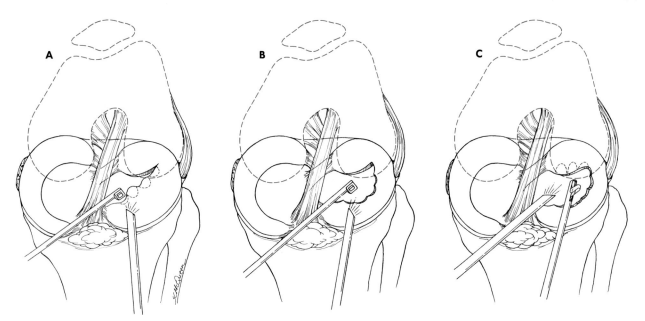

Fig. 59-39. Technique for discoid lateral meniscus. **A,** Anterior portion of discoid lateral meniscus removed with rotary basket forceps. **B,** Further contouring of anterior rim with 90-degree rotary basket forceps. **C,** Posterior discoid fragment removed with basket forceps.

beginning at its inner edge. Place the 30-degree viewing arthroscope in the anterolateral portal and the knee in a figure-four position. Begin the resection using basket forceps through the anteromedial portal. Bit by bit remove the inner edge (Fig. 59-39, *A*). Excision may be made easier by splitting the meniscus from its inner edge radially out into the discoid meniscus. This technique may improve the efficiency of the basket forceps. Usually the middle third of the discoid meniscus can be removed in this manner. Removal of the anterior third is best done by using the Acuflex rotary biting basket forceps through the anteromedial portal, since they cut 90 degrees to the long axis of the instrument (Fig. 59-39, *B*), or by moving the viewing arthroscope to the anteromedial portal and using a down-biting Kerrison rongeur. Contour the posterior third of the meniscus with basket forceps through the anterolateral portal (Fig. 59-39, *C*). When the desired amount of meniscal tissue is removed and the rim is balanced, the thickness of the inner edge will be much greater than that after routine partial meniscus excision. Thoroughly lavage and suction the joint.

ARTHROSCOPIC REPAIR OF TORN MENISCI

Tears within the vascular, outer 10% to 25% of the menisci have been shown to heal predictably when they are sutured and immobilized. Initially repair was reserved for relatively acute peripheral tears, but recent reports indicate that repair can be successful in chronic tears if the body of the meniscus does not contain additional tears. Arnoczky has shown experimentally in animals that tears outside the vascular zone may also heal with fibrovascular scar if a vascular access channel is created linking the tear to the peripheral vascular area. The results of repair attempts on tears in portions of the meniscus other than pe-

ripheral detachments in humans have not been encouraging. At the present time, it appears that meniscoplasty should be limited to the peripheral 10% to 25% of the meniscus.

To date, several reports document the merits of repair of peripheral tears of the meniscus using open arthrotomy techniques. Description of these techniques may be found in Chapter 56, p. 2319.

Instrumentation is being developed to permit repair of certain peripheral meniscal tears using arthroscopic techniques. Currently the instrumentation and techniques are not refined enough to be recommended for routine use and probably should be limited to use by only the most experienced arthroscopic surgeons. Arthroscopic meniscal repair has been described, using Keith needles, spinal needles, thin Kirschner wires with holes drilled through their tips, and single and double cannulated instrument systems through which thin needles and sutures are passed.

The first repair procedures using arthroscopic techniques involved passing the needle and suture with direct arthroscopic viewing from an inside-to-outside direction; that is, the needle and suture were pushed initially from within the joint, through the meniscus, across the tear, and exited the joint through the synovium and capsule. Without an incision and open exposure of the capsular exit point, the needle exited the joint "blindly." There were neurovascular structures near the exit sites posteromedially and posterolaterally, and some were injured even by the most experienced arthroscopic surgeons. The risk of these complications led some surgeons to advise an open posteromedial or posterolateral capsular exposure, so a retractor could be placed anterior to these important popliteal structures. In such instances, as the needles were pushed blindly through the meniscus and capsule, they would encounter the popliteal retractor and deflect away from the neurovascular structures. Most meniscal tears suitable for suture are torn posteriorly, so injury to these structures was a constant risk. The structure on the lateral side most frequently at risk is the common peroneal nerve; on the medial side, the saphenous nerve is most at risk, and the popliteal vessels in posterior meniscal tears are always at risk.

Meniscal suturing techniques involving inside-to-outside methods most frequently use either single- or double-barreled cannula systems for passing the needles through the joint. Techniques for meniscoplasties using cannula techniques will be described later in this section.

Because of the occasional neurovascular complication using the inside-to-outside techniques, Warren, Casscells, Johnson, and others developed an outside-to-inside technique. These arthroscopists believe that precise entry points with the needles are possible only when introduced from without and directed inward. A suture is passed through an ordinary spinal needle with approximately 2.5 cm protruding from the sharp tip and the remainder of the suture exiting the needle hub. This suture-loaded spinal needle is inserted through the capsule after a small posteromedial or posterolateral skin incision is made. The sharp point of the needle pierces the capsule and synovium from outside to inside. It is viewed through the arthroscope in an anterior portal. The needle and suture are then passed through the meniscus, and the suture is grasped and pulled to the outside through the anteromedial portal. A large knot is tied in its end. Tension on the opposite end of the suture exiting through the posterior incision brings the large knot back into the joint via the anteromedial portal, down to the meniscus, thus reducing it to the synovial capsular bed. Successive sutures so placed are tied over the capsule to each other. This technique will also be described.

Initially, regardless of the technique used, the exiting sutures were tied over a cotton bolster superficial to the skin. This produced potential tracts for infection of the knee joint, and some infections resulted. This can and should be avoided by making an appropriate skin incision in the area of the anticipated repair, dissecting down to the outer surface of the capsule so the sutures once passed can be tied over the capsule and buried beneath the skin.

Much controversy still exists concerning open versus arthroscopic meniscoplasty. Proponents for open techniques argue that (1) better preparation of the repair site is possible through an arthrotomy, (2) more precise suture placement is possible, (3) the sutures can be placed vertically through the meniscus only with open techniques and these hold better, (4) since an open incision is required to expose the capsule with arthroscopic techniques, these techniques have no advantage over open techniques, and (5) the immobilization required is the same for both open and arthroscopic techniques. Proponents for arthroscopic techniques claim that (1) results have now been proven to be equal to those of open techniques, (2) certain tears are easier to suture by arthroscopic techniques (i.e., posterolateral tears and tears central to the meniscosynovial junction—such tears 2 to 5 mm from the periphery cannot be exposed and sutured by open arthrotomy methods), and (3) morbidity is less after arthroscopic techniques.

We prefer to use the open arthrotomy technique for longitudinal peripheral tears or for tears being repaired at the same time that we perform a stabilizing ligamentous operation, for example, an anterior cruciate reconstruction. Arthroscopic techniques are used for (1) posterior tears of the lateral meniscus, (2) longitudinal tears more than 2 mm central to the peripheral attachment, and (3) tears deep to the tibial collateral ligament where exposure by open technique would be difficult.

With increased interest in arthroscopic techniques refinement in instrument design and operative techniques will surely be forthcoming. Currently, the average orthopaedic surgeon should repair most peripheral meniscal tears by the standard arthrotomy and suture techniques. The following will describe arthroscopic meniscoplasty using first the single cannula system, then a double cannula system with the instruments currently available.

Regardless of the arthroscopic technique preferred by the surgeon, arthroscopic meniscus repairs consist of three important steps:

1. Appropriate patient selection by documenting a single vertical longitudinal tear in the outer one third of the meniscus, which is able to heal
2. Tear debridement and local synovial, meniscal, and capsular abrasion to stimulate a proliferative fibroblastic healing response
3. Suture placement to reduce and stabilize the meniscus

Often we will combine the two basic arthroscopic techniques; that is, inside-to-outside cannula technique and outside-to-inside needle technique for a given repair. For instance, if a large bucket handle tear of the medial meniscus is suitable for repair, an initial stabilizing horizontal mattress suture in the midpoint of the tear near the posteromedial corner may be inserted with a single or double cannula technique, followed by additional sutures posteriorly—hence nearer neurovascular structures, using the outside-to-inside needle technique. The more anterior the tear in the meniscus, the more often a cannula technique will be used; the more posterior the tear, the more important it is for the sake of safety to use the outside-to-inside needle techniques.

If a patient has an unstable knee caused, for example, by an anterior cruciate ligament deficiency, and also a reparable meniscal lesion, we believe that generally a ligament reconstruction and meniscal repair both should be carried out at the same time. Certainly the risk of a retear is greater if no ligament stabilizing procedure is done.

TECHNIQUE (SINGLE CANNULA SYSTEM). Carry out a systematic and complete diagnostic arthroscopy. If a reparable meniscal lesion is noted after thorough probing to ensure that no additional meniscal damage is present, exsanguinate the extremity and inflate the tourniquet. It is also helpful to have a leg holder in place for stressing the knee. This will open up the compartment so that viewing the periphery of the meniscus is possible.

For repair of the medial meniscus, insert the 30-degree viewing arthroscope through the anterolateral or central portal, and view and probe the extent of the tear. If the tear is acute and within the vascular red zone of the periphery of the meniscus, minimal preparation of the rim

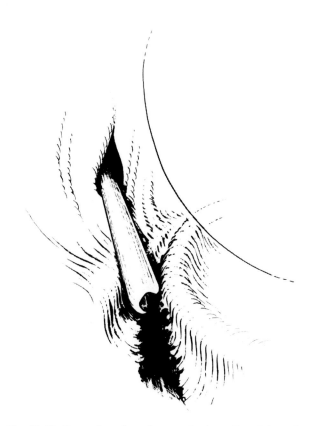

Fig. 59-40. Preparation of meniscocapsular tear of medial meniscus through accessory posteromedial portal. (From Rosenberg, T.D., et al.: Arthoscopy 2:14, 1986.)

before suturing is required. If the tear is clearly within the red vascular zone, do not resect that part peripheral to the tear. Resection of this material decompresses the meniscus from the peripheral side and has an effect similar to partial meniscectomy by narrowing the meniscus. If the tear is chronic, freshening and debridement of the torn surfaces, especially peripherally, are required. Again, limit the excision to no more than about 0.5 mm of meniscal tissue if possible. This debridement and preparation of the torn surfaces can be accomplished with basket forceps, the motorized shaver, curved meniscal knives, or small angled rasps introduced through the anteromedial, accessory medial, or posteromedial portals while the tear is viewed with the arthroscope through the anterolateral portal. The rasp is preferred for excoriating and abrading the surfaces (Fig. 59-40). Usually the anterior limit of the tear is readily seen with strong valgus stress and with the knee flexed 10 to 20 degrees. When the posterior peripheral limits of the tear cannot be viewed from the anterior portal, applying a small Wagner distraction device has been useful, one pin being inserted in the medial femoral epicondylar area and the other in the medial tibial metaphysis. If this mechanical distractor is used, exercise care not to distract enough to tear the tibial collateral ligament. Apply only enough distraction to view the posterior peripheral tear. Carry out further preparation by abrading and roughening the peripheral rim of the tear and the synovium superiorly and underneath the meniscus until vascular tissue is present for healing once the tear is reduced and sutured. Insert the

instruments to carry out this rim preparation alternately through the anteromedial, accessory medial, or posteromedial portals, depending on which allows the instruments to pass and work in the desired area of the tear (Fig. 59-41, *A*). Once this is completed, reduce the meniscus for suture. Any additional intraarticular procedures should be completed before the suturing begins.

The best angle for the single cannula and arthroscope depends on the location of the tear. If a straight cannula technique is employed, approach an anterior or middle third tear of the medial meniscus, or both, from the lateral portal, crossing under the arthroscope, which is in the central or anteromedial portal (Fig. 59-41, *B*). Approach posterior third tears of the medial meniscus for suturing by inserting the cannula through the anteromedial portal with the arthroscope located centrally or anterolaterally (Fig. 59-41, *C*). The cannula may be contoured so its presenting end approaches the area to be sutured more efficiently.

One may occasionally pass the curved single cannula through the anterolateral portal posterior to the ipsilateral tibial eminence. The needle enters the medial meniscus and is directed away from the popliteal structures by the curve in the cannula (Fig. 59-41, *D*). If you are repairing a peripheral tear that extends beyond the posteromedial corner of the knee posteriorly, it is best to first make a 5 to 7 cm incision over the posteromedial aspect of the knee, dissecting through the subcutaneous tissue down to the posteromedial corner of the knee. Identify the interval between the medial head of the gastrocnemius and the posterior capsule of the joint and retract the medial head of the gastrocnemius posteriorly off the posterior capsule. Place a flat, right-angled retractor in this interval, extending it laterally between the popliteal vessels and the posterior capsule. This gives the necessary protection for the vessels when the needles and suture material are passed from within the joint through the meniscus and capsule and out into the popliteal space. If the posterior limit of the peripheral tear does not extend beyond the posteromedial corner of the knee, it is not necessary to place the retractor. However, most tears that are being repaired extend sufficiently far posteriorly that this step will avoid potential disastrous complications. Keep the knee between 10 and 20 degrees of flexion as the sutures are passed through the posterior capsule. If the knee is positioned in greater flexion, the lax posterior capsule will be shortened and result in too much tension on the suture line when the knee extends. Also, the saphenous nerve is more likely to be injured when the sutures are passed with the knee flexed 45 to 90 degrees. Pass the cannula of the suturing instrumentation through the anteromedial portal, and place its tip near the posterior limit of the tear. Remove the needle cradle and have an assistant load the cradle with the first needle. Cover the end of the cannula to limit leakage of fluid. Then pass the needle through the cannula and the tear and out through the capsule. Remove the needle cradle after loosening the suture from the handle, and have the assistant then load the second needle while the cannula remains in the joint. While this is being done, move the cannula 2 to 3 mm in preparation for the second needle. Then pass this in a similar manner through the meniscal tear and out through the capsule. Obtain a firm bite of inner rim of the

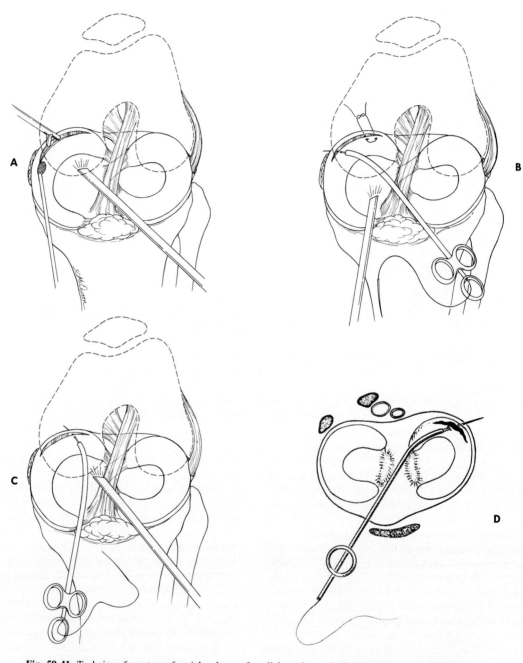

Fig. 59-41. Technique for suture of peripheral tear of medial meniscus. **A,** Peripheral tear of medial meniscus prepared with rasp or basket forceps before suturing. **B,** Suture of peripheral tear of medial meniscus using single cannula technique. Most posterior sutures are placed with cannula in ipsilateral portal. **C,** Suture of peripheral tear of medial meniscus, using single cannula technique. Anterolateral and midmedial sutures are inserted with cannula through contralateral portal. **D,** Suture of peripheral tear of medial meniscus, using single curved cannula technique. Anteromedial and midmedial sutures are inserted with cannula through contralateral portal. Cannula passed posterior to medial tibial eminence from contralateral portal. (From Rosenberg, T.D., et al.: Arthroscopy **2:**14, 1986.)

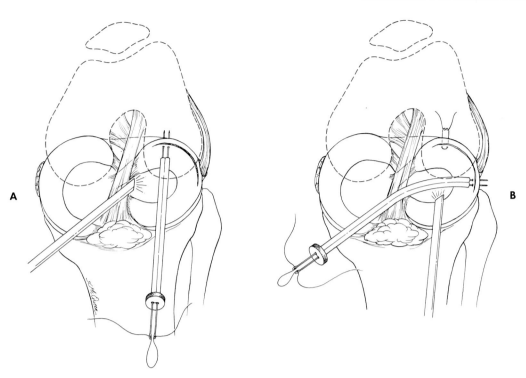

Fig. 59-42. Suture technique using double cannula system, lateral meniscus tear. **A,** Most posterior suture placements are through straight cannula; arthroscope anteromedial, cannula anterolateral. Popliteal vessels pose danger to positioning. **B,** Anterior limit of tear sutured with curved double cannula system through contralateral portal. Common peroneal nerve poses danger to positioning.

meniscus, and pass the needle through it and out through the capsule. Visibility is better if you place the second suture posteriorly rather than anteriorly with respect to the first suture. The needle may pierce the meniscus through its superior or inferior surface. Often horizontal mattress sutures are placed from both surfaces of the meniscus. If it is difficult to maintain reduction of a bucket handle tear, place the first mattress suture anteriorly to help hold the meniscus in place while subsequent sutures are passed. The number of mattress sutures required depends on the length of the tear. Usually one to four mattress sutures are required to adequately stabilize most medial meniscal tears. Generally 2-0 Vicryl suture is selected for meniscal repair, although any absorbable suture with a long tensile life would be suitable.

If the tear involves mainly the middle third of the medial meniscus and open exposure of the capsule posteriorly to protect the neurovascular elements has not been considered necessary, make an incision over the medial joint line, as you push the initial needles through the capsule and into the subcutaneous tissue. Expose the capsule parallel to the peripheral tear of the meniscus and essentially throughout its length. Exposure of this area before passing the sutures through the capsule lessens the likelihood of cutting the sutures in making the exposure. Once all sutures are passed into this medial incision, tie them over the capsule. It is important to be sure that the tear is closed and the meniscus is reduced as the sutures are tied. It is better to tie the sutures over the bridge of capsule, rather than bringing them all the way out to the skin and tying them

over buttons or bolsters, as was done in early menisco-plasty attempts. Then close the skin incision, burying the sutures. If the sutures are brought out through the skin and tied over bolsters or buttons they are not as secure technically, and their holes are potential tracts for infection of the knee.

Place the knee in a long leg cylinder cast or splint in nearly full extension. Permit the patient only touch-down weight bearing between two crutches for the first 4 weeks. Then apply a controlled motion brace, gradually allowing for increased flexion. At 6 to 8 weeks, remove all immobilization and begin a rehabilitative exercise program. The patient continues increasing weight bearing over the next 4 to 6 weeks, and is generally not unprotected in his weight bearing for 10 to 12 weeks postoperatively. No running, squatting, or vigorous stress is allowed for 6 months.

TECHNIQUE (DOUBLE CANNULA SYSTEM). A double lumen instrument cannula (Acuflex) has been developed for arthroscopic meniscal repair. These instruments consist of straight and curved double lumen cannulas through which 2.028 mm needles may be passed. A channel exists between the two lumens so that a single 2-0 Vicryl suture, passed between the two needles, may slip through the cannula. The following paragraphs outline the use of this double cannula system in repair of a posterolateral tear of the lateral meniscus.

Complete a systematic and thorough diagnostic arthroscopy. If a posterior tear of the lateral meniscus is found, carefully probe the location and extent of the tear with the

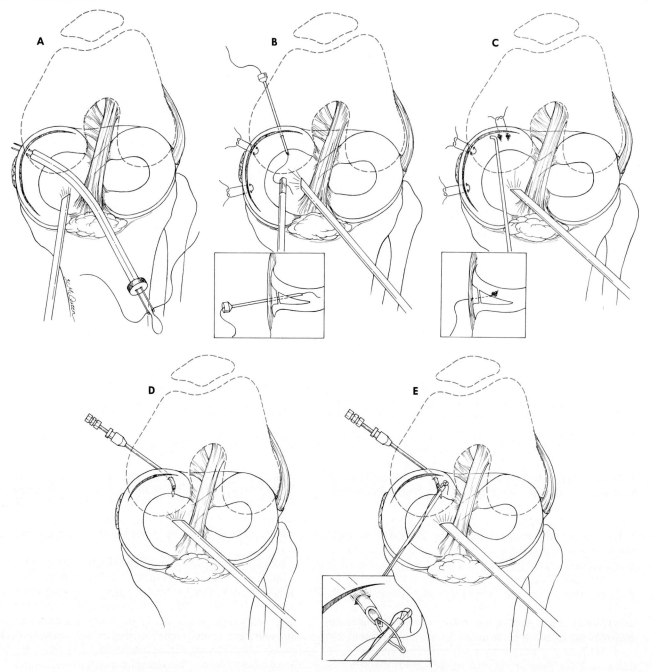

Fig. 59-43. Suture medial meniscus. **A** to **C**, Combination of cannula (inside-to-outside) and outside-to-inside needle technique. **A,** Suture placement midportion large bucket handle tear using curved double cannula technique. **B,** Outside-to-inside loaded needle technique for posterior suture. **C,** Stability of repair is probed. **D** to **H,** Outside-to-inside technique (Johnson). **D,** Curved needle shown penetrating posterior horn tear. Wire loop passes through needle and is viewed in joint. **E,** Suture passed through loop with miniature ligature holder.

30-degree viewing arthroscope in the anteromedial portal and a probe in the anterolateral portal. If the peripheral tear is determined to lie within the vascular 10% to 25% of the periphery of the meniscus and no additional tears within the body of the meniscus are found either open or arthroscopic repair may be suitable. If arthroscopic repair is elected, exsanguinate the leg and inflate the tourniquet. Then place the leg in the figure-four position, and advance the 30-degree viewing arthroscope through the anteromedial portal and into the anterolateral compartment.

Again probe the extent of the tear, and roughen and freshen the surfaces of the peripheral rim and adjacent surface of the meniscus using a basket forceps, a motorized shaver, curved meniscal blades, or a small angled rasp. These instruments are inserted through the appropriate anterolateral, accessory lateral, or posterolateral portal, as determined by which portal allows advancement of the instrument to the proper area of the tear. An alternate portal for the viewing arthroscope is the midpatellar lateral portal of Patel (p. 2553), which allows generally good views of

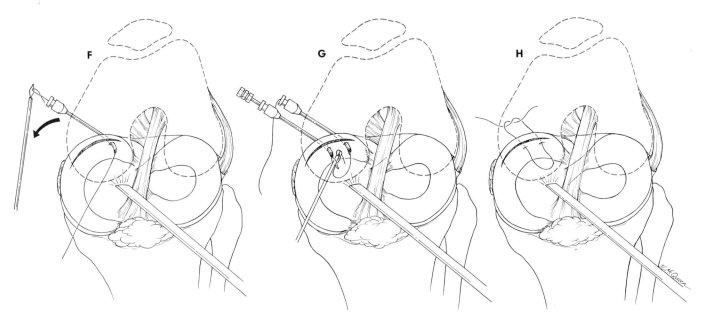

Fig. 59-43, cont'd. F, Loop pulled out of needle bringing suture to outside. **G,** Second needle penetrates meniscus tear; suture procedure repeated. **H,** Suture tied over capsule. (**D** to **H,** Redrawn from Johnson, L.: Meniscus Mender, Technique Brochure, Instrument Makar, Okemos, Mich.)

the tear. Once the peripheral rim is prepared, repair the most posterior aspect of the tear first by placing the curved cannula through the anterolateral portal. The cannula may be contoured to approach the meniscus more precisely if necessary. Then place the cannula against the meniscal body, and run the needles with the absorbable suture through the cannula, meniscal body, meniscal rim, and capsule, and out through a previously made skin incision over the posterolateral aspect of the knee (Fig. 59-42, *A*).

The safest position of the knee for suture of lateral meniscus tears is near 90 degrees of flexion. The peroneal nerve drops more inferiorly with flexion and out of harm's way. This is in contrast to the most optimal position for medial repairs, which are more safely done with the knee in 10 to 15 degrees of flexion.

If the posterior extent of the tear is near the midline, the popliteal vessels should be protected before bringing the needles through the capsule by placing a wide metallic retractor between them and the posterior capsule. Remember that the common peroneal nerve lies slightly posterior to the posterior aspect to the biceps femoris tendon. Therefore the needles must always exit anterior to the biceps tendon. It is much better, however, to make the posterior skin incision and expose the area of the posterior capsule and peroneal nerve before bringing the sutures through the posterior aspect of the capsule. Orient additional mattress sutures every 2 to 3 mm apart until the tear of the meniscus is apposed to the freshened peripheral rim. Place subsequent sutures with either the straight or the curved cannula, alternating between the anteromedial and anterolateral portals. The portal chosen depends on the area being sutured (Fig. 59-42, *B*). It may be necessary to place sutures through the meniscus beginning on its inferior and superior surfaces to secure it to the peripheral meniscosynovial attachments. Tie the multiple sutures over a small bridge of capsule, being sure that the torn surfaces

are accurately and snugly apposed as the sutures are tied.

Place the leg, with the knee extended, in a cylinder cast or splint and follow the guidelines for the postoperative care and rehabilitation given in the discussion of medial meniscus tears.

ARTHROSCOPIC REPAIR—OUTSIDE-TO-INSIDE TECHNIQUE

Morgan and Casscells and Warren have described a technique for arthroscopic meniscal repair in which a suture is introduced through a spinal needle that is inserted from outside to inside. We have used this technique and find it most appropriate and safe for tears located in the posterior aspects of either meniscus.

Common to repair of either meniscus a thorough knee examination is carried out through standard anterior portals. The longitudinal tear in the meniscus must be carefully probed to determine its extent, the stability of the meniscus, whether additional intrasubstance tears are also present, and the amount of meniscal tissue peripheral to the tear. For both acute and chronic lesions, the apposing surfaces along the tear are debrided of all fibrous tissue using a combination of basket forceps, motorized instruments, and small rasps. The surfaces are smoothed and the synovium on both the femoral and tibial sides of the meniscus in the region of the tear are abraded with the rasp to stimulate proliferative fibrovascular tissue which will be the source of healing.

TECHNIQUE FOR MEDIAL MENISCUS SUTURING (MORGAN AND CASSELLS). Carry out a systemic diagnostic arthroscopic examination, identify the meniscal tear, prepare the tear and surrounding synovial tissue for suturing, and position the knee in 10 to 15 degrees of flexion. A knee holder should be in place for applying a valgus stress on the joint to open up the medial compartment for better viewing. With the tear viewed arthroscopically, make a small 5 to 10 mm skin puncture posteromedially at the joint line, approximately 2 cm behind the readily palpable posteromedial corner of the knee. Maintain the knee in 5 to 10 degrees of flexion during the suturing procedure to avoid injury to the sartorial branch of the saphenous nerve at the posterior aspect of the medial meniscus. With the knee flexed to 90 degrees, this nerve lies at or near the joint line at the posteromedial corner. However, with the knee in extension the nerve lies anterior to the joint line by about 2.5 cm. Thread a single strand of 0-gauge absorbable suture (PDS or Vicryl) down the lumen of a standard 18-gauge spinal needle with about 5 cm of suture material protruding from the sharp end. Place this loaded needle through the previously created posteromedial puncture site and advance it through the capsule and meniscus tear from outside-to-inside with the needle directed under arthroscopic vision with the arthroscope in the standard anterolateral portal (Fig. 59-43, *B*). Once the needle and suture are seen, withdraw the needle approximately 0.5 cm, thus leaving a loop of suture which is grasped and brought out in front of the knee with a grasping instrument directed from the anteromedial portal. Tie three knots on themselves in the end of the suture. Then trim the tail of the knot flush with the knot surface. Draw the knot end of the suture back into the knee through the anteromedial portal by pulling the posteromedial puncture suture tail until the knot abuts the meniscus, always watching the progress of the suture through the arthroscope (Fig. 59-43, *C*). Apply sufficient tension on the suture to reduce and stabilize the meniscus. Repeat the process as many times as necessary to completely stabilize the medial meniscus tear. When a satisfactory number of sutures have been placed, tie them to themselves over the capsule through the posteromedial incision with the knee in full extension. Gently test the approximation of the torn edges and the stability of the repair before tying the sutures. This can be done by direct viewing, using a probe while tension is applied to the suture tails. Johnson has devised a similar outside-to-inside suturing technique, but loops of suture rather than knots reduce and stabilize the meniscus.

For large peripheral lesions on the medial side, such as a displaced peripheral bucket handle tear, a combination of inside-to-outside and outside-to-inside methods may be used. In this type of repair a single horizontal mattress suture using a cannulated technique is first placed in the midportion of the tear anterior to the posteromedial corner. This suture provides the necessary stability to the large bucket handle fragment and prevents gross displacement when the spinal needle loaded with suture material is placed through the posterior and anterior horn regions of the fragment (Fig. 59-43, *A*).

TECHNIQUE FOR LATERAL MENISCUS SUTURING (MORGAN AND CASSCELLS). The technique for suture placement on the lateral side is similar to that described for the medial side with the structure most at risk when suturing the posterior horn of the lateral meniscus being the common peroneal nerve. Keep the knee near 90 degrees of flexion when suturing the posterior horn of the lateral meniscus since in this position the nerve falls well below the joint line posterolaterally. With the knee in nearly 90 degrees of flexion or in the figure-four position, posterior and posterolateral suturing involves little risk of injury to the peroneal nerve

if the needles enter and exit the capsule superior to the palpable biceps femoris tendon.

Make a horizontal 1 to 2 cm incision through the skin and subcutaneous tissues down to the posterolateral capsule in the region of the anticipated meniscus repair. Through the arthroscope define the limits of the tear, carefully debride and prepare the meniscal surfaces for reapproximation and abrade the surrounding synovial tissue on both the femoral and tibial sides of the meniscus. The arthroscope should be in the anteromedial portal during this part of the procedure. Using an 18-gauge spinal needle loaded with a 0-gauge absorbable suture, pierce the capsule through the posterolateral incision with the point passing from outside to inside traversing the capsule and then the meniscus to be seen with the arthroscope in the anteromedial portal. Then grasp with a grasping instrument inserted through an anterolateral portal the 2.5 cm of suture protruding through the pointed end of the spinal needle in the lateral compartment and pull the suture through the compartment and out through the anterolateral portal. Then tie three knots stacked together in the end of the suture. Cut the tail of the suture flush with the knotted end and draw the suture back into the joint by gentle traction on its opposite end that passes through the posterolateral capsule and the posterolateral skin incision. By gentle traction on the suture, the knot abuts the meniscus and being larger than the needle hole reduces and stabilizes the meniscus by gentle tension. Place additional sutures in a similar manner until the full extent of the tear has been approximated and is stable. Gently examine the tear for accuracy of approximation and stability with a probe inserted through the anterolateral portal as gentle tension is maintained on the several sutures exiting the posterolateral incision. If approximation and stability have been achieved, tie the sutures to each other over appropriate bridges of posterolateral capsule. Tie the sutures with the knee in full extension. Immobilize the knee in a plaster cast or a commercial knee immobilizer with the knee in extension.

LOOSE BODIES IN KNEE JOINT

Removal of loose bodies from the knee joint is especially suitable for arthroscopic techniques. A loose body may be a singular isolated problem or multiple and represent part of a more complex pathologic process. Every attempt should be made to identify the underlying process.

Loose bodies may be classified into the following types:

1. Osteocartilaginous. These are composed of bone and cartilage and hence are detectable roentgenographically. Osteocartilaginous loose bodies may originate from several sources. The most common are osteochondritis dissecans, osteochondral fractures, osteophytes, and synovial osteochondromatosis.
2. Cartilaginous. These radiolucent loose bodies are usually traumatic and originate from the articular surfaces of the patella or the femoral or tibial condyle.
3. Fibrous. These radiolucent loose bodies are less frequent and result from hyalinized reactions originating usually from the synovium secondary to trauma or, more commonly, from chronic inflammatory conditions. Synovial villi become thickened and fibrotic,

may become pedunculated, and may detach and fall into the joint as loose bodies. Chronic inflammations, such as tuberculosis, may produce multiple fibrinous loose bodies known as "rice bodies."

4. Others. Intraarticular tumors, such as lipomas, and localized nodular synovitis may be pedunculated and by palpation feel like loose bodies or, in rare instances, drop free into the joint. Bullets, needles, and broken arthroscopic instruments may also appear as foreign loose bodies within the knee.

TECHNIQUE. Two techniques are generally chosen, based on the problem facing the surgeon. (1) Small loose bodies may be removed from the knee joint by suction and lavage of the joint. (2) Larger loose bodies are removed using triangulation techniques.

Insert the 30-degree viewing arthroscope through the anterolateral portal. Rarely is bleeding a problem in loose body removal; therefore, usually inflating the tourniquet is unnecessary. Carry out a complete systematic diagnostic arthroscopy; during this examination sequentially and systematically move through the joint to avoid missing the loose body or any others that may be present. If the loose body is large and radiopaque, you have a clue as to where to look; however, it may have moved since the roentgenogram was taken. Still, search the joint systematically for additional loose bodies, including the suprapatellar pouch, the medial and lateral gutters, the medial and lateral compartments, the intercondylar notch, and the posterior compartments.

If the loose body is in the suprapatellar pouch, it may float away from the arthroscope or grasping instrument. In addition, the slightest turbulence in the irrigation fluids, or the slightest touching with the grasper frequently will make it move away. This can be somewhat reduced by turning off the outflow of irrigating solution and inserting a small suction tip. Frequently the loose body will be drawn to the suction tip, where it may be held until a third instrument is brought into the knee to grasp it.

The loose body may also be trapped or stabilized by triangulating a spinal needle to it, piercing it with the needle, and holding it in place until a grasper is inserted, usually through a superolateral or superomedial portal (Fig. 59-44). Once within the jaws of the grasper, the loose body is slowly withdrawn to the portal entrance. If necessary the entrance may be enlarged so that the loose body can be extracted. It is better to enlarge the portal than to have the loose body slip from the grasper and become free again within the joint.

If multiple loose bodies are present, remove the smaller ones first. Removal of the largest one first, may require enlargement of the portal, and may result in significant leakage of irrigation solutions from the joint.

Once all loose bodies that can be seen are removed, suction the joint, especially the posterior compartments and the intercondylar notch. Occasionally this will pull small, previously unseen loose bodies into view. Finally, try to identify, if possible, the pathologic process producing the loose bodies, and treat it appropriately, that is, by biopsy, synovectomy, or chondroplasty.

Loose bodies that gravitate into the posterior compart-

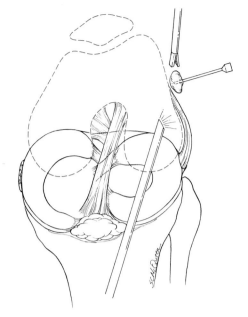

Fig. 59-44. Removal of loose body. Loose body impaled with needle and grasper inserted through superolateral portal.

ment may be seen with the viewing arthroscope by way of a posteromedial or a posterolateral portal, or by the central portal, using a 70-degree oblique viewing arthroscope. Triangulating a grasping instrument into either the posteromedial or posterolateral compartments, with the arthroscope also through a posteromedial or posterolateral portal, may be difficult due to crowding and collision of instruments. It is easier to pass the 70-degree oblique viewing arthroscope through the intercondylar notch into the appropriate posterior compartment, locate the loose body, then triangulate a grasping instrument through a posteromedial or posterolateral portal to remove it.

Loose bodies large enough to require a major incision to remove may be removed in smaller fragments by morcellation if desired. Do not use the delicate basket forceps or other arthroscopic instruments for this purpose, or severe damage to the instrument will result. It is better to use a Kerrison rongeur to break up larger loose bodies for removal.

Pedunculated "loose bodies" caused by disorders such as nodular synovitis may be removed using standard triangulation techniques after the restraining pedicle is cut with scissors.

Instrument breakage during arthroscopic procedures is not rare. Portions of such instruments may drop free into the joint. It is imperative, under these circumstances, to remain calm, turn off the irrigating solution, move the knee as little as possible, and always keep the fragment in view. Do not proceed with the intended surgical procedure until the instrument part is removed. The broken part may be stabilized using a small magnet (Dyonics Golden Retriever) inserted through an appropriate portal until it can be secured by a grasping instrument and removed.

SYNOVIAL PLICAE OF KNEE

Embryologically, the knee joint forms from three synovial compartments. Normally these fuse into a single synovial cavity with the intervening synovial partitions resolving. The important synovial plicae of the knee represent unresolved remnants of these partitions. These plicae are synovial folds, usually classified according to their anatomic relationship to the patella: suprapatellar, infrapatellar, medial patellar, and lateral patellar plicae. They vary in frequency, size, thickness, and clinical significance. Jackson et al. have suggested that the term "plica" or "shelf" be reserved to describe a normal synovial fold, and if the plica is believed to be contributing to the patient's symptomatology, it should be referred to as a "pathological plica".

The *infrapatellar plica,* or ligamentum mucosum, probably never produces symptoms but may cause difficulty in passing the arthroscope from one compartment to the other; if it is prominent, viewing of the anterior cruciate ligament can be difficult. It may vary in size from a thin band of synovium running from the back side of the fat pad into the intercondylar notch to a nearly complete synovial partition separating the medial and lateral compartments.

The *suprapatellar plica* is superior to the patella, partially dividing the suprapatellar pouch into two compartments. Rarely can it account for symptoms in the knee.

A *lateral patellar shelf* or *plica* has been described, but is exceedingly rare.

By far the most frequent of these plicae to be of clinical significance is the *medial patellar plica.* Its incidence has been reported as varying from 10% to over 50% in normal knees. The frequency of this medial patellar plicae and its possible role in the cause of anterior knee pain have been more greatly appreciated as diagnostic arthroscopy has developed.

The medial patellar plica begins just superior to the patella and sometimes continues with the distal extent of the suprapatellar plica, running distally along the medial sidewall of the joint and over the medial femoral condyle to insert onto the fat pad. This structure can account for symptoms only if it becomes thickened and inelastic from trauma or chronic inflammation. A common precipitating cause is a direct blow to the anteromedial knee region, traumatizing the plica. This results in swelling and inflammatory changes. Repetitive knee flexion and extension in such instances may result in thickening and hyalinization within the plica, leading to loss of elasticity. If this is accompanied by increased activities, the narrow, noncompliant structure could act as an abrasive band, rubbing across the medial femoral condyle instead of smoothly gliding over it. This abrasive action may with time result in chondromalacia of the medial femoral condyle. This plica, to be considered pathologic, should have a fairly thickened, rounded, fibrotic, and white inner border. Moreover, as the knee is moved from the extended position to the 90-degree flexed position, this pathologic plica should make firm contact with the underlying femoral condyle at approximately 30 to 40 degrees of flexion. Either a softened area of articular cartilage on the edge of the medial femoral condyle or a pannus of synovium growing over the edge of the condyle from the medial gutter are added clues that the plica may indeed be pathologic and responsible for the patient's symptoms, provided the examination and symptom complex are consistent.

Clinically, the patient usually describes striking the anteromedial aspect of the knee on a hard object, a fall on the anterior aspect of the knee, or some direct blow to this region. This is followed by a chronic aching discomfort in the anterior aspect of the knee, which is made worse by activities. The patient may also sense a clicking sensation during flexion and extension of the joint. Effusion is rarely noted. On examination, usually a locally tender area well above the joint line on the anteromedial aspect of the knee is found. On occasion one may, with active flexion and extension of the joint, note a popping of the plica over the medial femoral condyle, more commonly at about 30 to 40 degrees of flexion. Sometimes, this thickened fibrotic plica may be palpable along the medial border of the patella.

The initial treatment of pathologic medial plicae should be conservative. Modification of activities to reduce repetitive flexion and extension movements of the knee should be advised. The patient should avoid keeping the knee in the flexed position for prolonged periods of time, and quadriceps exercises consisting of isometric and stiff-legged exercises are advised, along with a short course of antiinflammatory medications. Occasional immobilization of the knee in the extended position for a few days will be of benefit. One should specifically avoid progressive resistive exercises of the quadriceps, since these repetitive flexion and extension movements of the knee will result in continual aggravation of the plica. Conservative measures are usually beneficial in medial plica syndromes of short duration. If the symptoms are chronic and these conservative measures have failed, then arthroscopic examination of the knee and resection of the pathologic plica may be required.

TECHNIQUE. A complete and systematic diagnostic arthroscopy is performed to rule out other intraarticular pathologic conditions. If a thickened, inelastic, rounded, and whitish plica is noted, then arthroscopic resection of the plica will probably relieve the symptoms. Viewing the medial patellar plica is usually easy from the standard anterolateral portal with the 30-degree viewing arthroscope. Further confirmation of the pathologic nature of the plica should be made through a superolateral portal with viewing of the structure from the superior aspect. If the plica is indeed found to be pathologic, it is better to resect a large portion of it rather than to simply cut it, as originally advised. With the viewing arthroscope in the anterolateral portal, insert scissors or a basket forceps through a superolateral portal, advance it to the medial sidewall, and beginning at the superior aspect of the plica, excise 1 to 2 cm of it. A saucerization of the plica down to the synovial sidewall should be the goal of treatment. Often the initial division of the plica is accompanied by a snapping apart of the structure and a wide separation of its cut ends, indicating that the plica was indeed under considerable tension. The motorized shaver or synovial resector may be inserted through the superolateral portal, and the remaining tags of synovium and plica are removed. Thoroughly lavage and suction the joint to remove any remaining debris.

OSTEOCHONDRITIS DISSECANS OF FEMORAL CONDYLES

Osteochondritis dissecans of the knee is a common disorder whose exact etiology is unknown. It is thought to result from ischemia of a localized area of subchondral bone, precipitated by infarction, trauma, or other causes. An area of subchondral bone becomes avascular, with subsequent changes occurring in the overlying articular cartilage. It must be differentiated from true osteochondral fractures and irregular ossification within the femoral condyles. While it is well established that undisplaced lesions in skeletally immature children will heal if immobilized, for osteochondritis dissecans in mature or almost mature patients, and for those who have partially or completely detached fragments, surgery may be indicated. Arthroscopic techniques are being applied increasingly to those requiring surgical treatment.

Osteochondritis dissecans of the femoral condyles has been classified roentgenographically, depending on the size and location of the lesion (Fig. 59-45, *A*). Lesions of the medial femoral condyle have been described as central, laterocentral, and inferocentral. Lesions of the lateral femoral condyle are usually inferocentral and posterior. More than standard anteroposterior and lateral roentgenograms of the knee are required to accurately assess these lesions.

Tomograms, weight-bearing lateral views (Fig. 59-45, *B*), and occasionally patellofemoral joint views are required. If the patient is skeletally immature, roentgenograms of the opposite knee are also needed. Bone age films to determine actual skeletal maturity are useful. Bone scans have been advocated, but their usefulness is not yet well defined. Classification of lesions of osteochondritis dissecans based on their arthroscopic appearance will be presented later, and are used by Guhl and others as a basis for treatment.

Lesions in skeletally immature patients are treated by immobilization for up to 3 to 4 months, the duration being determined by the age of the patient, the size of the lesion, and whether it involves a weight-bearing area. Small lesions in non-weight-bearing areas may be treated with restriction of activities, while smaller lesions in weight-bearing areas may be immobilized only for 3 to 4 weeks. Lesions of 1 cm or larger in a weight-bearing area are immobilized until some healing is noted on subsequent roentgenograms. Those destined to heal will show some signs of healing during this time. Those showing no evidence of healing are considered for either open or arthroscopic surgical treatment.

Guhl recommends arthroscopic evaluation and treatment of all patients who are 12 years or older as determined by

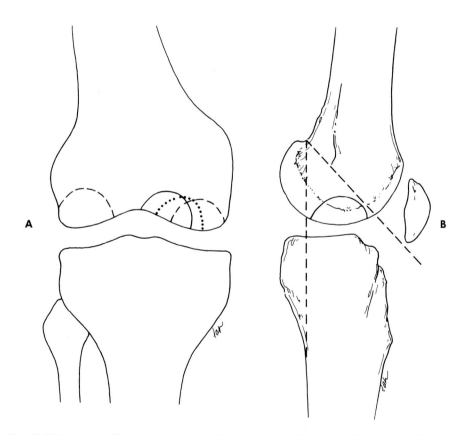

Fig. 59-45. Locations of lesions of osteochondritis dissecans. **A,** Locations of lesions of medial femoral condyle (central, centrolateral, or inferocentral) and of lateral femoral condyle (inferocentral and often posterior). **B,** Lateral view of medial femoral condyle showing common location of lesions. (From Shahriaree, H.: O'Connor's textbook of arthroscopic surgery, Philadelphia, 1984, J.B. Lippincott Co.)

bone age roentgenograms, and who have lesions larger than 1 cm in diameter located primarily in a weight-bearing area. Lesions that are massive, that is, over 3 cm in diameter, lesions having large or multiple loose bodies that are thought to be replaceable, or lesions that are inaccessible to arthroscopic techniques are best treated by open arthrotomy rather than arthroscopic techniques. Treatment of the lesion is based on the arthroscopic examination. The lesions are classified into one of the following groups: (1) intact lesions, (2) lesions showing signs of early separation, (3) partially detached lesions, and (4) craters with loose bodies (salvageable or unsalvageable).

The intact lesion presents only a minor irregularity of the articular surface, with no break in the continuity of the surface. This is determined by careful palpation and probing with the arthroscope probe. Guhl suggests treatment of these lesions by multiple holes drilled through the articular surface into the subchondral fragment and into the underlying vascular bone. Since the articular surface viewed arthroscopically may show little or no surface irregularity, the use of an image intensifier during this process may accurately locate the site for drilling. The early separated lesion presents an essentially intact smooth articular surface, but with greater irregularity than that of the intact lesion. The articular surface will show at some point a break in a small portion of the periphery of the lesion and the fragment can be noted to move significantly when probed. Guhl advocates treatment of these lesions by fixation with Kirschner wires after debridement of the break in the articular surface. The partially detached lesion presents a greater disruption in the articular surface, and with probing the lesion can be displaced or hinged on one edge. Guhl advocates gently turning back the lesion, curetting the base of the crater, debriding it of all fibrous tissue, replacing the hinged articular surface flap, and securing it with Kirschner wires. Occasionally, cancellous bone grafting in the crater base is required. When viewed arthroscopically, lesions that already have developed a loose body and a crater are treated by reconstruction of the crater, that is, by curettage and debridement to bleeding bone, and by contouring and smoothing the edges and walls of the crater. If the loose body has detached recently, as indicated by hemorrhage or a little fibrous material within the crater, and the loose body can be replaced congruously, it is secured back in the crater and held with multiple Kirschner wires. Most loose bodies, however, cannot be replaced congruously and therefore require removal and reconstruction of the crater base.

TECHNIQUE OF ARTHROSCOPIC DRILLING OF INTACT LESION OF FEMORAL CONDYLE. Carry out a complete and systematic diagnostic arthroscopy with the 30-degree viewing arthroscope in the anterolateral portal. Inspect carefully the articular surface of the medial femoral condyle. Vary the degree of flexion of the knee between 20 and 90 degrees to review the posterior extent of the lesion. The articular surfaces will appear smooth, except for a slightly raised irregularity at the borders of the lesion. Insert a probe through the anteromedial portal, and carefully probe this irregular line to be sure there is no break in the continuity of the articular surface overlying the subchondral bone lesion. If the lesion is determined to be intact perforate it with mul-

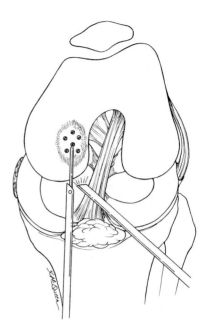

Fig. 59-46. Technique for drilling intact lesion of osteochondritis dissecans. Multiple perforations of lesion of medial femoral condyle, using Kirschner wire through anteromedial portal.

tiple holes using a .062 mm Kirschner wire. Position the Kirschner wire perpendicular to the articular surface, with the soft tissues protected by a sleeve or cannula over the Kirschner wire (Fig. 59-46). Access to drill inferocentral lesions of the medial femoral condyle is usually through the anteromedial portal; laterocentral lesions may be better approached bringing the Kirschner wire through the anterolateral portal while viewing through the anteromedial portal. Large lesions may require some drilling through both anteromedial and anterolateral portals. Penetrate the articular surface, the subchondral lesion, and the underlying bone to a depth of 1 to 1.5 cm to assure vascular access to the lesion. If the patient is not fully skeletally mature and the epiphyseal plate is open, take care not to penetrate too deeply and injure the plate. Thoroughly lavage and suction the joint, and remove the instruments.

Postoperative management consists of immobilization in a restricted motion brace, with the arc of motion controlled to prevent contact of the tibial articular surface with the lesion. Use of crutches with partial weight bearing is encouraged until early healing is noted roentgenographically. Four to six weeks of immobilization for young patients is common, whereas older patients with larger lesions continue the immobilization and avoid weight bearing until definite roentgenographic evidence of healing is noted.

TECHNIQUE OF PINNING OSTEOCHONDRITIS DISSECANS LESIONS IN MEDIAL FEMORAL CONDYLE. Early separated or partially detached lesions may be secured in their beds using Kirschner wires introduced by arthroscopic control.

After thorough diagnostic arthroscopy to rule out other pathologic conditions and removal of any loose bodies, insert the 30-degree viewing arthroscope through the anterolateral portal and a probe through the anteromedial portal. Carefully probe the area of osteochondritis dissecans in-

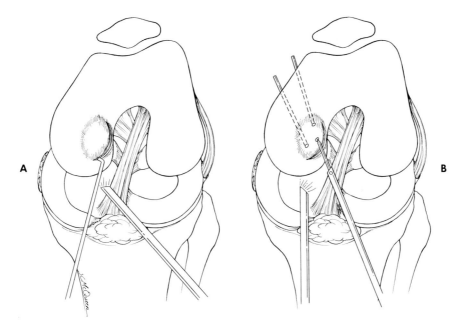

Fig. 59-47. Technique for pinning lesion of osteochondritis dissecans. **A,** Probing lesion of medial femoral condyle showing early detachment. **B,** Insertion of multiple Kirschner wires for fixation of early separated lesion of medial femoral condyle.

volving the medial femoral condyle (Fig. 59-47, *A*). If the surface is basically smooth, with only an area along the margin of the lesion fissured and loose, the disorder is classified as an early separated lesion. Pushing on the lesion with the arthroscope or probe will reveal only minor movement of the fragment where the articular surface defect is present. Carefully debride this defect in the articular surface with basket forceps or a small curet through the anteromedial portal.

Pass a .062 mm Kirschner wire through a small cannula to prevent winding up the soft tissues (Fig. 59-47, *B*). Place the tip of the cannula and the Kirschner wire through the capsule into the joint at an optimal position, so that the direction of the Kirschner wire is perpendicular to the surface of the fragment and directed superiorly and medially so that it will ultimately exit through the posteromedial aspect of the femoral condyle in the epicondylar area. To locate accessory puncture holes, insert an 18-gauge spinal needle through various locations until the proper location and direction are achieved. Make a small portal, and push the small cannula and sharp obturator through the capsule into the joint under direct view of the viewing arthroscope. Remove the sharp obturator from the sheath, and insert a .062 mm Kirschner wire through the cannula. Push the tip of the Kirschner wire into and through the articular cartilage layer by hand. When the desired position is achieved, gently tap the Kirschner wire with an instrument to seat it in the fragment. Apply a power drill to the distal end of the wire, and drill the wire out through the medial femoral condyle, exiting in the epicondylar area. When the tip of the wire is palpated under the skin in the epicondylar area, make a small skin incision over it and advance the wire. Remove the drill from the distal end of the wire and apply it to the proximal end. Then withdraw the wire retrograde

until only a few millimeters of its tip remain within the joint. Observe the lesion and the tip of the wire through the arthroscope as the wire is slowly withdrawn until its tip is flush or slightly below the articular cartilage surface. One to three wires are usually required, depending on the size of the lesion. The Kirschner wires should be slightly divergent, if possible, through the femoral condyle. Alternate the viewing arthroscope and cannula and wire portal sites to allow perpendicular insertion of the wires through the fragment as necessary. Cut off the proximal ends of the wires so they are prominent beneath the skin surface for easy location and removal 4 to 8 weeks later. Smooth .062 mm Kirschner wires are most often used. Kirschner wires with only the distal 3 cm having raised threads probably are more desirable, however.

If the osteochondritis dissecans lesion encountered is partially detached, it is usually hinged on an intact bridge of articular cartilage or on some of the fibers of the posterior cruciate ligament attachment near the intercondylar notch. Careful probing indicates that the flap can be lifted out of the bed, revealing a crater containing varying amounts of fibrous tissue. With the viewing arthroscope in the anterolateral portal, make an accessory portal for probe insertion, and insert the probe to hold the flap hinged out of its bed. With a small curet through the anteromedial portal clear the base of the crater of fibrous tissue down to bleeding cancellous bone (Fig. 59-48). Occasionally the base of the crater will be so sclerotic that it must be perforated by multiple holes made with a small drill or Kirschner wire inserted through a small protective cannula through the anteromedial portal. A small burr may also be useful in freshening the base of the crater. Be careful not to break the hinge of the flap, making reduction and fitting of the fragment into the prepared bed more difficult. Once

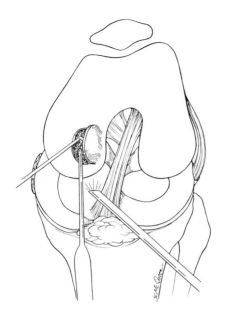

Fig. 59-48. Curettage of base of partially detached osteochondritis dissecans lesion of medial femoral condyle.

the base of the crater is clear, hinge the fragment back into place, and if there is no significant step-off between the junction of the fragment and the intact articular surface, insert one to three .062 mm Kirschner wires, similar to the treatment described for pinning early separated lesions (see Fig. 59-47, *B*). Minor debridement and smoothing of the edges where they fit together complete the fixation.

If there are multiple hinged fragments, that is, two or three, reducing these and placing Kirschner wires through each are the objectives. The more fragmented the flap, the more difficult are accurate reduction and fixation.

If a significant step-off is present once the fragment is reduced into its bed, occasionally packing cancellous bone grafts obtained from the femoral epicondylar area where the pins are to exit will correct this. Once the fragment can be reduced on top of the graft, pin it with one to three Kirschner wires. This type of defect is probably best treated by the open arthrotomy technique.

Postoperatively the patient remains in a restricted motion brace, allowing motion only through arcs that protect the osteochondritic lesion. Remove the transfixing pins after 6 to 8 weeks and allow protected weight bearing. Full weight bearing and increase in activity are forbidden until mature trabeculation is noted across the defect.

Osteochondritic loose bodies

Osteochondritis dissecans with loose bodies that are already completely detached and floating free within the joint usually is not suitable for reduction of the fragment and fixation or bone grafting. Only when one encounters a recently detached loose body with a fresh crater base are replacement and fixation possible. More often the loose body or bodies become rounded off and cannot be made to fit congruously back within the crater by either open or closed methods. In these incidences the loose bodies should be extracted from the joint, the base of the crater cleared of fibrous debris, the underlying eburnated and sclerotic bone perforated with multiple drill holes or abraded to bleeding cancellous bone, and the edges and walls of the crater contoured and smoothed without removing additional healthy articular cartilage.

In such instances the patient postoperatively is permitted immediate motion and weight bearing. Prolonged protection in these circumstances does not seem to improve coverage of the base of the crater with fibrocartilagenous tissue.

Bone grafting

Cancellous bone grafts may be packed into the base of the crater in partially detached lesions before reduction and fixation to obliterate step-off (as described previously) or they may be inserted down a channel through the medial femoral condyle behind the early separated or partially detached types of lesions. The latter technique may be useful in large deep radiolucent lesions in adults. A channel through the femoral condyle, of course, should not be created if the epiphyseal plate is open.

Arthroscopically, treat the articular surface as previously described. If the lesion is classified as an early separated lesion, insert a .062 mm Kirschner wire from the articular surface through the avascular fragment, through the femoral condyle, and out through the epicondylar area (Fig. 59-49, *A*). Make a small skin incision over the tip of the Kirschner wire, and insert a 4 to 5 mm cannulated reamer over the Kirschner wire. Carefully ream a channel toward the articular surface, taking great care not to penetrate the surface (Fig. 59-49, *B*). The use of an image intensifier aids in determining the proper depth of the channel. The objective is to penetrate with the channel the sclerotic bone opposite the subchondral avascular fragment. In early separated lesions, additional Kirschner wires to secure the fragment to the medial femoral condyle are inserted under arthroscopic control. Pack the cancellous bone grafts removed from the medial femoral epicondylar area down the previously reamed channel, so that fresh cancellous bone chips are immediately behind the avascular osteochondritic lesion. Secure the fragment with one to three Kirschner wires (Fig. 59-49, *C*).

In partially detached lesions thoroughly debride and drill the base of the crater. With the partially detached flap hinged out of the way, drill a .062 mm Kirschner wire from the articular surface at the base of the crater out through the medial femoral condyle. Insert a 4 to 5 mm cannulated reamer over the Kirschner wire, and ream a channel along the previously placed Kirschner wire to the base of the crater. Once this channel has been completed, remove the Kirschner wire. Reduce the partially detached flap and secure it in place with one to three Kirschner wires inserted from the articular surface into the femoral condyle as previously described. Pack the cancellous bone grafts taken from the medial epicondylar area down the reamed channel behind the osteochondritic defect. Take care to prevent the graft material from being forced through the articular surface or packed too tightly.

Rehabilitation after these bone grafting procedures is

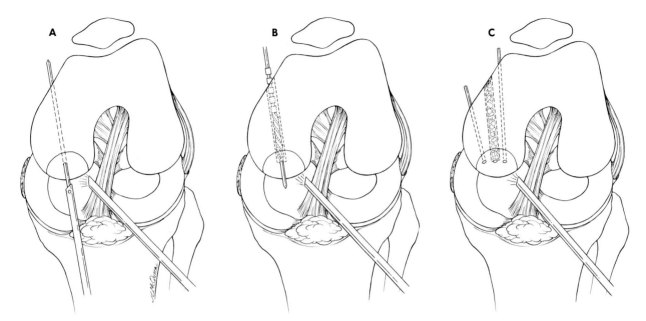

Fig. 59-49. Bone grafting of osteochondritis dissecans. **A,** Placement of Kirschner wire through center of lesion to be internally fixed and bone grafted. **B,** Cannulated reamer over wire creates tunnel through femoral condyle to point immediately behind osteochondritis dissecans fragment. **C,** Bone grafts packed down tunnel to defect. Fixation of fragment with multiple Kirschner wires.

similar to that described for internally fixed, partially detached lesions.

CHONDROMALACIA OF PATELLA SYNDROME

Release of the lateral retinacular or capsular structures has become a popular procedure for the syndrome of chondromalacia of the patella. Chondromalacia simply means softening, subsequent fibrillation, and degeneration of the articular cartilage. It, therefore, has multiple etiologies. Lateral releasing procedures should not be applied to every disorder producing anterior knee pain but should be reserved for those in which a definite clinical, roentgenographic, or arthroscopic abnormality of the tracking or dynamics of the patella is definable. Disorders for which it may be useful include lateral subluxation and dislocation, the lateral tracking abnormality where the patella cannot be proven to subluxate but is laterally riding and tilted on patellofemoral roentgenograms, and the lateral compression syndrome described by Ficat and Hungerford. Routine lateral retinacular release for undefined disorders of the anterior region of the knee should be discouraged.

The procedure may be done as a truly arthroscopic intraarticular procedure or, as is more commonly performed, by a percutaneous method. In the former method the synovium, capsule, and retinacular structures from near the tibial plateau along the lateral side of the patella and proximally into the muscular fibers of the vastus lateralis are cut with arthroscopic knives or by electocautery techniques. If the electrocautery method is used, the electrolyte irrigating solution must be removed from the joint and sterile water is used to distend and lavage the joint. The use of the cautery may allow cauterization of the cut ends of the superolateral geniculate vessels.

TECHNIQUE. View the patellofemoral joint with a 30-degree viewing arthroscope from the inferior or superior portal; either is adequate. With the arthroscope in the standard anterolateral portal and advanced into the patellofemoral joint the lens can be rotated upward and downward alternately to view the articular surfaces of the patella and the trochlear groove of the distal femur. Manual manipulation of the patella with the thumb and index finger usually allows complete viewing of the entire surface of the patella. The tracking of the patella and the dynamics of the patella and the patellofemoral joint can be viewed better from a superior portal. The patella, naturally, rides laterally with the knee in extension, and observation of it in this position does not confirm that the patella is subluxable or riding laterally. As the knee is carried from full extension into 30 to 40 degrees of flexion, the patella enters the trochlear groove and should become congruous and centered at this degree of flexion. Persistent lateral tilt or overhang of the lateral facet over the edge of the lateral femoral condyle with knee in this position suggests a lateral tracking phenomenon. Note the various degrees of chondromalacia of the patellar and trochlear articular surfaces and record them. Before performing the lateral retinacular release, carry out a complete and systematic examination of the knee for other pathologic entities and trim and shave severe patellar articular surface chondromalacic changes where appropriate. Extensive shaving of chondromalacic areas on the patellar or trochlear surface probably has only short-term effects; shaving should be kept to a minimum, emphasizing removal of only degenerative fibrillated material. The most significant objective is restoration of the proper dynamics of the extensor mechanism.

Once complete arthroscopic examination has been carried out and any chrondoplastic shaving finished, remove the arthroscopic instruments from the joint and evacuate

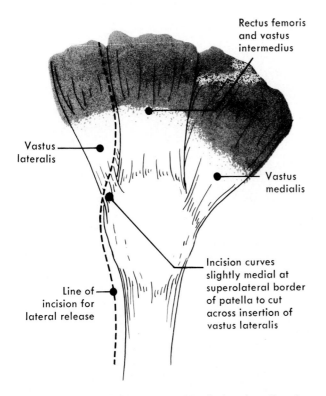

Rectus femoris
and vastus
intermedius

Vastus
lateralis

Vastus
medialis

Incision curves
slightly medial at
superolateral border
of patella to cut
across insertion of
vastus lateralis

Line of
incision for
lateral release

Fig. 59-50. Diagram of line of deep incision for lateral patellar release of right knee. (From Metcalf, R.W.: Operative arthroscopy of the knee. In American Academy of Orthopaedic Surgeons: Instructional course lectures, St. Louis, 1981, The C.V. Mosby Co.)

the irrigating fluids. Through a 1 cm incision at the lateral border of the patella, undermine the skin and subcutaneous tissue along the entire lateral border of the patella, along the lateral retinacular area, distally along the lateral border of the patellar tendon, and proximally along the insertion of the vastus lateralis muscle into the superolateral pole of the patella (Fig. 59-50). With a No. 15 Bard Parker blade make an incision at the lateral border of the patella through the retinacular, capsular, and synovial structures into the joint. Once the joint is identified, insert one tine of a curved Mayo scissors into this retinacular and capsular defect and push the scissors superiorly along the lateral edge of the patella and across the tendinous insertion of the vastus lateralis into the superolateral border of the patella. Repeat this maneuver distally along the lateral border of the patella and the patellar tendon to the level of the lateral tibial plateau. It is critical that the proximal release be carried well into the muscular fibers of the vastus lateralis or sufficient release will not have been accomplished.

Once these structures have been released proximally and distally, remove the scissors, and with the knee in full extension, grasp the patella between thumb and index finger and tilt it 90 degrees to the plane of the trochlear surface. If you are unable to tilt the patella, carefully inspect the release and carry it further if necessary. Place a thick sponge rubber pad over the superolateral aspect of the distal thigh just proximal to the patellar tendon to serve as a pressure pad over the cut superolateral geniculate vessels. This has reduced the incidence of troublesome hemarthrosis after release.

Postoperatively maintain the knee in an immobile extended position for 72 hours, then begin gentle range of motion exercises. Immobilization of the knee in extension longer than 48 to 72 hours may allow the edges of the lateral retinacular release to adhere and become ineffective. Early range of motion tends to spread the release. Encourage quadriceps isometric and stiff-leg exercises. Allow weight bearing as the patient's discomfort will permit.

OTHER APPLICATIONS OF ARTHROSCOPY OF KNEE

The following are additional, less frequent applications for arthroscopy of the knee. Many are refinements of principles and techniques previously described in this chapter, and most should be attempted only by surgeons with considerable arthroscopic experience. Many of these techniques have not been sufficiently reported on to determine the long-term results and these, therefore, will not be described in detail.

Arthroscopy in fractures about knee

Arthroscopic techniques have been used to evaluate fractures of the anterior intercondylar eminence of the tibia, to reduce such fractures, and once reduced, to fix the eminence by percutaneously inserted Kirschner wires. In addition, arthroscopy has been advocated to assess the degree of articular surface depression and the adequacy of reduction following tibial plateau fractures.

Arthrofibrosis

Arthroscopic techniques for lysis and excision of postoperative adhesions and adhesions in arthrofibrosis have been reported. Advocates of arthroscopic release of such adhesions prefer it over manual manipulation of the joint. Arthroscopic release and resection of extensive arthrofibrosis are some of the more difficult arthroscopic procedures and should probably be reserved only for the most experienced arthroscopists.

Evaluation before proximal tibial osteotomies

Conflicting reports concerning the merits of arthroscopic examination to assess the quality of the articular surfaces before proximal tibial osteotomies and the Maquet (p. 2480) procedures have been reported. Some surgeons recommend its routine use, whereas others report a series in which the condition of the articular surface in the contralateral compartment had no bearing on the eventual outcome following proximal tibial osteotomy.

Debridement of osteoarthrosis and abrasion arthroplasty

Numerous reports concern the merits of arthroscopic debridement in degenerative arthritis of the knee. Resection of mobile portions of degenerative menisci, resection of excessive synovial fronds or shaving of severe chondromalacic changes and removal of loose bodies are proved to have a place in the management of the degenerative arthritis of the knee. Recently Johnson has advocated the use of abrasion arthroplasty on articular surfaces where areas of the articular cartilage have deteriorated down to subchondral bone. Johnson's early experience suggests that abrading the eburnated subchondral bony surface sufficiently to permit capillary or petechial bleeding through the joint surface allows vascular access and hence covering of that surface with a fibrocartilage. Long-term results of this method have not yet been presented.

Synovectomy

Closed synovectomy is possible using arthroscopic techniques, but again this is one of the more difficult arthroscopic surgical exercises and should be reserved for experienced arthroscopic surgeons. Synovectomy in rheumatoid disease and other chronic inflammatory conditions and in hemophilia has been reported to produce less morbidity, shorter hospitalization, and more rapid return of function to the joint.

Drainage and debridement in pyarthrosis

Arthroscopic lysis of adhesions and decompression of compartmentalized inflamed areas in the infected knee are most effective. Fibrinoid material, infected debris, and purulent material may be removed and the joint thoroughly lavaged.

Arthroscopy of Ankle

While the techniques of diagnostic and operative arthroscopy of the knee are well accepted, arthroscopy of the ankle is less well established. The ankle is a much smaller and tighter joint than the knee or the shoulder; therefore arthroscopic examination is more difficult, and the available surgical procedures are more limited. Nevertheless, for the orthopaedic surgeon willing to patiently master the technique, excellent viewing of the joint can be achieved, and some articular surface and synovial surgical procedures can be carried out with minimal morbidity to the patient. Distraction of the joint by means of a fixed distraction device via pins in the os calcis and lower tibia facilitates viewing.

INDICATIONS

Ankle arthroscopy has been reported to be useful in several conditions, including (1) osteochondritis dissecans, (2) loose bodies, (3) chondromalacia, (4) rheumatologic disorders, (5) pyarthrosis, and (6) posttraumatic conditions.

Osteochondritis dissecans

Chronic ankle pain and disability secondary to osteochondritis dissecans of the talus may be appropriately evaluated arthroscopically. If a loose body develops secondary to an osteochondritic lesion, surgical treatment is generally accepted as appropriate. Osteochondritic fragments that have become separated may be retrieved with minimal morbidity to the patient by arthroscopic means. The stability and viability of the articular cartilage overlying nondisplaced osteochondritis dissecans may be appraised by arthroscopic examination and careful probing. Such examination may determine whether the lesion is stable and can be treated conservatively or whether its removal may be necessary.

Loose bodies

Chondral or osteochondral loose bodies noted by either roentgenographic or arthroscopic examination may be removed arthroscopically. Etiologic factors include posttrau-

matic synovial disorders and a variety of rheumatologic conditions. Parisien recommends arthroscopic examination of the unstable ankle before any ligamentous reconstruction to rule out intraarticular loose bodies and to assess the status of the articular surfaces. We have had no arthroscopic experience in this situation.

Chondromalacia

The articular surfaces of the talus and tibia may undergo chondromalacic changes similar to those in other joints. These areas can be evaluated, probed, and shaved using arthroscopic triangulation techniques, but rarely does the shaving of such areas significantly affect the long-term status of the joint.

Rheumatologic disorders

Arthroscopic examination for assessing the presence of intraarticular erosions and for selected biopsy of the synovial lining has been reported worthwhile before synovectomy of the ankle in rheumatoid arthritis. This permits more precise planning for the procedure. We have not used the arthroscope for this purpose.

Pyarthrosis

Arthroscopic irrigation and debridement of septic disorders of the ankle joint have been reported to have clinical usefulness, breaking up adhesions and partitions of infected materials. Again we have no experience with this indication.

Posttraumatic conditions

Diagnostic arthroscopy may be useful in unexplained pain in the ankle joint in young athletes with normal roentgenograms following failure of the usual conservative treatment. Articular surface defects, chondral fractures not apparent roentgenographically, and the "meniscoid" lesion have been reportedly noted arthroscopically. Diagnostic arthroscopy may be useful in evaluating chronic intraarticular symptoms. Intraarticular surgical procedures such as debridement of pathologic articular surfaces, drilling of exposed subchondral bony defects, and removal of loose bodies may be appropriate and useful in some instances.

TECHNIQUE. Unless it is contraindicated, we prefer to perform diagnostic or operative ankle arthroscopy procedures with the patient under general or spinal anesthesia. The potential difficulty in viewing the structures and the relative infrequency of ankle arthroscopy compared with arthroscopy of the knee dictate that a local anesthetic not be the anesthetic of choice in the average orthopaedists' hands. Place a tourniquet about the thigh but do not inflate it unless it is required. No leg-holding device is needed. View the anterior and posterior portions of the ankle joint from the anterior and posterior portals, respectively. As with arthroscopic examination of other joints, carefully delineate the bony landmarks before beginning the procedure. Precise placement of the arthroscopic portals means the difference between successful viewing and a frustrating, unsuccessful procedure. For anterior approaches, mark the tendons of the tibialis anterior, extensor hallucis longus, and extensor digitorum comminus muscles and the dorsalis pedis artery with a marking pencil.

Three anterior portals have been described (Fig. 59-51,

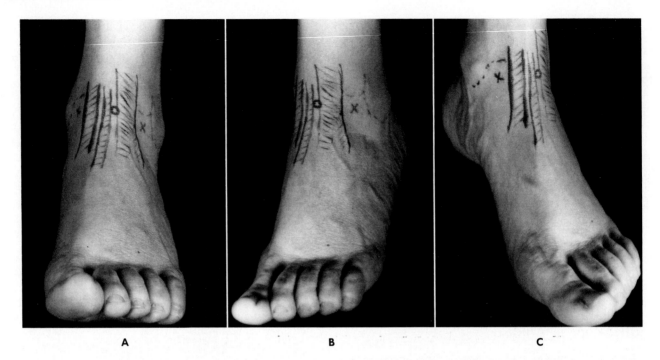

A   B   C

Fig. 59-51. A, Three anterior portals for ankle arthroscopy are marked in relation to tibialis anterior and other extensor tendons where they cross anterior aspect of ankle. **B,** Anterior central and anterolateral portal sites. **C,** Anteromedial portal site.

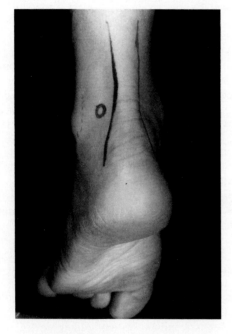

Fig. 59-52. Posterolateral portal site.

A). The anterolateral portal site is located lateral to the peroneus tertius tendon (Fig. 59-51, *B*). The anterocentral portal site is lateral to the extensor hallucis longus tendon and medial to the extensor digitorum comminus tendon and dorsalis pedis artery (Fig. 59-51, *A*). The third anterior portal, the anteromedial, is medial to the tibialis anterior tendon (Fig. 59-51, *C*).

Posteriorly place marks along the medial and lateral borders of the tendo calcaneus, over the peroneal tendons, and over the posterior tibial artery. The two useful posterior portals are the posterolateral (Fig. 59-52), located between the tendo calcaneus and peroneal tendons, and the posteromedial, located between the tendo calcaneus and the posterior tibial artery. Rarely is this posteromedial portal used because of its proximity to the neurovascular structures. Most often the arthroscopic portal to best view the suspected pathologic condition within the joint is the portal in the same area as the pathology. While all five of these portal sites may be required to evaluate the ankle, more commonly only the anteromedial, anterolateral, and posterolateral portals are necessary to perform a comprehensive arthroscopic examination of most joints.

Position yourself at the foot of the table while the assistant is positioned on the lateral side of the extremity to be examined. Use a suspended overhead irrigation system, as with arthroscopy of other joints, or a bolus syringe connected to the arthroscope sheath to intermittently distend and irrigate the joint. Because of the small volume of the ankle joint, the latter method often provides adequate irrigation and distention for most diagnostic and surgical procedures. A small-caliber arthroscope (2.2 to 4.0 mm,) is required, preferably with an angled lens. Several commercially available devices can distract the joint for better visualization.

Distend the ankle joint with 10 or 15 ml of irrigating solution using a large-gauge needle inserted from an anteromedial or anterolateral position. When the syringe is removed from the needle, a rush of irrigating solution from the needle confirms pressure distention of the joint. This needle may be connected to an outflow tubing. Attempt to judge where the most important finding within the joint might be and place the arthroscope and outflow needle accordingly. Localize the various parts of the joint by careful palpation during dorsiflexion and plantar flexion of the ankle. Maximum distention of the joint permits a good examination, and multiple poorly localized ports make maintenance of optimal distention difficult. If an anterolateral portal is selected, make a small incision in the skin just lateral to the peroneus tertius tendon. Using a hemostat, spread the soft tissues down to the anterior capsule. Then with an arthroscope sheath and sharp trocar, penetrate the anterior capsule. Confirm penetration of the joint by the rush of irrigating solution upon removal of the trocar. Insert the arthroscope into the sheath, and maintain joint distention by fluid injection through the arthroscope sheath.

If a pathologic disorder is suspected in the anteromedial compartment, insert the arthroscope anteromedially and place the distention and outflow needle anterolaterally. On the medial side, inspect the medial tibiotalar joint, the medial talomalleolar articulation, the medial malleolus, the medial synovial wall, and the deep portions of the deltoid ligament. On the lateral side, inspect the lateral tibiotalar joint, the distal tibiofibular joint, the lateral malleolus, the lateral talomalleolar articulation, and the lateral synovial wall, and view the anterior talofibular ligament. Carry out a systematic examination regardless of the approach. Initially, inspect the dome of the talus as well as the corresponding surface of the tibial plafond. Bring varying areas of the dome of the talus into view by plantar flexing and dorsiflexing the foot. Use distraction of the joint and an angled lens arthroscope to better view the other important structures. In a loose-jointed individual and with maximal distraction, occasionally the posterior compartment may be seen through an anterior portal. If this is not possible, complete the systematic and thorough examination of the ankle joint through the posterolateral entry lateral to the tendo calcaneus. If a posterolateral portal is required, turn the patient to the prone position or flex the knee and adduct the hip, exposing the posterolateral aspect of the ankle. Positioning the patient halfway between supine and lateral decubitus positions with sandbags (or an Air Vac bag) facilitates posterolateral viewing.

While awareness of nearby neurovascular structures is essential in all arthroscopic procedures, it is especially important about the ankle. A posteromedial portal, either for arthroscopic examination or as an accessory instrument portal, is probably not warranted because of the proximity to the posterior tibial artery and tibial nerve. With the posterolateral portal, care should be taken to avoid injury to the sural nerve and to the short saphenous vein during incision and trocar insertion. With the anterior portals, precise localization of the portal is necessary to avoid injury to the deep peroneal nerve and anterior tibial artery.

INTRAARTICULAR OPERATIVE ANKLE ARTHROSCOPY

The procedures listed earlier may be suitable for intraarticular synovial biopsy, adhesion lysis, chondroplasty procedures, loose body removal, curettage of articular erosions and defects, and drilling of certain articular surface

lesions. The technique for any of these procedures involves an initial thorough and systematic diagnostic arthroscopic procedure with the previously described portals and technique used. If intraarticular pathology is identified by direct viewing but requires intraarticular arthroscopic surgical procedures, accessory probing or cutting instruments are introduced through the previously described portals under direct vision. Initially a needle is inserted through the anticipated portal site, and its passage to the proposed area of pathology is observed under direct vision through the arthroscope. Once the optimal position is assured, an accessory instrument portal is made in the appropriate site, and a grasping or cutting instrument is inserted. As with all arthroscopic viewing, probing of the lesion for further delineation and clarification is generally desired. If a synovial biopsy is needed, this is carried out under direct vision using a small pituitary rongeur. If an articular surface defect requires debridement and curettage, this is carried out using the appropriate basket forceps and small curets. If a loose body or bodies require extraction, they are first viewed and then small loose bodies are removed through a suction cannula and larger ones are removed by insertion of grasping forceps using triangulation techniques. Accessory instrument portals should be near the optimal arthroscope portals previously described to avoid injury to underlying neurovascular structures.

REFERENCES

Aicroth, P.: Osteochondritis dissecans of the knee: a clinical study, J. Bone Joint Surg. **53-B:**440, 1971.

Aicroth, P.: Osteochondral fractures and their relationship to osteochondritis dissecans of the knee, J. Bone Joint Surg. **53-B:**448, 1971.

Alm, A., Gillquist, J., and Liljedahl, S.O.: The diagnostic value of arthroscopy of the knee joint, Injury, **5:**319, 1974.

Aritomi, H., and Yamamoto, M.: A method of arthroscopic surgery: clinical evaluation of synovectomy with the electric resectoscope and removal of loose bodies in the knee joint, Orthop. Clin. North Am. **10:**565, 1979.

Arnoczky, S.P.: The blood supply of the meniscus and its role in healing and repair. In American Academy of Orthopaedic Surgeons: Symposium on sports medicine: the knee, St. Louis, 1985, The C.V. Mosby Co.

Arnoczky, S.P., and Warren, R.F.: Microvasculature of the human meniscus, Am. J. Sports Med. **10:**90, 1982.

Arnoczky, S.P., and Warren, R.F.: The microvasculature of the meniscus and its response to injury. An experimental studdy in the dog, Am. J. Sports Med. **11:**131, 1983.

Arnoczky, S.P., Warren, R.F., and Kaplan, N.: Meniscal remodeling following partial meniscectomy: an experimental study in the dog, Arthroscopy **1:**247, 1985.

Bergstrom, R., Hamberg, P., Lysholm, J., and Gillquist, J.: Comparison of open and endoscopic meniscectomy, Clin. Orthop. **184:**133, 1984.

Betz, R.R., et al.: The percutaneous lateral retinacular release, Orthopedics **5:**57, 1982.

Bots, R.A.A., and Slooff, T.J.J.H.: Arthroscopy in the evaluation of operative treatment in osteochondritis dissecans, Orthop. Clin. North Am. **10:**685, 1979.

Cabaud, H.E., Rodkey, W.G., and Fitzwater, J.E.: Medial meniscus repairs: an experimental and morphologic study, Am. J. Sports Med. **9:**129, 1981.

Cameron, M., Piliar, R., and Macnab, I.: Fixation of loose bodies in joints, Clin. Orthop. **100:**309, 1974.

Carruthers, C.C., and Kennedy, M.: Knee arthroscopy: a follow-up of patients initially not recommended for further surgery, Clin. Orthop. **147:**275, 1980.

Carson, R.W.: Arthroscopic meniscectomy, Orthop. Clin. North Am. **10:**619, 1979.

Caspari, R.B., Hutton, P.M., Whipple, T.L.: The role of arthroscopy in the management of tibial plateau fractures, Arthroscopy **1:**76, 1985.

Casscells, S.W.: Arthroscopy of the knee joint: a review of 150 cases, J. Bone Joint Surg. **53-A:**287, 1971.

Casscells, S.W.: The arthroscope in the diagnosis of disorders of the patellofemoral joint, Clin. Orthop. **144:**45, 1979.

Casscells, S.W.: The place of arthroscopy in the diagnosis and treatment of internal derangement of the knee: an analysis of 1000 cases, Clin. Orthop. **151:**135, 1980.

Casscells, S.W.: The place of 35 mm still photography in arthroscopic surgery, Arthroscopy **1:**116, 1985.

Cassidy, R.E., and Shaffer, A.J.: Repairs of peripheral meniscus tears: a preliminary report, Am. J. Sports Med. **9:**209, 1981.

Clancy, W.G., Jr.: The role of arthrography and arthroscopy in the acutely injured knee, Med. Times **109:**20, 1981.

Clancy, W.G., Jr., and Graf, B.K.: Arthroscopic meniscal repair, Orthopedics **6:**1125, 1983.

Cox, J.S., Nye, C.E., Schaefer, W.W., and Woodstein, I.J.: The degenerative effects of partial and total resection of the medial meniscus in dogs' knees, Clin. Orthop. **109:**178, 1975.

Crabtree, S.D., Bedford, A.F., and Edgar, M.A.: The value of arthrography and arthroscopy in association with a sports injuries clinic: a prospective and comparative study of 182 patients, Injury **13:**220, 1981.

Curran, W.P., Jr., and Woodward, E.P.: Arthroscopy: its role in diagnosis and treatment of athletic knee injuries, Am. J. Sports Med. **8:**415, 1980.

Dandy, D.J.: Arthroscopic surgery of the knee, Br. J. Hos. Med. **17:**360, 1982.

Dandy, D.J.: The bucket handle meniscal tear: a technique detaching the posterior segment first, Orthop. Clin. North Am. **13:**369, 1982.

Dandy, D.J., Flanagan, J.P., and Steenmeyer, V.: Arthroscopy and the management of the ruptured anterior cruciate ligament. Clin. Orthop. **167:**43, 1982.

Dandy, D.J., and Jackson, R.W.: The impact of arthroscopy on the management of disorders of the knee, J. Bone Joint Surg. **57-B:**346, 1975.

Dandy, D.J., and O'Carroll, P.F.: Arthroscopic surgery of the knee, Br. Med. J. (Clin. Res.) **285:**1256, 1982.

Dandy, D.J., and O'Carroll, P.F.: The removal of loose bodies from the knee under arthroscopic control, J. Bone Joint Surg. **64-B:**473, 1982.

Daniel, D., Daniels, E., and Aronson, D.: The diagnosis of meniscus pathology, Clin. Orthop. **163:**218, 1982.

DeHaven, K.E.: Diagnosis of acute knee injuries with hemarthrosis, Am. J. Sports Med. **8:**9, 1980.

DeHaven, K.: Meniscus repair: open versus arthroscopic, Arthroscopy **1:**173, 1985.

DeHaven, K.E., and Collins, H.R.: Diagnosis of internal derangements of the knee: the role of arthroscopy, J. Bone Joint Surg. **57-A:**802, 1975.

DeLee, J.C.: Complications of arthroscopy and arthroscopic surgery: results of a national survey, Arthroscopy **1:**214, 1985.

DiNubile, N.A., and Joyce, J.J., III: Arthroscopy of the postmeniscectomy knee, Orthopedics **6:**1301, 1983.

DiStefano, V.J., and Bizzle, P.: A technique of arthroscopic meniscoplasty, Orthopedics **6:**1135, 1983.

Dorfmann, H., Orengo, P., and Amarenco, G.: Pathology of the synovial folds of the knee: value of arthroscopy, Rev. Rhum. Mal. Osteoartic. **49:**67, 1982.

Drez, D., Guhl, J.F., and Gollehon, D.L.: Ankle arthroscopy, technique and indications, Clin. Sports Med. **1:**35, 1982.

Eriksson, E., and Sebik, A.: A comparison between the transpatellar tendon and the lateral approach to the knee joint during arthroscopy: a cadaver study, Am. J. Sports Med. **8:**103, 1980.

Eriksson, E., and Sebik, A.: Arthroscopy and arthroscopic surgery in a gas versus a fluid medium, Orthop. Clin. North Am. **13:**293, 1982.

Ferkel, R.D., et al.: Arthroscopic partial medial meniscectomy: analysis of unsatisfactory results, Arthroscopy **1:**44, 1985.

Ficat, R.P., and Hungerford, D.S.: Disorders of the patellofemoral joint, Baltimore, 1977, The Williams & Wilkins Co.

Fox, J.M., Sherman, O.H., and Markolf, K.: Arthroscopic anterior cruciate ligament repair: preliminary results and instrumented testing for anterior instability, Arthroscopy **1:**175, 1985.

Fujisawa, Y., Masuhara, K., and Shiomi, S.: The effect of high tibial osteotomy on osteoarthritis of the knee: an arthroscopic study of 54 knee joints, Orthop. Clin. North Am. **10:**585, 1979.

Gillies, H., and Seligson, D.: Precision in the diagnosis of meniscal lesions: a comparison of clinical evaluation, arthrography, and arthroscopy, J. Bone Joint Surg. **61-A:**343, 1979.

Gillquist, J., and Boeryd, B.: Endoscopic total one-piece medial meniscectomy: its effect on the medial collateral ligament, Acta Orthop. Scand, **53:**619, 1982.

Gillquist, J., and Hagberg, G.: A new modification of the technique of arthroscopy of the knee joint, Acta Chir. Scand. **142:**123, 1976.

Gillquist, J., and Hagberg, G.: Findings at arthroscopy and arthrography in knee injuries, Acta Orthop. Scand. **49:**398, 1978.

Gillquist, J., Hagberg, G., and Oretorp, N.: Arthroscopic examination of the posteromedial compartment of the knee joint, Int. Orthop. **3:**13, 1979.

Gillquist, J., Hagberg, G., and Oretorp, N.: Arthroscopic visualization of the posteromedial compartment of the knee joint, Orthop. Clin. North Am. **10:**545, 1979.

Gillquist, J., Hagberg, G., and Oretorp, N.: Arthroscopy in acute injuries of the knee joint, Acta Orthop. Scand. **48:**190, 1977.

Gillquist, J., and Karpf, P.M.: Arthroscopic knee surgery, Fortschr. Med. 21 **100:**51, 1982.

Gillquist, J., and Oretorp, N.: Different techniques for diagnostic arthroscopy: a randomized comparative study. Acta Orthop. Scand. **52:**353, 1981.

Gillquist, J., and Oretorp, N.: Arthroscopic partial meniscectomy: technique and long-term results, Clin. Orthop. **167:**29, 1982.

Gillquist, J., and Oretorp, N.: The technique of endoscopic total meniscectomy, Orthop. Clin. North Am. **13:**363, 1982.

Glinz, W.: Diagnostic arthroscopy and arthroscopic surgery: experiences with 500 knee arthroscopies, Helv. Chir. Acta **46:**25, 1979.

Glinz, W.: Indications for arthroscopy after injuries of the knee joint, Z. Unfallmed. Berufskr. **75:**133, 1982.

Glinz, W., Segantini, P., and K''agi, P.: Arthroscopy in acute trauma of the knee joint, Endoscopy **12:**269, 1980.

Gollehon, D.L., and Drez, D., Jr.: Ankle arthroscopy: approaches and technique, Orthopedics **6:**1150, 1983.

Grana, W.A., Connor, S., and Hollingsworth, S.: Partial arthroscopic meniscectomy: a preliminary report. Clin. Orthop. **164:**78, 1982.

Green, W.T., and Banks, H.H.: Osteochondritis dissecans in children. J. Bone Joint Surg. **35-A:**26, 1953.

Guhl, J.F.: Arthroscopic treatment of osteochondritis dissecans: preliminary report, Orthop. Clin. North Am. **10:**671, 1979.

Guhl, J.F.: Arthroscopic treatment of osteochondritis dissecans, Clin. Orthop. **167:**65, 1982.

Guhl, J.F.: Excision of flap tears, Orthop. Clin. North Am. **13:**387, 1982.

Guhl, J.F.: Operative arthroscopy, Am. J. Sports Med. **7:**328, 1979.

Guten, G.: Methylene blue staining of the articular cartilage during arthroscopy, Orthop. Rev. **6:**60, 1977.

Hamberg, P., Gillquist, J., and Lysholm, J.: Suture of new and old peripheral meniscus tears, J. Bone Joint Surg. **65-A:**193, 1983.

Hamberg, P., Gillquist, J., and Lysholm, J.: A comparison between arthroscopic meniscectomy and modified open meniscectomy: a prospective randomised study with emphasis on postoperative rehabilitation, J. Bone Joint Surg. **66-B:**189, 1984.

Hamberg, P., Gillquist, J., Lysholm, J., and Oberg, B.: The effect of diagnostic and operative arthroscopy and open meniscectomy on muscle strength in the thigh, Am. J. Sports Med. **11:**289, 1983.

Harty, M., and Joyce, J.J., III: Synovial folds in the knee joint, Orthop. Rev. **10:**91, 1977.

Heller, A.J., and Vogler, H.W.: Ankle joint arthroscopy, J. Foot Surg. **21:**23, 1982.

Henning, C.E.: Arthroscopic repair of meniscus tears, Orthopedics **6:**1130, 1983.

Hershman, E.B., and Nisonson, B.: Arthroscopic meniscectomy: a follow-up report, Am. J. Sports Med. **11:**253, 1983.

Highgenboten, C.L.: Arthroscopy synovectomy, Orthop. Clin. North Am. **13:**399, 1982.

Highgenboten, C.L.: Arthroscopic synovectomy, Arthroscopy **1:**190, 1985.

Hotchkiss, R.N., Tew, W.P., and Hungerford, D.S.: Cartilaginous debris in the injured human knee: correlation with arthroscopic findings, Clin. Orthop. **168:**133, 1982.

Hughston, J.C., Stone, M., and Andrews, J.R.: The suprapatellar plica: its role in internal derangement of the knee, J. Bone Joint Surg. **55-A:**1318, 1973.

Hughston, J.C., Whatley, G.S., Dodelin, R.A., and Stone, M.M.: The role of the suprapatellar plica in internal derangement of the knee, Am. J. Orthop. 5:24, 1963.

Iino, S.: Normal arthroscopic findings of the knee joint in adults, J. Jpn. Orthop. Assoc. 14:467, 1939.

Ikeuchi, H.: Meniscus surgery using the Watanabe arthroscope, Orthop. Clin. North Am. 10:629, 1979.

Ikeuchi, H.: Trial and error in the development of instruments for endoscopic knee surgery, Orthop. Clin. North Am. 13:255, 1982.

Ikeuchi, H.: Arthroscopic treatment of the discoid lateral meniscus: technique and long-term results, Clin. Orthop. 167:19, 1982.

Ireland, J., Trickey, E.L., and Stoker, D.J.: Arthroscopy and arthrography of the knee: a critical reivew, J. Bone Joint Surg. 62-B:3, 1980.

Ivey, F.M., Jr.: Evaluating acute knee injuries, Am. Fam. Physician 25:122, 1982.

Ivey, F.M., Blazina, M.E., Fox, J.M., and Del Pizzo, W.: Arthroscopy of the knee under general anesthesia: an aid to the determination of ligamentous instability, Am. J. Sports Med. 8:235, 1980.

Jackson, R.W.: The role of arthroscopy in the management of the arthritic knee, Clin. Orthop. 101:28, 1974.

Jackson, R.W.: Current concepts review: arthroscopic surgery, J. Bone Joint Surg. 65-A:416, 1983.

Jackson, R.W.: The septic knee, arthroscopic treatment, Arthroscopy 1:194, 1985.

Jackson, R.W., and Abe, I.: The role of arthroscopy in the management of disorders of the knee: an analysis of 200 consecutive examinations, J. Bone Joint Surg. 54-B:310, 1972.

Jackson, R.W., and Dandy, D.J.: Arthroscopy of the knee, New York, 1976, Grune & Stratton, Inc.

Jackson, R.W., and DeHaven, K.E.: Arthroscopy of the knee, Clin. Orthop. 107:87, 1975.

Jackson, R.W., Marshall, D.J., and Fujisawa, Y.: The pathological medial shelf, Orthop. Clin. North Am. 13:307, 1982.

Jackson, R.W., and Rouse, D.W.: The results of partial arthroscopic meniscectomy in patients over 40 years of age, J. Bone Joint Surg. 64-B:481, 1982.

Jennings, J.E.: Arthroscopic management of tibial plateau fractures, Arthroscopy 1:160, 1985.

Johnson, L.L.: Comprehensive arthroscopic examination of the knee, St. Louis, 1977, The C.V. Mosby Co.

Johnson, L.L.: Diagnostic and surgical arthroscopy: the knee and other joints, ed. 2, St. Louis, 1981, The C.V. Mosby Co.

Johnson, L.L.: Surgical arthroscopy: principles and practice, ed. 3, St. Louis, 1986, The C.V. Mosby Co.

Johnson, L.L.: Creating the proper environment for arthroscopic surgery, Orthop. Clin. North Am. 13:283, 1982.

Johnson, L.L.: Impact of diagnostic arthroscopy in the clinical judgement of an experienced arthroscopist, Clin. Orthop. 167:75, 1982.

Johnson, L.L., et al.: Two per cent glutaraldehyde: a disinfectant in arthroscopy and arthroscopic surgery, J. Bone Joint Surg. 64-A:237, 1982.

King, D.: The healing of semilunar cartilages, J. Bone Joint Surg. 18:333, 1936.

Korn, M.W., Spitzer, R.M., and Robinson, K.E.: Correlations of arthrography with arthroscopy, Orthop. Clin. North Am. 10:535, 1979.

Koshino, T., Okamoto, R., Takamura, K., and Tsuchiya, K.: Arthroscopy in spontaneous osteonecrosis of the knee, Orthop. Clin. North Am. 10:609, 1979.

Kreft, E.: Arthroscopy: its place in the diagnosis of knee lesions, J. Bone Joint Surg. 57-B:255, 1975.

Lindenbaum, B.L.: Complications of knee joint arthroscopy, Clin. Orthop. 160:158, 1981.

Lindholm, S., and Pylkkanen, P.: Internal fixation of the fragments of osteochondritis dissecans of the knee by means of a bone pin, Acta Chir. Scand. 140:626, 1974.

Lipscomb, P.R., Jr., Lipscomb, P.R., Sr., and Bryan, R.S.: Osteochondritis dissecans of the knee with loose fragments: treatment by replacement and fixation with readily removed pins, J. Bone Joint Surg. 60-A:235, 1978.

Lysholm, J.: Arthroscopic surgery, Acta Orthop. Belg. 48:517, 1982.

Lysholm, J., and Gillquist, J.: Arthroscopic examination of the posterior cruciate ligament, J. Bone Joint Surg. 63-A:363, 1981.

Lysholm, J., and Gillquist, J.: Endoscopic meniscectomy, Int. Orthop. 51:265, 1981.

Lysholm, J., Gillquist, J., and Liljedahl, S.D.: Arthroscopy in the early diagnosis of injuries to the knee joint, Acta Orthop. Scand. 52:111, 1981.

Mariani, P.P., and Gillquist, J.: The blind spots in arthroscopic approaches, Int. Orthop. 5:257, 1982.

Marshall, S., Levas, M.G., and Harrah, A.: Simple arthroscopic partial meniscectomy associated with anterior cruciate–deficient knees, Arthroscopy 1:22, 1985.

Matsui, N., Moriya, H., and Kitahara, H.: The use of arthroscopy for follow-up in knee joint surgery, Orthop. Clin. North Am. 10:713, 1979.

McGinty, J.B.: Arthroscopic surgery in sports injuries, Orthop. Clin. North Am. 11:787, 1980.

McGinty, J.B.: Arthroscopic removal of loose bodies, Orthop. Clin. North Am. 13:313, 1982.

McGinty, J.B., and Freedman, P.A.: Arthroscopy of the knee, Clin. Orthop. 121:173, 1976.

McGinty, J., Guess, L., and Marvin, R.: Partial or total meniscectomy, J. Bone Joint Surg. 59-A:763, 1977.

McGinty, J.B., and Matza, R.A.: Arthroscopy of the knee: evaluation of an out-patient procedure under local anesthesia, J. Bone Joint Surg. 60-A:787, 1978.

McLennan, J.G.: The role of arthroscopic surgery in the treatment of fractures of the intercondylar eminence of the tibia, J. Bone Joint Surg. 64-B:477, 1982.

Metcalf, R.W.: Operative arthroscopy of the knee. In American Academy of Orthopaedic Surgeons: Instructional course lectures, vol. 30, St. Louis, 1981, The C.V. Mosby Co.

Metcalf, R.W.: An arthroscopic method for lateral release of the subluxating or dislocating patella, Clin. Orthop. 167:9, 1982.

Miller, G.K., Maylahn, D.J., and Drennan, D.B.: The treatment of idiopathic osteonecrosis of the medial femoral condyle with arthroscopic debridement, Arthroscopy 2:21, 1986.

Miller, G.K., et al.: The use of electrosurgery for arthroscopic subcutaneous lateral release, Orthopaedics 5:309, 1982.

Mital, M.A., and Karlin, L.I.: Diagnostic arthroscopy in sports injuries, Orthop. Clin. North Am. 11:771, 1980.

Morgan, C.D., and Casscells, W.: Arthroscopic meniscus repair: a safe approach to the posterior horns, Arthroscopy 2:3, 1986.

Morrissy, R.T., Eubanks, R.G., Park, J.P., and Thompson, S.B., Jr.: Arthroscopy of the knee in children, Clin. Orthop. 162:103, 1982.

Mulhollan, J.S.: Swedish arthroscopic system, Orthop. Clin. North Am. 13:349, 1982.

Muse, G.L., Grana, W.A., and Hollingsworth, S.: Arthroscopic treatment of medial shelf syndrome, Arthroscopy 1:63, 1985.

Ngo, I.U., Hamilton, W.G., Wichern, W.A., and Andree, R.A.: Local anesthesia with sedation for arthroscopic surgery of the knee, Arthroscopy 1:237, 1985.

Nole, R., Munson, N.M., and Fulkerson, J.P.: Bupivacaine and saline effects on articular cartilage, Arthroscopy 1:123, 1985.

Northmore-Ball, M.D., and Dandy, D.J.: Long-term results of arthroscopic partial meniscectomy, Clin. Orthop. 167:34, 1982.

Northmore-Ball, M.D., Dandy, D.J., and Jackson, R.W.: Arthroscopic, open partial, and total meniscectomy: a comparative study, J. Bone Joint Surg. 65-B:400, 1983.

Noyes, F.R., Bassett, R.W., Grood, E.S., and Butler, D.L.: Arthroscopy in acute traumatic hemarthrosis of the knee: incidence of anterior cruciate tears and other injuries, J. Bone Joint Surg. 62-A:687, 1980.

Noyes, F.R., and Spievack, E.S.: Extraarticular fluid dissection in tissues during arthroscopy: a report of clinical cases and a study of intraarticular and thigh pressures in cadavers, Am. J. Sports Med. 10:346, 1982.

O'Connor, R.L.: Arthroscopy in the diagnosis and treatment of acute ligament injuries of the knee, J. Bone Joint Surg. 56-A:333, 1974.

O'Connor, R.L.: Arthroscopy, Philadelphia, 1977, J.B. Lippincott Co.

O'Connor, R.L.: Arthroscopy of the knee. Surg. Annu. 9:265, 1977.

Oretorp, N.: On the diagnosis and treatment of meniscus and ligament injuries in the knee, especially on the medial side, Stockholm, 1978, A.B. Linkopings Tryckeri.

Oretorp, N., and Gillquist, J.: Transcutaneous meniscectomy under arthroscopic control, Int. Orthop. 3:19, 1979.

Parisien, J.S.: Arthroscopy of the ankle: state of the art, Contemp. Orthop. 5:21, 1982.

Parisien, J.S., and Shereff, M.J.: The role of arthroscopy in the diagnosis and treatment of disorders of the ankle, Foot Ankle 2:144, 1981.

Patel, D.: Arthroscopy of the plicae-synovial folds and their significance, Am. J. Sports Med. **6:**217, 1978.

Patel, D.: Proximal approaches to arthroscopic surgery of the knee, Am. J. Sports Med. **9:**296, 1981.

Patel, D.: Superior lateral-medial approach to arthroscopic meniscectomy, Orthop. Clin. North Am. **13:**299, 1982.

Pettrone, F.A.: Meniscectomy: arthrotomy versus arthroscopy, Am. J. Sports Med. **10:**355, 1982.

Pipkin, G.: Knee injuries: the role of the suprapatellar plica and suprapatellar bursa in simulating internal derangements, Clin. Orthop. **74:**161, 1971.

Pipkin, G.: Lesions of the suprapatellar plica, J. Bone Joint Surg. **32-A:**363, 1950.

Poehling, G.G., Bassett, F.H., and Goldner, J.L.: Arthroscopy: its role in treating non-traumatic and traumatic lesions of the knee, South. Med. J. **70:**465, 1977.

Pritsch, M., Horoshovski, H., and Farine, I.: Ankle arthroscopy, Clin. Orthop. **184:**137, 1984.

Rosenberg, T.D., and Wong, H.C.: Arthroscopic knee surgery in a free-standing outpatient surgery center, Orthop. Clin. North Am. **13:**277, 1982.

Rosenberg, T.D., et al.: Arthroscopic meniscal repair evaluated with repeat arthroscopy, Arthroscopy **2:**14, 1986.

Scapinelli, R.: Studies on the vasculature of the human knee joint, Acta Anat. **70:**305, 1968.

Schonholtz, G.J.: Arthroscopy and arthroscopic surgery, Md. State Med. J. **30:**56, 1981.

Schonholtz, G.J., and Ling, B.: Arthroscopic chondroplasty of the patella, Arthroscopy **1:**92, 1985.

Shahriaree, H.: O'Connor's textbook of arthroscopic surgery, Philadelphia, 1984, J.B. Lippincott Co.

Shneider, D.A.: Peripheral detachment of the meniscus: arthroscopic and clinical correlations, Orthop. Rev. **6:**55, 1977.

Shneider, D.: Arthroscopy and arthroscopic surgery in patellar problems, Orthop. Clin. North Am. **13:**407, 1982.

Sim, F.H.: Complications and late results of meniscectomy. In American Academy of Orthopaedic Surgeons: Symposium on the athlete's knee, surgical repair and reconstruction, St. Louis, 1980, The C.V. Mosby Co.

Smillie, I.: Treatment of osteochondritis dissecans, J. Bone Joint Surg. **39-B:**248, 1957.

Smith, M.: Arthroscopic treatment of the septic knee, Arthroscopy **2:**30, 1986.

Sprague, N.F., III: Arthroscopic debridement for degenerative knee joint disease, Clin. Orthop. **160:**118, 1981.

Sprague, N.F., III: The bucket handle meniscal tear: a technique using two incisions, Orthop. Clin. North Am. **13:**337, 1982.

Sprague, N.F., III: Operative arthroscopy, Clin. Orthop. **167:**4, 1982.

Sprague, N.F., III, O'Connor, R.L., and Fox, J.M.: Arthroscopic treatment of postoperative knee fibroarthrosis, Clin. Orthop. **166:**165, 1982.

Stone, R.G.: Peripheral detachment of the menisci of the knee: a preliminary report, Orthop. Clin. North Am. **10:**643, 1979.

Stone, R.G., and Miller, G.A.: A technique of arthroscopic suture of torn menisci, Arthroscopy **1:**226, 1985.

Tippett, J.W.: Arthroscopy and the Maquet proximal tibial osteotomy, Orthopedics **6:**1145, 1983.

Warren, R.F.: Arthroscopic meniscus repair, Arthroscopy **1:**170, 1985.

Whipple, T.L.: Posterior peripheral detachment of the lateral meniscus: pathogenesis with respect to the popliteus tendon, Contemp. Orthop. **4:**533, 1982.

Whipple, T.L., and Bassett, F.H.: Arthroscopic examination of the knee: polypuncture technique with percutaneous intraarticular manipulation, J. Bone Joint Surg. **60-A:**444, 1978.

Yerys, P.: A technique for lateral retinacular release, Arthroscopy **1:**233, 1985.

Zarins, B.: Arthroscopic surgery in a sports medicine practice, Orthop. Clin. North Am. **13:**415, 1982.

Zarins, B.: Knee arthroscopy: basic technique, Contemp. Orthop. **6:**63, 1983.

Zarins, B.: Technique of arthroscopic medial meniscectomy, Contemp. Orthop. **6:**19, 1983.

Ziv, I., and Carroll, N.C.: The role of arthroscopy in children, J. Pediatr. Orthop. **2:**243, 1982.

CHAPTER 60

Arthroscopy of shoulder and elbow

T. David Sisk

Diagnostic and surgical arthroscopy have been used less frequently in the upper extremity than in the lower. Disorders of the joints of the upper extremity are less frequent and therefore arthroscopy was rarely used in the upper extremity before 1980. With modern equipment, all joints of the upper extremity have been arthroscoped; however, only in the shoulder and elbow joints is the use of arthroscopy practical and frequently indicated. The indications and techniques for arthroscopy of these two joints are discussed in this chapter.

SHOULDER

Although arthroscopy of the shoulder was performed more than 50 years ago, little attention was paid to arthroscopy of this joint until the late 1970s. As orthopaedists gained experience and confidence with arthroscopy of the knee, confirming its importance in diagnosis and treatment, it was inevitable that the procedure would be applied to other joints as well. Continued improvements in the arthroscope and arthroscopic instrument design have aided this effort.

Painful syndromes, altered function, and signs and symptoms of instability and internal derangement are frequent in the shoulder. The causes of such dysfunctions can be difficult to prove. The underlying cause can often be established by a careful history and physical examination combined with appropriate roentgenographic evaluation of the shoulder girdle, cervical spine, and thoracic cavity; special roentgenographic studies, such as stress roentgenograms, arthrography, and arthrotomography; computed tomography with and without contrast materials; and electromyographic and nerve conduction studies when appropriate. Although arthroscopy should not become a routine diagnostic aid for minor derangements of the shoulder, if other diagnostic aids fail to establish the cause of a chronic shoulder problem, direct observation of the interior of the shoulder joint may be invaluable.

Arthroscopy of the shoulder affords an enormous opportunity to better understand the anatomy and pathophysiology of the joint. Although its use has been less firmly established than arthroscopy of the knee, several reports have confirmed its merits. Andrews et al. recently reported that arthroscopic examination of chronic painful shoulders revealed one or more abnormalities in 88% of the patients.

Indications

There are no absolute indications for arthroscopy of the shoulder. In all of the following disorders arthroscopy may prove useful to the experienced arthroscopist in diagnostic evaluation and treatment. As a general rule arthroscopy, which requires an anesthetic and a surgical incision, should be used as a last resort rather than before other common diagnostic procedures; these latter will make the diagnosis in most disorders. Thus it should be used for diagnostic problems rather than for routine complaints.

ARTHRITIDES

Arthroscopy may be useful in evaluating a variety of rheumatologic conditions. The synovium and joint surfaces can be clearly viewed, articular erosions and chondromalacic changes can be evaluated, localized osteophytes and loose bodies can be removed and the joint debrided, and selected synovial biopsies and synovectomies can be performed. Patients with arthritis may experience significant relief of symptoms from the lavage alone even if no intraarticular operative procedure is carried out.

DISLOCATIONS

Arthroscopy may be valuable in dislocations of the shoulder in the absence of roentgenographic documentation as to the direction of the dislocation. If surgical reconstruction is contemplated and physical examination, stress roentgenograms, and examination under anesthesia do not establish the direction of the instability, arthroscopy may demonstrate the location of the pathology—capsular, labral, or articular. Even today, without arthroscopy, too many recurrent posterior dislocations and subluxations are subjected to anterior capsulorraphy procedures.

SUBLUXATIONS

Painful shoulder syndromes, especially in young athletes, may be the result of undetectable instability and mild subluxations. Stress roentgenograms, arthrograms, and arthrotomograms may not establish the diagnosis accurately. Arthroscopy may demonstrate the labral or capsular separation confirming the diagnosis.

LOOSE BODIES

Once they have been clearly viewed on standard roentgenograms, loose bodies may be seen and removed arthroscopically. Loose bodies may develop in any of the rheumatologic conditions, in synovial proliferation, following instabilities, and in other disorders. Occasionally they may become impinged within the joint and require removal. Most will gravitate to the inferior pouch or axillary part of the joint. Small loose bodies may be removed by suction through the irrigation cannula; larger ones may be extracted using triangulation techniques with appropriate grasping instruments. Arthroscopic removal greatly reduces the morbidity compared with an open arthrotomy.

RUPTURE OF BICEPS TENDON

In chronic bicipital tenosynovitis involving the tendon of the long head or in chronic impingement syndromes, the tendon may rupture intraarticularly or more commonly within the bicipital groove beneath the transverse humeral ligament. Following such ruptures, the chronic symptoms may subside if the underlying cause is treated adequately. In some patients continued symptoms of persistent pain within the glenohumeral joint, catching, and popping may be caused by to the retained insertion of the tendon. If the biceps tendon ruptures within the bicipital groove, a significant segment of tendon may remain attached to the supraglenoid tubercle and become a pedunculated mass of collagen, which can produce continued joint derangement and pain. Patients whose pain persists despite adequate treatment of the primary pathology may benefit from arthroscopic removal of any retained tendon. Using arthroscopic triangulation techniques, any retained portion of the tendon may be resected using a variety of power or other cutting instruments.

TEARS AND AVULSIONS OF GLENOID LABRUM

Tears and avulsions of the fibrocartilaginous glenoid labrum are being recognized and documented as frequent causes of chronic shoulder problems. Separation of the labrum and the accompanying capsule have long been recognized as the pathogenesis of recurrent subluxations and instability syndromes (Plate 6, *A*). Increased experience with the arthroscope has shown that disorders of the labrum produce problems in addition to and apart from instability syndromes.

Longitudinal tears within the glenoid labrum may become pedunculated and be a source of impingement and loose body formation, or they may occasionally act like a meniscus derangement within the knee, producing popping, catching, and other symptoms of internal derangement. Many arthroscopists have noted a bucket-handle, meniscal-type lesion involving the glenoid labrum.

According to Andrews and associates, avulsion of the anterosuperior portion of the glenoid labrum can produce chronic anterior shoulder pain in the throwing athlete. They postulated that the strong pull of the long head of the biceps tendon on its attachment to the supraglenoid tubercle in direct continuity with the glenoid labrum results in this pathologic condition. They used arthroscopy to examine painful shoulders in throwing athletes and found tearing, fraying, and a partial avulsion of the anterosuperior labrum (Plate 6, *B*). Short-term results of arthroscopic debridement of this torn and frayed labral tissue are encouraging. Increased tearing or separation of the labrum can progress to anterior shoulder instability in such patients.

TEARS OF ROTATOR CUFF

Large rotator cuff tears can generally be diagnosed by a careful history and physical examination and can be documented by a careful arthrographic examination of the shoulder. If the rotator cuff tear is chronic, it may become sealed with synovium or other tissue, preventing gross leakage of the contrast media into the subacromial bursa. Careful arthroscopic examination of the undersurface of the superior rotator cuff may reveal areas of irregularities in its contour, tags or flaps of ruptured tendon, or local fibrosis and hemorrhage, indicating a disruption in that portion of the rotator cuff. The undersurface of the supraspinatus and infraspinatus and the posterior surface of the subscapularis can be clearly seen arthroscopically from a posterior portal. The anterior or deep surface of the teres minor can be clearly viewed from an anterior portal. The outer surface of the rotator cuff may be viewed with the scope in the subacromial bursa. Adhesions or inflammation within the bursa may make viewing difficult, however. If the tear in the rotator cuff is small, with frayed and fibrotic tissue seen on the undersurface, then arthroscopic debridement of this impinging tissue and any surrounding inflammatory reaction using the power cutter and shaver may relieve the symptoms sufficiently.

FROZEN SHOULDER

The cause and pathogenesis of the frozen shoulder syndrome have been controversial. Some arthroscopists believe that arthroscopic examination with distention and lavage of the joint followed by instillation of a steroid preparation is the treatment of choice for this difficult problem. Most accept the fact that the underlying precipitating event is an inflammatory one that produces a synovitis and subsequent fibrosis within the pericapsular tissues. Several authors, including Wiley and Older, have reported that few intraarticular adhesions are actually noted during arthroscopic examination in the frozen shoulder syndrome. Restriction of either active or passive motion, or both, and the inability to instill a significant volume of fluid into the joint are hallmarks supporting this diagnosis. The shoulder will normally hold 50 to 60 ml of saline, but in this syndrome often only 20 or 30 ml can be instilled. Although this limits the possible synovial and capsular distention and the restricted motion makes arthroscopic examination more difficult, good viewing can generally be achieved. A variety of abnormalities have been reported: tears and fissures of the labrum, chronic synovitis, degenerative changes of the articular surfaces, and chronic tears of the rotator cuff. Wiley and Older suggest that fibrosis and adhesions with obliteration of the subscapular bursa may be a significant causative factor in the development of this syndrome.

Other indications

As increased clinical experience and skill are gained and reported in the literature, this list of potential chronic shoulder disorders treatable by arthroscopic procedures will expand. Early success with arthroscopic stable capsulorraphy for instability, release of the coracoacromial ligament, and acromioplasty procedures have been reported.

Diagnostic technique

Thorough diagnostic arthroscopy of the shoulder and arthroscopic surgical procedures should be performed with the patient under general endotracheal anesthesia. After the anesthetic is administered, the shoulder should be examined, testing its range of motion and stability and comparing it with the opposite normal shoulder. The patient is then positioned in a lateral decubitus position maintained by a Vac-Pac. The upper extremity to be examined is placed in a skin traction apparatus connected to an overhead pulley and traction rope, which is secured by a suspended weight and pulley system (Fig. 60-1). The weight on the traction may be adjusted later to produce the amount of distraction needed for maneuvering the arthroscopic instruments within the joint. The suspended upper extremity is positioned so that the arm is in approximately 70 degrees of abduction and 15 degrees of forward flexion

(Fig. 60-2). Care should be taken not to lift the patient's head off the table by the distraction for fear of producing a traction neurapraxia of the brachial plexus.

The shoulder is then prepared and draped to allow access to both the anterior and posterior aspects of the joint. The shoulder should be draped with a surgical barrier (an adhesive-type waterproof draping) to seal off the shoulder from any unsterile area. The bony anatomic landmarks are identified and outlined with a skin-marking pen. These are the anterior, lateral, and posterior corners or borders of the acromion, the spine of the scapula, the distal clavicle, the coracoid process, and the humeral head (Fig. 60-3).

The preferred approach to begin the diagnostic arthroscopy is through a posterior portal located approximately 2 to 3 cm inferior and slightly medial to the posterolateral tip of the acromion. Do not place this portal more than 3 cm inferior to the acromion or the axillary nerve may be damaged. Proper location of this posterior portal can be aided by palpating the coracoid process anteriorly with the index finger and feeling with the thumb for a posterior soft spot that makes up the interval between the infraspinatus and teres minor muscles. As the suspended arm is internally and externally rotated, the humeral head can be palpated beneath the thumb and the exact location of the glenohumeral joint can be confirmed. An 18-gauge needle is inserted through this posterior soft spot and directed anteriorly and medially toward the coracoid process. When the needle has been placed in the desired position a 50 ml syringe containing saline is connected to it and 40 to 50 ml of saline solution is injected to distend the joint. If there is significant capsulitis, the joint may accept far less solution. The syringe is disconnected from the needle, and the presence of free backflow will confirm correct placement of the needle.

The 18-gauge needle is removed and a small skin incision is made with a No. 11 knife blade through the skin

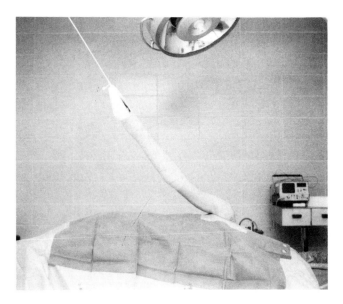

Fig. 60-1. Traction suspension system for shoulder arthroscopy.

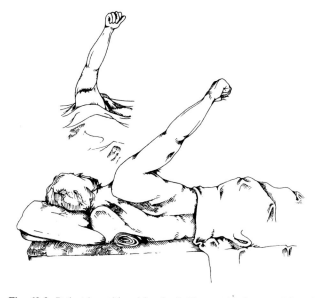

Fig. 60-2. Patient is positioned involved side up, with the arm abducted 45 to 60 degrees and forward flexed about 15 degrees. (From Matthews, O.: Advances in Arthroscopic Surgery, Baltimore, 1984, The Williams and Wilkins Co.)

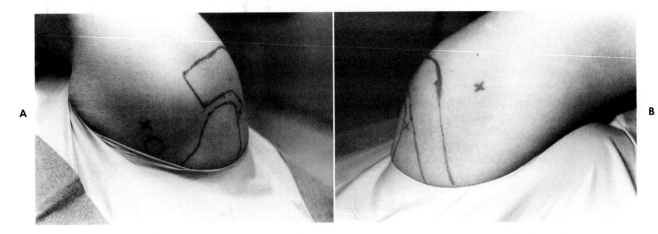

Fig. 60-3. Bony landmarks identified and outlined with a marking pin. **A,** Anterior landmarks for shoulder arthroscopy showing acromion, clavicle, coracoid, and anterior and superior portal sites marked with x. **B,** Posterior landmarks for shoulder arthroscopy showing posterior acromion, spine of scapula, and posterior portal site marked with x.

and subcutaneous tissue at the point of the needle insertion. A cannula and sharp trocar are then inserted along the path taken by the needle anteriorly and medially toward the coracoid process. The use of a sharp trocar to pierce the deltoid and posterior rotator cuff interval is safer than the use of a No. 11 knife blade. Attempts to incise the portal track with a knife blade increase the risk of damage to neurovascular structures. Once the sharp trocar pierces the musculotendinous capsule, it is removed and a free backflow of saline confirms penetration of the capsule. The sharp trocar is replaced by the blunt trocar, and the sheath and trocar are inserted further into the interior of the joint. The blunt trocar is then removed and the arthroscope is inserted. The use of a 30-degree arthroscope facilitates viewing the entire interior of the shoulder joint. We normally use the 5 to 6 mm diagnostic arthroscope for routine shoulder arthroscopy, although on certain occasions a smaller scope in the 2.2 to 2.7 mm size may be better.

An anterior portal is located one-half the distance between the coracoid process and the anterolateral edge of the acromion. A spinal needle is inserted through this second portal through the capsule under direct view from the arthroscope previously inserted in the posterior portal. The spinal needle should ideally enter the capsule just medial to the tendon of the long head of the biceps. Once proper placement of the needle is confirmed, its direction and course are memorized and the needle is removed. With a No. 11 knife blade, a small skin and subcutaneous incision is made in the site where the needle had been, and the anterior portal is entered in the same way as the posterior portal. This cannula is connected to a continuous inflow of saline solution introduced into the joint by gravity flow from a large fluid bag elevated 1 to 2 meters above the level of the patient. With inflow running through the anterior portal and outflow through the sheath of the arthroscope, maximum distention of the joint can be maintained throughout the procedure (Fig. 60-4). A superior portal is frequently needed during intraarticular surgery. It accommodates an inflow cannula, the anterior cannula serving for instrument passage.

The amount of joint distraction required for easy viewing and maneuverability of the instruments can be adjusted by means of the rope and traction apparatus. No more distraction than what is required for clear viewing should be used.

Additional portals, either anterior, posterior, or superior may be established by initially directing a spinal needle through the soft tissues and capsule, confirming its entry into the joint through the capsule by direct arthroscopic viewing, memorizing the direction and course of the needle, and then making an additional arthroscopic or instrument portal along this same path. Many of the instruments can be exchanged between the posterior and anterior portals as needed during the procedure.

Maneuvering the arthroscope and arthroscopic instruments during shoulder arthroscopy is more difficult than during knee arthroscopy because of the thickness of the soft tissues through which they pass before entering the joint. This large soft tissue fulcrum makes the passage and manipulation of the instruments more difficult. With care and practice, these maneuvers can be mastered, however.

Arthroscopic anatomy

As with arthroscopy of other joints, a thorough knowledge of the major anatomic structures about the shoulder is necessary. The surgeon must be familiar with the normal to identify the abnormal or pathologic processes seen (Fig. 60-5). Once the joint has been entered, the most helpful landmark is the point at which the long head of the biceps tendon passes the humeral head. This tendon is the key to maintaining proper orientation during the arthroscopic procedure. If one becomes disoriented during the procedure, returning to the biceps tendon and then proceeding will often clear the confusion. Once the biceps tendon has been seen initially, successful diagnostic evaluation must proceed in a systematic order, identifying the biceps tendon, (Plate 6, *C*) the articular surface of the humeral head, the

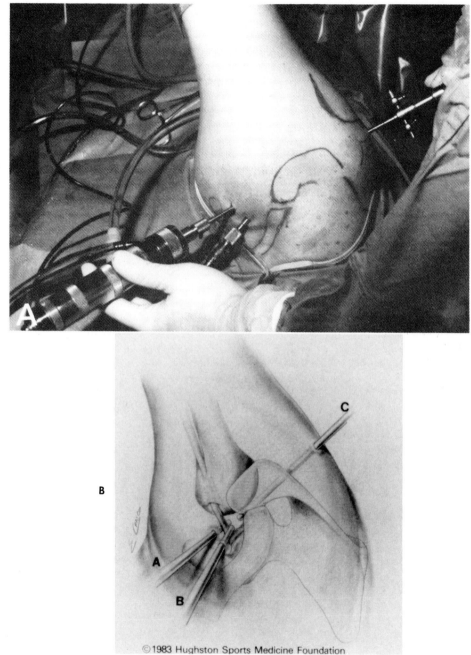

© 1983 Hughston Sports Medicine Foundation

Fig. 60-4. Technique of operative shoulder arthroscopy. **A,** Operative arthroscopy performed with a motorized instrument and inflow cannula through two portals. Arthroscope is placed posteriorly. **B,** Anterior instruments are placed medial *(a)* and lateral *(b)* to the biceps tendon. Arthroscope enters through the posterior portal *(c).* (From Andrews, J.R., et al.: Am. J. Sports Med. **12**(1):1, 1984.)

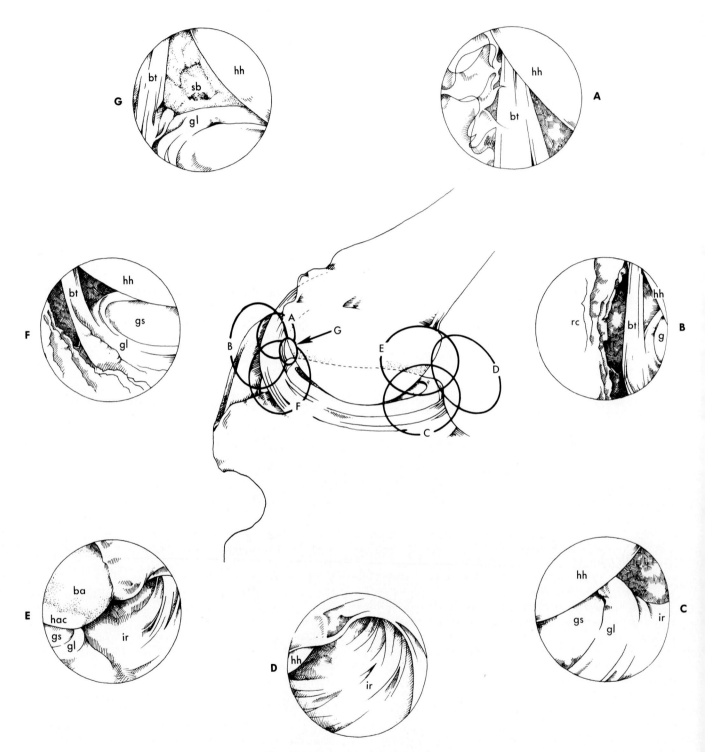

Fig. 60-5. For legend see opposite page.

Fig. 60-5. Overview of arthroscopic anatomy of normal right shoulder. *Ellipses* indicate perspectives of **A** to **G** and correspond to typical views in systematic examination of joint described in text. **A,** Initial orienting view of biceps tendon, which disappears into bicipital groove above; *hh,* humeral head; *bt,* biceps tendon. **B,** Withdrawing scope slightly and viewing superiorly, synovium overlying those tendons of rotator cuff that course to greater tuberosity can be inspected: *hh,* humeral head; *g,* glenoid with edging labrum; *bt,* biceps tendon; *rc,* rotator cuff area. **C,** Withdrawing and swinging inferiorly, glenoid surface and posteroinferior glenoid labrum are seen: *hh,* humeral head; *gs,* glenoid articular surface; *gl,* glenoid labrum; *ir,* inferior recess. **D,** Further inferiorly, inferior recess is lined by synovium, which sweeps from edge of glenoid labrum up to anatomic neck of humeral head; *hh,* humeral head; *ir,* inferior recess. **E,** Again withdrawing and then turning the scope to view superiorly, humeral head is inspected. Note large bare area between articular cartilage and attachment of synovially lined capsule. This is normal and should not be confused with Hill-Sachs type lesion: *hac,* humeral articular cartilage; *ba,* bare area; *gs,* glenoid surface; *gl,* glenoid labrum, *ir,* inferior recess. **F,** Bringing arthroscope superolaterally, anterior glenoid labrum is visualized. Note blended appearance of biceps tendon with glenoid labrum where tendon attaches to supraglenoid tubercle: *hh,* humeral head; *gs,* glenoid surface; *gl,* glenoid labrum; *bt,* biceps tendon. **G,** Intraarticular triangle, bounded by humeral head, *hh;* biceps tendon, *bt;* and glenoid labrum, *gl.* Floor of triangle is anterior capsule, including opening into subscapularis bursa, *sb.* Tendon of subscapularis muscle, although not shown in this illustration, often traverses, medial to lateral, in floor of intraarticular triangle. It should not be confused with biceps tendon, which it resembles. An anterior portal should enter joint in this triangle. (From Matthews, O., et al.: Advances in orthopaedic surgery, Baltimore, 1984, The Williams & Wilkins Co.)

---

anterior glenoid labrum, (Plate 6, *D*) the glenohumeral ligaments of the anterior capsule, the posterior surface of the subscapularis tendon and recess, the undersurface of the rotator cuff muscles (supraspinatus and infraspinatus), the superior recess and the surfaces of the glenoid cavity, the inferior pouch (Plate 6, *E*), and the posterior glenoid labrum. Finally, the undersurface of the teres minor and posterior capsule can be viewed by switching the arthroscope to the anterior portal and directing the fore lens posteriorly and superiorly.

The long head of the biceps tendon can be traced to its attachment to the supraglenoid tubercle at the superior margin of the glenoid cavity and is in direct continuity with the glenoid labrum. Rotation of the suspended arm by the first assistant makes further examination of the intraarticular portion of the biceps tendon easier. Externally rotating the arm makes it possible to see the biceps tendon anteriorly to the bicipital groove.

After inspecting the biceps tendon, most portions of the articulating surface of the humeral head can be examined using a 30-degree arthroscope. This examination is aided by rotating the humeral head into internal and external rotation. The glenoid surface should be seen in its entirety with adequate distraction of the humeral head, keeping in mind the biceps tendon insertion superiorly on the supraglenoid tubercle. Next, the anterior glenoid labrum is examined; by beginning at the insertion of the biceps tendon in continuity with the superior portion of the labrum and sweeping the arthroscope anteriorly and inferiorly, this fibrocartilaginous structure may be followed along its anterior and inferior limits. Again, distraction of the humeral head by the traction will aid in viewing the inferior portion of the glenoid rim. The 30-degree fore lens is directed anteriorly and inferiorly during this sweep of the arthroscope. The posterior glenoid labrum is viewed by retracting the arthroscope tip to near its portal of entry through the posterior capsule and directing the fore angle lens posteriorly and inferiorly.

The course of the glenoid labrum can be followed from inferior to superior using this technique. Care must be taken to prevent inadvertently withdrawing the arthroscope tip through the capsule and out of the joint. Further examination of the posterior glenoid labrum and posterior capsular structures can be accomplished later in the procedure by switching the arthroscope to the anterior portal. Derangements or abnormalities of the labrum may be appropriately probed through additional portals made by first directing the spinal needle to the appropriate location and then inserting the probe or other instrument accordingly. Examination by probing of the anterior labrum is done by inserting the probe through a supplemental anterior portal; conversely, probing of the posterior labrum is done by inserting the probe through an accessory posterior portal.

The glenohumeral ligaments can be viewed by bringing the arthroscope tip back to its original position, orienting the field of view to the long head of the biceps tendon, and then advancing the arthroscope. Great variations in the configuration and prominence of the glenohumeral ligaments are present from patient to patient. In one patient they may be quite prominent and in others they may blend almost imperceptibly with the capsule and posterior surface of the subscapularis. The subscapularis recess may be found in the anterior aspect of the shoulder joint and is most often in the area of the middle glenohumeral ligament; however, great variations in the size and location of this recess may occur. The posterosuperior edge of the subscapularis tendon may be seen lying between the superior and middle glenohumeral ligaments, although it may be obscured by a prominent middle glenohumeral ligament, or may appear to blend with that ligament. When the subscapularis recess is large, the posterosuperior edge of the tendon may be seen through this recess.

The arthroscope should be returned to its original orientation, again using the long head of the biceps tendon. The arthroscope with its 30-degree lens should be rotated or directed superiorly and slightly toward the humeral head. The undersurface of the supraspinatus tendon can be seen just superior to the long head of the biceps tendon. The infraspinatus and the upper edge of the teres minor may be seen by directing the arthroscope posteriorly and superiorly. The superior recess is located superior and slightly anterior to the superior edge of the glenoid cavity and to the insertion of the biceps tendon. The inferior pouch is next examined by directing the arthroscope posterior to the humeral head and in an inferoanterior direction. With the lens directed anteriorly, the extent of the inferior or axillary pouch of the joint can be examined for loose bodies or other abnormalities.

Arthroscopic surgical procedures

As in all other joints, any intraarticular arthroscopic surgical procedure begins with a systematic and complete diagnostic examination. Attempts to perform delicate intraarticular arthroscopic surgical procedures before developing experience and skill in diagnostic shoulder arthroscopy will result in poor surgical procedures and frequently in harm to the joint. As in the knee, a good surgical procedure performed through an arthrotomy is preferable to a poorly performed arthroscopic procedure. Once sufficient diagnostic acumen is achieved, the same accessory arthroscopic surgical instruments and triangulation techniques used in knee procedures apply to the shoulder. Intraarticular arthroscopic surgical procedures commonly performed today are: (1) removal of loose bodies, (2) debridement of labral lesions (frayed areas, pedunculated flaps, and bucket handle tears), (3) resection of retained ruptured biceps tendon stumps, (4) chondroplasty procedures, (5) synovial biopsy, and (6) debridement of frayed, degenerated, inferior surface tears of the rotator cuff.

Again common to all of the above procedures is a thorough systematic diagnostic examination. Since the surgical procedures begin with the diagnostic arthroscopy, the reader is referred to the section on diagnostic arthroscopy technique (p. 2611).

REMOVAL OF LOOSE BODIES

Loose bodies encountered during routine diagnostic arthroscopy may be removed either by suctioning through large-caliber inflow and outflow cannulas, which will remove small ones, or by triangulating a grasping forceps into the area for grasping and extracting larger ones. Applying suction to the 4 to 5 mm inflow cannula will evacuate loose bodies that will pass through it. Larger loose bodies tend to gravitate into the axillary pouch of the joint or occasionally into the subscapularis recess. Those gravitating into the axillary pouch are usually removed easily using triangulation techniques. Once the loose body is within the field of vision, an 18-gauge spinal needle is triangulated to the loose body by trial-and-error penetrations. This becomes readily accomplishable as skill in triangulation is acquired. Once the tip of the needle can be placed next to the loose body, the direction and orientation of the needle's path is memorized, an accessory portal is made, and the grasping instrument is inserted. Loose bodies tend to bob like apples in a rain barrel; turning off the inflow at this time may make it easier to grasp the loose body. Once the loose body is securely grasped, it should be extracted in a slow, twisting movement to decrease the likelihood of its slipping from the jaws of the grasper. The accessory portal may be enlarged if necessary to prevent pulling the loose body from the jaws of the grasper. If the loose body floats away, a suction tip may be inserted or

suction may be applied to the outflow cannula, which will often pull the loose body to the cannula, stabilize it, and thereby allow the grasping instrument to grasp it.

Loose bodies that are noted anteriorly on roentgenograms but are not readily visible arthroscopically, are frequently hidden within the subscapularis bursa and may be ''milked'' from the bursa through the opening in the subscapularis recess by palpating in the subcoracoid area. Once they are milked and maneuvered into the joint, they are grasped and removed by the technique just described.

DEBRIDEMENT OF LABRAL LESIONS

Following thorough diagnostic arthroscopy, pathologic conditions involving the glenoid labrum, such as frayed areas, pedunculated flaps, or bucket handle tears, may be debrided in the following manner. If the anterior glenoid labrum is the site of the pathology encountered, it is viewed with the arthroscope through the posterior portal with inflow and accessory instrument portals placed anteriorly and superiorly in the manner previously described. The use of the 18-gauge needle to direct portal placement and capsular entry again ensures accurate portal placement. Abnormal fraying, pedunculated flaps, or bucket handle tears may be resected by any of the accessory cutting arthroscopic instruments: basket forceps, scissors, or motorized cutting and shaving instruments. More often the motorized cutter and shaver is used for cutting, morselization, and suction removal of the abnormal tissue. If the motorized cutter is selected, it is passed through the previously placed inflow cannula or through an accessory anterior portal located initially by passing an 18-gauge needle and subsequently entering the joint using a sheath and sharp trocar. A superior location for the inflow cannula may be selected if the instrument is passed through the anterior cannula. The rotary motorized cutter is then passed through the positioned sheath to the area to be debrided, and the frayed area, pedunculated flap, or bucket handle flap is resected with the cutter. Before removal, the area in question should be carefully probed to determine the extent of the pathology and the limits to the tissues that should be removed. If basket forceps or scissors are selected for cutting such flaps, they are passed in a manner similar to the motorized cutter. The tissues are amputated and then removed by means of suction, or if the flaps are large, by means of a second grasping instrument.

RESECTION OF RETAINED BICEPS TENDON STUMP

The long head of the biceps tendon may become frayed and ruptured in chronic impingement syndrome, bicipital tenosynovitis, or degenerative conditions about the shoulder joint. It may rupture in the bicipital groove, leaving a frayed proximal segment attached to the supraglenoid tubercle. Popping and pain within the joint may be caused by impingement of this proximal stump of tendon between the glenoid cavity and humeral head. A resection of the retained stump can be carried out easily by intraarticular arthroscopic surgical techniques. Following systematic examination of the shoulder with the arthroscope in the posterior portal, with the supraglenoid tubercle area in view, an accessory anterior portal is selected by triangulating an 18-gauge needle through the anterior capsule. Once optimal passage of this needle to the ruptured biceps tendon stump is seen, the course and direction of the needle are memorized and an accessory anterior portal is created. The motorized cutter and shaver sheath with a sharp trocar is used to penetrate the anterior capsule, and then the anterior and superior aspects of the joints are entered. The sharp trocar is removed and a blunt trocar is substituted in the sheath. The tip of the blunt trocar is brought under direct vision to the supraglenoid tubercle and then the blunt trocar is removed. The motorized cutter and shaver is inserted through the sheath, and its tip is brought into view at the supraglenoid tubercle. The pedunculated retained stump of the ruptured biceps tendon can be removed using the motorized suction cutter, the stump being morcellized and removed from the joint. The attachment site on the supraglenoid tubercle is trimmed and smoothed until no fragment is present of sufficient size to impinge between the glenoid and humeral articulating surfaces.

CHONDROPLASTY AND SYNOVIAL BIOPSY

Although chondroplasty procedures alone are rarely required in the shoulder, smoothing of grossly irregular flaps on the articular surfaces of the glenoid cavity or humeral head may be required as a part of other arthroscopic procedures. In a variety of rheumatologic conditions, selected synovial biopsy may help establish a definitive diagnosis. The entire synovium may not be uniformly affected, especially early in the course of certain of these conditions, and arthroscopy can direct one to the most suitable area for biopsy.

Chondroplasty and biopsy procedures, again, follow a thorough examination and a diagnostic evaluation of the joint. The optimal placement of the arthroscope depends on the area to be treated, but the arthroscope is usually inserted through the posterior portal. The biopsy procedure is usually carried out through an accessory anterior portal using the techniques previously described for portal location and the insertion of a basket forceps, a pituitary rongeur, or another biting instrument. The instrument is directed to the area of synovial involvement and a generous bite of synovial and subsynovial tissue is taken and submitted for pathologic evaluation. Chondroplasty procedures to resect severe chondromalacic areas are required for large articular flaps that have peeled from the glenoid or from the head; they are usually carried out by means of accessory anterior portals through which basket forceps or the motorized cutter and shaver is inserted.

DEBRIDEMENT OF ROTATOR CUFF TEARS

Degenerative tears of the undersurface of the rotator cuff may be debrided. They often look like ''crab meat'' hanging near the supraspinatus or infraspinatus insertion. They are locally debrided with the motorized cutter and shaver through appropriate portals.

Complications

Complications following diagnostic shoulder arthroscopy or intraarticular arthroscopic surgical techniques are as uncommon as they are in other joints. However, the potential for serious complications does exist. The less frequent use of shoulder arthroscopy by the average orthopaedic surgeon often results in an increased incidence of complications. Placing and maneuvering the arthroscope

and instruments in the shoulder joint are much more difficult than in the knee, largely because there are fewer well-defined bony landmarks for portals and because the joint is surrounded by thick layers of musculotendinous cuff and capsular tissue. Difficulties in shoulder arthroscopy and intraarticular arthroscopic surgical procedures are often directly related to poor portal placement caused by poor bony landmark identification and localization. The fact that the instruments must traverse thick layers of deltoid muscle and other soft tissues makes the fulcrum around the instrument much thicker and increases the difficulty of placing and maneuvering the instruments once they are inserted. This may result in increased scuffing or scoring of the articular surfaces of the glenoid cavity and humeral head leading to secondary degenerative arthritic changes that must be considered a direct complication of the invasive procedure. Careful localization of the optimum sites for portal placements will minimize this possible complication. Difficulty in maneuvering instruments within the joint can result in increased instrument breakage and difficult retrieval procedures. Even arthrotomy may be required if a small cutting instrument is broken and lost within the joint.

Infections should be at a minimum because of the limited exposure, the rich vascularity about the joint, and the dilutional effect of the irrigating solution, but nevertheless they can occur with gross violations of good technique. Careful preparation and draping will minimize fluid leakage and contamination through the drapes to unsterile areas.

The axillary nerve can be injured as it horizontally traverses the deep surface of the deltoid muscle or in the axillary area. The cephalic vein may be lacerated or injured if accessory anterior portals are required. To minimize neurovascular lacerations, only the skin portal site should be incised; the trocar should be used for gently pushing through the soft tissues exterior to the joint capsule. Neurologic deficits about the shoulder can also be caused by extravasation of large amounts of fluid or by overdistraction of the joint. As with other arthroscopic procedures, fluids for irrigation and distention are a necessity, but the surgeon must be aware that the numerous bursal connections about the shoulder allow for greater extravasation of solutions into the surrounding tissues than normally occurs in the other joints. Tremendous amounts of fluids may be extravasated into the soft tissues if excessively long procedures are undertaken or if any pump mechanism is used for joint distention. (Pump mechanisms are not needed and should be condemned in shoulder arthroscopy.) Distraction of the joint is necessary for adequate arthroscopic diagnosis and surgical procedures. The use of distraction by an assistant pulling on the soft tissues about the lower arm, elbow, and forearm is generally less than optimally effective, produces potential local soft tissue contusions and neurovascular problems, and is generally not consistent because of fatigue. Therefore, skin traction using a rope and pulley arrangement is not only more effective but is probably safer. The amount of joint distraction should be the minimum that allows for adequate vision and maneuverability of the instruments. Excessive distraction of the joint has caused significant traction neurapraxia involving various components of the brachial plexus. The anesthesiologist should remain generally aware of the stretch on the patient's neck and should remind the surgeon if it becomes excessive. Serious neurologic defects caused by overdistraction of the joint, excessive traction on the brachial plexus, and excessive pressures from extravasation of large amounts of fluid may produce problems far greater than the chronic shoulder problem for which the procedure was performed.

ELBOW

Arthroscopy of the elbow was described by Burman in the early 1930s, but the tight confines of this joint and the larger size of the arthroscopes made adequate viewing difficult. Although significant improvements in optics and instrumentation, and especially the development of smaller arthroscopes, have improved the ability to examine this joint, even today experience is limited.

Fewer diagnostic and therapeutic problems treatable by arthroscopic techniques are seen in the elbow than in the knee or shoulder. This added to the technical difficulties has resulted in few surgeons developing skills in elbow arthroscopy. Nevertheless, with careful attention to the bony landmarks and technical details, much of the joint can be seen anteriorly with a 5 mm arthroscope. The posterior aspect is examined best with the smaller arthroscopes.

Indications

Theoretically, arthroscopy could be used to examine the elbow joint in any or all of the disorders one might use it for in any other joint, such as rheumatologic conditions or trauma. From a practical standpoint, however, arthroscopy of the elbow is currently most often indicated for evaluation of osteochondritis dissecans and similar lesions, osteochondral fractures of the capitellum and radial head, and removal of loose bodies.

Technique

Arthroscopy of the elbow may be done with axillary block, intravenous regional, or general anesthesia. For all but the most experienced arthroscopists, local anesthesia is probably not indicated. A pneumatic tourniquet is placed around the upper arm, but it is not inflated unless required. Some surgeons prefer to suspend the extremity by a rope and pulley mechanism, abducting the shoulder, and thus gain access to both the lateral and medial sides of the elbow joint. Access to the anterior aspect as well as the posterior is possible. Traction on the forearm to distract the joint by way of the suspension system is not required. The extremity from the tourniquet to the wrist is prepared and draped with waterproof drapes, thereby sealing the operative field from the unsterile areas.

If the suspected pathologic condition is in the posterior or olecranon fossa area, then this part of the joint should be viewed initially. Maximum distention is required for optimum viewing here. If the anterior joint is viewed initially, leakage of the irrigating fluids through the anterior portals may make distention suboptimal posteriorly.

The bony landmarks are marked on the overlying skin with a marking pen (Fig. 60-6). The location of the radial head can be palpated and marked by pronation and supination of the forearm. The superior aspect of the radiocapitellar interval can be palpated and marked along with the outline of the capitellar surface. The anterolateral portal site, just anterior to the lateral humeral condyle and slightly superior and anterior to the radial head, is marked. The outlines of the medial epicondyle and ulnar nerve are marked. The optimum medial portal is slightly superior and anterior to the medial epicondyle. The posterior aspect of the joint is best entered through a posterolateral portal. With the elbow maximally distended, a posterolateral bulge can be palpated between the posterior aspect of the lateral humeral condyle and the lateral aspect of the olecranon.

With an 18-gauge needle connected to a 20 ml syringe and inserted through the anterolateral portal site previously marked with a marking pen, the joint is distended with irrigating solution. Reflux of solution into the syringe confirms the presence of the needle within the joint. Then the needle is removed from the joint. If the pathology suspected or noted on roentgenograms, for instance a loose body, is located anteriorly, examination of this aspect of the joint is now undertaken. If the location is unknown or suspected to be posterior, the posterior aspect of the joint should be examined first. Examination of the posterior compartment requires maximum joint distention and is best done before making anterior portals. Leakage of solution through posterior portals generally does not prevent subsequent adequate anterior compartment distention for examination. Thus, once the joint is distended from the anterolateral site, the elbow joint may be entered either anteriorly or posteriorly as dictated by the suspected location of the abnormality.

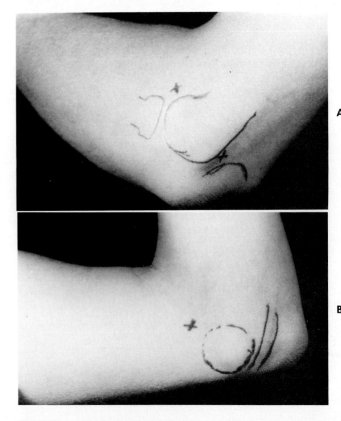

Fig. 60-6. A, Standard anterolateral and posterolateral portals. **B,** Standard anteromedial portal.

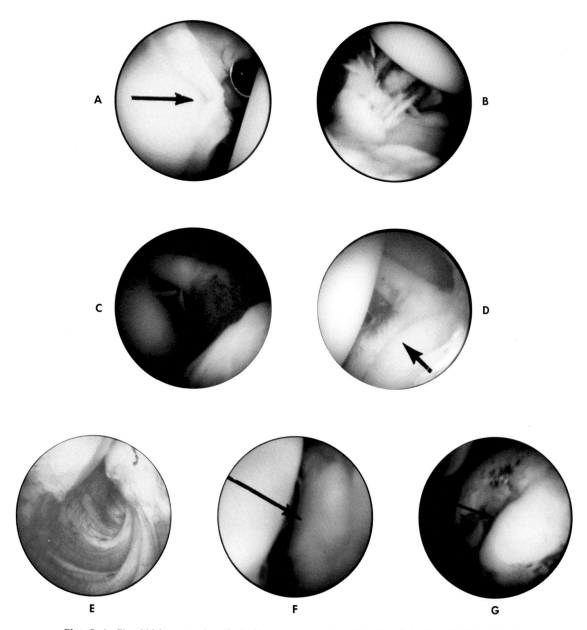

Plate 8. A, Glenoid labrum tear in patient with recurrent anterior subluxation of shoulder. **B,** Marked fraying of glenoid labrum near insertion of biceps tendon in throwing athlete with anterior shoulder pain. **C,** Arthroscopic view of biceps tendon. **D,** Arthroscopic view of anterior glenoid labrum. **E,** Arthroscopic view of inferior pouch of shoulder joint. **F,** Arthroscopic view of radial head at its capitellar articulation showing moderate degenerative changes of radial head. **G,** Arthroscopic view showing posteromedial osteophyte on olecranon.

Arthroscopic approaches
ANTERIOR APPROACHES

The anterior compartment of the elbow joint may be approached with the arthroscope or accessory instruments through either an anterolateral or an anteromedial portal site, as previously described (Fig. 60-7). As a general rule, the anteromedial intraarticular structures, such as the synovium, the coronoid process of the ulna, and the trochlear notch of the humerus, can best be viewed from the lateral side, whereas the radial head and its articulation with the capitellum can best be viewed from the anteromedial portal (Plate 6, *F*). Again, the joint should be maximally distended before either of the portals is used.

TECHNIQUE. With a No. 11 knife blade, make a small skin incision at the previously marked portal site (site of the previous needle penetration for distention of the joint). Penetrate only the skin and subcutaneous tissue with the knife blade. With an arthroscope sheath and sharp trocar, penetrate the underlying soft tissues and gently force the sheath and trocar through the lateral capsule slightly superior and anterior to the radial head. Once the sharp trocar is removed, the reflux of irrigating solution confirms the entry into the joint. Exchange the sharp trocar for the blunt trocar, and gently penetrate farther into the depths of the joint. Now remove the blunt trocar and insert a 30-degree arthroscope through the positioned sheath. Connect the inflow tubing from the suspended irrigation solutions to the inflow stopcock on the arthroscope sheath. Now open the stopcock and maximally distend the joint again. Advance the arthroscope farther into the anterior compartment of the joint; by rotation of the 30-degree lens, inspect the coronoid area of the olecranon and the trochlear notch of the humerus, aided by maximum distention of the anterior capsule. The anterior synovium may obliterate the

view of these structures; if so, assure maximum distention of the joint by turning off the outflow stopcock and flexing the elbow joint. The flexed position allows the anterior capsule to relax and be further distended. Now the articular surfaces of the trochlear portion of the humeral condyle and a part of the articular surface of the coronoid process can be viewed. Loose bodies in the anterior part of the joint tend to settle into this anterior capsular pouch region. If probing of articular surface abnormalities or extraction of loose bodies from the anterior compartment is required, insert the probe or accessory grasping or cutting instruments through an accessory anteromedial portal. Select the optimal site for the accessory portal by inserting an 18 gauge needle through the skin, subcutaneous tissues, and capsule under direct vision with the arthroscope in the anterolateral portal. This is usually near the marked anteromedial portal just superior and anterior to the medial epicondyle. If the tip of the needle can be brought to the desired spot within the joint, it should be possible to make a portal and carry the appropriate instrument to that same spot. Once the position is determined, make a small accessory anteromedial portal and pass the probe or the operating instrument under direct vision into the anteromedial aspect of the joint. If a loose body must be retrieved, insert a grasper, grasp the loose body, and extract it with a slow twisting movement to prevent dislodging it as it exits through the capsule. Enlargement of the portal about the neck of the grasping instrument will reduce the chances of dislodging the loose body from the grasper. If a cutting instrument is required for local synovectomy or marsupialization of adhesions, insert the small-tipped rotary cutter and shaver through a similar anteromedial portal under direct vision. Remove the pathologic tissue with suction and cutting. Take extreme care when using these portals to

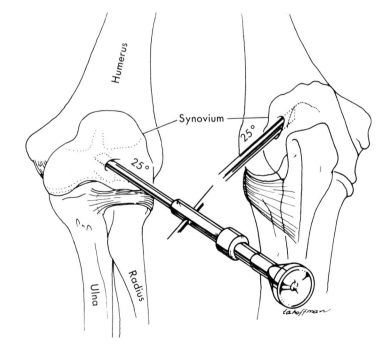

Fig. 60-7. Anterolateral and posteromedial portals. (From Shahriaree, H.: O'Connor's textbook of arthroscopic surgery, Philadelphia, 1984, J.B. Lippincott Co.)

avoid injuring the motor branch of the radial nerve laterally and the ulnar nerve in the region of the medial epicondyle medially.

ANTEROMEDIAL APPROACH

If the pathologic condition is suspected to be in the anterolateral aspect of the joint, the anteromedial portal is selected for arthroscopic viewing.

TECHNIQUE. Note the previously marked site just superior and anterior to the medial epicondyle; following maximum joint distention, make an anteromedial portal by incising the skin and subcutaneous tissues with a No. 11 knife blade, penetrating the anteromedial capsule with a sheath and sharp trocar, advancing the sharp trocar, substituting a blunt trocar for the sharp trocar, and advancing the sheath across toward the lateral aspect of the joint. Then insert the 30-degree arthroscope. Connect the inflow and outflow irrigation tubes as previously described. View the capitellar articular surfaces, the radiohumeral joint, and the articular surface of the radial head by rotating the 30-degree scope. Gently flex and extend the elbow, and pronate and supinate the forearm to bring various portions of the articular surfaces into view. Distraction on the joint will rarely produce a large enough opening to advance the scope into the radiocapitellar joint. If articular fragments on the capitellum or abnormalities of the radial head require probing or removal, insert the probe and the accessory instruments through the anterolateral portal under direct arthroscopic vision to accomplish this task. Carry out the procedures as described for anterolateral viewing.

POSTERIOR APPROACHES

The posterior aspect of the joint and olecranon fossa are best viewed with the arthroscope in a posterolateral position.

TECHNIQUE. Maximally distend the joint, and if the pathologic tissue is suspected to be in the posterior compartment, view this compartment first to maintain the distention. Distention of the joint aids in localizing the posterolateral portal. A bulge can generally be palpated between the humerus and the olecranon laterally. Insert an 18-gauge needle into the proposed site and confirm entry into the posterolateral pouch by the reflux of irrigating solution. Make a small skin incision and through it insert the sheath and sharp trocar of a small-caliber scope. Enter the posterolateral capsular area slightly anteriorly and approach obliquely posteriorly and superiorly at approximately a 25-degree angle. Degenerative changes within the olecranon notch, loose bodies, or impinging osteophytes may be seen by carefully maneuvering the arthroscope (Plate 6, *G*). Note any small loose bodies and remove them through a suction cannula inserted into the olecranon fossa; remove any larger loose bodies with a small grasper. Because of the tight confines of the olecranon fossa, insert suction or accessory instruments from the posterolateral aspect near the portal for the arthroscope and determine the entry point by positioning a needle in the joint and into the visual field of the arthroscope. Once the needle is correctly positioned, make an accessory portal and insert the suction device or accessory grasping instrument. Placing acccessory portals posteromedially is ill advised; the risk of injury to the ulnar nerve is too great.

OTHER UPPER EXTREMITY JOINTS

Arthroscopy of the wrist and finger joints has been carried out by a few arthroscopists. Using maximum joint distention and distraction by means of traction, these joints can be penetrated and viewed through a small-caliber arthroscope. The indications and uses for the method in these joints are yet to be clearly delineated; such procedures are not recommended for routine use by the average orthopaedic surgeon. Perhaps in the future, arthroscopy of the wrist and smaller joints may be refined enough to provide insight into some of the difficult diagnostic problems, such as chondral fractures and intercarpal disassociations.

REFERENCES

Andrews, J.R., Carson, W.G., and Ortega, K.: Arthroscopy of the shoulder: technique and normal anatomy, Am. J. Sports Med. **12:**1, 1984.

Andrews, J.R., and Carson, W.G.: Shoulder joint arthroscopy, Orthopedics **6:**1157, 1983.

Burman, M.S.: Arthroscopy or the direct visualization of joints: an experimental cadaver study, J. Bone Joint Surg. **13:**669, 1931.

Caspari, R.B.: Shoulder arthroscopy: a review of the present state of the art, Contemp. Orthop. **4:**523, 1982.

Ha'eri, G.B., and Maitland, A.: Arthroscopic findings in the frozen shoulder, J. Rheumatol. **8:**149, 1981.

Johnson, L.L.: Arthroscopy of the shoulder, Orthop. Clin. North Am. **11:**197, 1980.

Lombardo, S.J.: Arthroscopy of the shoulder, Clin. Sports Med. **2:**309, 1983.

Matthews, L.S., Vetter, W.L., and Helfet, D.L.: Arthroscopic surgery of the shoulder, Advances Orthop. Surg. **7:**203, 1984.

O'Connor, R.L.: Arthroscopy, Philadelphia, 1977, J.B. Lippincott Co.

Wiley, A.M., and Older, M.W.J.: Shoulder arthroscopy, Am. J. Sports Med. **8:**31, 1980.

PART XV

Congenital Anomalies

CHAPTER 61

Congenital anomalies of lower extremity

James H. Beaty

In this chapter are discussed congenital anomalies of the lower extremities exclusive of the hip. Those of the hip are discussed in Chapter 62. Also discussed is lower limb length discrepancy from any cause.

CONSTRICTURES OF LEG

A congenital circumferential constricture of the soft tissues of the leg is rare. It is seen at birth as a depression in the soft tissues completely encircling the limb (Fig. 61-

1). Often the foot is also deformed. The skin, subcutaneous tissue, and deep fascia may all be affected, and usually the lymphatics and superficial circulation are partially obstructed. Distal to the constricture is a persistent pitting edema that can be cured only by excising the constricture and in most instances the edematous tissues distal to it. Fractures of the tibia and fibula at the level of the constricture have been reported. In marked contrast to congenital pseudarthrosis, after successful treatment of the constricture, the fractures heal promptly without surgery.

An operation to eliminate a constricture must include a Z-plasty; if it is simply excised, the constricture usually recurs.

TECHNIQUE (FROM COZEN AND BROCKWAY). Lengthen the constricted tissues in stages; at least three Z-plastic operations are usually required. In each, first make the middle limb of the Z in the cleft of the constricture. Then make the superior and inferior limbs of the Z each at an angle of 60 degrees to the middle limb. Deepen all three incisions through the subcutaneous tissue and fascia and undermine widely the two triangular flaps thus created. Transpose each flap to the original bed of the opposite flap, and suture the free edges of the skin.

Repeat the operation two or more times, allowing the wound to heal after each, until the area of constricture has been lengthened throughout its circumference.

TECHNIQUE (PEET). Remove the entire constricture by circumferential excision of the skin and subcutaneous tissue down to the deep fascia (Fig. 61-2). If the limb tapers, curve the distal incision in a serpentine line so that its length is about the same as that of the proximal one. Then undermine the skin and subcutaneous tissue on each side of the excised area. Approximate the deep tissues with interrupted sutures. Approximate the skin edges with interrupted mattress sutures except in one area; in this area lengthen the edges of the skin with one or more Z-plasties, the limbs of which are approximately 2 cm long. Raise and transpose the triangular flaps and suture them in position with small interrupted sutures.

AFTERTREATMENT. A pressure bandage is applied from proximal to the area of surgery to the distal end of the limb. With young children a cast or plaster splint is applied and worn until the incision has healed.

ANOMALIES OF TOES

The most common anomaly of the toes is polydactyly, that is, the presence of supernumerary digits; others are syndactyly (webbed toes), macrodactyly (enlarged toes),

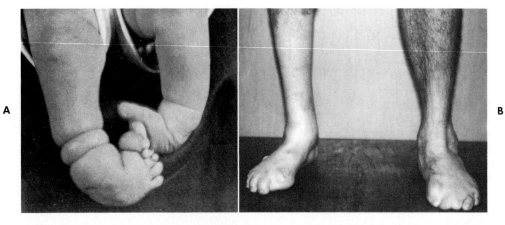

Fig. 61-1. A, Congenital constrictures of one leg and great toe and bilateral clubfoot. **B,** Adult with loss of several toes caused by congenital constrictures.

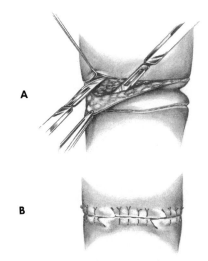

Fig. 61-2. Congenital constricture. **A,** Excision of constricture and undermining of skin edges. **B,** Skin edges have been sutured except in two areas where Z-plastic incisions have been made. (Redrawn from Peet, E.W.: In Rob, C., and Smith, R., editors: Operative surgery, Part 10, London, 1959, Butterworth & Co., Ltd.)

and congenital contracture or angulation. Any of these may require surgery.

When surgery is being contemplated for anomalies of the toes, several factors must be considered, including cosmesis, pain, and difficulty in fitting shoes. A satisfactory clinical result should correct all of these problems.

Polydactyly

Polydactyly of the toes may occur in established genetic syndromes, but occurs most commonly as an isolated trait with an autosomal dominant inheritance pattern and variable expression (Fig. 61-3). The overall incidence of polydactyly is approximately two cases per 1000 live births.

Surgical treatment of polydactyly is amputation of the accessory digit. Preoperative roentgenograms should be obtained to detect any extra metatarsal articulating with the digit.

TECHNIQUE OF AMPUTATING EXTRA TOE. At the base of the toe to be amputated make an oval or racquet-shaped incision through the skin and fascia (Fig. 61-4). Draw the tendons distally as far as possible and divide them. Incise the capsule of the metatarsophalangeal joint transversely, dissect it from the metatarsal, and disarticulate the joint. With an osteotome or bone-cutting forceps resect any bone that may have protruded from the metatarsal head to support the articular surface of the amputated phalanx. If the roentgenogram has revealed an extra metatarsal, resect it after continuing the incision proximally on the lateral or dorsal aspect of the foot.

Syndactyly

Syndactyly of the toes rarely interferes with function, and surgery is indicated for cosmetic reasons only. The same technique is used as for the fingers (Chapter 16).

Macrodactyly

Macrodactyly occurs when one or more toes or fingers have hypertrophied and are significantly larger than the surrounding toes or fingers (Fig. 61-5). The most common associated condition is neurofibromatosis, with occasional hemangiomatosis or plantar hamartomatous fat. Surgery is indicated to relieve functional symptoms, primarily pain or difficulty in fitting shoes. The cosmetic goal is to alter the grotesque appearance of the toes and foot and to achieve a foot similar in size to the opposite foot.

Many operative procedures have been described for the treatment of macrodactyly, including reduction syndactyly, soft tissue debulking combined with ostectomy or epiphysiodesis, toe amputation, and ray amputation. Reduction syndactyly may be used as a primary operative procedure when macrodactyly involves the great toe and second toe. Soft tissue debulking combined with ostectomy or epiphysiodesis may be used in the initial treatment of a single digit with macrodactyly. Unfortunately, recurrence following this technique is virtually 100%. Ray amputation is indicated in patients with massive enlargement of the bone and soft tissues and, of course, is not followed by recurrence. Ray amputation is also the procedure of choice for

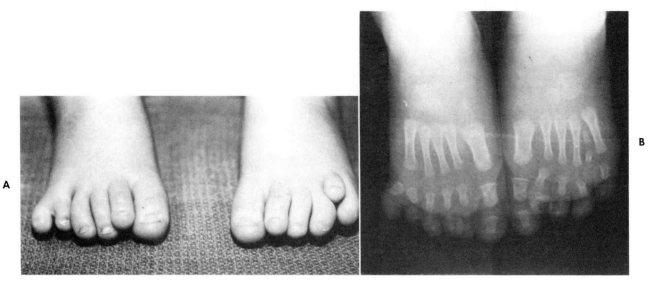

Fig. 61-3. Polydactyly. **A,** Preoperative photograph of feet with polydactyly. **B,** Preoperative roentgenogram of same feet.

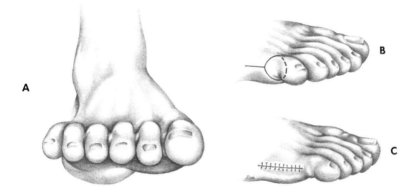

Fig. 61-4. Polydactyly. **A,** Frontal view of foot with polydactyly. **B,** Outline of incision passing through web space between fifth and sixth toes and extending in racquet-shaped incision along lateral border of foot. **C,** Surgical excision of supernumerary digit completed and incision closed.

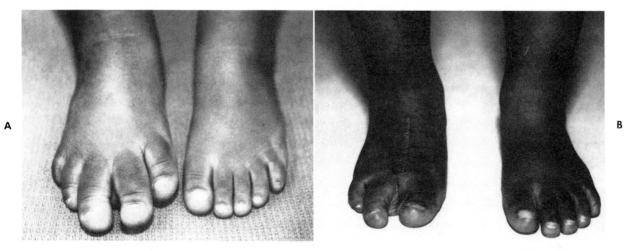

Fig. 61-5. Macrodactyly. **A,** Preoperative foot with macrodactyly. **B,** Foot after excision of second and third rays.

recurrence after reduction syndactyly or soft tissue debulking.

TECHNIQUE (DIAMOND AND GOULD). With their apices at the bases of the first and second metatarsals, make identical V-shaped incisions on the dorsal and plantar aspects of the foot and extend them distally in the midsagittal plane of the great and second toes (Fig. 61-6). Now deepen the incisions and remove a central wedge of tissue as a block, including the skin and the underlying parts of the phalanges and metatarsals that are in line with the incisions. If necessary realign the first metatarsal by a distal osteotomy to decrease the space between the first and second rays; transfix the osteotomy with a Kirschner wire. Next excise any bony prominences along the remainder of both metatarsals. Appose the bone and soft tissue surfaces with deep interrupted sutures. Also suture together the adjacent

capsules of the metatarsophalangeal joints. Excise any nail beds that interfere with skin closure or might cause pressure on an adjoining toe. Next secure hemostasis and close the skin and subcutaneous tissues with interrupted sutures. Apply a bulky dressing and a heavy plaster splint.

AFTERTREATMENT. After the skin has healed, a short leg cast is applied and is worn until any osteotomy has healed.

TECHNIQUE OF RAY AMPUTATION. Outline the ray to be amputated with skin flaps to include amputation from the tip of the toe to the base of the metatarsal. Make dorsal and plantar incisions starting over the metatarsophalangeal joint with connecting incisions in the web space of adjacent toes. Continue the incisions proximally, both dorsally and plantarward, to the base of the metatarsal to be resected (Fig. 61-7). Amputate the metatarsal and its associated phalanges, as well as any surrounding hypertrophied

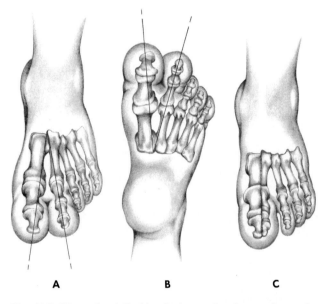

A   B   C

Fig. 61-6. Diamond and Gould reduction syndactyly operation to decrease size of great and second toes. **A** and **B,** Dorsal and plantar views of foot showing identical V-shaped incisions (see text). **C,** Dorsal view after reduction syndactyly operation. (Redrawn from Diamond, L.S., and Gould, V.E.: South. Med. J. **67:**645, 1974. Reprinted by permission from the Southern Medical Journal.)

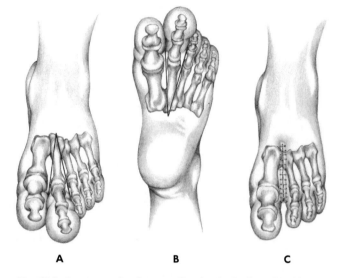

A   B   C

Fig. 61-7. Ray amputation for macrodactyly. **A,** Outline of incision on dorsal surface of foot. **B,** Plantar incision. **C,** Closed incision after amputation.

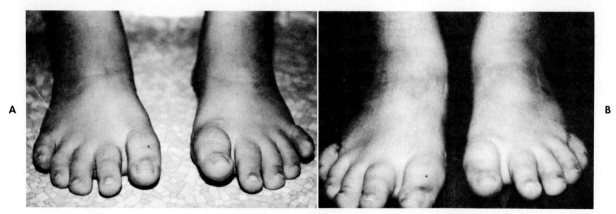

Fig. 61-8. Congenital contracture of fifth toe. **A,** Preoperative photograph of congenital contracture of the fifth toes. **B,** Postoperative photograph following Lapidus procedure for correction of dorsal overlapping of toes.

soft tissue. Take care to protect the neurovascular bundles that supply adjacent toes. After adequate resection of tissue, close the wound with interrupted sutures in the usual manner.

AFTERTREATMENT. A short leg cast is applied to protect the wound until healing occurs at 3 weeks.

Contracture or angulation

Congenital hammertoe and claw toe can be treated by the techniques described in Chapters 35 and 66.

Congenital contracture, angulation, or subluxation of the fifth toe is a fairly common familial deformity but causes disability in only about half of the patients concerned. The phalanges of the fifth toe are externally rotated, and the metatarsophalangeal joint is dorsally contracted so that the fifth toe overlaps the fourth (Fig. 61-8, *A*). It may also be somewhat adducted at the proximal interphalangeal joint. The anomaly is rarely disabling, and surgery is usually indicated only to improve the appearance of the foot. The direction of angulation of the fifth toe determines the operative procedure.

Lapidus described an operation for correction of hyperextension of the fifth toe when it is in either neutral position otherwise or overlapping the fourth toe (Fig. 61-8, *B*).

TECHNIQUE (LAPIDUS). Make a longitudinal bayonet-shaped incision, coursing first along the dorsomedial aspect of the fifth toe from the distal interphalangeal joint to the web between the fifth and the fourth toes, then laterally over the dorsum of the fifth metatarsophalangeal joint, and then proximally along the lateral aspect of the head of the fifth metatarsal. Flex the toe to tighten its long extensor tendon. Now make a second incision dorsally and transversely 1 cm long over the middle of the fifth metatarsal. Through this second incision identify the long extensor tendon, cut it transversely, and retract its distal part through the first incision. Then completely free this part of the tendon distally to its insertion on the distal phalanx.

By blunt dissection expose the capsule of the fifth metatarsophalangeal joint and incise it transversely on its dorsal and medial aspects to relieve the contracture of the capsule and of the medial collateral ligament. Now make a channel through the soft tissues; start it near the distal interphalangeal joint on the dorsomedial aspect of the fifth toe, wind it around the plantar aspect of the toe proximally and laterally, and end it on the plantar lateral aspect of the fifth metatarsophalangeal joint. Pass the end of the freed tendon proximally through this tunnel. Split the abductor and short flexor of the fifth toe longitudinally and then suture the long extensor tendon through these two tendons under enough tension to correct all components of the deformity. Close the skin with interrupted sutures, shifting its edges as necessary to correct any severe contracture.

AFTERTREATMENT. The toe is immobilized for 3 to 4 weeks on a short aluminum splint loosely applied. Walking is allowed in a shoe cut out over the fifth toe.

• • •

In another technique McFarland resected the base of the proximal phalanx and after excising enough skin produced an artificial syndactyly between the fourth and fifth toes. Scrase of Birmingham, England, reported 39 good results in 42 patients so treated. Kelikian et al. also have found the procedure satisfactory.

TECHNIQUE (KELIKIAN ET AL.). Fashion cruciate incisions between the two toes to be syndactylized (Fig. 61-9). Begin the first incision on the dorsal surface of the web proximal

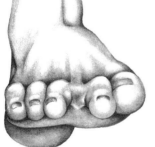

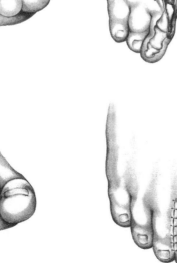

Fig. 61-9. Technique of Kelikian, Clayton, and Loseff, similar to McFarland's, for creating artificial syndactyly in contracture or angulation of toes. **A,** Skin incisions have been made and triangular flaps of plantar skin will be excised from adjacent surfaces of each toe (see text). **B,** Base of proximal phalanx of each toe has been excised. **C,** Skin edges are being approximated. **D,** Surgical syndactyly has been completed. (Redrawn from Kelikian, H., Clayton, L., and Loseff, H.: Clin. **19:**208, 1961.)

to the base of the toes and carry it between the toes over the middle of the web and then proximally on the plantar surface of the foot to the level of the metatarsal heads. Then on the adjacent surfaces of the two toes make longitudinal incisions that bisect the first incision. Carry these incisions to the tips of the toes if the deformity to be corrected involves the distal interphalangeal joints. Now resect triangular flaps of plantar skin from the adjacent surfaces of each toe. Excise as much of the base of the proximal phalanx of the deformed toe or of both toes as is necessary for easy closure (Fig. 61-9, *B*). Secure hemostasis and suture the dorsal and plantar skin margins to produce an artificial syndactyly (Fig. 61-9, *C* and *D*).

AFTERTREATMENT. A pressure dressing is applied. At 2 weeks the sutures are removed, and 2 or 3 days later weight bearing is allowed.

Straub reports that congenital subluxation of the fifth toe (Fig. 61-10, *A*) can be consistently and satisfactorily corrected by the technique of Ruiz-Mora.

TECHNIQUE (RUIZ-MORA). Excise an elliptic segment of skin and subcutaneous tissue from the plantar surface of the fifth toe and the adjacent metatarsal area as shown in Fig. 61-10, *B*. Curving the proximal end of the ellipse medially makes the fifth toe approximate the fourth more closely after operation. Now excise the proximal phalanx and close the deep tissues by two subcutaneous sutures. Then close the skin by three interrupted sutures placed as shown in Fig. 61-10, *C*.

Janecki and Wilde reported that the shortening of the fifth toe produced by excision of the entire proximal pha-

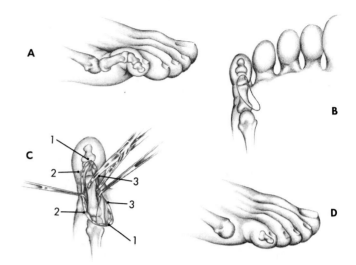

Fig. 61-10. Ruiz-Mora operation to correct congenital contracture of fifth toe. **A,** Deformity. **B,** Ellipse of skin has been excised from plantar surface of toe and foot. **C,** Proximal phalanx of toe is being excised. In closing skin, point *1* is sutured to point *1*, *2* to *2*, and *3* to *3*. **D,** Appearance of toe after surgery. (Redrawn from Straub, L.R.: In Cecil, R.L., editor: The specialties in general practice, Philadelphia, 1951, W.B. Saunders Co.)

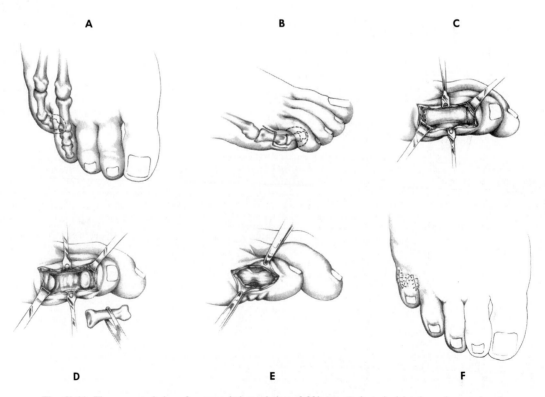

Fig. 61-11. Thompson technique for congenital angulation of fifth toe. Z-plasty incision is made over dorsal aspect of toe, proximal phalanx is excised, and skin flaps are rotated and closed. (Redrawn from Thompson, T.C.: J. Bone Joint Surg. **46-A:**1117, 1964.)

lanx resulted in a painful prominence of the head of the fifth metatarsal in 23% of these feet. In 32% a painful hammertoe deformity of the fourth toe developed. Consequently they recommend excising only the head and neck of the proximal phalanx.

Cockin of Oxford, England, reported good results in 70 feet in which Butler's operation for dorsally adducted fifth toe was performed. A double-handle racquet incision is made about the base of the fifth toe, one handle being longitudinal and dorsal and the other longitudinal and plantar. Dorsal and plantar capsulotomies of the metatarsophalangeal joint, tenotomy of the extensor tendon of the toe at the metatarsophalangeal joint, and plastic closure of the racquet incision are carried out.

For fifth toe plantar constrictures, Thompson recommends making a Z-plasty skin incision over the dorsal aspect of the fifth toe, excising the proximal phalanx, and rotating and closing the skin flaps (Fig. 61-11).

Congenital hallux varus

Hallux varus is a deformity in which the great toe is angulated medially at the metatarsophalangeal joint. It should not be confused with varus deformity of the first metatarsal (metatarsus primus varus) in which the metatarsophalangeal joint is not deformed. The varus deformity of the toe varies in severity from only a few degrees to as much as 90 degrees.

Hallux varus is usually unilateral and is associated with one or more of the following: (1) a short, thick first metatarsal, (2) accessory bones or toes, (3) varus deformity of one or more of the four lateral metatarsals, and (4) a firm fibrous band that extends from the medial side of the great toe to the base of the first metatarsal.

The explanation for this anomaly is that two great toes originate in utero but the medial or accessory one fails to develop. Later the rudimentary medial toe together with the band of fibrous tissue acts like a taut bowstring and gradually pulls the more fully developed great toe into a varus position.

The proper treatment for congenital hallux varus depends on the severity of the deformity and the rigidity of the contracted soft structures. The Farmer technique is effective in correcting mild or moderate deformity (Fig. 61-12). The operation of Kelikian et al. is also satisfactory (Fig. 61-13). When the deformity is complicated by traumatic arthritis of the metatarsophalangeal joint, arthrodesis of this joint as described by McKeever (p. 886) is indicated. When the deformity is too severe to be either corrected or fused, amputation is indicated.

TECHNIQUE (FARMER). Raise a broad Y-shaped flap of skin and subcutaneous tissue from the dorsal surface of the web between the first and second toes; base the flap dorsally in the space between the first and second metatarsals and include in it the skin contiguous with the web distally along

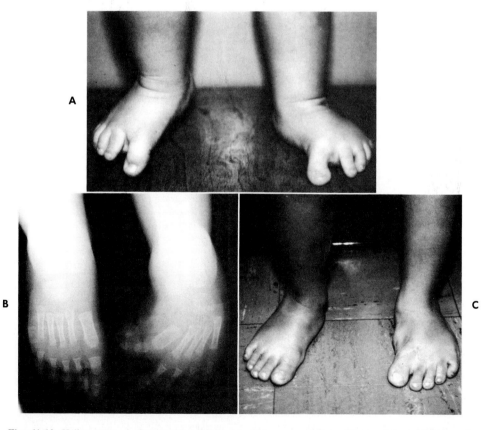

Fig. 61-12. Hallux varus. **A,** Preoperative photograph. Note varus position of the great toe with increased web space between great and second toes. **B,** Preoperative roentgenogram. **C,** Photograph following Farmer procedure.

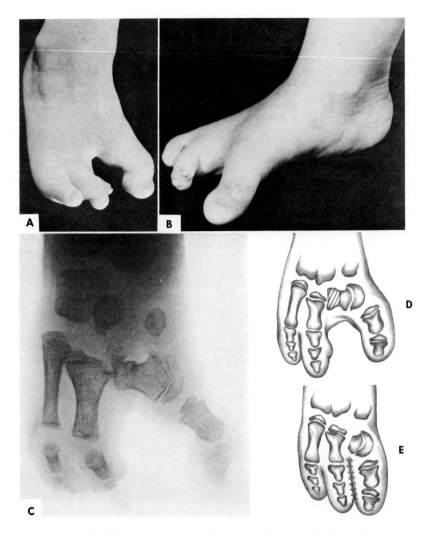

Fig. 61-13. Operation of Kelikian, Clayton, and Loseff to create artificial syndactyly as applied to congenital hallux varus. **A** and **B,** Photographs of foot before surgery. **C,** Anteroposterior roentgenogram of foot before surgery. **D,** Tracing of roentgenogram showing segment *(striped)* of first metatarsal to be resected. **E,** Drawing of foot after resection of segment of first metatarsal and creation of syndactyly between medial two toes. (From Kelikian, H., Clayton, L., and Loseff, H.: Clin. Orthop. **19:**208, 1961.)

the two toes for one third their length (Fig. 61-14). From the medial edge of the base of the flap curve the incision medially and slightly distally across the medial aspect of the first metatarsophalangeal joint. Deepen this incision transversely through the medial part of the capsule of the first metatarsophalangeal joint. Then move the great toe laterally against the second toe and create a syndactyly between these two toes by suturing the apposing skin edges together. Excise any accessory phalanx or hypertrophic soft tissue from the great toe through a separate dorsomedial incision. Now swing the Y-shaped flap of skin and subcutaneous tissue medially and suture it in place to cover the defect in the skin on the dorsal and medial aspects of the first metatarsophalangeal joint.

Farmer described an alternative technique in which the Y-shaped flap of skin and subcutaneous tissue is raised from the plantar surface of the foot (Fig. 61-15); the same procedure is then performed, the flap being swung medi-

ally to cover the defect in the skin at the first metatarsophalangeal joint. Any defect that cannot be closed by the flap is either left open to heal secondarily or is covered by a full-thickness skin graft.

AFTERTREATMENT. The foot is immobilized in a cast. At 3 weeks the cast is removed, and full activities are allowed.

ANOMALIES OF FOOT
Congenital metatarsus adductus

Metatarsus adductus consisting of adduction of the forefoot in relation to the midfoot and hindfoot (Fig. 61-16) is a fairly common anomaly, often causing in-toeing in children. It may occur as an isolated anomaly or in association with clubfoot. Of those with metatarsus adductus, 1% to 5% also have congenital hip or acetabular dysplasia.

Clinically, metatarsus adductus may be classified as mild, moderate, or severe. In the mild form the forefoot

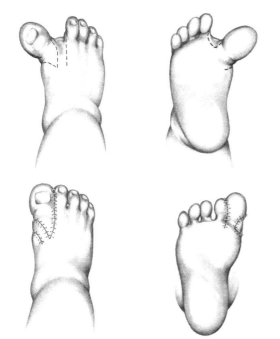

Fig. 61-14. Farmer operation for congenital hallux varus (see text). (From Farmer, A.W.: Am J. Surg. **95**:274, 1958.)

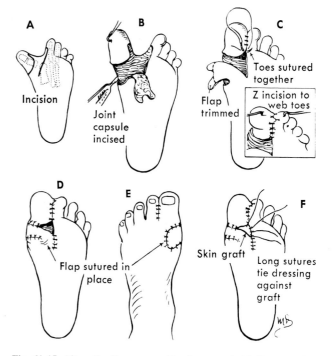

Fig. 61-15. Alternative Farmer operation for congenital hallux varus (see text). (From Farmer, A.W.: Am. J. Surg. **95**:274, 1958.)

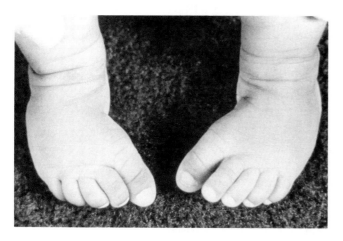

Fig. 61-16. Metatarsus adductus in 6 month old child.

can be clinically abducted to the midline of the foot and beyond. The moderate form has enough flexibility to allow abduction of the forefoot to the midline, but usually not beyond. In rigid metatarsus adductus, the forefoot cannot be abducted at all. There may also be a transverse crease on the medial border of the foot or an enlargement of the web space between the great and second toes. In general, mild metatarsus adductus will resolve without treatment. Moderate or severe metatarsus adductus is best treated initially by serial stretching and casting until the foot is clinically flexible.

As already mentioned metatarsus adductus may be seen as a residual deformity in patients previously treated for congenital clubfoot, either surgically or nonsurgically.

This residual metatarsus adductus may be rigid, indicating a fixed positioning of the forefoot on the midfoot and hindfoot, or it may be dynamic caused by imbalance of the tibialis anterior tendon during gait. The rigidity or flexibility of the forefoot should be determined before undertaking any surgical correction in the older child.

SURGICAL TREATMENT

In the young child surgery is not indicated until conservative treatment has failed. Once a child passes the appropriate age for serial stretching and casting, surgery becomes a reasonable option. The indications for surgery include pain, objectional appearance, or difficulty in fitting shoes because of residual forefoot adduction.

Numerous soft tissue and bony procedures have been described for correction of metatarsus adductus. We prefer to tailor the surgery to the age and deformity of the particular child.

Lichtblau described division of the abductor hallucis tendon for early correction of metatarsus adductus, especially following treatment for clubfoot. This procedure is indicated infrequently because one can rarely be confident that release of the tendon will correct the deformity. In 1958 Heyman, Herndon, and Strong described mobilization of the tarsometatarsal and intermetatarsal joints by capsular release for correction of metatarsus adductus. This is the procedure of choice in a preschool age child. Potential complications of the procedure include subluxation of the bases of the metatarsals and injury to the small joints of the midfoot and forefoot.

In children 5 years old and older with a residual rigid metatarsus adductus, metatarsal osteotomy is the procedure of choice. Berman and Gartland described dome-shaped osteotomies made at the bases of the metatarsals for this situation. Full correction may also require small lateral closing wedge osteotomies.

For children with dynamic metatarsus adductus from imbalance of the tibialis anterior tendon, especially after treatment for congenital clubfoot, we recommend either a split transfer of the tibialis anterior tendon or transfer of the entire tendon to the middle cuneiform if symptoms are sufficient to require surgery.

TECHNIQUE (LICHTBLAU). Make a medial longitudinal incision 2.5 cm long over the head and neck of the first metatarsal. Next abduct the forefoot to place the tendon of the abductor hallucis under tension and make it prominent. Slip a small hemostat beneath the entire tendon. Next di-

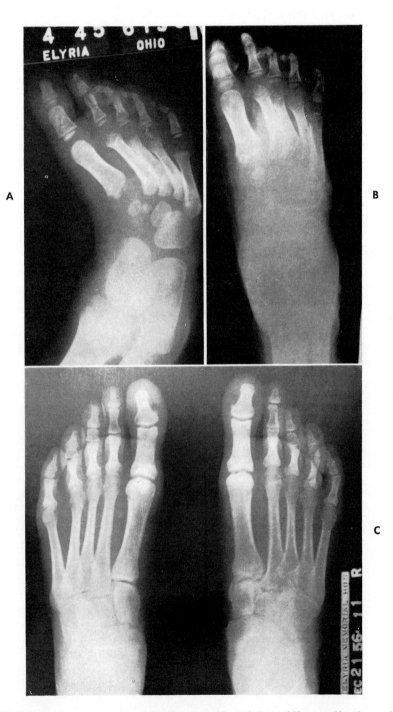

Fig. 61-17. Congenital metatarsus varus of right foot treated by technique of Heyman, Herndon, and Strong. **A,** Right foot of 5-year-old boy before surgery. **B,** Same foot 7 weeks after surgery. **C,** Both feet 11 years and 4 months after surgery. (From Heyman, C.H., Herndon, C.H., and Strong, J.M.: J. Bone Joint Surg. **40-A:**299, 1958.)

vide the tendon distally and again abduct the forefoot to be sure that all of the fibers of the tendon have been cut; do not disturb the muscle itself. Close the wound with interrupted sutures and apply a plaster cast with the foot in the corrected position.

AFTERTREATMENT. The cast is worn from 3 to 10 weeks. Following removal of the cast, the foot may be held corrected in straight-last shoes for 6 months.

• • •

In 1970 Kendrick, Sharma, Hassler, and Herndon reviewed 80 feet treated by capsular releases at the metatarsal bases, and the result was good or excellent in 92%. They recommend the operation for children 3 to 8 years of age. The indications for the operation are (1) residual adduction of the forefoot after correction of the varus deformity of the hindfoot and equinus deformity of the ankle in clubfoot and (2) recurrent or untreated deformity in pa-

tients in this age group (Fig. 61-17). The operation may also be indicated to correct adduction of the forefoot in a serpentine foot as a second procedure after correction of the deformity in the hindfoot.

TECHNIQUE (KENDRICK ET AL.). Make a curved dorsal incision across the full width of the foot just distal to the tarsometatarsal joints. Two straight incisions may be used instead, one between the first and second metatarsals and the second in line with the fourth metatarsal (Fig. 61-18, *A*). With gentle care for the skin edges free the extensor hallucis longus and the extensor digitorum longus of the second toe and retract them medially and laterally, respectively. Protect the neurovascular bundle between the bases of the first and second metatarsals. Now identify the intermetatarsal space by probing with a small hemostat and sharply divide the intermetatarsal ligament between the first and second metatarsals from distally to proximally. Locate and divide the dorsal capsule of the first tarsometa-

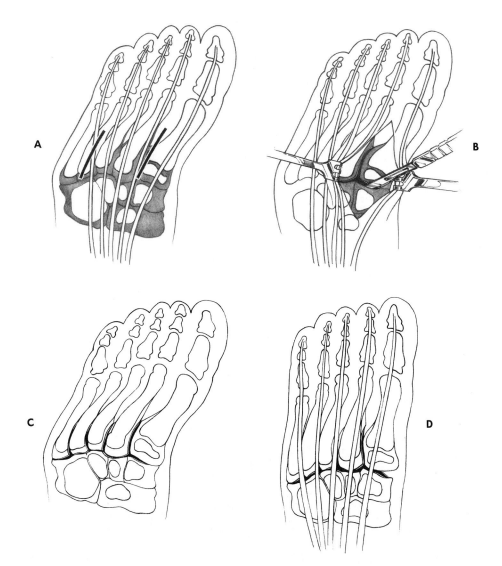

Fig. 61-18. Technique of Kendrick, Sharma, Hassler, and Herndon for correcting congenital metatarsus adductus (see text). (Redrawn from Kendrick, R.E., Sharma, N.K., Hassler, W.L., and Herndon, C.H.: J. Bone Joint Surg. **52-A:**61, 1970.)

tarsal joint, avoiding damage to the articular surfaces of the bones. Protect the tibialis anterior tendon and divide sharply the medial capsule of the first tarsometatarsal joint, leaving only the plantar capsule of this joint intact (Fig. 61-18, *B*). Next identify the second tarsometatarsal joint a little proximal to the first and divide its dorsal capsule. Dissect longitudinally over the third metatarsal, protecting the neurovascular bundles and the extensor tendons, to reach the intermetatarsal space between the second and third metatarsals. Divide the intermetatarsal ligament here also and incise the dorsal capsule of the third tarsometatarsal joint. By similar incisions free the bases of the other metatarsals, leaving the plantar capsules intact (Fig. 61-18, *C*). Preserve the lateral capsule of the fifth tarsometatarsal joint to serve as a hinge and to prevent lateral displacement of the base of the fifth metatarsal. While plantar flexing each metatarsal and applying traction, and using care not

to damage the articular surfaces, divide the medial two thirds of the plantar capsule of each joint, leaving the lateral one third intact. Enough stability should be retained to prevent displacement of the metatarsal bases when the bones are properly aligned. Now abduct the metatarsals to their normal positions (Fig. 61-18, *D*), but do not be concerned tht the articular surfaces are irregular because they will remodel with time. Next secure hemostasis and close the incision. Apply a well-molded short leg cast with the foot in the corrected position. When the metatarsal bases are unstable, we have used Kirschner wires to fix the first metatarsal base to the first cuneiform and the fifth to the cuboid. Thus position will not be lost during changes of the cast.

AFTERTREATMENT. At 3 weeks when the wound has healed, the cast is changed and the sutures are removed. A carefully molded short leg cast should be worn for about

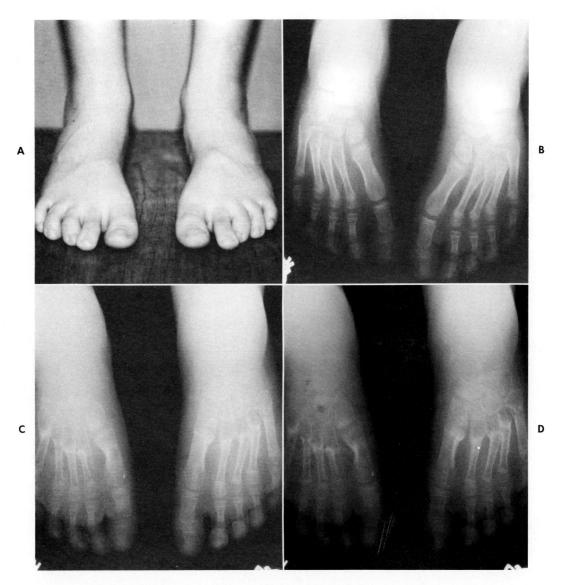

Fig. 61-19. Metatarsus adductus. **A,** Metatarsus adductus in 8-year-old child. **B,** Roentgenogram before metatarsal osteotomies. **C** and **D,** Roentgenograms after metatarsal osteotomies.

4 months. Complications after surgery have been few. Occasionally there is slight dorsal subluxation of the proximal end of the first metatarsal or lateral prominence of the base of the fifth metatarsal. Preservation of one third of each plantar capsule should prevent these deformities. Damage to the articular surfaces must be avoided to minimize early stiffening of the forefoot and osteoarthritis in later life.

• • •

Berman and Gartland have recommended dome-shaped osteotomies for all five metatarsal bases for resistant forefoot adduction in children 5 years of age or older regardless of the cause (Fig. 61-19).

For the mature foot with uncorrected metatarsus varus, because all of the medial structures are shortened, they recommend a laterally based closing wedge osteotomy through the bases of the metatarsals and through the cuneiforms and the cuboid. Correcting the alignment without shortening the lateral border of the foot will cause excessive tension on the skin on the medial border or on the neurovascular bundle posterior to the medial malleolus. Steinmann pins inserted parallel to the medial and lateral borders of the foot are usually necessary to hold the foot in the corrected position until the osteotomy has healed. Without internal fixation the tight structures on the medial side may cause recurrence of deformity and nonunion of the osteotomy.

TECHNIQUE (BERMAN AND GARTLAND). Approach all five metatarsal bases dorsally. Make two longitudinal dorsal incisions, one between the first and second metatarsals and the other overlying the fourth. Protect the extensor tendons and superficial nerves and preserve the superficial veins as much as possible. Next expose subperiosteally the proximal metaphysis of each metatarsal and with a small power drill make a dome-shaped osteotomy in each with the apex of the dome proximally (Fig. 61-20). Avoid the epiphyseal plate at the base of the first metatarsal. When adequate correction cannot be obtained by these osteotomies, resect small wedges of bone based laterally at the osteotomies as needed. Align the metatarsals and transfix the foot in the corrected position with small unthreaded Steinmann pins

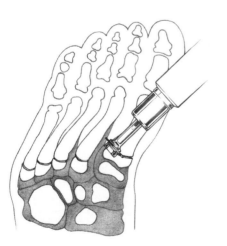

Fig. 61-20. Berman and Gartland technique for metatarsal osteotomy. Dome-shaped osteotomy is being completed at base of each metatarsal.

inserted proximally through the shafts of the first and fifth metatarsals and across the osteotomies in these bones. Prevent dorsal or volar angulation and overriding of the fragments. Before closing the wound check the placement of the pins and position of the osteotomies by roentgenograms.

AFTERTREATMENT. A short leg cast is applied with the foot in the corrected position. At 6 weeks the cast and pins are removed and weight bearing is begun, commonly in a walking cast for a few weeks. Complications from this operation have been few. Exposure is better through a single curved incision, but small skin sloughs occasionally occur, so we prefer two dorsal longitudinal incisions.

Congenital clubfoot (equinovarus foot)

The incidence of congenital clubfoot is approximately 1 in every 1,000 live births. Although most cases are sporadic occurrences, families have been reported with clubfoot presenting as an autosomal dominant trait with incomplete penetrance. Bilateral deformities occur in 50% of patients.

Several theories have been proposed regarding the cause of clubfoot. One is that a primary germ plasm defect in the talus causes continued plantar flexion and inversion of this bone with subsequent soft tissue changes in the joints and musculotendinous complexes. Another theory is that primary soft tissue abnormalities within the neuromuscular units cause secondary bony changes. Clinically children with clubfoot have a hypotrophic anterior tibial artery, in addition to the obvious atrophy of the musculature about the calf, in both the anterior and posterior compartments. The abnormal foot may be as much as a half to one size smaller in both length and width.

The pathologic changes caused by congenital clubfoot (equinovarus foot) must be understood if the anomaly is to be treated effectively. The deformity varies in severity from one in which the entire foot is in an equinus and varus position, the forefoot is in adduction, and there is a cavus deformity to one much less severe in which the foot is in only a mild equinus and varus position (Fig. 61-21). It is often accompanied by internal tibial torsion. In a typical clubfoot changes in the soft structures consist chiefly of contractures of the more medially located plantar ligaments, the deltoid ligament, the tibialis posterior tendon, the abductor hallucis, the tendo calcaneus, the medial and plantar parts of the capsules of the tarsometatarsal and tarsal joints (including the plantar calcaneonavicular [spring] ligament and the master knot of Henry where the flexor hallucis longus and flexor digitorum longus cross), the posterior part of the ankle joint capsule, the posterior capsule of the subtalar joint, and commonly the tibialis anterior tendon. Sometimes one or more tendons, such as the tibialis anterior or the peroneals, are inserted abnormally so that they exert deforming forces.

The chief deformities of the tarsals involve the talus, calcaneus, navicular, and cuboid. The calcaneus is in a varus position and its distal end is displaced medially. Its proximal end is displaced upward and laterally. The talus is deviated medially and plantarward, sometimes so severely that part of its articular surface lies outside the ankle mortise. The navicular is displaced medially and is rotated

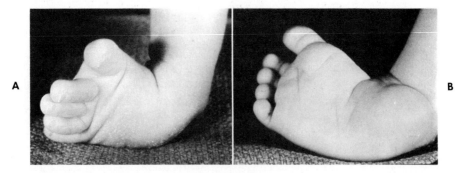

Fig. 61-21. Congenital clubfoot. **A,** Newborn with left clubfoot. Note forefoot supination and adduction as well as increased web space between great and second toes. **B,** Plantar view. Note transverse crease at junction of midfoot and forefoot indicating rigidity. Note inversion and plantar flexion of the calcaneus with skin cleft proximal to calcaneus.

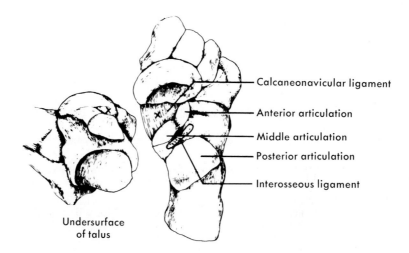

Fig. 61-22. Talocalcaneonavicular joint (see text). (From Turco, V.J.: In American Academy of Orthopaedic Surgeons: Instructional course lectures, vol. 24, St. Louis, 1975, The C.V. Mosby Co.)

so that it articulates only with the inferior and medial aspects of the head of the talus. It may abut against the medial malleolus and form a false joint. In turn the head of the talus is prominent subcutaneously on the dorsum of the foot. The cuboid may be displaced medially on the calcaneus so that its surface, which would normally articulate with the calcaneus, abuts instead against the medial nonarticular surface of the distal end of the bone; contracture of the soft structures may fix the cuboid in this position and alter the contour of the distal end of the calcaneus. Most of the joints of this complex of four tarsal bones and their supporting ligaments and capsules have been termed the talocalcaneonavicular joint (Fig. 61-22). As described by Turco, there are three talocalcaneal articulations: the anterior, middle, and posterior. The talocalcaneal interosseous ligament divides the anterior and posterior compartments of the subtalar joint. The posterior compartment is occupied by the convex posterior facet of the calcaneus and the concave articulation beneath the body of the talus. The anterior compartment includes the anterior and middle facets of the calcaneus and the plantar calcaneonavicular

(spring) ligament, supporting the head of the talus. This is a ball-and-socket complex, and most of the movement in the talocalcaneonavicular joint occurs here. The articulation is unusual in that the head of the talus remains fixed and is the pivotal point around which the concave surface of the inferior part of this complex moves. This socket for the head of the talus includes dorsomedially the navicular, the talonavicular capsule, the diltoid ligament, and the tibialis posterior tendon. Plantarward there is the plantar calcaneonavicular (spring) ligament and laterally the bifurcated (Y) ligament that extends from the calcaneus to the cuboid and navicular. Posteriorly the socket is completed by the talocalcaneal interosseous ligament. In the equinovarus position this bone and soft tissue socket is displaced medially and plantarward and the soft tissues contract, making the socket smaller. The socket is then not large enough to accommodate the head of the talus unless it is enlarged by passive stretching or by soft tissue release.

The metatarsals often are also deformed. They may deviate at their tarsometatarsal joints, or these joints may be

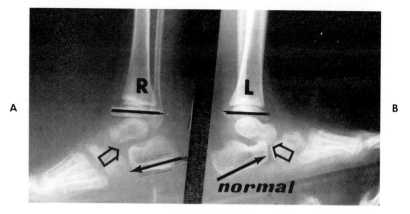

Fig. 61-23. Lateral roentgenogram of foot held in dorsiflexion. Lines drawn parallel to articular surface of distal tibia and through long axis of calcaneus. **A,** Clubfoot. Dorsiflexion of calcaneus is absent, two lines are almost parallel, and head of talus and distal end of calcaneus do not overlap. **B,** Normal foot. Dorsiflexion of calcaneus is present, two lines are not nearly parallel, and head of talus and distal end of calcaneus overlap. (From Turco, V.J.: In American Academy of Orthopaedic Surgeons: Instructional course lectures, vol. 24, St. Louis, 1975, The C.V. Mosby Co.)

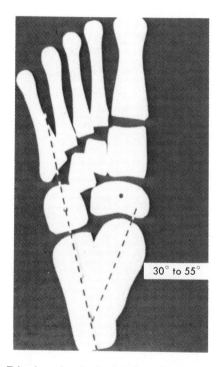

Fig. 61-24. Talocalcaneal angle. Angle is formed by lines drawn through long axis of talus and calcaneus. It normally varies from 30 to 55 degrees. (From LeNoir, J.L.: Orthop. Rev. **5**:35, February 1976.)

normal and the shafts of the metatarsals themselves may be adducted.

If the clubfoot is allowed to remain deformed, many other late adaptive changes occur in the bones. These changes depend on the severity of the soft tissue contractures and the effects of walking. Some of the joints may spontaneously fuse, or they may develop degenerative changes secondary to the contractures.

The initial examination of the foot and the progress of treatment should depend on both clinical judgment and roentgenographic examination. A standard roentgenographic technique is essential, and the technician should be carefully instructed in its use.

ROENTGENOGRAPHIC EVALUATION

Roentgenograms should be included as part of the evaluation of clubfoot, before, during, and after treatment. In the nonambulatory child, standard roentgenograms include anteroposterior and stress dorsiflexion lateral roentgenograms of both feet.

Important angles to consider in the evaluation of clubfoot are the talocalcaneal angle on the anteroposterior roentgenogram (Fig. 61-23), the talocalcaneal angle on the lateral roentgenogram, the tibiocalcaneal angle on the stress lateral roentgenogram (Fig. 61-24), and the talometatarsal angle. The anteroposterior talocalcaneal angle in the normal child ranges from 30 to 55 degrees. In clubfoot, this angle progressively decreases with increasing heel varus. On the lateral stress dorsiflexion roentgenogram the talocalcaneal angle in the normal foot varies from 25 to 50 degrees; in clubfoot, this angle progressively decreases with the severity of the deformity to an angle of zero. The sum of these two angles (anteroposterior talocalcaneal and lateral talocalcaneal) is known as the talocalcaneal index and should be at least 40 degrees. The tibiocalcaneal angle on the stress lateral roentgenogram is 5 to 15 degrees in the normal foot. In clubfoot this angle is generally negative, indicating equinus of the calcaneus in relation to the tibia. Finally, the talometatarsal angle is a roentgenographic measurement of forefoot adduction. This is useful in the treatment of metatarsus adductus alone, but is equally important in the treatment of clubfoot to evaluate the position of the forefoot. In a normal foot, this angle is 5 to 15 degrees; in clubfoot, it is zero or negative, indicating adduction of the forefoot.

The importance of the roentgenographic findings and

the measurement of angles in clubfoot cannot be overstated. The angles correlate well with the clinical appearance of the foot and with the result following nonsurgical and surgical treatment. Adequate roentgenograms must be obtained during treatment to be certain that the foot is not only corrected clinically but roentgenographically as well.

NONSURGICAL METHODS OF TREATMENT

The initial treatment of clubfoot is nonsurgical. Various treatment regimens have been proposed, including the use of corrective splinting, taping, and casting. Our treatment consists of weekly serial manipulation and casting during the first 6 weeks of life (Fig. 61-25), followed by manipulation and casting every other week until the foot is clinically and roentgenographically corrected.

In our experience about 50% of clubfeet can be treated successfully by serial manipulation and casting, with the remainder requiring surgical release. With experience, the clinician is able to predict which feet will respond to nonsurgical treatment. The more rigid the initial deformity, the more likely it is that surgical treatment will be required.

The order of correction by serial manipulation and casting should be: first, correction of forefoot adduction; next correction of heel varus; and finally, correction of hindfoot equinus. Correction should be pursued in this order so that a rocker-bottom deformity will be prevented by dorsiflexing the foot through the hindfoot rather than the midfoot. The casting program initially outlined by Kite and modified by Lovell has been successful.

If the clubfoot is corrected between birth and 6 months of age this should be documented by both the clinical appearance and repeated anteroposterior and dorsiflexion lateral stress roentgenograms. Following this, the foot may be placed in a series of holding casts that can be used part-time on children with compliant families. Continued casting or bracing is an effort to prevent recurrence. The first sign of recurrence is usually progressive contracture of the tendo calcaneus. In children between 6 and 18 months of age, a Phelps brace fitted with an inside bar and outside T-strap on a hightop shoe may be used as a holding device during the day. A Denis Browne splint may be used at night for both correction of residual internal tibial torsion associated with clubfoot and continued maintenance of the foot in the corrected position.

SURGICAL METHODS OF TREATMENT

Surgery in clubfoot is indicated for deformities that do not respond to the conservative treatment by serial manipulation and casting. We often see children with a significant rigid clubfoot deformity in which the forefoot has been corrected by conservative treatment but the hindfoot remains fixed in both varus and equinus. We also see children whose clubfoot has been corrected and who return with recurrence of deformity. Surgery in the treatment of clubfoot must be tailored to the age of the child and to the deformity to be corrected. In the child aged 6 to 12 months whose deformity has not been corrected by a conservative program the treatment of choice is a one-stage surgical release (Fig. 61-26). The technique described here is the Turco posteromedial release.

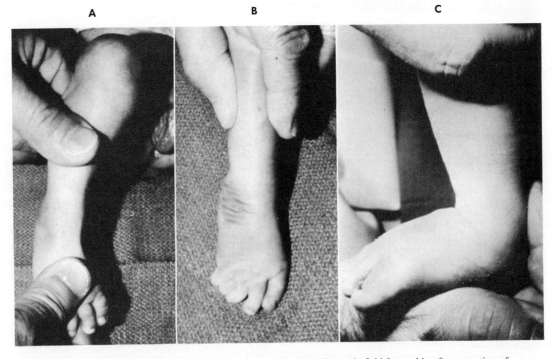

Fig. 61-25. Serial manipulation and stretching of clubfoot in newborn. **A,** Initial stretching for correction of metatarsus adductus. **B,** Forefoot stretched to corrected position at initial examination. Note redundant skin on anterolateral border of foot and ankle. **C,** Initial manipulation of hindfoot to correct a heel valgus. Note placement of palm under hindfoot rather than at midfoot or forefoot level. (Courtesy Dr. Wood Lovell.)

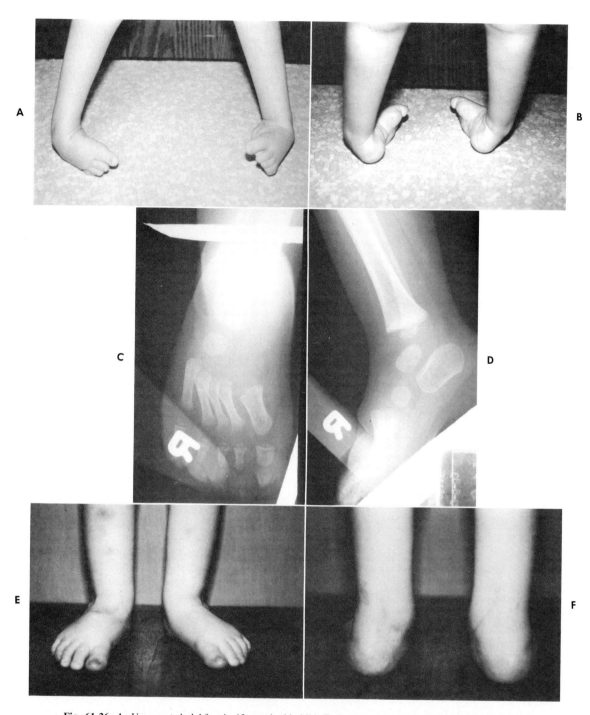

Fig. 61-26. A, Uncorrected clubfeet in 12-month-old child. **B,** Posterior view showing uncorrected forefoot adduction and heel varus and equinus. **C,** Preoperative anteroposterior roentgenogram of feet showing residual forefoot adduction and heel varus. **D,** Preoperative dorsi flexion lateral stress roentgenogram of feet illustrating lack of correction of heel varus and residual equinus of hind foot. **E,** After Turcopostero medial release. **F,** Posterior view postoperatively showing correction of heel varus and equinus.

Continued.

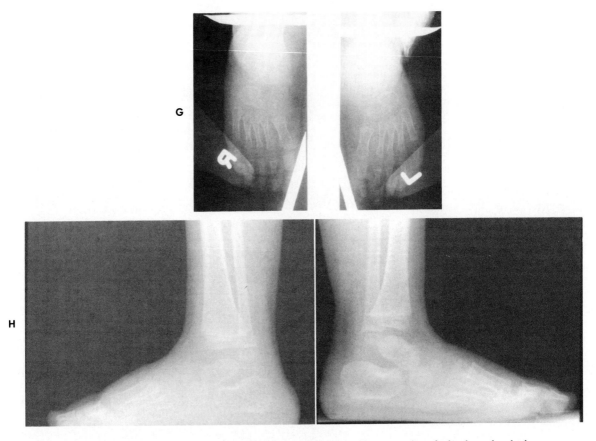

Fig. 61-26, cont'd. G, Postoperative roentgenogram of both feet. Note correction of talocalcaneal and talo-metatarsal angles bilaterally. **H,** Standing lateral roentgenogram of both feet.

Clubfoot surgery in older children should be directed at correction of either the complete deformity of the forefoot and hindfoot or any specific remaining deformity or deformities: forefoot adduction, heel varus, or equinus of the hindfoot.

For correction of the forefoot with residual metatarsus adductus, surgery is similar to that described for correction of isolated metatarsus adductus: tarsometatarsal capsulotomy (p. 2633) in preschool children or as we prefer, metatarsal osteotomies (p. 2635) in children 5 years old or older with residual metatarsus adductus and troublesome symptoms. Correction of residual heel varus can be accomplished by three different surgical techniques. The first is a soft tissue release, as recommended by Turco; the heel varus is corrected by extensive subtalar joint release, which corrects the deformity at the site of the pathology. The second technique is the Dwyer calcaneal osteotomy, to which we add a lateral closing wedge osteotomy. The third technique is triple arthrodesis in children 12 years old or older with its included hindfoot osteotomies.

Finally, any correction of residual heel equinus is by soft tissue procedures. Tendo calcaneus lengthening and posterior ankle and subtalar capsulotomies are used in younger children. In older children a fixed equinus not correctible by soft tissue releases can be corrected by a Lambrinudi procedure (p. 2955) or triple arthrodesis (p. 2935).

Special attention should be given to two specific problems in clubfoot. The first is residual hindfoot equinus in children age 6 to 12 months who have obtained adequate correction of forefoot adduction and hindfoot varus. This equinus can be corrected adequately by tendo calcaneus lengthening and posterior capsulotomy of the ankle and subtalar joints without an extensive one-stage posteromedial release. However one must be certain that the heel varus has been corrected adequately if tendo calcaneus lengthening and posterior capsulotomy alone are to be used (Fig. 61-27).

The second specific problem is dynamic metatarsus adductus caused by overpull of the tibialis anterior tendon in older children whose clubfeet have been corrected. In a symptomatic child, the treatment of choice is transfer of the tibialis anterior tendon, either as a split transfer or as a transfer of the entire tendon to the middle cuneiform. The forefoot must be flexible for a tendon transfer to succeed. A stress anteroposterior abduction roentgenogram of the forefoot, in addition to the clinical findings, can assist in this evaluation.

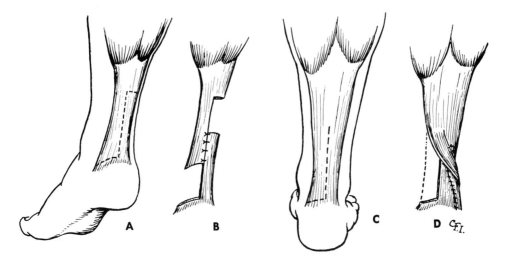

Fig. 61-27. Stewart technique of lengthening tendo calcaneus or transposing its medial part laterally. **A,** Tendon is contracted. Note that its insertion is more medial than normal and extends anteriorly on medial surface of calcaneus. **B,** Tendon has been lengthened by Z-plasty in which medial half is freed from calcaneus. **C,** Tendon is not contracted. *Broken line,* incision to be made in tendon to transpose medial part of its insertion laterally. **D,** Medial part has been transposed (see text). (After Stewart, S.F.: J. Bone Joint Surg. **33-A:**577, 1951.)

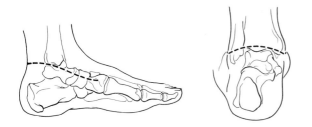

Fig. 61-28. Possible medial extensions of Cincinnati incision, superimposed over tarsal bones and malleoli. Incision may be extended laterally to same extent as medially, depending on needs of surgeon. (From Crawford, A.H., Marxen, J.L., and Osterfeld, D.L.: J. Bone Joint Surg. **64-A:**1355, 1982.)

POSTEROMEDIAL RELEASE

One option available in performing a one-stage posteromedial release is the use of the transverse, or "Cincinnati," incision. In our experience, this incision provides excellent exposure of the subtalar joint and is useful in patients with a severe internal rotational deformity of the calcaneus. One potential problem with this incision is tension on the suture line when attempting to dorsiflex the foot to apply the postoperative cast. To avoid this, the foot may be placed in mild plantar flexion in the immediate postoperative cast, and dorsiflexed to the corrected position at the first cast change when the wound has healed (Fig. 61-28).

TECHNIQUE (TURCO). Make a medial incision 8 to 9 cm long extending from the base of the first metatarsal to the tendo calcaneus, curving it slightly just inferior to the medial malleolus (Fig. 61-29, *A*). Do not undermine the skin. Next expose and mobilize by careful dissection the tendons of the tibialis posterior, flexor digitorum longus, and flexor

hallucis longus and the posterior tibial neurovascular bundle; also expose the tendo calcaneus (Fig. 61-29, *B*). Incise the sheaths of the tendons as they are exposed. Next free the posterior tibial neurovascular bundle and retract it posteriorly. Now by continuing the incision in the sheaths of the flexor digitorum longus and flexor hallucis longus, divide the master knot of Henry beneath the navicular. Divide the calcaneonavicular (spring) ligament and the abnormal origin of the abductor hallucis.

Of the remaining contractures, release the posterior ones first. Lengthen the tendo calcaneus by Z-plasty technique, detaching the medial half of its tendinous insertion on the calcaneus (Fig. 61-29, *C*). Now retract the neurovascular bundle and the flexor hallucis longus anteriorly and expose the posterior aspect of the ankle and subtalar joints. Incise the posterior capsule of the ankle joint under direct vision (Fig. 61-29, *D*). If necessary divide the posterior talofibular ligament at this time. Next identify the posterior capsule of the subtalar joint and divide this along with the calcaneofibular ligament. This ligament is usually contracted in older children.

Retract the neurovascular bundle posteriorly and divide the tibiocalcaneal part of the deltoid ligament. Do this by merely extending the incision in the posterior capsule of the subtalar joint medially and anteriorly. Next release the deep medial structures. Retract the neurovascular bundle and lengthen by Z-plasty the tibialis posterior tendon just proximal to the medial malleolus. Use its distal end as a retractor of the navicular. Now pull on the distal end of the tendon and mobilize the navicular by opening the talonavicular joint and excising that part of the deltoid ligament that inserts on this bone. Incise the talonavicular capsule but avoid damaging any articular surfaces. Next free the tibialis posterior attachment to the sustentaculum tali

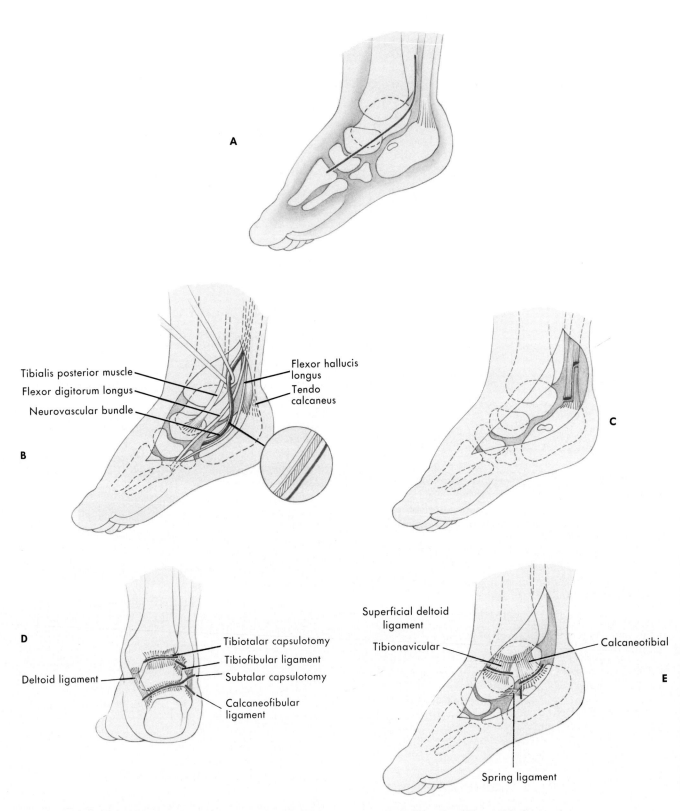

Tibialis posterior muscle

Flexor digitorum longus

Neurovascular bundle

Flexor hallucis longus

Tendo calcaneus

Tibiotalar capsulotomy

Tibiofibular ligament

Subtalar capsulotomy

Calcaneofibular ligament

Deltoid ligament

Superficial deltoid ligament

Tibionavicular

Calcaneotibial

Spring ligament

Fig. 61-29. Turco technique for releasing soft tissues (see text). (Redrawn from Turco, V.J.: In American Academy of Orthopaedic Surgeons: Instructional course lectures, vol. 24, St. Louis, 1975, The C.V. Mosby Co.)

and the spring ligament and detach the spring ligament from the sustentaculum (Fig. 61-29, *E*).

Now return to the posterior part of the incision and evert the foot. Release the superficial layer of the deltoid ligament from the calcaneus posteriorly under direct vision. Do not incise the deep layer of this ligament that extends from the body of the talus to the medial malleolus because this would cause a flatfoot deformity. The only remaining structures to be released are the subtalar ligaments. Evert the foot, expose the talocalcaneal interosseous ligament, and cut the ligament under direct vision. Now divide the bifurcated (Y) ligament that extends from the calcaneus to the lateral border of the navicular and to the medial border of the cuboid. This completes the mobilization of the navicular.

Reduce the navicular onto the head of the talus, and this will properly align the other tarsal bones. Avoid pushing the navicular too far laterally on the head of the talus. Make sure that the relationship of the calcaneus and the navicular to the talus is correct. Next insert a Kirschner wire percutaneously from the dorsum of the first metatarsal shaft across the medial cuneiform and the navicular and into the talus, transfixing the talonavicular joint. A second Kirschner wire may be used to fix the subtalar joint. The foot now should remain corrected without external force.

Repair the tendo calcaneus with one or two interrupted sutures after it has been lengthened enough to allow dorsiflexion of the ankle to a right angle. Do not lengthen the tendon too much. Suture the tibialis posterior tendon. Now close the subcutaneous tissues and skin with interrupted sutures. Bend the wire as it lies just outside the skin so that it does not migrate, and place a sterile piece of felt between the wire and the skin for protection. Apply a well-padded long leg cast with the knee in slight flexion and the ankle dorsiflexed only to the neutral position. Excessive dorsiflexion will cause too much tension on the skin and subcutaneous tissues.

AFTERTREATMENT. At 3 weeks the cast is changed with the patient under general anesthesia, but the sutures are not removed. A new long leg cast is applied with the foot in more dorsiflexion. At 6 weeks the cast, the sutures, and the Kirschner wire are removed. A new long leg cast is applied with the foot held in full correction. This cast is worn until 4 months after surgery. Pronator shoes are then worn during the day and are attached to a Denis Browne splint at night.

TRANSFER OF TIBIALIS ANTERIOR TENDON

Garceau and Peabody believed that clubfoot is caused by prenatal muscle imbalance in which the pronators and extensors of the foot are weak, that often the peroneals are permanently weak, and that when this weakness can be demonstrated in recurrent clubfoot, lateral transfer of the tibialis anterior tendon is indicated. Weakness of the peroneals is suggested clinically when a varus deformity of the foot can be corrected passively but not actively and when roentgenograms show the osseous deformity to have been corrected. Transfer of the tibialis anterior tendon is most successful when performed between the third and sixth years but then only after parts of the deformity have been corrected.

Some surgeons have been displeased with the results of this operation. They have noted that it can result in such deformities as too great a valgus position of the forefoot and hindfoot, in an equinus position of the first metatarsal, in clawing of the great toe, and in an equinus position of the heel. Care should be taken then to use it only in feet suitable for it. As described by Garceau, it is indicated only (1) when the forefoot supinates and adducts during the swing phase of gait, (2) when the tibialis anterior tendon bowstrings across the ankle joint, and (3) when the peroneal muscles are profoundly weak or apparently do not function at all after the foot has been maintained in a corrected or nearly corrected position long enough to allow their strength to be determined. When the peroneal muscles are normal, the operation is contraindicated because the force of the normal peroneals would be augmented by that of the transferred tibialis anterior and the evertors, then being too strong, would pull the foot into too great a valgus position. Furthermore, the strong peroneus longus would act unopposed on the first metatarsal, pulling it into an equinus deformity and causing callosities beneath its head and clawing of the great toe. Many surgeons believe the tendon should not be transferred as far laterally as the base of the fifth metatarsal but only as far as the middle cuneiform.

Garceau in 1972 reviewed 94 feet treated by the operation. In 32 the patients had reached skeletal maturity since surgery, and those still immature had been followed for at least 7 years. Twenty-six of the 38 feet in the mature group and 49 of the 56 feet in the immature group were either good or excellent. Overcorrection was present in only two feet. There were no other complications.

TECHNIQUE (GARCEAU). Make an incision 2.5 cm long over the tibialis anterior tendon just proximal to the ankle. Then through a short longitudinal incision over the first cuneiform expose and free the insertion of the tendon. Now pull the tendon out through the proximal incision. Pass a curved hemostat from the proximal incision distally and laterally deep to the cruciate crural ligament to the base of the fifth metatarsal. Next expose the base of the fifth metatarsal through a short longitudinal incision and drill a hole plantarward in it. Place a silk suture in the free end of the tibialis anterior tendon, pass the tendon through the tunnel made with the hemostat and the hole drilled in the bone, and anchor it securely. A Bunnell pull-out suture is useful in anchoring the tendon, which often is short (Fig. 61-30).

AFTERTREATMENT. With the foot in the corrected position a boot cast is applied. At 2 weeks the cast and stitches are removed, and a new cast is applied. Immobilization is continued for at least 8 weeks; a walking tread may be applied to the cast during the last few weeks. After the cast has been removed, the transferred tendon is reeducated by an exercise program.

OSTEOTOMY OF CALCANEUS FOR PERSISTENT VARUS DEFORMITY OF HEEL

In 1955 Dwyer reported osteotomy of the calcaneus for cavus deformity in children. He noted that the deformity is progressive and that it is usually characterized by (1) equinus deformity of the forefoot, (2) contracture of the

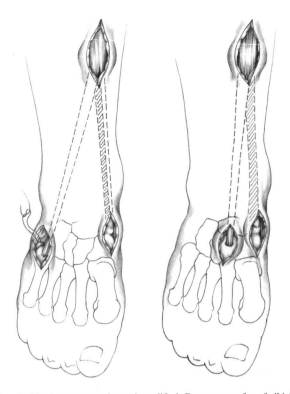

Fig. 61-30. Garceau transfer and modified Garceau transfer of tibialis anterior tendon for recurrent clubfoot.

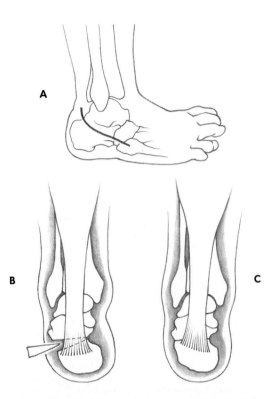

Fig. 61-31. Modified Dwyer osteotomy. **A,** Laterally based incision beginning posterior to fibula and ending at base of fifth metatarsal. **B,** Closing wedge removed from lateral aspect of calcaneus. **C,** Osteotomy is closed with calcaneus placed in neutral position.

plantar fascia, (3) clawing of the toes, and (4) gradually developing varus deformity of the heel and forefoot. He pointed out that with the onset of varus deformity the tendo calcaneus becomes an inverter of the foot, that part of the pull of the tendo calcaneus is transmitted to the thickened medial part of the plantar fascia, that the child tends to walk on the lateral border of the foot and thus to increase the deformity, and that because the heel is in a varus position the plantar fascia is not stretched during weight bearing and consequently becomes contracted. After the varus deformity of the heel has been corrected and the weight-bearing alignment has been restored by osteotomy of the calcaneus, the varus deformity of the forefoot gradually disappears. The technique of osteotomy of the calcaneus for cavus deformity is described on p. 2942.

In 1963 Dwyer reported osteotomy of the calcaneus for relapsed clubfoot. In it an opening wedge osteotomy is made medially to increase the length and height of the calcaneus. The osteotomy is held open by a wedge of bone taken from the tibia. The ideal age for the operation is 3 to 4 years, but there is really no upper age limit. He had performed the operation on 56 feet in 48 patients, and the result was good in 27 and fair in 29. Repeating the operation was necessary in 6 feet because correction had been insufficient at the first operation.

In our experience an opening wedge osteotomy of the calcaneus has been followed too often by sloughing of the tight skin along the incision over the calcaneus. Conse-

quently, although some height of the calcaneus is lost after a closing wedge osteotomy, this is our preference (Fig. 61-31). Weseley and Barenfeld in a report of 50 osteotomies of the calcaneus advised against simultaneous posterior release of the soft tissues and medial opening wedge osteotomy because they cause too much tension on the skin. They recommend instead that the release be performed as a separate technique.

TECHNIQUE (DWYER, MODIFIED). Expose the calcaneus through a lateral incision over the calcaneus, cuboid, and base of the fifth metatarsal (Fig. 61-31, *A*). Strip the lateral surface of the bone subperiosteally and with a wide osteotome resect a wedge of bone based laterally large enough, when removed, to permit correction of the heel varus (Fig. 61-31, *B*). Take care not to injure the peroneal tendons. Remove the wedge of bone, pull the heel into the corrected position (Fig. 61-31, *C*), and close the incision with interrupted sutures. If necessary, fix the osteotomy with a Kirschner wire.

RESECTION AND ARTHRODESIS OF CALCANEOCUBOID JOINT
(EVANS PROCEDURE)

Evans believes that in congenital clubfoot the basic deformity is at the midtarsal joints, that all other deformities are adaptive, and that fully correcting the deformity at the midtarsal joints and releasing all contracted soft structures medially will result in a reasonably normal foot. He devised an operation that shortens the lateral side of the foot by resecting a wedge of bone including the calcaneocuboid joint and releases the medial side by dividing the contracted soft structures. The navicular can then be placed in its normal relation with the talus so that the longitudinal axis of the first metatarsal is in line with that of the talus. The calcaneus is then allowed to fuse with the cuboid to hold the foot in the corrected position. We have had little experience with this operation.

The procedure may be used in older children with uncorrected clubfoot in which the lateral border of the foot is longer roentgenographically.

CORRECTION OF TIBIAL TORSION IN CLUBFOOT

After a clubfoot deformity has been corrected, any moderate or severe internal tibial torsion should also be corrected. Otherwise as the patient walks, the internally rotated foot is dynamically adducted and inverted, and adduction of the forefoot, inversion of the heel, and cavus deformity may all recur. Sell, who studied the relation of internal tibial torsion to the recurrence of deformity in clubfoot, concluded that torsion of as much as 15 degrees should be corrected surgically. The technique of correction by derotational osteotomy of the tibia is described in Chapter 66.

CORRECTION OF PERSISTENT OR UNTREATED CLUBFOOT

Davis in 1892 described a wedge resection of bone from the midtarsal area to correct persistent varus deformities of the foot. The base of the wedge is dorsolateral; the distal cut is made through the cuboid and the proximal part of the cuneiforms, and the proximal cut is made through the distal part of the calcaneus and the neck of the talus. This resection is still part of most operations used to correct these varus deformities.

The earlier the deformity is corrected, the more resilient and normal is the foot when growth is complete. Furthermore, in a young child after the deformity has been corrected, the soft structures, especially the gastrocnemius and soleus muscles, develop more rapidly and eventually the contour of the leg becomes almost normal. In an older child or adolescent, however, after the deformity has been corrected, the gait is inelastic because little motion will have been preserved in the remaining tarsal joints. In an adult, especially one with severe deformity, much bone must be resected to align the foot; the foot will then be much smaller than normal, but function will be improved and an ordinary shoe can be worn.

Many operations have been devised to correct old clubfoot deformities in patients 8 years of age or older. Several procedures are usually combined as follows.

TECHNIQUE. Make an incision along the medial side of the foot parallel with the inferior border of the calcaneus. Free the attachments of the plantar fascia and of the short flexors of the toes from the plantar aspect of the calcaneus as in the Steindler operation (p. 2941). Now by manipulation correct the cavus deformity as much as possible. Next through an anterolateral approach (p. 28), a Kocher approach (p. 29), or an Ollier approach (p. 29) expose the midtarsal and subtalar joints. Then resect a laterally based wedge of bone to include the midtarsal joints (Fig. 61-32). Resect enough bone to correct the varus and adduction deformities of the forefoot.

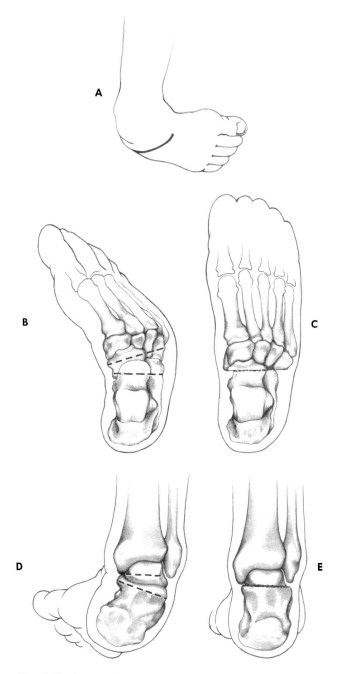

Fig. 61-32. Operation for persistent or untreated clubfoot. *Between broken lines*, amount of bone removed from midtarsal region and subtalar joint in moderate, fixed deformity. In severe deformity, wedge may include large part of talus and calcaneus and even part of cuneiforms.

Next through the same incision resect a wedge of bone, again laterally based, to include the subtalar joint. Resect enough bone to correct the varus deformity of the calcaneus. If necessary include in the first wedge the entire navicular and most of the cuboid and the third cuneiform as well as the anterior part of the talus and calcaneus and in the second wedge much of the superior part of the calcaneus and the inferior part of the talus. Finally lengthen the tendo calcaneus by Z-plasty (p. 2952) and perform a posterior capsulotomy of the ankle joint. Then by manipulating the ankle correct the equinus deformity.

AFTERTREATMENT. With the foot in the corrected position and the knee flexed 30 degrees, a cast is applied from the base of the toes to the groin. At 2 weeks the cast is removed, and any remaining deformity of the foot is corrected; care must be taken to avoid a rocker-bottom deformity with bone prominent in the sole of the foot. A short leg walking cast is then applied, and walking is begun with the aid of crutches. At 8 to 12 weeks a short leg brace with a freely moving ankle joint and an outside T-strap is fitted, and the lateral border of the shoe sole is elevated. Usually all support can be discarded after 6 months but not before fusion has occurred among the tarsal bones. The foot should be examined periodically for 2 years. Fig. 61-33 shows the results of tarsal reconstruction for untreated clubfeet.

• • •

Herold and Torok have managed 44 untreated clubfeet in 33 older children and adults by operations carried out in two stages with an intermediate period of manipulations. In the first stage the contracted structures of the medial side of the foot are released and the tendo calcaneus is lengthened, and in the second stage further correction is obtained if necessary by operations on the bones. They emphasize that many of these patients have refused previous treatment for such reasons as fear of an operation or religious beliefs. They also emphasize that many get along quite well without surgery and that correction of the deformity may result in little functional improvement. Consequently they advise psychologic evaluation before surgery to be certain that the patient is willing to be treated essentially for cosmetic reasons alone.

TECHNIQUE (HEROLD AND TOROK). Begin a skin incision at the posteromedial aspect of the tendo calcaneus and pass it distally beneath the medial malleolus to the base of the proximal phalanx of the great toe. Section the tibialis posterior tendon near its insertion on the navicular and detach the insertion of the abductor hallucis from the proximal phalanx of the great toe. In older patients totally excise the abductor hallucis muscle. Next divide the master knot of

Henry to free the tendons of the flexor digitorum longus and flexor hallucis longus and the neurovascular bundle. Retract these structures dorsally and release subperiosteally from the calcaneus the short flexor muscles and the plantar fascia. Resect all joint capsules on the medial side of the foot, including the metatarsophalangeal joint of the great toe, the first tarsometatarsal joint, the naviculocuneiform joint, the talonavicular joint, and the medial aspect of the subtalar joint. Leave intact the tibiotalar ligament, which is the deep part of the deltoid ligament.

Next incise the tibiocalcaneal and tibionavicular parts of the deltoid ligament. Lengthen the tendo calcaneus by Z-plasty, releasing its calcaneal attachment medially. Now resect the capsules of the subtalar joint medially and of the ankle joint posteriorly. Manipulate the foot toward the corrected position but close the skin without tension. Apply a long leg plaster cast with the foot in a partially corrected position.

When the wound has healed at 10 to 14 days, remove the sutures and apply a second plaster cast with the patient sedated, improving the position of the foot but without placing too much tension on the skin. Repeat the manipulation and casting at reasonable intervals until the deformity is corrected as much as possible. If satisfactory correction is impossible, then perform as the second stage of the procedure a calcaneocuboid wedge resection, a tarsal wedge osteotomy, or a triple arthrodesis as indicated. Additional operations may be needed for deformities distal to the midtarsal joint such as metatarsal osteotomies (p. 2635) to correct forefoot adduction. Or a derotational osteotomy of the tibia may be indicated.

• • •

We have found talectomy (p. 3029) to be a salvaging operation for untreated clubfoot. It relaxes the soft tissues enough to allow correction of equinus and varus deformities of the hindfoot and midfoot. However, adduction of the forefoot is not corrected, and an additional operation on this part of the foot may be necessary.

In persistent or recurrent clubfoot in which the dome of the talus is flat, the equinus deformity cannot be corrected completely by lengthening of the tendo calcaneus and pos-

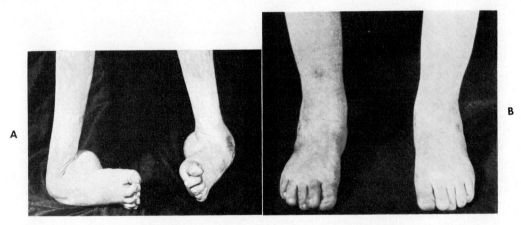

Fig. 61-33. A, Severe untreated clubfeet in adult. **B,** After correction by tarsal reconstruction.

terior capsulotomy of the ankle joint. In these instances, Garceau performed a Lambrinudi operation, which corrects the deformities except for some residual equinus deformity of the talus.

Congenital vertical talus

Congenital vertical talus, rocker-bottom flatfoot, or congenital rigid flatfoot (Fig. 61-34) must be distinguished from flexible pes planus commonly seen in the infant and pediatric population. Many neuromuscular disorders are often associated with congenital vertical talus, including arthrogryposis and myelomeningocele.

Congenital vertical talus can usually be detected at birth by the presence of a rounded prominence of the medial and plantar surfaces of the foot produced by the abnormal location of the head of the talus. The talus is so distorted plantarward and medially as to be almost vertical. Thus it is in a severe equinus position. The calcaneus is in an equinus position also but to a lesser degree. The forefoot is dorsiflexed at the midtarsal joints and the navicular lies on the dorsal aspect of the head of the talus. The sole is convex, and there are deep creases on the dorsolateral aspect of the foot anterior and inferior to the lateral malleolus. As the foot develops and weight bearing is begun, adaptive changes occur in the tarsals. The talus becomes shaped like an hourglass but remains in so marked an equinus position that its longitudinal axis is almost the same as that of the tibia, and only the posterior one third of its superior articular surface articulates with the tibia. The calcaneus remains in an equinus position also and becomes displaced posteriorly, and the anterior part of its plantar surface becomes rounded. Callosities develop beneath the anterior end of the calcaneus and along the medial border of the foot superficial to the head of the talus. When full weight is borne, the forefoot becomes severely abducted, and the heel does not touch the floor. Adaptive changes, of course, also occur in the soft structures. All of the capsules, ligaments, and tendons on the dorsum of the foot become contracted. The tendons of the tibialis posterior and peroneus longus and brevis may come to lie anterior to the malleoli and act as dorsiflexors rather than plantar flexors.

Congenital vertical talus may be difficult to distinguish from severe pes planus. This can be accomplished easily by the use of appropriate stress roentgenograms. Routine roentgenograms should include anteroposterior and dorsiflexion and plantar flexion stress lateral roentgenograms. The plantar flexion stress lateral roentgenogram will confirm the diagnosis of congenital vertical talus.

Rocker-bottom flatfoot is difficult to correct. It tends to recur, especially after conservative treatment. However, gentle manipulations followed by immobilization in casts is beneficial in that the skin, the fibrous tissue structures, and the tendons on the anterior aspect of the foot and ankle are stretched. Reduction of the talonavicular joint is rarely possible by conservative means alone, and consequently an open reduction is usually necessary.

The exact surgery indicated is determined by the age of the child and the severity of the deformity. Children 1 to 4 years old are generally best treated by open reduction and realignment of the talonavicular and subtalar joints. Children 4 to 8 years old may be treated by open reduction and soft tissue procedures combined with extraarticular subtalar arthrodesis. Children 12 years old and older are best treated by triple arthrodesis for permanent correction of the deformity. In any operation for congenital vertical talus other than triple arthrodesis the bones must be fixed in proper position by Kirschner wires or Steinmann pins before the incisions are closed.

Thus for a young child with a mild or moderate deformity the technique of Kumar, Cowell, and Ramsey is recommended. This may be supplemented by transfer of the tibialis anterior tendon through the neck of the talus. For an older child with a more severe deformity or recurrent deformity the technique of Coleman et al. that includes a Grice extraarticular subtalar fusion is recommended. For an even older child (12 years old or older) a triple arthordesis (p. 2935), as already mentioned, is preferred.

TECHNIQUE (KUMAR, COWELL, AND RAMSEY). Make the first of three incisions on the lateral side of the foot centered over the sinus tarsi (Fig. 61-35, *A*). Expose the extensor digitorum brevis and reflect it distally to expose the anterior part of the talocalcaneal joint. Next, identify the calcaneocuboid joint and release all tight structures around it, in-

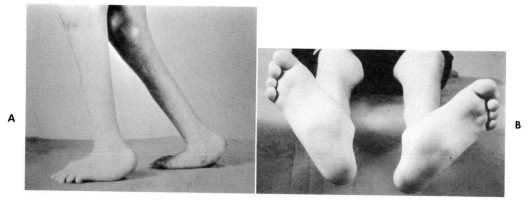

Fig. 61-34. Untreated congenital vertical talus in 10-year old child. **A,** Rocker bottom appearance of foot bilaterally. **B,** Plantar view showing weight-bearing stress on medial aspect of foot bilaterally. (Courtesy Dr. S.J. Kumar.)

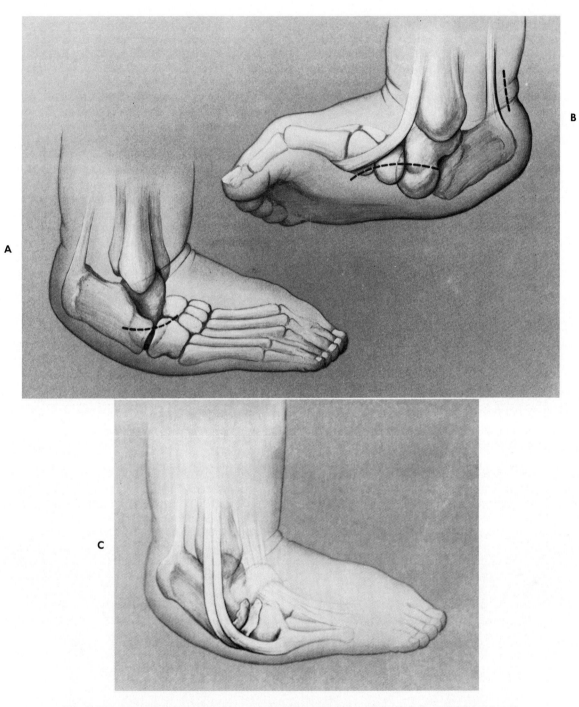

Fig. 61-35. Kumar, Cowell, and Ramsey technique for congenital vertical talus. **A,** Lateral incision. **B,** Medial and posterior incisions. **C,** Calcaneocuboid ligament has been divided and calcaneocuboid joint opened. (From Kumar, S.J., Cowell, H.R., and Ramsey, P.L.: In American Academy of Orthopaedic Surgeons: Instructional course lectures, vol. 31, St. Louis, 1982, The C.V. Mosby Co.)

cluding the calcaneocuboid ligament (Fig. 61-35, *C*). Next, make the second incision on the medial side of the foot centered over the prominent head of the talus. (Fig. 61-35, *B*) This exposes the head of the talus and medial part of the navicular. The tibialis anterior tendon is also exposed. Release all tight structures on the medial and dorsal aspects of the head of the talus and the navicular. Free also the anterior part of the talus from its ligamentous attachments to the navicular and calcaneus. This includes releasing the dorsal talonavicular ligament, the plantar calcaneonavicular ligament, and the anterior part of the superficial deltoid ligament. If necessary, divide part of the talocalcaneal interosseous ligament so that the talus can be easily maneuvered into position by a blunt instrument.

Next, make a third incision, one inch (2.5 cm) long on the medial side of the tendo calcaneus (Fig. 61-35, *B*). Lengthen this tendon by Z-plasty, and if necessary, carry out a capsulotomy of the posterior ankle and subtalar joints. The talus and calcaneus can now be placed in the corrected position and the forefoot reduced on the hindfoot. If the tibialis anterior is to be transferred, drill a small hole in the neck of the talus from the superior surface to the inferior surface. Release two thirds of the tibialis anterior tendon from its insertion and thread it through this hole and suture it to itself. This forms a sling to hold the talus in the reduced position (Fig 61-36). Now pass a smooth Steinmann pin through the navicular and into the neck of the talus to maintain the reduction. Make an at-tempt to reconstruct the talonavicular ligament and close the wound in layers. Apply a long-leg cast with the knee flexed and the foot in proper position.

AFTERTREATMENT. At 8 weeks the cast and Steinmann pin are removed. A new long-leg cast is applied, and this type of cast is worn for 3 months. A short leg cast is worn for an additional month. Then the foot is supported in an ankle-foot orthosis for another 6 months.

TECHNIQUE (COLEMAN ET AL.). Stretch the skin and tendons over the dorsum of the foot by plantar flexion wedging casts for 4 to 6 weeks before surgery. Then make an oblique incision centered over the sinus tarsi, extending posteriorly to the peroneal tendons and medially to the tibialis anterior tendon (Fig. 61-37, *A*). Next retract the extensor digitorum longus, extensor hallucis longus, and tibialis anterior tendons medially and completely evacuate the sinus tarsi, including the talocalcaneal interosseous ligament (Fig. 61-37, *B*). Lengthen the above-listed tendons by Z-plasty technique (Fig. 61-37, *C*). Now carry out a complete talonavicular and calcaneocuboid capsulotomy to permit reduction of the talonavicular joint (Fig. 61-37, *D*). Position the navicular properly on the talus and fix the talonavicular joint with a Kirschner wire (Fig. 61-37, *E*). Through a longitudinal incision over the distal fibula (Fig. 61-37, *A*) resect a full-thickness piece of fibula 2.5 cm long (Fig. 61-37, *B*) and perform a subtalar extraarticular arthrodesis (p. 2963). Now apply a long leg cast. At 6 to 8 weeks remove the cast and through an approach on the

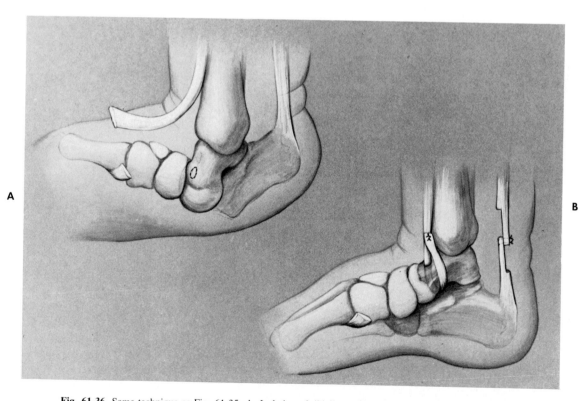

Fig. 61-36. Same technique as Fig. 61-35. **A,** Isolation of tibialis anterior tendon and placement of drill hole in talar neck. Depending on size of tendon, either whole tendon or preferably only two thirds of it is detached. **B,** Tendon threaded through drill hole and sutured to itself. (From Kumar, S.J., Cowell, H.R., and Ramsey, P.L.: In American Academy of Orthopaedic Surgeons: Instructional course lectures, vol. 31, St. Louis, 1982, The C.V. Mosby Co.)

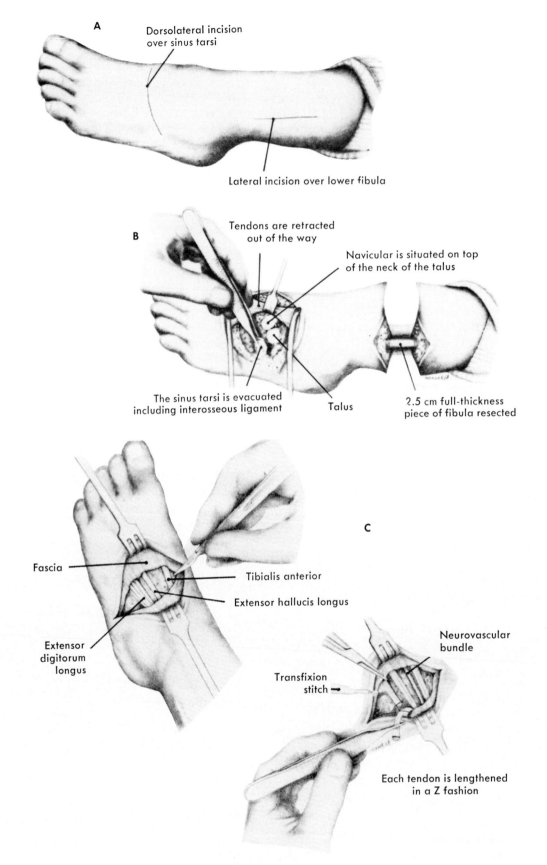

Fig. 61-37. Technique of Coleman et al. for correcting rocker-bottom flatfoot (see text). (From Coleman, S.S., Stelling, F.H., III, and Jarrett, J.: Clin. Orthop. **70**:62, 1970.)

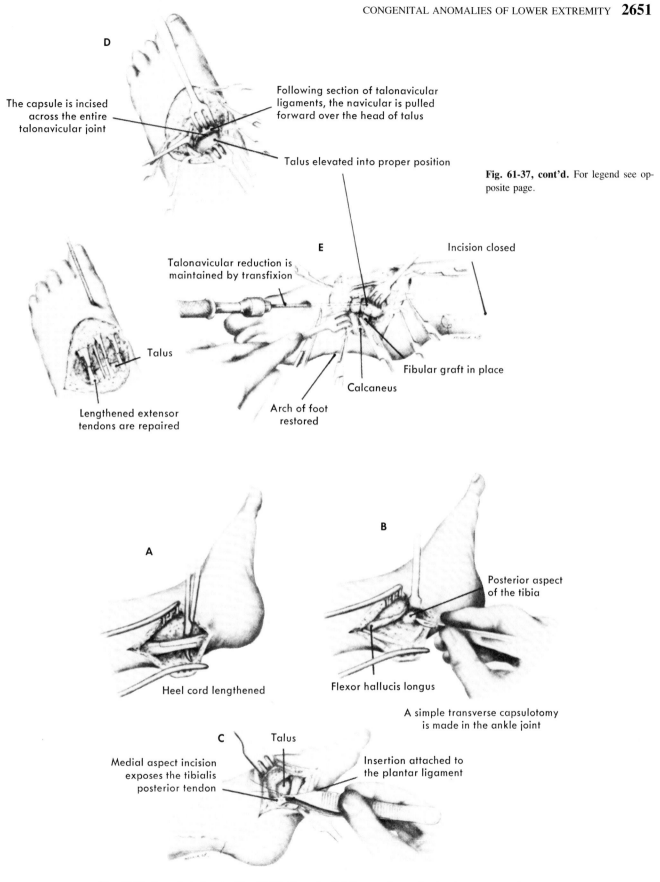

D

The capsule is incised across the entire talonavicular joint

Following section of talonavicular ligaments, the navicular is pulled forward over the head of talus

Talus elevated into proper position

Fig. 61-37, cont'd. For legend see opposite page.

Talus

Lengthened extensor tendons are repaired

E

Talonavicular reduction is maintained by transfixion

Incision closed

Fibular graft in place

Calcaneus

Arch of foot restored

A

Heel cord lengthened

B

Posterior aspect of the tibia

Flexor hallucis longus

A simple transverse capsulotomy is made in the ankle joint

C

Talus

Medial aspect incision exposes the tibialis posterior tendon

Insertion attached to the plantar ligament

Fig. 61-38. Same technique as Fig. 61-37. Once the tibialis posterior tendon has been properly freed, it is advanced to the plantar aspect of the talus and navicular. (See text). (From Coleman, S.S., Stelling, F.H., III, and Jarrett, J.: Clin. Orthop. **70:**62, 1970.)

medial side of the foot and ankle (Fig. 61-38, *A*) lengthen the tendo calcaneus, release the posterior capsular structures of the ankle, plicate the calcaneonavicular ligament, and advance the tibialis posterior tendon to the plantar surface of the navicular (Fig. 61-38, *B* and *C*).

AFTERTREATMENT. At 6 weeks the cast is removed, and a double upright spring-loaded foot-drop brace is fitted and is worn for about 2 months.

TECHNIQUE (GRICE). First expose the medial aspect of the ankle joint and midtarsal area through an S incision; beginning just anterior to the medial malleolus, extend it plantarward, then curve it distally over the dorsal aspect of the foot to the first metatarsocuneiform joint, and then curve it again plantarward. Elevate the skin and subcutaneous tissue down to the capsular and ligamentous structures. Divide transversely the abnormal joint capsule between the tibia and navicular dorsally, leaving a large cuff of capsule attached to the navicular. Free the navicular medially from the tibia and inferiorly from the superior aspect of the talus. Free the insertion of the tibialis anterior tendon. Now the navicular can be brought inferiorly into normal relation with the talus. Next make a second incision, a curved lateral one, over the sinus tarsi and reflect the skin and subcutaneous tissue. Incise the transverse tarsal ligament, the capsule of the subtalar joint, and the ligaments in the sinus tarsi. Now plantar flex, invert, and adduct the foot so that the talus is aligned normally with the other tarsals. Fix the foot in this position with two Kirschner wires, one inserted parallel with the sole of the foot through the navicular and into the talus and the other through the sole superiorly through the calcaneus and into the talus. Now redirect the severed tibialis anterior tendon along the medial aspect of the neck of the talus, then through the joint capsule beneath the head of the talus, and then distally along the plantar calcaneonavicular (spring) ligament and fix it to the plantar aspect of the navicular. Close the skin and apply a cast with the ankle in as much dorsiflexion as possible.

AFTERTREATMENT. When the wounds have healed, the sutures and cast are removed, the foot is placed in as much dorsiflexion as possible, and a new cast is applied. With repeated manipulation and with wedging and changes of cast, the equinus deformity can often be corrected conservatively. If not, then lengthening of the tendo calcaneus and posterior capsulotomy of the ankle joint should be performed. At about 12 weeks the Kirschner wires are removed, and ambulation is begun in corrective shoes.

CONGENITAL SKELETAL LIMB DEFICIENCIES

Classification of congenital skeletal limb deficiencies must be standardized for proper understanding of reports of various authors and for proper prescription of prosthetic devices. The classification now used is that developed by O'Rahilly as outlined in Table 61-1. Fig. 61-39 shows the dermatome relationships of congenital limb deficiences. How an injury produces a terminal or intercalcary deficiency is shown in Fig. 61-40. Diagrams depicting the various congenital skeletal limb deficiencies are shown in Fig. 60-41.

Another classification of congenital limb deficiencies has been adopted by the American Society for Surgery of

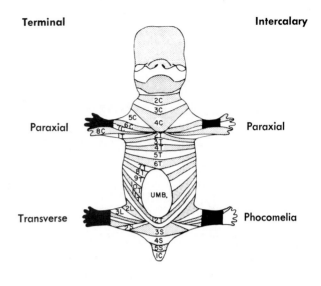
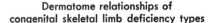

Dermatome relationships of
congenital skeletal limb deficiency types

Fig. 61-39. Dermatome relationships of congenital skeletal limb deficiencies. Cephalad to caudad somitic arrangement extends into limbs and may be divided into preaxial and postaxial elements. This lamination of embryonic arm or leg lends itself to deficiencies that may occur transversely across elements or longitudinally in those elements that lie in preaxial or postaxial aspect of arm. (From Hall, C.B., Brooks, M.B., and Dennis, J.F.: JAMA **181**:590, 1962.)

the Hand and the International Federation of Societies for Surgery of the Hand. This classification, proposed by Swanson, is based on the result of the insult to the embryonic limb and is as follows:

1. Failure of formation of parts (arrest of development)
   a. Transverse deficiencies
   b. Longitudinal deficiencies
2. Failure of differentiation (separation) of parts
3. Duplication
4. Overgrowth (gigantism)
5. Undergrowth (hypoplasia)
6. Congenital constriction band syndrome
7. Generalized skeletal abnormalities

Although experience with this classification is accumulating, the classification is not yet as widely known as that of Frantz and O'Rahilly. For this reason the former classification is retained in this chapter.

Cleft foot (partial adactylia)

Cleft foot (lobster foot) is an anomaly in which usually a single cleft extends proximally into the foot, sometimes even as far as the tarsus. Usually one or more toes and parts of their metatarsals are absent, and often the tarsals are abnormal. Although the deformity varies in degree and type, the first and fifth rays are usually present (Fig. 61-42). If a metatarsal is partially or completely absent, its respective toe is always absent.

Any surgery for cleft foot should improve function; improving appearance is of secondary importance. When the cleft extends proximally between the metatarsals, the skin

Table 61-1. Classification of congenital skeletal limb deficiencies*†

Transverse (−)	Longitudinal (∕)
Terminal (T)	
1. *Amelia* (absence of limb) 2. *Hemimelia* (absence of forearm and hand or leg and foot) 3. *Partial hemimelia* (part of forearm or leg is present) 4. *Archeiria or apodia* (absence of hand or foot) 5. *Complete adactylia* (absence of all five digits and their metacarpals or metatarsals) 6. *Complete aphalangia* (absence of one or more phalanges from all five digits)	1. *Complete paraxial hemimelia* (complete absence of one of the forearm or leg elements and of the corresponding portion of the hand or foot)—R, U, TI, or FI‡ 2. *Incomplete paraxial hemimelia* (similar to above but part of defective element is present)—r, u, ti, or fi‡ 3. *Partial adactylia* (absence of one to four digits and their metacarpals or metatarsals): 1,2,3,4,or 5 4. *Partial aphalangia* (absence of one or more phalanges from one to four digits): 1,2,3,4,or 5
Intercalary (I)	
1. *Complete phocomelia* (hand or foot attached directly to trunk) 2. *Proximal phocomelia* (hand and forearm, or foot and leg, attached directly to trunk) 3. *Distal phocomelia* (hand or foot attached directly to arm or thigh)	1. *Complete paraxial hemimelia* (similar to corresponding terminal defect but hand or foot is more or less complete)—R, U, TI, or FI‡ 2. *Incomplete paraxial hemimelia* (similar to corresponding terminal defect but hand or foot is more or less complete—r, u, ti, or fi‡ 3. *Partial adactylia* (absence of all or part of a metacarpal or metatarsal): 1 or 5 4. *Partial aphalangia* (absence of proximal or middle phalanx or both from one or more digits): 1,2,3,4, or 5

*From Frantz, C.H., and O'Rahilly, R.: J. Bone Joint Surg. **43-A:**1202, 1961.
†List of symbols used:

− transverse	R or r, radial
∕ longitudinal	T, terminal
: 1,2,3,4, or 5 denote digital ray involved	TI or ti, tibial
FI or fi, fibular	U or u, ulnar
I, intercalary	

A line below a numeral denotes upper-limb involvement, for example, T-2 represents terminal transverse hemimelia of the upper limb.

A line above a numeral denotes lower-limb involvement, for example, I-1 represents intercalary tranverse complete phocomelia of the lower limb.

‡In capital letters when the paraxial hemimelia is complete; in small letters when the defect is incomplete.

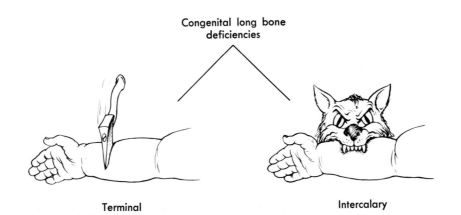

Fig. 61-40. Illustrations of terminal and intercalary skeletal limb deficiencies. Should injury completely sever limb, terminal amputation is produced. Should injury cut through only preaxial or postaxial somites and areas distal to injury fail to develop, remainder of limb develops as paraxial deformity. In intercalary deficiencies, areas proximal and distal to injury survive and continue to develop. Should injury completely transect limb, terminal part survives foreshortened to its base at trunk and produces phocomelia. Should injury merely remove segment of preaxial or postaxial elements, somites survive distally and proximally, continue to develop, and paraxial intercalary deficiency results. (From Hall, C.B., Brooks, M.B., and Dennis, J.F.: JAMA **181:**590, 1962.)

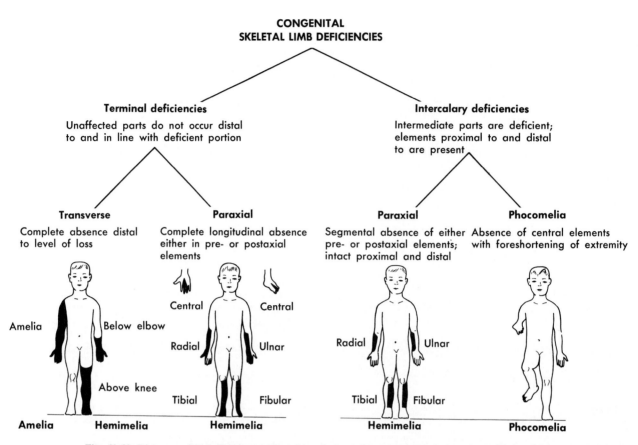

Fig. 61-41. Diagrams of Hall, Brooks, and Dennis to depict terminal and intercalary types of skeletal limb deficiencies. (Adapted from O'Rahilly, R.: Am. J. Anat. **89:**135, 1951; from Hall, C.B., Brooks, M.B., and Dennis, J.F.: JAMA **181:**590, 1962.)

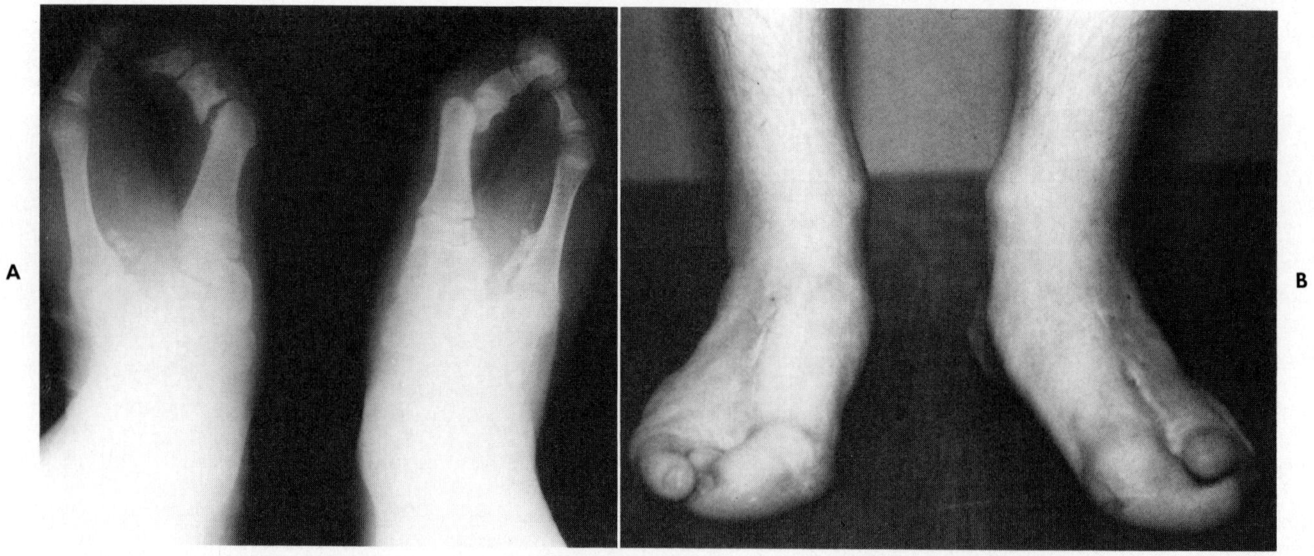

Fig. 61-42. A, Standing anteroposterior roentgenograms of bilateral cleft foot in 8-year-old child. **B,** Eight years after surgery.

of the apposing surfaces within the cleft is excised, but leaving dorsal and plantar flaps that will close the cleft when sutured together. If a metatarsal has no corresponding toe, it is resected and the cleft is closed as just described. (Fig. 61-43)

Congenital absence of part or all of long bone

Congenital absence of part or all of a long bone may be treated by reconstruction such as transplantation of a whole bone from the same limb or from another, by amputation, or by a combination of these operations. Usually the limb affected is so short that to make the limbs match either by shortening the normal bone or by lengthening the defective one would be impossible. Whether amputation is wisest should be decided by comparing the function anticipated after amputation and fitting with a prosthesis with that anticipated after bone grafting. The function anticipated after any operation should never be compared with that of a normal limb; no surgery can result in a normal limb. But now that lighter and more versatile prostheses are available, amputation in early childhood, even earlier than walking would normally begin, has become more helpful and thus more common.

Congenital amputations are caused by total or partial absence of the long bones of an extremity. According to the O'Rahilly classification, these absences may be transverse or longitudinal, and terminal or intercalary. The deformity that results depends on the bones involved and on the degree of absence of bone. Intercalary and longitudinal losses are discussed here for the fibula, tibia, and femur. Those of the radius and ulna are discussed in Chapter 16. To obtain maximum functional use of the remainder of the extremity, part of it may require amputation (conversion surgery), or the limb may be reconstructed even though a less than normal function may be expected.

The limb deficiencies resulting in congenital amputation are the terminal transverse ones. The treatment is essentially the same as that for acquired amputations, and surgery may or may not be required for prosthetic fitting. When the distal epiphysis of a bone is absent at the end of a stump, the stump will become progressively shorter than the growing bone on the normal side. Consequently in revising a congenital amputation a disarticulation is usually better than an amputation proximal to the epiphysis. Disarticulation provides a strong and wide base for weight bearing, preserves length, and usually eliminates terminal overgrowth. As in all amputation surgery, that for congenital amputations should preserve as much length as possible. Because a child's healing ability is superior, closure of the skin under tension, covering the stump with a skin graft, and even strong skin traction to aid in closure when skin length is questionable may be attempted when the situation demands. Terminal overgrowth, bony spurs, stump scarring, terminal neuromas, and limb pain are all problems in acquired juvenile amputations but not usually in congenital amputations. These complications may occur, however, after conversion surgery. Bursal formation can be bothersome and is best treated by excision.

In transverse terminal deficiencies, amelia, and phocomelia, revision of the stump is rarely necessary. Although function in the remaining terminal parts is impaired because of the shortened lever arm on which they work, they

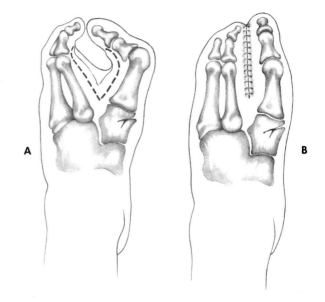

Fig. 61-43. Cleft foot. **A,** Outlines of skin incisions along cleft between abnormal rays of foot. **B,** Artificial syndactyly created after excision of skin cleft and apposition of rays.

should seldom be amputated. Function in the retained part may be used to mechanically initiate activity in an externally powered prosthesis and thus may be valuable in rehabilitation. For a congenital amputation an appropriate apparatus should be designed around the deformity in such a way that maximum function can be obtained from the remaining parts. The problems of acquired amputations in children are discussed in Chapter 22.

FIBULA

The fibula is partially or completely absent more often than is any other long bone. It is also often congenitally shortened. In a review of 291 patients with congenital unilateral shortening of an extremity, Pappas, Hanawalt, and Anderson found shortening of the fibula of 10% or more in 44% of the patients. Many excellent studies of absence of the fibula have been made, and it is now possible to predict with some accuracy the shortening and other deformities likely to develop in this anomaly.

As Kite points out, one cannot be sure that the fibula is completely absent until after the fifth year because before then an epiphysis may be present that roentgenograms cannot show because bone has not yet begun to form. Coventry and Johnson classify the anomaly into three types. In type 1 (Fig. 61-44) the fibula is partially absent unilaterally, and the leg is mildly or moderately short. But there is little if any anterior bowing of the tibia or deformity of the foot, and no other anomalies are present. Except for inequality in leg length, this type causes little if any disability. In (Fig. 61-45) the fibula is almost or completely absent unilaterally; the extremity is severely short; the tibia is bowed anteriorly at the junction of its middle and distal thirds, and the skin is dimpled but not adherent over the apex of the bow; and the foot is in an equinus and valgus position, and some of its bones may be deformed or absent. Often the ipsilateral femur is also short, and devel-

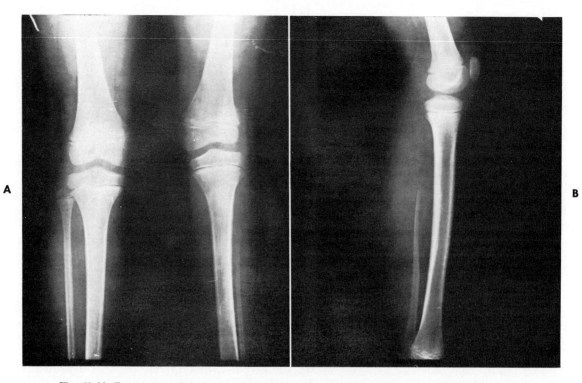

Fig. 61-44. Type 1 congenital absence of fibula (intercalary longitudinal incomplete paraxial hemimelia: fibular) in girl 5 years of age. **A,** Anteroposterior roentgenogram of both lower limbs showing absence of proximal fibula on one side. Affected limb is 1½ inches (4 cm) shorter than other. **B,** Lateral view of affected limb. (From Coventry, M.B., and Johnson, E.W., Jr.: J. Bone Joint Surg. **34-A:**941, 1952.)

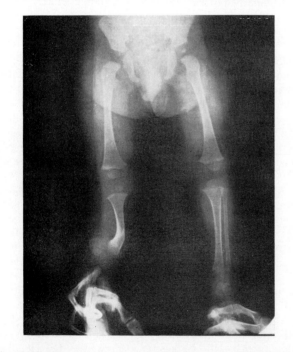

Fig. 61-45. Type 2 congenital absence of fibula (terminal longitudinal complete paraxial hemimelia: fibular) in boy 1 month of age. There is anteromedial bowing of tibia, calcaneovalgus deformity of foot, and absence of two rays. (From Coventry, M.B., and Johnson, E.W., Jr.: J. Bone Joint Surg. **34-A:**941, 1952.)

opment of the capital femoral epiphysis is delayed. In this type, even after expert treatment, the prognosis for function is only fair and that for appearance is poor. In type 3 (Fig. 61-46) the anomaly is either unilateral or bilateral and is associated with other severe anomalies. In this type, of course, the prognosis is poorest.

Kruger and Talbott, in a review of 48 patients with congenital absence of the fibula, found deformity of type 1 in one patient, of type 2 in 28, and of type 3 in 19. Thus the type 2 deformity (that is, unilateral absence of the fibula, anterior bowing of the tibia, and equinovalgus deformity of the foot) is the most common. Calcaneovalgus and equinovarus deformity of the foot and varus deformity of the ankle have also been reported in congenital absence of the fibula.

When part or all of the fibula is absent, treatment varies with the age of the patient when first seen, the severity of the deformity, the tightness of the soft structures, and whether the anomaly is unilateral or bilateral. In type 1 when there is little if any deformity of the foot or anterior bowing of the tibia, the only treatment necessary is lengthening of the tibia by an appropriate technique (p. 2699), epiphyseal arrest of the opposite limb to equalize the leg lengths (p. 2687) if practical, or elevation of the shoe on the affected side. In type 2, which includes equinovalgus deformity of the foot and anterior bowing of the tibia, surgery is usually indicated because conservative treatment is rarely effective. The anteromedial bowing of the tibia, as seen in this anomaly, does not indicate any relationship to

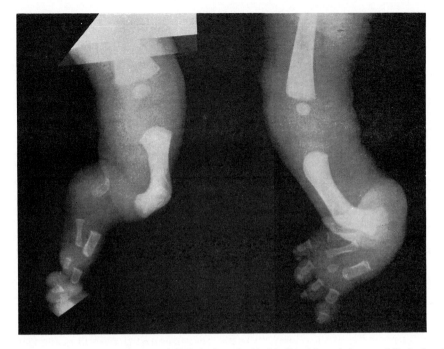

Fig. 61-46. Type 3 congenital absence of fibula in 2-week-old girl. Note bilateral absence of fibula, bowing of tibia, and deformity of foot. (From Coventry, M.B., and Johnson, E.W., Jr.: J. Bone Joint Surg. **34-A:**941, 1952.)

congenital pseudarthrosis of the tibia (p. 2670). Prompt healing usually follows osteotomies of the tibia in congenital absence of the fibula. In type 3 the treatment depends on the severity of the deformities of the feet and legs and on the nature of the associated anomalies. The rest of this section is a discussion of the surgical treatment of type 2.

When the fibula is absent, the foot is in an equinovalgus position, and the tibia is bowed anteriorly; the presence of a tight band of fibrous or fibrocartilaginous tissue that replaces the absent fibula was once thought to be the chief cause of continuing or increasing deformity. Freund as well as Harmon and Fahey mentioned this band, and according to Freund, Haudek discussed it in 1896. It received little attention, however, until the reports first of Thompson, Straub, and Arnold (1957) and then of Arnold (1959) and of Farmer and Laurin (1960). In the experience of Thompson et al. and later of Arnold, this band, when searched for, was found in almost every leg having the deformities of type 2. It is of course invisible on roentgenograms unless it contains bits of bone or calcified cartilage. It extends from the lateral border of the proximal tibia to the posterolateral aspect of the calcaneus. Excision of the band, once considered helpful, is now rarely carried out.

Several operations have been used in the past to stabilize the ankle in congenital absence of the fibula. Wiltse has devised an osteotomy to correct valgus deformity of the ankle, either congenital or acquired, that does not produce abnormal prominence of the medial malleolus or shortening of the limb as occurs after a closing wedge osteotomy (Fig. 61-47). The osteotomy is indicated when skeletal growth is complete or almost so. When significant growth

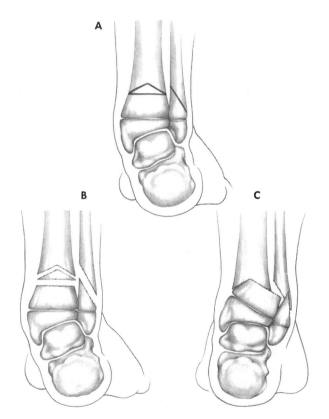

Fig. 61-47. Wiltse osteotomies for correcting valgus deformity of ankle. **A,** Lines of osteotomies. **B,** Triangular segment of tibia is resected, and fibula is cut obliquely. **C,** Distal fragments of tibia and fibula are shifted as shown to align ankle joint properly. (Redrawn from Wiltse, L.L.: J. Bone Joint Surg. **54-A:**595, 1972.)

potential remains in the distal tibial epiphysis, Wiltse recommends epiphyseal stapling medially. After alignment of the foot and ankle the chief deformity remaining is shortening of the extremity, usually involving both the tibia and the femur. The shortening may be minimal, but usually by the time of skeletal maturity the discrepancy is between 7.5 and 17.5 cm.

Jansen and Andersen in studying 29 patients found an average growth deficiency in the femur of 2 mm per year with a range of 0 to 6 mm; the average in the tibia was 4 mm per year with a range of 1 to 9 mm. An epiphyseal arrest on the normal side is contraindicated unless it will equalize the length of the legs; sacrificing height is never justified if an elevated shoe or a prosthesis must still be worn. But when a short tibia or femur or both can be lengthened enough that epiphyseal arrest on the normal side will equalize the length of the legs without sacrificing too much height, then such an arrest is indicated.

Kawamura et al. state that lengthening an extremity more than 10% of the length of the involved bone or bones should not be considered. Which operation is best—several reconstructive operations or early amputation—is usually determined by the anticipated final shortening of the affected limb. Kruger and Talbott found that when all five rays are present in the affected foot, the discrepancy is likely to be greater than when only three or four are present. Farmer and Laurin recommend early amputation if inequality of more than 7.5 cm can be anticipated. Before amputation, however, any anterior bowing of the tibia must be corrected by osteotomy. The Syme amputation (p. 609) is recommended because it preserves the distal tibial epiphysis and the heel pad and an endbearing prosthesis can be worn (Fig. 61-48). If amputation is not performed earlier, the patient may request amputation at adolescence because the leg and the elevated shoe look so unsightly. Aitken recommends disarticulation at the ankle with clo-sure as in a Syme amputation. This produces a comfortable end-bearing below-knee stump that is satisfactory cosmetically and functionally.

When congenital absence of the fibula of type 2 is first seen after the age of 5 or 6 years, any indicated amputation should be preceded by osteotomy to correct anterior bowing of the tibia. If the decision is not to amputate, then the soft structures should be released and bowing of the tibia should be corrected.

TIBIA

The tibia is partly or wholly absent less often than is the fibula. The deformity may be unilateral or bilateral and is often accompanied by others in the same limb: dysplasia of the hip, shortness of the femur, ill-formed femoral condyles that consist merely of a broadening of the distal shaft, absence of the fibula, and absence of one or more bones of the foot. The deformity of the foot may be the most severe one present in the limb.

Congenital deficiency of the tibia, including tibial hemimelia, aplasia, and dysplasia, is rare. In this condition, the fibula is usually intact, but the tibia is aplastic or markedly dysplastic. At birth marked shortening and bowing of the involved leg is apparent. Flexion contracture of the knee and a skin dimple overlying the proximal tibial region are commonly present. The foot is often rigid in a varus and supinated position, pointing toward the perineum. The first metatarsal is markedly shortened in combination with other medial ray defects (Fig. 61-49).

Congenital deficiency of the tibia has been classified into three types: type I—total absence of the tibia, type II—distal tibial aplasia, and type III—dyplasia of the distal tibia and diastasis of the distal tibiofibular syndesmosis.

The recommended treatment for this anomaly is surgical. For the type I deficiency (Fig. 61-50) the options are transfer of the fibula by the Brown technique of knee re-

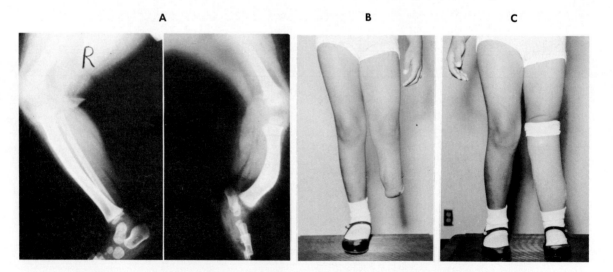

Fig. 61-48. A, Congenital absence of left fibula (terminal longitudinal complete paraxial hemimelia) at 14 months of age. Tibia is bowed, foot is deformed, and limb is short. Right leg is normal. **B,** At 6 years of age, after Syme amputation. Treatment had already consisted of excision of fibrocartilaginous band, lengthening of tendo calcaneus and of peroneal tendons, multiple plaster casts, and brace. Limb was 11.3 cm short. **C,** Molded plastic Syme prosthesis has been fitted. Note absence of any straps. (From Wood, W.L., Zlotsky, N., and Westin, G.W.: J. Bone Joint Surg. **47-A:**1159, 1965.)

construction (Fig. 61-51) or disarticulation of the knee. The presence of a significant flexion contracture of the knee or recurrence of a flexion contracture after multiple reconstructive procedures is an indication for knee disarticulation rather than reconstruction.

For type II deficiency (Fig. 61-52) the treatment of choice is tibiofibular fusion to stabilize the knee. In a young child this can be accomplished by a modified Putti procedure with placement of the proximal fibula in the car-

tilaginous analog of the tibia. In an older child a side-to-side tibiofibular synostosis can be performed (Fig. 61-53). In addition, if the foot cannot be placed in a plantigrade position by soft tissue releases and repositioning, the treatment of choice is an ankle disarticulation or a modified Boyd amputation, implanting the distal fibula within the body of the calcaneus. Below-knee amputation should be avoided to prevent bony overgrowth in a below-knee stump in a growing child.

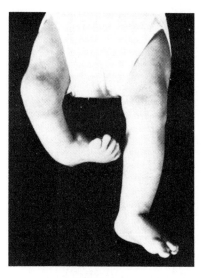

Fig. 61-49. Typical appearance of child with congenital tibial deficiency. Flexion contracture of knee and medial deviation of deformed foot are apparent. Distal fibula is prominent. (From Kalamchi, A., and Dawe, R.V.: J. Bone Joint Surg. **67-B:**581, 1985.)

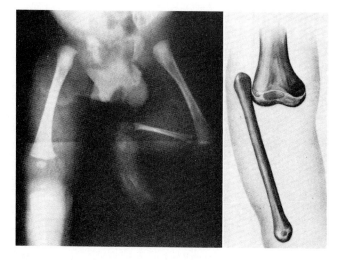

Fig. 61-50. Roentgenogram and diagram of type I deformity demonstrating total absence of tibia. Roentgenogram also shows foot deformity with missing medial rays and absence of distal femoral epiphysis. (From Kalamchi, A., and Dawe, R.F.: J. Bone Joint Surg. **67-B:**581, 1985.)

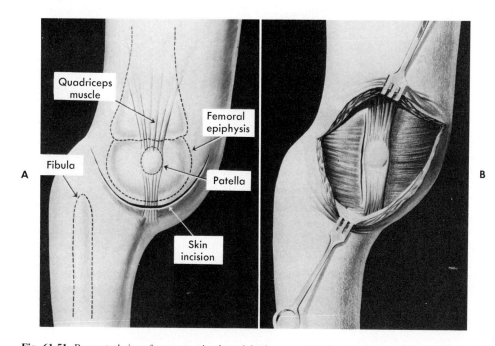

Fig. 61-51. Brown technique for constructing knee joint in congenital absence of entire tibia. **A,** Diagram of anterior aspect of knee. U-shaped skin incision is made from immediately proximal to proximal end of fibula to distal femoral epiphysis and then medially and proximally to point opposite to beginning of incision. **B,** Skin flaps are retracted and longitudinal incision is made lateral to patella, extending throughout length of exposure. Note that patella is abnormally small.

Continued.

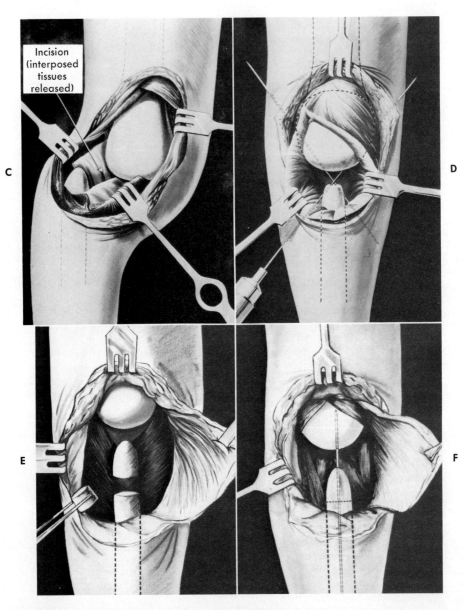

Fig. 61-51, cont'd. C, Soft tissues are dissected to expose distal end of femur and proximal end of fibula. Soft tissue between ends of bones is incised. **D,** About 1 cm of fibular epiphysis is resected to provide flat surface, fibula is positioned in proper weight-bearing alignment beneath femur, and two Kirschner wires are inserted to engage both epiphyses. **E,** If fibula cannot be fully aligned with femur, segmental resection of proximal fibular shaft is carried out. **F,** Fibular fragments and new knee joint are fixed with medullary Kirschner wire. (**A** to **D** modified from Brown, F.W.: J. Bone Joint Surg. **47-A:**695, 1965; **E** and **F** courtesy Dr. F.W. Brown.)

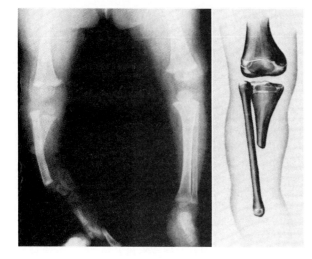

Fig. 61-52. Roentgenogram and diagram of type II deformity. Proximal tibia is present and knee is well preserved. There is less proximal migration of fibula, but foot is displaced. (From Kalamchi, A., and Dawe, R.F.: J. Bone Joint Surg. **67-B:**581, 1985.)

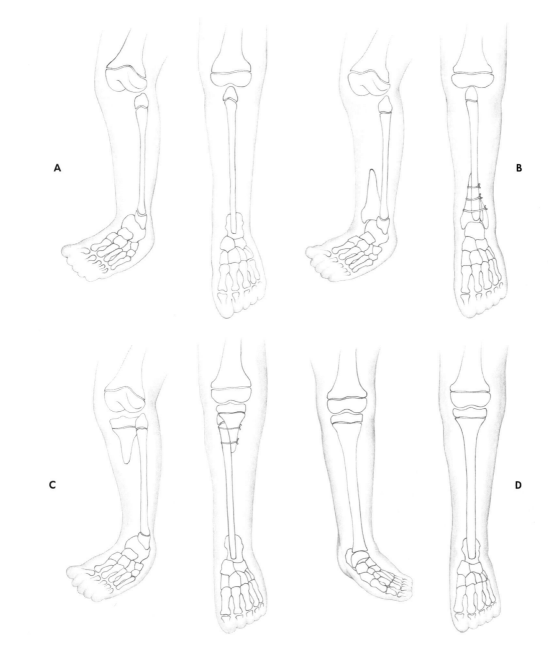

Fig. 61-53. Putti operations for congenital absence of tibia or fibula. **A,** Complete absence of tibia. **B,** Partial absence of tibia. **C,** Partial absence of tibia. **D,** Complete absence of fibula. (Redrawn from Putti, V.: Chir. Organi. Mov. **13:**513, 1929.)

For type III deficiency (Fig. 61-54) treatment should include calcaneofibular fusion with placement and stabilization of the heel in a plantigrade position. If this is not possible, treatment options include ankle disarticulartion or a modified Boyd amputation.

TECHNIQUE (BROWN). Make a U-shaped skin incision on the anterior aspect of the knee. Begin it laterally just proximal to the proximal end of the fibula, carry it distally inferior to the distal femoral epiphysis, and curve it medially and proximally to a point opposite the level of the beginning of the incision (Fig. 61-51, *A*). Retract the skin flaps and make a longitudinal incision through the capsular structures lateral to the patella (Fig. 61-51, *B*). Next separate the vastus lateralis insertion from the quadriceps tendon. Trace the patellar tendon as far distally as possible and divide it at its most distal point. Next release by sharp dissection the tissues lying deep between the proximal fibula and the distal femur and any soft tissue attachments to the fibula that would prevent positioning it in weight-bearing alignment beneath the femur (Fig. 61-51, *C*). If the fibula can be fully aligned with the femur in all directions, fix it to the femur with crossed Kirschner wires (Fig. 61-51, *D*). If the fibula cannot be fully aligned with the femur, carry out a segmental resection of enough of the proximal fibular shaft to allow such alignment (Fig. 61-51, *E*). Next from the osteotomy drive a Kirschner wire distally in the medullary canal of the fibula and out through the distal end of the bone at the ankle joint. Reduce the two fragments of the fibula and drive the Kirschner wire proximally to the knee. Now with the reconstructed fibula in full extension at the knee and the knee in otherwise proper alignment, drive the Kirschner wire across the joint and into the distal femur (Fig. 61-51, *F*). Reattach the distal end of the patellar tendon to the proximal fibula to provide an extensor mechanism. Close the wounds and apply either a posterior molded plaster splint or a long leg cast.

AFTERTREATMENT. At 4 to 6 weeks the Kirschner wire is extracted distally to below the knee joint. If the fibular osteotomy has not united, the Kirschner wire is left in the fibula but not across the knee until the fibula has united. Then the Kirschner wire is removed and passive motion of the new knee joint is begun.

TECHNIQUE (PUTTI)—FIRST STAGE. Make an oblique anterolateral incision from proximal to the femoral condyles laterally and distally to the lateral aspect of the leg at the junction of its middle and proximal thirds. Then isolate and protect the common peroneal nerve. Next open the capsule of the knee to expose the femoral condyles and divide that part of the capsule that lies between the femur and the proximal fibula. Detach the biceps femoris tendon from the fibular head and mobilize the proximal third of the fibula. Then by abducting and flexing the leg insert the proximal end of the fibula into the intercondylar notch of the femur (Fig. 61-53). Now two courses are possible: either leave the cartilaginous surfaces of the proximal fibula and distal femur undisturbed so that a joint is created or roughen these apposing surfaces so that they will eventually fuse. Because the posterior soft structures are so short, completely extending the fibula on the femur is not feasible; often it must be left flexed 30 degrees to 40 degrees.

AFTERTREATMENT. A single spica cast is applied from the nipple line to the toes on the affected side. Successive casts applied at monthly intervals may be required to align the fibula with the femur and to correct the varus deformity of the foot. At 6 months the cast is removed, and a long leg brace with a leather corset is fitted to hold the thigh and leg as straight as possible and the foot in an extreme equinus position. The shoe is elevated to compensate for shortness, and the child is taught to walk.

TECHNIQUE (PUTTI)—SECOND STAGE. In the second stage, performed 1 year or more after the first, the distal fibula is implanted into the talus (Fig. 61-53). The foot is usually fixed in an extreme equinus position to increase the length of the limb. Weight is then borne almost entirely on the metatarsal heads and on the toes, and therefore the toes must be made to dorsiflex to 90 degrees by successive changes of cast.

Through an anterolateral approach (p. 28) expose the distal fibula and its articulation with the tarsus, mobilize it, and maneuver it until it is directly superior to the talus. After alignment has been obtained, with an osteotome split the talus longitudinally (or if this bone is absent, the calcaneus) to form a cleft into which the distal fibula can be fixed. Then roughen the distal fibula, insert it into the cleft, and fix it with two screws or threaded wires.

AFTERTREATMENT. With the foot in an equinus position, a single spica cast is applied from the iliac crest to the toes on the affected side. The cast is changed each month for 3 months. A long leg brace with a leather corset is then fitted, and the sole of the shoe is elevated. Any remaining flexion deformity of the knee may be treated by a supracondylar osteotomy of the femur (p. 689).

TECHNIQUE (BOYD). Expose the ankle through a curved lateral Kocher incision (p. 29) and remove the talus by the

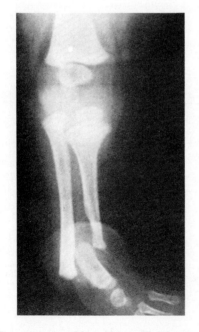

Fig. 61-54. Roentgenogram of leg with type III deformity showing hypoplasia of distal tibia and diastasis of tibiofibular syndesmosis. (From Kalamchi, A., and Dawe, R.F.: J. Bone Joint Surg. **67-B:**581, 1985.)

method of Whitman (p. 3029). Excise any remaining tarsal bones with the exception of the calcaneus. Remove the articular cartilage from the superior surface of the calcaneus and from the entire mortise of the ankle joint. Then shift the calcaneus anteriorly until the weight-bearing surface of the heel is directly beneath the long axis of the leg and is accurately fitted into the ankle mortise. This requires removal of a portion of the sustentaculum tali. Strip the periosteum from the surfaces of the calcaneus in contact with the malleoli and abrade the cortex. Remove the anterior surface of the calcaneus and approximately 1 cm of the contiguous bone. The plantar skin flap should be sufficiently long to cover the anterior portion of the calcaneus. The resulting scar passes just below the lateral malleolus and around the front of the ankle joint.

FEMUR

Complete absence of the femur (intercalary transverse complete phocomelia: femoral) is extremely rare. A diagnosis of this anomaly cannot be made before the age of 10 years because a rudimentary femoral epiphysis may be present, but it is invisible on roentgenograms if ossification has not begun. King, after a review of roentgenograms of over 100 proximal femoral deficiencies collected from several juvenile amputee clinics, concluded that if all elements of the acetabulum are present on the affected side, a femoral head epiphysis will appear even though its ossification is delayed.

Absence or malformation of part of the femur, usually the proximal part (proximal femoral focal deficiency), is much more common. Proximal femoral focal deficiency varies in type and severity and is difficult to treat. It is often accompanied by other abnormalities in the same limb, such as a defective acetabulum or subluxation or dislocation of the hip, absence of the patella and fibula, absence of part of the tibia, or anomalies elsewhere in the body. Ipsilateral fibular hemimelia has been found in 69% of 45 patients with proximal femoral focal deficiencies. Aitken described four types of this deficiency. In each type, of course, a residual femoral shaft is present. In type A the acetablum is competent and contains an ossified femoral head. The defect between the femoral shaft and head is composed of elements that gradually ossify with the result that the proximal femur is bony at skeletal maturity. However, the bone is severely angulated in a varus position at the subtrochanteric level, and pseudarthrosis may be present also (Fig. 61-55). In type B the acetabulum is variously dysplastic but contains an ossified femoral head. The femoral shaft is displaced proximally such that its proximal end lies well proximal to the femoral head.

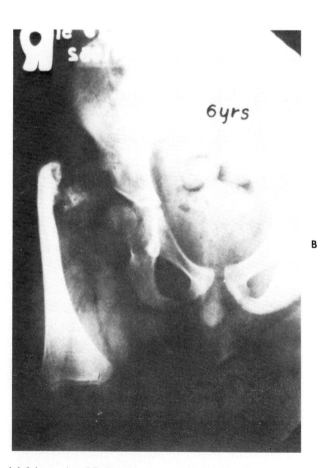

Fig. 61-55. Aitken type A proximal femoral focal deficiency. **A** and **B,** Drawing and roentgenogram showing features of abnormality (see text). (From Aitken, G.T.: In American Academy of Orthopaedic Surgeons: Instructional course lectures, vol. 24, St. Louis, 1975, The C.V. Mosby Co.)

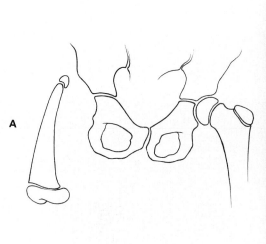

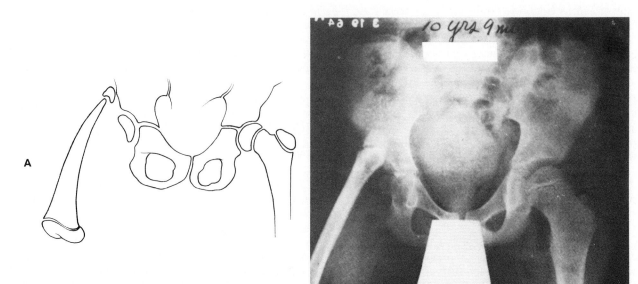

Fig. 61-56. Aitken type B proximal femoral focal deficiency. **A** and **B,** Drawing and roentgenogram showing features of abnormality (see text). (From Aitken, G.T.: In American Academy Of Orthopaedic Surgeons: Instructional course lectures, vol. 24, St. Louis, 1975, The C.V. Mosby Co.)

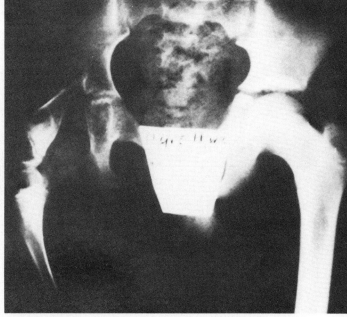

Fig. 61-57. Aitken type C proximal femoral focal deficiency. **A** and **B,** Drawing and roentgenogram showing features of abnormality (see text). (From Aitken, G.T.: In American Academy of Orthopaedic Surgeons: Instructional course lectures, vol. 24, St. Louis, 1975, The C.V. Mosby Co.)

Although a small tuft of ossified tissue is usually present at the proximal end of the shaft, ossification does not occur between the shaft and the head (Fig. 61-56). In type C the acetabulum is variously dysplastic and does not contain an ossified femoral head. Again, as in type B, a small tuft of ineffective ossified tissue is present at the proximal end of the shaft. Bony stability is always absent between the dysplastic acetabulum and the proximal end of the femoral shaft (Fig. 61-57). In type D the acetabulum is almost completely absent and contains no ossified femoral head. No tuft of ossified tissue is present at the proximal end of the shaft (Fig. 61-58). In types C and D the femoral head never ossifies, and whether a cartilaginous model of it is present is unknown. In any of these types the roentgenographic appearance varies with the amount of bone that has formed by the time the patient is first seen. It must be remembered that if all elements of the acetabulum are present, the epiphysis for the femoral head will eventually ossify. In fact, King's treatment of the anomaly is based on this assumption.

The treatment of proximal femoral focal deficiency depends, of course, on the deformity in the specific patient. The aim of treatment is to properly align the part or parts of the femur present, thus stabilizing the pelvis on the femur, and to create a satisfactory skeletal lever with sufficient strength to control a prosthesis. King has outlined as follows a treatment plan for each of the four types as classified by Aitken. However, before proceeding with surgery, the individual patient must be carefully considered because reconstructive surgery may not be justified and amputation or bracing may be more reasonable.

Type A. The femur is aligned by subtrochanteric osteotomy stabilized by some type of internal fixation.

Type B. The fragments of the femur are aligned and fixed internally to create a skeletal lever (Fig. 61-59). Often the knee is arthrodesed. Often, too, a Syme amputation

is carried out, allowing the distal tibial epiphysis to continue its growth. Thus a stump suitable for weight bearing is created. The length of the stump should be such that the knee joint of a prosthesis will be about level with the knee of the normal limb.

Type C. The knee is fused to create a skeletal lever. No stability between the femur and pelvis exists or can be provided. Usually the ankle lies at a level distal to the knee of the normal limb. Then the affected limb is amputated below the knee so that the knee joint of a prosthesis will be level with the normal knee, but because the tibia and fibula may overgrow, amputation should be delayed until near skeletal maturity.

Type D. The pelvis is stabilized on the femur by a Chiari osteotomy of the pelvis (p. 2748). Then the femoral fragment is fixed to the pelvis, and the knee joint serves as a hip joint. Later the ankle is disarticulated so that a conventional prosthesis can be worn. Fixsen and Lloyd-Roberts use five methods to stabilize an unstable hip or repair a pseudarthrosis as follows.

1. A tibial or fibular graft to bridge the gap between the proximal ossified femur and the cartilaginous femoral head. When coxa vara is present or develops later, a subtrochanteric abduction osteotomy is perfomed after the grafts have incorporated.
2. Impaction of the shaft into the femoral head as advised by King. The femoral shaft is sharpened into a spike and is inserted into a hole drilled in the head. It is stabilized with a large medullary Kirschner wire, and cancellous bone grafts are added.
3. Cancellous onlay bone grafting and medullary fixation for persisting subtrochanteric pseudarthrosis.
4. Open reduction of a dislocated hip.
5. Pelvifemoral arthrodesis, either directly (Fig. 61-60) or with a fibular bone graft extending from the proximal femur into the acetabulum.

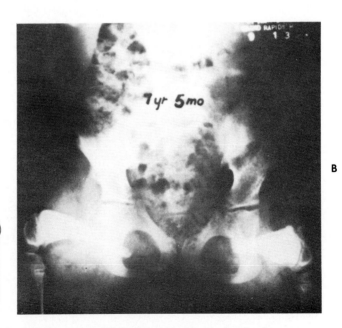

Fig. 61-58. Aitken type D proximal femoral focal deficiency. **A** and **B,** Drawing and roentgenogram showing features of abnormality (see text). (From Aitken, G.T.: In American Academy of Orthopaedic Surgeons: Instructional course lectures, vol. 24, St. Louis, 1975, The C.V. Mosby Co.)

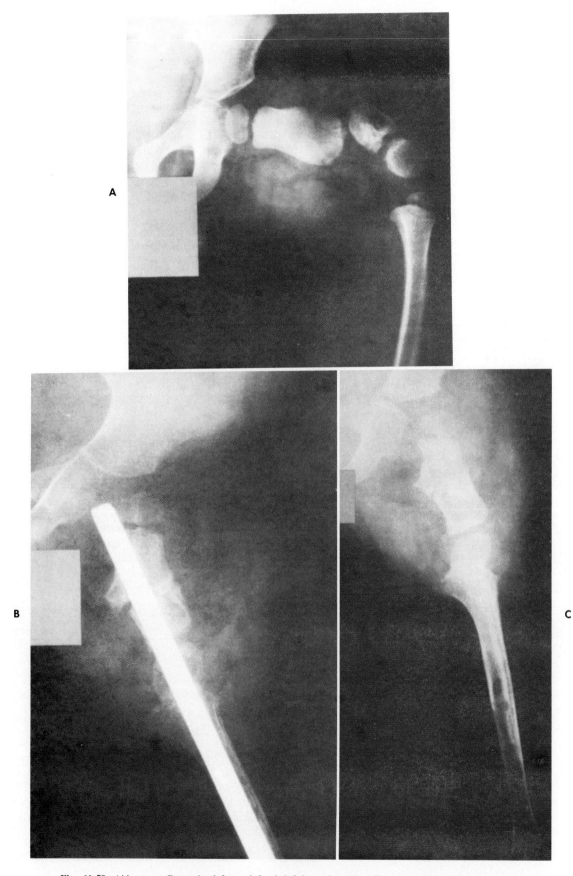

Fig. 61-59. Aitken type B proximal femoral focal deficiency in patient 2½ years old. **A,** Roentgenogram before surgery. **B,** Area of pseudarthrosis between femoral neck and elements of distal femur and its epiphysis was removed, knee was fused, and Küntscher nail was used for fixation. **C,** At 2½ months knee fusion was solid, nail was removed, and ankle was disarticulated. End of stump was at level of opposite knee.

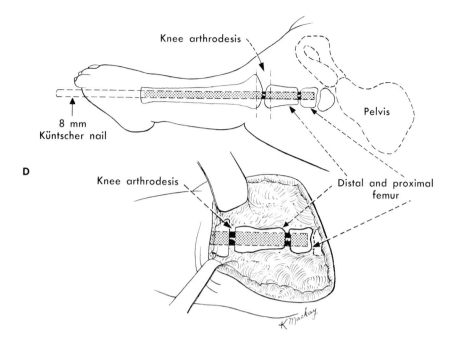

Fig. 61-59, cont'd. D, Drawings to show details of operation to fix femoral fragments and fuse knee joint. (**A** to **C** reproduced from King, R.E.: In Aitken, G.T., editor: *Proximal Femoral Focal Deficiency* (1969), pages 40 and 49, with the permission of the National Academy of Sciences, Washington, D.C.; **D** courtesy Dr. R.E. King.)

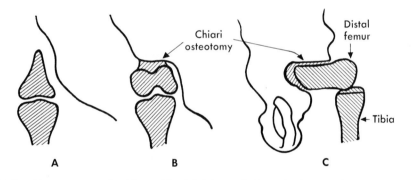

Fig. 61-60. Aitken type D proximal femoral focal deficiency. **A,** Femur is short and limb is unstable. **B** and **C,** Chiari innominate osteotomy is made, and femur is fused to pelvis. (Courtesy Dr. R.E. King.)

Van Nes has described his experiences with Borggreve's method of rotating the limb 180 degrees in proximal femoral focal deficiency. Then the heel points anteriorly, and the dorsum of the foot points posteriorly, and the ankle joint is used to control the knee joint of a prosthesis. Therefore after reconstruction, which should be performed at or near skeletal maturity, the level of the ankle on the affected side must be near that of the knee on the normal side. Because of the danger of ischemia after a one-stage operation, rotating the limb the entire 180 degrees by means of at least two operations may be advisable. Hall and Bochmann reported 20 patients in whom this technique was used and concluded that for a limb too short to be lengthened, the operation is valuable and allows more efficient prosthetic fitting (Fig. 61-61). The requirements

for the operation are (1) an ankle joint with essentially normal motion and motor power and (2) a leg length discrepancy that would place the ankle on the affected side at the level of the opposite knee. The operation should not be performed before the child is 12 years old in order to avoid repeated operations to rotate the tibia. It is worth considering before performing a Syme amputation and fitting a knee disarticulation type of prosthesis.

TECHNIQUE (BORGGREVE, HALL). At the level of the anticipated osteotomy make an oblique incision across the limb so directed that the wound opens up during rotation. If necessary to bring the ankle joint level with the knee joint of the normal limb, resect the distal femur and proximal tibia. If such resection is unnecessary, osteotomize the tibia. Resect a part of the fibula and at the osteotomy insert

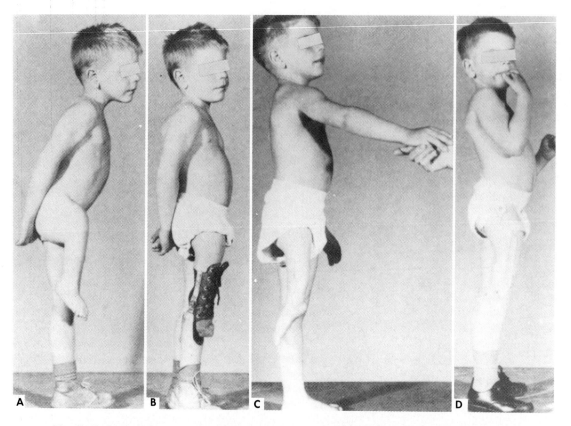

Fig. 61-61. Proximal femoral focal deficiency treated by Borggreve limb rotation operation. **A,** Unilateral deformity with short, flexed thigh. **B,** Original prosthesis with passive knee joint below heel. **C,** After one-stage tibial rotational osteotomy (Borggreve). **D,** Final prosthesis with good cosmetic appearance and active knee control from full extension to 75 degrees of flexion. (Reproduced from Hall, J.E., and Bochmann, D.: In Aitken, G.T., editor: *Proximal Femoral Focal Deficiency* (1969), page 91, with permission of the National Academy of Sciences, Washington, D.C.)

it into the medullary canal of the proximal and distal fragments. Rotate the distal fragments as desired and fix the fragments by a staple inserted through holes drilled in the bone. Stabilization of the pelvis on the femur or fusion of the knee may precede rotational osteotomy, or part of the desired rotation may be obtained during one of these operations. However, stabilization of the pelvis on the femur is not absolutely necessary when the Borggreve rotational osteotomy is used.

OTHER TECHNIQUES. The following operations might also be useful, either alone or in combination, depending on the requirements of the individual patient.

1. Multiple osteotomies to lengthen the femur in lateral bowing of the subtrochanteric region. The technique of Sofield (p. 1070) is useful in correcting lateral bowing.
2. Tibial or femoral lengthening operations (p. 2702) in simple femoral or tibial hypoplasia. The femur should be lengthened cautiously because a subluxation or dislocation of the hip can develop even when acetabular dysplasia is mild.
3. Arrest of one or more epiphyses of the opposite limb (p. 2693) to equalize the leg lengths in femoral hypoplasia.

4. Stabilization of the femur when its proximal end is absent or malformed (Fig. 61-60). The acetabulum is shelved or otherwise reconstructed, and a Vitallium cup is placed on the proximal end of the malformed femur and is inserted into the acetabulum. This operation may stabilize the limb enough to permit satisfactory control of a prosthesis later.

PATELLA

Absence of the patella as an isolated anomaly is extremely rare. It is usually absent as part of a syndrome, most commonly hereditary arthro-onycho-dysplasia (nail-patella syndrome). It usually causes no disability. The femoral condyles and the tibial tuberosity are often larger than normal, the quadriceps is strong, and the extensor mechanism is well developed and glides in the patellar groove between the femoral condyles. Occasionally, however, absence of the patella without any other osseous anomaly is accompanied by severe lateral dislocation of the extensor mechanism. In these instances placing the mechanism in the groove between the femoral condyles, transplanting the tibial tuberosity medially, and transferring one or more of the medial hamstring tendons to the extensor mechanism usually result in satisfactory function.

Usually, however, congenital absence of the patella is only one of several anomalies such as dislocation of the knee, genu recurvatum, anomalies of the femur and fibula, clubfoot, or dislocation of the hip. In these instances the treatment of any disability about the knee depends primarily on its chief cause, for example, genu recurvatum. It is this anomaly that should be treated; the absence of the patella is of minor importance and requires no specific treatment.

CONGENITAL ANGULAR DEFORMITIES OF LEG

Congenital angular deformities of the leg are of two chief kinds: those in which the apex of the angulation is anterior and those in which it is posterior. In each of these two kinds the tibia is often bowed not only anteriorly or posteriorly but also medially or laterally; Badgley, O'Connor, and Kudner have therefore suggested the term "congenital kyphoscoliotic tibia" for both these deformities. Their work and that of Heyman and Herndon have increased our understanding of these deformities, especially in regard to the prognosis for each kind. Kyphoscoliosis of the tibia is commonly associated with neurofibromatosis, but there is not an absolutely established causal relationship between the two.

Posterior angular deformities of the tibia usually tend to improve with growth. A limb length discrepancy may also be present that can range from several millimeters to several centimeters. Children with these deformities should be examined yearly for any potential limb length discrepancy that may require limb equalization, usually by an appropriately timed epiphysiodesis.

In contrast, anterior angular deformities of the tibia are more worrisome because of their potential association with congenital pseudarthrosis of the tibia. If these tibias maintain a normal medullary canal and show no evidence of narrowing or the sclerotic "high-risk tibia," they are usually only observed. If any indication of narrowing of the medullary canal develops in an anteriorly bowed tibia, especially in patients with neurofibromatosis, the limb should be braced until skeletal maturity.

CONGENITAL PSEUDARTHROSIS

Congenital pseudarthrosis is a specific type of nonunion that at birth is either present or incipient. Its cause in unknown, but it occurs often enough in patients with either neurofibromatosis or related stigmata to suggest that neurofibromatosis is closely related to congenital pseudarthrosis if not its cause (see the discussion in Chapter 34). Congenital pseudarthrosis most commonly involves the distal half of the tibia and often that of the fibula in the same limb. Sometimes, but more rarely, it involves other bones of chondral origin, including the first rib, the clavicle, the humerus, the radius, the ulna, and the femur. In this section congenital pseudarthrosis of the fibula and tibia is discussed.

Fibula

Congenital pseudarthrosis of the fibula often precedes or accompanies the same condition in the ipsilateral tibia. Several grades of severity of this pseudarthrosis are seen: bowing of the fibula without pseudarthrosis, fibular pseud-

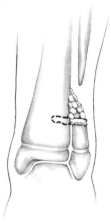

Fig. 61-62. Langenskiöld technique of creating synostosis between distal tibial and fibular metaphyses to prevent valgus deformity of ankle in congenital pseudarthrosis of fibula (see text). (Redrawn from Langenskiöld, A.: J. Bone Joint Surg. **49-A:**463, 1967.)

arthrosis without ankle deformity, fibular pseudarthrosis with ankle deformity, and fibular pseudarthrosis with latent pseudarthrosis of the tibia. Sometimes it even develops between the time of successful bone grafting of a pseudarthrosis of the tibia and skeletal maturity. Then, because the lateral malleolus becomes displaced proximally, a progressive valgus deformity of the ankle develops. (As just noted, pseudarthrosis of the fibula can occur without an ankle deformity, and in this instance treatment is not required because the fibula bears almost no weight.)

Until skeletal maturity is reached, the ankle can be stabilized by a brace with an inside T-strap. At maturity any significant deformity can be treated by supramalleolar osteotomy made through essentially normal bone, and union of the osteotomy can be expected. But Langenskiöld has devised an operation for children to prevent this valgus deformity or halt its progression. He creates a synostosis between the distal tibial and fibular metaphyses. Because in congenital pseudarthrosis securing union by bone grafting may be as difficult in the fibula as in the tibia, an operation that prevents the ankle deformity without grafting in fibular pseudarthrosis is useful.

TECHNIQUE (LANGENSKIÖLD). Make a longitudinal incision anteriorly over the distal fibula. Then divide the fibula 1 to 2 cm proximal to the level of the distal tibial epiphyseal plate and excise the cone-shaped part of the distal fibular shaft. In the lateral surface of the tibia at the level of the cut surface of the fibula and at the attachment of the interosseous membrane make a hole as wide as the diameter of the fibula. Then proximal to the hole remove the periosteum and interosseous membrane from the tibia over an area of several square centimeters. From the ilium obtain a bone graft the same width as that of the hole in the tibia and long enough to extend from the lateral surface of the fibula into the spongy bone of the tibial metaphysis. Insert the graft perpendicular to the long axis of the limb so that it rests on the cut surface of the fibula and extends into the slot in the tibial cortex (Fig. 61-62). Then pack spongy iliac bone in the angle between the proximal surface of the graft and the lateral surface of the tibia. Apply a cast from below the knee to the base of the toes.

AFTERTREATMENT. At 2 months full weight bearing in the cast is allowed, and at 4 months the cast is discarded.

Tibia

Congenital pseudarthrosis of the tibia is rare, with an incidence of approximately 1 in 250,000 live births. A relationship between congenital pseudarthrosis of the tibia and neurofibromatosis seems to exist, although it is not absolute. Most large series report 50% to 90% association of this disorder with the stigmata of neurofibromatosis, including skin and osseous lesions.

Congenital pseudarthrosis of the tibia has been classified by Boyd into six different types.

Type I pseudarthrosis occurs with anterior bowing and a defect in the tibia present at birth. Other congenital deformities may also be present, and these may affect the management of the pseudarthrosis.

Type II pseudarthrosis occurs with anterior bowing and an hourglass constriction of the tibia present at birth. Spontaneous fracture, or fracture following minor trauma, commonly occurs before age 2 years. This is the so-called high-risk tibia. The bone is tapered, rounded, and sclerotic, and the medullary canal is obliterated. This type is the most frequent, is often associated with neurofibromatosis, and has the poorest prognosis. Recurrence of the fracture is common during the growth period but decreases in frequency with age and ceases to occur after skeletal maturation (Fig. 61-63).

Type III pseudarthrosis develops in a congenital cyst, usually near the junction of the middle and distal thirds of the tibia. Anterior bowing may precede or follow the development of a fracture. Recurrence of the fracture after treatment is less frequent than in type II and excellent results after only one operation have been reported to last well into adulthood (Fig. 61-64).

Type IV pseudarthrosis originates in a sclerotic segment of bone in the classic location without narrowing of the tibia. The medullary canal is partially or completely obliterated. An ''insufficiency'' or ''march'' fracture develops in the cortex of the tibia and gradually extends through the sclerotic bone (Fig. 61-65). With completion of the fracture, healing fails to occur, and the fracture site widens and becomes a pseudarthrosis. The prognosis for this type is generally good, especially when treated before the insufficiency fracture becomes complete.

Type V pseudarthrosis of the tibia occurs with a dysplastic fibula. A pseudarthrosis of the fibula or tibia or both may develop. The prognosis is good if the lesion is confined to the fibula. If the lesion progresses to a tibial pseudarthrosis, the natural history usually resembles that of type II.

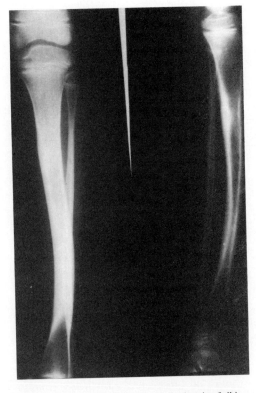

Fig. 61-63. Type II congenital pseudarthrosis of tibia.

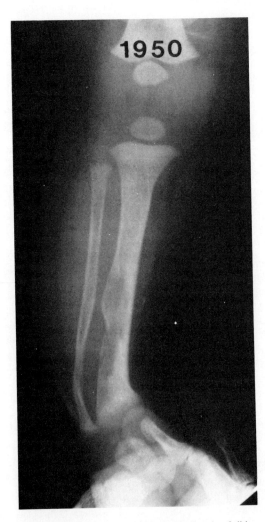

Fig. 61-64. Type III congenital pseudarthrosis of tibia.

Type VI pseudarthrosis occurs as an intraosseous neurofibroma or Schwannoma that results in a pseudarthrosis. This is extremely rare. The prognosis depends on the aggressiveness and treatment of the intraosseous lesion.

Treatment of congenital pseudarthrosis of the tibia depends on the age of the patient and the type of pseudarthrosis. A true congenital pseudarthrosis of the tibia will not heal when treated by casting alone. Initially, the decision must be made whether to attempt to secure union or if amputation is the treatment of choice. Factors favoring amputation include anticipated shortening of more than 2 or 3 inches (5 to 7.5 cm), a history of multiple failed surgical procedures, and stiffness and decreased function of a limb that would be more useful after an amputation and fitting with a prosthesis.

For the tibia with a cyst in the medullary canal, prophylactic curettage and autogenous iliac bone grafting are recommended. The limb is immobilized in plaster until the grafts have united, and then a brace, preferably of the patellar tendon–bearing type, is worn until skeletal maturity.

A tibia with anterior bowing and the narrow sclerotic canal of the high-risk tibia will generally fracture during the first 12 to 18 months of life. Initially, bracing may be beneficial for an anterolaterally bowed tibia with a narrow

canal in which a fracture has not developed. Once a fracture does develop the treatment is usually surgical. Occasionally treatment by pulsating electromagnetic fields may be indicated.

TREATMENT OF ESTABLISHED PSEUDARTHROSIS

Established congenital pseudarthrosis of the tibia has been treated in the past by bone grafting or amputation. Unfortunately sometimes grafting fails and must be followed by amputation.

Osseous union is probably more difficult to obtain in this condition than in any other. Consequently mature judgment is needed to choose the proper treatment. The age of the patient, the difficulty in obtaining union, and should union be obtained, the anticipated residual shortening and other deformities of the tibia must all be considered. In an infant or young child bone grafting is indicated as early as feasible. Even though the likelihood of obtaining union increases with increasing age, especially after puberty, the longer grafting is delayed the shorter and more poorly developed the leg will be and the more deformed and smaller the foot will be. When union is obtained in a young child, weight bearing in a brace results in more normal development of the limb. The child's par-

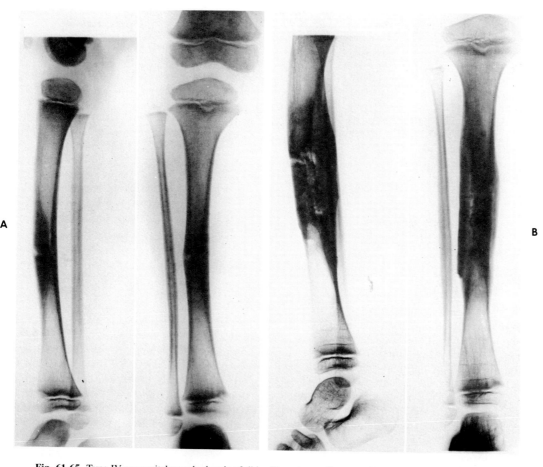

Fig. 61-65. Type IV congenital pseudarthrosis of tibia. There is specific type of insufficiency or stress fracture of tibia. **A,** Before treatment. Cortex is sclerotic, medullary canal is narrow, and bone is bowed only slightly. **B,** One year after treatment by dual onlay bone grafting.

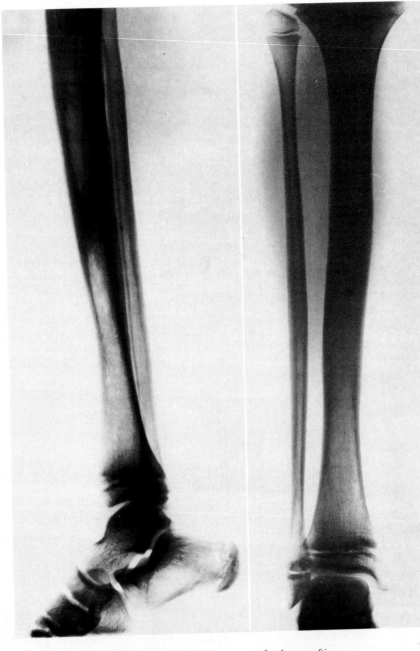

Fig. 61-65, cont'd. C, Seven years after bone grafting.

ents should be told that treatment often consists of several operations and that even then amputation may be necessary later because of failure to obtain union. If grafting is indicated but for some reason must be delayed, the limb should be braced to prevent increase in angulation at the pseudarthrosis. In an older child bone grafting is indicated unless shortness or other deformity of the limb is such that function would be better after amputation and fitting with a prosthesis.

Current studies are evaluating the use of pulsating electromagnetic fields externally and constant direct current implanted internally in the treatment of congenital pseudarthrosis of the tibia, and the results are promising. The use of a free vascularized fibular graft from the contralateral extremity is also promising (Fig. 61-66).

Surgical procedures that have been used commonly in recent years include the Boyd dual onlay bone graft, the McFarland bypass graft, the Sofield technique of multiple osteotomies, and insertion of medullary nail with or without the implantation of an electric stimulation device.

The Boyd dual onlay bone graft is the treatment of choice in patients with stress fractures that proceed to pseudarthrosis but do not have a wide gap between the bone ends.

For patients with a more established pseudarthrosis of the tibia, we recommend that the bone be straightened and

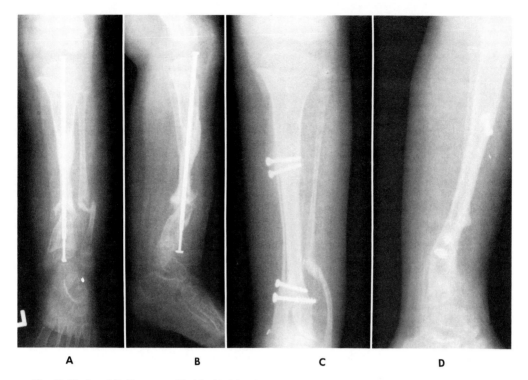

Fig. 61-66. **A** and **B,** Two-year-old girl with failed insertion of medullary nail and Sofield procedure. **C** and **D,** Same patient age 4 years at 18 months after excision of middle third of tibia and insertion of vascularized fibular graft.

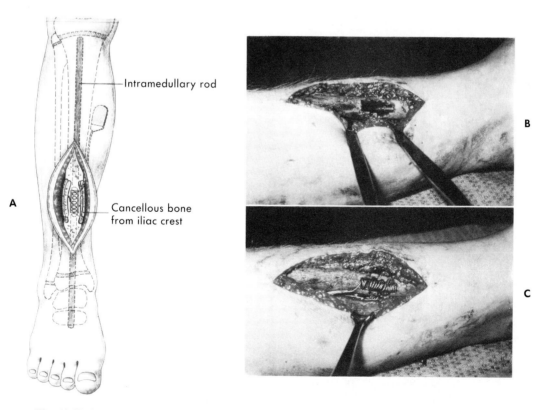

Fig. 61-67. **A,** Paterson procedure for congenital pseudarthrosis of tibia consisting of insertion of medullary rod, cancellous bone grafts, and constant direct current stimulator. **B,** Pseudarthrosis of tibia with medullary nail in canal and defect in cortical bone. **C,** Constant direct current stimulator placed in medullary canal. (Courtesy Sir Dennis Paterson.)

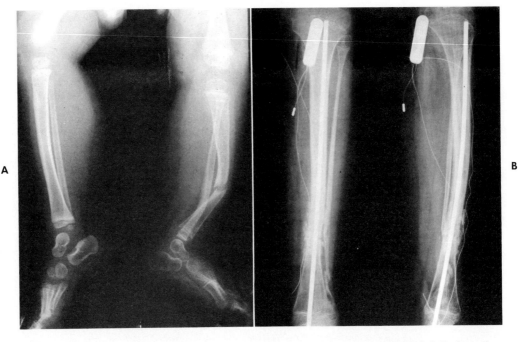

Fig. 61-68. A, Congenital pseudarthrosis of tibia at junction of middle and distal thirds of shaft. **B,** Immediately after insertion of medullary pin, cancellous bone grafts, and constant direct current stimulator. (Courtesy Sir Dennis Paterson.)

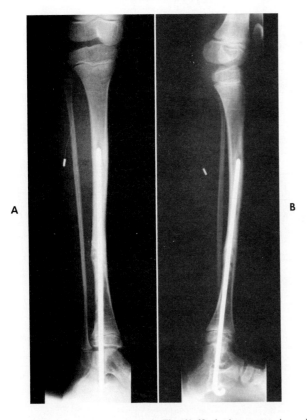

Fig. 61-69. Same patient as shown in Fig. 61-68. **A,** Anteroposterior and **B,** lateral roentgenograms made after clinical union was obtained and stimulator was removed. (Courtesy Sir Dennis Paterson.)

held in position with a medullary rod. We also recommend the use of a large quantity of autogenous iliac cancellous bone. Paterson reports a 75% union rate from his technique of inserting a medullary nail plus bone grafting and the implantion of an electric stimulation device in the medullary canal (Figs. 61-67 to 61-69).

Elvenny first called attention to the heavy cuff of tissue surrounding the bone at the pseudarthrosis and advised that it be completely excised before grafting. He reasoned that the presence of this tissue, whether congenital or secondary to the fracture, may decrease bone production and consequently healing. Since first reading McElvenny's interesting report we have found this thick tissue about the ends of the bone at every operation for this condition. It is consistent microscopically with that described by Aegerter as hamartomatous proliferation of fibrous tissue. Any operation for congenital pseudarthrosis should include complete excision of this tissue.

TECHNIQUE OF APPLYING DUAL GRAFTS (BOYD). Prepare two cortical tibial grafts 11 cm long and 2 cm wide and remove the endosteal bone from each. Have available an ample supply of cancellous bone in addition to that removed from the tibial grafts. When autogenous grafts are used cancellous bone is easily obtained from the proximal metaphysis of the donor tibia.

Expose the pseudarthrosis through a long anterior longitudinal incision. Excise all thickened periosteum and constricting fibrous tissue to healthy muscle and subcutaneous tissue. Resect all sclerotic bone from the ends of the fragments, but take care to preserve as much length of the bone as possible. Then with a drill open the medullary canal of each fragment. If necessary to correct anterior bowing of the tibia, lengthen the tendo calcaneus through

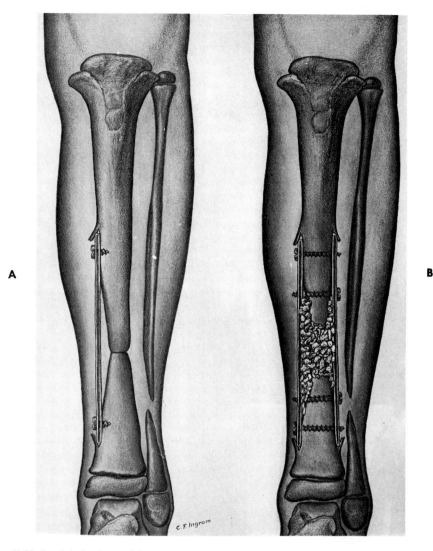

Fig. 61-70. Boyd dual onlay graft for congenital pseudarthrosis. **A,** First graft is held in position temporarily by two short screws. **B,** Subsequently both grafts are fixed in position by screws that pass through both grafts and intervening bone. Temporary screws have been removed and replaced by permanent screws, and trough has been filled with cancellous bone. (From Boyd, H.B.: J. Bone Joint Surg. **23:**497, 1941.)

a second incision (p. 2952). Osteotomizing the fibula is usually unnecessary because apposition of the tibial fragments is not needed and the intact fibula adds stability to the grafted tibia.

Next prepare beds for the grafts on the medial and lateral surfaces of the tibial fragments. Shave away enough bone from each side to create a flat surface for maximum contact between the grafts and the tibia. Remove more bone from the expanded areas of the tibia proximally and distally than from the region of pseudarthrosis. In fact, considerable space may remain between the tibia and the grafts near the pseudarthrosis, especially if the ends of the fragments are conical. This is not a disadvantage if the space is filled with cancellous bone. Place the graft as far distally on the tibia as possible without damaging the distal tibial epiphysis and also as far proximally as possible—the longer the graft the better. In small children it may extend to the proximal tibial epiphysis. Begin applying the grafts by placing one on the medial or lateral surface of the tibia and temporarily fixing it in position by two short screws (Fig. 61-70). Then apply the second graft on the opposite side of the bone and transfix both grafts and the proximal and distal tibial fragments by two long screws. Then remove the two short screws one at a time and replace them with similar long screws. Place the screws as far as practicable from the pseudarthrosis because they may predispose the tibia to fracture later.

Finally pack the space between the two grafts and about the pseudarthrosis with cancellous bone. Completely fill these areas both anteriorly and posteriorly. This is an important step in the operation because cancellous bone is necessary for union. With interrupted sutures close only the skin and subcutaneous tissues; make no effort to close the deep fascia.

AFTERTREATMENT. Apply a long leg cast or, if needed for adequate immobilization in a small obese child, a spica cast. At 10 to 14 days the cast is usually changed and should be changed again thereafter as often as necessary to ensure immobilization until the bone has united. A cast is usually necessary for a total of 4 to 6 months or more. After the last cast has been discarded, a long leg brace with a leather corset or a PTB brace is fitted and is worn until maturity. Because the tibia usually tends to angulate anteriorly, the brace recommended by Kite is excellent: the leather corset laces posteriorly rather than anteriorly so that a solid, well-molded piece of leather, rather than lacing, supports the anterior surface of the leg.

• • •

Boyd noted that even after osseous union has been obtained refracture is likely, and that if it occurs, a condition similar to the original pseudarthrosis quickly develops. Why bone is absorbed so rapidly from about the fracture is unknown. The hamartomatous tissue already mentioned may be responsible not only for causing bone to be absorbed but also for preventing new bone from forming, because it may strangle and narrow the area that needs remodeling. In one of our patients a fatigue fracture (sometimes called a march fracture, that is, one without displacement and resulting from some inadequacy in the bone to meet normal stress) gradually began to develop at the site of the original pseudarthrosis years after the bone had united; it differed from the usual march fracture, however, in that no callus formed about it. It so weakened the bone that a minor injury completed the fracture even though the patient was wearing a brace at the time, another typical pseudarthrosis resulted, and amputation was finally chosen.

Because refracture is so likely, it is important that bracing be continued until skeletal maturity. The patient should also be periodically examined for early evidence of an incipient march fracture, of recurrence of sclerosis in the area of previous pseudarthrosis, or of narrowing of a previously formed medullary canal. When one or more of these conditions is discovered, operation is indicated to excise all fibrous tissue and to reinforce the tibia by further grafting before a fracture occurs.

Of 22 patients we have operated on for congenital pseudarthrosis, 15 have reached skeletal maturity. Osseous union has been obtained in 12 of the 15, even though all 15 required more than one operation. This experience suggests that with patience and care the likelihood of union is good (Fig. 61-71).

Umber and Coleman have used medullary nailing of

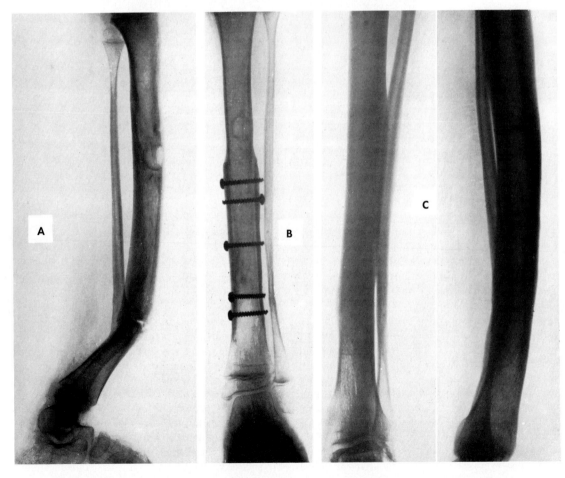

Fig. 61-71. A, Congenital pseudarthrosis in patient 7 years of age. **B,** Four months after dual bone grafting. **C,** Seven years after dual grafting.

both the tibia and fibula, autogenous iliac bone grafting, and immobilization in a spica cast. Union was obtained in four of six patients. The tibial pin crossed the ankle and subtalar joints to transfix the talus and the calcaneus. None of the patients had reached skeletal maturity at the time of their report.

McFarland described an ingenious grafting operation for congenital pseudarthrosis. In it he makes no attempt to correct the deformity; rather, he places a single graft so as to span the pseudarthrosis posteriorly (Fig. 61-72). His operation seems especially applicable in anterior angulation of the tibia with impending fracture. Of 11 procedures McFarland has reported, 9 were successful. The patients followed for a long time showed remarkable correction of angulation as well as incorporation and hypertrophy of the graft. We have used this technique in three patients; in two union was achieved and in one the operation failed because of infection in the wound after surgery. Four years later angulation of the two united tibias remained.

TECHNIQUE (McFARLAND AS DESCRIBED BY BOYD). Make a straight incision along the medial side of the tibia long enough for the contemplated graft and with the apex of the angulation opposite the middle of the incision. Now divide the subcutaneous tissue down to the hamartomatous periosteum and expose the periosteum circumferentially proximally and distally until normal periosteum is reached at each end. Resect all of the hamartomatous tissue. The bone for grafting, whether autogenous or homogenous, should be almost as wide as the tibia and long enough to reach normal periosteum proximally and distally. Raise an osteoperiosteal flap on the posterior aspect of both the proximal and distal tibia and taper each end of the graft to wedge snugly under the flaps (Fig. 61-72). Then insert the graft. If the graft is unstable, make transverse slots through the full thickness of the posterior cortex of the tibia at the appropriate levels and wedge the graft into them. Next fill the triangular space between the tibia and the graft with cancellous bone chips. With interrupted sutures close only

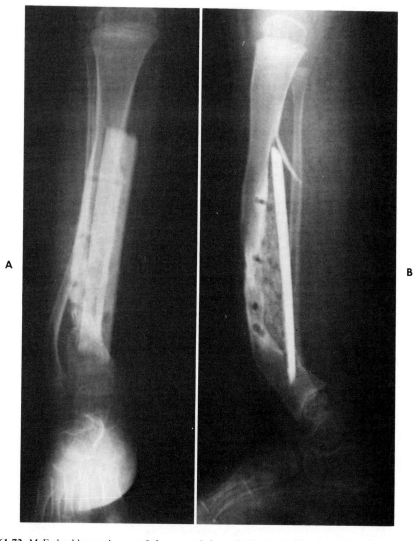

Fig. 61-72. McFarland bypass bone graft for congenital pseudarthrosis of tibia. **A** and **B,** Anteroposterior and lateral roentgenograms of tibia after removal of screws and insertion of bypass graft of homogenous freeze-dried bone. Space between tibia and graft is filled with cancellous bone.

the skin incision. Apply a long leg cast with the knee flexed 60 degrees.

AFTERTREATMENT. At 6 weeks weight bearing is started in a long leg cast and is continued until the graft has united to the tibia. Immobilization is then continued in a long leg brace with pressure applied in a posterior direction over the apex of the angulated tibia.

• • •

In a small series of patients with congenital pseudarthrosis of the tibia, Sofield successfully used a technique of multiple osteotomies and internal fixation with a medullary nail (Chapter 37). We have found it to be most useful when the distal fragment is too short to be held efficiently between dual grafts. Paterson has modified the method.

TECHNIQUE (PATERSON). Calculate preoperatively the amount of diseased bone to be excised from tracings made of recent anteroposterior and lateral roentgenograms. Approach the fibula through a lateral incision and perform an osteotomy to allow correction of the tibial deformity. Then approach the tibia through an anterior longitudinal incision. The exact amount of bone to be removed varies, but union is most likely when the whole sclerotic segment is excised and good quality bone is left in contact at each end. Such extensive excision, however, often leaves an unacceptable shortening (leg length discrepancy of up to 8 cm is acceptable). Sometimes the sclerotic segment is so long that some of it must be left in place, but union still occurs in most instances. Remove all abnormal, thick, fibrous tissue including the periosteum from the area of the defect. Choose a medullary rod (Steinmann pin or Küntscher nail) of the largest diameter that can be inserted. If the tibial medullary canal is quite small, a Rush nail can be used. Insert the rod in a retrograde fashion, beginning

at the defect and proceeding through the tibia, ankle joint, the talus, and the calcaneus to emerge through a small incision on the bottom of the heel. Take care to avoid any inversion, eversion, or equinus deformity of the foot. Then hammer the rod upwards into the proximal tibia to just below the epiphysis (Fig. 61-67, *A*). Cut off the distal end of the rod at the base of the calcaneus. Then insert the electrical bone growth stimulator according to the manufacturer's instructions (Fig. 61-67, *B* and *C*). Pack the area with cancellous bone grafts from the iliac crest, close the wound with absorbable sutures, and apply a long leg cast.

AFTERTREATMENT. The cast is changed at 2 weeks and weight bearing is encouraged once the skin has healed. The patient is examined every 2 months, and at 6 months the cast is removed with the patient under general anesthesia and union is assessed both clinically and roentgenographically. It is important to test for rotation of the distal tibial fragment around the medullary rod.

CONGENITAL HYPEREXTENSION AND DISLOCATION OF KNEE

Congenital hyperextention of the knee is only the first of three degrees of severity of a single abnormality. These degrees are (1) congenital hyperextension, (2) congenital hyperextension with anterior subluxation of the tibia on the femur, and (3) congenital hyperextension with anterior dislocation of the tibia on the femur (Fig. 61-73).

Congenital hyperextension or dislocation of the knee is usually associated with skeletal abnormalities elsewhere in the extremity. Katz, Grogono, and Soper in a study of 155 children with congenital dislocation of the knee treated in 17 Shriner's hospitals found other musculoskeletal abnormalities in 82%; 45% had congenital dislocation of the hip. Curtis and Fisher in a study of 15 knees with congen-

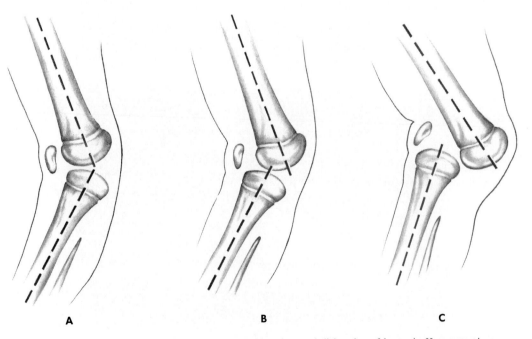

Fig. 61-73. Stages of congenital hyperextension, subluxation, and dislocation of knee. **A,** Hyperextension. **B,** Subluxation. **C,** Dislocation. (Redrawn from Curtis, B.H., and Fisher, R.L.: J. Bone Joint Surg. **51-A:**225, 1969.)

ital hyperextension and anterior subluxation of the tibia in 11 patients found an abnormality of the hip in each.

Katz et al. found the cruciate ligaments in five knees to be either markedly attenuated or absent and postulated that the basic defect in congenital dislocation of the knee is absence or hypoplasia of these ligaments. However, other investigators consider these findings secondary to the dislocation. Middleton has suggested that congenital hyperextension of the knee is caused by degeneration of the quadriceps muscles in utero, a form of myodystrophia fetalis. This may be the cause in some instances, but in most that respond rapidly, satisfactorily, and permanently to conservative stretching, the cause is probably malposition in utero. Often congenital hyperextension of the knee is one manifestation of arthrogryposis multiplex.

The pathology usually varies with the severity of the deformity, but always the anterior capsule of the knee and the quadriceps mechanism are contracted. As the severity of the anterior displacement of the tibia increases, other findings include intraarticular adhesions and other abnormalities within the joint and hypoplasia or absence of the patella. Curtis and Fisher noted fibrosis and loss of bulk of the vastus lateralis muscle. Furthermore, the suprapatellar pouch was obliterated by the adherent quadriceps tendon, and in over half of the knees the patella was displaced laterally. In severe anterior dislocation the collateral ligaments coursed anteriorly from their femoral attachments, and the hamstring muscles in some patients were subluxated anteriorly to function as extensors of the knee in the deformed position. In two small children whom we have treated surgically, the tibia and the patella were displaced laterally, and the iliotibial band and the lateral intermuscular septum were extremely hypertrophic.

The treatment of congenital hyperextension of the knee depends on the severity of the subluxation or dislocation and the age of the patient. In the newborn with mild to moderate hyperextension or subluxation, conservative treatment methods such as the use of the Pavlik harness for posturing of the knee in a continued position and serial casting to increase knee flexion are most likely to succeed. In children who do not respond to conservative measures the use of skeletal traction for correction is an option. The traction may allow the soft tissues to stretch enough to permit continuation of the serial casting technique. In older children with a moderate to severe subluxation or dislocation, surgery is indicated. In a child with both congenital dislocation of the knee and congenital dislocation of the hip, surgical correction of the knee first is advisable.

TECHNIQUE. Through an anteromedial approach (p. 37) expose the quadriceps tendon, the patella, and the patellar tendon. Lengthen the quadriceps tendon by Z-plasty and flex the knee as much as possible. Then divide any adhesions within the joint. Divide also the anterior part of the joint capsule. Steindler recommended suturing flaps of fat over the defect in the capsule.

AFTERTREATMENT. The knee is held in 90 degrees of flexion by a splint for 8 weeks. Then a brace with a stop at the knee joint that prevents the last 5 degrees of extension is fitted, and physical therapy is begun. The brace should be worn for at least 1 year or until it seems probable that the deformity will not recur. After the brace has been discarded, a splint holding the knee in some flexion should be worn at night.

Because the contours of the joint remain abnormal, the deformity may recur. Even if it does not, motion is usually limited. To correct recurrent hyperextension, osteotomy of the distal femur or proximal tibia is indicated when feasible; operations on the soft structures alone usually fail.

An operation necessary to reduce a congenital dislocation should be performed before the patient reaches the age of 2 years. It is similar to that for congenital hyperextension just described, but the anterior structures about the knee must be dissected more widely to permit reduction of the joint (Fig. 61-74).

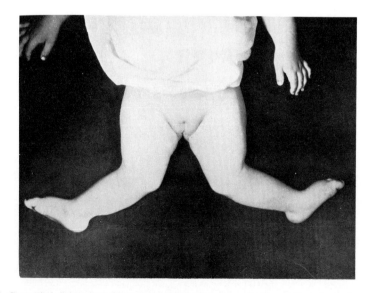

Fig. 61-74. Congenital dislocation of both knees treated by open reduction. Patient also had open reduction and shelf operation for congenital dislocation of right hip. Dislocation of left hip was treated conservatively.

TECHNIQUE (NIEBAUER AND KING). The operation of Niebauer and King is well illustrated in Fig. 61-75. After reduction the joint remains unstable because the contours of the bone are abnormal. To remedy this instability they recommend transferring the insertion of the anterior cruciate ligament distally on the tibia, but they warn that transferring it too far distally may produce a flexion contracture. They often transfix the femur and tibia with Steinmann pins and keep them in place for several weeks after surgery.

AFTERTREATMENT. With the knee flexed 30 degrees, a long leg cast is applied. At 8 weeks the cast is removed, the alignment of the joint is checked by roentgenograms, and the limb is measured for a long leg brace with a stop at the knee joint that will prevent hyperextension. A new long leg cast is then applied and is worn for 4 weeks. The brace is then fitted and is worn for at least a year or until it seems likely that dislocation will not recur. Because the articular surfaces of the knee are irrregular, function can be only fair and may deteriorate until fusion becomes necessary, or when growth is complete, arthroplasty may be done.

TECHNIQUE (CURTIS AND FISHER). Make a long anterior incision starting superomedially at the level of the lesser trochanter and extending inferolaterally to the tibial tuberosity. Expose the anterior thigh muscles and divide the quadriceps mechanism superior to the patella by either an inverted V-shaped incision (Fig. 61-76) or a Z-plasty. The former incision provides a tongue of tissue superior to the patella suitable for attachment of the proximal muscle mass after the extensor mechanism has been lengthened. Next divide the arterior capsule transversely and extend the

incision posteriorly to the tibial and fibular collateral ligaments. Mobilize and displace these ligaments posteriorly as the knee is flexed. If the patella is displaced laterally, release the lateral part of the patellar tendon so that the patella may be moved to its proper location on the femoral condyles. Now release any tight iliotibial band and lengthen the fibular collateral ligament if needed. Mobilize all normal-appearing quadriceps muscle and align it in the long axis of the femur to exert a direct pull on the patella. Suture the lengthened quadriceps mechanism with the knee

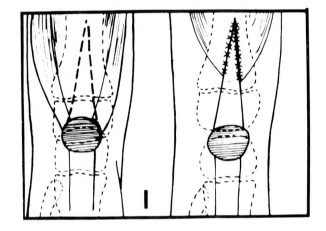

Fig. 61-76. Curtis and Fisher technique for congenital subluxation of knee. Quadriceps mechanism superior to patella is divided by inverted V-shaped incision. (From Curtis, B.H., and Fisher, R.L.: J. Bone Joint Surg. **51-A:**255, 1969.)

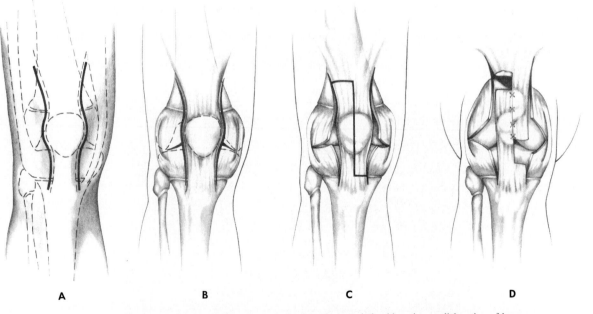

Fig. 61-75. Niebauer and King technique of open reduction of congenital subluxation or dislocation of knee. **A,** Capsule has been incised on each side of quadriceps tendon, patella, and patellar tendon. **B,** Capsule is incised transversely at joint level both medially and laterally. **C,** Technique of Z-plasty lengthening of quadriceps and patellar tendons. **D,** Z-plasty division has been carried out and tendon is sutured; division of capsule medially and laterally is adequate. (Redrawn from Niebauer, J.J., and King, D.E.: J. Bone Joint Surg. **42-A:**207, 1960.)

flexed 30 degrees. Close the wound and apply a long leg cast with the knee flexed 30 degrees.

AFTERTREATMENT. At 4 to 6 weeks the cast is removed, and active and passive exercises are begun. At 10 to 12 weeks weight bearing is permitted after optimal strength and range of motion are achieved. In older patients to prevent hyperextension of the knee, a long leg brace is worn after the cast is removed.

CONGENITAL DISLOCATION OF PATELLA

Congenital dislocation of the patella is often familial and bilateral. Occasionally it is accompanied by other abnormalities, especially arthrogryposis multiplex congenita and Down syndrome. It is persistent and irreducible, and there are usually abnormalities of the quadriceps mechanism; the vastus lateralis may be absent, and the patella may be attached to the anterior aspect of the iliotibial band. Often the patella is small and misshapen and in an abnormal location in the quadriceps mechanism. Genu valgum and external rotation of the tibia on the femur commonly develop. The capsule on the medial side of the knee is stretched, the lateral femoral condyle is flattened, or the insertion of the patellar tendon is located more laterally than normally. Stanisavljevic et al. postulate that the precursors of the quadriceps muscle and patella fail to internally rotate during the first trimester of fetal life and consequently the muscle remains on the anterolateral aspect of the thigh and the patella is permanently dislocated laterally.

The diagnosis of congenital dislocation of the patella is difficult to make before the patient is 3 to 4 years old. Because the severity of the deformity is directly related to the length of time that the deformity is allowed to remain uncorrected, surgery should be carried out as soon as the diagnosis is made.

Stanisavljevic et al. have described on operation to correct malrotation of the quadriceps muscle by medially rotating the muscle mass, the patella, and the lateral half of the patellar tendon.

TECHNIQUE (STANISAVLJEVIC ET AL.). Make a skin incision along the lateral aspect of the thigh, beginning proximally 4 cm inferior to the greater trochanter, curving anteriorly over the lateral femoral condyle, and ending 4 or 5 cm inferior to the medial tibial condyle (Fig. 61-77, *A*). Incise the subcutaneous tissues and expose the fascia lata and the anterior and medial aspects of the knee, including the pes anserinus. Next excise as much of the fascia lata from the lateral aspect of the thigh as possible and preserve it in a saline solution. Separate the vastus lateralis muscle from the lateral intermuscular septum and expose the periosteum on the lateral aspect of the femur (Fig. 61-77, *B*). Now incise the periosteum of the femur longitudinally 1 to 2 cm anterior to the lateral intermuscular septum. Incise the lateral capsule of the knee joint distally alongside the dislo-

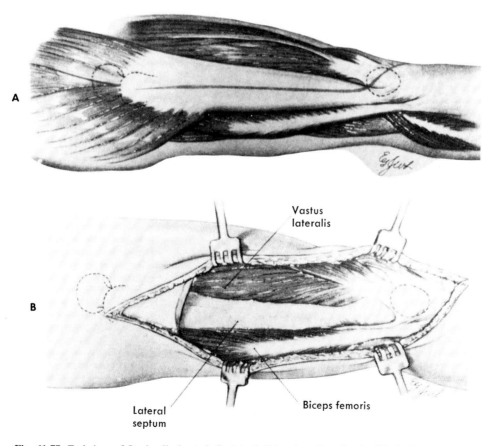

Fig. 61-77. Technique of Stanisavljevic et al. for lateral dislocation of patella. **A,** Skin incision. **B,** Vastus lateralis is separated from lateral intermuscular septum to expose periosteum of femur.

Continued.

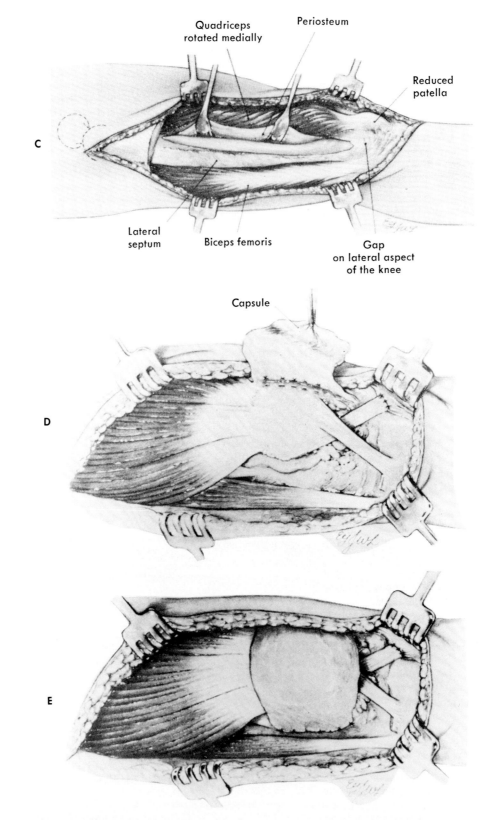

Fig. 61-77, cont'd. C, Periosteum of lateral aspect of femur and lateral joint capsule are incised longitudinally, and periosteum and quadriceps muscle are elevated from femur and rotated medially, carrying patella with them. **D,** Patellar tendon is divided longitudinally and its lateral half is detached from tibial tuberosity, is carried beneath medial half, and is sutured to tibia. **E,** Remaining medial flap of capsule is carried anteriorly and laterally and sutured to lateral edge of patella. (From Stanisavljevic, S., Zemenick, G., and Miller, D.: Clin. Orthop. **116:**190, 1976.)

cated patella and the patellar tendon to the tibial tuberosity. Next elevate the periosteum and the quadriceps muscle from the lateral and anterior aspects of the femur and rotate them medially, carrying with them the patella (Fig. 61-77, *C*). If necessary for adequate rotation of the soft tissues, incise the periosteum along the anterior aspect of the knee just proximal to the distal femoral epiphysis. Next expose the knee joint and correct any other pathologic conditions found. Make a medial parapatellar incision in the capsule to allow anatomic reduction of the patella. Next divide the patellar tendon longitudinally, detach its lateral half from the tibial tuberosity, carry this half beneath the remaining medial half, and suture it to the tibia near the insertion of the tibial collateral ligament (Fig. 61-77, *D*). Now place the patella in normal position beneath the thickened medial capsule and suture its medial border to this structure. Draw the remaining flap of medial capsule anteriorly and laterally over the patella and suture it to the lateral edge of the bone (Fig. 61-77, *E*). To prevent a synovial fistula cover the defect in the lateral retinaculum between the biceps femoris and the patella with the fascia lata that was previously excised. Close the incision and apply a long leg cast with the knee flexed 5 degrees to 10 degrees.

AFTERTREATMENT. At 5 to 6 weeks the long leg cast is removed, and active and passive exercises are started.

LOWER LIMB LENGTH DISCREPANCY

The treatment of lower limb length discrepancy involves children and adults, with congenital, developmental, paralytic, inflammatory, neoplastic, and posttraumatic disorders. Accurate assesment of growth in children and mature judgment are necessary if treatment is to be proper. In children the limb length equality desired or attainable at maturity must determine the type of treatment: shoe lift, brace, limb shortening, limb lengthening, or combinations of these. One must remember that all patients are not candidates for limb length equalization but may be better treated with a permanent orthosis or by amputation and fitting with a prosthesis, for example, proximal femoral focal deficiency with fibular hemimelia.

Developmental patterns

Shapiro reviewed the lower extremity length discrepancy in 803 children followed to skeletal maturity at the Growth Study Unit of the Children's Hospital Medical Center in Boston over a 40-year period and found that not all length discrepancies increase continually with time. Rather, several different patterns of developmental discrepancy occur, depending on the nature of the condition causing the discrepancy and on the time and place of their occurrence. Patients included in the study were followed in the unit for at least 5 years and, excepting those with fracture of the femur, had a discrepancy of at least 1.5 cm. Limb lengths were measured by standard roentgenographic methods and skeletal age by Todd's atlas and later by that of Greulich and Pyle, and were recorded on the Green and Anderson tibial and femoral length, growth remaining, and growth inhibition charts.

Five different developmental patterns of lower-extremity length discrepancy were observed. (Fig. 61-78).

Type I discrepancies have an upward slope pattern (Fig. 61-79), in which the discrepancy develops and increases continually with time, at the same proportionate rate or otherwise in a straight line. In its most severe manifestation this pattern is seen in proximal femoral focal deficiency (Fig. 61-79, *B*), epiphyseal destruction and enchondromatosis (Ollier's disease), and less severely in anisomelia (Fig. 61-79, *A*) (hemiatrophy or hemihypertrophy, and hemangiomatosis. It may also be seen in more severe forms of congenitally short femur, including coxa vara, but nearly two-fifths of such patients exhibit a different pattern. Approximately two-thirds of patients with poliomyelitic paralysis of the lower extremity muscles exhibited type I discrepancy patterns, and former studies have demonstrated a good but variable correlation between shortening and the severity of involvement. Upward slope patterns may also be seen in neurofibromatosis, juvenile rheumatoid arthritis, and Legg-Calvé-Perthes disease.

Type II discrepancies have an upward slope-deceleration pattern (Fig. 61-80) in which the discrepancy increases regularly and progressively for a time and then a decremental rate of increase occurs that varies with the patient and the condition under observation. This is the most dif-

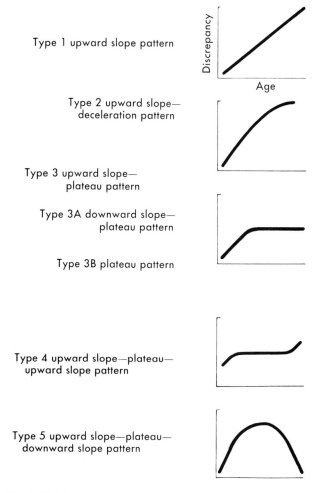

Fig. 61-78. Five patterns of leg length discrepancy observed by Shapiro at Growth Study Unit of Children's Medical Center in Boston.

ficult pattern to project, and thus requires the most careful monitoring. This type of discrepancy curve is sometimes seen after poliomyelitis, hemangiomatosis, in milder instances of congenitally short femur, septic arthritis of the hip, fractured femur, anisomelia, neurofibromatosis, and juvenile rheumatoid arthritis.

Type III discrepancies have an upward slope, plateau pattern (Fig. 61-81). This pattern typically was seen in overgrowth of the femur following anatomic reduction of a diaphyseal fracture, and once the plateau was reached, the discrepancy did not change throughout the remaining period of growth in the 116 fractures of the femur studied. In type IIIB the discrepancy is detected after it has developed and remains unchanged with further growth. Type III

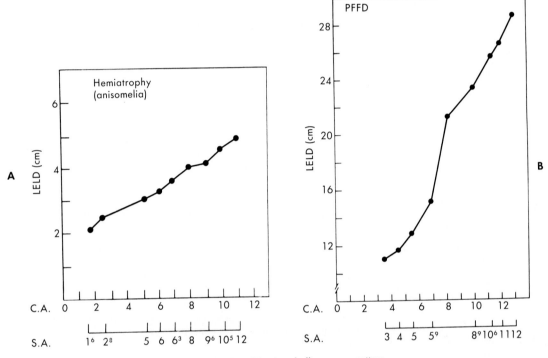
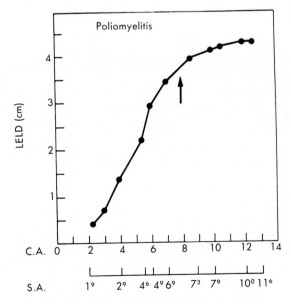

Fig. 61-79. Type I leg length discrepancy pattern.

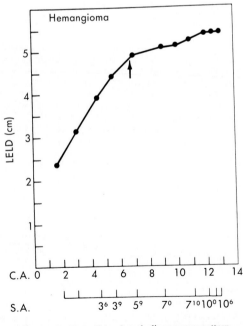

Fig. 61-80. Type II leg length discrepancy pattern.

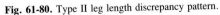

Fig. 61-81. Type III leg length discrepancy pattern.

developmental growth patterns are also seen in certain patients with congenitally short femur, after poliomyelitis, after osteomyelitis, and in hemiparetic cerebral palsy, anisomelia, hemangiomatosis, neurofibromatosis, juvenile rheumatoid arthritis, and Legg-Calvé-Perthes disease.

Type IV discrepancies have an upward slope-plateau-upward slope pattern (Fig. 61-82) in which the discrepancy develops, increases steadily for a while, stabilizes for a variable time, then increases again toward the end of the growth period. This curve pattern is characteristically seen after hip disease in childhood affecting the proximal femoral capital epiphysis such as septic arthritis of the hip with mild or moderate damage, Legg-Calvé-Perthes disease, and avascular necrosis of the femoral head with or without arrested growth of the epiphysis.

Type V discrepancies have an upward slope-plateau-downward slope pattern, (Fig. 61-83) in which the discrepancy undergoes spontaneous correction with growth and inactivation or correction of the causative pathologic process such as Legg-Calvé-Perthes disease, juvenile rheu-

matoid arthritis, and occasionally in hemiparetic cerebral palsy, hemangiomatosis, and neurofibromatosis.

The demonstration of these patterns of growth discrepancy and the identification of the various clinical entities in which they occur serve again to emphasize the importance of serial observations carried out at 6-month intervals at first and later annually with teleoroentgenograms of patients younger than 5 years of age and orthoroentgenograms for all older children, correlated with chronologic and skeletal age and recorded on tibial and femoral length, growth remaining, and growth inhibition charts. In this manner the orthopaedic surgeon collects maximum information on which he may then base his decision concerning the timing and the nature of the surgical procedure needed to equalize lower limb lengths.

Treatment

The treatment of a limb for an anticipated shortening in a child differs completely from that of a limb with an established shortening in an adult. In a child growth in the

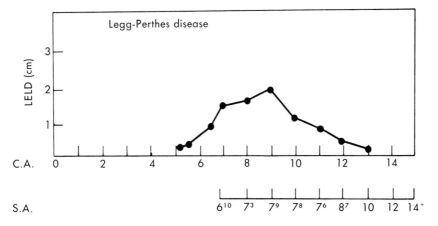

Fig. 61-82. Type IV leg length discrepancy pattern.

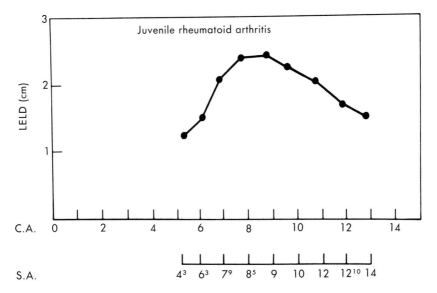

Fig. 61-83. Type V leg length discrepancy pattern.

longer limb may be retarded by operations on the epiphyseal plates at the appropriate age. As is mentioned later, operations designed to accelerate epiphyseal growth of the shorter limb have not been successful.

In an adult a discrepancy in limb length severe enough to warrant surgery is treated by resecting an appropriate segment of the femur or of the tibia and fibula of the longer limb or by surgical lengthening of the shorter limb.

Before any operation designed to equalize partially or completely the length of the lower extremities, it is important that the measurement of difference in their lengths be accurate. Many orthopaedic surgeons merely measure with tape the distance between the anterosuperior iliac spine and the medial malleolus, but White, Gill and Abbot, and Green and Anderson, and Moseley have described practical roentgenographic methods that are much more accurate. In a growing child the *rates* of growth of the two extremities are just as important as the difference in the lengths, and they should be plotted regularly against the child's skeletal age (Green and Anderson). Only by these data can the final difference in the lengths be anticipated and the ability of the shorter extremity to respond to epiphysiodesis of the longer one be predicted.

The various operations for correcting discrepancy in length of the lower extremities are discussed later. Remarkable discrepancies can be corrected accurately. The individual operations are based on different principles; therefore several methods are available, each of which has its advantages and disadvantages. As pointed out by Wag-

ner, it is the duty of the surgeon to select the proper operation or combination of operations best suited for a given patient. Therefore the surgeon must fully understand the cause and extent of the patient's disability and the magnitude and possible complications of all the operations available to be able to advise the patient properly.

In considering a treatment program it is important to realize that discrepancy in limb length of 2 cm or less can be satisfactorily camouflaged by conservative means; therefore surgery for discrepancy of 2 cm or less is rarely indicated. Further, if in addition to the shortening the extremity is so deformed that it will require a brace permanently, then surgical lengthening is probably not indicated because usually the brace can also be made to correct for shortening. When a decision has been made to correct discrepancy in length of the limbs by surgery, the surgeon must consider the value of a relatively simple procedure such as shortening of the healthy limb as opposed to an extensive operation such as lengthening of the pathologic limb.

Surgical lengthening corrects the shortening directly and can result in complete restoration of length of the limb. However, shortening operations usually leave the original deformity untouched while producing a symmetric duplication of the deformity, reducing total height of the body, and disturbing significantly the proportions of the body. This may be relatively unimportant in tall patients but is quite important in shorter ones, especially in females. Composite photography developed by Wagner (Fig. 61-84)

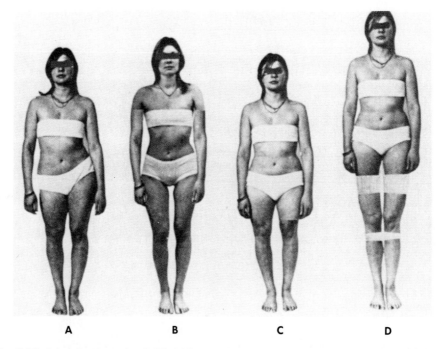

A   B   C   D

Fig. 61-84. Composite photos showing body disproportions after limb shortening operations. **A,** Woman, 24 years old, with marked shortening of right lower limb caused by right hip joint sepsis during infancy, with varus deformity of left knee after Blount epiphysiodesis of distal femur and proximal tibia; residual shortening of right femur of 8.5 cm. **B,** Result of operative lengthening of right femur by 8.5 cm (unretouched photograph). **C,** Composite photograph showing results if left femur had been shortened by 8.5 cm. **D,** Composite photograph showing results if epiphysiodesis had not been performed and total limb discrepancy had been fully corrected by a lengthening operation. (From Wagner, H.: Reprint from Hungeford, D.S., editor: Progress in orthopaedic surgery, vol. 1, Berlin, 1977, Springer-Verlag.)

demonstrates that when the lower extremities are shortened, the torso and upper limbs seem to be loo long; this is especially true if the shortening is below the knees.

The disadvantages of lengthening operations must be weighed against the advantages of shortening operations as follows. (1) Lengthening operations require a long period of hospitalization. Depending on the severity of the inequality, hospitalization may be required for 6 weeks to 6 months as compared with only about 2 weeks required for shortening operations. Bony consolidation after lengthening requires up to 8 months, whereas that following shortening usually requires only 3 to 4 months. Most patients with lengthening operations require cancellous bone grafting, which is almost never required in shortening operations. (2) Lengthening osteotomies are difficult in patients over 20 years of age because the osteotomy does not heal rapidly. Lengthening operations after the age of 40 years are contraindicated, whereas shortening operations can be performed at any age. (3) Lengthening operations are technically difficult to perform; they may require three or four stages (osteotomy, osteosynthesis by internal fixation, cancellous bone grafting, and removal of metallic implants). Further, in lengthening operations additional surgery is often needed such as lengthening of the tendo calcaneus, adductor tenotomy, and lengthening of the flexors of the knee. Shortening operations, on the other hand, are usually technically easy and may require only one or two stages (osteotomy and removal of metallic implants). Furthermore, additional surgery is rarely required after shortening operations. (4) Lengthening operations often produce tension on the soft tissues, resulting in temporary restriction of motion of adjacent joints. Shortening operations, on the other hand, although they may occasionally result in muscular weakness, do not produce restriction of motion of joints. These factors are listed in Table 61-2 developed by Wagner; these should be carefully considered by both the surgeon and the patient before a definite decision is made.

Surgical shortening is indicated more often in the femur because shortening in the tibia is associated with a relatively high incidence of complications. In the experience of Wagner, whereas it is technically possible to lengthen a limb by amounts up to 22 cm, esthetic considerations and the presence of excessive amounts of soft tissue and of muscular insufficiencies after surgery limit shortening operations to 10 cm.

In summary, whereas the variety of choices of operations makes the selection of the appropriate one more difficult, it also allows the selection of the proper combination that will be appropriate in any given patient.

Limb shortening

The long limb may be shortened either by epiphyseal arrest or by resecting a segment of the femur or of the tibia and fibula. For a child with a growth expectancy of several years, epiphyseal arrest is a simple but effective method of equalizing the limb lengths. For adults shortening the long limb may be preferable to lengthening the shorter one. There are obvious disadvantages in shortening the normal limb. Complications from the operation could be catastrophic, but are no more likely to occur than after other elective operations. The chief disadvantage is that the total height of the body is decreased; as already mentioned, in patients of average height or taller, this is not a major consideration, but in shorter ones it may cause continued dissatisfaction even though the limb lengths have been equalized.

EPIPHYSEAL ARREST

Before 1933, when Phemister introduced his method of arresting the longitudinal growth of bones, little could be done to correct inequality in the length of the limbs in growing children. His operation and the others that have

Table 61-2. Advantages and disadvantages of leg lengthening and leg shortening operations*

Leg lengthening	Leg shortening
+ Surgery on the affected limb	− Operation of the uninvolved limb
+ Correction of concomitant deformities of the involved limb	− Operation on both legs necessary if concomitant deformities have to be corrected
+ Correction of deformity (restitutio ad integrum)	− Compensation of deformity
+ Preservation of body length	− Diminution of body weight
+ Normalization of body proportions	− Interference with body proportions
+ Can be done on femur and/or tibia	− Leg operations may lead to complications
+ Gain of length up to 22 cm	− Limitation of correction up to approximately 10 cm
+ Shortening of uninvolved limb usually not necessary	− Lengthening of the shortened limb frequently necessary
− Long hospitalization (6 weeks-6 months)	+ Short hospitalization (3 weeks)
− Slow consolidation (8 weeks-8 months)	+ Quick bony consolidation (8-12 weeks)
− Cancellous grafting frequently necessary	+ No cancellous bone graft at osteotomy site
− Increasing problems with advancing age	+ Age of no importance
− Operation technically difficult	+ Operation technically easy
− Three- to four-stage surgery necessary (osteotomy, osteosynthesis, spongiosa grafting, metallic implant removal)	+ Two-stage operation (osteotomy, removal of metallic implants)
− Concomitant surgery frequently necessary (achillotenotomy, knee flexor lengthening)	+ No concomitant surgery required
− Temporary restriction of motion of adjacent joints caused by soft tissue tension	+ No restriction of joint motion

*From Wagner, H.: Reprint from Hungerford, D.S., editor: Progress in orthopaedic surgery, vol. 1, Berlin, 1977, Springer-Verlag.

followed consist of fusing one or more of the epiphyses of the longer limb to retard the growth of this limb; because the growth of the shorter limb is allowed to continue, the length of the two limbs may be equal (or nearly so, as desired) at maturity. These operations, of course, are effective only when done several years before maturity. They are relatively simple and involve little risk either to the limb or to life; however, unless carefully timed, they will fail to achieve the desired correction, and unless carefully done, they will result in complications.

GROWTH PREDICTION

Several important facts should be noted about timing epiphyseal arrests and predicting the final correction they are to produce.

1. Although the operation inhibits the growth of the longer limb, its effect on the relative lengths of the limbs is determined by the growth potential of the shorter one; when this potential is abnormal, the amount of shortening desired in the longer one must be adjusted accordingly.

2. Skeletal age is much more important than chronologic age in determining the relative maturity of a child and in timing epiphyseal arrests. Skeletal age may be determined from Todd's atlas or from that of Greulich and Pyle.

3. The average skeletal age at which the distal femoral and proximal tibial epiphyses close, according to Green and Anderson, is 15¼ years in girls and 17¼ years in boys. In their studies the epiphyses closed within 1 year of these skeletal ages in every instance, but the chronologic ages at the time of closure varied over a range of 4 to 5 years.

4. The average annual growth at the distal femoral epiphysis is ⅜ inch (0.9 cm) and at the proximal tibial and fibular epiphyses ¼ inch (0.6 cm), according to White; these values are about the same as those found by Green and Anderson.

In 1957 Anderson and Green devised a new growth prediction chart (Fig. 61-85) to replace those of 1947 and 1951. It is based on 50 boys and 50 girls, each "being represented at every consecutive skeletal age"; the 1950 edition of the Greulich and Pyle atlas was used to determine the skeletal ages. The chart shows the amount of growth remaining in the normal distal femoral and proximal tibial epiphyses at the various skeletal ages. Because the chart is based on normal growth, adjustments must be made for the individual patient when using it to predict the correction to be derived from epiphyseal arrest, as follows.

1. *Percent of growth inhibition in the short limb.* When this percentage is high, adjustment should be made toward the lower value on the chart for the given age.

2. *Extreme variations in bone lengths.* For a tall child with long legs adjustments should be made toward the upper value and for a short child with short legs toward the lower.

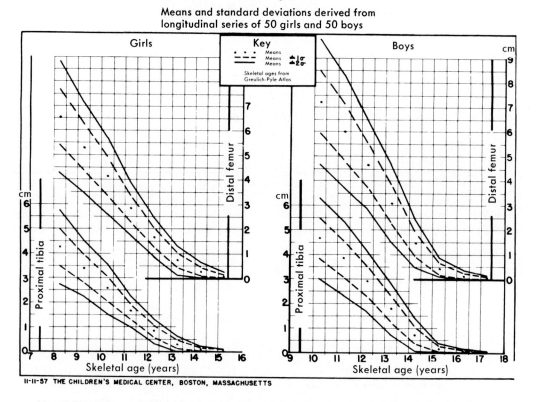

Growth remaining in normal distal femur and proximal tibia following consecutive skeletal age levels

Means and standard deviations derived from longitudinal series of 50 girls and 50 boys

11-11-57 THE CHILDREN'S MEDICAL CENTER, BOSTON, MASSACHUSETTS

Fig. 61-85. Anderson and Green revised growth prediction chart showing amount of growth potential in normal distal femoral and proximal tibial epiphyses at various skeletal ages. Since it is based on normal growth, adjustment must be made for individual patients in predicting correction to be derived from epiphyseal arrest (From Anderson, M., Green, W.T., and Messner, M.B.: J. Bone Joint Surg. **45-A:**1, 1963.)

3. *The child's individual pattern of skeletal maturation.*

The reader is referred to the work of Green and Anderson for the technique involved in using their chart. We now use the Moseley straight-line graph (Fig. 61-86) that makes easier the recording and interpretation of data in patients with discrepancy in limb lengths. The method predicts future growth and automatically takes into account the child's growth percentile and the degree of growth inhibition in the short limb. It can be used to predict the effects of corrective operations and thus establish the proper timing of epiphysiodesis. Moseley carefully studied 30 patients who had been treated by epiphysiodesis and had been followed to skeletal maturity and found that his straight-line graph method was significantly more accurate than the growth-remaining graph method, especially in patients with growth inhibition.

Two new concepts distinguish this method from the traditional one. The first is that the growth of the limbs can be represented by straight lines by a suitable manipulation of the scale of the abscissa. The second is that a nomogram relating limb length to skeletal age provides a correction factor for the growth percentile that is easily applied to these growth lines.

Regarding the first concept, it should be emphasized that this is purely a mathematical principle and is neither concerned with the nature of the data at hand nor involves an approximation of the data or the selection of an ideal case. In the straight-line graph method, the length of the long lower extremity is represented by a straight line because the method of plotting points defines it so. The following consequences result.

1. Growth of the short limb is also represented by a straight line that lies below that of the long limb on the graph and will have a different slope depending on its rate of growth.

2. The discrepancy in limb lengths is represented by the vertical distance on the graph between the two lines.

3. The percentage of inhibition of growth of the short limb is represented by the difference in slope of the two growth lines, designating the slope of the normal limb as 100%.

4. The growth line of a lower limb that has undergone surgical lengthening thereafter approximates a straight line of the same slope but is displaced upward on the graph by an amount equal to the lengthening accomplished.

5. The length of the lower limb that has been treated by epiphysiodesis thereafter approximates a straight line of

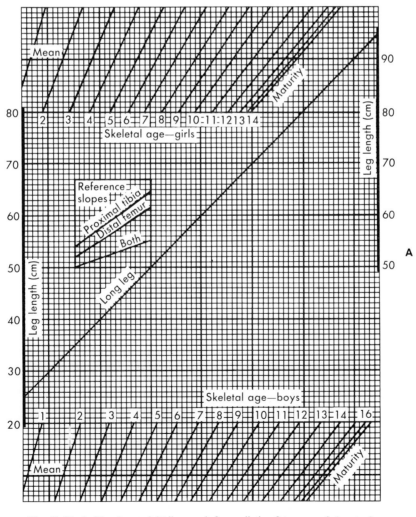

Fig. 61-86. A, Moseley straight-line graph for predicting future growth (see text).

Continued.

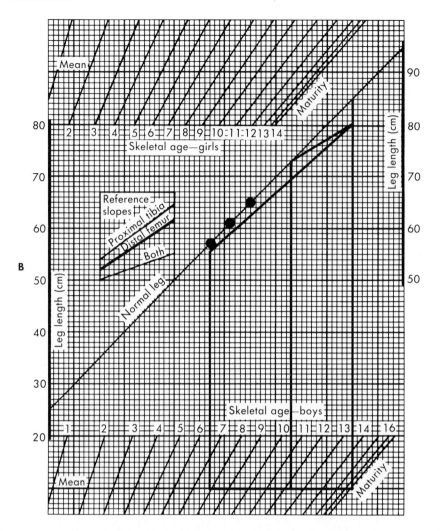

Fig. 61-86, cont'd. B, Moseley graph demonstrating static limb length discrepancy and planned result of distal epiphysiodesis.

decreased slope where the decrease in slope (the normal being defined as 100%) exactly equals the percentage contribution that the fused epiphyseal plate would otherwise have made to the total growth of the limb. Because the contributions of the proximal tibial and distal femoral epiphyseal plates are approximately 28% and 37%, respectively, of the total growth of the limb, the amount of inhibition to be introduced by epiphysiodesis can be predicted. The growth line of the limb operated on in tibial, femoral, or combined epiphysiodesis will thereafter have a slope of 72%, 63%, or 35%, respectively. This new growth line will be parallel to one of the three reference lines drawn on the graph for the specific slopes.

Regarding the second concept, in the straight-line graph method a nomogram is used to obtain a correction factor for growth percentile since skeletal age data are plotted with reference to sloping lines whose positions are based on the growth data of Anderson and Green. The inaccuracies of single estimates of skeletal age are circumvented by making use of all longitudinal data plotted on the nomogram to predict the length of the normal lower limb at

maturity. This gives a representation of the percentile in which a child's growth plot belongs and allows placement on the graph of a vertical line representing the cessation of growth. This line serves as a guide not only to predict the child's final discrepancy but also to estimate the final results of surgery to correct the discrepancy.

The straight-line graph method thus provides a means of assessing clearly and accurately the pattern of past growth of the limbs and allows the prediction of a pattern of growth and of the end point of future growth. The growth lines on the graph can be manipulated either by displacing the line of the short limb upward for a limb lengthening procedure or by decreasing the slope of the normal line of the long limb for an epiphysiodesis in such a way that the two growth lines will converge at cessation of growth.

Certain assumptions are implied in this method and in the traditional methods of prediction of future growth.

1. That the method of comparing roentgenograms of the patient's hand with standards permits the skeletal age of the patient studied to be determined at any chronologic age with precision. This is not true.

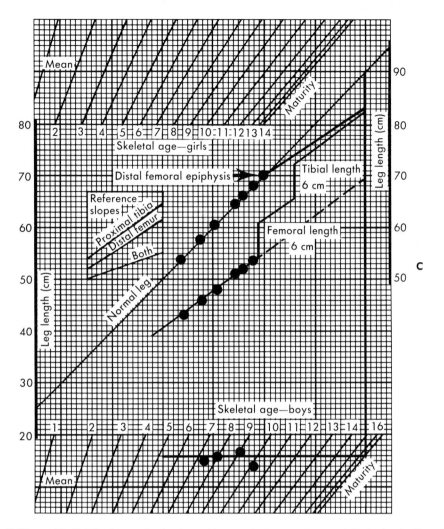

Fig. 61-86, cont'd. C, Moseley graph of patient with congenitally short femur and fibular hemimelia and demonstrating plan of femoral lengthening, tibial lengthening, and distal femoral epiphysiodesis. (From Moseley, C.F.: J. Bone Joint Surg. **59-A:**174, 1977.)

2. That skeletal age as defined by Greulich and Pyle correlates perfectly with growth. This also is not true.

3. That the growth line of the short lower limb is straight and can be plotted on the same graph as the normal limb. This is obviously false in recent poliomyelitis, and the method would not take into account any alteration in the growth rate of the shorter limb resulting from metabolic diseases and other factors.

4. That the individual child remains constantly in the same percentile as regards growth with respect to skeletal age. This is open to question.

5. That the length of the lower limbs of all children of a certain skeletal age is the same proportion of the limb lengths as those people when they reach adulthood regardless of their growth percentiles or chronologic ages. This is unlikely for children of different races or with markedly different familial habitus.

We have had moderate experience with this method, and it has certain advantages when compared with traditional ones. The margin of error is decreased because the number of measurements and mathematical calculations required is kept to a minimum. Perhaps its greatest advantage is that it demonstrates clearly the presence of growth inhibition and automatically takes it into account when making decisions regarding the timing of surgery. Fig. 61-87 shows use of the graph clinically in the depiction of past growth, the prediction of future growth, the effect of surgery, the timing of surgery, and examination after surgery.

Fries in 1976, using the growth charts of Anderson, Green, and Messner, developed four simple straight-line equations representing the mean values of these growth charts. They predict the growth remaining in an epiphyseal plate at any given age, are easily memorized, and can be used for rapid calculations.

Male
Distal femur: cm + 1½ age = 23
Proximal tibia: cm + age = 15

Female
Distal femur: cm + 1¼ age = 17
Proximal tibia: cm + age = 13

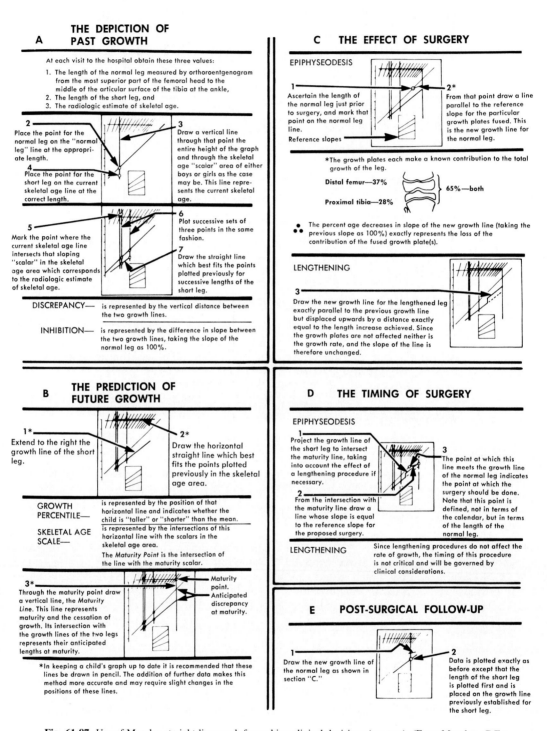

A THE DEPICTION OF PAST GROWTH

At each visit to the hospital obtain these three values:

1. The length of the normal leg measured by orthoroentgenogram from the most superior part of the femoral head to the middle of the articular surface of the tibia at the ankle,
2. The length of the short leg, and
3. The radiologic estimate of skeletal age.

2 Place the point for the normal leg on the "normal" line at the appropriate length.

4 Place the point for the short leg on the current skeletal age line at the correct length.

3 Draw a vertical line through that point the entire height of the graph and through the skeletal age "scalar" area of either boys or girls as the case may be. This line represents the current skeletal age.

5 Mark the point where the current skeletal age line intersects that sloping "scalar" in the skeletal age area which corresponds to the radiologic estimate of skeletal age.

6 Plot successive sets of three points in the same fashion.

7 Draw the straight line which best fits the points plotted previously for successive lengths of the short leg.

DISCREPANCY— is represented by the vertical distance between the two growth lines.

INHIBITION— is represented by the difference in slope between the two growth lines, taking the slope of the normal leg as 100%.

B THE PREDICTION OF FUTURE GROWTH

1* Extend to the right the growth line of the short leg.

2* Draw the horizontal straight line which best fits the points plotted previously in the skeletal age area.

GROWTH PERCENTILE— is represented by the position of that horizontal line and indicates whether the child is "taller" or "shorter" than the mean.

SKELETAL AGE SCALE— is represented by the intersections of this horizontal line with the scalars in the skeletal age area.

The *Maturity Point* is the intersection of the line with the maturity scalar.

3* Through the maturity point draw a vertical line, the *Maturity Line*. This line represents maturity and the cessation of growth. Its intersection with the growth lines of the two legs represents their anticipated lengths at maturity.

Maturity point.
Anticipated discrepancy at maturity.

*In keeping a child's graph up to date it is recommended that these lines be drawn in pencil. The addition of further data makes this method more accurate and may require slight changes in the positions of these lines.

C THE EFFECT OF SURGERY

EPIPHYSEODESIS

1 Ascertain the length of the normal leg just prior to surgery, and mark that point on the normal leg line.
Reference slopes

2* From that point draw a line parallel to the reference slope for the particular growth plates fused. This is the new growth line for the normal leg.

*The growth plates each make a known contribution to the total growth of the leg.

Distal femur—37%
Proximal tibia—28%
65%—both

The percent age decreases in slope of the new growth line (taking the previous slope as 100%) exactly represents the loss of the contribution of the fused growth plate(s).

LENGTHENING

3 Draw the new growth line for the lengthened leg exactly parallel to the previous growth line but displaced upwards by a distance exactly equal to the length increase achieved. Since the growth plates are not affected neither is the growth rate, and the slope of the line is therefore unchanged.

D THE TIMING OF SURGERY

EPIPHYSEODESIS

1 Project the growth line of the short leg to intersect the maturity line, taking into account the effect of a lengthening procedure if necessary.

2 From the intersection with the maturity line draw a line whose slope is equal to the reference slope for the proposed surgery.

3 The point at which this line meets the growth line of the normal leg indicates the point at which the surgery should be done. Note that this point is defined, not in terms of the calendar, but in terms of the length of the normal leg.

LENGTHENING

Since lengthening procedures do not affect the rate of growth, the timing of this procedure is not critical and will be governed by clinical considerations.

E POST-SURGICAL FOLLOW-UP

1 Draw the new growth line of the normal leg as shown in section "C."

2 Data is plotted exactly as before except that the length of the short leg is plotted first and is placed on the growth line previously established for the short leg.

Fig. 61-87. Use of Moseley straight-line graph for making clinical decisions (see text). (From Moseley, C.F.: J. Bone Joint Surg. **59-A:**174, 1977.)

Centimeters in these formulas represent the remaining growth at each epiphysis within 0.5 cm. The ages used are skeletal ages as determined by comparing roentgenograms of the hand with the atlas of Gruelich and Pyle.

Fig. 61-88 shows the approximate contribution of each epiphysis to longitudinal growth.

EPIPHYSIODESIS

Epiphysiodesis is generally the treatment of choice for anticipated shortening of 2 to 10 cm. Many authors use 5 cm as the upper limit of epiphysiodesis and the lower limit to consider limb lengthening. We have been pleased with these guidelines, but will extend the use of epiphysiodesis to a maximum of 10 cm.

White reported his experiences with epiphyseal arrest in 279 patients; in 198, the distal femoral epiphysis alone was arrested; in 40, the proximal tibial and fibular epiphyses, in 41, all three. In 46 patients who had the distal femoral epiphysis arrested and who were followed to maturity, the average limb length discrepancy was only 1.7 cm. White recommended that arrest of the distal femoral epiphysis be deferred until at least the age of 8 years and of the proximal tibial and fibular epiphyses until at least the age of 10 years. He reserved arrest of all three epiphyses for those patients seen too late or those whose discrepancies were increasing too rapidly to expect equalization from femoral arrest alone. In planning arrest of all three, it may be wise to perform only the femoral arrest initially and to observe the patient for 1 or 2 years before arresting the other two epiphyses; this safeguards against overcorrection should the rate of growth in the affected limb change.

Menelaus reported his experiences with epiphyseal arrest in 96 patients, 44 of whom had become skeletally mature before the study. Timing of the arrests had been based on the assumptions that the average annual growth at the distal femoral epiphysis is 1.1 cm and at the proximal tibial and fibular epiphyses is 0.7 cm (White), and that these epiphyses close at age 14 years in girls and 16 years in boys. Of the 44 patients studied, 52% showed correction within 0.7 cm of the predicted amount and 93% within 2 cm. In the remaining 7% a discrepancy of more than 2 cm remained. Calculated another way, 80% obtained correction within 1.2 cm of the predicted amount; this figure should be compared with the 89.6% obtained by Green and Anderson using their method of predicting growth (p. 2688).

Abbott and Gill developed approaches to the epiphyseal plates about the knee and ankle that do little damage to the soft tissues.

LATERAL EXPOSURE OF DISTAL FEMORAL, PROXIMAL TIBIAL, AND PROXIMAL FIBULAR EPIPHYSEAL PLATES (ABBOTT AND GILL). Support the knee in 30 degrees flexion so that the landmarks

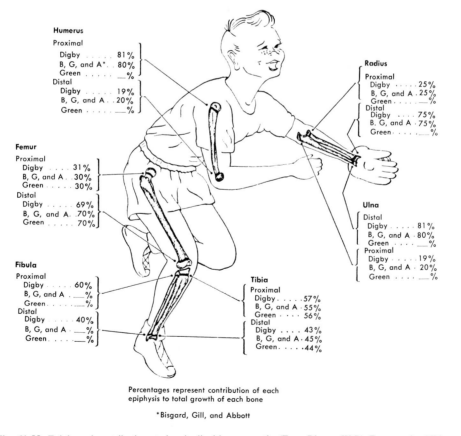

Percentages represent contribution of each
epiphysis to total growth of each bone

*Bisgard, Gill, and Abbott

Fig. 61-88. Epiphyseal contributions to longitudinal bone growth. (From Blount, W.P.: Fractures in children, Baltimore, 1954, The Williams & Wilkins Co. © 1954, The Williams & Wilkins Co., Baltimore, Md., 21202, U.S.A.)

are prominent and the hamstrings are relaxed. Beginning 6.5 cm proximal to the lateral femoral condyle, incise the skin over the interval between the biceps tendon and the iliotibial band, proceed distally and posteriorly to the head of the fibula, and then gently curve anteriorly to the lateral surface of the leg (Fig. 61-89, *B*). We have found that two short incisions 2.5 cm in length separated by a bridge of skin and subcutaneous tissue result in less noticeable scars. Image intensification may be used to center the incision over the epiphyses. Expose the lateral intermuscular septum to the linea aspera and retract the vastus lateralis muscle anteriorly. This exposes the lateral surface of the femur at its junction with its condyle, the site of the epiphyseal plate. Divide and ligate the superior lateral genicular vessels. Then in the periosteum make a longitudinal I-shaped incision across the epiphyseal plate. By subperiosteal dissection raise flaps of periosteum anteriorly and posteriorly to expose the epiphyseal plate, which appears as a thin white transverse line.

Now develop the distal incision and expose the proximal tibial and fibular epiphyses as follows. Identify and isolate the common peroneal nerve medial to the biceps tendon. Then make an incision directly down to the head of the fibula over its anterolateral aspect and expose the epiphyseal plate by subperiosteal dissection. Expose the lateral aspect of the proximal tibial epiphysis by reflecting the origin of the extensor muscles from the arcuate line.

MEDIAL EXPOSURE OF DISTAL FEMORAL AND PROXIMAL TIBIAL EPIPHYSEAL PLATES (ABBOTT AND GILL). Make a curved medial longitudinal incision 12.5 cm long as follows. Begin proximal to the adductor tubercle, proceed distally across it and the femoral condyle, and gently curve anteriorly in line with the tendon of the sartorius (Fig. 61-89, *A*). Or as we prefer, along this line of incision make two incisions 2.5

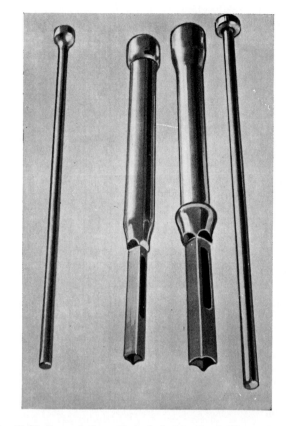

Fig. 61-90. Square hollow chisels devised by Dr. J. Warren White to make epiphysiodesis easier; obturators for each chisel are also shown.

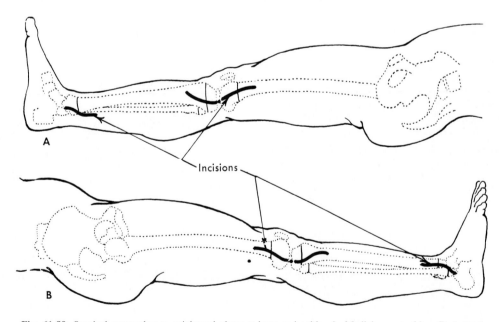

Fig. 61-89. Surgical approaches to epiphyseal plates at knee and ankle. **A,** Medial aspect of leg. **B,** Lateral aspect of leg. (From Abbott, L.C., and Gill, G.G.: Arch. Surg. **46:**591, 1943.)

cm long separated by a bridge of intact skin and subcutaneous tissue. Incise the deep fascia over the medial aspect of the femur, follow the anterior surface of the medial intermuscular septum to the bone, and retract the vastus medialis anteriorly. The epiphyseal plate is overlapped by the attachment of the capsule and the reflected synovial membrane of the knee joint. Ligate and divide the superior medial genicular vessels, expose the epiphyseal plate at the adductor tubercle through a longitudinal incision in the periosteum, and increase the exposure by subperiosteal dissection.

Expose the medial aspect of the proximal tibial epiphysis by incising the deep fascia at the anterior margin of the sartorius tendon; idenfity and retract posteriorly the anterior edge of the tibial collateral ligament. Through a longitudinal incision directly anterior to this ligament expose the epiphyseal plate, which is located about 1 to 2 cm distal to the articular surface of the tibia.

TECHNIQUES OF EPIPHYSIODESIS

Before arrest of the distal femoral and proximal tibial and fibular epiphyses, anteroposterior roentgenograms of the knee should be made to determine the exact contour of the epiphyses. In a child the epiphyseal plates do not lie in a plane exactly transverse to the longitudinal axis of the bones. The distal femoral epiphysis is usually shaped like a shallow V when viewed from the front and the proximal tibial epiphysis is somewhat like an inverted V. The planes of the epiphyseal plates become transverse at maturity.

TECHNIQUE (WHITE). White used a hollow chisel that resembles an apple corer in principle and is made from a woodworker's mortising chisel about 1.2 cm square (Fig. 61-90). An obturator is made from a rod small enough to fit loosely in the chisel. We use White's technique because it makes the operation easier and shorter, permits better access to the epiphyseal plate, makes plugging of the bony defect more secure, allows better closure of the periosteum, and causes less local reaction.

After exposing the epiphyseal plate medially and laterally, accurately determine its direction by probing with an ordinary straight needle if desired. Then straddle the plate on one side with the mortising chisel diagonally so that two of its four points are forced into the plate and one each into the metaphysis and the epiphysis; drive the chisel 1 to 2 cm into the bone. Loosen and extract the chisel, which removes a plug of bone with it; leave this plug in the chisel until needed. With a small curet remove the contiguous plate to a depth of 2.5 cm and leave the debris in the hole created by removing the plug. Do not curet the epiphyseal plate to its peripheral margin. Then with the obturator push the plug from the chisel, rotate it 90 degrees, and replace it in its original bed so that the epiphyseal plate in the plug is in the longitudinal axis of the leg. Tap the plug into place with a mallet. Repeat these maneuvers on the opposite side.

The plugs of bone fuse first; the pressure that results from this fusion then causes growth to cease in the entire plate, and fusion occurs in about 3 months.

AFTERTREATMENT. The extremity is immobilized in a long leg night splint or a gutter splint for 3 weeks. Full weight bearing may usually be allowed in 1 month.

Canale et al. have reported preliminary clinical results of percutaneous epiphysiodesis using pneumatic reamers and burrs under image intensification control. The results included 13 children who demonstrated epiphyseal closure following the procedure.

TECHNIQUE. Place the child supine on the fracture table or an operating table that will allow image intensification in two planes by rotation of the image intensifier rather than rotation of the child's leg. Identify, with the aid of the image intensifier, the epiphyseal plate to be obliterated and make a small vertical stab wound 0.5 to 1 cm in length medially and laterally. Introduce a small Kirschner wire into the epiphyseal plate, proceeding to the midportion of the bone (Fig. 61-91). After this is secured, introduce a 4 mm cannulated reamer over the Kirschner wire and ream the epiphyseal plate to the midportion of the bone (Fig. 61-92). Remove the reamer and the wire and insert various sizes and angles of pneumatic burrs up to 3 mm in size (for example, dental drill and Hall air drills). Completely burr and obliterate the epiphyseal plate for about 6 cm or to the midline of the epiphyseal plate. Attention to the undulation of the epiphyseal plate is mandatory. It is important to drill not only from outside to the middle, but also from cephalad to caudad and anterior to posterior. It should be remembered that the object is to create a bony

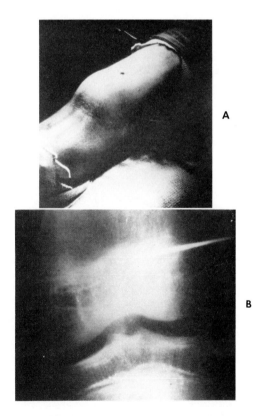

Fig. 61-91. A and **B,** Introduction and placement of the Kirschner wire into epiphyseal plate (From Canale, S.T. et al.: J. Pediatr. Orthop. **6:**150, 1986.)

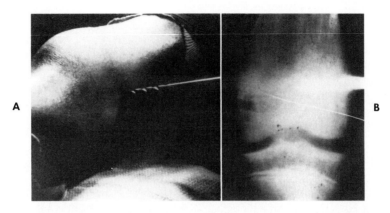

Fig. 61-92. A and **B,** Cannulated reamer being passed over Kirschner wire into eipihyseal line. (From Canale, S.T. et al.: J. Pediatr. Orthop. **6:**150, 1986.)

bridge as a central core of the epiphyseal plate from medial to lateral (periphery) and that the entire epiphyseal plate anterior and posterior, espcially as seen on the lateral image, does not need to be obliterated. Following partial obliteration of the epiphyseal plate, irrigate the wound copiously with saline, and with one small stitch close the skin. To epiphysiodese the proximal fibula, insert a small Kirschner wire in an anteroposterior direction and use the 4-mm cannulated reamer to destroy the epiphysis. Avoid the peroneal nerve by not penetrating the posterior cortex of the fibula. Do not use a burr on the proximal fibular epiphyseal plate to avoid overheating or damaging the peroneal nerve.

AFTERTREATMENT. A knee immobilizer or cylinder cast is applied, which is worn for about 3 weeks. Weight bearing is allowed 5 days after surgery.

COMPLICATIONS OF EPIPHYSIODESIS

Green and Anderson in a study of 147 epiphyseal arrests in 105 patients with poliomyelitis found a deformity at the knee in 7 patients (5%); 6 required a secondary operation, but in the seventh the deformity was not severe enough to justify surgery. In 4 patients in whom overcorrection seemed imminent an arrest was made on the originally short side. More recently (1957) Green and Anderson studied a series of 237 epiphyscal arrests in 173 patients. Twenty-two patients (9.3%) had complications that they considered significant: asymmetric fusion occurred in six, slow fusion in five, infection in two, neuromuscular dysfunction in two, and overcorrection of the discrepancy in seven. Nineteen secondary operations were either performed or recommended, an incidence of 8% for the series; four had osteotomies to correct a deformity, one declined a recommended osteotomy, five had arrest on the originally short limb to prevent overcorrection, and six had the epiphyseal arrest repeated on one or both sides of the epiphyses when there was evidence of incomplete fusion. The final result in those who required secondary operations was rated as good to excellent.

Stamp and Lansche (1960) reviewed the experience of the staff of the St. Louis Unit of the Shriners Hospital for Crippled Children. Only 61 of a total of 102 epiphyseal arrests controlled growth to within 2 cm of the desired length; in 41 the residual discrepancy exceeded this amount. Genu valgum occurred in four patients, progressive shortening in two, and genu varum in one. The causes of failure of epiphyseal arrest were as follows. The arrest was made too late in 18 instances, the opposite epiphyseal plate closed prematurely because of immobilization or disease in 10, the epiphyseal plate was narrowed at the time of the arrest in two, technical error was made at surgery in one, and the cause of failure was unknown in 10. These figures indicated that epiphyseal arrest must be well thought out in advance if complications are to be kept to a minimum.

ARREST OF EPIPHYSEAL GROWTH BY STAPLING

If epiphyseal stapling would temporarily arrest growth until the discrepancy in limb lengths had been overcome, and if after removal of the staples growth would resume at a predictable rate, then the operation would merit enthusiastic use. Unfortunately, experience has shown that this chain of events does not always take place. Furthermore, several significant complications have been reported after epiphyseal stapling. Evidence available to date indicates that epiphysiodesis is a safer and more reliable method of equalizing the length of the limbs. The reader is referred to the works of Blount for details of stapling.

RESECTION OF TIBIA

As a rule femoral shortening is preferred to tibial shortening for the following reasons: (1) only one bone is involved, and it is both protected and concealed by being deeply embedded in the musculature of the thigh; (2) delayed union and nonunion are less common in the femur than in the tibia after shortening; and (3) the muscles of the thigh regain their strength and tension more quickly than do the muscles of the leg.

According to Wagner, surgical shortening of the tibia is indicated in patients with unilateral pathologic elongation of the bone resulting from fractures, infections, hemihypertrophy, or vascular disease. Thus the operation is performed on the affected limb to fully equalize the limb lengths. Wagner prefers diaphyseal tibial osteotomy except when correction of angular or rotational deformity is re-

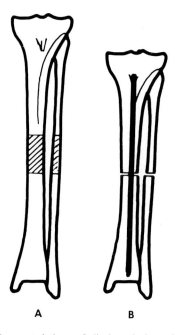

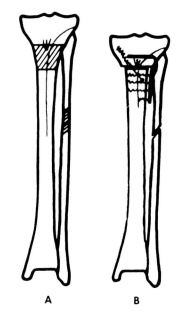

Fig. 61-93. Wagner technique of diaphyseal shortening of tibia. **A,** *Shaded areas,* segments of bone to be resected. **B,** Bone has been resected and tibia is stabilized by medullary nail. (From Wagner, H.: Reprint from Hungerford, D.S., editor: Progress in orthopaedic surgery, vol. 1, Berlin, 1977, Springer-Verlag.)

Fig. 61-94. Wagner technique of metaphyseal shortening of tibia. **A,** *Shaded areas,* segments of bone to be resected. **B,** Bone has been resected and proximal tibia is stabilized by compression plate and screws. (From Wagner, H.: Reprint from Hungerford, D.S., editor: Progress in orthopaedic surgery, vol. 1, Berlin, 1977, Springer-Verlag.)

quired and then metaphyseal osteotomy is the method of choice. Furthermore, Wagner prefers medullary nail fixation of the tibia, reserving the use of plates and screws for patients in whom deformity of the tibia would preclude medullary fixation, in whom inflammatory changes in the bone make medullary reaming inadvisable, and in whom growth is incomplete and the medullary nail might damage an epiphyseal plate.

No more than 5 cm should be removed from the tibia; otherwise the muscles of the leg may be so relaxed that their normal tension and strength are never regained. In a few instances ischemic necrosis of the muscles in the anterior compartment of the leg has followed tibial shortening of more than 5 cm.

TECHNIQUE OF DIAPHYSEAL SHORTENING. Make a longitudinal incision 15 cm long over the anteromedial aspect of the tibia. Split the periosteum throughout the length of the incision and divide the bone in the middle of the incision with a Gigli saw or with a motor saw that has a reciprocating blade. Remove the medial half of the proximal fragment and the lateral half of the distal fragment to form a step cut; the lengths of the fragments removed will depend on the amount of shortening desired. Put the resected bone in a sterile pan for use as grafts. Then make a second longitudinal incision over the junction of the middle and distal thirds of the fibula; split the periosteum for 5 cm and divide the bone. Overlap the fibular fragments and appose the raw surfaces of the tibia. Now from the lateral side fix the tibial fragments with two screws; cut the tibial fragments into toothpick grafts and place them across the osteotomy on the lateral and posterior surfaces of the tibia.

AFTERTREATMENT. A cast is applied from the groin to the toes, with the knee in flexion and the foot in slight equinus position; to allow for swelling a window is cut in the cast from above the knee to the toes. At 3 to 4 weeks the cast is changed. If union is firm at 8 weeks, the cast is removed, and a brace with a drop lock catch at the knee and a leather lacer corset that completely encases the lower leg is fitted. Weight bearing is then gradually resumed, and active and passive exercises of the knee and ankle are started. Usually all support may be discarded after 4 to 6 months. Although the muscles may show some residual weakness for a few months, they will recover satisfactorily unless the leg has been shortened too much.

TECHNIQUE OF DIAPHYSEAL SHORTENING (WAGNER). Make a longitudinal incision 3 or 4 mm lateral to the tibial crest and expose the tibia subperiosteally. Through a lateral incision resect an appropriate segment of fibula at the junction of its proximal and middle thirds. Next make a longitudinal incision proximal to the tibial tuberosity, split the patellar tendon longitudinally, broach the cortex of the tibia, and ream the medullary canal of the bone. Resect the desired amount of tibia from its middle third by stepcut osteotomy (Fig. 61-93, *A*). Now insert a snugly fitting medullary nail, stabilizing the fragments in proper alignment after the bone has been shortened (Fig. 61-93, *B*). Apply a long leg cast.

AFTERTREATMENT. At 1 month the cast is removed and a long leg walking cast is applied and is worn until union is complete.

TECHNIQUE OF METAPHYSEAL SHORTENING (WAGNER). Make a longitudinal incision over the fibula, identify the junction of its proximal and middle thirds, and resect an appropriate segment of bone. Next expose the proximal tibial metaphysis through a longitudinal anterior incision and outline the site for proximal osteotomy just distal to the tibial tuberosity. Next outline the site for distal osteotomy and resect the desired amount of bone by dividing the bone proximally and distally (Fig. 61-94, *A*). Appose the raw surfaces at the osteotomy and fix the bone with a small angled plate or a T plate using compresssion (Fig. 61-94, *B*). Apply a long leg cast.

AFTERTREATMENT. At 6 weeks the cast is removed and a long leg walking cast is applied and is worn until union is complete.

RESECTION OF FEMUR

By resecting the femur an extremity may be shortened 7 to 10 cm without permanently weakening the muscles. Femoral shortening has been established as a safe method of equalizing limb lengths. However, when considering femoral shortening in a child, the fact must be weighed that the operation itself will often stimulate growth by as much as 1.7 cm. Thus either this operation should be deferred until skeletal maturity or appropriate epiphyseal arrests should be made at the same time.

When Wagner desires to shorten the femur he prefers either proximal metaphyseal shortening or diaphyseal shortening and fixation with a medullary nail to distal metaphyseal shortening. Whereas the stability and efficiency of supracondylar osteotomy may be equal to that of proximal femoral osteotomy, it has several disadvantages. Since it is performed near the knee joint where soft tissue mobility is important, complications of wound healing or infection can cause adhesions and thus interfere with motion of the knee. Further, surplus soft tissues resulting from shortening can create cosmetically undesirable changes in the contour of the thigh. Also because the osteotomy is performed within an area of free movement of the quadriceps, the resulting redundancy of the quadriceps can cause weakness of extension of the knee. Therefore supracondylar osteotomies for shortening are advisable only if correction of angular or rotational deformity near the knee is also necessary. When femoral shortening is required without correction of axial deformity, Wagner recommends diaphyseal shortening with resection of the desired amount of bone and internal fixation with a medullary nail. He has found that fixation is better, the nail withstands the abnormal stresses at the osteotomy better, and thus weight bearing can be permitted earlier than when fixation is by plates and screws. The many complications previously reported by others in using medullary fixation for limb shortening have apparently not been a problem in his patients. Thus Wagner recommends medullary nails in all situations in which their use is anatomically feasible. Plates are recommended for diaphyseal osteotomies only if the use of a medullary nail is contraindicated, as, for example, in healed osteomyelitis, in marked deformity of a bone that precludes insertion of a nail, or in children or adolescents in whom a nail might damage an epiphyseal plate.

TECHNIQUE OF DIAPHYSEAL SHORTENING (WAGNER). Expose the tip of the greater trochanter through a short incision, enter the medullary canal at this point, and ream the canal large enough to accommodate a heavy medullary nail that will fit snugly within the femur for the desired distance.

Next expose the femur through a lateral longitudinal incision at the middle third of the thigh, split the fascia longitudinally, detach the vastus lateralis muscle from the intermuscular septum and linea aspera, and expose the femur. Demarcate proximally and distally the sites of osteotomy on the middle of the femoral shaft (Fig. 61-95, *A*). Make longitudinal marks in the bone superiorly and inferiorly so that rotation of the fragments after fixation will be correct. Now resect the outlined segment of bone in a stepcut or a straight transverse fashion. Next strip the soft tissues from the linea aspera for about 5 cm at each end of the two fragments to allow mobility of the soft tissues after the shortening. Approximate the fragments and insert a medullary nail from the trochanter distally in a routine manner (Fig 61-95, *B*).

AFTERTREATMENT. The limb is suspended in a Thomas splint for 2 weeks while quadriceps exercises are carried out. Then walking on crutches with partial weight bearing is started and is continued until union is complete. Quadriceps exercises are continued for several months.

TECHNIQUE OF PROXIMAL METAPHYSEAL SHORTENING (WAGNER). Expose the proximal femur through a midlateral incision that splits the fascia lata longitudinally. Detach the vastus lateralis muscle from the lateral aspect of the proximal femur and from the linea aspera and expose the femur subperiosteally. Next make a hole in the lateral cortex of the greater trochanter for seating a plate bent at a right angle; then insert the blade of the plate into the area of the trochanter and neck. When shortening alone is required, the blade is inserted at a right angle to the femoral shaft; if angular deformity must be corrected, then the blade is inserted as required to correct the deformity. Next outline the amount of bone to be resected and mark the bone lon-

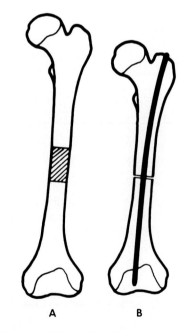

Fig. 61-95. Wagner technique of diaphyseal shortening of femur. **A,** *Shaded area,* segment of bone to be resected. **B,** Bone has been resected and femur has been stabilized by medullary nail. (From Wagner, H.: Reprint from Hungerford, D.S., editor: Progress in orthopaedic surgery, vol. 1, Berlin, 1977, Springer-Verlag.)

gitudinally so that rotation of the fragments will be proper after the osteotomy. With a saw osteotomize the bone proximally and distally in a transverse fashion but proximally leave a spike of medial cortex in continuity with the lesser trochanter (Fig. 61-96, *A*); this creates bony surfaces for wide contact. Now appose the fragments and fix the plate to the femur by screws (FIg. 61-96, *B*). As an alternative the bone fragment may be fixed with a hip compression screw as would be used for subtrochanteric femur fracture.

AFTERTREATMENT. Aftertreatment is about the same as after internal fixation of trochanteric fractures (p. 1734).

TECHNIQUE OF DISTAL METAPHYSEAL SHORTENING (WAGNER). Expose the supracondylar area of the femur through a mid-lateral longitudinal incision, splitting the fascia lata. Detach the vastus lateralis muscle and retract it anteriorly. Now expose entirely the distal femoral metaphysis without entering the knee joint. Next prepare the site for insertion in the lateral femoral condyle of the blade of a plate and outline the segment of bone to be resected (Fig. 61-97, *A*). Now with the saw divide the bone proximally in a transverse manner and distally also transversely but leave the medial cortex intact (Fig. 61-97, *B*). This type of osteotomy results in a wide area of bony contact for healing. Now insert the blade of the plate into the femoral condyles and fix the plate to the shaft with screws.

AFTERTREATMENT. The limb is suspended in a Thomas splint for 2 weeks. Then partial weight bearing on crutches is started and is continued until union is complete.

We have preferred proximal metaphyseal shortening to segmental resection of bone and internal fixation with a medullary nail. However, preliminary reports of shortening of the femur and the insertion of a medullary nail by closed techniques are appealing.

Limb lengthening
STIMULATION OF EPIPHYSEAL GROWTH

Of all the possible methods of equalizing limb lengths, stimulating the growth of the short limb is theoretically the most desirable. The search for a reliable and safe way of stimulating growth of a limb was begun by von Langenbeck in 1869; no such way has yet been found. The creation of an arteriovenous fistula in the thigh to stimulate growth of the extremity has been discontinued because the results of this procedure are so unpredictable. Castle has attempted epiphyseal stimulation by plugging of the medullary canal, and Jenkins, Cheng, and Hodgson and Chan and Hodgson have attempted to accomplish this by periosteal stripping of the femur or tibia or both; again the results have been so unpredictable that the search for a safe and reliable method of stimulating growth of a limb must continue.

OSTEOTOMY AND DISTRACTION

Operations to lengthen limbs by osteotomy and distraction may be followed by numerous and sometimes severe complications. As Compere has said, ''Interest in the successful cases has sometimes detracted from the lessons that could be learned from the failures.''*

---

*From Compere, E.L.: Indications for and against the leg lengthening operation, J. Bone Joint Surg. **18:**692, 1936

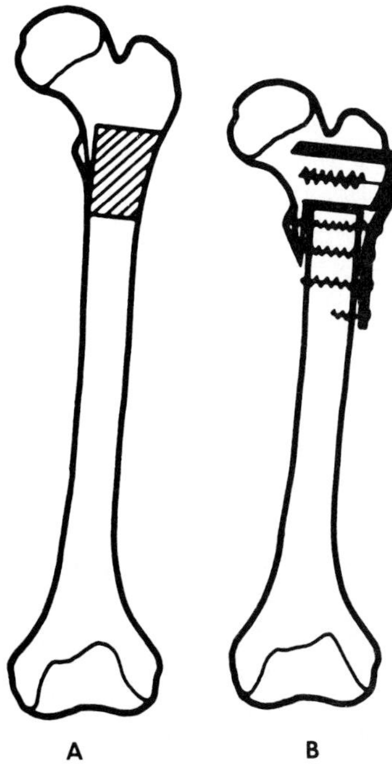

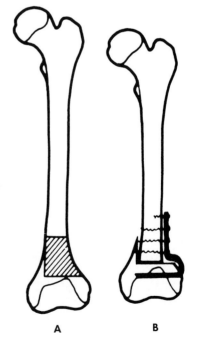

Fig. 61-96. Wagner technique of proximal metaphyseal shortening of femur. **A,** *Shaded area,* bone to be resected. **B,** Bone has been resected and proximal femur is stabilized by blade plate and screws. (From Wagner, H.: Reprint from Hungerford, D.S., editor: Progress in orthopaedic surgery, vol. 1, Berlin, 1977, Springer-Verlag.)

Fig. 61-97. Wagner technique of distal metaphyseal shortening of femur. **A,** *Shaded area,* segment of bone to be resected. **B,** Bone has been resected and distal femur is stabilized by blade plate and screws. (From Wagner, H.: Reprint from Hungerford, D.S., editor: Progress in orthopaedic surgery, vol. 1, Berlin, 1977, Springer-Verlag.)

The complications of leg lengthening listed by Abbott and Saunders are as follows.

1. *Deformities of the foot.* Valgus, equinus, equinovalgus, and calcaneovalgus deformities, usually caused by failure of the deep fascia, intermuscular septa, interosseous membrane, periosteum, tendons, and the tendinous content of the muscles to lengthen as much as do the bones. Valgus deformity was the most serious complication in a series of 71 cases of leg lengthening reported by W.V. Anderson.

2. *Deformities of the knee.* Genu valgum, flexion contracture, and relaxation of the ligaments.

3. *Deformities of the tibia.* Anterior and medial bowing of the fragments with malunion or nonunion.

4. *Limitation of ankle motion.* This is probably caused by traumatic arthritis from pressure on the articular surfaces of the joint. B.H. Moore noted that the usual change is flattening of the dome of the talus beneath the tibia.

5. *Weakening of the leg muscles.*

6. *Nerve complications.* Paralysis or weakening of the muscles or disturbance of sensation. These usually disappear spontaneously.

7. *Circulatory disturbance.* Chronic swelling of the leg is usually neither serious nor permanent. Campbell, however, observed complete gangrene of a leg distal to the area of lengthening.

8. *Infection.* This usually occurred in the operative wound or in pin tracts.

Among other complications Compere noted that avascular necrosis of the fragments may occur if the periosteum is stripped too extensively. McCarroll noted delayed union, nonunion, and late fracture. Allan encountered the latter complication in 2 of 101 patients; he also encountered pressure sores.

According to McCarroll, any attempt at lengthening the femur requires prolonged hospitalization and constant attention to detail and at least 1 year of the patient's life; these disadvantages also apply in some respects to lengthening of the tibia.

Wilk and Badgley reported the development of hypertension in one patient during femoral lengthening; the blood pressure returned to normal after the lengthening was complete. They noted that on two occasions Crego had also observed this complication. Yosipovitch and Palti reported increases in blood pressure of more than 20 mm Hg in 20 to 24 children during tibial lengthening by the Anderson method; again the blood pressure returned to normal within a few days after the lengthening was complete. They concluded after experimental tibial lengthenings in dogs that the hypertension is a reflex response to traction exerted on the sciatic nerve in the proximal thigh.

Despite these reported complications the search for an improved apparatus with which to lengthen bones has continued.

Wagner has modified the Anderson apparatus and has developed his own technique of diaphyseal lengthening. In his procedure a transverse osteotomy is made in the middle of the shaft of the bone, the apparatus is attached to Schanz screws anchored in the proximal and distal metaphyses, and the bone is lengthened by slow distraction. The distraction apparatus and its fixation in bone are so stable that additional external fixation is unnecessary. The limb can be moved freely and the patient can walk with Canadian crutches 2 or 3 days after surgery (Fig. 61-98). The elongation is carried out by the patient himself or in the hospital by turning a serrated screw connected to a worm gear that distracts the square bars of the apparatus, resulting in a steady increase in the distance between the

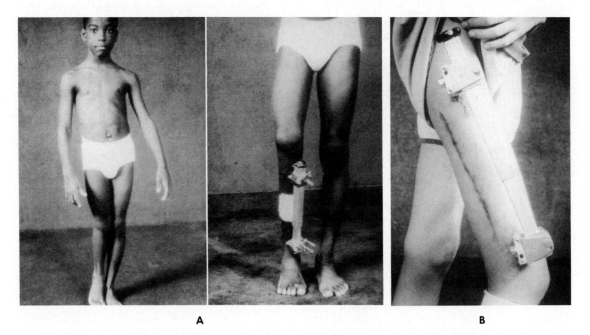

A   **B**

Fig. 61-98. A, Wagner apparatus on medial aspect of tibia. **B,** Wagner apparatus on posterolateral femur. Note scarring from posterolateral incisions and pin tracts. (Courtesy A.I. duPont Institute.)

two bony fragments; distraction of 1 cm per week or 1.5 mm per day is usually possible. After the desired distraction has been obtained the fragments are fixed with a plate with at least four screws in each fragment. If the formation of callus is delayed, then autogenous cancellous iliac bone grafts are inserted at the osteotomy. After the wound has healed the patient is followed as an outpatient and is allowed to walk on crutches.

According to Wagner, this procedure despite its magnitude has several advantages when compared to bone shortening. The lengthening is carried out at the site of shortening, where normal anatomic conditions can be recreated, and remarkable amounts of lengthening can be obtained. In more than 150 operations he has been able to obtain a maximum lengthening of 20 cm in a lower limb, 15.2 cm in a femur, and 8 cm in a tibia. He has also lengthened a humerus 19 cm. Wagner reported the complications in his first 75 patients in whom 88 osteotomies for lengthening were carried out, as shown in Table 61-3. This table reveals that the use of new and improved mechanical devices has greatly reduced the morbidity and complications in this type of surgery.

In surgical limb lengthening technical and physiologic problems may develop, which if not managed successfully can cause several complications, some quite serious.

In particular, lengthening of congenitally short limbs is especially difficult. The soft tissues are "programmed" to be the length of the shortened extremity. Tension on the musculotendinous and neurovascular structures begins as soon as the lengthening is begun, and becomes clinically troublesome at 5 cm of lengthening. Lengthening of traumatically short limbs is somewhat easier, since the soft tissues were "programmed" to be longer and may be more accommodating.

Tension on the soft tissues may become excessive. Because the two fragments can be separated more rapidly

than the surrounding soft tissues can stretch, tension frequently develops in the muscles. The muscles do elongate but more slowly than the bone. When tension is excessive, motion in the joint distal to the lengthening device is limited and the joint may be damaged. In tibial lengthening an equinus contracture of the ankle develops. Active exercises and partial weight bearing on the forefoot will usually correct or prevent this complication; if not, lengthening of the tendo calcaneus may be required. In femoral lengthening if the elongation is more than 6 or 8 cm, motion in the knee is always limited. This may be corrected by active exercises, but if not, lengthening of the hamstring tendons or adductor tenotomy may be neccessary. Tension on the soft tissues is especially difficult to manage in severe shortening caused by congenital hypoplasia of the femur or hypoplasia of the tibia with fibular hemimelia because in these situations muscles may be replaced by dense fibrous tissue. On the contrary, in surgical lengthening after fractures, epiphyseal arrests, osteomyelitis, or infectious arthritis of the hip, tension on the soft tissues usually causes no major difficulty. The neurologic and vascular complications relatively common in previous techniques have been eliminated by the Wagner technique. In the first 88 lengthening operations carried out by Wagner only two instances of transient peroneal nerve palsy occurred and no significant circulatory disturbance was present.

DISTRACTION EPIPHYSEOLYSIS

Distraction epiphyseolysis as a method of limb lengthening was described by Zivyalov and Plaskin in 1968, by Ilizarov and Soybelmon in 1969, by Eydelshtein and associates in 1973, and by Fischencko et al. in 1976. In 1981 Monticelli and Spinelli reported successful experimental limb lengthening in sheep using this technique, and encouraged by such results, performed the procedure on 16 children between the ages of 13 and 15 years, successfully obtaining tibial lengthening from 5 to 10 cm in all. The operation consists of the transfixion of the epiphysis and of the metaphysis by three pairs of Kirschner wires, their secure fixation to a distraction apparatus, and as a result of gradual distraction, a fracture is produced at the metaphyseal side of the epiphyseal plate. Distraction proceeds gradually until the desired lengthening is obtained, while the immobilization is maintained by the original apparatus until bone consolidation has occurred. It is then removed and a long leg cast is worn until the bone has healed and its cortex is at least 70% as solid as that of opposite tibia.

Because the epiphyseal plate cannot with certainty be expected to resume normal growth at the conclusion of this procedure, it should be done near the time of epiphyseal closure, but not after closure. Thus tomographic roentgenograms should be made to demonstrate that the growth plate is open before proceeding. Transient peroneal palsy developed in two patients after 6 or 7 cm of lengthening had occurred. It subsided when the rate of lengthening was slowed. Dependent swelling of the foot was common after 4 or 5 cm of lengthening was achieved. In one instance the epiphyseal Kirschner wire broke, resulting in a loss of 2.5 cm of length.

Table 61-3. Summary of 88 limb-lengthening procedures*†

Complications resulting from technique

Refractures at Z-osteotomies	5
Pressure necrosis of skin caused by the bone ends	1
Temporary peroneal nerve paralysis caused by traction	1
Temporary peroneal nerve paralysis resulting from positioning	2
Thermal sequestra caused by pin	1
Excessive periosteal reaction	2
Yielding of traction apparatus	1

Complications not resulting from technique

Mild soft tissue infection cleared after removal of device	5
Infection of bone healed after sequestrectomy	1
Refracture after removal of metal	2
Fatigue fracture at end of metal plate	1
Fatigue fracture	1
Bending of bone in congenital shortening	2
Infection at Schanz screws	1
Breaking or loosening of metal during delayed union	2
Bending of metal caused by accidental overload	1

*From Wagner, H.: Der Chirurg. 42:260, 1971.
†In 75 patients (50 females, 25 males); 88 osteotomies (56 femurs, 32 tibias).

While we have had no experience with this method it is included here for completeness and because it represents a new and interesting approach to a major problem. An obvious area for improvement is in the distraction apparatus itself, likely by modification of one of the existing external skeletal fixation devices.

TECHNIQUE (MONTICELLI AND SPINELLI). The apparatus used is derived from the design of Ilizarov and Soybelman, consisting of three C-shaped elements made of duraluminium alloy (inner diameter 17 cm, width 3 cm, thickness 5 mm) in which nine holes (diamter 6.5 mm) have been drilled at regular intervals. It has three threaded bars (6 mm thick), varying in length from 25 to 35 cm according to the amount of bone lengthening required; 18 nuts (6mm hole); three pairs of Kirschner wires (30 cm long, 2.5 mm thick); and 12 clamps holding the wire ends against the aluminum elements. Two wrenches are used to turn the nuts. When assembled, the apparatus holds the bone fragments (epiphysis and diaphysis) firmly.

With the patient under general anesthesia, insert the Kirschner wires using image intensifier control. Pass three pairs of wires through the bone at different levels—one pair through the epiphysis, one pair through the middle portion of the diaphysis, and one pair through the distal portion of it. The last two pairs guarantee the stability of the diaphysis and prevent any lateral displacement with respect to the epiphysis. Take care to avoid damaging the common peroneal nerve by inserting the pins from the lateral aspect of the leg. In addition, pass one of the third pair of wires through the diaphysis of the fibula to avoid producing a valgus condition of the foot caused by an upward dislocation of the fibula itself, which might otherwise be produced by traction of the tibia. Cross each pair of Kirschner wires within the bone and attach the wires to the C-shaped elements by means of the clamps. Connect the C-shaped elements to each other by means of the longitudinal threaded bars. Produce traction by turning the nuts of the epiphyseal C-shaped element along the longitudinal bars in such a way as to increase the distance between this and the diaphyseal elements. One complete turn increases this distance by 1 mm. Produce fibular epiphysiolysis by passing a wire through the upper portion of the fibular epiphysis or through the fibular collateral ligament (often the top of the fibula is lower than the epiphyseal plate of the tibia) (Fig. 61-99).

The apparatus attached to the bones (Fig. 61-100) comprises a stable exoskeleton capable of not only mobilizing the fragment but also of assuming the supporting function of the tibia once it has undergone epiphysiolysis.

AFTERTREATMENT. During the first 3 or 4 days after the application of the distraction apparatus, the patient becomes familiar with it and learns to walk assisted by crutches without direct weight bearing. The nuts holding the epiphyseal element are then unscrewed in such a way as to withdraw the element 0.25 mm from the diaphyseal elements (Fig. 61-101). This procedure is carried out four times a day. The lengthening process is checked by roentenography (Fig. 61-102), computed tomography, and any other method desired.

TIBIAL LENGTHENING

The indications for tibial lengthening listed by Anderson are (1) a predictable shortening of at least 4 cm in a child 8 to 12 years old and (2) weakness in the leg severe enough that little power can be lost by lengthening. Additional indications listed by Coleman and Noonan are (1) age sufficient during skeletal immaturity so that satisfactory equalization cannot be obtained by epiphyseal arrest or inequality such that shortening of bone on the long side would not produce satisfactory equalization, and (2) the likelihood that an amputation or some form of prosthesis will be needed if acceptable equalization cannot be obtained. According to Coleman, leg lengthening should not be considered if the shortening is expected to be less than 4 cm or greater than 15 cm. Further, a bone should not be lengthened more than 20% of its total length, and ideally the foot should be flexible, the ankle should be stable, and the muscles controlling the ankle should be acceptable.

Wagner has modified the Anderson method by designing a distraction apparatus useful in lengthening either the femur or the tibia. The principle of the apparatus is essentially the same as that of Anderson except that two threaded Schanz screws are inserted percutaneously in both

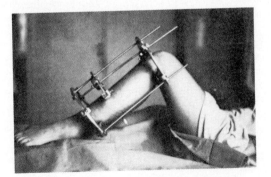

Fig. 61-99. Distraction apparatus applied to patient's leg. (From Monticelli, G., and Spinelli, R.: Clin. Orthop. **154:**274, 1981.)

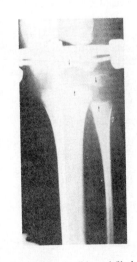

Fig. 61-100. Epiphysiolysis of both tibia and fibula as seen 10 days after separation. (From Monticelli, G., and Spinelli, R.: Clin. Orthop. **154:**274, 1981.)

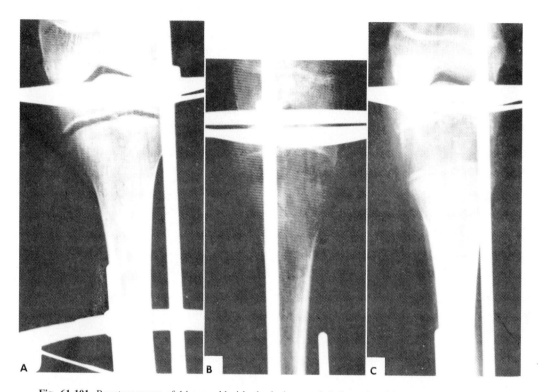

Fig. 61-101. Roentgenogram of 14-year-old girl who had congenital shortening (12 cm) of left leg, absence of fibula, talus, fourth and fifth metatarsal bones and toes, and moderate instability and subluxation of knee. **A,** Separation of epiphysis. **B,** After 20 days. **C,** After 40 days. (From Monticelli, G., and Spinelli, R.: Clin. Orthop. **154:**274, 1981.)

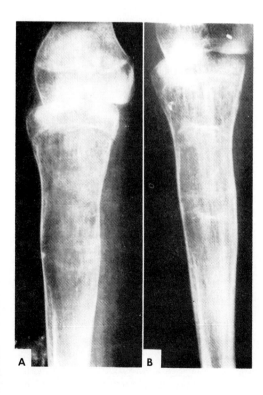

Fig. 61-102. Patient in Fig. 61-101, 11 months after distraction. **A,** Full weight-bearing without cast. **B,** After 2 years. (From Monticelli, G., and Spinelli, R.: Clin. Orthop. **154:**274, 1981.)

the proximal and the distal metaphysis. The apparatus and its attachments to bone are so stable that no additional external fixation is required during the period of lengthening and the patient may walk on crutches the second or third day after surgery.

TECHNIQUE (WAGNER). Make a longitudinal incision 5 cm long over the lateral aspect of the middle third of the fibula. Split the deep fascia longitudinally and free and retract the peroneal muscles from the fibula. Retract the deep structures away from the interosseous membrane and expose the tibia. Then insert two cortical screws through the fibula and tibia 1.5 cm apart. At a point 1 cm proximal to the most proximal screw osteotomize the fibula obliquely and close the wound. Now make two puncture wounds medially over the proximal tibial metaphysis and using a guide template drill two holes in the bone 3.6 mm in diameter, parallel to the proximal articular surface of the tibia. Now again using the template insert two Schanz self-threading screws 6 mm in diameter. Using the same technique insert two similar screws in the distal tibial metaphysis parallel to the articular surface of the tibia. The use of an image intensifier makes it easier to insert the screws properly. Now expose the middle of the tibia by a longitudinal incision 3 to 4 mm lateral to its anterior crest. Incise and elevate the periosteum and with an oscillating saw osteotomize the tibia transversely. Now insert a drain and close the wound. Attach the distraction apparatus to the Schanz screws on the medial aspect of the leg (Fig. 61-103, *A*). If much length is to be gained, lengthen the tendo calcaneus with the distraction apparatus in place to prevent equinus contracture of the ankle. Tension on the calf muscles may bend the Schanz screws, allowing anterior bowing of the tibial fragments; this can result in pressure necrosis of the overlying skin. If indicated, correct the bowing by realigning the Schanz screws at their connections to the distraction apparatus.

AFTERTREATMENT. Slow distraction is carried out by the patient. The distraction apparatus is operated by a knob that has a marker for every complete turn (Fig. 61-103, *B*). Each turn produces a lengthening of 1.5 mm, and the limb should be lengthened by this amount each day, or approximately 1 cm per week. If the limb is to be lengthened more than 6 cm, especially in older patients, soft tissue tension develops and lengthening is carried out to a lesser extent several times each day. The patient is cautioned to increase the lengthening to a point just short of pain. The drainage tubes are removed on the second or third day and the patient is allowed to walk with crutches. The foot of the operated limb is allowed to bear weight up to 5 kg; this partial loading is practiced, using a weight scale. Further, active exercises of all the joints are encouraged. The screw tracts are protected by dry sterile bandages during the first few days and later by an antibiotic powder or spray. During the period of lengthening, traction may cause necrosis of the skin or pain at the Schanz screws. To treat this complication the puncture wounds may be lengthened under local anesthesia so that the skin is relaxed at the screws. When the desired lengthening has been obtained, the fragments are fixed by a metal plate with four screws in each end and the apparatus is removed. If sufficient callus is demonstrated on roentgenograms, the wound is simply closed over drains. However, if callus formation is insufficient, the distracted area is filled with autogenous iliac bone grafts (Fig. 61-103, *B*), and the wound is closed over drains. No immobilization is required. The patient resumes walking on crutches after a few days and when the wound has healed is followed as an outpatient. Roentgenograms are obtained at intervals of about 8 weeks; partial weight bearing can usually be allowed after 8 weeks and full weight bearing after 16 to 24 weeks. After 6 to 8 months when the bone appears normal and the medullary canal has been reestablished, the plate and screws may be removed.

FEMORAL LENGTHENING

For most patients with inequality in the length of the lower limbs the best treatment is epiphysiodesis of the longer limb at the distal femur or proximal tibia or both, at the appropriate age. However, some patients, because they are short or because of special circumstances, should be considered for lengthening of the femur of the shorter limb. This procedure may cause serious complications and therefore it should be performed only in a hospital where proper apparatus is available and where the patient can be carefully observed.

Codivilla in 1905 osteotomized the femur and applied traction through the calcaneus to lengthen the femur. Magnuson in 1913 attempted to lengthen the femur several inches by distraction at the time of surgery, but the results were often disastrous. Putti in 1921 applied traction and countertraction to pins fixed in the bone being lengthened.

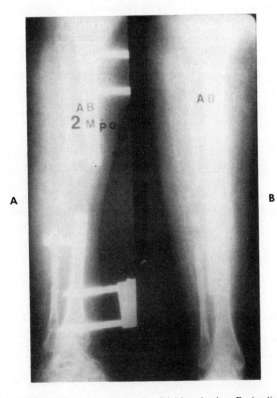

Fig. 61-103. A, Wagner apparatus for tibial lengthening. **B,** Application of plate and bone grafts to strengthen tibia and removal of Wagner apparatus.

McCarroll in 1950 used a slotted plate and traction. Bost and Larsen in 1956 reported using a medullary nail to maintain alignment of the femur while traction and countertraction were applied. Allan in 1963 reported simultaneous lengthening of the femur and tibia. Westin in 1967 described a technique of lengthening the femur over a medullary nail using a periosteal sleeve to cover the gap in the bone as advised by Bost. He reported 18 lengthenings in 17 patients, and the average increase in length was 4.1 cm. The most common complication was infection in pin tracts that occurred to some extent in all patients; all cleared without permanent damage. The chief disadvantage of this technique, however, is its morbidity. The patient must be in a spica cast for at least 6 to 9 months. During this time he is confined to bed, much of the time in the hospital. As a result, many orthopaedic surgeons attempted to use the Anderson tibial lengthening apparatus for femoral lengthening but found it cumbersome, uncomfortable, and mechanically inefficient.

Wagner modified the Anderson tibial lengthening apparatus, and his modification is not only more efficient but results in fewer complications. The morbidity is decreased because immobilization in plaster is not required.

TECHNIQUE OF DIAPHYSEAL LENGTHENING (WAGNER). Place the patient prone on the operating table and make two puncture wounds laterally over the distal femoral metaphysis. Using a guide template drill two holes in the bone with a bit 3.6 mm in diameter. Again using the guide template insert two Schanz self-threading screws 6 mm in diameter (Fig. 61-104, A). Now using the same technique insert two similar screws in the proximal femur just distal to the greater trochanter and parallel to the distal pair of screws. Use of the image intensifier simplifies this part of the operation. Next make a lateral longitudinal incision 6 to 8 cm long. Split the fascia lata longitudinally, retract the

vastus lateralis muscle anteriorly, and expose the femur. With an oscillating saw make a longitudinal groove in the femur at the predetermined site of osteotomy to use as a guide in aligning rotation of the fragments. Now again using the oscillating saw cut the femur transversely. Close the wound over a drain and attach the distraction apparatus to the two sets of Schanz screws so that it is 1 to 2 cm lateral to the thigh. Distract the apparatus immediately 5 or 6 mm to prevent painful crepitation at the ends of the bones and to stabilize the soft tissues.

AFTERTREATMENT. The distraction is carried out by the patient. The apparatus is operated by a knob that is marked for each complete turn, and each turn lengthens the femur 1.5 mm. Lengthening should be about 1.5 mm per day or about 1 cm per week. The patient is instructed to increase the lengthening to a point just short of pain. If necessary, repeated lesser lengthenings can be carried out each day. If pain develops, distraction may be discontinued for a few days. The drains are removed on the second or third day and the patient is allowed to walk on crutches. A load of approximately 5 kg of weight is permitted on the foot on the affected side, and active exercises of all joints are encouraged. The screw tracts are protected by dry sterile bandages during the first few days and then by an antibiotic powder or spray. Pain almost always develops from pressure of the screws against the skin; if so the puncture wounds may be lengthened under local anesthesia to relax the skin. When the desired length has been obtained, the patient is carried to the operating room and placed prone on the operating table with the distraction apparatus in place. The femoral shaft is exposed through the previous incision, and the fragments are fixed with a wide heavy metal plate with at least four screws in each fragment. If the roentgenograms show insufficient callus, the defect is filled with autogenous iliac grafts (Fig. 61-104, B). The distraction apparatus is then removed, and the wound is closed over a drain. After the wound has healed the patient is followed in the clinic. Roentgenograms are made at intervals of 6 to 8 weeks. Partial weight bearing of up to 5 kg is allowed on the foot on the affected side. As union becomes more solid, weight bearing is increased. When the appearance of the femur is normal and the medullary canal has been reestablished, the plate and screws are removed.

TECHNIQUE OF METAPHYSEAL FEMORAL LENGTHENING IN ONE STAGE (WAGNER). A metaphyseal lengthening osteotomy carried out in one stage should be considered only if an angular or rotational deformity must be corrected at either the proximal or distal end of the femur. Otherwise diaphyseal lengthening is preferred. The most common indication for metaphyseal lengthening is the presence of a valgus deformity of the distal femur with shortening (Fig. 61-105, A).

Through a lateral longitudinal incision divide the fascia lata longitudinally, retract the vastus lateralis muscle anteriorly, and identify the supracondylar part of the femur. Next expose the distal femoral metaphysis without entering the knee and prepare the site for insertion of the blade of a bent plate in the lateral femoral condyle. Now make a supracondylar osteotomy parallel to the distal articular surface of the femur, leaving the medial cortex intact. Correct

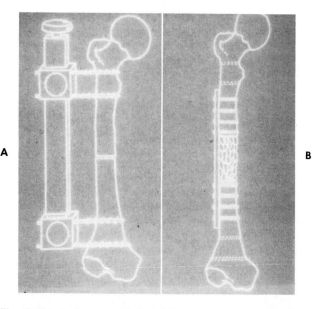

A   B

Fig. 61-104. A, Proper positioning of Shanz screws and osteotomy for femoral lengthening. B, Removal of Wagner device and application of plate and bone grafts to strengthen femur.

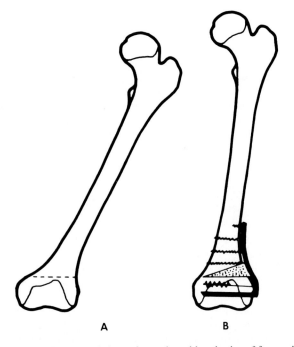

Fig. 61-105. Wagner technique of metaphyseal lengthening of femur. **A,** Femur is short and valgus deformity at distal femur is present. **B,** Osteotomy has been made and opened, bent blade plate is applied, and bone grafts are inserted. (From Wagner, H.: Reprint from Hungerford, D.S., editor: Progress in orthopaedic surgery, Berlin, 1977, Springer-Verlag.)

the valgus deformity by opening an appropriate wedge laterally and creating a greenstick fracture medially. Insert the blade of the plate in the femoral condyles and fix the plate to the femur with screws. Fill the osteotomy with autogenous cancellous iliac bone (Fig. 61-105, *B*) and close the wound.

REFERENCES
Constrictures of leg

Cozen, L., and Brockway, A.: Z-plasty procedure for release of constriction rings. In Operative orthopedic clinics, Philadelphia, 1955, J. B. Lippincott Co.

Peet, E.W.: Congenital constriction bands. In Rob, C., and Smith, R., editors: Operative surgery, part 10, Philadelphia, 1959, F.A. Davis Company.

Sarnat, B.G., and Kagan, B.M.: Prenatal constricting band and pseudoarthrosis of the lower leg, Plast. Reconstr. Surg. **47:**547, 1971.

Anomalies of toes

Cockin, J.: Butler's operation for an over-riding fifth toe, J. Bone Joint Surg. **50-B:**78, 1968.

Diamond, L.S., and Gould, V.E.: Macrodactyl of the foot: surgical syndactyly after wedge resection, South. Med. J. **67:**645, 1974.

Farmer, A.W.: Congenital hallux varus, Am. J. Surg. **95:**274, 1958.

Goodwin, F.C., and Swisher, F. M.: The treatment of congenital hyperextension of the fifth toe, J. Bone Joint Surg. **25:**193, 1943.

Horwitz, M.T.: Unusual hallux-varus deformity and its surgical correction, J. Bone Joint Surg. **19:**828, 1937.

Janecki, C.J., and Wilde, A.H.: Results of phalangectomy of the fifth toe for hammertoe: the Ruiz-Mora procedure, J. Bone Joint Surg. **58-A:**1005, 1976.

Kelikian, H., Clayton, L., and Loseff, H.: Surgical syndactylia of the toes, Clin. Orthop. **19:**209, 1961.

Lantzounis, L.A.: Congenital subluxation of the fifth toe and its correction by periosteocapsuloplasty and tendon transplantation, J. Bone Joint Surg. **22:**147, 1940.

Lapidus, P.W.: Transplantation of the extensor tendon for correction of the overlapping fifth toe, J. Bone Joint Surg. **24:**555, 1942.

Leonard, M.H., and Rising, E.E.: Syndactylization to maintain correction of overlapping 5th toe, Clin. Orthop. **43:**241, 1965.

McElvenny, R.T.: Hallux varus, Q. Bull. Northwestern Univ. Med. School **15:**277, 1941.

McFarland, B.: Congenital deformities of the spine and limbs. In Platt, H., editor: Modern trends in orthopaedics, New York, 1950, Paul B. Hoeber, Inc.

Ruiz-Mora, J.: Personal communication to L.R. Straub, May, 1954.

Ruiz-Mora, J.: Plastic correction of overriding fifth toe, vol. 6, Orthopaedic Letters Club, 1954.

Scrase, W.H.: The treatment of dorsal adduction deformities of the fifth toe, J. Bone Joint Surg. **36-B:**146, 1954.

Straub, L.R.: Orthopaedic surgery. In Cecil, R.L., editor: The specialties in general practice, Philadelphia, 1951, W.B. Saunders Co.

Thompson, T.C.: Surgical treatment of disorders of the fore part of the foot, J. Bone Joint Surg. **46-A:**1117, 1964.

Thomson, S.A.: Hallux varus and metatarsus varus: a five-year study (1954–1958), Clin. Orthop. **16:**109, 1960.

Wilson, J.N.: V-Y correction for varus deformity of the fifth toe, Br. J. Surg. **41:**133, 1953.

Wilson, J.N.: Discussion of paper by W.H. Scrase, British Orthopaedic Association Meeting, October 1953, J. Bone Joint Surg. **36-B:**146, 1954.

Anomalies of foot

Altchek, M.: Treatment of clubfeet by molding the talus, Orthop. Rev. **3:**54, May 1974.

Ashby, M.E.: Roentgenographic assessment of soft tissue medial release operations in club foot deformity, Clin. Orthop. **90:**146, 1973.

Attenborough, C.G.: Severe congenital talipes equinovarus, J. Bone Joint Surg. **48-B:**31, 1966.

Attenborough, C.G.: Early posterior soft-tissue release in severe congenital talipes equinovarus, Clin. Orthop. **84:**71, 1972.

Barenfeld, P.A., and Weseley, M.S.: Surgical treatment of congenital clubfoot, Clin. Orthop. **84:**79, 1972.

Barenfeld, P.A., Weseley, M.S., and Shea, J.M.: The congenital cavus foot, Clin. Orthop. **79:**119, 1971.

Basile, C.J., Waldrop, W.L., Voshell, A.F., and Gellman, M.: Subtalar arthrorhisis for certain types of flat foot, Exhibit, American Academy of Orthopaedic Surgeons, Chicago, 1946.

Becker-Andersen, H., and Reimann, I.: Congenital vertical talus: reevaluation of early manipulative treatment, Acta Orthop. Scand. **45:**130, 1974.

Bényi, P.: A modified Lambrinudi operation for drop foot, J. Bone Joint Surg. **42-B:**333, 1960.

Berman, A., and Gartland, J.J.: Metatarsal osteotomy for the correction of adduction of the fore part of the foot in children, J. Bone Joint Surg. **53-A:**498, 1971.

Björnness, T.: Congenital clubfoot: a follow-up of 95 persons treated in Sweden from 1940–1945 with special reference to their social adaption and subjective symptoms from the foot, Acta Orthop. Scand. **46:**848, 1975.

Blount, W.P.: Forward transference of posterior tibial tendon for paralytic talipes equinovarus, Personal communication, July 1954.

Blumenfeld, I., Kaplan, N., and Hicks, E.O.: The conservative treatment of congenital talipes equinovarus, J. Bone Joint Surg. **28:**765, 1946.

Bost, F.C., Schottstaedt, E.R., and Larsen, L.J.: Plantar dissection: an operation to release the soft tissues in recurrent or recalcitrant talipes equinovarus, J. Bone Joint Surg. **42-A:**151, 1960.

Carpenter, E.B., and Huff, S.H.: Selective tendon transfers for recurrent club foot, South. Med. J. **46:**220, 1953.

Coleman, S.S., Martin, A.F., and Jarrett, J.: Congenital vertical talus: pathomechanics and treatment, J. Bone Joint Surg. **48-A;**1442, 1966.

Coleman S.S., Stelling, F.H., III, and Jarrett, J.: Pathomechanics and treatment of congenital vertical talus, Clin. Orthop. **70:**62, 1970.

Colton, C.L.: The surgical management of congenital vertical talus, J. Bone Joint Surg. **55-B:**566, 1973.

Cowell, H.R.: Tarsal coalition: review and update. In American Academy of Orthopaedic Surgeons: Instructional course lectures, vol. 31, St. Louis, 1982, The C.V. Mosby Co.

Cowell, H.R., and Elener, V.: Rigid painful flatfoot secondary to tarsal coalition, Clin. Orthop. **177:**54, 1983.

Crawford, A.H., Marxen, J.L., and Osterfeld, D.L.: The Cincinnati incision: a comprehensive approach for surgical procedures of the foot and ankle in childhood, J. Bone Joint Surg. 64-A:1355, 1982.

Dekel. S., and Weissman, S.L.: Osteotomy of the calcaneus and concomitant plantar stripping in children with talipes cavo-varus, J. Bone Joint Surg. 55-B:802, 1973.

De Langh, R., et al.: Treatment of clubfoot by posterior capsulectomy, Clin. Orthop. 106:248, 1975.

Duckworth, T., and Smith, T.W.D.: The treatment of paralytic convex pes valgus, J. Bone Joint Surg. 56-B:305, 1974.

Dunn, H.K., Samuelson, K.M.: Flat-top talus: a long-term report of twenty club feet, J. Bone Joint Surg. 56-A:57, 1974.

Dwyer, F.C.: A new approach to the treatment of pes cavus, Sixième Congrès de Chirurgie orthopédique, Berne, 1954, Sociéeté Internationale de Chirurgie Orthopédique et de Traumatologie, Bruxelles, 1955, Imprimerie Lielens.

Dwyer, F.C.: Osteotomy of the calcaneum for pes cavus, J. Bone Joint Surg. 41-B:80, 1959.

Dwyer, F.C.: The treatment of relapsed club foot by the insertion of a wedge into the calcaneum, J. Bone Joint Surg. 45-B:67, 1963.

Dwyer, F.C.: The present status of the problem of pes cavus, Clin. Orthop. 106:254, 1975.

Ellis, J.N., and Scheer, G.E.: Congenital convex pes valgus, Clin. Orthop. 99:168, 1974.

Evans, D.: Relapsed club foot, J. Bone Joint Surg. 43-B:722, 1961.

Eyre-Brook, A.: Congenital vertical talus, J. Bone Joint Surg. 49-B:618, 1967.

Fisher, R.L., and Shaffer, S.R.: An evaluation of calcaneal osteotomy in congenital clubfoot and other disorders. Clin. Orthop, 70:141, 1970.

Fliegel, O.: Congenital pes adductus, Bull. Hosp. Joint Dis.16:65, 1955.

Fripp, A.T.: The relapsed clubfoot, Proc. R. Soc. Med. 44:873, 1951.

Fripp, A.T.: The problem of the relapsed club foot (editorial), J. Bone Joint Surg. 43-B:626, 1961.

Fripp, A.T., and Shaw, N.E.: Club-foot, Edinburgh, 1967, E. & S. Livingstone, Ltd.

Garceau, G.J.: Anterior tibial tendon transposition in recurrent congenital club-foot, J. Bone Joint Surg. 22:932, 1940.

Garceau, G.J.: Talipes equino-varus. In American Academy of Orthopaedic Surgeons: Instructional course lectures, vol. 7, Ann Arbor, 1950, J.W. Edwards.

Garceau, G.J.: Recurrent clubfoot, Bull Hosp. Joint Dis. 15:143, 1954.

Garceau, G.J.: Talipes equino-varus. In American Academy of Orthopaedic Surgeons: Instructional course lectures, vol. 12, Ann Arbor, 1955, J.W. Edwards.

Garceau, G.J.: Anterior tibial tendon transfer for recurrent clubfoot, Clin. Orthop. 84:61, 1972,

Garceau, G.J., and Manning, K.R.: Transposition of the anterior tibial tendon in the treatment of recurrent congenital club-foot, J. Bone Joint Surg. 29:1044, 1947.

Garceau, G.J., and Palmer, R.M.: Transfer of the anterior tibial tendon for recurrent club foot: a long-term follow-up, J. Bone Joint Surg. 49-A:207, 1967.

Gartland, J.J.: Posterior tibial transplant in the surgical treatment of recurrent club foot: a preliminary report, J. Bone Joint Surg. 46-A:1217, 1964.

Goldner, J.L.: Surgical correction of foot deformities in children, Spectator Letter, January 1959 (mimeographed).

Gordon, S.L., and Dunn, E.J.: Peroneal nerve palsy as a complication of clubfoot treatment, Clin. Orthop. 101:229, 1974.

Grice, D.S.: An extra-articular arthrodesis of the subastragalar joint for correction of paralytic flat feet in children, J. Bone Joint Surg. 34-A:927, 1952.

Grice, D.S.: Further experience with extra-articular arthrodesis of the subtalar joint, J. Bone Joint Surg. 37-A:246, 1955.

Grice, D.S.: The role of subtalar fusion in the treatment of valgus deformities of the feet. In American Academy of Orthopaedic Surgeons: Instructional course lectures, vol. 16, St. Louis, 1959, The C.V. Mosby Co.

Hadidi, H.: Management of congenital talipes equinovarus, Orthop. Clin. North Am. 5:53, 1974.

Handelsman, J.E., Youngleson, J., and Malkin, C.: A modified approach to the Dwyer os calcis osteotomy in club foot, S. Afr. Med. J. 39:989, 1965.

Hark, F.W.: Rocker-foot due to congenital subluxation of the talus, J.Bone Joint Surg. 32-A:344, 1950.

Harrold, A.J.: Congenital vertical talus in infancy, J.Bone Joint Surg. 49-B:634, 1967.

Harrold, A.J.: The problem of congenital verticle talus, Clin. Orthop. 97:133, 1973.

Herndon, C.H., and Heyman, C.H.: Problems in the recognition and treatment of congenital convex pes valgus, J. Bone Joint Surg. 45-A:413, 1963.

Herold, H.Z., and Torok, G.: Surgical correction of neglected club foot in the older child and adult, J. Bone Joint Surg. 55-A:1385, 1973.

Hersh, A., and Fuchs, L.A.: Treatment of the uncorrected clubfoot by triple arthrodesis, Orthop. Clin. North Am. 4:103, 1973.

Heyman, C.H.: The surgical release of fibrous tissue structures resisting correction of congenital clubfoot and metatarsus varus. In American Academy of Orthopaedic Surgeons: Instructional course lectures, vol. 16, St. Louis, 1959, The C.V. Mosby Co.

Heyman, C.H., Herndon, C.H., and Strong, J.M.: Mobilization of the tarsometatarsal and intermetatarsal joints for the correction of resistant adduction of the fore part of the foot in congenital clubfoot or congenital metatarsus varus, J. Bone Joint Surg. 40-A:299, 1958.

Ingram, A.J.: Pollex varus or the thumb clutched hand. Thesis submitted to the American Orthopaedic Association, February 1957.

Irani, R.N., and Sherman, M.S.: The pathological anatomy of club foot, J. Bone Joint Surg. 45-A:45, 1963.

Johanning, K.: Excochleatio ossis cuboidei in the treatment of pes equino-varus, Acta Orthop. Scand. 27:310, 1957-1958.

Jørring, K., and Christiansen, L.: Congenital clubfoot: a follow-up of 58 children treated during 1964–1969, Acta Orthop. Scand. 46:152, 1975.

Judet, J.: New concepts in the corrective surgery of congenital talipes equinovarus and congenital and neurologic flatfeet, Clin. Orthop. 70:56, 1970.

Kandel, B.: Treatment of congenital clubfoot, Bull. Hosp. Joint Dis. 19:20, 1958.

Kendrick, R.E., Sharma, N.K., Hassler, W.L., and Herndon, C.H.: Tarsometatarsal mobilization for resistant adduction of the fore part of the foot: a follow-up study, J. Bone Joint Surg. 52-A:61, 1970.

Kite, J.H.: The treatment of congenital club-feet, Surg. Gynecol. Obstet. 61:190, 1935.

Kite, J.H.: Principles involved in treatment of club foot, J. Bone Joint Surg. 21:595, 1939.

Kite, J.H.: Congenital metatarsus varus (a study based on four hundred cases). In American Academy of Orthopaedic Surgeons: Instrcutional course lectures, vol. 7, Ann Arbor, 1950, J. W. Edwards.

Kite, J.H.: Errors and complications in treating foot conditions in children, Clin. Orthop. 53:31, 1967.

Kite, J.H.: Conservative treatment of the resistant recurrent clubfoot, Clin. Orthop. 70:93, 1970.

Kuhlmann, R.F.: A survey and clinical evaluation of the operative treatment for congenital talipes equinovarus, Clin. Orthop. 84:88, 1972.

Kuhlmann, R.F., and Bell, J.F.: A clinical evaluation of operative procedures for congenital talipes equinovarus, J. Bone Joint Surg. 39-A:265, 1957.

Kumar, S.J., Cowell, H.R., and Ramsey, P.L.: Foot problems in children. Part I. Vertical and oblique talus. In American Academy of Orthopaedic Surgeons: Instructional course lectures, vol. 31, St. Louis, 1982, the C.V. Mosby Co.

Lambrinudi, C.: New operation on drop-foot, Br. J. Surg. 15:193, 1927.

Lambrinudi, C.: A method of correcting equinus and calcaneus deformities at the sub-astragaloid joint, Proc. R. Soc. Med. 26:788, 1933.

Lamy, L., and Weissman, L.: Congenital convex pes valgus, J. Bone Joint Surg. 21:79, 1939.

Lange, M.: Orthopädisch-chirurgische operationslehre, München, 1951, J.F. Bergmann.

LeNoir, J.L.: The long undescribed inverted clubfoot. South. Med. J. 64:199, 1971.

LeNoir, J.L.: Propedeutics of clubfoot radiology, Orthop. Rev. 5:35, February 1976.

Lichtblau, S.: A medial and lateral release operation for club foot: a preliminary report, J. Bone Joint Surg. 55-A:1377, 1973.

Lichtblau, S.: Section of the abductor hallucis tendon for correction of metatarsus varus deformity, Clin. Orthop. 110:227, 1975.

Lloyd-Roberts, G.C., and Clark, R.C.: Ball and socket ankle joint in metatarsus adductus varus (S-shaped or serpentine foot), J. Bone Joint Surg. 55-B:193, 1973.

Lloyds-Roberts, G.C., Swann, M., and Catterall, A.: Medial rotational osteotomy for severe residual deformity in club foot: a preliminary report on a new method of treatment, J. Bone Joint Surg. **56-B**:37, 1974.

Lovell, W.W., and Hancock, C.I.: Treatment of congenital talipes equinovarus, Clin. Orthop. **70**:79, 1970.

Lowe, L.W., and Hannon, M.A.: Residual adduction of the forefoot in treated congenital club foot, J. Bone Joint Surg. **55-B**:809, 1973.

MacEwen, G.D., Scott, D.J., Jr., and Shands, A.R., Jr.: Follow-up survey of club foot: treated at the Alfred I. du Pont Institute with special reference to the value of plaster therapy instituted during earliest signs of recurrence, and the use of night splints to prevent or minimize the manifestations, JAMA **175**:427, 1961.

Marciniak, W.: Early surgical correction of residual congenital equinovarus deformities in infants, Am. Dig. Foreign Orthop. Lit. 4th qtr: 25, 1971.

Mayer, L.: Orthopaedic surgery of childhood—a review of 25 years at the Joint Disease Hospital, Bull. Hosp. Joint Dis. **9**:110, 1948.

McCauley, J.C., Jr.: Treatment of clubfoot. In American Academy of Orthopaedic Surgeons: Instructional course lectures, vol. 16, St. Louis, 1959, The C.V. Mosby Co.

McCauley, J.C., Jr., Lusskin, R., and Bromley, J.: Recurrence in congenital metatarsus varus, J. Bone Joint Surg. **46-A**:525, 1964.

McCormick, D.W., and Blount, W.P.: Metatarsus adductovarus: "skewfoot," JAMA **141**:449, 1949.

McKay, D.W.: New concept of and approach to clubfoot treatment. Section I. Principles and morbid anatomy, J. Pediatr. Orthop. **2**:347, 1982.

McKay, D.W.: New concept of and approach to clubfoot treatment. Section II. Correction of clubfoot, J. Pediatr. Orthop. **3**:10, 1983.

McKay, D.W.: New concept of and approach to clubfoot treatment. Section III. Evaluation and results, J. Pediatr. Orthop. **3**:141, 1983.

McKeever, D.C.: Arthrodesis of the first metatarsophalangeal joint for hallux valgus, halux rigidus, and metatarsal primus varus, J. Bone Joint Surg. **34-A**:129, 1952.

Meyerding, H.W., and Upshaw, J.E.: Heredofamilial cleft foot deformity (lobster-claw or splitfoot), Am. J. Surg. **74**:889, 1947.

Ober, F.R.: An operation for the relief of congenital equino-varus deformity, J. Bone Joint Surg. **2**:558, 1920.

O'Donoghue, D.H.: Controlled rotation osteotomy of the tibia, South Med. J. **33**:1145, 1940.

Ono, K., and Hayashi, H.: Residual deformity of treated congenital club foot: a clinical study employing frontal tomography of the hind part of the foot, J. Bone Surg. **56-A**:1577, 1974.

O'Rahilly, R.: A survey of carpal and tarsal anomalies, J. Bone Joint Surg. **35-A**:626, 1953.

Outland, T., and Sherk, H.H.: Congenital vertical talus, Clin. Orthop. **16**:214, 1960.

Parrish, T.F.: Congenital convex pes valgus accompanied by previously undescribed anatomic derangements, South. Med. J. **60**:983,1967.

Patterson, W.R., Fitz, D.A., and Smith, W.S.: The pathologic anatomy of congenital convex pes valgus: post mortem study of a newborn infant with bilateral involvement, J. Bone Joint Surg. **50-A**:459, 1968.

Peabody, C.W.: Discussion of paper by Garceau, G.J.: Transposition of the anterior tibial tendon in the treatment of recurrent congenital clubfoot, J. Bone Joint Surg. **29**:1044, 1947.

Peabody, C.W., and Muro, F.: Congenital metatarsus varus, J. Bone Joint Surg. **15**:171, 1933.

Ponseti, I.V., and Becker, J.R.: Congenital metatarsus adductus: the results of treatment, J. Bone Joint Surg. **48-A**:702, 1966.

Ponseti, I.V., and Smoley, E.N.: Congenital club foot: the results of treatment, J. Bone Joint Surg. **45-A**:261, 1963.

Reimann, I., and Becker-Anderson H.: Early surgical treatment of congenital clubfoot, Clin. Orthop. **102**:200, 1974.

Reimann, I., and Werner, H.H.: Congenital metatarsus varus: on the advantages of early treatment, Acta Orthop. Scand. **46**:857, 1975.

Richardson, T.A.: Calcaneo-talar bar in a club foot, vol. 7, Orthopaedic Letters Club, 1956 (mimeographed).

Rocher, H.L., and Pouyanne, L.: Pied plat congénital par subluxation sous-astragalienne congénitale et orientation verticale de l'astragale, Bordeaux Chir. **5**:249, 1934. (Cited in Lamy, L., and Weissman, L.: Congenital convex pes valgus, J. Bone Joint Surg. **21**:79, 1939.)

Sell, L.S.: Tibial torsion accompanying congenital club-foot, J. Bone Joint Surg. **23**:561, 1941.

Silk, F.F., and Wainwright, D.: The recognition and treatment of congenital flat foot in infancy, J. Bone Joint Surg. **49-B**:628, 1967.

Silver, C.M., Simon, S.D., and Litchman, H.M.: Long term follow-up observations on calcaneal osteotomy, Clin. Orthop. **99**:181, 1974.

Simons, G.W.: Complete subtalar release in club feet. Part. I. A preliminary report, J. Bone Joint Surg. **67-A**:1044, 1985.

Simons, G.W.: Complete subtalar release in club feet. Part II. Comparison with less extensive procedures, J. Bone Joint Surg. **67-A**:1056, 1985.

Singer, M.: Tibialis posterior transfer in congenital club foot, J. Bone Joint Surg. **43-B**:717, 1961.

Singer, M., and Fripp, A.T.: Tibialis anterior transfer in congenital club foot, J. Bone Joint Surg. **40-B**:252, 1958.

Somppi, E., and Sulamaa, M.: Early operative treatment of congenital club foot, Acta Orthop. Scand. **42**:513, 1971.

Sotirow, B.: Radiological analysis of talipes planovalgus and equinovarus, Am. Dig. Foreign Orthop. Lit. 4th qtr:35, 1971.

Stewart, S.F.: Club-foot: its incidence, cause and treatment: an anatomical-physiological study, J. Bone Joint Surg. **33-A**:577, 1951.

Stone, K.H. (for Lloyd-Roberts, G.C.): Congenital vertical talus: a new operation (abstract), Proc. R. Soc. Med. **56**:12, 1963.

Tachdjian, M.O.: Congenital convex pes valgus, Orthop. Clin. North Am. **3**:131, 1972.

Turco. V.J.: Surgical correction of the resistant club foot: one-stage posteromedial release with internal fixation: a preliminary report, J. Bone Joint Surg. **53-A**:477, 1971.

Turco, V.J.: Resistant congenital clubfoot. In American Academy of Orthopaedic Surgeons: Instructional course lectures, vol. 24, St. Louis, 1975, The C.V. Mosby Co.

Weseley, M.S., and Barenfeld, P.A.: Mechanism of the Dwyer calcaneal osteotomy, Clin. Orthop. **70**:137, 1970.

Weseley, M.S., Barenfeld, P.A., and Barrett, N.: Complications of the treatment of clubfoot, Clin. Orthop. **84**:93, 1972.

White, R.K., and Kraynick, B.M.: Surgical uses of the peroneus brevis tendon, Surg. Gynecol. Obstet. **108**:117, 1959.

Wynne-Davies, R.: Talipes equinovarus: a review of eighty-four cases after completion of treatment, J. Bone Joint Surg. **46-B**:464, 1964.

Zimbler, S.: Practical considerations in the early treatment of congenital talipes equinovarus, Orthop. Clin. North Am. **3**:251, 1972.

Congenital absence of part or all of long bone

Aitken, G.T.: Amputation as a treatment for certain lower-extremity congenital anomalies, J. Bone Joint Surg. **41-A**:1267, 1959.

Aitken, G.T.: Proximal femoral focal deficiency. In Swinyard, C.A., editor: Limb development and deformity: problems of evaluation and rehabilitation, Springfield, Ill., 1969, Charles C. Thomas, Publisher.

Aitken, G.T.: Congenital lower limb deficiencies. In American Academy of Orthopaedic Surgeons: Instructional course lectures, vol. 24, St. Louis, 1975, The C.V. Mosby Co.

Amstutz, H.C., and Wilson, P.D., Jr.: Dysgenesis of the proximal femur (coxa vara) and its surgical management, J. Bone Joint Surg. **44-A**:1, 1962.

Arnold, W.D.: Congenital absence of the fibula, Clin. Orthop. **14**:20, 1959.

Badgley, C.E.: Primary and secondary-congenital deformities. In American Academy of Orthopaedic Surgeons: Instructional course lectures, vol. 10, Ann Arbor, 1953, J.W. Edwards.

Bevan-Thomas, W.H., and Millar, E.A.: A review of proximal focal femoral deficiencies, J. Bone Joint Surg. **49-A**:1376, 1967.

Borggreve, J.: Arch. Orthop. Chir. **28**:175, 1930. (Cited in van Nes, C.P.: Rotation-plasty for congenital defects of the femur, making use of the ankle of the shortened limb to control the knee joint of a prosthesis, J. Bone Joint Surg. **32-B**:12, 1950.)

Brown, F.W.: Construction of a knee joint in congenital total absence of the tibia (paraxial hemimelia tibia): a preliminary report, J. Bone Joint Surg. **47-A**:695, 1965.

Brown, F.W.: Personal communication, 1976.

Coventry, M.B., and Johnson, E.W., Jr.: Congenital absence of the fibula, J. Bone Joint Surg. **34-A**:941, 1952.

Davidson, A.J., and Horwitz, M.T.: Congenital club-hand deformity associated with absence of the radius; its surgical correction, J. Bone Joint Surg. **21**:462, 1939.

Farmer, A.W., and Laurin, C.A.: Congenital absence of the fibula, J. Bone Joint Surg. **42-A**:1, 1960.

Fixsen, J.A., and Lloyd-Roberts, G.C.: The natural history and early treatment of proximal femoral dysplasia, J. Bone Joint Surg. **56-B**:86, 1974.

Frantz, C.H.: Lower extremity anomaly, Spectator Letter, January 1959 (mimeographed).

Frantz, C.H., and O'Rahilly, R.: Congenital skeletal limb deficiencies, J. Bone Joint Surg. **43-A**:1202, 1961.

Freund, E.: Congenital defects of femur, fibula and tibia, Arch. Surg. **33**:349, 1936.

Gaenslen, F.J.: Congenital defects of the tibia and fibula, Am. J. Orthop. Surg. **12**:453, 1915.

Hall, C.B., Brooks, M.B., and Dennis, J.F.: Congenital skeletal deficiencies of the extremities: classification and fundamentals of treatment JAMA **181**:590, 1962.

Hall, J.E.: Rotation of congenitally hypoplastic lower limbs to use the ankle joint as a knee: a preliminary report, Inter-Clin. Inform. Bull. **6**:3, November 1966.

Hall, J.E., and Bochmann, D.: The surgical and prosthetic management of proximal femoral focal deficiency. In Aitken, G.T., editor: Proximal femoral focal deficiency: a symposium, Washington, D.C., 1969, National Academy of Sciences.

Harmon, P.H., and Fahey, J.J.: The syndrome of congenital absence of the fibula, Surg. Gynecol. Obstet. **64**:876, 1937.

Haslam, E.T.: The management of patients with skeletal limb deficiencies of the foot and ankle, Clin. Orthop. **85**:23, 1972.

Jansen, K., and Andersen, K.S.: Congenital absence of the fibula, Acta Orthop. Scand. **45**:446, 1974.

Kalamchi, A., and Dawe, R.V.: Congenital deficiency of the tibia, J. Bone Joint Surg. **67-B**:581, 1985.

Karchinov, K.: Congenital deplopodia with hypoplasia or aplasia of the tibia: a report of six cases, J. Bone Joint Surg. **55-B**:604, 1973.

Kawamura, B., et al.: Limb lengthening by means of subcutaneous osteotomy: experimental and clinical studies, J. Bone Joint Surg. **50-A**:851, 1968.

Kiil-Nielsen, K.: Case of congenital absence of the patella and its treatment. Acta Orthop. Scand. **15**:49, 1944.

King, R.E.: Some concepts of proximal femoral focal deficiency, Personal communication, 1969.

King, R.E.: Some concepts of proximal femoral focal deficiency. In Aitken, G.T., editor: Proximal femoral focal deficiency: a symposium, Washington, D.C., 1969, National Academy of Sciences.

Kostuik, J.P., Gillespie, R., Hall, J.E., and Hubbard, S.: Van Nes rotational osteotomy for treatment of proximal femoral focal deficiency and congenital short femur, J. Bone Joint Surg. **57-A**:1039, 1975.

Kruger, L.M., and Talbott, R.D.: Amputation and prosthesis as definitive treatment in congenital absence of the fibula, J. Bone Joint Surg. **43-A**:625, 1961.

Lewin, P.: Congenital absence or defects of bones of extremities, Am. J. Roentgen. **4**:431, 1917.

McCullough, F.H., Jr.: The congenital short femur, Duke Trainees Orthopaedic Correspondence Club Letter, February 1953.

Murat, J.E., Guilleminet, M., and Descamps, R.: Long-term results of rotation-plasty in two patients with subtotal aplasia of the femur, Am. J. Surg. **113**:676, 1967.

Nutt, J.J., and Smith, E.E.: Total congenital absence of the tibia, Am. J. Roentgen. **46**:841, 1941.

Ober, F.R.: Congenital anomalies of upper extremity and shoulder girdle. In Bancroft, F.W., and Marble, H.C.: Surgical treatment of the motor-skeletal system, ed. 2, Philadelphia, 1951, J.B. Lippincott Co.

Ollerenshaw, R.: Congenital defects of the long bones of the lower limb: a contribution to the study of their causes, effects, and treatment, J. Bone Joint Surg. **7**:528, 1925,

O'Rahilly, R.: Morphological patterns in limb deficiences and duplications, Am J. Anat. **89**:135, 1951.

Pappas, A.M., Hanawalt, B.J., and Anderson, M.: Congenital defects of the fibula, Orthop. Clin. North Am. **3**:187, 1972.

Peabody, C.W.: Congenital absence of the radius, Orthopaedic Correspondence Club Letter, 1947.

Putti, V.: The treatment of congenital absence of the tibia or fibula, Int. Abstr. Surg. **50**:42, 1930. (Abstracted from Chir. Organi. Mov. **7**:513, 1929.)

Ring, P.A.: Congenital short femur: simple femoral hypoplasia, J. Bone Joint Surg. **41-B**:73, 1959.

Steindler, A.: Post-graduate lectures on orthopedic diagnosis and indications, vol. 1, sect. B. Congenital deformities and disabilities, Springfield, Ill., 1950, Charles C Thomas, Publisher.

Swanson, A.B.: A classification for congenital limb malformations, J. Hand Surg. **1**:8, 1976.

Thompson, T.C., Straub, L.R., and Arnold, W.D.: Congenital absence of the fibula, J. Bone Joint Surg. **39-A**:1229, 1957.

Van Nes, C.P.: Rotation-plasty for congenital defects of the femur, making use of the ankle of the shortened limb to control the knee joint of a prosthesis, J. Bone Joint Surg. **32-B**:12, 1950.

Wiltse, L.L.: Valgus deformity of the ankle: a sequel to acquired or congenital abnormalities of the fibula, J. Bone Joint Surg. **54-A**:595, 1972.

Wood, W.L., Zlotsky, N., and Westin, G.W.: Congenital absence of the fibula: treatment by Syme amputation—indications and technique, J. Bone Joint Surg. **47-A**:1159, 1965.

Congenital angular deformities of leg and congenital pseudarthrosis

Aegerter, E.E.: The possible relationship of neurofibromatosis, congenital pseudarthrosis, and fibrous dysplasia. J. Bone Joint Surg. **32-A**:618, 1950.

Alldred, A.J.: Congenital pseudarthrosis of the clavicle, J. Bone Joint Surg. **45-B**:312, 1963.

Andersen, K.S.: Congenital angulation of the lower leg and congenital pseudarthrosis of the tibia in Denmark, Acta Orthop. Scand. **43**:539, 1972.

Andersen, K.S.: Radiological classification of congenital pseudarthrosis of the tibia, Acta Orthop. Scand. **44**:719, 1973.

Andersen, K.S.: Operative treatment of congenital pseudarthrosis of the tibia: factors influencing the primary result, Acta Orthop. Scand. **45**:935, 1974.

Andersen, K.S.: Congenital pseudarthrosis of the tibia and neurofibromatosis, Acta Orthop. Scand. **47**:108, 1976.

Badgley, C.E., O'Connor, S.J., and Kudner, D.F.: Congenital kyphosocoliotic tibia, J. Bone Joint Surg. **34-A**:349, 1952.

Baldwin, D.M., and Weiner, D.S.: Congenital bowing and intraosseous neurofibroma of the ulna: a case report, J. Bone Joint Surg. **56-A**:803, 1974.

Barber, C.G.: Congenital bowing and pseudarthrosis of the lower leg: manifestations of von Recklinghausen's neurofibromatosis, Surg. Gynecol. Obstet. **69**:618, 1939.

Baw, S.: The transarticular graft for infantile pseudarthrosis of the tibia: a new technique, J. Bone Joint Surg. **57-B**:63, 1975.

Birkett, A.N.: Note on pseudarthrosis of the tibia in childhood, J. Bone Joint Surg. **33-B**:47, 1951.

Boyd, H.B.: Congenital pseudarthrosis: treatment by dual bone grafts, J. Bone Joint Surg. **23**:497, 1941.

Boyd, H.B., and Fox, K.W.: Congenital pseudarthrosis: follow-up study after massive bone-grafting, J. Bone Joint Surg. **30-A**:274, 1948.

Boyd, H.B., and Sage, F.P.: Congenital pseudarthrosis of the tibia, J. Bone Joint Surg. **40-A**:1245, 1958.

Camurati, M.: Le pseudartrosi congenite della tibia, Chir. Organi Mov. **15**:1, 1930.

Charnley, J.: Congenital pseudarthrosis of the tibia treated by the intramedullary nail, J. Bone Joint Surg. **38-A**:283, 1956.

Compere, E.L.: Localized osteitis fibrosa in the new-born and congenital pseudarthrosis, J. Bone Joint Surg. **18**:513, 1936.

Dooley, B.J., Menelaus, M.B., and Paterson, D.C.: Congenital pseudarthrosis and bowing of the fibula. J. Bone Joint Surg. **56-B**:739, 1974.

Evans, E.B., and Eggers, G.W.N.: Nonrigid fixation in the treatment of childhood pseudarthrosis of the tibia, Am. J. Surg. **28**:510, 1962.

Eyre-Brook, A.L., Baily, R.A.J., and Price, C.H.G.: Infantile pseudarthrosis of the tibia: three cases treated successfully by delayed autogenous by-pass graft: with some comments on the causative lesion, J. Bone Joint Surg. **51-B**:604, 1969.

Garth, W.P., Jr., and Canale, S.T.: Congenital pseudarthroses of the ulna associated with neurofibromatosis: a report of two cases and review of the literature, Staff meeting report, Campbell Clinic, Memphis, 1977.

Gibson, D.A., and Carroll, N.: Congenital pseudarthrosis of the clavicle, J. Bone Joint Surg. **52-B**:629, 1970.

Green, W.T., and Rudo, N.: Pseudarthrosis and neurofibromatosis, Arch. Surg. **46**:639, 1943.

Greenberg, L.A., and Schwartz, A.: Congenital pseudarthrosis of the distal radius, South. Med. J. **68:**1053. 1975.

Henderson, M.S.: Congenital pseudarthrosis of the tibia, J. Bone Joint Surg. **10:**483, 1928.

Henderson, M.S., and Clegg, R.S.: Pseudarthrosis of tibia: report of one case, Mayo Clin. Proc. **16:**769, 1941.

Herman, S.: Congenital bilateral pseudarthrosis of the clavicles, Clin. Orthop. **91:**162, 1973.

Heyman, C.H., and Herndon, C.H.: Congenital posterior angulation of the tibia. J. Bone Joint Surg. **31-A:**571, 1949.

Heyman, C.H., Herndon, C.H., and Heiple, K.G.: Congenital posterior angulation of the tibia with talipes calcaneus: a long-term report of eleven patients, J. Bone Joint Surg. **41-A:**476, 1959.

Hsu, L.C.S., O'Brien, J.P., Yau, A.C.M.C., and Hodgson, A.R.: Valgus deformity of the ankle in children with fibular pseudarthrosis: results of treatment by bone-grafting of the fibula, J. Bone Joint Surg. **56-A:**503, 1974.

Inglis, K.: The pathology of congenital pseudarthrosis of the tibia, J. Coll. Surg. Australasia **1:**194, 1928.

Ingram, A.J.: Personal communication, 1978.

Kite, J.H.: Congenital pseudarthrosis of tibia and fibula, South. Med. J. **34:**1021, 1941.

Kite, J.H.: Congenital deformities of the lower extremities. In Bancroft, F.W., and Marble, H.C.: Surgical treatment of the motor-skeletal system, ed. 2, Philadelphia, 1951, J.B. Lippincott Co.

Krida, A.: Congenital posterior angulation of the tibia: a clinical entity unrelated to congenital pseudarthrosis, Am. J. Surg. **28:**98, 1951.

Langenskiöld, A.: Pseudarthrosis of the fibula and progressive valgus deformity of the ankle in children: treatment by fusion of the distal tibial and fibular metaphyses: review of three cases, J. Bone Joint Surg. **49-A:**463, 1967.

Lawsing, J.F., III, et al.: Congenital pseudarthrosis of the tibia: successful one stage transposition of the fibula into the distal tibia: a case report, Clin. Orthop. **110:**201, 1975.

Lloyd-Roberts, G.C., Apley, A.G., and Owen, R.: Reflections upon the aetiology of congenital pseudarthrosis of the clavicle: with a note on cranio-cleido dysostosis, J. Bone Joint Surg. **57-B:**24, 1975.

Lloyd-Roberts, G.C., and Shaw, N.E.: The prevention of pseudarthrosis in congenital kyphosis of the tibia, J. Bone Joint Surg. **51-B:**100, 1969.

Makin, A.S.: Congenital pseudarthrosis of tibia treated by twin grafts, Proc. R. Soc. Med. **38:**71, 1944.

Masihuz-Zaman: Pseudarthrosis of the radius associated with neurofibromatosis: a case report, J. Bone Joint Surg. **59-A:**977, 1977.

Masserman, R.L., Peterson, H.A., and Bianco, A.J., Jr.: Congenital pseudarthrosis of the tibia: a review of the literature and 52 cases from the Mayo Clinic, Clin. Orthop. **99:**140, 1974.

McElvenny, R.T.: Congenital pseudo-arthrosis of the tibia, Q. Bull. Northwestern Univ. Med. School **23:**413, 1949.

McFarland, B.: "Birth fracture" of the tibia, Br. J. Surg. **27:**706, 1939.

McFarland, B.: Congenital deformities of the spine and limbs. In Platt, H., editor: Modern trends in orthopaedics, New York, 1950, Paul B. Hoeber, Inc.

McFarland, B.: Pseudarthrosis of the tibia in childhood, J. Bone Joint Surg. **33-B:**36, 1951.

McKellar, C.C.: Congenital pseudarthrosis of the tibia: treatment by tibial lengthening and corrective osteotomy seven years after successful bone graft: a case report, J. Bone Joint Surg. **55-A:**193, 1973.

Milgram, J.E.: Impaling (telescoping) operation for pseudarthrosis of long bones in childhood, Bull. Hosp. Joint Dis. **17:**152, 1956.

Moore, B.H.: Some orthopaedic relationships of neurofibromatosis, J. Bone Joint Surg. **23:**109, 1941.

Moore, J.R.: Pseudarthrosis of the tibia and fibula in children, Int. Surg. **9:**7, 1946.

Moore, J.R.: Delayed autogenous bone graft in the treatment of congenital pseudarthrosis, J. Bone Joint Surg. **31-A:**23, 1949.

Morris, H.D.: Amputation as a tool in managing congenital deformities. Movie presented at The Russell A. Hibbs Society, April 1961, New Orleans.

Owen, R.: Congenital pseudarthrosis of the clavicle, J. Bone Joint Surg. **52-B:**644, 1970.

Paterson, D.: Treatment of nonunion with a constant direct current: a totally implantable system, Orthop. Clin. North Am. **15:**47, 1984.

Purvis, G.D., and Holder, J.E.: Dual bone graft for congenital pseudarthrosis of the tibia: variations of technic, South. Med. J. **53:**926, 1960.

Rathgeb, J.M., Ramsey, P.L., and Cowell, H.R.: Congenital kyphoscoliosis of the tibia, Clin. Orthop. **103:**178, 1974.

Richin, P.F., Kranik, A., Van Herpe, L., and Suffecool, S.L.: Congenital pseudarthrosis of both bones of the forearm: a case report, J. Bone Joint Surg. **58-A:**1032, 1976.

Rose, G.K.: Restraint in the treatment of a bowed tibia associated with neurofibromatosis, Acta Orthop. Scand. **46:**704, 1975.

Scaglietti, O.: Il perone in posto della tibia, Boll. Mem. Soc. Emiliano-Romagnola Chir. **2:** No. 2, 1936.

Sofield, H.A.: Congenital psuedarthrosis of the tibia, Clin. Orthop. **76:**33, 1971.

Sofield, H.A., and Millar, E.A.: Fragmentation realignment, and intramedullary rod fixation of deformities of the long bones in children: a ten-year appraisal, J. Bone Joint Surg. **41-A:**1371, 1959.

Sprague, B.L., and Brown, G.A.: Congenital pseudarthrosis of the radius, J. Bone Joint Surg. **56-A:**191, 1974.

Umber, J.S., and Coleman, S.S.: Congenital pseudoarthrosis of the tibia (abstract), Orthop. Transactions, **2:**212, November 1978.

Van Nes, C.P.: Congenital pseudarthrosis of the leg, J. Bone Joint Surg. **48-A:**1467, 1966.

Wall, J.J.: Congenital pseudarthrosis of the clavicle, J. Bone Joint Surg. **52-A:**1003, 1970.

Wellwood, J.M., Bulmer, J.H., and Graff, D.J.C.: Congenital defects of the tibia in siblings with neurofibromatosis, J. Bone Joint Surg. **53-B:**314, 1971.

Williams, R.E.: Two congenital deformities of the tibia: congenital angulation and congenital pseudoarthrosis, Br. J. Radiol. **16:**371, 1943.

Wilson, P.D.: A simple method of two stage transplantation of the fibula for use in cases of complicated and congenital pseudarthrosis of the tibia, J. Bone Joint Surg. **23:**639, 1941.

Congenital hyperextension and dislocation of knee

Charif, P., and Reichelderfer, T.E.: Genu recurvatum congenitum in the newborn: its incidence, course, treatment, prognosis, Clin. Pediatr. **4:**587, 1965.

Curtis, B.H., and Fisher, R.L.: Congenital hyperextension with anterior subluxation of the knee: surgical treatment and long-term observations, J. Bone Joint Surg. **51-A:**255, 1969.

Ferrone, J.D., Jr.: Congenital deformities about the knee, Orthop. Clin. North Am. **7:**323, 1976.

Finder, J.G.: Congenital hyperextension of the knee, J. Bone Joint Surg. **46-B:**783, 1964.

Katz, M.P., Grogono, B.J., and Soper, K.C.: The etiology and treatment of congenital dislocation of the knee, J. Bone Joint Surg. **49-B:**112, 1967.

Laurence, M.: Genu recurvatum congenitum, J. Bone Joint Surg. **49-B:**121, 1967.

Mayer, L.: Congenital anterior subluxation of the knee, Am. J. Orthop. Surg. **10:**411, 1913.

McFarland, B.L.: Congenital dislocation of the knee, J. Bone Joint Surg. **11:**281, 1929.

Middleton, D.S.: The pathology of congenital genu recurvatum, Br. J. Surg. **22:**696, 1935.

Niebauer, J.J., and King, D.E.: Congenital dislocation of the knee, J. Bone Joint Surg. **42-A:**207, 1960.

Provenzono, R.W.: Congenital dislocation of the knee. N. Engl. J. Med. **236:**360, 1947.

Steindler, A.: Congenital dislocation of the knee, In Abt, I.A., editor: Pediatrics, vol. 5, Philadelphia, 1924, W.B. Saunders Co.

Congenital dislocation of patella

Conn, H.R.: A new method of operative reduction for congenital luxation of the patella, J. Bone Joint Surg. **7:**370, 1925.

Green, J.P., and Waugh, W.: Congenital lateral dislocation of the patella, J. Bone Joint Surg. **50-B:**285, 1968.

Green, W.T., Jr.: Painful bipartite patellae: a report of three cases, Clin. Orthop. **110:**197, 1975.

McCarroll, H.R., and Schwartzmann, J.R.: Lateral dislocation of the patella: correction by simultaneous transplantation of the tibial tubercle and semitendinosus tendon, J. Bone Joint Surg. **27:**446, 1945.

Mumford, E.B.: Congenital dislocation of the patella: case report with history of four generations, J. Bone Joint Surg. **29:**1083, 1947.

Stanisavljevic, S., Zemenick, G., and Miller, D.: Congenital, irreducible, permanent lateral dislocation of the patella, Clin. Orthop. **116:**190, 1975.

Storen, H.: Congenital complete dislocation of patella causing serious disability in childhood: the operative treatment, Acta Orthop. Scand. **36:**301, 1965.

Lower limb length discrepancy

Abbott, L.C.: The operative lengthening of the tibia and fibula. J. Bone Joint Surg. **9:**128, 1927.

Abbott, L.C., and Gill, G.G.: Surgical approaches to the epiphyseal cartilages of the knee and ankle joint, Arch. Surg. **46:**591, 1943.

Abbott, L.C., and Saunders, J.B. deC.M.: The operative lengthening of the tibia and fibula, preliminary report on further development of principles and technic, Ann. Surg. **100:**961, 1939.

Allan, F.G.: Leg-lengthening, Br. Med. J. **1:**218, 1951.

Allan, F.G.: Simultaneous femoral and tibial lengthening, J. Bone Joint Surg. **45-B:**206, 1963.

Anderson, M., and Green, W.T.: Length of femur and tibia; norms derived from ortho-roentgenograms of children from 5 years of age until epiphyseal closure, Am. J. Dis. Child. **75:**279, 1948.

Anderson, M., Green., W.T., and Messner, M.B.: Growth and predictions of growth in the lower extremities, J. Bone Joint Surg. **45-A:**1, 1963.

Anderson, M., Messner, M.B., and Green, W.T.: Distribution of lengths of the normal femur and tibia in children from one to eighteen years of age, J. Bone Joint Surg. **46-A:**1197, 1964.

Barr, J.S., and Ober, F.R.: Leg lengthening in adults, J. Bone Joint Surg. **15:**674, 1933.

Bisgard, J.D., and Bisgard, M.E.: Longitudinal growth of long bones, Arch. Surg. **31:**568, 1935.

Blount, W.P.: Blade-plate internal fixation for high femoral osteotomies, J. Bone Joint Surg. **25:**319, 1943.

Blount, W.P.: Kontrolle der Knochenlänge bei epiphysärer Klammerung. Verhandlungen der Deutschen Orthopädischen Gesellschaft 40 Kongress, Wiesbaden, 1952.

Blount, W.P.: Unequal leg length. In American Academy of Orthopaedic Surgeons: Instructional course lectures, vol. 17, St. Louis, 1960, The C.V. Mosby Co.

Blount, W.P., and Clark, G.R.: Control of bone growth by epiphyseal stapling, preliminary report, J. Bone Joint Surg. **31-A:**464, 1949.

Blount, W.P., and Zeier, F.: Control of bone length, JAMA **148:**451, 1952.

Bost, F.C.: Operative lengthening of the bones of the lower extremity. In American Academy of Orthopaedic Surgeons: Instructional course lectures, vol. 1, Ann Arbor, 1944, J.W. Edwards.

Bost, F.C., and Larsen, L.J.: Experiences with lengthening of the femur over an intramedullary rod, J. Bone Joint Surg. **38-A:**567, 1956.

Brockway, A., and Fowler, S.B.: Experience with 105 leg lengthening operations, Surg. Gynecol. Obstet. **75:**252, 1942.

Brockway, A., Craig, W.A., and Cockrell, B.R., Jr.: End result study of sixty-two stapling operations, J. Bone Joint Surg. **36-A:**1063, 1954.

Canale, S.T., Russell, T.A., and Holcomb, R.L.: Percutaneous epiphysiodesis: an experimental study and preliminary clinical results, J. Pediatr. Orthop. **6:**150, 1986.

Carpenter, E.B., and Dalton, J.B., Jr.: A critical evaluation of epiphyseal stimulation, J. Bone Joint Surg. **38-A:**1089, 1956.

Castle, M.E.: Epiphyseal stimulation, J. Bone Joint Surg. **53-A:**326, 1971.

Chan, K.P., and Hodgson, A.R.: Physiologic leg lengthening: a preliminary report, Clin. Orthop. **68:**55, 1970.

Codivilla, A.: On the means of lengthening, in the lower limbs, the muscles and tissues which are shortened through deformity, Am. J. Orthop. Sur. **2:**353, 1905.

Coleman, S.S.: Current concepts of tibial lengthening, Orthop. Clin. North Am. **3:**201, 1972.

Coleman, S.S., and Noonan, T.D.: Anderson's method of tibial-lengthening by percutaneous osteotomy and gradual distraction: experience with thirty-one cases, J. Bone Joint Surg. **49-A:**263, 1967.

Compere, E.L.: Indications for and against the leg lengthening operation, J. Bone Joint Surg. **18:**692, 1936.

Dalton, J.B., Jr., and Carpenter, E.B.: Clinical experiences with epiphyseal stapling, South. Med. J. **47:**544, 1954.

d'Aubigne, R.M., and Dubousset, J.: Surgical correction of large length discrepancies in the lower extremities of children and adults: an analysis of twenty consecutive cases, J. Bone Joint Surg. **53-A:**411, 1971.

Eydelshtein, B.M., Udalova, F., and Bochkarev, G.F.: Dynamics of reparative regeneration after lengthening by the method of distraction epiphysiolysis, Acta Chir. Plast. **15:**149, 1973.

Eyre-Brooke, A.L.: Bone shortening for inequality of leg lengths, Br. Med. J. **1:**222, 1951.

Fischenko, P.J., Karimova, L.F., and Pilipenko, N.P.: Distraction epiphysiolysis in congenital shortening of lower extremity, Ortop. Traumatol. Protez. (Russian) **37:**44, 1976.

Fries, I.B.: Growth following epiphyseal arrest: a simple method of calculation, Clin. Orthop. **114:**316, 1976.

Gill, G.G., and Abbott, L.C.: Practical method of predicting the growth of the femur and tibia in the child, Arch. Surg. **45:**286, 1942.

Green, W.T., and Anderson, M.: Discrepancy in length of the lower extremities. In American Academy of Orthopaedic Surgeons: Instructional course lectures, vol. 8, Ann Arbor. 1951, J.W. Edwards.

Green, W.T., and Anderson, M.: Epiphyseal arrest for the correction of discrepancies in length of the lower extremities, J. Bone Joint Surg. **39-A:**853. 1957.

Green, W.T., and Anderson, M.: Skeletal age and the control of bone growth. In American Academy of Orthopaedic Surgeons: Instruction course lectures, vol. 17, St. Louis, 1960, The C.V. Mosby Co.

Green, W.T., Wyatt, G.M., and Anderson, M.: Orthoroentgenography as a method of measuring the bones of the lower extremity. J. Bone Joint Surg. **28:**60, 1946.

Greulich, W.W., and Pyle, S.I.: Radiographic atlas of skeletal development of the hand and wrist, Stanford, Calif. 1950, Stanford University Press.

Haas, S.L.: Longitudinal osteotomy, JAMA **92:**1656, 1929.

Haas, S.L.: Mechanical retardation of bone growth, J. Bone Joint Surg. **30-A:**506, 1948.

Harmon, P.H., and Krigsten, W.H.: The surgical treatment of unequal leg length, Surg. Gynecol. Obstet. **71:**482, 1940.

Howorth, M.B.: Leg-shortening operation for equalizing leg length, Arch. Surg. **44:**543, 1942.

Ilizarov, G.A., and Soybelman, L.M.: Some clinical and experimental data concerning bloodless lengthening of lower extremities, Eksp. Khir. Anesthesiol. **4:**27, 1969.

Jenkins, D.H.R., Cheng, D.H.F., and Hodgson, A.R.: Stimulation of bone growth by periosteal stripping: a clinical study, J. Bone Joint Surg. **57-B:**482, 1975.

McCarroll, H.R.: Trials and tribulations in attempted femoral lengthening, J. Bone Joint Surg. **32-A:**132, 1950.

McGibbon, K.C., Deacon, A.E., and Raisbeck, C.C.: Experiences in growth retardation with heavy Vitallium staples, J. Bone Joint Surg. **44-B:**86, 1962.

Macnicol, M.F., and Catto, A.M.: Twenty-year review of tibial lengthening for poliomyelitis, J. Bone Joint Surg. **64-B:**607, 1982.

Magnuson, P.B.: Lengthening shortened bones of the leg by operation Surg. Gynecol. Obstet. **17:**63, 1913.

May, V.R., Jr., and Clements, E.L.: Epiphyseal stapling: with special references to complications, South. Med. J. **58:**1203, 1965.

Menelaus, M.B.: Correction of leg length discrepancy by epiphysial arrest, J. Bone Joint Surg. **48-B:**336, 1966.

Montgomery, W.S., and Ingram, A.J.: Experimental studies and clinical evaluation of linear growth stimulation. South. Med. J. **49:**793, 1956.

Montecelli, G., and Spinelli, R.: Distraction epiphysiolysis as a method of limb lengthening. III. Clinical applications. Clin. Orthop. **154:**274, 1981.

Moore, B.H.: A critical appraisal of the leg lengthening operation, Am. J. Surg. **52:**415, 1941.

Moseley, C.F.: A straight-line graph for leg-length discrepancies, J. Bone Joint Surg. **59-A:**174, 1977.

Petty, W., Winter, R.B., and Felder, D.: Arteriovenous fistula for treatment of discrepancy in leg length, J. Bone Joint Surg. **56-A:**581, 1974.

Phalen, G.S., and Chatterton, C.C.: Equalizing the lower extremities: a clinical consideration of leg lengthening versus leg shortening, Surgery **12:**768, 1942.

Phemister, D.B.: Operative arrestment of longitudinal growth of bones, in the treatment of deformities, J. Bone Joint Surg. **15:**1, 1933.

Pilcher, M.F.: Epiphyseal stapling: thirty-five cases followed to maturity, J. Bone Joint Surg. **44-B:**82, 1962.

Poirier, H.: Epiphysial stapling and leg equalization, J. Bone Joint Surg. **50-B:**61, 1968.

Putti, V.: The operative lengthening of the femur, JAMA **77:**934, 1921.

Putti, V.: Operative lengthening of the femur, Surg. Gynecol. Obstet. **58:**318, 1934.

Regan, J.M., and Chatterton, C.C.: Deformities following surgical epiphyseal arrest, J. Bone Joint Surg. **28:**265, 1946.

Shapiro, F.: Devlopmental patterns in lower extremity length discrepancies, J. Bone Joint Surg. **64-A:**639, 1982.

Sofield, H.A., Blair, S.J., and Millar, E.A.: Leg-lengthening: a personal follow-up of forty patients some twenty years after the operation, J. Bone Joint Surg. **40-A:**311, 1958.

Stamp, W.G., and Lansche, W.E.: Treatment of discrepancy in leg length, South. Med. J. **53:**764, 1960.

Straub, L.R., Thompson, T.C., and Wilson, P.D.: The results of epiphyseodesis and femoral shortening in relation to equalization of limb length, J. Bone Joint Surg. **27:**254, 1945.

Thompson, T.C., Straub, L.R., and Campbell, R.D.: An evaluation of femoral shortening with intramedullary nailing, J. Bone Joint Surg. **36-A:**43, 1954.

Thornton, L.: A method of subtrochanteric limb shortening, J. Bone Joint Surg. **31-A:**81, 1949.

Todd, T.W.: Atlas of skeletal maturation, St. Louis, 1937, The C.V. Mosby Co.

Trueta, J.: The influence of the blood supply in controlling bone growth, Bull. Hosp. Joint Dis. **14:**147, 1953.

Tupman, G.S.: Treatment of inequality of the lower limbs: the results of operations for stimulation of growth, J. Bone Joint Surg. **42-B:**489, 1960.

von Langenbeck, B.: Ueber krankhaftes Längenwachsthum der Röphrenknocken und seine Verwerthung für die chirurgische Praxis, Berlin. Klin. Wschr. **6:**265, 1869, Cited in Pease, C.N.: Local stimulation of growth of long bones, a preliminary report, J. Bone Joint Surg. **34-A:**1, 1952.

Wagner, H.: Operative beinverlägerung, Der Chirurg. **42:**260, 1971.

Wagner, H.: Surgical lengthening or shortening of femur and tibia: technique and indications. Reprint from Hungerford, D.S., editor: Progress in orthopaedic surgery, Berlin, 1977, Springer-Verlag.

Westin, G.W.: Femoral lengthening using a periosteal sleeve. Report of twenty-six cases, J. Bone Joint Surg. **49-A:**836, 1967.

White, J.W.: A simplified method for tibial lengthening, J. Bone Joint Surg. **12:**90, 1930.

White, J.W.: Femoral shortening for equalization of leg length, J. Bone Joint Surg. **17:**597, 1935.

White, J.W.: A practical graphic method of recording leg length discrepancies, South Med. J. **33:**946, 1940.

White, J.W.: Leg-length discrepancies. In American Academy of Orthopaedic Surgeons: Instructional course lectures, vol. 6, Ann Arbor, 1949, J.W. Edwards.

Wilk, L.H., and Badgley, C.E.: Hypertension, another complication of the leg-lengthening procedure: report of a case, J. Bone Joint Surg. **45-A:**1263, 1963.

Wilson, P.D., and Thompson, T.C.: A clinical consideration of the methods of equalizing leg length, Ann. Surg. **110:**992, 1939.

Yosipovitch, Z.H., and Palti, Y.: Alterations in blood pressure during leg-lengthening, a clinical and experimental investigation, J. Bone Joint Surg. **49-A:**1352, 1967.

Zavijalov, P.V., and Plaskin, J.T.: Distraction epiphysiolysis in lengthening of the lower extremity in children. Khirurgija **44:**121, 1968.

CHAPTER 62

Congenital anomalies of hip and pelvis

James H. Beaty

In this chapter are discussed congenital dislocation of the hip, congenital and developmental coxa vara, and extrophy of the bladder.

CONGENITAL DISLOCATION OF HIP

Congenital dislocation of the hip generally includes subluxation and dysplasia as well as dislocation of the hip. The term "subluxation" denotes that the femoral head lies within the true acetabulum, but is partially dislocated from it. The term "dysplasia" is generally used to describe abnormal acetabular development. A true congenital dislocation of the hip in the newborn produces findings that include the ability to dislocate or reduce the femoral head into and out of the true acetabulum. In the older child, the femoral head remains dislocated from the true acetabulum and secondary changes develop.

The incidence of congenital dislocation of the hip is approximately 1 in 1000 live births. The left hip is more commonly involved than the right, and bilateral involvement is more common than involvement of the right hip alone. Several risk factors should arouse suspicion of congenital dislocation of the hip. The disorder is more common in females than in males, in many series as much as 5 times more common. Breech deliveries comprise approximately 3% to 4% of all deliveries, and the incidence of congenital dislocation of the hip is significantly increased in this patient population. MacEwen and Ramsey in a study of 25,000 infants found the combination of female infants and breech presentation to result in congenital dislocation of the hip in 1 out of 35 births. Congenital dislocation of the hip is more common in firstborn children than in subsequent siblings. A family history of congenital dislocation of the hip increases the likelihood of this condition to approximately 10%. Ethnic background plays

some role in that congenital dislocation of the hip is more common in Caucasian children than in black children. Other reported examples include the high incidence among the Navajo Indians and the relatively low incidence among the Chinese. A strong association also exists between congenital dislocation of the hip and other musculoskeletal abnormalities, such as skull and facial abnormalities, congenital torticollis, metatarsus adductus, and talipes calcaneovalgus.

Several theories regarding the cause of congenital dislocation of the hip have been proposed, including mechanical factors, hormone-induced joint laxity, primary acetabular dysplasia, and genetic inheritance. Breech delivery, with the mechanical forces of abnormal flexion of the hips, can easily be seen as a cause of posterior dislocation of the femoral head.

Ligamentous laxity has been proposed as a contributing factor in congenital dislocation of the hip by several authors. The theory is that the influence of the maternal hormones that produce relaxation of the pelvis during delivery may cause enough ligamentous laxity in the child in utero and during the neonatal period to allow dislocation of the femoral head.

Wynne-Davies described a familial occurrence of shallow acetabulum defined as a "dysplasia trait" in proposing primary acetabular dysplasia as one of the risk factors for congenital dislocation of the hip. The risk of a genetic influence was noted by Ortolani, who reported a 70% incidence of a positive family history in children with congenital dislocation of the hip.

Diagnosis and clinical presentation

The clinical presentation of congenital dislocation of the hip varies according to the age of the child. In the newborn (up to 6 months) it is especially important to perform a careful clinical examination, since roentgenograms are not absolutely reliable in making the diagnosis of congenital dislocation of the hip in this age group. Routine clinical screening should include both the Ortolani test and the provocative maneuver of Barlow. The Ortolani test is performed by gently abducting and adducting the flexed hip to detect any reduction into or dislocation of the femoral head from the true acetabulum. The provocative maneuver of Barlow detects any potential subluxation or posterior dislocation of the femoral head by direct pressure on the longitudinal axis of the femur while the hip is in adduction. Both of these tests require a relaxed and pacified child (Fig. 62-1). However, a child may be born with ac-

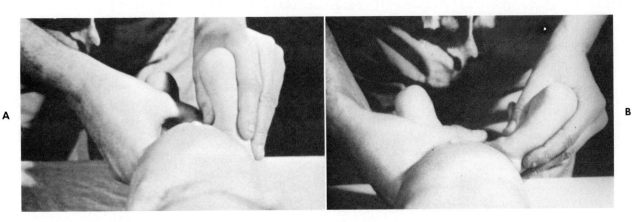

Fig. 62-1. A, Barlow and **B,** Ortolani maneuvers for routine screening of congenital dislocation of hip. Note that examiner stabilizes infants left hip and lower extremity and places left hand around right thigh and index and middle fingers over greater trochanter.

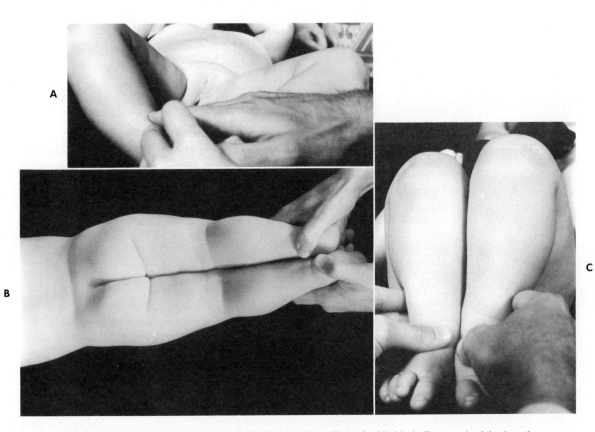

Fig. 62-2. Clinical signs of congenital dislocation of hip in a 13-month-old girl. **A,** Decrease in abduction of right hip with adduction contracture. **B,** Asymmetric skin fold with difference in level of popliteal and gluteal skin clefts. **C,** Positive Galeazzi sign with apparent shortening of right lower extremity.

etabular dysplasia without dislocation of the hip, and the latter may develop weeks or months later.

As the child reaches the age of 3 to 6 months, several factors in the clinical presentation change. Once the femoral head is dislocated and the ability to reduce it by abduction has disappeared, several other clinical signs become obvious. The first and most reliable is a decrease in the ability to abduct the dislocated hip because of a contracture of the adductor musculature (Fig. 62-2, A). Asymmetric skin folds (Fig. 62-2, B) are commonly mentioned as a sign to look for, but unfortunately, this sign is not reliable in that normal children may have asymmetric skin folds, and children with a dislocated hip may have symmetric folds. The Galeazzi sign is noted when the femoral head not only becomes displaced laterally, but proximally as well, causing an apparent shortening of the femur on the side of the dislocated hip (Fig. 62-2, C).

In the child of walking age with an undetected dislocated hip, families describe a "waddling" type of gait, indicating dislocation of the femoral head and a Trendelenburg gait pattern. Mothers may also describe difficulty in abducting the hip during diaper changes.

Although roentgenograms are not always helpful in making the diagnosis of congenital dislocation of the hip in the newborn, screening roentgenograms may reveal any acetabular dysplasia or teratologic dislocation. As the child with a dislocated hip ages and the soft tissues become contracted, the roentgenograms become more reliable and helpful in the diagnosis and treatment (Fig. 62-3). The most commonly used lines of reference are Perkins' vertical line and Hilgenreiner's horizontal line, both used to assess the position of the femoral head. In addition, Shenton's line will be disrupted in the older child with a dislocated hip. Reference lines for the evaluation of the acetabulum include the acetabular index and the CE angle of Wiberg. Normally, the metaphyseal beak of the proximal femur will lie within the inner lower quadrant of the reference lines noted by Perkins and Hilgenreiner. The acetabular index in a newborn is generally 30 degrees or less. Any significant increase in this measurement may be a sign of acetabular dysplasia. The CE angle of Wiberg is especially useful in older children in evaluating coverage of the femoral head by the acetabulum, and will measure 15 to 30 degrees.

Treatment

The treatment of congenital dislocation of the hip is age-related and tailored to the specific pathologic condition.

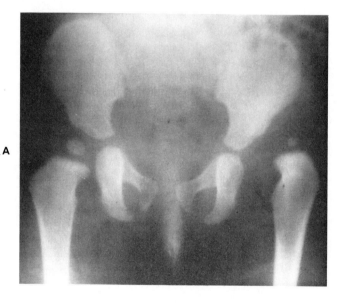

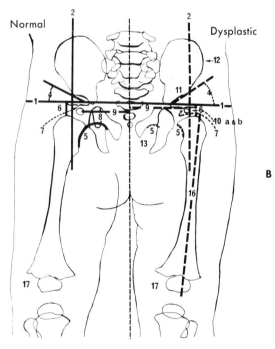

Fig. 62-3. A, Thirteen-month-old child with congenital dislocation of left hip. **B,** Roentgenographic signs of congenital hip dislocation. *1,* Horizontal Y line (Hilgenreiner's line). *2,* Vertical line (Perkins' line). *3,* Quadrants (formed by lines *1* and *2*). *4,* Acetabular index (Kleinberg and Lieberman). *5,* Shenton's line. *6,* Upward displacement of the femoral head. *7,* Lateral displacement of the femoral head. *8,* U figure of teardrop shadow (Kohler). *9,* Y coordinate (Ponseti). *10,* Capital epiphyseal dysplasia: a) delayed appearance of the center of ossification of the femoral head, b) irregular maturation of the center of ossification. *11,* Bilification (furrowing of the acetabular roof in late infancy (Ponseti). *12,* Hypoplasia of the pelvis (ilium). *13,* Delayed fusion (ischiopublic juncture). *14,* Absence of a shapely, defined, well-ossified acetabular margin, caused by delayed ossification of the cartilage of the roof of the socket. *15,* Femoral shaft-neck angle. *16,* Adduction attitude of the extremity. *17,* Development of the epiphyses of other joints (knee, wrists, and lumbosacral spine). *18,* Radiolucent acetabular roof, limbus, joint capsule (arthrographic studies). (**B** From Hart, V.: Congenital dysplasia of the hip joint and sequelae, Springfield, Ill., 1952, Charles C Thomas.)

Five treatment groups related to age have been designated: (1) newborn, birth to 6 months of age, (2) infant, 6 to 18 months of age, (3) toddler, 18 to 36 months of age, (4) child, 3 to 8 years of age, and (5) juvenile, beyond 8 years of age.

NEWBORN (BIRTH TO 6 MONTHS OF AGE)

From birth to approximately 6 months of age, treatment is directed at stabilizing the hip that has a positive Ortolani or Barlow test or to reducing the dislocated hip with a mild to moderate adduction contracture. Both the Pavlik harness and von Rosen splint have been used in this age group, but our current choice is the Pavlik harness (Fig. 62-4). A success rate of 85% to 95% has been reported in children treated in the Pavlik harness during the first few months of life. As the child ages and soft tissue contractures develop, along with secondary changes in the acetabulum, the success rate of the Pavlik harness decreases. Attention to detail is required in the use of this harness since the potential complications include avascular necrosis of the femoral head.

When properly applied and maintained, the Pavlik harness is a dynamic flexion abduction orthosis that can produce excellent results in the treatment of dysplastic, subluxable, and dislocated hips in infants up to 6 months of age. Once the diagnosis has been made, either clinically or roentgenographically, it is essential to carefully evaluate the direction of dislocation, the stability, and the reducibility of the hip before treatment. If a teratologic dislocation is present, the Pavlik harness should not be used.

The Pavlik harness consists of a chest strap, two shoulder straps, and two stirrups. Each stirrup has an anteromedial flexion strap and a posterolateral abduction strap.

The harness is applied with the child supine. The chest strap is fastened first, allowing enough room for a hand to be placed between the chest and the harness. The shoulder straps are buckled to maintain the chest straps at the nipple line. The feet are then placed in the stirrups one at a time. The hip is reduced in flexion (90 to 120 degrees) by the clinician, and the anterior flexion strap is tightened to maintain this position. Finally, the lateral strap is loosely fastened to limit adduction—not to force abduction. The knees should be 3 to 5 cm apart at full adduction in the harness (Fig. 62-5).

The Barlow test should be performed within the limits of the harness to assure adequate stability. The child is then placed in the prone position and the greater trochanters are palpated; if asymmetry is noted, a persistent dislocation is present. A roentgenograph of the patient in the harness must be obtained to confirm that the hip has been reduced and the femoral neck is directed toward the triradiate cartilage.

Four basic patterns of persistent dislocation have been observed following application of the Pavlik harness: superior, inferior, lateral, and posterior. If the dislocation is superior, additional flexion of the hip is indicated. If the dislocation is inferior, a decrease in flexion is indicated. A lateral dislocation in the Pavlik harness should be observed initially. As long as the femoral neck is directed toward the triradiate cartilage, the head should gradually reduce

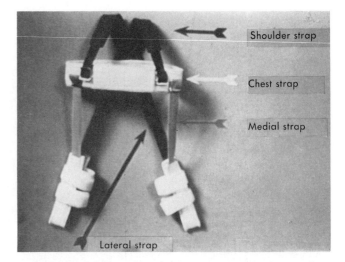

Fig. 62-4. Pavlik harness. (Courtesy Alfred I. duPont Institute.)

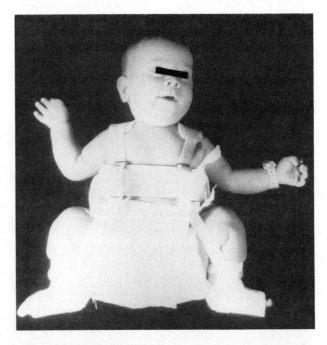

Fig. 62-5. Pavlik harness. (Courtesy Alfred I. duPont Institute.)

into the acetabulum. A persistent posterior dislocation is difficult to treat and is usually accompanied by tight hip adductor muscles. This type of dislocation may be diagnosed by palpation of the greater trochanter posteriorly.

If any of the above patterns of dislocation or subluxation persist for more than 6 to 8 weeks, treatment in the Pavlik harness should be discontinued and a new program initiated; in most patients, this consists of traction, closed reduction, and casting. The Pavlik harness should be worn full-time until stability is attained, as determined by a negative Barlow test. During this time, the patient is clinically examined every week, and the harness straps are adjusted to accommodate growth. The harness may be removed for bathing 1 month after stability has been documented. Outpatient visits should continue at 1- to 2-week intervals for the remainder of the treatment program.

The duration of treatment depends on the patient's age at diagnosis and the degree of hip instability. For example, the duration of full-time harness wear for a patient with a dislocated hip is approximately equal to the age at which stability is attained plus 2 months. Weaning is then started by removing the harness for 2 hours each day. This time is doubled every 2 to 4 weeks until the device is worn only at night. Night bracing may be continued until the hip is normal roentgenographically. Roentgenographic documentation should be used throughout the treatment period to verify the position of the hip. Roentgenograms are indicated at least at the following times: immediately after the initiation of treatment, following any major adjustment in the harness, 1 month after weaning begins, at 6 months of age, and at 1 year of age.

INFANT (6 TO 18 MONTHS OF AGE)

Once a child reaches crawling age, (approximately 6 months), the success with the Pavlik harness decreases significantly. The child with a dislocated hip aged 6 to 18 months will probably require either closed manipulation or open reduction.

Children in this age group often are initially seen with a shortened extremity, limited passive abduction, and a positive Galeazzi sign. If the child is walking, a Trendelenburg gait will be present. Roentgenographic changes include delayed ossification of the femoral head, lateral and proximal displacement of the femoral head, and a shallow acetabulum.

With persistent dysplasia, the femoral head eventually moves superiorly and laterally with weight bearing. The capsule becomes permanently elongated, and anteriorly the psoas tendon may obstruct reduction of the femoral head into the true acetabulum. The acetabular limbus may fold and invert into the acetabulum, and the ligamentum teres hypertrophies and elongates. The femoral head becomes reduced in size with a posteromedial flattening, and coxa valga and excessive anteversion are noted. The true acetabulum is characteristically shallow and at surgery appears small because of the anterior capsular constriction and the inverted limbus.

Treatment in this age group should follow a detailed regimen, which includes adequate preoperative traction, adductor tenotomy, closed reduction and arthrogram, or open reduction in children with a failed closed reduction. Adequate preoperative traction, adductor tenotomy, and gentle reduction are especially helpful in the prevention of avascular necrosis of the femoral head. No effort should be spared to avoid this complication.

PREOPERATIVE TRACTION

In children with compliant and educated parents, we have had success with the use of a home skin traction program that spares the expense of hospitalization and allows the child to stay in traction in a home environment (Fig. 62-6). Skeletal traction in the hospital is used if home traction is impossible. The objectives of traction are to bring the laterally and proximally displaced femoral head down

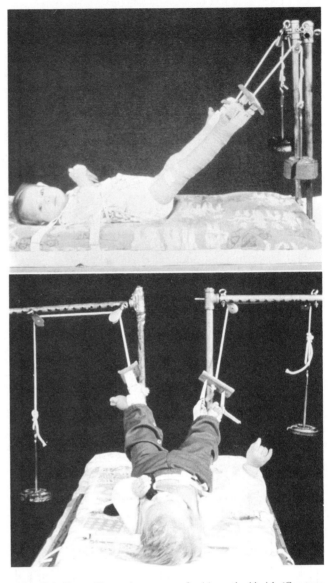

Fig. 62-6. Home skin traction program for 14-month-old girl. (Courtesy Alfred I. duPont Institute.)

to and below the level of the true acetabulum to permit a more gentle reduction.

ADDUCTOR TENOTOMY

A percutaneous adductor tenotomy under sterile conditions may be performed for a mild adduction contracture. For an adduction contracture of long duration, an open adductor tenotomy is preferable (Fig. 62-7).

CLOSED REDUCTION AND ARTHROGRAM

Gentle closed reduction is accomplished with the patient under general anesthesia.

The interposition of soft tissue in the acetabulum may be suggested by lateralization of the femoral head. Because the roentgenogram of the hip in an infant or young child cannot yield all of the information desired in diag-

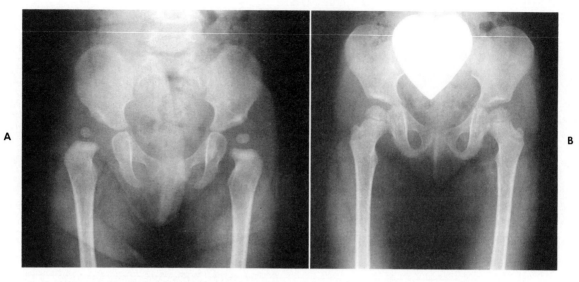

Fig. 62-7. Congenital dislocation of hip in 8-month-old girl. **A,** Before adductor tenotomy, closed reduction, and application of spica cast. **B,** At age 2 years, femoral head appears normal with excellent acetabular remodeling.

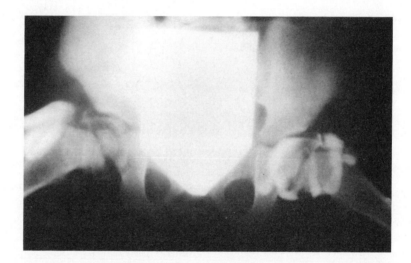

Fig. 62-8. Arthrography of normal hips at autopsy. Note positive "thorn sign" outlining normal labrum, cartilaginous anlage of normal acetabulum, and small amount of dye pooling medially.

nosing or treating congenital dysplasia, arthrography is often helpful in determining (1) whether mild dysplasia is present, (2) whether the femoral head is subluxated or dislocated, (3) whether manipulative reduction has been or can be successful, (4) to what extent any soft structures within the acetabulum may interfere with complete reduction of the dislocation, (5) what is the condition and position of the acetabular labrum (the limbus), and (6) whether the acetabulum and femoral head are developing normally during treatment. Because arthrograms are not always easy to interpret well, the surgeon must be thoroughly familiar with the normal and abnormal signs they may reveal and with the technique of making arthrograms (Figs. 62-8 to 62-10).

We make an arthrogram of the hip in all children, re-

gardless of age, who are given a general anesthetic for closed reduction and in whom we think the reduction may be incomplete. It is most helpful when manipulative reduction is unstable or when the femoral head fails to become progressively more deeply and concentrically seated within the acetabulum during conservative treatment. The use of image intensifier television fluoroscopy makes placement of the needle much easier. The danger of damaging the articular surfaces by the needle is decreased, and the possibility of injecting the contrast medium directly into the ossific nucleus or the epiphyseal plate is prevented. This type of fluoroscopy decreases the radiation exposure of both the examiner and the patient. When such equipment is not available, brief but careful use of an ordinary fluoroscope can aid in centering the needle properly. The most

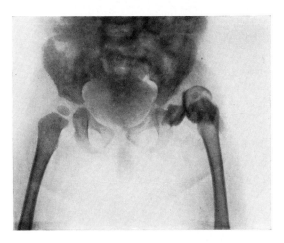

Fig. 62-9. Arthogram of hip demonstrating inverted limbus of medium size, giving appearance often described as hourglass constriction of capsule. (From Somerville, E.W.: J. Bone Joint Surg. **35-B**:363, 1953.)

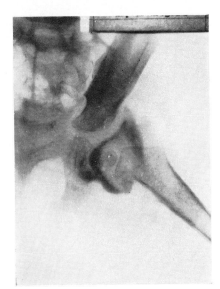

Fig. 62-10. Arthrogram of hip demonstrating very large inverted limbus that almost forms a diaphragm. Femoral head has been deformed by pressing on limbus. (From Somerville, E.W.: J. Bone Joint Surg. **35-B**:363, 1953.)

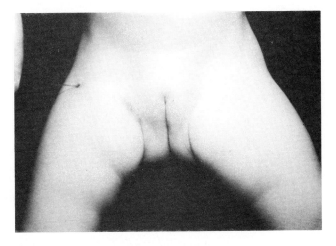

Fig. 62-11. Insertion of 22-gauge spinal needle one fingerbreadth lateral to femoral artery and immediately inferior to anterosuperior iliac spine for arthrography.

common cause of failure is extravasation of the contrast medium. This usually occurs because the needle is not in the hip joint or because when it is in, the bevel of the needle may be so long that a part of the contrast medium leaks outside the capsule. In addition, when too much of the medium is used, some of it may be forced into the soft tissue through the hole made by the needle. But when image intensifier television fluoroscopy is used for localizing the needle, when a needle with a short bevel is used, and when a small volume of contrast medium is injected, these complications can usually be avoided.

The findings of the clinical examination and of arthrography at the time of attempted closed reduction determine if the hip will be stable or may require open reduction.

Clinical findings that usually result in an acceptable closed reduction include the sensation of a ''clunk'' as the femoral head reduces in the true acetabulum. The ''safe zone'' concept of Ramsey, Lasser, and MacEwen can be used in determining the zone of abduction and adduction in which the femoral head remains reduced in the acetabulum. A wide safe zone is preferred and a narrow safe zone implies a possibly unstable or unacceptable closed reduction.

Arthrography permits analysis of the cartilaginous anlage of the femoral head and acetabulum. Factors that help determine the success or failure of closed reduction include the amount of dye pooling in the medial joint space, inversion of the acetabular limbus, or an ''hourglass'' constriction obstructing reduction.

TECHNIQUE. With the patient under general anesthesia, place him supine. Then perform sterile preparation and draping of the hip or hips. With a gloved fingertip locate the hip joint immediately inferior to the middle of the inguinal ligament and one fingerbreadth lateral to the pulsating femoral artery, (Fig. 62-11). With the assistance of image intensification insert a 22-gauge needle, to which is attached a 5 ml syringe filled with normal saline solution, until it enters the hip joint; resistance will be met as the needle passes through the joint capsule. Then inject the

saline solution into the joint; this is easy at first but becomes more difficult as the joint becomes distended. Release the plunger of the syringe; if the joint has been successfully entered, the saline solution that is under pressure in it will reverse the plunger and fluid will escape into the syringe. Then aspirate the saline solution from the joint and remove the syringe from the needle. Next fill the syringe with 5 ml of a 25% strength Hypaque solution and inject 3.5 to 5 ml through the needle into the joint. Then rapidly withdraw the needle, and while the hip is still unreduced, have an arthrogram made. Before developing it gently reduce the hip into a stable position and have a second arthrogram made. Enough dye will remain in the hip during manipulation for the second arthrogram to be

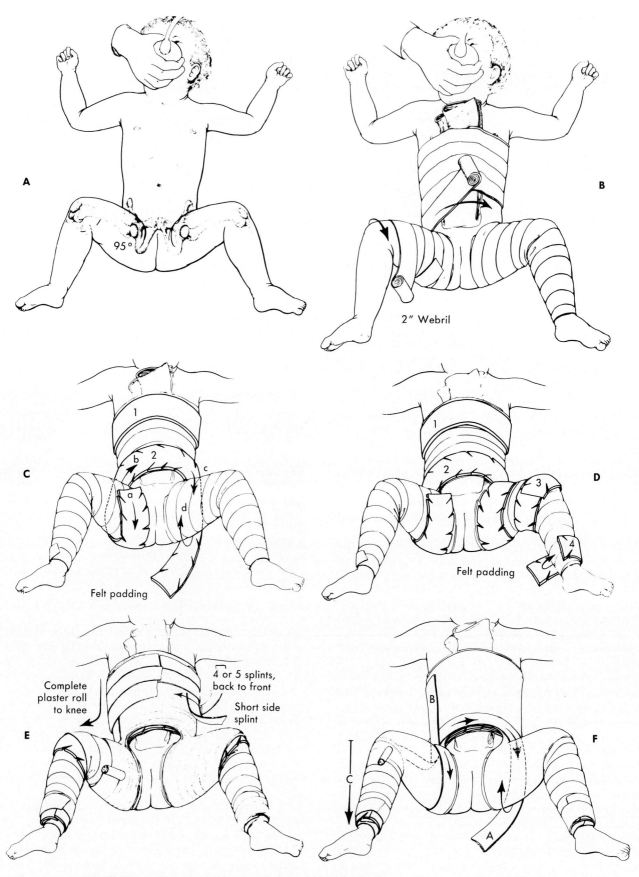

Fig. 62-12. Technique of application of spica cast for congenital dislocation of hip. Note positioning of patient in "human" position. (From Kumar, S.J.: J. Ped. Orthop. **1:**97, 1981.)

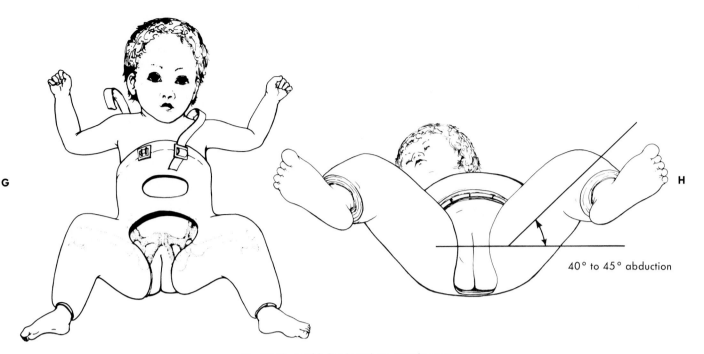

G

H

40° to 45° abduction

Fig. 62-12, cont'd. For legend see opposite page.

satisfactory. Maintain reduction until both arthrograms have been developed and studied.

When arthrograms are to be made of both hips, insert a needle into each, being sure that both are within the joints before either joint is injected. Then inject both hips as described here and make arthrograms of both on the same cassette.

APPLICATION OF HIP SPICA

After confirmation of a stable reduction, a hip spica cast is applied. The desired position of the hip joint is 95 degrees of flexion and 40 to 45 degrees of abduction. Studies have indicated that the "human position" is best for maintaining hip stability and minimizing the risk of avascular necrosis. Kumar has described an easily reproducible and simple technique for applying a hip spica cast.

TECHNIQUE (KUMAR). Anesthetize the child and place him on the spica frame. Abduct the hip to 40 to 45 degrees and flex it to about 95 degrees (Fig. 62-12, *A*). Excessive abduction should be avoided, since it may hamper the circulation to the femoral head. The amount of hip flexion and abduction required to keep the hip in the most stable position should be determined clinically and checked by roentgenograms.

After the hip is reduced and the correct position of flexion and abduction for stability is determined, place a small towel in front of the abdomen. Then roll 2-inch (5 cm) Webril from the level of the nipples down to the ankles (Fig. 62-12, *B*). Pad around the bony points with 2 inch (5 cm) standard felt. Apply the first pad over the proximal end of the spica, near the nipple line (Fig. 62-12, *C*). Start a second piece of the same sized felt at the level of the right groin and carry it posteriorly across the gluteal fold, over the right iliac crest, in front of the abdomen, over the

lateral aspect of the left thigh, and then to the left inguinal area (Fig. 62-12, *C*). Apply a third piece of felt over the knee (Fig. 62-12, *D*) and a fourth piece above the ankle over the distal leg (Fig. 62-12, *D*). Place similar pieces of felt over the opposite knee and leg.

Apply the plaster in two sections: a proximal section from the nipple line to the knees and a distal section from the knees to the ankles. Apply a single layer of 4-inch (10 cm) plaster roll from the nipple line to the level of the knees on both sides. Apply four or five plaster splints back to front from the nipple line to the back of the sacrum to reinforce the back of the cast. At the same time apply a short, thick splint over the anterolateral aspect of the inguinal area (Fig. 62-12, *E*). Apply another splint: starting from the right inguinal area, carry it posteriorly across the gluteal region, the iliac crest, the front of the abdomen, and back the same way on the opposite thigh (Fig. 62-12, *E*). This is a reinforcing splint that attaches the thigh to the upper segment. Apply another long splint from the level of the knee across the anterolateral aspect of the inguinal area and up the chest wall (Fig. 62-12, *F*). This splint is one of the main anchors of the thigh to the body segment. Follow this by a roll of 4-inch (10 cm) plaster from the nipple line to the knees. This completes the proximal section of the spica.

Then complete the cast from the knees down to the ankles. Do this by applying on both sides a single roll of 3-inch (7.5 cm) plaster from the knee to the ankle level, and reinforce this by two splints over the medial and lateral aspects of the thigh, knee, and leg. Follow this by another roll of 3 inch (7.5 cm) plaster. Then apply shoulder straps to prevent pistoning of the child in the cast (Fig. 62-12, *G*).

Since the cast is reinforced laterally around the hips, a wide segment can be removed from the front of the hips

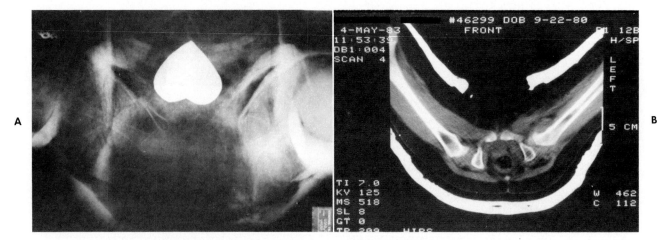

Fig. 62-13. A, Anteroposterior roentgenogram of pelvis obtained with patient in spica cast following closed reduction. Note difficulty in assessing position of femoral head. **B,** Computed tomography scan of pelvis to document reduction of femoral head into true acetabulum.

without weakening the cast. This permits better roentgenograms of the hips (Fig. 62-12, *G*).

The final view of the spica from inferiorly should appear as shown in Fig. 62-12, *H*, with about 40 to 45 degrees of abduction. The amount of abduction is determined by the position of hip stability. Once again it is emphasized that excessive abduction should be avoided since it may damage the circulation of the femoral head.

AFTERTREATMENT. Spica cast immobilization is continued for 4 months. The cast is changed with the patient under general anesthesia at 2 months. Roentgenograms or arthrograms are mandatory to be sure that the femoral head is reduced anatomically into the acetabulum (Fig. 62-13). Clinical and roentgenographic follow-up is essential until the hip is considered normal.

OPEN REDUCTION

In a child under 18 months of age in whom efforts to reduce a dislocation without force have failed, open reduction is indicated to remove the offending soft tissue structures and to reduce the femoral head concentrically in the acetabulum. An anterior approach using a transverse "bikini" skin incision and careful iliofemoral dissection, as described by Somerville, may be used. Sequential technical steps must be performed: psoas tenotomy, complete capsulotomy medially including the transverse acetabular ligament, excision of the hypertrophied ligamentum teres, and reduction of femoral head into the true acetabulum. As much of the labrum as possible should be preserved.

TECHNIQUE (SOMERVILLE). This operation should be preceded by closed reduction in which the head is placed as concentrically as possible within the acetabulum; operation is then indicated only if concentric reduction is impossible.

Place a sandbag beneath the affected hip. Make a straight skin incision, beginning anteriorly inferior and medial to the anterosuperior spine and coursing obliquely superiorly and posteriorly to the middle of the iliac crest (Fig. 62-14, *A*). Deepen the incision to expose the crest.

Then reflect the abductor muscles subperiosteally from the iliac wing distally to the capsule of the joint. Increase exposure of the capsule by separating the tensor fasciae latae from the sartorius for about 2.5 cm inferior to the anterosuperior spine. Next expose the reflected head of the rectus femoris and separate it from the acetabulum and capsule, leaving the straight head attached to the anteroinferior spine (Fig. 62-14, *B*). The straight head may be detached to increase exposure. Near the acetabular rim make a small incision in the capsule and extend it anteriorly to a point deep to the rectus and posteriorly to the posterosuperior margin of the joint (Fig. 62-14, *C*). Exert enough traction on the limb to distract the cartilage of the femoral head from that of the acetabulum about 0.7 cm. Examine the inside of the acetabulum visually (Fig. 62-14, *D*). If no inverted limbus is seen, insert a blunt hook and palpate the joint for the free edge of an inverted limbus. If one is found, place the tip of the hook deep to the limbus and force it through its base; then separate from its periphery that part of the limbus lying anterior to the hook until the hook comes out (Fig. 62-14, *E*). Then with Kocher forceps grasp the limbus by the end thus freed and excise it with strong curved scissors, or make radial T-shaped incisions to evert the limbs and allow reduction of the femoral head. Reduce the head into the acetabulum by abducting the thigh 30 degrees and internally rotating it. Hold the joint in this position and close the capsule. Reattach the muscles to the iliac crest, close the skin, and apply a spica cast.

AFTERTREATMENT. A spica cast is worn for 8 weeks. Subsequently the patient is allowed free movement in bed (Fig. 62-15)

• • •

An alternative to anterior open reduction is open reduction through the medial approach (Ludloff) popularized by Ferguson. It is especially useful when closed reduction can be achieved only in an extreme nonphysiologic position. This approach allows direct access to the psoas tendon and the constricted anteromedial capsule with less major dis-

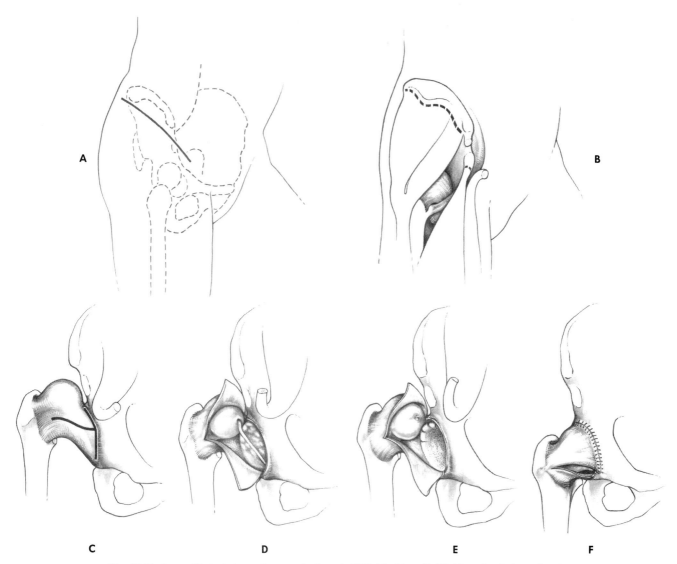

Fig. 62-14. Somerville technique of open reduction. **A,** Bikini incision. **B,** Division of sartorius and rectus femoris tendons and iliac epiphysis. **C,** T-shaped incision of capsule. **D,** Capsulotomy of hip and use of ligamentum teres to find true acetabulum. **E,** Radial incisions in acetabular labrum and removal of all tissue from depth of true acetabulum. **F,** Capsulorrhaphy after excision of redundant capsule.

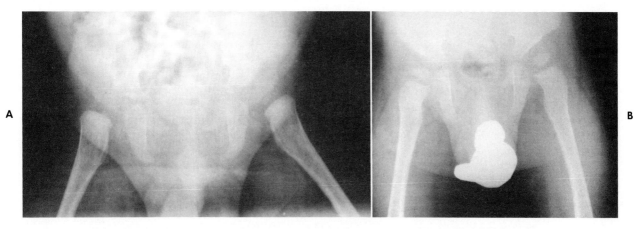

Fig. 62-15. A, Bilateral congenital dislocation of hip in 8-month-old boy immediately before surgery. **B,** At age 19 months following bilateral open reduction through anterior iliofemoral approach. Note residual acetabular dysplasia.

section. It is, however, a technically difficult procedure requiring meticulous dissection to avoid injury to the medial femoral circumflex artery. Various authors have reported avascular necrosis of the femoral head following this approach ranging from 10% to 15%. We have included it here for completeness.

TECHNIQUE BY MEDIAL APPROACH (FERGUSON). Preliminary traction in an infant younger than 2 years old is not necessary. Place the patient supine with the affected hip abducted and flexed 90 degrees. Make a straight incision along the posterior margin of the adductor longus beginning at its origin and extending distally. Incise the deep fascia in line with the skin incision and by blunt dissection with the finger separate the adductor longus anteriorly from the adductor magnus and gracilis posteriorly (Fig. 62-16, *A*). Extend the dissection posterior to the adductor brevis and palpate the lesser trochanter. Next push the pericapsular fat medially so that the psoas tendon can be seen (Fig. 62-16, *B*). With a curved hemostat isolate this tendon and divide it transversely. As the tendon retracts superiorly

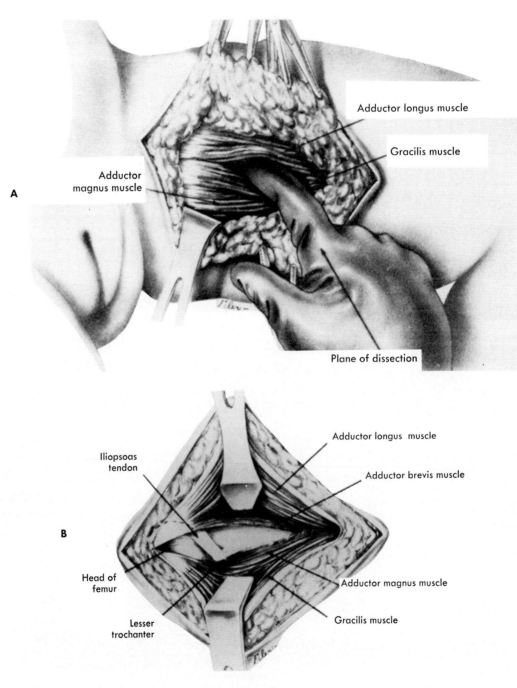

Fig. 62-16. Ferguson open reduction of congenital dislocation of hip through medial approach. **A,** Adductor longus anteriorly is separated from adductor magnus and gracilis posteriorly. **B,** Psoas tendon is exposed by dissecting posterior to adductor brevis. (From Ferguson, A.B., Jr.: J. Bone Joint Surg. **55-A:**671, 1973.)

push the fat from the anterior capsule of the hip joint. This exposes an hourglass constriction of the capsule that has been formed by the taut psoas tendon. Now pass a retractor over the capsule superior to the femoral head. Incise the capsule in line with the femoral neck and extend the incision anteriorly as far as necessary to permit the femoral head to enter the acetabulum with ease. After the dislocation has been reduced, the capsular incision spreads and cannot be closed. Suturing the adductors is unnecessary. Close the skin in a routine manner.

AFTERTREATMENT. A spica cast is applied with both hips in 10 degrees of flexion, 30 degrees of abduction, and 10 to 20 degrees of internal rotation. The cast is molded posterior to the affected hip to press anteriorly on the greater trochanter, thus preventing redislocation. A spica cast with the hips in this position is worn for at least 4 months after surgery.

TODDLER (18 TO 36 MONTHS OF AGE)

Because of widespread screening of newborns, it is becoming uncommon for congenital dislocation of the hip to be undetected beyond the age of 1 year. The older child with this condition presents with a wide perineum, shortened lower extremity, and hyperlordosis of the lower spine secondary to femoropelvic instability. For these children with well-established hip dysplasia, open reduction with femoral or pelvic osteotomy or both is often required. Persistent dysplasia can be corrected by a redirectional proximal femoral osteotomy, such as the MacEwen and Shands osteotomy, Wagner's blade plate technique, or the lag screw technique of Lloyd-Roberts et al. If the primary dysplasia is acetabular, pelvic redirectional osteotomy alone, such as the Salter innominate osteotomy, is more appropriate. However, these patients will require both femoral and pelvic osteotomies if significant deformity is present on both sides of the joint.

FEMORAL OSTEOTOMY IN DYSPLASIA OF HIP

Many surgeons recommend that dysplasia of the hip after conservative treatment or no treatment be treated first by femoral osteotomy to correct either anteversion or valgus deformity of the femoral neck. Some believe that the operation should correct the valgus deformity alone and consequently that only a varus osteotomy is indicated. Others, however, believe that correction of anteversion alone is desirable. Still others believe that both the valgus deformity and anteversion should be corrected simultaneously by one osteotomy at the subtrochanteric level. Most surgeons who recommend femoral osteotomies advise an operation on the pelvic side of the joint only after the femoral head has been concentrically seated in the dysplastic acetabulum by such an osteotomy, the joint has failed to develop satisfactorily, and the growth potential of the acetabulum no longer exists. Opinions differ widely as to the age at which the acetabulum loses its ability to develop satisfactorily over a femoral head concentrically located; Kasser, Bowen, and MacEwen reported consistently good results in patients less than 4 years old at the time of femoral osteotomy. Remodeling of the acetabulum occurred through the age of 8 years, but 4 of 13 hips in patients between the ages of 4 and 8 showed persistent dysplasia despite the operation. The results were less predictable as the patients approached the age of 8 years. No benefit was derived from femoral osteotomy alone in 10 of 11 hips in patients older than 8 years of age.

The degree of anteversion was once impossible to measure precisely, although efforts had been made to obtain this information in several ways. In 1953, however, Dunlap et al. and Ryder and Crane independently reported extensive studies on the measurement of true anteversion. They devised methods that have proved accurate. Dunlap et al. have shown that at birth the femoral neck is normally anteverted about 30 degrees and that anteversion decreases progressively until at maturity it averages about 10 degrees (Fig. 62-17). In 1956 Magilligan described a technique for measuring true anteversion that does not require a special apparatus and uses the anteroposterior and lateral roentgenographic views of Laage et al. and a graph.

TECHNIQUE FOR MEASURING ANTEVERSION (MAGILLIGAN). Place the patient supine on either a fracture table or a roentgenographic table with the femur held parallel to it and in neutral rotation and comfortable abduction; maintain the hip in this position throughout the examination. First make an anteroposterior roentgenogram; from this determine the

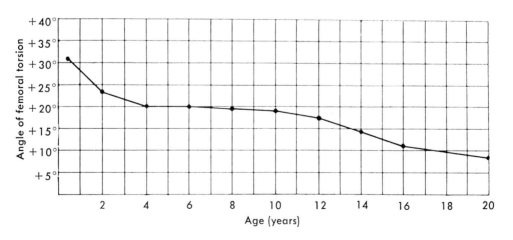

Fig. 62-17. Graph showing amount of femoral anteversion according to age. (From Dunlap, K., et al.: J. Bone Joint Surg. **35-A**:289, 1953.)

cervicofemoral angle designated α (Fig. 62-18, *A*). Next make a lateral roentgenogram with the tube between the thighs and aimed directly at the hip joint; place the cassette against the lateral side of the trunk, absolutely vertical and parallel to the long axis of the femoral neck (Fig. 62-18, *B*). From this roentgenogram determine the angle of anteversion designated β (Fig. 62-18, *C*). Now with the graph of Magilligan that uses the trigonometric function of the α angles and β angles (Fig. 62-18, *D*), determine the true

angle of anteversion designated β′. The true anteversion, angle β′, always equals or exceeds angle β.

We have recently used computerized tomography to determine femoral anteversion. A scan through the femoral neck and femoral condyles gives an exact measurement of true femoral anteversion.

From a practical standpoint clinically, if anteversion is severe enough to cause the hip to be subluxated or dislocated when the thigh is in the neutral position or in slight

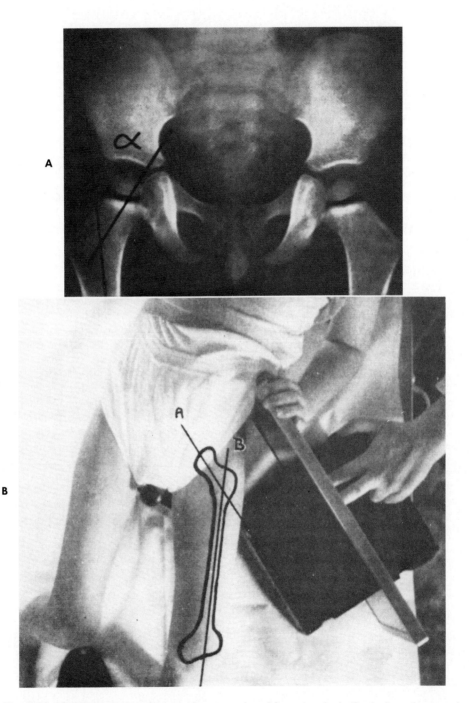

Fig. 62-18. Magilligan technique for measuring anteversion of femoral neck. **A,** Cervicofemoral or α angle is measured as shown. **B,** Lateral roentgenogram is made with cassette vertical and parallel to long axis of femoral neck.

external rotation, it should be corrected surgically. Whether it is this severe should be determined at the time of closed or open reduction, and if it is, rotational osteotomy of the femur should be performed after an appropriate period of immobilization, usually 4 to 8 weeks.

Rotational osteotomy of the femur may be made in either the subtrochanteric or the supracondylar region, and

several methods are available by which the fragments can be controlled after it. The level of the osteotomy and the method of controlling the fragments are a matter of choice. The trochanteric or subtrochanteric level is used much more frequently than the supracondylar. Regardless of the type of internal fixation used, the fragments must be controlled after surgery. Usually immobilization in a spica

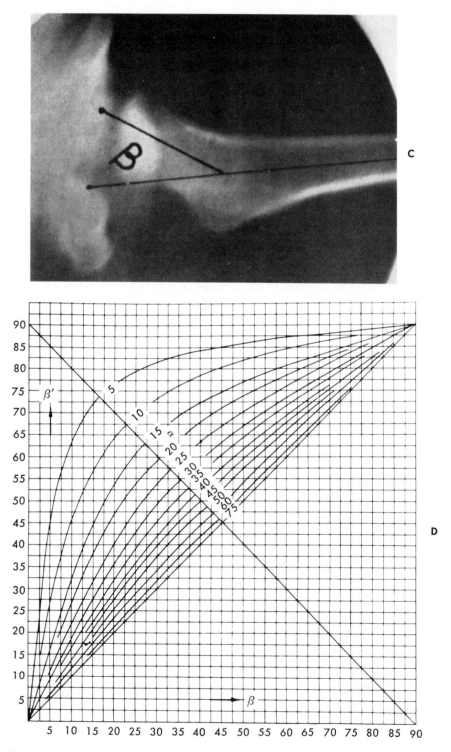

Fig. 62-18, cont'd. C, Angle of anteversion or β angle is measured as shown. **D,** From graph true angle of anteversion or β′ is determined. (From Magilligan, D.J.: J. Bone Joint Surg. **38-A:**1231, 1956.)

cast is necessary until union is solid. We always make a subtrochanteric osteotomy and fix the fragments internally with either plates and screws or some type of lag screw–plate fixation. Both anteversion and varus deformity of the femoral neck are usually corrected at the same time.

DISTAL FEMORAL DEROTATIONAL OSTEOTOMY

TECHNIQUE (CREGO). After the patient has been anesthetized and the cast has been removed, have an assistant hold the affected limb in internal rotation while the patient is prepared and draped for surgery. Then with the limb in this position drill a threaded Kirschner wire transversely through the femur 7.5 cm proximal to the distal femoral epiphysis and parallel with the floor. Apply a traction bow to the wire. Next make a lateral longitudinal incision 5 cm long just distal to the wire and through it make a transverse supracondylar osteotomy. Then while the proximal fragment remains internally rotated, externally rotate the distal fragment until the knee, ankle, and foot are aligned with the anterosuperior iliac spine. With the distal fragment in this corrected position apply a single spica cast that incorporates the wire and traction bow.

AFTERTREATMENT. At 2 months the cast and Kirschner wire are removed, and the patient is allowed to use the

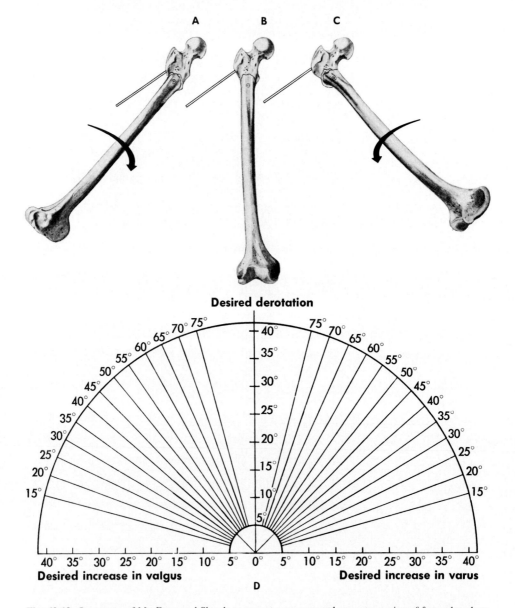

Fig. 62-19. Osteotomy of MacEwen and Shands to correct coxa vara and any retroversion of femoral neck or coxa valga and any anteversion of femoral neck. Osteotomy has been made from anterosuperior to posterinferior. **A,** Abduction of distal fragment produces internal rotation of this fragment and increase in angle of neck with shaft. **B,** Position before adduction or abduction of distal fragment. **C,** Adduction of distal fragment produces external rotation of this fragment and decrease in angle of neck with shaft. **D,** Graph of d'Aubigne and Vaillant used to determine angle of osteotomy as related to long axis of femur. Desired degree of change in angle of neck with shaft is plotted along ordinate; desired degree of change in retroversion or anteversion of neck is plotted on abscissa. Intersection of these lines determines angle of proposed osteotomy.

limb as soon as tolerated. Motion in the hip is usually satisfactory by 8 to 12 weeks.

PROXIMAL FEMORAL VARUS DEROTATIONAL OSTEOTOMY

TECHNIQUE (MACEWEN AND SHANDS). Before surgery determine the angle of the osteotomy necessary to correct the valgus deformity and any anteversion of the femoral neck. Use the graph of d'Aubigne and Vaillant to determine the angle (Fig. 62-19). The desired number of degrees of change in the angle between the shaft and neck is plotted along the ordinate, and the desired number of degrees of change in rotation is plotted on the abscissa. The point of intersection of these two values determines the plane of the osteotomy in relation to the long axis of the femur. As already mentioned we have recently used computed tomography as a more exact technique for determination of femoral anteversion (Fig. 62-20).

Expose the trochanteric region and proximal shaft of the femur through a lateral longitudinal approach (p. 57). Then rotate the limb so that the neck of the femur is in the frontal plane. Next to control the position of the proximal fragment insert a heavy Steinmann pin through the greater trochanter into the neck. Drill several holes along the line of the proposed osteotomy that extends from anterosuper-

ior to posteroinferior and complete the osteotomy with an osteotome or electric saw. Then adduct the distal fragment while maintaining the osseous surfaces in contact, thus correcting both angulation and rotation. Finally insert a screw across the osteotomy and check the position of the fragments by roentgenograms. Apply a one and one-half spica cast incorporating the Steinmann pin.

Lloyd-Roberts et al. have recommended a trochanteric osteotomy controlled by a lag screw and plate (the Coventry or Campbell apparatus).

TECHNIQUE (LLOYD-ROBERTS ET AL.). Place the patient supine on the operating table, elevate the affected hip with a small sandbag beneath the buttock, and drape the extremity free. Make a lateral approach to the proximal shaft and trochanteric region of the femur (p. 57) 10 or 12 cm long. With the hip fully rotated internally, drill a 3 mm hole through the lateral cortex just distal to the greater trochanter and insert a guide pin into the femoral neck, parallel with its long axis in both planes. Be sure the guide pin is small enough in diameter for the screw and tapper (barrel) to fit over it. Take care that the guide pin does not cross the capital femoral epiphyseal plate; its end should be just distal to it. Next confirm the placement of the pin by anteroposterior and lateral roentgenograms or image intensifica-

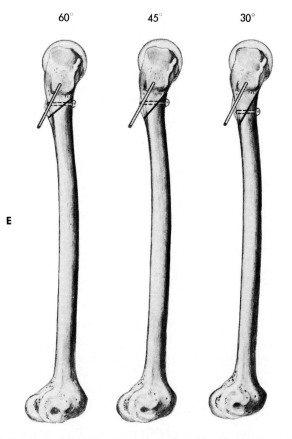

Fig. 62-19, cont'd. E, Lateral view of femur showing various obliquities of osteotomy that result in varying amounts of rotation of distal fragment for set number of degrees of change in angle of neck with shaft. Osteotomy made at 60 degrees to long axis of shaft produces more rotation, whereas osteotomy made at 30 degrees produces less rotation. (Modified from MacEwen, G.D., and Shands, A.R., Jr.: J. Bone Joint Surg. **49-A:**345, 1967.)

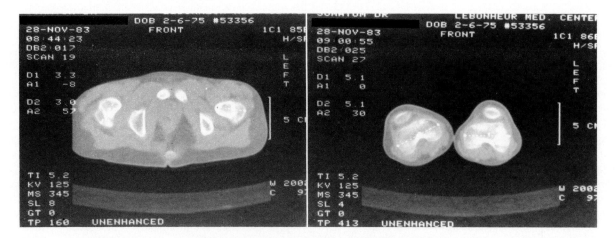

Fig. 62-20. Computed tomography for assessment of femoral anteversion. Note scan of right and left hips to determine anatomic angles through femoral necks and intertrochanteric regions as well as transverse plane of femoral condyles.

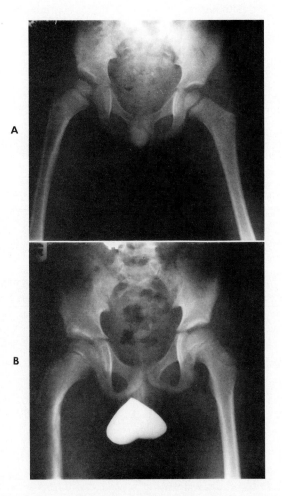

Fig. 62-21. A, Three-year-old boy with right hip dysplasia before varus derotational osteotomy. **B,** At age 9 years after removal of Campbell screws.

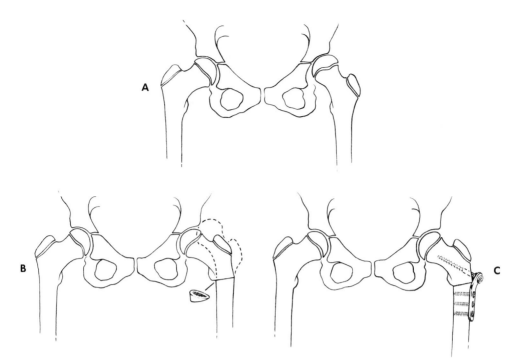

Fig. 62-22. A, Persistent valgus and subluxation of left hip. **B,** Centralization of femoral head in acetabulum following medial wedge closing osteotomy in subtrochanteric region. **C,** Fixation with Campbell device.

tion. When placement of the pin is satisfactory, advance the tapper over the pin. Next remove the tapper and with the lag screw inserter insert the appropriate screw. Now confirm the position of the screw by anteroposterior and lateral roentgenograms or image intensification. Next bend the side plate to the desired angle and place its proximal hole over the screw. Place the self-retaining nut loosely on the screw over the plate. Now rotate the plate out of the way and perform the desired osteotomy in the trochanteric area (Fig. 62-22). Take care that the osteotomy is not too far distally; otherwise the proximal hole in the plate will be too near the osteotomy. After the distal fragment has been appropriately rotated or adducted or both, position the side plate on the femoral shaft. Hold it against the shaft just distal to the osteotomy with clamps. Now catch the lag screw with a wrench so that it does not rotate and tighten the self-locking nut. Finally fix the plate to the distal fragment with screws. Close the wound and apply a spica cast.

AFTERTREATMENT. When roentgenograms show solid union of the osteotomy, usually at 6 to 12 weeks, the cast is removed and the hip is mobilized by exercises. When the limb can be controlled, graduated weight bearing on crutches is allowed.

PELVIC OSTEOTOMY

Operations on the pelvis, either alone or combined with open reduction, are useful in congenital dysplasia or dislocation of the hip to ensure or to increase stability of the joint. Those most often used are (1) osteotomy of the innominate bone, (2) acetabuloplasty, (3) osteotomies that free the acetabulum (triple or double innominate osteotomy or dial acetabular osteotomy), (4) shelf operation, and (5) innominate osteotomy with medial displacement of the acetabulum. In an older child one of these operations may be combined with femoral osteotomy to correct valgus deformity or anteversion of the femoral neck or to shorten the femur to allow reduction of the dislocation without undue pressure on the femoral head.

Osteotomy of the innominate bone, an operation devised by Salter, is useful only when any subluxation or dislocation has been reduced or can be reduced by open reduction at the time of osteotomy in a child 18 months of age or older. In it the entire acetabulum together with the pubis and ischium is rotated as a unit, the symphysis pubis acting as a hinge. The osteotomy is held open anterolaterally by a wedge of bone, and thus the roof of the acetabulum is shifted more anteriorly and laterally.

Acetabuloplasty is also useful only when any subluxation or dislocation has been reduced or can be reduced by open reduction at the time of operation in children at least 1 year old. In it the inclination of the acetabular roof is decreased by an osteotomy of the ilium made superior to the acetabulum. In the earlier acetabuloplasties the osteotomy is made through the lateral cortex only, and a medially based flap of bone consisting of the acetabular roof is turned distally. But in the one devised by Pemberton and called *pericapsular osteotomy of the ilium* the osteotomy is made through the full thickness of the bone from just superior to the anteroinferior iliac spine anteriorly to the triradiate cartilage posteriorly; the triradiate cartilage acts as a hinge on which the acetabular roof is rotated anteriorly and laterally. Acetabuloplasty, as is noted later, includes several procedures that have been called shelf operations.

Osteotomies that free the acetabulum have been devised by Steel, Sutherland and Greenfield, and Eppright. These operations free part of the pelvis, creating a movable segment of bone that includes the acetabulum. They are indicated in older children with residual dysplasia and subluxation in whom remodeling of the acetabulum can no longer be anticipated. They are useful because they place articular cartilage over the femoral head. On the other hand, the shelf operations, and the operation of Chiari, interpose capsular fibrous tissue between the femoral head and the reconstructed acetabulum. In the triple innominate osteotomy (Steel), the ischium, the superior pubic ramus, and the ilium superior to the acetabulum are all divided, and the acetabulum is repositioned and is stabilized by a bone graft and metal pins. In the double innominate osteotomy

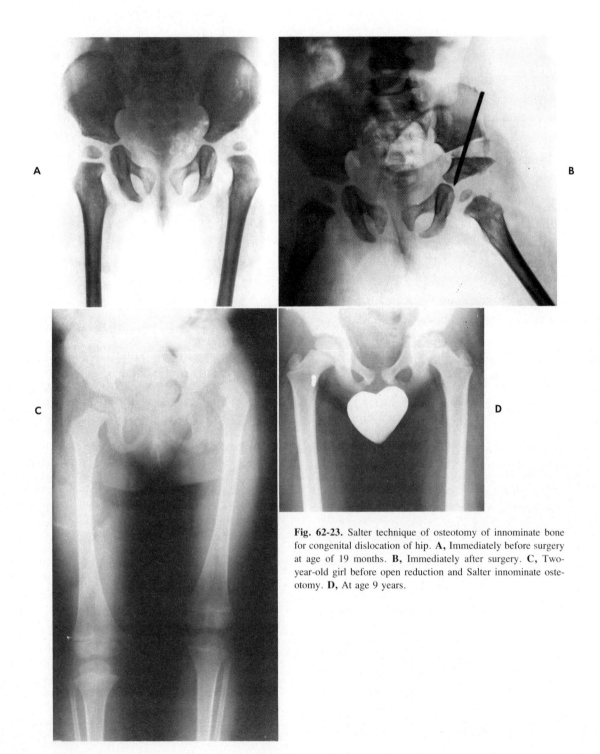

Fig. 62-23. Salter technique of osteotomy of innominate bone for congenital dislocation of hip. **A,** Immediately before surgery at age of 19 months. **B,** Immediately after surgery. **C,** Two-year-old girl before open reduction and Salter innominate osteotomy. **D,** At age 9 years.

(Sutherland and Greenfield), the ilium is osteotomized superior to the acetabulum, the pubic rami are osteotomized just lateral to the symphysis pubis, and the acetabulum is repositioned and stabilized by a bone graft and Kirschner wires. In the dial osteotomy of the acetabulum (Eppright), the entire acetabulum superiorly, posteriorly, inferiorly, and anteriorly is freed by osteotomy and as a single segment of bone is redirected to appropriately cover the femoral head.

A *shelf operation* is useful for subluxations, dislocations that have been reduced but that have later become subluxations. In a classical shelf operation the acetabular roof is extended laterally, posteriorly, or anteriorly, either by a graft or by turning distally over the femoral head the acetabular roof and part of the lateral cortex of the ilium superior to it.

Innominate osteotomy with medial displacement of the acetabulum, an operation devised by Chiari for patients over 4 years old, is a modified shelf operation that places the femoral head beneath a surface of bone and joint capsule and corrects the pathologic lateral displacement of the femur. An osteotomy is made at the level of the acetabulum, and the femur and the acetabulum are displaced medially. The inferior surface of the proximal fragment forms a roof over the femoral head.

The operations devised by Salter and by Pemberton have resulted in many mechanically efficient hip joints in which severe osteoarthritis is unlikely to develop later. In patients in whom we have properly performed Salter's osteotomy of the innominate bone, the results have been pleasing (Fig. 62-23). As in any operation errors in technique can occur. Pemberton's pericapsular osteotomy is technically more difficult to perform but is equally as satisfactory. Each operation has its indications and advantages.

OSTEOTOMY OF INNOMINATE BONE

During open reduction of congenital dislocations of the hip, Salter observed that the entire acetabulum faces more anterolaterally than it should. Thus when the hip is extended, the femoral head is insufficiently covered anteriorly, and when it is adducted, there is insufficient cover superiorly. His osteotomy of the innominate bone redirects the entire acetabulum so that its roof covers the head both anteriorly and superiorly. Any dislocation or subluxation must have been reduced completely before this operation is performed, or if not, then open reduction is carried out at the time of osteotomy. During the operation any contractures of the adductor or iliopsoas muscles are released by tenotomy, and in dislocations when the capsule is elongated, a capsulorrhaphy is carried out. Salter recommends his osteotomy in the primary treatment of congenital dislocation of the hip between the ages of 18 months and 6 years and of congenital subluxation as late as early adulthood. He also recommends it in the secondary treatment of any residual or recurrent dislocation or subluxation after other methods of treatment within the age limits described.

The following prerequisites are necessary for this operation to be successful:

1. The femoral head must be pulled inferiorly to the level of the acetabulum. This may require a period of traction before surgery.

2. Any contractures of the iliopsoas and adductor muscles must be released. This is indicated in subluxations as well as dislocations.
3. The femoral head must be reduced into the depth of the true acetabulum completely and concentrically. This may require careful open reduction and excision of any debris, exclusive of the labrum, from the acetabulum.
4. The joint must be reasonably congruous so that degenerative arthritis of the hip joint is unlikely.
5. The range of motion of the hip must be good, especially in abduction, internal rotation, and flexion.
6. The age of the patient must be between 18 months and 6 years.

In the absence of any of these prerequisites the operation as described by Salter is contraindicated.

Preliminary skeletal traction is indicated in almost all children 18 months old or older to bring the femoral head inferiorly to the level of the acetabulum. Skin traction with adhesive tape in a child younger than 3 years old may be sufficient, but in older children skeletal traction is usually required.

TECHNIQUE, INCLUDING OPEN REDUCTION (SALTER). Have whole blood available and start an intravenous infusion. Place the patient supine on the operating table with the thorax on the affected side elevated by a sandbag. Drape the trunk on the affected side to the midline anteriorly and posteriorly and to the lower rib cage superiorly. Drape the lower extremity so that it can be moved freely during the operation. Now release the adductor muscles by subcutaneous tenotomy. Then make a skin incision beginning just inferior to the middle of the iliac crest, extending anteriorly to just inferior to the anterosuperior iliac spine, and continuing to about the middle of the inguinal ligament (Fig. 62-24). Decrease bleeding by applying pressure with sponges to the wound edges. Bluntly dissect between the tensor fasciae latae laterally and the sartorius and rectus femoris medially and expose the anterosuperior iliac spine. Next dissect the rectus femoris from the underlying joint capsule and release its reflected head. Make a deep inci-

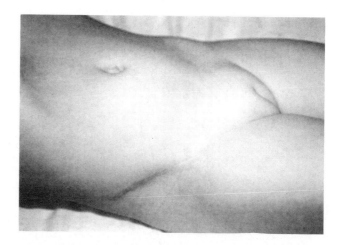

Fig. 62-24. Healed incision following Salter osteotomy. Note position of incision immediately inferior to curve of iliac spine and extending along inguinal ligament into anterior thigh.

sion that splits the iliac epiphysis along the crest from the posterior end of the skin incision posteriorly to the anterosuperior iliac spine anteriorly and then turns distally to the anteroinferior iliac spine.

Reflect the lateral part of the iliac epiphysis and the periosteum from the lateral surface of the iliac wing in a continuous sheet inferiorly to the superior edge of the acetabulum and posteriorly to the greater sciatic notch. Free any adhesions of the joint capsule from the lateral surface of the ilium and from any false acetabulum. Expose the capsule anteriorly and laterally by dissecting bluntly the interval between it and the abductor muscles.

Now pack the dissected spaces with large sponges to control bleeding and to increase the interval between the reflected periosteum and the sciatic notch. If concentric reduction of the femoral head into the acetabulum is impossible, open the capsule superiorly and anteriorly, parallel with and about 1 cm distal to the rim of the acetabulum.

Excise the ligamentum teres only if it is hypertrophied.

Now gently reduce the femoral head into the acetabulum. Never excise the limbus. Now incise the distal flap of capsule at right angles to the first incision, thus creating a T-shaped incision, and resect the inferolateral triangular flap so created. Now test the stability of the joint; if the head becomes displaced superiorly from the acetabulum when the hip is adducted or anteriorly when it is extended or externally rotated, then osteotomy of the innominate bone is indicated.

Next allow the hip to redislocate. Then strip the medial half of the iliac epiphysis from the anterior half of the iliac crest and the periosteum from the medial surface of the ilium posteriorly and inferiorly to expose the entire medial aspect of the bone to the sciatic notch. Pack the surfaces thus exposed with sponges, again to control the loss of blood and to enlarge the interval between the periosteum and the bone. Next expose the tendinous part of the iliopsoas muscle at the level of the pelvic brim. With scissors separate the tendinous part from the muscular part and divide the former while protecting the muscle beneath it.

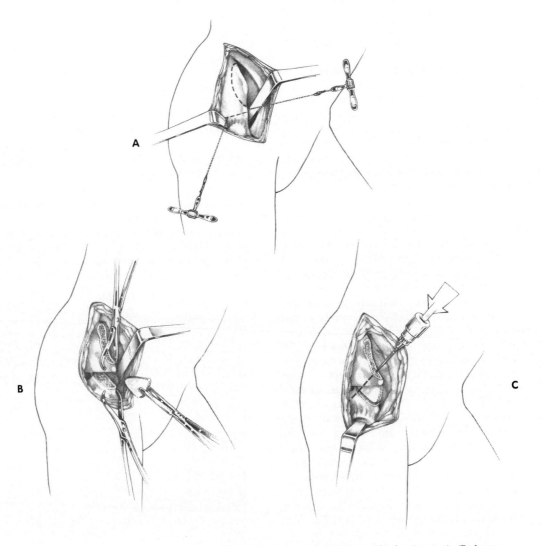

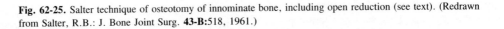

Fig. 62-25. Salter technique of osteotomy of innominate bone, including open reduction (see text). (Redrawn from Salter, R.B.: J. Bone Joint Surg. **43-B:**518, 1961.)

Then pass a curved forceps subperiosteally medial to the ilium into the sciatic notch and with it grasp one end of a Gigli saw.

Retract the tissues medially and laterally from the ilium and divide the bone with the saw in a straight line from the sciatic notch to the anteroinferior spine. Now remove a full-thickness graft from the anterior part of the iliac crest (Fig. 62-25, *A*) and trim it to the shape of a wedge. Make the base of the wedge about as wide as the distance between the anterosuperior and anteroinferior iliac spines. With towel clips grasp each fragment of the osteotomized ilium. Next insert a curved elevator into the sciatic notch and by levering it anteriorly and by exerting traction on the towel clip that grasps the inferior fragment, shift this fragment anteriorly, inferiorly, and laterally to open the ostoetomy anterolaterally. Be sure that the osteotomy remains closed posteriorly (Fig. 62-25, *B*).

Do not apply traction in a cephalad direction on the proximal fragment because this may dislocate the sacroiliac joint. Now insert the bone graft into the osteotomy and release the traction on the inferior fragment. Drill a strong Kirschner wire through the remaining superior part of the ilium, through the graft, and into the inferior fragment (Fig. 62-25, *C*). Be sure that the Kirschner wire does not enter the acetabulum but that it does traverse all three fragments. Now drill a second Kirschner wire parallel with the first, using the same precautions. Next reduce the femoral head again into the acetabulum and reevaluate its stability. Reduction should now be stable with the hip either in adduction or in slight external rotation. While closing the wound have an assistant hold the knee flexed and the hip slightly abducted, flexed, and internally rotated. Next obliterate any residual pocket of capsule by performing a capsulorrhaphy.

Move the distal half of the lateral flap of capsule medially beyond the anteroinferior iliac spine. This brings the capsular edges together and increases the stability of reduction by keeping the hip internally rotated. Now repair the capsule with interrupted sutures. Suture together over the iliac crest the two halves of the iliac epiphysis. Cut the Kirschner wires so that their anterior ends lie within the subcutaneous fat. Now close the skin with a continuous subcuticular suture. With the hip held in the same position as during closure, apply a single spica cast.

AFTERTREATMENT. At 6 weeks the spica cast is removed, and with general or local anesthesia the Kirschner wires are also removed. The position of the osteotomy and of the hip is checked by roentgenograms. Bilateral long leg casts are then applied and are held in abduction and internal rotation by two bars. These casts will allow flexion and extension of the hips. After 4 weeks the casts are removed, and walking with crutches is started under the supervision of a physical therapist or nurse. The crutches are discontinued when the ostoetomy is secure and when muscle power has been regained. Rotational osteotomy of the femur has not been found necessary.

ERRORS IN OPERATIVE TECHNIQUE. As in any operation, not all surgeons are as successful in its use as the one who devised it. Therefore Salter has listed the errors made in performing the osteotomy and associated procedures as re-

lated to him by other surgeons. In addition to errors in judgment in selecting patients and mistakes in management before surgery, the following errors in operative technique have been made:

1. Failure to perform a subcutaneous adductor tenotomy to release an adduction contracture
2. Insufficient operative exposure
3. Failure to obtain a concentric reduction of the femoral head within the true acetabulum
4. Mistaking the false acetabulum for the true acetabulum
5. Failure to release the iliopsoas tendon
6. Failure to perform an adequate capsulorrhaphy
7. Insufficient exposure of the sciatic notch
8. Failure to stay within the periosteum
9. Failure to use the Gigli saw for making the osteotomy, using instead an osteotome or power saw
10. Using a mechanical spreader to open the osteotomy
11. Allowing the osteotomy to remain open posteriorly
12. Displacement of the distal fragment of the osteotomy posteriorly and medially
13. Failure to rotate the distal fragment
14. The use of small Kirschner wires for fixation and insufficient penetration of the wires into the distal fragment.
15. Allowing the Kirschner wires to enter the hip joint
16. Insertion of the Kirschner wires from inferiorly to superiorly
17. Performing a bilateral innominate osteotomy during a single operative session

CHILD (3 TO 8 YEARS OF AGE)

The management of untreated congenital dislocation of the hip in the child over 3 years of age is quite difficult. By this age adaptive shortening of the periarticular structures and structural alterations in both the femoral head and the acetabulum have occurred. Most dislocated hips in this age group require open reduction. Preoperative skeletal traction should not be used. Schoenecker and Strecker reported a 54% incidence of avascular necrosis and a 31% incidence of redislocation after the use of skeletal traction in patients older than 3 years. Open reduction combined with femoral shortening resulted in no avascular necrosis and only an 8% incidence of redislocation. Coleman reported an 8% incidence of avascular necrosis in his series of femoral shortening. Although femoral shortening aids in the reduction and decreases the potential for complications, it is technically difficult (Fig. 62-26).

OPEN REDUCTION AND FEMORAL SHORTENING

Klisić and Jankovic have devised an operation in which open reduction and femoral shortening are combined with operations on the acetabulum as indicated. The operation is used for both unilateral and bilateral dislocations. In younger children open reduction and femoral shortening are combined with either a Salter osteotomy of the innominate bone (p. 2733) or a Pemberton acetabuloplasty (p. 2738).

TECHNIQUE (KLISIĆ AND JANKOVIC). Place the patient supine on the operating table. Begin a curved incision at the an-

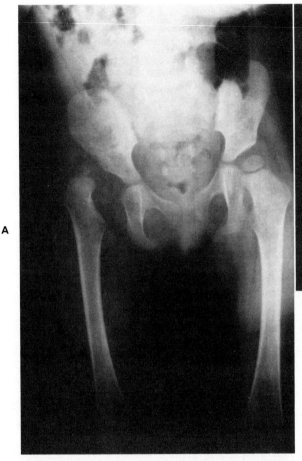

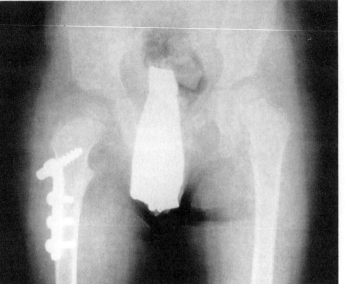

Fig. 62-26. A, Three-year-old girl before primary open reduction, femoral shortening, and Salter innominate osteotomy. **B,** One year after surgery.

terosuperior iliac spine, carry it toward the greater trochanter, and then curve it distally along the femoral shaft for about 12 cm. Two incisions may be used, one anterior and one lateral. Incise the fascia lata in line with the skin incision. Now mobilize the anterior fascial flap and reflect it anteriorly. Incise the posterior fascial flap transversely for about 2 cm. Now dissect the vastus lateralis from the lateral surface of the femur and reflect it anteriorly. Next incise the periosteum along the lateral surface of the femoral shaft proximally to the base of the trochanter and carry the incision anteriorly and posteriorly over the trochanter. Strip the periosteum from the entire circumference of the femoral shaft. With an oscillating saw osteotomize the femur at the level of the distal border of the lesser trochanter (Fig. 62-27, *A*).

Next determine the distance between the superior surface of the femoral head and the roof of the true acetabulum by measuring this on an anteroposterior roentgenogram made before surgery. Now using this measurement shorten the femur appropriately by making another osteotomy distal to the first and removing a segment of bone. Grasp the proximal fragment firmly and abduct it. Now starting at the lesser trochanter incise the periosteum along the medial border of the femur. Identify the trochanteric insertion of the iliopsoas tendon, tag it with a heavy nonabsorbable suture, and free it from its insertion. Dissect the iliopsoas from the fat on the inferior part of the joint capsule and pull it anteriorly (Fig. 62-27, *B*).

Next dissect medially from the inferior joint capsule the pericapsular fatty tissue containing a branch of the medial femoral circumflex artery. Incise the capsule along its inferior surface parallel to the femoral neck. At the medial end of this incision divide the transverse acetabular ligament. Retract the capsular flaps and excise the ligamentum teres. At this point place the femoral head in the acetabulum. Next dissect between the tensor fasciae latae and the gluteal muscles and expose the superior aspect of the joint capsule proximally to the point where it begins to be reflected inferiorly. Free the adherent part of the capsule from the iliac wing down to its insertion on the true acetabulum. This opens the capsule over the false acetabulum. Now incise the periosteum of the ilium just proximal to the true acetabulum, strip it from the entire circumference of the bone, and retract it by means of two grooved elevators that cross in the greater sciatic notch. The pelvic osteotomy, generally a Salter or Pemberton, is performed as described on pp. 2733 and 2738.

Now drill two holes through both cortices of the proximal femoral fragment 5 cm proximal to the ostoetomy, and pass the ends of the suture tagging the iliopsoas tendon through these holes from medially to laterally. Reduce the femoral head into the acetabulum (Fig. 62-27, *C*) and reat-

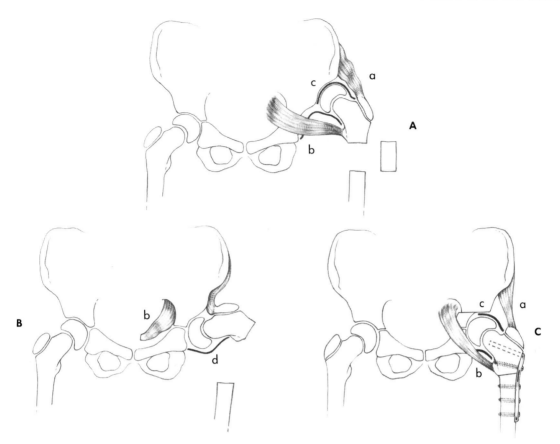

Fig. 62-27. Klisić technique of open reduction of dislocation, femoral shortening, and Chiari innominate osteotomy. **A,** Femoral head is dislocated. Gluteal muscles, *a,* are wrinkled and shortened. Iliposas muscle, *b,* is intact. Capsule, *c,* is interposed between femoral head and ilium. Segment of femur is resected. **B,** Proximal femur is abducted. Iliopsoas tendon, *b,* is divided. Capsule, *d,* is incised on inferior surface parallel to femoral neck. **C,** Operation is complete. Gluteal muscles, *a,* are tight. Iliopsoas muscle, *b,* is reattached. Superior capsule, *c,* is interposed between femoral head and superior surface of iliac osteotomy. Femoral fragments are fixed with plate and screws.

tach the iliopsoas muscle to the femur by tying the tagging suture. Next with the femoral head properly oriented in the frontal plane clamp the two femoral fragments together with the distal one so rotated that the supracondylar axis of the femur lies in the frontal plane parallel to the femoral neck and the angle between the femoral shaft and neck is adjusted to 115 to 120 degrees. Check the position of the fragments by palpation and roentgenograms. Now fix the femoral fragments together by a plate and four screws. Suture the periosteum over the plate if possible. Now reattach the vastus lateralis in its original position and close the wound in layers. Apply a double spica cast with the affected limb in abduction and neutral rotation.

AFTERTREATMENT. After the osteotomy has healed, at about 2 months, the cast is removed and physical therapy is begun. Exercises are continued, but weight bearing is not allowed until at least 4 months. With unilateral dislocation discrepancy in leg lengths is observed.

ACETABULOPLASTY

The term ''acetabuloplasty'' designates operations that redirect the inclination of the acetabular roof by an oste-

otomy of the ilium superior to the acetabulum followed by levering of the roof inferiorly.

Pemberton has devised an acetabuloplasty that he calls pericapsular osteotomy of the ilium in which an osteotomy is made through the full thickness of the ilium, using the triradiate cartilage as the hinge about which the acetabular roof is rotated anteriorly and laterally. After a review of 115 hips in 91 patients followed for at least 2 years after surgery, he recommends it for any dysplastic hip in patients between the age of 1 year and the age when the triradiate cartilage becomes too inflexible to serve as a hinge (about 12 years of age in girls and 14 in boys), provided that any subluxation or dislocation has been reduced or can be reduced at the time of osteotomy (Fig. 62-28). When the hip is not dislocated, he recommends it if, when the thigh is extended and rotated externally, the femoral head can be felt to thrust anterior to the anterior acetabular rim and if on roentgenograms the acetabular index has not improved during a period of 6 months while the femoral head has been held in the acetabulum by abduction. Furthermore, he recommends it when the femoral head is obviously too big to be covered by the acetabulum. In his

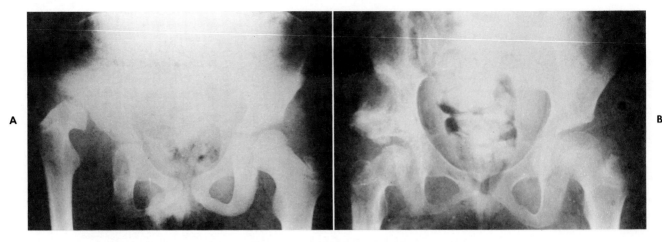

Fig. 62-28. A, Pelvis and hips of 10-year-old child. **B,** At age 12 following open reduction, primary femoral shortening, and Pemberton osteotomy.

experience anteversion of the femoral neck is not a threat to continued stability after surgery.

After a recent review of his operation Pemberton recommends that the capsule be opened routinely. In high dislocations he recommends traction before surgery to prevent coxa plana; however, to avoid excessive softening of the bone it should be used for no more than 3 weeks. He also recommends that when the femoral head cannot be pulled easily to the level of the acetabulum, the iliopsoas tendon should be divided. In addition any significant anteversion of the femoral neck should not be corrected by derotational osteotomy until after the pericapsular osteotomy has been performed.

Coleman in a review of pericapsular and innominate osteotomies noted that one advantage of the former operation is the lack of need for internal fixation and thus a second but minor operation is avoided. Furthermore, a greater degree of correction can be achieved with less rotation of the acetabulum in the pericapsular osteotomy because the fulcrum, the triradiate cartilage, is nearer the site of desired correction. According to him, however, Pemberton's operation is technically more difficult to perform. In addition it alters the configuration and capacity of the acetabulum and may result in an incongrous relationship between it and the femoral head; consequently some remodeling of the acetabulum may be required. On the other hand, in the innominate osteotomy since its shape is not changed, remodeling of the acetabulum is unnecessary.

TECHNIQUE (PEMBERTON). Place the patient supine with a small sandbag beneath the affected hip and expose the hip joint through an anterior iliofemoral approach (p. 59). Make the superior part of the incision distal to and parallel with the iliac crest and extend it from the anterosuperior spine anteriorly to the middle of the crest posteriorly. Extend the distal part of the incision from the anterosuperior spine inferiorly for 10 to 12 cm parallel with the anterior border of the tensor fasciae latae. Beginning at the crest, strip the glutei and the tensor fasciae latae subperiosteally from the anterior third of the ilium distally to the joint capsule and posteriorly until the greater sciatic notch is

exposed. Now with a sharp elevator separate the iliac epiphysis with its attached abdominal muscles from the anterior third of the iliac crest. Then strip the muscles subperiosteally from the medial aspect of the ilium until the sciatic notch is again exposed. At this point open the capsule of the hip and remove any soft tissue that restricts reduction. Reduce the hip under direct vision and be sure that it is well seated; then redislocate it until the osteotomy has been made and propped open with a graft.

Now insert two flat retractors subperiosteally into the sciatic notch, one along the medial surface of the ilium and one along the lateral to keep the anterior third of the ilium exposed both medially and laterally. With a narrow curved osteotome cut through the lateral cortex of the ilium as follows. First start slightly superior to the anteroinferior iliac spine and curve the osteotomy posteriorly about 1 cm proximal to and parallel with the joint capsule until the osteotome is seen to be well anterior to the retractor resting in the sciatic notch.

From this point when driven farther, the blade of the osteotome disappears from sight, and it is therefore important to direct its tip sufficiently inferiorly so that it does not enter the sciatic notch but instead enters the ilioschial rim of the triradiate cartilage at its midpoint. After directing the osteotome properly, drive it 1.5 cm farther to complete the osteotomy of the lateral cortex of the ilium. With the same osteotome make a corresponding cut in the medial cortex of the ilium, starting anteriorly at the same point just superior to the anteroinferior iliac spine. Direct this cut posteriorly parallel with that in the lateral cortex until it reaches the triradiate cartilage (Fig. 62-29, *A*).

The direction in which the acetabular roof becomes displaced after the osteotomy is controlled by varying the position of the posterior part of the osteotomy of the medial cortex. The more anterior this part of the osteotomy the less the acetabular roof rotates anteriorly; conversely, the more posterior this part of the osteotomy the more the acetabular roof rotates anteriorly. After completing the osteotomy of the two cortices, insert a wide curved osteotome into the anterior part of the osteotomy and lever the distal

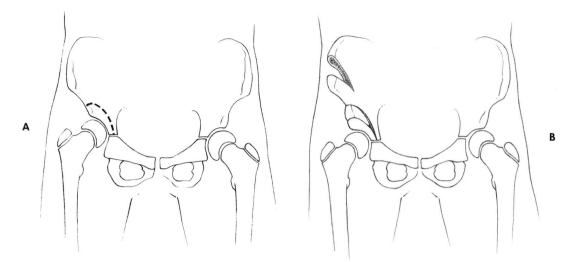

Fig. 62-29. Pemberton pericapsular osteotomy of ilium. **A,** Line of osteotomy beginning slightly superior to anterosuperior iliac spine and curving into triradiate cartilage. **B,** Completed osteotomy with acetabular roof in corrected position and wedge of bone impacted into open osteotomy site.

fragment distally until the anterior edges of the two fragments are at least 2.5 to 3 cm apart.

The acetabular roof should be turned inferiorly far enough to result in an estimated acetabular index of 0 degrees. Next cut a narrow groove in the anteroposterior direction in each raw surface of the ilium. Resect a wedge of bone from the anterior part of the iliac wing, including the anterosuperior spine. Then with a laminectomy spreader separate the fragments and place the wedge of bone in the grooves made in the surfaces of the ilium; drive the wedge into place and impact it firmly (Fig. 62-29, *B*). The acetabular roof should then remain fixed in the corrected position. If the hip has remained dislocated during the osteotomy, reduce it at this time. Close the capsule, overlapping if possible any edges so that it will be fairly snug and will hold the head within the acetabulum. Suture the iliac epiphysis over the remaining ilium and close the wound.

AFTERTREATMENT. With the hip in neutral position (or in slight abduction and internal rotation if this has been found the most favorable position for closure of the wound), a spica cast is applied from the nipple line to the toes on the affected side and to above the knee on the opposite side. At 2 months the cast is removed, and the osteotomy is checked by roentgenograms. If it has united solidly, walking is allowed. No further protection or treatment is needed. Within a month after the cast is discarded, the patient should be able to walk fairly well.

• • •

The Pemberton pericapsular osteotomy is limited by the mobility of the triradiate cartilage, and by hinging on this cartilage may cause premature epiphyseal closure. Though the Salter innominate osteotomy may be used in older patients, its results depend on the mobility of the symphysis pubis and the amount of femoral head coverage is limited. Other, more complex osteotomies, such as those of Steel, Sutherland and Greenfield, and Eppright, can provide

more correction and improve femoral head coverage. These reconstructive procedures are technically difficult and should be performed only by an experienced hip surgeon.

In the *triple innominate osteotomy* developed by Steel, the ischium, the superior pubic ramus, and the ilium superior to the acetabulum are all divided, and the acetabulum is repositioned and is stabilized by a bone graft and metal pins. Its goal is to establish a stable hip in anatomic position for dislocation or subluxation of the hip in older children when this is impossible by any one of the other osteotomies (Salter's, Pemberton's, or Chiari's). For the operation to be successful the articular surfaces of the joint must be congruous or become so once the acetabulum has been redirected so that a functional, painless range of motion will be achieved and a Trendelenburg gait will be absent. Steel has reviewed 45 patients in whom 52 of his operations had been performed. The results were satisfactory in 40 hips and unsatisfactory in 12. The unsatisfactory hips were painful and easily fatigued; in two the Trendelenburg test was positive, and in one significant motion had been lost.

Before surgery skeletal traction must be used until the femoral head is brought distally to the level of the acetabulum; if necessary any contracted muscles about the hip are released surgically.

TECHNIQUE (STEEL). Place the patient supine on the operating table and flex the hip and knee 90 degrees. Keep the hip in neutral abduction, adduction, and rotation. First drape the posterior aspect of the proximal thigh and the buttock, leaving the ischial tuberosity exposed. Make a transverse incision perpendicular to the long axis of the femoral shaft 1 cm proximal to the gluteal crease. Retract the gluteus maximus laterally and expose the hamstring muscles at their ischial origin. By sharp dissection free the biceps femoris, the most superficial muscle in the area, from the ischium and expose the interval between the semimembranosus and the semitendinosus. The sciatic nerve lies far enough laterally not be endangered. Now pass a curved hemostat in the interval between the origins of the semimembranosus and the semitendinosus deep to the ischium and into the obturator foramen. Elevate the origins of the obturator internus and externus and bring the tip of the hemostat out at the inferior margin of the ischial ramus. Be sure the hemostat remains in contact with the bone during its passage deep to the ramus. Now with an osteotome directed posterolaterally and 45 degrees from the perpendicular divide the ischial ramus completely. Allow the origin of the biceps femoris to fall into place. Next suture the gluteus maximus to the deep fascia and close the skin.

Change gowns, gloves, and instruments and begin in the iliopubic area the second stage of operation. Carry out a full skin preparation medially to the midline and superiorly to the costal margin and drape the extremity free. Through an anterior iliofemoral approach (p. 59) reflect the iliac and gluteal muscles from the wing of the ilium. Detach the sartorius and the lateral attachments of the inguinal ligament from the anterosuperior iliac spine and reflect them medially. Now reflect the iliacus and psoas muscles subperiosteally from the inner surface of the pelvis; this protects the femoral neurovascular bundle. Next divide the tendinous part of the origin of the iliopsoas and expose the pectineal tubercle. Detach the pectineus muscle superiosteally from the superior pubic ramus and expose the bone 1 cm medial to the pubic tubercle. Pass a curved hemostat superior to the superior pubic ramus into the obturator foramen near the bone. With it penetrate the obturator fascia so that its tip is brought out inferior to the ramus. If the bone is especially thick, pass a second hemostat inferior to the ramus and direct it superiorly to contact the first one.

Now direct an osteotome posteromedially and 15 degrees from the perpendicular and osteotomize the pubic ramus.

The obturator artery, vein, and nerve are protected by the hemostat. Now using the technique as described by Salter for innominate osteotomy (p. 2753), divide the ilium with a Gigli saw. When this osteotomy has been completed, free the periosteum and fascia from the medial wall of the pelvis to free the acetabular segment (Fig. 62-30, *A*). If the femoral head is subluxated or dislocated, open the capsule at this time and remove any tissue obstructing reduction. Reduce the femoral head as near as possible to the center of the triradiate cartilage and close the capsule.

Next with a towel clip grasp the anteroinferior iliac spine and rotate the acetabular segment in the desired direction, usually anteriorly and laterally, until the femoral head is covered. In an older child use a laminectomy spreader to open the osteotomy because the sacroiliac joint is usually more stable in this age group and is not likely to be damaged. With the acetabular fragment in proper position, stabilize it with a triangular bone graft removed from the superior rim of the ilium. Transfix the graft with two pins that penetrate the inner wall of the ilium (Fig. 62-30, *B*). Now allow the pectineus and iliopsoas to fall into place. Reattach the sartorius and the lateral end of the inguinal ligament to the anterosuperior iliac spine and close the wound in layers.

AFTERTREATMENT. A spica cast is applied with the hip in 20 degrees of abduction, 5 degrees of flexion, and neutral rotation. At 8 to 10 weeks the cast and pins are removed, and active and passive motion of the hip is started. All three osteotomies will probably unite by 12 weeks after surgery. At 12 to 14 weeks, when the ostoetomies have

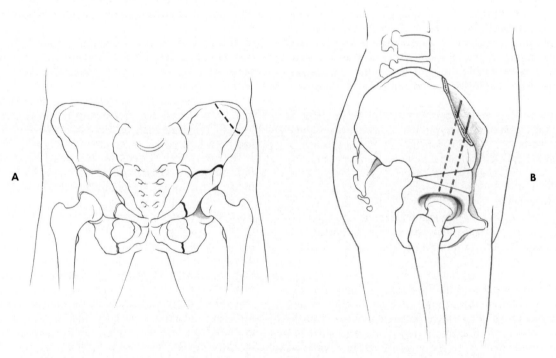

Fig. 62-30. Steel triple innominate osteotomy. **A,** Osteotomies to be performed in iliac wing and superior and inferior pubic rami. Note wedge of bone to be taken as graft from most superior portion of iliac. **B,** Lateral view showing graft in place and fixation with two Kirschner wires.

united, weight bearing on crutches is started. By 6 months the patient should be walking independently (Fig. 62-31).

• • •

In the *double innominate osteotomy* described by Sutherland and Greenfield the ilium is divided superior to the acetabulum, the pubic rami are divided just lateral to the symphysis pubis, and the acetabulum is repositioned and is stabilized by a bone graft and Kirschner wires. More rotation of the acetabulm and consequently more coverage of the femoral head can be achieved by this operation than by a single innominate osteotomy. Furthermore, the removal of a section of bone from the pubis allows more medial displacement of the hip. The operation is recommended for children 6 years of age and older and for adolescents and young adults. It is indicated in a subluxated or dislocated hip that is reducible and is free from severe degenerative changes in which the range of motion is good. It may be combined with other operations such as osteotomy of the femur.

TECHNIQUE (SUTHERLAND AND GREENFIELD). Have the patient's bladder emptied or insert a catheter before surgery. Place the patient supine with the affected hip elevated by a folded towel or sandbag placed beneath the buttock. First perform an osteotomy of the innominate bone as described by Salter (p. 2733). Next make a transverse incision in the suprapubic area through the skin and fat down to the periosteum of the symphysis pubis. On the affected side retract laterally the spermatic cord in the male or the round ligament in the female. Next release the rectus abdominis and pyramidalis muscles from the superior border of the symphysis. Free the tendon of the adductor longus from the anterior surface of the pubis. Now insert a hypodermic needle in the symphysis and make a roentgenogram to localize accurately the site for osteotomy. Then elevate the periosteum from the pubis and protect the soft tissues by passing Chandler retractors anteriorly and posteriorly around the bone. Take care during the periosteal dissection to avoid damaging the internal pudendal artery along the medial margin of the inferior pubic ramus. Also be careful when stripping the periosteum at the inferior margin of the symphysis pubis to avoid damaging the deep dorsal vein, artery, or nerve of the penis, for they pierce the urogenital diaphragm near the arcuate ligament of the pubis in the midline. Now with a small rongeur resect a wedge of bone 7 to 13 mm wide just lateral to the symphysis pubis and parallel to it (Fig. 62-32, *A*).

As the inferior aspect of the pubis is reached, elevate with a towel clip the lateral pubic segment and carefully free the inferior part of the periosteum and the urogenital diaphragm. Now complete the osteotomy with a rongeur and curet. Next with the towel clip displace the lateral segment medially, posteriorly, and superiorly (Fig. 62-32, *B*). At the site of the Salter osteotomy displace the acetabular fragment distally and anteriorly and insert a triangular graft (Fig. 62-32, *D*). Traction on the acetabular segment must be distal, not lateral.

In contrast to the standard Salter procedure, a medial projection of the distal innominate fragment is to be expected because the segment of bone at the pubis has been removed. Obtain optimum rotation by simultaneously displacing the acetabular fragment at both osteomies as described. Transfix the pubic osteotomy with one or two medium-sized threaded Steinmann pins. Next transfix the iliac osteotomy and the graft with two heavy threaded Kirschner wires passed through the proximal fragment of the ilium across the graft and into the distal fragment (Fig. 62-32, *B* and *D*). Insert suction drainage tubes and close the wound. Apply a spica cast.

AFTERTREATMENT. At 24 to 48 hours the drainage tubes are removed. At 6 weeks in children the spica cast and the pins are removed; at 8 weeks with adults the cast is removed, but the pins are left in place until the osteotomies have united.

• • •

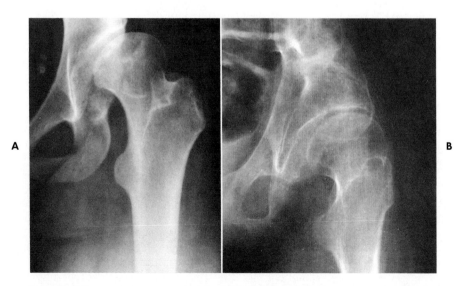

Fig. 62-31. A, Primary acetabular dysplasia in a 16-year-old girl before Steel osteotomy. **B,** One year postoperatively. (Courtesy Dr. H. Steel and Dr. R. Betz.)

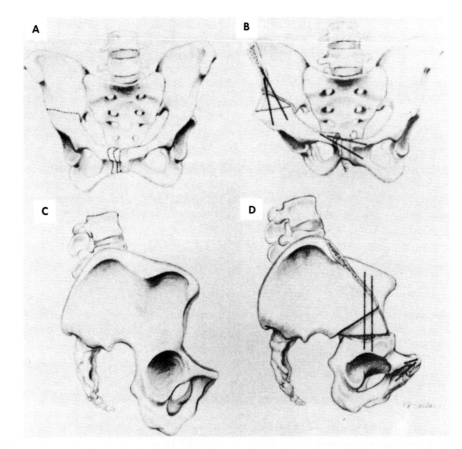

Fig. 62-32. Sutherland and Greenfield double innominate osteotomy. **A,** Lines of osteotomies. **B** and **D,** Osteotomies are made, bone graft is inserted, and Steinmann pins and Kirschner wires are used for fixation (see text). **C,** Lateral view of pelvis before osteotomies. (From Sutherland, D.H., and Greenfield, R.: J. Bone Joint Surg. **59-A:**1082, 1977.)

In the *dial osteotomy* of the acetabulum, developed by Eppright, the entire acetabulum superiorly, posteriorly, inferiorly, and anteriorly is freed by osteotomy and as a single segment of bone is redirected to appropriately cover the femoral head. It was devised to treat residual dysplasia in older children or young adults in whom the hip is painful, is easily fatigued, and feels unstable and in whom the Trendelenburg test is positive. It is indicated only in a truly dysplastic hip in which the head is concentrically located but the CE angle of Wiberg is less than 15 to 20 degrees (Fig. 62-33). In addition, the thickness of the cartilaginous surfaces should be almost normal, and motion in the hip should be normal except for some limitation of external rotation. Eppright reported the use of this operation in 11 patients. There were no sciatic nerve palsies or other serious complications.

TECHNIQUE (EPPRIGHT). Place the patient supine on the operating table over a roentgenographic cassette holder to allow roentgenograms to be made in the anteroposterior direction if needed during surgery or use an image intensifier. Drape the lower limb so that it can be moved freely during the operation. Now expose the hip through an anterior iliofemoral incision (p. 59), modifying it slightly by extending it farther distally. Now divide prox-

imally the lateral femoral cutaneous nerve and separate the sartorius muscle from the tensor fasciae latae. Reflect the muscles from the lateral aspect of the iliac crest subperiosteally. Next reflect the iliac epiphysis, if present, medially from the anterior half of the iliac crest and strip the periosteum from the medial wall of the ilium. Divide the tendon of the rectus femoris at the anteroinferior iliac spine and reflect it medially and distally. Expose the capsule of the hip joint adjacent to the acetabulum over as much of its circumference as possible.

Now with a curved periosteal elevator carefully remove the periosteum from the posterior aspect of the ilium and the acetabulum down to the ischium. The sciatic nerve commonly lies near the ilium posteriorly. Consequently strip the periosteum posteriorly, and when indicated during the operation, place a finger posterior to the acetabulum to protect the nerve. Now flex the hip slightly and remove the iliopsoas tendon and muscle from the lesser trochanter. This allows additional medial retraction so that the iliopubic eminence can be exposed medially and inferiorly. To prevent injuring the femoral nerve and artery keep the knee and hip flexed 20 degrees or more while retracting the iliopsoas. Next incise the capsule of the hip joint in line with the femoral neck. Retract the capsule superiorly and

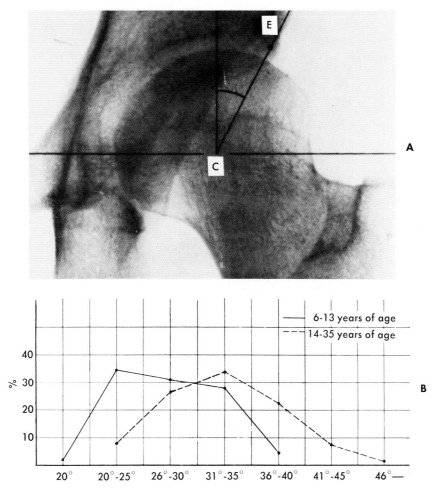

Fig. 62-33. CE angle of Wiberg. **A,** Angle is formed between line through center of head, *C,* parallel with longitudinal axis of body and another through center of head, *C,* extending to lateral margin of acetabulum, *E.* **B,** Relative frequency of different CE angles in two age groups obtained from measurements in 400 hips. (From Severin, E.: Acta Chir. Scand. Suppl. 63, 1941.)

inferiorly, locate precisely the acetabular margins, and determine the condition of the cartilage on the femoral head.

With a 1.3 cm osteotome outline the osteotomy anteriorly (Fig. 62-34, *A*). Start it at the anteroinferior iliac spine, extend it medially and inferiorly as close as possible to the iliopectineal line, and then curve it inferiorly and laterally. Ideally take 1 cm of bone with the acetabular cartilage to avoid a fracture into the articular surface. Now continue the osteotomy straight posteriorly until it approaches the posterior surface of the ilium. Place a finger posterior to the acetabulum to protect the sciatic nerve and continue the osteotomy through the posterior cortex of the ilium until the point of the osteotome can be felt. Now dissect inferior to the capsule of the hip. Retract the obturator externus posteriorly and inferiorly and extend the osteotomy through the posterior aspect of the ischium. After the osteotomy has been completed, place gentle traction on the leg to allow the acetabular fragment to be dialed to the desired position over the femoral head. If the anterior part of the acetabulum is deficient, take a bone graft from the

exposed ilium and wedge it in anteriorly, thus tilting the entire acetabulum posteriorly. Now abduct the hip and release the traction; the acetabulum should now be held in place by the tension of the soft structures. However, if better fixation is needed, transfix the fragment with a Steinmann pin.

Now hold the hip in slight abduction through the rest of the procedure. Close the capsule and attach the iliopsoas tendon to the periosteum on the medial side of the proximal femur. Reattach the tendon of the rectus femoris proximal to the osteotomy on the anteroinferior iliac spine and replace the iliac epiphysis. Close the subcutaneous tissues with interrupted absorbable sutures and the skin with a continuous subcuticular suture. With the hip in slight abduction, 10 degrees of flexion, and neutral rotation, apply a spica cast to the toes on the affected side and to above the knee on the opposite side.

AFTERTREATMENT. At 6 weeks the spica cast is removed, and roentgenograms are made. Active motion of the hip and knee is encouraged. As soon as the patient has active control of the limb and passive flexion of the hip allows

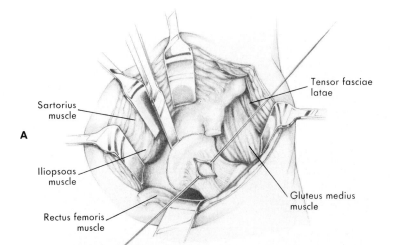

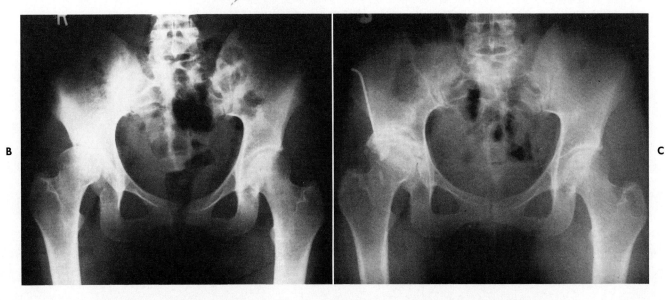

Fig. 62-34. Eppright dial osteotomy. **A,** Line of osteotomy for rotation of acetabular fragment. **B,** Roentgenogram of 16-year-old female before Dial osteotomy. **C,** Postoperative roentgenogram. (**B** and **C** courtesy Dr. R.H. Eppright.)

him to sit, crutch walking with partial weight bearing is started. Full weight bearing is not permitted until active abduction of the hip can be carried out against gravity; this is usually at 4 to 6 weeks after the cast has been removed.

SHELF OPERATIONS

Shelf procedures have commonly been performed by enlarging the volume of the acetabulum; however, pelvic redirectional and displacement osteotomies have largely replaced this operation. The redirectional osteotomies are inappropriate in hips in which the femoral head and acetabulum are misshapen but still congruent because redirection may cause incongruity. Staheli has described a slotted acetabular augmentation procedure to create a congruous acetabular extension in which the size and position of the augmentation can be easily controlled. A deficient acetab-

ulum that cannot be corrected by redirectional pelvic osteotomy is the primary indication for this operation. Contraindications include dysplastic hips with spherical congruity suitable for redirectional osteotomy, hips requiring concurrent open reduction that must have supplementary stability, and patients unsuited for spica cast immobilization.

TECHNIQUE (STAHELI). Preoperatively, the CE angle of Wiberg is determined from anteroposterior standing pelvic roentgenograms and a normal CE angle (about 35 degrees) is drawn on the film. The additional width necessary to extend the existing acetabulum to achieve the normal angle is measured (Fig. 62-35). This determines the width of the augmentation; this measurement added to the depth of the slot gives the total graft length. If the patient is small or easily moved, the procedure is performed on a standard operating table with the affected side elevated 15 degrees

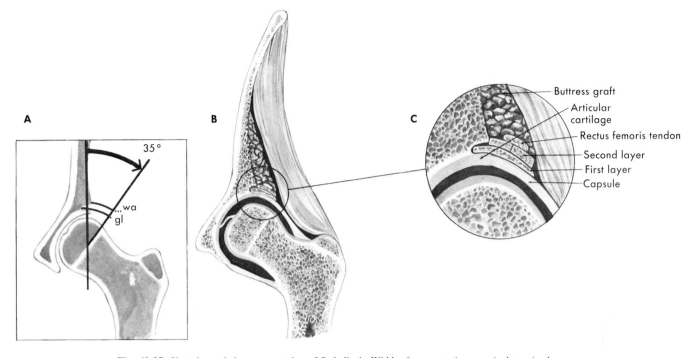

Fig. 62-35. Slotted acetabular augmentation of Staheli. **A,** Width of augmentation, *wa,* is determined preoperatively from standing anteroposterior roentgenogram of pelvis. CE angle and 35-degree angle are drawn. Graft length, *gl,* is sum of *wa* and slot depth. **B,** Objective of procedure is to provide congruous extension of acetabulum. **C,** Details of extension. (From Staheli, L.T.: J. Pediatr. Orthop. **1:**321, 1981.)

on a pad. For heavier patients, a fracture table is used and the involved limb is draped free.

Make a straight "bikini" skin incision 2 to 3 cm below and parallel to the iliac crest. Expose the hip joint through a standard iliofemoral approach. Divide the tendon of the reflected head of the rectus femoris anteriorly and displace it posteriorly (Fig. 62-36). If the capsule is abnormally thick (greater than 6 to 7 mm), thin it by "filleting" with a scalpel.

The placement of the acetabular slot is the most critical part of the procedure; the slot must be created *exactly* at the acetabular margin (Fig. 62-37). Determine the position of the slot by placing a probe into the joint to palpate the position of the acetabulum. Next place a drill in the selected site and make an anteroposterior roentgenogram to verify correct position. The floor of the slot should be acetabular articular cartilage and little bone; the end and roof of the slot should be cancellous bone. The slot should be 1 cm deep.

Make the slot by drilling a series of holes with a ⁵⁄₃₂-inch (4.5 mm) bit and join them with a narrow rongeur. Determine the length of the slot intraoperatively by the need for coverage. If excessive femoral anteversion is present, extend the slot anteriorly. If the acetabulum is deficient posteriorly, extend the slot in that direction.

Take thin strips of cortical and cancellous bone from the lateral surface of the ilium; cut these as long as possible (Fig. 62-38). Extend the shallow decortication inferiorly from the iliac crest to the superior margin of the slot to ensure rapid fusion of the graft to the ilium. Do not re-move the inner table of the ilium because this may change the contour of the pelvis.

Now measure the depth of the slot and add this to the width of the augmentation as determined preoperatively. Select thin strips (1 mm) of cancellous bone and cut them into rectangles about 1 cm wide and of the appropriate length. Assemble these rectangular pieces on a moist sponge, cutting enough to provide a single layer the length of the augumentation. Apply the first layer radially from the slot with the concave side down to provide a congruous extension (Fig. 62-39).

Select longer cancellous strips for the second layer and cut them to the length of the extension. Place these at right angles to the first layer and parallel to the acetabulum. They may be a little thicker (2 mm), especially the most lateral strip, to provide a well-defined lateral margin of the extension. Both layers must be of appropriate width and length. The augmentation should not extend too far anteriorly to avoid blocking hip flexion.

Secure these two layers of cancellous grafts by bringing the reflected head of the rectus femoris forward over the graft and suturing it back in its original position. A capsular flap may be substituted if this tendon is not available. Cut the remaining grafts into small pieces and pack them above but not beyond the initial layer. They are held in place by the reattached abductor muscles. Confirm the position and width of the graft by roentgenograms. After closure, apply a single hip spica cast with the hip in 15 degrees of abduction, 20 degrees of flexion, and neutral rotation (Fig. 62-40).

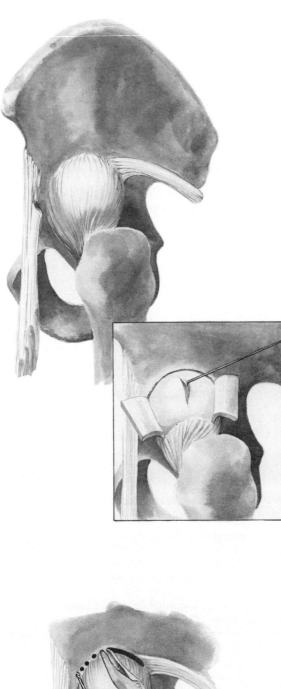

Fig. 62-36. Slotted acetabular augmentation of Staheli, cont'd. Reflected head of rectus femoris is detached anteriorly and reflected. *Inset,* If rectus femoris is not available, capsular flap may be fashioned to cover graft. (From Staheli, L.T.: J. Pediatr. Orthop. **1:**321, 1981.)

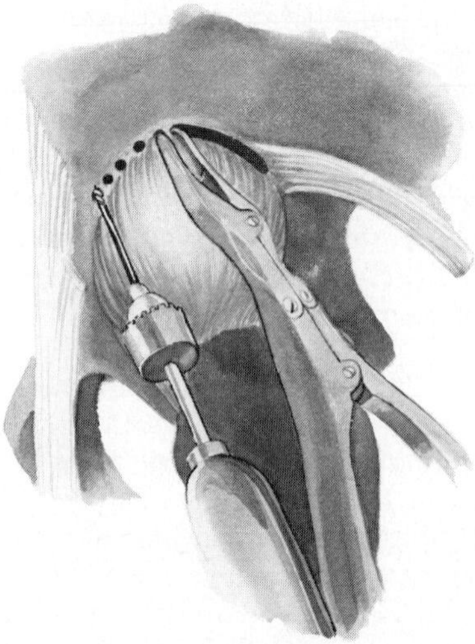

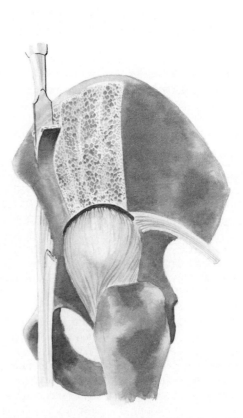

Fig. 62-37. Slotted acetabular augmentation of Staheli, cont'd. Slot is created exactly at acetabular margin, approximately 5 mm wide and 10 mm deep. (From Staheli, L.T.: J. Pediatr. Orthop. **1:**321, 1981.)

Fig. 62-38. Slotted acetabular augmentation of Staheli, cont'd. Cortical and cancellous bone is taken from lateral surface of ilium. (From Staheli, L.T.: J. Pediatr. Orthop. **1:**321, 1981.)

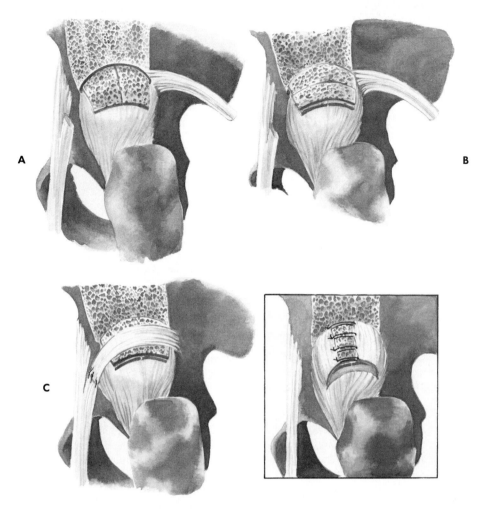

Fig. 62-39. Slotted acetabular augmentation of Staheli, cont'd. Steps in augmentation. **A,** First layer is placed radially. **B,** Second layer is placed parallel to acetabular margin. **C,** Both layers are held in place by reattached reflected head of rectus femoris. *Inset,* Capsular flaps closed over graft. (From Staheli, L.T.: J. Pediatr. Orthop. **1:**321, 1981.)

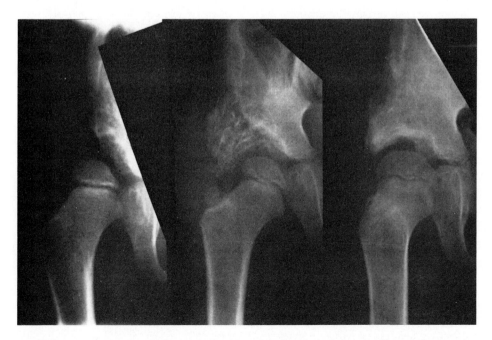

Fig. 62-40. Severe congenital acetabular dysplasia in 4-year-old girl. **A,** Before slotted acetabular augmentation. **B,** Immediately after operation. **C,** Six months after operation. (From Staheli, L.T.: J. Pediatr. Orthop. **1:**321, 1981.)

AFTERTREATMENT. The cast is removed after 6 weeks, and crutch walking is permitted with one-fifth body weight bearing on the affected side until the graft is incorporated, usually at 3 to 4 months.

INNOMINATE OSTEOTOMY WITH MEDIAL DISPLACEMENT OF ACETABULUM

The Chiari osteotomy is a capsular interposition arthroplasty and should be considered only in those instances when other reconstructions are impossible: when the femoral head cannot be centered adequately in the acetabulum by abduction and internal rotation or in painfully subluxated hips with early signs of osteoarthritis. This procedure deepens the deficient acetabulum by medial displacement of the distal pelvic fragment and improves superolateral femoral coverage. Excessive medial displacement of the distal fragment, osteotomy performed too high or too low, and injury to the sciatic nerve are technical pitfalls that may lead to a poor result.

Betz reported 89% good results, and Mitchell reported relief of pain in 88% of patients.

The Chiari procedure is an operation that uses no bone grafts, places the femoral head beneath a surface of spongy bone with the capacity for regeneration, and corrects the lateral pathologic displacement of the femur. The pelvis is osteotomized at the superior margin of the acetabulum, and the pelvis inferior to the osteotomy along with the femur is displaced medially (Fig. 62-41). The superior fragment of the osteotomy then becomes a shelf, and the capsule is interposed between it and the femoral head. After using this operation on more than 600 patients, 400 of whom have been observed for more than 2 years, Chiari recommends the operation as follows:

1. For all congenital subluxations in patients 4 to 6 years old or older, including adults. These include subluxations persisting after conservative treatment of dislocations and those never treated before.
2. For untreated congenital dislocations in patients over 4 years old, soon after open or closed reduction.
3. For dysplastic hips with osteoarthritis, including those with severe involvement.

4. For paralytic dislocations caused by muscular weakness or spasticity.
5. For coxa magna after Perthes' disease or after forced orthopaedic treatment of congenital dislocation with resultant avascular necrosis.

These indications are broader than those usually accepted in this country. For a young child under about 10 years of age we do not recommend the osteotomy in subluxations or in dislocations that can be reduced either surgically or conservatively and in which osteotomy of the innominate bone, acetabuloplasty, or osteotomies that free the acetabulum would result in a competent acetabulum. Some surgeons recommend the operation for patients in the second and later decades who have symptomatic early subluxation of the hip with acetabular dysplasia too severe to be treated by other pelvic osteotomies; for them innominate osteotomy with medial displacement is preferred to a shelf operation. The procedure has also been used in older children with underlying neuromuscular disorders and acetabular dysplasia.

Chiari's operation is a capsular arthroplasty because the capsule is interposed between the newly formed acetabular roof and the femoral head. Because the biomechanics of the hip are improved by displacing the hip nearer the midline, a Trendelenburg limp is often eliminated.

TECHNIQUE (CHIARI). Place the patient supine on a fracture table with the feet fastened to the traction plate. Now slightly abduct and externally rotate the affected hip. Make an anterolateral approach about 10 cm long, beginning slightly lateral to the iliac crest, extending anteriorly past the anterosuperior iliac spine, and continuing distally along the tensor fasciae latae. Develop the interval between the tensor fasciae latae and the sartorius and retract the former laterally. Now incise the iliac epiphysis in line with the iliac crest. With a periorsteal elevator detach the lateral half of the epiphysis along with the tensor fasciae latae and the anterior part of the gluteus medius.

Now dissect these muscles subperiosteally and retract them posteriorly. Insert a periosteal elevator between the capsule of the hip and the gluteus minimus. Dissect subperiosteally posteriorly to the point where the pelvis curves

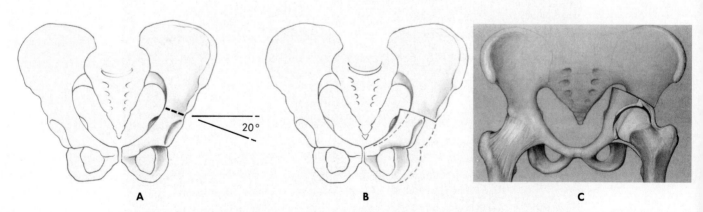

Fig. 62-41. Chiari medial displacement osteotomy. **A,** Line of osteotomy extending from immediately superior to lip of acetabulum into sciatic notch. **B,** Completed osteotomy with medial displacement of distal fragment for interpositional capsular arthroplasty. **C,** Chiari osteotomy with medial displacement of distal fragment and capsular arthroplasty. (Courtesy Alfred I. duPont Institute.)

inferiorly. Now with a curved periosteal elevator dissect subperiosteally farther posteriorly until the sciatic notch is reached. Replace this elevator with a flexible metal ribbon retractor 3 cm wide. This completes the dissection posteriorly. Now return anteriorly to the medial aspect of the ilium. With a periosteal elevator strip the iliacus muscle and the underlying periosteum posteriorly to the sciatic notch.

Once the sciatic notch is reached, replace the elevator with a flexible metal ribbon retractor that touches and overlaps the ribbon retractor already in the notch. With curved scissors separate the rectus muscle and its reflected head from the capsule of the hip joint. Now divide the reflected head. The osteotomy should be made precisely between the insertion of the capsule and the reflected head of the rectus, following the capsular insertion in a curved line and ending distal to the anteroinferior iliac spine anteriorly and in the sciatic notch posteriorly. Do not open or damage the capsule of the joint. After the line of the osteotomy has been determined, start the osteotomy with a straight, narrow osteotome, opening the lateral table of the ilium along this line.

At the beginning determine the exact position of the osteotome by image intensifier television fluoroscopy or by roentgenograms. Direct the osteotomy superiorly approximately 20 degrees toward the inner table of the ilium. Change the position of the osteotome as necessary to make the osteotomy curved superiorly. Do not direct the osteotomy more than 20 degrees superiorly because it might then enter the sacroiliac joint. Furthermore, do not splinter the inner cortex of the ilium.

When the osteotomy has been completed, displace the hip medially by releasing the traction on the extremity and by forcing the limb into abduction. The distal fragment then displaces medially, hinging at the symphysis pubis. However, if the adductor muscles are extremely relaxed, manually forcing the head medially or displacing the distal fragment with an instrument may be necessary. Be sure the distal fragment is displaced far enough medially so that the proximal fragment covers the femoral head. Separation of the bony surfaces must be prevented.

After the displacement has been completed, decrease the abduction of the limb to about 30 degrees. If the capsule is loose, perform a capsulorrhaphy. Now check the position of the hip and the osteotomy by image intensifier television fluoroscopy or by roentgenograms (Fig. 62-42). Replace and suture the iliac epiphysis and close the wound. Apply a spica cast with the hip in 20 to 30 degrees of abduction, neutral rotation, and neutral extension.

AFTERTREATMENT. In children and adults the cast is removed at 3 weeks, and active and passive exercises of the hip are started. If motion in the hip is restricted and does not improve during rehabilitation, the joint is manipulated. At 4 weeks partial weight bearing on crutches is allowed.

JUVENILE AND YOUNG ADULT (OLDER THAN 8 TO 10 YEARS OF AGE)

In children older than 8 to 10 years of age or in young adults when the femoral head cannot be pulled distally to the level of the acetabulum, only palliative salvaging operations are possible. With a bone graft a shelf or buttress can be created on the iliac wing over the femoral head as near the acetabulum as possible. This type of operation is always mechanically unsound, but as a salvage operation it may be useful. Rarely a femoral shortening combined with a pelvic osteotomy could be considered. After a few years degenerative arthritic changes develop in the hip joint. When these changes cause enough pain or limitation of motion to require additional surgery, a reconstructive operation such as a total hip arthroplasty (Chapter 41) may be indicated at the appropriate age. Arthrodesis (Chapter 38) is now rarely indicated for an old unreduced dislocation. The Schanz or Lorenz osteotomy is likewise rarely indicated except in paralytic dislocations. In bilateral dislocations in this age group the hips should be left unreduced, and total hip arthroplasties should be carried out later.

CONGENITAL AND DEVELOPMENTAL COXA VARA

The term "congenital coxa vara" has been applied to two types of coxa vara seen in infancy and childhood. The first type is present at birth, is rare, and is associated with

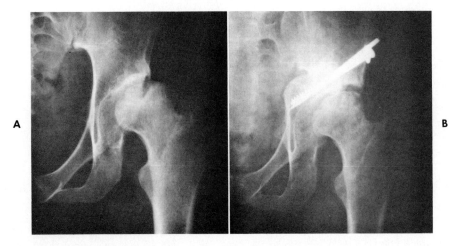

Fig. 62-42. A, Before Chiari osteotomy. **B,** After surgery. Note that internal fixation has been used in this patient. (Courtesy Dr. R. Betz.)

other congenital anomalies such as proximal femoral deficiency or anomalies in other parts of the body such as cleidocranial dysostosis. The second type, usually not discovered until walking is begun, is more common than the first and is associated with no other abnormality except possibly a torsional deformity of the same femur or coxa vara of the opposite femur. Whether this second type is congenital or developmental is unknown; thus it is often called coxa vara infantatum or developmental coxa vara. In the rest of this section we use the term "developmental coxa vara" to designate the more common type, that is, that associated with no other deformities.

Developmental coxa vara, often bilateral, is characterized by a progressive decrease in the angle between the femoral neck and shaft, a progressive shortening of the limb, and the presence of a defect in the medial part of the neck. Microscopically, the tissue in this defect consists of cartilage that, because the columnar arrangement of its cells is irregular and ossification within it is atypical, resembles an abnormal epiphyseal plate. The adjacent metaphyseal bone is osteoporotic, its trabeculae being atrophic, and occasionally it contains large groups of cartilage cells. Much connective tissue may be seen in the irregularly arranged cartilage and bone. Pylkkänen, after a histologic study of tissue removed from the defect in 25 hips of children, concluded that the cause of developmental coxa vara (coxa vara infantum) is a disturbance in ossification and growth originating in the medial part of the. proximal femoral epiphyseal plate. This disturbance results in delay of ossification, in deposition of groups of cartilage cells within the metaphyseal bone of the neck, and consequently in weakness of the neck. When walking is begun, the forces that the femoral neck must withstand are of course increased, and because the neck is weak, varus deformity gradually develops.

Conservative treatment is of little or no value in developmental coxa vara. As the patient becomes older and

heavier, the deformity increases until the greater trochanter eventually lies superior to the femoral head; furthermore, pseudarthrosis of the femoral neck may develop. In adults the trochanter may come to lie several inches superior to the head, and when pseudarthrosis is present, the head may be widely separated from the neck. Thus the deformity should be corrected by surgery as early as possible. After the age of 8 years the likelihood of obtaining a hip whose function approaches normal diminishes rapidly.

The treatment of choice for correction of developmental coxa vara is trochanteric or subtrochanteric osteotomy to place the femoral neck and head in an appropriate valgus position with the shaft of the femur. Surgery is indicated when the neck-shaft angle is 110 degrees or less.

Numerous techniques have been described for femoral osteotomy in coxa vara. Two techniques are commonly used. One is a trochanteric or subtrochanteric osteotomy fixed internally with either a blade-plate or screw-plate combination (Fig. 62-43). Although biomechanically this may provide enough rigid internal fixation to eliminate the need for postoperative immobilization, we recommend a spica cast until union is almost complete. The other technique is the oblique trochanteric osteotomy, as described by MacEwen and Shands with correction of the coxa vara and associated retroversion of the femoral neck. With this technique, two long flat surfaces of bone remain in opposition, and the fragments are fixed by removable Steinmann pins and a pins-and-plaster type of cast. This technique allows removal of the internal fixation at the time of cast removal, avoiding a secondary procedure for plate removal.

Regardless of the method of osteotomy, the deformity can recur and children should be examined periodically after surgery until their growth is complete. In addition, a significant number of children with coxa vara have associated femoral hypoplasia, which may ultimately require limb equalization in unilateral involvement.

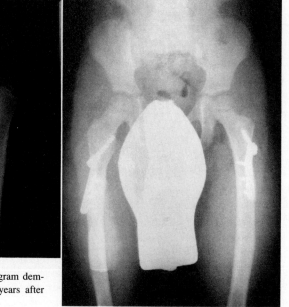

Fig. 62-43. Congenital coxa vara. **A,** Preoperative roentgenogram demonstrating neck-shaft angle less than 100 degrees. **B,** Two years after surgery demonstrating correction of neck-shaft angle.

Valgus osteotomy for developmental coxa vara

TECHNIQUE. Before surgical exposure of the lateral border of the femur, perform an adductor tenotomy through a separate incision. Then expose the trochanteric region and proximal shaft of the femur through a lateral longitudinal approach (p. 57). Then using roentgenographic control insert the blade of a blade plate into the trochanter, neck, and femoral head after having bent the plate to a predetermined angle. Then divide the femur transversely at the level of the lesser trochanter. Now use the plate as a lever to place the proximal fragment in the desired valgus position; because of contracture of the soft tissues this stage of the operation is often difficult. As an alternative a coventry or Campbell screw plate may be used for internal fixation to correct the neck-shaft angle to 135 degrees or more.

The femoral shaft may be shortened moderately to allow placement of the fragments in sufficient valgus. Combined with an adductor tenotomy, this will make positioning significantly easier. Then fix the plate to the femoral shaft with screws.

AFTERTREATMENT. If the deformity corrected has been severe, a spica cast is applied from the nipple line to the toes on the affected side and to above the knee on the opposite unless the operation has been bilateral, and then a double spica cast is necessary. The cast is worn for 8 to 12 weeks until roentgenographic union is achieved.

TECHNIQUE (MACEWEN AND SHANDS). Before surgery determine the angle of the osteotomy necessary to correct the varus deformity and any retroversion of the femoral neck. The closer the plane of the osteotomy approaches a plane perpendicular to the long axis of the femur, the greater will be the correction of retroversion (see Fig. 62-19, E). Use the graph of d'Aubigne and Vaillant to determine the angle (see Fig. 62-19, D). The desired number of degrees of change in the angle between the shaft and neck is plotted along the ordinate, and the desired number of degrees of change in rotation is plotted on the abscissa. The point of intersection of these two values determines the plane of the osteotomy in relation to the long axis of the femur.

Expose the trochanteric region and proximal shaft of the femur through a lateral longitudinal approach (p. 57). Then rotate the limb so that the neck of the femur is in the frontal plane. Next to control the position of the proximal fragment insert a heavy Steinmann pin through the greater trochanter into the neck. Drill several holes along the line of the proposed osteotomy that extends from anterosuperior to posteroinferior and complete the osteotomy with an osteotome or electric saw. Then abduct the distal fragment while maintaining the osseous surfaces in contact, thus correcting both angulation and rotation. Finally insert a screw across the osteotomy and check the position of the fragments by roentgenograms. Apply a one and one-half spica cast incorporating the Steinmann pin.

AFTERTREATMENT. At 3 weeks the Steinmann pin is removed, and usually at 6 weeks the cast is removed.

EXSTROPHY OF BLADDER

Exstrophy of the bladder causes several problems because of a congenital failure of fusion of the tissues of the midline of the body. The major anomaly is a maldevelopment of the lower part of the abdominal wall and the anterior wall of the bladder so that the anterior surface of the

posterior wall of the bladder is exposed to the exterior. Hernias and other defects of the anterior abdominal wall may also be present more proximally. However, as noted by O'Phelan, the orthopaedic surgeon becomes involved in treatment because of the diastasis of the symphysis pubis, the lateral flare of the innominate bones, and the resultant lateral displacement and external rotation of the acetabula that, if left uncorrected, would result in a wide-based, waddling, externally rotated gait (Fig. 62-44).

Because most of the urologic structures are present or bifid, reconstruction is possible. However, unless the symphysis pubis is approximated, urologic reconstruction is followed by complications such as the formation of fistulae or infection. These complications seem to be caused by tension placed on the soft tissues during closure, and this tension can be relieved by repair of the symphysis pubis. O'Phelan in 1963 and O'Phelan et al. in 1977 described the results of bilateral posterior iliac osteotomies and approximation of the symphysis in a large number of patients. First osteotomies of the iliac bones near the sacroiliac joints are made. Then 1 week later the symphysis pubis is approximated by heavy wire sutures. O'Phelan has altered his wiring technique because in his earlier patients the wire tended to break or cut through the pubic rami. After the symphysis pubis has been reduced and fixed, the urologic structures can be reconstructed without undue tension, and the gait is improved.

In our experience, after posterior iliac osteotomy and approximation of the symphysis pubis, the most common complication is cutting of the wire through the symphysis pubis and into the neck of the reconstructed urethra. Because of this possibility, we recommend a generous posterior iliac osteotomy to allow the wings of the ilium to be rotated without tension on the symphysis pubis anteriorly. We use preoperative computed tomography scans to outline the three-dimensional anatomy of the pelvis and help determine how much rotation of the iliac wings will be required to allow adequate apposition of the symphysis pubis (Fig. 62-45).

Preliminary reports of the use of an external fixator to substitute for wire fixation have appeared. We have no experience with this technique, but it sounds promising as a method of stabilizing the pelvic osteotomy and anterior reconstruction.

TECHNIQUE (O'PHELAN). Plan the procedure in two separate stages. In the first use endotracheal anesthesia and place the patient prone on the operating table. On one side make a curved incision starting along the lateral part of the posterior iliac crest, extending inferiorly toward the posterosuperior iliac spine, and turning caudally for a short distance along the sacroiliac joint. Identify the fascial plane between the sacrospinalis, the quadratus lumborum, and the oblique abdominal muscles medially and superiorly and the gluteal muscles inferiorly. Then detach the gluteal muscles from the ilium by subperiosteal dissection and retract them laterally to expose the posterior surface of the ilium and the greater sciatic notch. Release the soft tissue attachments on the iliac crest and the cartilaginous epiphysis to expose the anteroposterior thickness of the ilium. Then clear the medial surface of the pelvis down to the sciatic notch. Identify the sciatic notch and carefully insert a blunt retractor into it to provide counterpressure during

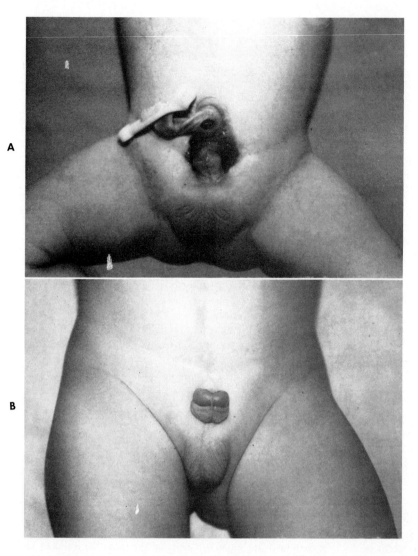

Fig. 62-44. Exstrophy of bladder. **A,** Newborn boy with exstrophy of bladder. **B,** After iliac osteotomies and anterior reconstruction.

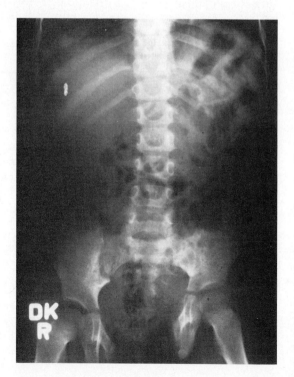

Fig. 62-45. Same patient as in Fig. 62-44, 12 years after surgery.

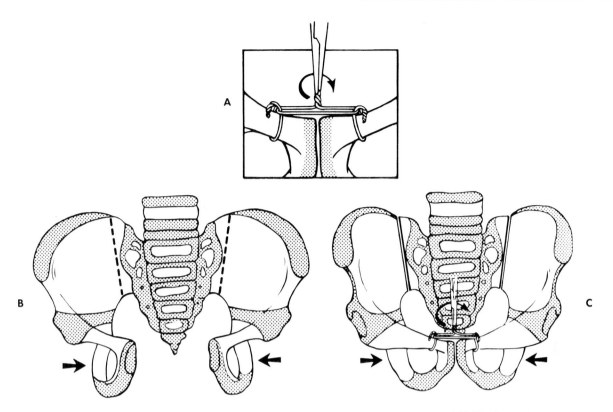

Fig. 62-46. Technique of Furnas, Haq, and Somers for reconstruction in exstrophy of bladder (see text). (From Furnas, D.W., Haq, M.A., and Somers, G.: Plast. Reconstr. Surg. **56**:61, 1975.)

the osteotomy and to prevent injury to the neurovascular structures. Now with a small osteotome make a vertical osteotomy about 2.5 cm lateral to the sacroiliac joint from the crest of the ilium to the sciatic notch (Fig. 62-46, *B*). Divide the bone completely, including both cortices, and use a bone or a lamina spreader to separate the fragments. Unless both cortices are divided, the deformity will recur. Now perform the same procedure on the opposite side. After both sides have been osteotomized, forcibly manipulate the pelvis by applying pressure in a medial and anterior direction on both sides to bring the pubic rami together.

If the posterior iliac osteotomies allow easy apposition of the pubic symphysis anteriorly, the anterior reconstruction may be done in the same operative procedure; otherwise, within a week perform the second stage of the operation with the help of a urologic surgeon. Place the patient supine and have the urologic surgeon suitably prepare the operative field and carefully identify the abnormal bladder and urethral structures. When these structures are ready for reconstruction, expose the symphysis pubis and the pubic rami by subperiosteal and subperichondral dissection. Then approximate the symphysis pubis by pushing the pelvis medially on both sides (Fig. 62-46, *C*). Circle each superior pubic ramus with a heavy wire loop and tighten each; then place a third wire through each of the first two loops and with the symphysis approximated tighten this wire appropriately (Fig. 62-46, *A*). After the urologic surgeon has repaired the genitourinary tissues and the abdominal wall, place the patient immediately in a

well-molded bilateral spica cast with the hips in internal rotation to keep the bone and soft structures anteriorly approximated as well as possible.

AFTERTREATMENT. The cast is worn until there is conclusive evidence roentgenographically that the osteotomies have healed with solid mature bone. This may require 10 to 16 weeks. Then the cast is removed, and a small pelvic support or brace is applied to allow the patient to walk. After the child has been walking for a short time the wire loops used to fix the symphysis pubis should be removed because otherwise they may erode into the urethra; they may be removed at the time of a cystoscopic checkup.

REFERENCES
Congenital dislocation of hip

Abbott, L.C.: The treatment of old congenital dislocation of the hip, Arch. Surg. **12**:983, 1926.

Albee, F.H.: The bone graft wedge: its use in the treatment of relapsing, acquired, and congenital dislocation of the hip, N.Y. Med. J. **102**:433, 1915.

Allison, N.: The open operations for congenital dislocation of the hip. In The Robert Jones birthday volume, London, 1928, Oxford University Press.

Alvik, I.: Increased anteversion of the femoral neck as sole sign of dysplasia coxae, Acta Orthop. Scand. **29**:301, 1960.

Anderson, M.E., and Bickel, W.H.: Shelf operation for congenital subluxation and dislocation of the hip, J. Bone Joint Surg. **33-A**:87, 1951.

Artz, T.D., et al.: Neonatal diagnosis, treatment and related factors of congenital dislocation of the hip, Clin. Orthop. **110**:112, 1975.

Ashley, K.R., Larsen, L.J., and James, P.M.: Reduction of dislocation of the hip in older children: a preliminary report, J. Bone Joint Surg. **54-A**:545, 1972.

d'Aubigne, R.M.: Reposition with arthroplasty for congenital dislocation of the hip in adults, J. Bone Joint Surg. **34-B**:22, 1952.

Barlow, T.G.: Early diagnosis and treatment of congenital dislocation of the hip, J. Bone Joint Surg. **44-B:**292, 1962.

Bell, B.T.: Pelvic support osteotomy, Surg. Clin. North Am. **33:**1719, 1953.

Betz, R.R., Palmer, C., Kumar, S., and MacEwen, G.D.: Long-term follow-up of Chiari pelvic osteotomies for dysplastic hips (abstract), Orthop. Trans. **8:**394, 1984.

Bickel, W.H., and Breivis, J.S.: Shelf operation for congenital subluxation and dislocation of the hip, Clin. Orthop. **106:**27, 1975.

Bjerkreim, I.: Congenital dislocation of the hip joint in Norway. Acta Orthop. Scand. Suppl. 157, 1974.

Bjøro, K.: Shelf operation in the treatment of congenital dysplasia and subluxation of the hip-joint in adults with special reference to the prevention of secondary osteoarthritis, Acta Orthop. Scand. **25:**190, 1956.

Blount, W.P.: Proximal osteotomies of the femur. In American Academy of Orthopaedic Surgeons: Instructional course lectures, vol. 9, Ann Arbor, 1952, J.W. Edwards.

Bosworth, D.M., Fielding, J.W., Ishizuka, T., and Ege, R.: Hip-shelf operation in adults, J. Bone Joint Surg. **43-A:**93, 1961.

Bowen, J., and Kassar, J.: The Pelvic harness (pamphlet), Wilmington, 1982, A.I. duPont Institute.

Brewer, B.J.: Controlled closed rotation osteoclasis of the femur, Clin. Orthop. **77:**128, 1971.

Bucholz, R.W., and Ogden, J.A.: Patterns of ischemic necrosis of the proximal femur in nonoperatively treated congenital hip disease. In The Hip: Proceedings of the sixth open scientific meeting of The Hip Society, St. Louis, 1978, The C.V. Mosby Co.

Caffey, J., et al.: Contradiction of the congenital dysplasia-predislocation hypothesis of congenital dislocation of the hip through a study of the normal variation in acetabular angles at successive periods in infancy, Pediatrics **17:**632, 1956.

Calot, F.: Treatment of congenital luxations and subluxations of the hip and their recurrence, Monde Med., Paris **44:**1, 1934.

Canale, S.T.: Personal communication, 1978.

Canale, S.T., Hammond, N.L., III, Cotler, J.M., and Snedden, H.E.: Pelvic displacement osteotomy for chronic hip dislocation in myelodysplasia, J. Bone Joint Surg. **57-A:**177, 1975.

Chakirgil, G.S.: Personal communication, 1978.

Chandler, F.A.: Congenital dislocation of the hip, Surg. Clin. North Am. **13:**1141, 1933.

Chapchal, G.: Indications for the various types of pelvic osteotomy, Clin. Orthop. **98:**111, 1974.

Chiari, K.: Pelvic osteotomy as shelf operation, Neuvième Congrès Internationale de Chirurgie Orthopédique, Wien (Hofburg), 1963.

Chiari, K.: Medial displacement osteotomy of the pelvis, Clin. Orthop. **98:**55, 1974.

Chuinard, E.G.: Early weight-bearing and corection of anteversion in the treatment of congenital dislocation of the hip, J. Bone Joint Surg. **37-A:**229, 1955.

Chuinard, E.G.: Femoral osteotomy in the treatment of congenital dysplasia of the hip, Orthop. Clin. North Am. **3:**157, 1972.

Chuinard, E.G., and Logan, N.D.: Varus-producing and derotational subtrochanteric osteotomy in the treatment of congenital dislocation of the hip, J. Bone Joint Surg. **45-A:**1397, 1963.

Cohen, J.: Congenital dislocation of the hip: case report of an unusual complication and unusual treatment, J. Bone Joint Surg. **53-A:**1007, 1971.

Cole, W.H.: The open treatment of congenital dislocation of the hip, J. Bone Joint Surg. **17:**18, 1935.

Coleman, S.S.: Diagnosis of congenital dysplasia of the hip in the newborn infant, JAMA **162:**548, 1956.

Coleman, S.S.: Congenital dysplasia of the hip in the Navajo infant, Clin. Orthop. **56:**179, 1968.

Coleman, S.S.: The incomplete pericapsular (Pemberton) and innominate (Salter) osteotomies: a complete analysis, Clin. Orthop. **98:**116, 1974.

Coleman, S.S.: Treatment of congenital dislocation of the hip in the older child. In Ahstrom, J.P., editor: Current practice in orthopaedic surgery, vol. 6, St. Louis, 1975, The C.V. Mosby Co.

Coleman, S.S.: Congenital dysplasia and dislocation of the hip, St. Louis, 1978, The C.V. Mosby Co.

Coleman, S.S., and MacEwen, G.D.: Congenital dislocation of the hip in infancy. In American Academy of Orthopaedic Surgeons: Instructional course lectures, vol. 21, St. Louis, 1972, The C.V. Mosby Co.

Colonna, P.C.: An arthroplastic operation for congenital dislocation of the hip—a two stage procedure, Surg. Gynecol. Obstet. **63:**777, 1936.

Colonna, P.C.: Arthroplasty of the hip for congenital dislocation in children, J. Bone Joint Surg. **29:**711, 1947.

Colonna, P.C.: Capsular arthroplasty for congenital dislocation of the hip: a two-stage procedure, J. Bone Joint Surg. **35-A:**179, 1953.

Colonna, P.C.: Care of the infant with congenital subluxation of the hip, JAMA **166:**715, 1958.

Colonna, P.C.: Capsular arthroplasty for congenital dislocation of the hip: indications and technique: some long-term results, J. Bone Joint Surg. **47-A:**437, 1965.

Colton, C.L.: Chiari osteotomy for acetabular dysplasia in young subjects, J. Bone Joint Surg. **54-B:**578, 1972.

Compere, E.L., and Schnute, W.J.: Treatment of congenital dislocation of the hip, J. Bone Joint Surg. **28:**555, 1946.

Conrad, M.B.: Congenital dislocation of the hip. In American Academy of Orthopaedic Surgeons: Instructional course lectures, vol. 18, St. Louis, 1961, The C.V. Mosby Co.

Crego, C.H., Jr., and Schwartzmann, J.R.: Follow-up study of the early treatment of congenital dislocation of the hip, J. Bone Joint Surg. **30-A:**428, 1948.

Crellin, R.Q.: Innominate osteotomy for congenital dislocation and subluxation of the hip: a follow-up study, Clin. Orthop. **98:**171, 1974.

Dameron, T.B., Jr.: Complications of the innominate osteotomy, South. Med. J. **64:**204, 1971.

Dega, W., Król, J., and Polakowski, L.: Surgical treatment of congenital dislocation of the hip in children: a one-stage procedure, J. Bone Joint Surg. **41-A:**920, 1959.

De Godoy Moreira, R., and De Godoy Moreira, F.E.: Congenital dysplasia of the hip: Pemberton operation, Spectator Correspondence Club Letter, August 1963 (mimeographed).

Denton, J.R., and Ryder, C.T.: Radiographic follow-up of Salter innominate osteotomy for congenital dysplasia of the hip, Clin. Orthop. **98:**210, 1974.

Dickson, F.D.: Davis method for closed reduction of congenital dislocation of the hip, J. Bone Joint Surg. **7:**873, 1925.

Dickson, F.D.: The shelf operation in the treatment of congenital dislocation of the hip, J. Bone Joint Surg. **17:**43, 1935.

Dooley, B.J.: Osteochondritis in congenital dislocation and subluxation of the hip, J. Bone Joint Surg. **46-B:**198, 1964.

Dunlap, K., et al.: A new method for determination of torsion of the femur, J. Bone Joint Surg. **35-A:** 289, 1953.

Emnéus, H.: A note on the Ortolani–Von Rosen–Palmén treatment of congenital dislocation of the hip, J. Bone Joint Surg. **50-B:**537, 1968.

Eppright, R.H.: Dial osteotomy of the acetabulum, J. Bone Joint Surg. **58-A:**283, 1976.

Epstein, G.J., and Epstein, N.S.: König's operation in the treatment of congenital dislocation of the hip, J. Bone Joint Surg. **17:**309, 1935.

Esteve, R.: Congenital dislocation of the hip: a review and assessment of results of treatment with special reference to frame reduction as compared with manipulative reduction, J. Bone Joint Surg. **42-B:**253, 1960.

Eyre-Brook, A.L., Jones, D.A., and Harris, F.C.: Pemberton's acetabuloplasty for congenital dislocation or subluxation of the hip, J. Bone Joint Surg. **60-B:**18, 1978.

Fairbank, H.A.T.: Congenital dislocation of the hip with special reference to anatomy, Br. J. Surg. **17:**380, 1930.

Farill, J.: Personal therapeutic conduct in the treatment of congenital dislocation of the hip in children, An. Ortop Traumatol. Montevideo **3:**281, 1950. (Abstracted in Steindler, A.: Orthopedic seminar notes, vol. 1, sect. C, 1950-1951.)

Farill, J.: The treatment of the congenital dislocation of the hip, joint arthrography and open reduction, Orthopaedic Correspondence Club Letter, September, 1951.

Ferguson, A.B., Jr.: Primary open reduction of congenital dislocation of the hip using a median adductor approach. J. Bone Joint Surg. **55-A:**671, 1973.

Ferré, R.L., and Schächter, S.: Congenital dislocation of the hip: innominate osteotomy, Clin. Orthop. **98:**183, 1974.

Francillon, M.R.: Colonna arthroplasty of the hip in the treatment of congenital dislocation of the hip, Z. Orthop. **84:**177, 1954.

Frank, G.R., and Michael, H.R.: Treatment of congenital dislocation of the hip: results obtained with the Pemberton and Salter osteotomies, South. Med. J. **60:**975, 1967.

Frankel, C.J.: Results of treatment of irreducible congenital dislocation of the hip by arthrodesis, J. Bone Joint Surg. **30-A:**422, 1948.

Fredensborg, N.: Observations in children with congenital dislocation of the hip, Acta Orthop. Scand. **47:**175, 1976.

Gaenslen, F.J.: The Schanz subtrochanteric osteotomy for irreducible dislocation of the hip, J. Bone Joint Surg. **17:**76, 1935.

Gage, J.R., and Winter, R.B.: Avascular necrosis of the capital femoral epiphysis as a complication of closed reduction of congenital dislocation of the hip: a critical review of twenty years' experience at Gillette Children's Hospital, J. Bone Joint Surg. **54-A:**373, 1972.

Galeazzi, R.: Uber die Torsion des verrenkten oberen Femurendes und ihre Beseitigung, Verhandl. d. Deutsch. Gesellsch F. Orthop. Chir., p. 334, 1910.

Galloway, H.P.H.: The open operation for congenital dislocation of the hip. J. Bone Joint Surg. **2:**390, 1920.

Galloway, H.P.H.: The open operation for congenital dislocation of the hip: special reference to results, J. Bone Joint Surg. **8:**539, 1926.

Ghormley, R.K.: Use of the anterior superior spine and crest of ilium in surgery of the hip joint, J. Bone Joint Surg. **13:**784, 1931.

Gill, A.B.: Plastic construction of an acetabulum in congenital dislocation of the hip—the shelf operation, J. Bone Joint Surg. **17:**48, 1935.

Gill, A.B.: End results of bloodless reduction of congenital dislocation of the hip, J. Bone Joint Surg. **25:**1, 1943.

Gill, A.B.: The end result of early treatment of congenital dislocation of the hip, J. Bone Joint Surg. **30-A:**442, 1948.

Gill, A.B.: The operative treatment of congenital dislocation of the hip: indications and methods. In American Academy of Orthopaedic Surgeons: Instructional course lectures, vol. 4, Ann Arbor, 1948, J.W. Edwards.

Groves, E.W.H.: Some contributions to the reconstructive surgery of the hip, Br. J. Surg. **14:**486, 1926-1927.

Groves, E.W.H.: The treatment of congenital dislocation of the hip-joint, with special reference to open operative reduction. In The Robert Jones birthday volume, London, 1928, Oxford University Press.

Haas, S.L.: The treatment of congenital dislocation of the hip-joint, Am. J. Surg. **13:**235, 1931.

Haas, S.L.: Pin fixation in dislocation of the hip joint, J. Bone Joint Surg. **14:**346, 1932.

Harris, L.E., Lipscomb, P.R., and Hodgson, J.R.: Early diagnosis of congenital dysplasia and congenital dislocation of the hip: value of the abduction test, JAMA **173:**229, 1960.

Harris, L.E., Lipscomb, P.R., and Hodgson, J.R.: Hilgenreiner measurements of the hip: roentgenograms in 247 normal infants 6 and 7 months of age: follow-up of deviations from ''normal,'' J. Pediatr. **56:**478, 1960.

Harris, N.H., Lloyd-Roberts, G.C., and Gallien, R.: Acetabular development in congenital dislocation of the hip: with special reference to the indications for acetabuloplasty and pelvic or femoral realignment osteotomy, J. Bone Joint Surg. **57-B:**46, 1975.

Hart, V.L.: Primary genetic dysplasia of the hip with or without classical dislocation, J. Bone Joint Surg. **24:**753, 1942.

Hart, V.L.: Congenital dislocation of the hip in the newborn and in early post-natal life, JAMA **143:**1299, 1950.

Hass, J.: Bifurcation operation of Lorenz. In Twenty-sixth report of progress in orthopedic surgery. (Abstracted from Z. Orthop. Chir. **43:**481, 1924.)

Hass, J.: A subtrochanteric osteotomy for pelvic support, J. Bone Joint Surg. **25:**281, 1943.

Hass, J.: Congenital dislocation of the hip, Springfield, Ill., 1951, Charles C Thomas, Publisher.

Henard, D.C., and Calandruccio, R.A.: Experimental production of roentgenographic and histological changes in the capital femoral epiphysis following abduction, extension and internal rotation of the hip (abstract), J. Bone Joint Surg. **52-A:**601, 1970.

Heublein, G.W., Greene, G.S., and Conforti, V.P.: Hip joint arthrography, Am. J. Roentgen. **68:**736, 1952.

Heyman, C.H.: Long-term results following a bone-shelf operation for congenital and some other dislocations of the hip in children, J. Bone Joint Surg. **45-A:**1113, 1963.

Hiertonn, T., and James, U.: Congenital dislocation of the hip: experiences of early diagnosis and treatment, J. Bone Joint Surg. **50-B:**542, 1968.

Hilgenreiner, H.: Zur Fruhdiagnose und Fruhbehandlung der angeborenen Huftgelenkverrenkung, Med. Clin. **21:**1385, 1925.

Hoffman, D.V., Simmons, E.H., and Barrington, T.W.: The results of the Chiari osteotomy, Clin. Orthop. **98:**162, 1974.

Howorth, M.B.: Shelf stabilization of the hip, J. Bone Joint Surg. **17:**945, 1935.

Howorth, M.B.: Congenital dislocation of the hip: technic of open reduction, Ann. Surg. **135:**508, 1952.

Hoyt, W.A., Jr., Weiner, D.S., and O'Dell, H.W.: Congenital dislocation of the hip: an investigation into the efficacy of pre-manipulative traction: the prevention of aseptic necrosis of the hip (abstract), J. Bone Joint Surg. **54-A:**1799, 1972.

Ilfeld, F.W., et al.: Congenital dislocation of the hip: prognostic signs and methods of treatment with results, Clin. Orthop. **86:**21, 1972.

Ingram, A.J., and Farrar, E.L., Jr.: Congenital dysplasia of the hip: recognition and treatment, Pediatr. Clin. North Am. **2:**1081, 1955.

Jacobs, J.E.: Metatarsus varus and hip dysplasia, Clin. Orthop. **16:**203, 1960.

Jakobsson, ÅA.: The shelf operation: an evaluation of results in congenital dysplasia, subluxation, and dislocation of the hip joint, Acta Orthop. Scand. Suppl. 15, 1954.

Jones, A.R.: Congenital dislocation of the hip. In Platt, H., editor: Modern trends in orthopaedics, New York, 1950, Paul B. Hoeber, Inc.

Jones, D.A.: Sub-capital coxa valga after varus osteotomy for congenital dislocation of the hip: a report of six cases with a minimum follow-up of nine years, J. Bone Joint Surg. **59-B:**152, 1977.

Jones, E.: The operative treatment of irreducible paralytic dislocation of the hip joint, J. Orthop. Surg. **2:**183, 1920.

Jones, R., and Lovett, R.W.: Orthopedic surgery, New York, 1924, William Wood & Co.

Kalamchi, A., and MacEwen, G.D.: Avascular necrosis following treatment of congenital dislocation of the hip, J. Bone Joint Surg. **62-A:**876, 1980.

Kalamchi, A., and MacFarlane, R., III: The Pavlik harness: results in patients over three months of age, J. Pediatr. Orthop. **2:**3, 1982.

Kasser, J.R., Bowen, J.R., and MacEwen, G.D.: Varus derotation osteotomy in the treatment of persistent dysplasia in congenital dislocation of the hip, J. Bone Joint Surg. **67-A:**195, 1985.

Kenin, A., and Levine, J.: A technique for arthrography of the hip, Am. J. Roentgen. **68:**107, 1952.

Kidner, F.C.: Open reduction of congenital dislocation of the hip, J. Bone Joint Surg. **13:**799, 1931.

Kidner, F.C.: Comparative analysis of the results of open and closed reductions in congenital dislocation of the hip, J. Bone Joint Surg. **17:**25, 1935.

Kirmission, E.: De l'osteotomie sous-trochanterienne appliqué à certains cas de luxation congenitale de la hanche, Rev. Orthop. **5:**137, 1894. (Cited in Blount, W.P.: Proximal osteotomies of the femur. In American Academy of Orthopaedic Surgeons: Instructional course lectures, vol. 9, Ann Arbor, 1952, J.W. Edwards.)

Kite, J.H.: Osteochondritic changes in the head of the femur after reduction of congenital dislocation of the hip, South. Med. J. **52:**945, 1959.

Klisić, P., and Jankovic, L.: Combined procedure of open reduction and shortening of the femur in treatment of congenital dislocation of the hips in older children, Clin. Orthop. **119:**60, 1976.

Krida, A.: Congenital dislocation of the hip: the effect of anterior distortion: a procedure for its correction, J. Bone Joint Surg. **10:**594, 1928.

Krida, A.: A new departure in the treatment of congenital dislocation of the hip, J. Bone Joint Surg. **13:**811, 1931.

Kumar, S.J.: Hip spica application for the treatment of congenital dislocation of the hip, J. Pediatr. Orthop. **1:**97, 1981.

Laage, H., et al.: Horizontal lateral roentgenography of the hip in children: a preliminary report, J. Bone Joint Surg. **35-A:**387, 1953.

Lange, B.: Closed reduction of congenital dislocation of the hip, Münch. Med. Wochenschr. **51:**872, 1904.

Lange, F.: Congenital dislocation of the hip, Münch. Med. Wochenschr. **75:**2001, 1928.

Lange, F.: Need for improvement of therapeutic methods in congenital dislocation of hip, Arch. Ortop. **49:**273, 1933.

Lange, M.: Bloodless treatment of congenital dislocation of hip, Prakt. Arzt. **16:**129, 1931.

Langenskiöld, F.: Technical aspects of the operative reduction of congenital dislocation of the hip, Acta Orthop. Scand. **20:**8, 1950.

Laurenson, R.D.: The acetabular index: a critical review, J. Bone Joint Surg. **41-B:**702, 1959.

Laurent, L.E.: Capsular arthroplasty (Colonna's operation) for congenital dislocation of the hip: results of 102 operations, Acta Orthop. Scand. **34:**66, 1964.

Lauritzen, J.: Treatment of congenital dislocation of the hip in the newborn, Acta Orthop. Scand. **42:**259, 1971.

Leveuf, J.: Primary congenital subluxation of the hip, J. Bone Joint Surg. **29:**149, 1947.

Leveuf, J.: Results of open reduction of "true" congenital luxation of the hip, J. Bone Joint Surg. **30-A:**875, 1948.

Lloyd-Roberts, G.C.: Address on proximal femoral osteotomy for congenital dislocation of the hip. Delivered at the International Symposium on Congenital Hip Pathology, William Beaumont Hospital, Royal Oak, Michigan, September 1974.

Lloyd-Roberts, G.C., and Swann, M.: Pitfalls in the management of congenital dislocation of the hip, J. Bone Joint Surg. **48-B:**666, 1966.

Lorenz, A.: Über die Behandlung der irreponiblen angeborenen Hüftluxation und der Schenkelhals pseudarthrosen mittels Gabelung (Bifurkation des oberen Femurendes), Wien, Klin. Wochenschr. **32:**997, 1919. (Cited in Blount, W.P.: Proximal osteotomies of the femur. In American Academy of Orthopaedic Surgeons: Instructional course lectures, vol. 9, Ann Arbor, 1952, J.W. Edwards.)

Lorenz, A.: A new method of treatment of irreducible, acquired or congenital hip dislocations, N.Y. Med. J. **117:**130, 1923.

Ludloff, K.: The open reduction of the congenital hip dislocation by an anterior incision, Am. J. Orthop. Surg. **10:**438, 1912-1913.

MacEwen, G.D., and Ramsey, P.L.: The hip. In Lovell, W.W., and Winter, R.B., editors: Pediatric orthopaedics, Philadelphia, 1978, J.B. Lippincott.

MacKenzie, I.G., Seddon, H.J., and Trevor, D.: Congenital dislocation of the hip, J. Bone Joint Surg. **42-B:**689, 1960.

Magilligan, D.J.: Calculation of the angle of anteversion by means of horizontal lateral roentgenography, J. Bone Joint Surg. **38-A:**1231, 1956.

Massie, W.K., and Howorth, M.B.: Congenital dislocation of the hip: Part I. Method of grading results, J. Bone Joint Surg. **32-A:**519, 1950.

Massie, W.K., and Howorth, M.B.: Congenital dislocation of the hip: Part II. Results of open reduction as seen in early adult, J. Bone Joint Surg. **33-A:**171, 1951.

Massie, W.K., and Howorth, M.B.: Congenital dislocation of the hip: Part III. Pathogenesis, J. Bone Joint Surg. **33-A:**190, 1951.

Mau, H., Dorr, W.M., Henkel, L., and Lutsche, J.: Open reduction of congenital dislocation of the hip by Ludloff's method, J. Bone Joint Surg. **53-A:**1281, 1971.

McCarroll, H.R.: Early management of congenital dislocation of the hip: classification of congenital dislocation of the hip with the treatment of each type from infancy to age of eight years. In American Academy of Orthopaedic Surgeons: Instructional course lectures, vol. 4, Ann Arbor, 1948, J.W. Edwards.

McCarroll, H.R.: Primary anterior congenital dislocation of the hip, J. Bone Joint Surg. **30-A:**416, 1948.

McCarroll, H.R.: Personal communication, April 1954.

McCarroll, H.R., and Crego, C.H., Jr.: Primary anterior congenital dislocation of the hip, J. Bone Joint Surg. **21:**648, 1939.

McKay, D.W.: A comparison of the innominate and the pericapsular osteotomy in the treatment of congenital dislocation of the hip, Clin. Orthop. **98:**124, 1974.

McSweeney, A.: A comment from the periphery on inonominate osteotomy, Clin. Orthop. **98:**195, 1974.

Medbo, I.: Early diagnosis and treatment of hip joint dysplasia, Acta Orthop. Scand. **31:**282, 1961.

Medbo, I.: Follow-up study of hip joint dysplasia treated from the newborn stage, Acta Orthop. Scand. **35:**338, 1965.

Mitchell, G.P.: Arthrography in congenital displacement of the hip, J. Bone Joint Surg. **45-B:**88, 1963.

Mitchell, G.P.: Problems in the early diagnosis and management of congenital dislocation of the hip, J. Bone Joint Surg. **54-B:**4, 1972.

Mitchell, G.P.: Chiari medial displacement osteotomy, Clin. Orthop. **98:**146, 1974.

Monticelli, G.: Intertrochanteric femoral osteotomy with concentric reduction of the femoral head in treatment of residual congenital acetabular dysplasia, Clin. Orthop. **119:**48, 1976.

Morel, G.: The treatment of congenital dislocation and subluxation of the hip in the older child, Acta Orthop. Scand. **46:**364, 1975.

Mueller, F.: A new primary position in the bloodless treatment of congenital hip joint dislocation, JAMA **48:**282, 1907.

Muller, G.M., and Seddon, H.J.: Late results of treatment of congenital dislocation of the hip, J. Bone Joint Surg. **35-B:**342, 1953.

Müller, M.E., Allgöwer, M., and Willenegger, H.: Manual of internal fixation, Berlin, 1970, Springer-Verlag.

Müller, M.E., Allgöwer, M., and Willenegger, H.: Manual der osteosyntheses, 2, aufl., Berlin, 1977, Springer-Verlag.

Nalebuff, E.A., and Norton, P.L.: Congenital dislocation of the hip: studies in the early walking group, JAMA **172:**1245, 1960.

Oh, W.H.: Dislocation of the hip in birth defects, Orthop. Clin. North Am. **7:**315, 1976.

Ortolani, M.: Congenital hip dysplasia in the light of early and very early diagnosis, Clin. Orthop. **119:**6, 1976.

Ozonoff, M.B.: Controlled arthrography of the hip: a technic of fluoroscopic monitoring and recording, Clin. Orthop. **93:**260, 1973.

Packer, J.W., Lefkowitz, L.A., and Ryder, C.T.: Habitual dislocation of the hip treated by innominate osteotomy: a report of three cases, Clin. Orthop. **83:**184, 1972.

Palmén, K., and von Rosen, S.: Late diagnosis dislocation of the hip joint in children, Acta Orthop. Scand. **46:**90, 1975.

Paterson, D.C.: Innominate osteotomy: its role in the treatment of congenital dislocation and subluxation of the hip joint, Clin. Orthop. **98:**198, 1974.

Pauwels, F.: Des affections de la hanche d'origine mécanique et de leur traitement par l'ostéotomie d'adduction (Mechanical disabilities of the hip and their treatment by adduction osteotomy), Rev. Chir. Orthop. **37:**22, 1951.

Pauwels, F.: Adduction osteotomy ("Varisierung"). Personal communication to Dr. W.P. Blount, November 1954.

Pavlik, A.: Functional treatment with a harness as a principle for the conservative treatment of congenital hip dislocations in infants, Z. Orthop. **89:**341, 1957.

Pemberton, P.A.: Pericapsular osteotomy of the ilium for treatment of congenital subluxation and dislocation of the hip, J. Bone Joint Surg. **47-A:**65, 1965.

Pemberton, P.A.: Pericapsular osteotomy of the ilium for the treatment of congenitally dislocated hips, Clin. Orthop. **98:**41, 1974.

Pérez, A., and Noguera, J.G.: Experience with innominate osteotomy (Salter) and medial displacement osteotomy (Chiari) in the treatment of acetabular dysplasia: preliminary report of 82 operations, Clin. Orthop. **98:**133, 1974.

Perkins, G.: Signs by which to diagnose congenital dislocation of the hip, Lancet **1:**648, 1928.

Platou, E.: Open operation for congenital dislocation of the hip: results in 44 cases (50 hip joints), J. Bone Joint Surg. **32-B:**193, 1950.

Platou, E.: Rotation osteotomy in the treatment of congenital dislocation of the hip, J. Bone Joint Surg. **35-A:**48, 1953.

Platou, E.: Luxatio coxae congenital: a follow-up study of four hundred six cases of closed reduction, J. Bone Joint Surg. **35-A:**843, 1953.

Platt, H.: Congenital dislocation of the hip (editorial), J. Bone Joint Surg. **35-A:**339, 1953.

Poggi, A.: The classic: contribution to the radical treatment of congenital unilateral coxo-femoral dislocation, Clin. Orthop. **98:**5, 1974.

Ponseti, I.: Pathomechanics of the hip after the shelf operation, J. Bone Joint Surg. **28:**229, 1946.

Ponseti, I.: Non-surgical treatment of congenital dislocation of the hip, J. Bone Joint Surg. **48-A:**1392, 1966.

Ponseti, I., and Frigerio, E.R.: Results of treatment of congenital dislocation of the hip, J. Bone Joint Surg. **41-A:**823, 1959.

Prevention of congenital dislocation of the hip joint in Sweden: efficiency of early diagnosis and treatment. Symposium held at the annual meeting of the Swedish Orthopaedic Association in Stockholm, April 1967, Acta Orthop. Scand. Suppl. 130, 1970.

Putti, V.: Early treatment of congenital dislocation of the hip, J. Bone Joint Surg. **11:**798, 1929.

Putti, V., and Zanoli, R.: Forty-seventh report of progress in orthopedic surgery. (Abstracted from Chir. Organi. Mov. **16:**1, 1931.)

Radin, E.L., and Paul, I.L.: The biomechanics of congenital dislocated hips and their treatment, Clin. Orthop. **98:**32, 1974.

Ramsey, P.L., and Hensinger, R.N.: Congenital dislocation of the hip associated with central core disease, J. Bone Joint Surg. **57-A:**648, 1975.

Ramsey, P.L., Lasser, S., and MacEwen, G.D.: Congenital dislocation of the hip: use of the Pavlik harness in the child during the first six months of life, J. Bone Joint Surg. **58-A:**1000, 1976.

Ring, P.A.: The treatment of unreduced congenital dislocation of the hip in adults, J. Bone Joint Surg. **41-B:**299, 1959.

Ritter, M.A., and Wilson, P.D.: Colonna capsular arthroplasty: a long-term follow-up of forty hips, J. Bone Joint Surg. **50-A:**1305, 1968.

Roth, A., Gibson, D.A., and Hall, J.E.: The experience of five orthopedic surgeons with innominate osteotomy in the treatment of congenital dislocation and subluxation of the hip, Clin. Orthop. **98:**178, 1974.

Ryder, C.T.: Congenital dislocation of the hip in the older child: surgical treatment, J. Bone Joint Surg. **48-A:**1404, 1966.

Ryder, C.T., and Crane, L.: Measuring femoral anteversion: the problem and a method, J. Bone Joint Surg. **35-A:**289, 1953.

Salter, R.B.: Innominate osteotomy in the treatment of congenital dislocation and subluxation of the hip, J. Bone Joint Surg. **43-B:**518, 1961.

Salter, R.B.: Role of innominate osteotomy in the treatment of congenital dislocation and subluxation of the hip in the older child, J. Bone Joint Surg. **48-A:**1413, 1966.

Salter, R.B.: Specific guidelines in the application of the principle of innominate osteotomy, Orthop. Clin. North Am. **3:**149, 1972.

Salter, R.B.: Editorial comment: osteotomy of the pelvis, Clin. Orthop. **98:**2, 1974.

Salter, R.B., and Dubos, J.P.: The first fifteen years' personal experience with innominate osteotomy in the treatment of congenital dislocation and subluxation of the hip, Clin. Orthop. **98:**72, 1974.

Salter, R.B., Hansson, G., and Thompson, G.H.: Innominate osteotomy in the management of residual congenital subluxation of the hip in young adults, Clin. Orthop. **182:**53, 1984.

Salvati, E.A., and Wilson, P.D.: Treatment of irreducible hip subluxation by Chiari's iliac osteotomy: a report of results in 19 cases, Clin. Orthop. **98:**151, 1974.

Scaglietti, O., and Calandriello, B.: Open reduction of congenital dislocation of the hip, J. Bone Joint Surg. **44-B:**275, 1962.

Schanz, A.: Zur Behandlung der veralteten angeborenen Hüftverrenkung, Münch. Med. Wochenschr. **69:**930, 1922.

Schede: Cited by Bade in Krida, A.: Congenital dislocation of the hip: the effect of anterior distortion: a procedure for its correction, J. Bone Joint Surg. **10:**594, 1928.

Schoenecker, P.L., and Strecker, W.B.: Congenital dislocation of the hip in children: comparison of the effects of femoral shortening and of skeletal traction in treatment, J. Bone Joint Surg. **66-A:**21, 1984.

Schwartz, D.R.: Acetabular development after reduction of congenital dislocation of the hip: a follow-up study of fifty hips, J. Bone Joint Surg. **47-A:**705, 1965.

Scott, J.C.: Frame reduction and congenital dislocation of the hip, J. Bone Joint Surg. **35-B:**372, 1953.

Seddon, H.J.: Congenital dislocation of the hip: intermediate-late results of standard methods of treatment, J. Bone Joint Surg. **33-B:**281, 1951.

Serafinov, L.: Biomechanical influence of the innominate osteotomy on the growth of the upper part of the femur, Clin. Orthop. **98:**39, 1974.

Severin, E.: Arthrography in congenital dislocation of the hip, J. Bone Joint Surg. **21:**304, 1939.

Severin, E.: Contribution to the knowledge of congenital dislocation of the hip joint: late results of closed reduction and arthrographic studies of recent cases, Acta Chir. Scand. **84**(Suppl. 63):1, 1941.

Severin, E.: Congenital dislocation of the hip: development of the joint after closed reduction, J. Bone Joint Surg. **32-A:**507, 1950.

Shenton, E.W.A.: Diseases in bone, London, 1911, Macmillan.

Siffert, R.S., Ehrlich, M.G., and Katz, J.F.: Management of congenital dislocation of the hip, Clin. Orthop. **86:**28, 1972.

Smaill, G.B.: Congenital dislocation of the hip in the newborn, J. Bone Joint Surg. **50-B:**524, 1968.

Smith, A.R.: Shelving operation as adjunct to open reduction in congenital dislocated hip and its use in paralytic and pathologic dislocations, Ann. Surg. **106:**278, 1937.

Smith, W.S., Badgley, C.E., Orwig, J.B., and Harper, J.M.: Correlation of postreduction roentgenograms and thirty-one-year follow-up in congenital dislocation of the hip, J. Bone Joint Surg. **50-A:**1081, 1968.

Somerville, E.W.: Development of congenital dislocation of the hip, J. Bone Joint Surg. **35-B:**568, 1953.

Somerville, E.W.: Open reduction in congenital dislocation of hip, J. Bone Joint Surg. **35-B:**363, 1953.

Somerville, E.W.: Persistent foetal alignment of the hip, J. Bone Joint Surg. **39-B:**106, 1957.

Somerville, E.W.: Results of treatment of 100 congenitally dislocated hips, J. Bone Joint Surg. **49-B:**258, 1967.

Somerville, E.W.: A long-term follow-up of congenital dislocation of the hip, J. Bone Joint Surg. **60-B:**25, 1978.

Somerville, E.W., and Scott, J.C.: The direct approach to congenital dislocation of the hip, J. Bone Joint Surg. **39-B:**623, 1957.

Sommer, J.: Atypical hip click in the newborn, Acta Orthop. Scand. **42:**353, 1971.

Staheli, L.T.: Technique: slotted acetabular augmentation, J. Pediatr. Orthop. **1:**321, 1981.

Steel, H.H.: Triple osteotomy of the innominate bone, J. Bone Joint Surg. **55-A:**343, 1973.

Steindler, A., Kulowski, J., and Freund, E.: Congenital dislocation of the hip: statistical analysis, JAMA **104:**302, 1935.

Sutherland, D.H., and Greenfield, R.: Double innominate osteotomy, J. Bone Joint Surg. **59-A:**1082, 1977.

Swett, P.P.: An operation for the reduction of certain types of congenital dislocation of the hip, J. Bone Joint Surg. **10:**675, 1928.

Thompson, F.R.: The early diagnosis and early treatment of congenital dislocation of the hip, N.Y. J. Med. **44:**1095, 1944.

Thomson, J.E.M.: The Jan Zahradnicek surgical approach to the problem of congenital hip dislocation, Clin. Orthop. **8:**237, 1956.

Trevor, D.: Treatment of congenital dislocation of the hip (editorial), J. Bone Joint Surg. **39-B:**611, 1957.

Trevor, D.: Treatment of congenital hip dysplasia in older children: president's address, Proc. R. Soc. Med. **53:**481, 1960.

Trevor, D., Johns, D.L., and Fixsen, J.A.: Acetabuloplasty in the treatment of congenital dislocation of the hip, J. Bone Joint Surg. **57-B:**167, 1975.

Utterback, T.D., and MacEwen, G.D.: Comparison of pelvic osteotomies for the surgical correction of the congenital hip, Clin. Orthop. **98:**104, 1974.

von Baeyer, H.: Behandlung von nicht-reponerbaren angeborenen Hüftverrenkungen, Münch. Med. Wochenschr. **65:**1216, 1918. (Cited in Blount, W.P.: Proximal osteotomies of the femur. In American Academy of Orthopaedic Surgeons: Instructional course lectures, vol. 9, Ann Arbor, 1952, J.W. Edwards.)

von Rosen, S.: Early diagnosis and treatment of congenital dislocation of the hip joint, Acta Orthop. Scand. **26:**136, 1957.

von Rosen, S.: Diagnosis and treatment of congenital dislocation of the hip joint in the newborn, J. Bone Joint Surg. **44-B:**284, 1962.

von Rosen, S.: The long-term results of early diagnosis and treatment of congenital dislocation of the hip, Dixième Congrès Internationale de Chirurgie Orthopédique et de Traumatologie, Paris, September 1966.

von Rosen, S.: Further experience with congenital dislocation of the hip in the newborn, J. Bone Joint Surg. **50-B:**538, 1968.

Wagner, H.: Osteotomies for congenital hip dislocation. In The Hip Society: Proceedings of the fourth open scientific meeting of The Hip Society, 1976, St. Louis, 1976, The C.V. Mosby Co.

Wagner, H.: Femoral osteotomies for congenital hip dislocation. In Weil, V.H., editor: Progress in orthopaedic surgery, vol. 2, Berlin, 1978, Springer-Verlag.

Watanabe, R.S.: Embryology of the human hip, Clin. Orthop. **98:**8, 1974.

Congenital and developmental coxa vara

Amstutz, H.C.: Developmental (infantile) coxa vara: a distinct entity. Report of two patients with previously normal roentgenograms, Clin. Orthop. **72:**242, 1970.

Amstutz, H.C., and Wilson, P.D., Jr.: Dysgenesis of the proximal femur (coxa vara) and its surgical management, J. Bone Joint Surg. **44-A:**1, 1962.

Babb, F.S., Ghormley, R.K., and Chatterton, C.C.: Congenital coxa vara, J. Bone Joint Surg. **31-A:**115, 1949.

Barr, J.S.: Congenital coxa vara, Arch. Surg. **18:**1909, 1929.

Becton, J.L., and Diamond, L.S.: Persistent limp in congenital coxa vara, South. Med. J. **60:**921, 1967.

Blount, W.P.: The valgus position in osteotomies. Personal communication, December 1954.

Borden, J., Spencer, G.E., Jr., and Herndon, C.H.: Treatment of coxa vara in children by means of a modified osteotomy, J. Bone Joint Surg. **48-A:**1106, 1966.

Calhoun, J.D., and Pierre, G.: Infantile coxa vara. Am. J. Roentgen. **115:**561, 1972.

Cleveland, M., Bosworth, D.M., and Della Pietra, A.: Subtrochanteric osteotomy and spline fixation for certain disabilities of the hip joint, J. Bone Joint Surg. **33-A:**351, 1951.

Duncan, G.A.: Congenital and developmental coxa vara, Surgery **3:**741, 1938.

Fairbank, H.A.T.: Infantile or cervical coxa vara. In The Robert Jones birthday volume, London, 1928, Oxford University Press.

Fisher, R.L., and Waskowitz, W.J.: Familial developmental coxa vara, Clin. Orthop. **86:**2, 1972.

Golding, F.C.: Congenital coxa vara and the short femur, Proc. R. Soc. Med. **32:**641, 1938.

Golding, F.C.: Congenital coxa vara, J. Bone Joint Surg. **30-B:**160, 1948.

Haas, S.L.: Lengthening of the femur with simultaneous correction of coxa vara, J. Bone Joint Surg. **15:**219, 1933.

Horwitz, T.: Treatment of congenital (or developmental) coxa vara, Surg. Gynecol. Obstet. **87:**71, 1948.

Johanning, K.: Coxa vara infantum: II. Treatment and results of treatment, Acta Orthop. Scand. **22:**100, 1952.

LeMesurier, A.B.: Developmental coxa vara, J. Bone Joint Surg. **30-B:**595, 1948.

LeMesurier, A.B.: Developmental coxa vara (letter to the editor), J. Bone Joint Surg. **33-B:**478, 1951.

LoCoco, S.J., Pusateri, W.M., and Newman, W.H.: Intramedullary fixation after subtrochanteric osteotomy for coxa vara and coxa valga deformities in children, South. Med. J. **66:**1379, 1973.

MacEwen, G.D., and Shands, A.R., Jr.: Oblique trochanteric osteotomy, J. Bone Joint Surg. **49-A:**345, 1967.

Pauwels, F.: The operative management of infantile coxa vara, Verh. Dtsch. Orthop. Ges. (30 Kongress), 1935.

Pauwels, F.: The "Y-osteotomy" in congenital coxa vara. Personal communication to Dr. W.P. Blount, November 1954.

Peabody, C.W.: Subtrochanteric osteotomy in coxa vara, Arch. Surg. **46:**743, 1943.

Pylkkänen, P.V.: Coxa vara infantum, Acta Orthop. Scand. Suppl. **48,** 1960.

Roberts, W.M.: End result study of congenital coxa vara: treated by the Haas trochanteric osteotomy, South. Med. J. **43:**389, 1950.

Wedge, J.H., and Salter, R.B.: Innominate osteotomy: its role in the arrest of secondary degenerative arthritis of the hip in the adult, Clin. Orthop. **98:**214, 1974.

Werndorff, R.: Axillary abduction in the treatment of congenital dislocation of the hip, Z. Orthop. Chir. **13:**765, 1904.

Wiberg, G.: Shelf operation in congenital dysplasia of the acetabulum and in subluxation and dislocation of the hip, J. Bone Joint Surg. **35-A:**65, 1953.

Wilkinson, J.A.: A post-natal survey for congenital displacement of the hip, J. Bone Joint Surg. **54-B:**40, 1972.

Wilkinson, J., and Carter, C.: Congenital dislocation of the hip: the results of conservative treatment, J. Bone Joint Surg. **42-B:**669, 1960.

Wilson, J.C., Jr.: Surgical treatment of the dysplastic acetabulum in adolescence, Clin. Orthop. **98:**137, 1974.

Wynne-Davies, R.: Acetabular dysplasia and familial joint laxity: two etiological factors in congenital dislocation of the hip: a review of 589 patients and their families, J. Bone Joint Surg. **52-B:**704, 1970.

Zadek, I.: Congenital coxa vara, Arch. Surg. **30:**62, 1935.

Exstrophy of bladder

Aadlen, R.J., et al.: Exstrophy of the bladder: long-term results of bilateral posterior iliac osteotomies and two-stage anatomic repair, Clin. Orthop. **151:**193, 1980.

Aadalen, R.J., O'Phelan, H., Sweetser, T.H., Jr., Chisholm, T.C., and McParland, F.A., Jr.: Exstrophy of the bladder: long term results of bilateral posterior iliac osteotomies and two stage anterior repair (abstract), Orthop. Trans. **1:**93, May 1977.

Chisholm, T.C.: Exstrophy of the bladder. In Benson, C.C., et al.: editors: Pediatric surgery, vol. 2, Chicago, 1962, Year Book Medical Publishers, Inc.

Cracciolo, A., III, and Hall, C.B.: Bilateral iliac osteotomy: the first stage in repair of exstrophy of the bladder, Clin. Orthop. **68:**156, 1970.

Furnas, D.W., Haq, M.A., and Somers, G.: One-stage reconstruction for exstrophy of the bladder in girls, Plast. Reconstr. Surg. **56:**61, 1975.

Grotte, G., and Sevastikoglou, J.A.: A modified technique for pelvic reconstruction in the treatment of exstrophy of the bladder, Acta Orthop. Scand. **37:**197, 1966.

O'Phelan, E.H.: Iliac osteotomy in exstrophy of the bladder, J. Bone Joint Surg. **45-A:**1409, 1963.

Sweetser, T.H., et al.: Exstrophy of the urinary bladder: its treatment by plastic surgery, J. Urol. **75:**448, 1956.

Trendelenburg, F.: The treatment of ectopia vesicae, Ann. Surg. **44:**281, 1906.

CHAPTER 63

Congenital anomalies of trunk and upper extremity

James H. Beaty

In this chapter are discussed congenital torticollis, congenital elevation of the scapula, and congenital pseudarthrosis of the clavicle, radius, and ulna. Congenital anomalies of the hand and certain others of the forearm are discussed in Chapter 16.

CONGENITAL TORTICOLLIS OR WRYNECK

Congenital torticollis or wryneck is caused by fribromatosis within the sternocleidomastoid muscle. As is true of all fibromatoses, its cause is unknown. The tumor either is palpable at birth or becomes so usually during the first 2 weeks. It is more common on the right than on the left. It may involve the muscle diffusely, but more often it is localized near the clavicular attachment of the muscle. It attains maximum size within 1 or 2 months and then may remain the same size or become smaller; usually it diminishes and disappears within a year. If it fails to disappear, then the muscle becomes permanently fibrotic and contracted and causes torticollis that is also permanent unless treated.

There is a reported incidence of congenital dislocation of the hip or dysplasia of the acetabulum ranging from 7% to 20% in children with torticollis. Careful screening, and if necessary, roentgenographic examination is indicated.

When congenital torticollis is seen in early infancy, it is impossible to tell whether the tumor causing it will disappear spontaneously. Consequently during infancy only conservative treatment is indicated. The parents should be instructed to stretch the sternocleidomastoid muscle by manipulating the head manually and by positioning it during sleep. Excising the lesion during infancy is unjustified; surgery should be delayed until evolution of the fibromatosis is complete, and then, if necessary, the muscle may be released at one or both ends or may be excised. Coventry and Harris, in a study of 35 infants with congenital torticollis seen at the Mayo Clinic, found that conservative treatment at home by the family produced excellent results

in 30. In only 5 was surgical release of the muscle necessary. They believe that if the muscle is still contracted after the age of 1 year it should be released, but they also believe that surgery at any age up to 12 years would produce as good a result as operation earlier because asymmetry of the face and skull could still correct itself during the remaining period of growth.

Canale et al. evaluated 57 patients with congenital torticollis who were treated between 1941 and 1977 at this clinic. The average follow-up was 18.9 years. They found that if congenital torticollis persisted beyond the age of 1 year, it did not resolve spontaneously. Children with torticollis who were treated during the first year of life had better results than those treated later, and an exercise program was more likely to be successful when the restriction of motion was less than 30 degrees and there was no facial asymmetry or the facial asymmetry was noted only by the examiner. Nonoperative therapy after the age of 1 year was rarely successful. Regardless of the type of treatment, established facial asymmetry and limitation of motion of more than 30 degrees at the beginning of treatment usually precluded a good result. While these 57 patients had little functional abnormality at follow-up (some of those with a persistent head tilt had mild, asymptomatic compensatory scoliosis), noticeable cosmetic deformity was present in approximately 31% of the patients.

Any permanent torticollis becomes worse during growth. The head becomes inclined toward the affected side and the face toward the opposite side. When the deformity is severe, the ipsilateral shoulder becomes elevated, and the frontooccipital diameter of the skull may become shorter than normal. Such severe deformity could and should be prevented by surgery during childhood. Unfortunately many patients are first seen only after the deformities have become fixed and the remaining growth potential is insufficient to correct them.

Several operations have been devised to release the sternocleidomastoid muscle at the clavicle. Subcutaneous tenotomy of the clavicular attachment of the muscle has been successful but is condemned because it is inaccurate and dangerous. Anomalies of the external jugular vein and of the clavicular attachment of the muscle are common, and the vein or even the phrenic nerve could be severed during this procedure. Operations have also been devised to excise the muscle or to free its attachment on the mastoid process.

Ling, in a review of 103 patients treated for torticollis, found that open tenotomy of the sternocleidomastoid muscle could be followed by tethering of the scar to the deep structures, reattachment of the clavicular head or the sternal head of the sternocleidomastoid muscle, loss of contour of the muscle, failure to correct the tilt of the head, or failure of facial asymmetry to correct. Because tethering of the scar to the deep structures is common before the age of 1 year, he recommends that the operation be delayed until later. In children treated surgically between the ages of 1 and 4 years, tilt of the head and facial asymmetry were usually corrected satisfactorily and motion of the neck was improved. In children over 5 years old correction of the secondary deformities became less certain, and the complications of loss of countour of the sternocleidomastoid muscle, disfiguring scarring, or reattachment of the muscle were more common. He concluded that the best time for surgery is between the ages of 1 and 4 years.

TECHNIQUE. Make an incision 5 cm long just superior to and parallel to the medial end of the clavicle (Fig. 63-1, A) and deepen it to the tendons of the sternal and clavicular attachments of the sternocleidomastoid muscle. Incise the tendon sheath longitudinally and pass a hemostat or other blunt instrument posterior to the tendons. Then by traction on the hemostat draw the tendons outside the wound (Fig. 63-1, B) and then superior and inferior to the hemostat clamp them and resect 2.5 cm of their inferior ends. If contracted, divide the platysma muscle and adjacent fascia. Then with the head turned toward the affected side and the chin depressed, explore the wound digitally for any remaining bands of contracted muscle or fascia, and if any are found, divide them under direct vision until the deformity can, if possible, be overcorrected. If after this procedure overcorrection is not possible, then make a small transverse incision inferior to the mastoid process and carefully divide the muscle near the bone. Take care to avoid damaging the spinal accessory nerve (Fig. 63-2).

Close the wound or wounds and apply a bulky dressing that holds the head in the overcorrected position.

AFTERTREATMENT. At 1 week physical therapy, including manual stretching of the neck to maintain the overcorrected position, is begun, Manual stretching should be continued three times daily for 3 to 6 months. During this time the patient may sleep with halter traction on the head. The use of plaster casts or braces is usually unnecessary (Fig. 63-3).

• • •

Surgical correction in older children or after failed operation usually requires a bipolar release of the sternocleidomastoid muscle. Ferkel et al. described a modified bipolar release and Z-plasty of the muscle for use in these circumstances.

TECHNIQUE (FERKEL ET AL.). Make a short transverse proximal incision behind the ear (Fig. 63-4, A) and divide the sternocleidomastoid muscle insertion transversely just distal to the tip of the mastoid process. With this limited incision the spinal accessory nerve is avoided, although the possibility that the nerve may take an anomalous route is always borne in mind. Then make a distal incision, 4 to 5 cm long in line with the cervical skin creases one fingerbreadth proximal to the medial end of the clavicle and the sternal notch. Never make the skin incision superficial to the clavicle because according to Ferkel et al., a scar located here may spread to a cosmetically unacceptable extent. Divide the subcutaneous tissue and platysma muscle, exposing the clavicular and sternal attachments of the sternocleidomastoid muscle. Carefully avoid the anterior and external jugular veins and the carotid vessels and sheath during the dissection. Then cut the clavicular portion of the muscle transversely and perform a z-plasty on the sternal attachment so as to preserve the normal v-contour of

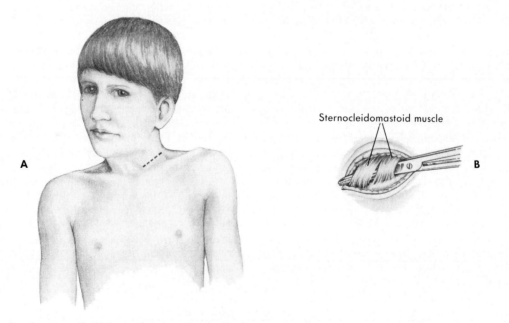

Fig. 63-1. Operation for torticollis. **A,** Line of skin incision. **B,** Clavicular and sternal attachments of sternocleidomastoid muscle withdrawn from wound and divided.

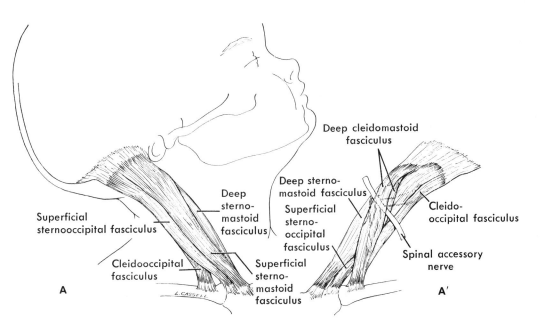

Fig. 63-2. Anatomy of sternocleidomastoid muscle. **A,** External view and, **A′,** deep view of right sternoclei-domastoid muscle showing muscle bellies and their relation to spinal accessory nerve. (Modified from Chandler, F.A., and Altenberg, A.: JAMA **125:**476, 1944.)

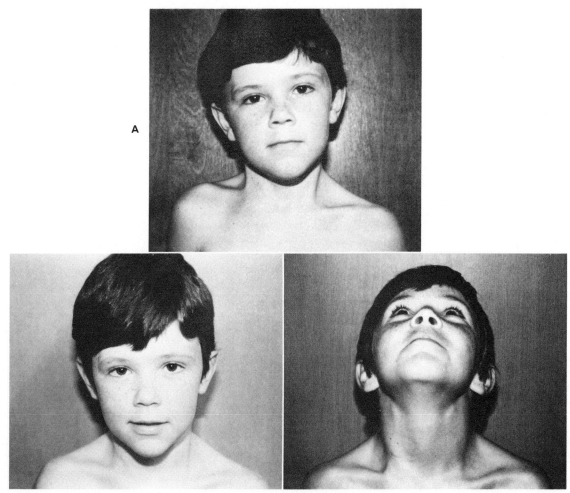

Fig. 63-3. Seven-year-old male with right torticollis. **A,** Before unipolar supraclavicular release. **B,** After unipolar supraclavicular release. **C,** Note scar 1 to 2 finger breadths superior to clavicle in transverse line of skin creases.

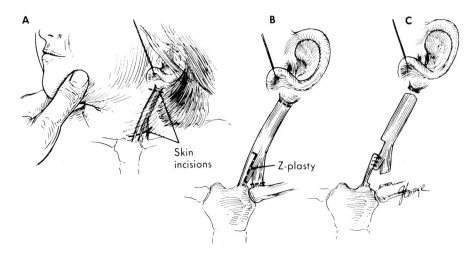

Fig. 63-4. Z-plasty operation for torticollis. **A,** Location of skin incisions. **B,** Clavicular and mastoid attachments of sternocleidomastoid muscle are cut and Z-plasty is performed on sternal origin. **C,** Completed operation is shown. Note that medial portion of sternal attachment is preserved. (From Ferkel, R.D., et al.: J. Bone Joint Surg. **65-A:**894, 1983.)

the sternocleidomastoid muscle in the neckline (Fig. 63-4, *B* and *C*). Obtain the desired degree of correction by manipulating the head and neck during the release. Occasionally, release of additional contracted bands of fascia or muscle is necessary before closure. Close both wounds with subcuticular sutures.

AFTERTREATMENT. Head-halter traction is used for 2 to 4 weeks, followed by the use of a Plastizote cervical collar in an overcorrected position for 3 to 4 months. Physical therapy consisting of stretching and muscle-strengthening exercises is then instituted.

CONGENITAL ELEVATION OF SCAPULA (SPRENGEL'S DEFORMITY)

In Sprengel's deformity, the scapula lies more superiorly than it should in relation to the thoracic cage and is usually hypoplastic and misshapen. Usually other congenital anomalies are present such as cervical ribs, malformations of ribs, and anomalies of the cervical vertebrae (Klippel-Feil syndrome); rarely one or more scapular muscles are partly or completely absent. Disability is never severe unless the deformity too is severe. When the deformity is mild, the scapula is only slightly elevated and is a bit smaller than normal, and its motion is only mildly limited, but when it is severe, the scapula is very small and may be so elevated that it almost touches the occiput. The patient's head is often deviated toward the affected side. In about one third of the patients an extra ossicle, the omovertebral bone, is present: this is a rhomboidal plaque of cartilage and bone, lying in a strong fascial sheath, that extends from the superior angle of the scapula to the spinous process, lamina, or transverse process of one or more lower cervical vertebrae. Sometimes a well-developed joint is found between it and the scapula; sometimes it is attached to the scapula by fibrous tissue only; rarely it makes a solid osseous ridge between the spinal column and the scapula.

When deformity and disability are mild, no treatment is indicated; when they are more severe, surgery may be indicated, depending on the age of the patient and the severity of any associated deformities. The results of surgery are occasionally disappointing because the deformity is never simply elevation of the scapula alone; it is always complicated by malformations and contractures of the soft structures of the region.

An operation to bring the scapula inferiorly to near its normal position may be attempted after about 3 years of age; before then the operation is probably too extensive. However, the earlier surgery is performed after 3 years of age, the better are the results because as the child grows the operation becomes more difficult and ultimately impossible. In older children an attempt to bring the scapula inferiorly to its normal level may seriously stretch and damage the brachial plexus.

Numerous operations have been described to correct Sprengel's deformity. Two surgical techniques are commonly used. Green described surgical release of muscles from the scapula along with excision of the supraspinatus portion of the scapula and any omovertebral bone. The scapula is them moved inferiorly to a more normal position and the muscles are reattached. Woodward described transfer of the origin of the trapezius muscle to a more inferior position on the spinous processes. We have had more experience with the Woodward procedure, and have been pleased with the results.

Brachial plexus palsy is the most severe complication of surgery for Sprengel's deformity. The scapula in this deformity is hypoplastic compared with the normal scapula. At surgery attention should be directed at placing the spine of the scapula at the same level as that on the opposite side, rather than aligning exactly the inferior angle of the scapulae. Several authors have recommended morcellation of the clavicle on the ipsilateral side as a first step in the operative treatment of Sprengel's deformity to avoid bra-

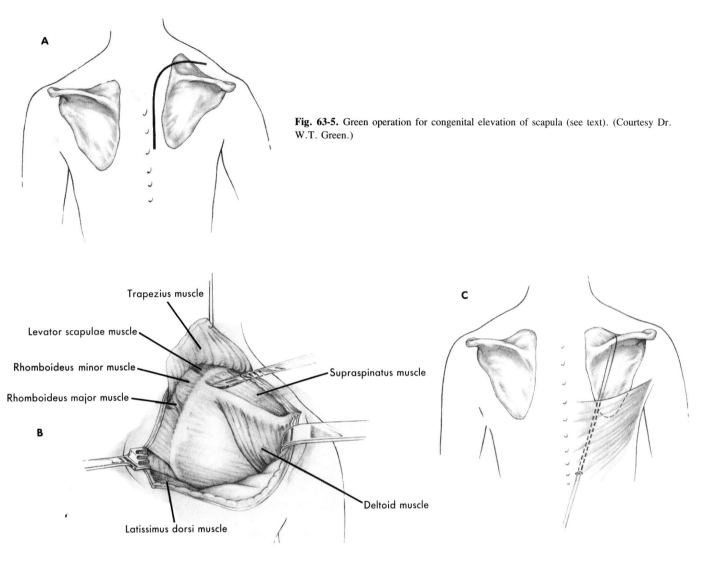

Fig. 63-5. Green operation for congenital elevation of scapula (see text). (Courtesy Dr. W.T. Green.)

chial plexus palsy. We have not included this as a routine part of our surgical treatment, but recommend it in severe deformity or in children who show signs of brachial plexus palsy following surgical correction.

TECHNIQUE (GREEN). Make a skin incision beginning one fingerbreadth superior to the middle of the scapular spine, coursing medially parallel with the spine to the medial margin of the bone, then curving distally parallel with and one thumbbreadth medial to this margin, and ending about 5 cm distal to the inferior angle (Fig. 63-5, *A*). Next reflect the deep fascia to expose the insertion of the trapezius on the scapular spine; free this insertion extraperiosteally, and as will all other muscles freed in this operation, place silk sutures in its freed end to mark it for reattachment later. Now reflect the trapezius medially to expose the levator scapulae, the rhomboideus major and minor, and the supraspinatus (Fig. 63-5, *B*). By extraperiosteal dissection free the supraspinatus from its fossa laterally to the scapular notch and retract it laterally. Carefully avoid the suprascapular nerve and transverse scapular artery that pass through this notch. Again extraperiosteally dissect the rhomboideus major and minor from the medial margin of

the scapula and the levator scapulae from the superior margin. Now again by extraperiosteal dissection separate from the anterior surface of the bone that part of the subscapularis that lies superior to the level of the scapular spine. Retract posteriorly the superior margin of the scapula to expose the anterior surface of the bone superior to the level of its spine. With an osteotome or bone-cutting forceps divide the scapula along the base of its spine laterally to the scapular notch. Then remove the supraspinous part of the scapula along with its periosteum. Next extraperiosteally excise any omovertebral bone. Now, again extraperiosteally, free the serratus anterior from its insertion along the medial margin of the scapula; before freeing it from the inferior angle, divide the origin of the latissimus dorsi from the spinous processes distally to a level just inferior to the most inferior fibers of origin of the trapezius. Then free the serratus anterior from the inferior angle. Divide any heavy fibrous bands extending from the inferior angle to the chest wall. These fibers lie close to the serratus anterior and must be completely divided before the scapula can be displaced enough distally. Next at the junction of its medial two thirds and lateral one third drill a hole in the base of the scapular spine. Through this hole insert a heavy wire about 90 cm long. Direct the two free ends of the wire posterior to the scapula and the infraspinatus and deep to the latissimus dorsi to emerge through the skin about 7.5 cm inferior to the anticipated position of the inferior angle of the scapula and pointing toward the middle of the buttock on the opposite side (Fig. 63-5). Now displace the scapula distally to the desired position with its inferior angle lying deep to the latissimus dorsi. Reattach the muscles as follows. Attach the supraspinatus to the scapular spine. Reattach the serratus anterior in line with the natural pull of its fibers in a new position more superior on the scapula. Using the same principle, reattach the levator scapulae and the rhomboideus major and minor; if necessary, lengthen the levator scapulae. Next reattach the inferior part of the trapezius tightly to the scapular spine 2 to 3 cm farther laterally than the spot from which it was removed. This increases its tension both inferiorly and medially so that it will hold the scapula in the distal position. Now reattach the superior part of the trapezius 2.5 cm more medial than before; this results in a relative lengthening of the superior fibers of the muscle. Then lap the divided part of the latissimus dorsi over the distal part of the trapezius and reattach it to the spinous processes at its normal level or, if necessary to better cover the inferior angle of the scapula, advance its attachment to a higher level on the spinous processes. Finally suture the superior edge of the latissimus dorsi to the inferior lateral edge of the trapezius. Place the patient in a previously prepared bivalved spica cast incorporating the leg opposite the side of the affected scapula. Fix a spring scale to the free ends of the wire attached to the scapula. Distally attach the scale by a strap to a ring in the spica. Cut a small groove in the cast to protect the scale and adjust the amount of pull as desired (usually about 3 pounds or 1.35 kg).

AFTERTREATMENT. At 4 or 5 days exercises to preserve and increase motion in the affected shoulder are begun. At about 3 weeks the cast and wire are removed without anesthesia. The limb is then protected in a sling between exercise periods for a few weeks. The exercises are continued until motion in the shoulder girdle is as near normal as possible; at 3 months overhead trapeze work and other strenuous abduction exercises are encouraged.

TECHNIQUE (WOODWARD). Place the patient prone on the operating table and prepare and drape the shoulder so that both the involved shoulder girdle and the arm can be manipulated. Make a midline incision from the spinous process of the first cervical vertebra distally to that of the ninth dorsal. Undermine the skin and subcutaneous tissues laterally to the medial border of the scapula. Next identify the lateral border of the trapezius in the distal end of the incision and by blunt dissection separate it from the underlying latissimus dorsi muscle. By sharp dissection free the fascial sheath of origin of the trapezius from the spinous processes. Identify the origins of the rhomboideus major and minor muscles and by sharp dissection free them from the spinous processes. Now free the rhomboids and the superior part of the trapezius from the muscles of the chest wall anterior to them. Retract the freed sheet of muscles laterally to expose any omovertebral bone of fibrous bands attached to the superior angle of the scapula (Fig. 63-6,

B). By extraperiosteal dissection excise any omovertebral bone, or if the bone is absent, excise any fibrous band or contracted levator scapulae; avoid injuring the spinal accessory nerve, the nerves to the rhomboids, or the transverse cervical artery. If the supraspinous part of the scapula is deformed, resect it along with its periosteum; this releases the levator scapulae (if not already excised), allowing the shoulder girdle to move more freely. Divide transversely the remaining narrow attachment of the trapezius at the level of the fourth cervical vertebra. Now displace the scapula along with the attached sheet of muscles distally until its spine lies at the same level as that of the opposite scapula. While holding the scapula in this position, reattach the aponeuroses of the trapezius and rhomboids to the spinous processes at a more inferior level (Fig. 63-6, *C* and *D*). In the distal part of the incision create a fold in the origin of the trapezius and either excise the excess tissue or incise the fold and overlap and suture in place the resultant free edges.

AFTERTREATMENT. A Velpeau bandage is applied and is worn for about 2 weeks. Figs. 63-7 and 63-8 show Sprengel's deformity in one patient and status after surgery in another.

TECHNIQUE OR MORCELLATION OF CLAVICLE (ROBINNSON ET AL., CHUNG AND FARAHVAR). Make a straight incision directly over the clavicle extending from 1.5 cm lateral to the sternoclavicular joint to 1.5 cm medial to the acromioclavicular joint. Expose the clavicle subperiosteally. Now divide the bone 2 cm from each end, remove it, and cut it into small pieces (morcellate). Then replace the pieces in the periosteal tube and close the tube with interrupted sutures. Close the subcutaneous tissues and skin in a routine manner. Then place the patient prone and perform the operation on the scapula itself.

CONGENITAL RADIOULNAR SYNOSTOSIS

Congenital radioulnar synostosis usually involves the proximal ends of the bones, fixing the forearm in pronation (Fig. 63-9). It is more often bilateral than unilateral. Often there is a familial predisposition, and the deformity seems to be transmitted on the paternal side of the family. Wilkie has noted two types. In the first the medullary canals of the radius and ulna are joined. The proximal end of the radius is malformed and is fused to the ulna for a distance of several centimeters. The radius is longer and larger than the ulna, and its shaft arches anteriorly more than normally. In the second type the radius is fairly normal, but its proximal end is dislocated either anteriorly or posteriorly and is fused to the proximal ulnar shaft; the fusion is neither as extensive nor as intimate as in the first type. Wilkie states that the second type is often unilateral and that sometimes other deformity, such as a supernumerary thumb, absence of the thumb, or syndactylism, is also present.

Congenital radioulnar synostosis is for several important reasons difficult to treat. The fascial tissues are short and their fibers are abnormally directed, the interosseous membrane is narrow, and the supinator muscles may be abnormal or absent. The anomalies in the forearm may be so widespread that sometimes no rotation is possible, even after the radius and ulna have been separated and the in-

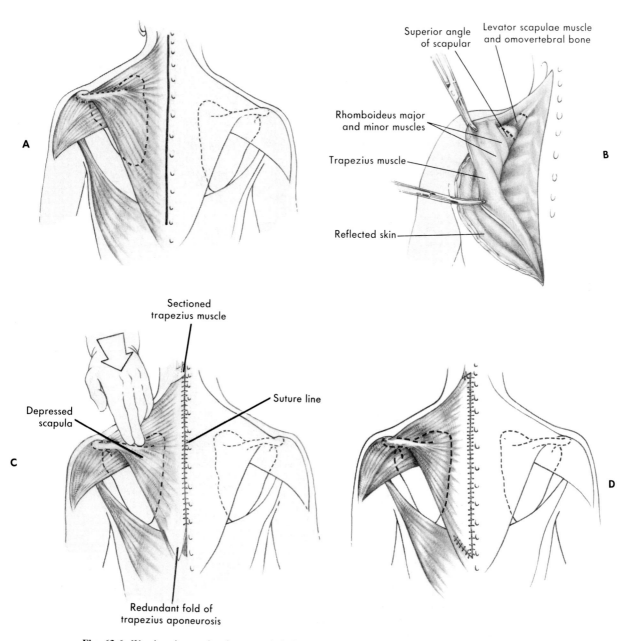

Fig. 63-6. Woodward operation for congenital elevation of scapula. **A,** Elevation of scapula and extensive origin of trapezius, and skin incision are shown. **B,** Skin has been incised in midline. Origins of trapezius and of rhomboideus major and minor have been freed from spinous processes, and these muscles have been retracted laterally. Levator scapulae, any omovertebral bone, and any deformed superior angle of scapula are to be excised. **C,** Remaining narrow attachment of trapezius superiorly has been divided at level of C-4. Scapula and attached sheet of muscles have been displaced inferiorly, and aponeuroses of trapezius and rhomboids have been reattached to spinous processes at more inferior level. Thus a redundant fold of trapezius aponeurosis is formed inferiorly. **D,** Fold of trapezius aponeurosis has been incised, and resultant free edges have been overlapped and sutured in place. Free superior edge of trapezius has also been sutured. (Modified from Woodward, J.W.: J. Bone Joint Surg. **43-A:**219, 1961.)

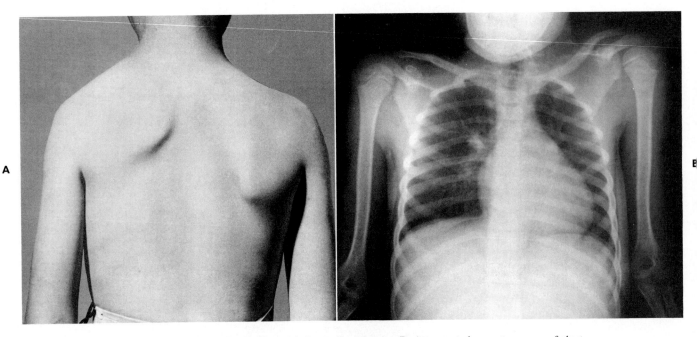

Fig. 63-7. A, Five-year-old male with left Sprengel's deformity. **B,** Anteroposterior roentgenogram of chest and arms demonstrating congenital elevation of left scapula.

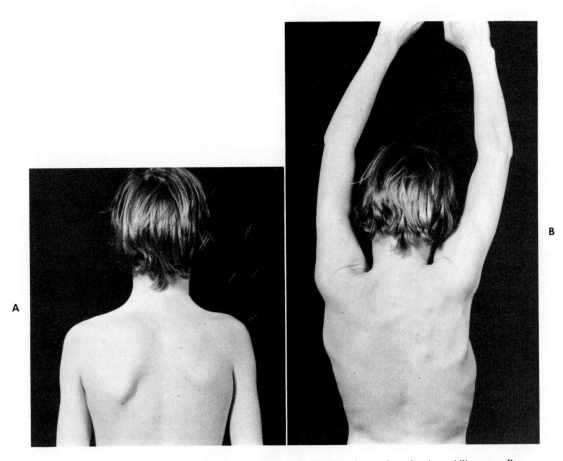

Fig. 63-8. Sixteen-year-old male after operation. **A,** After Woodward procedure showing midline scar. **B,** Active abduction of shoulders and scapulae.

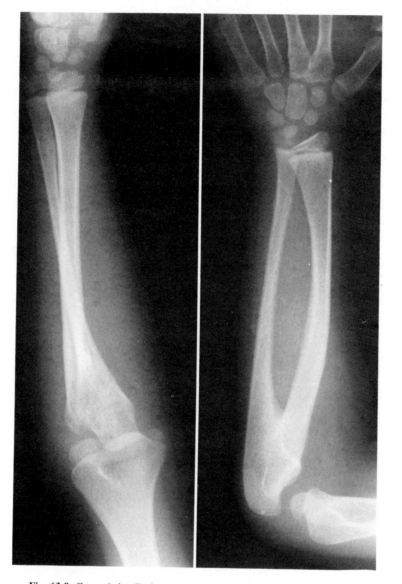

Fig. 63-9. Congenital radioulnar synostosis, involving proximal ends of bones.

terosseous membrane has been split throughout its length. Simply excising the fused part of the radius never improves function. We think it inadvisable to perform any operation with the hope of obtaining pronation and supination. Fortunately most patients are not disabled enough to justify an extensive operation. Any disabling pronation deformity should be corrected by osteotomy; then motion of the shoulder, especially when the elbow is extended, compensates well for the deformity.

CONGENITAL DISLOCATION OF RADIAL HEAD

Congenital dislocation of the radial head is rare but should be suspected when the head has been dislocated for a long time but there is no evidence that the ulna has been fractured. The roentgenographic findings are fairly characteristic (Fig. 63-10). The radial shaft is abnormally long, and the ulna is usually abnormally bowed. The radial head is dislocated, usually anteriorly, is rounded, showing little

if any depression for articulation with the capitulum, and is usually smaller than normal; occasionally there is an area of ossification in the tissues about it. The capitulum may also be small, and the radial notch of the ulna that should articulate with the radial head may be small or absent.

Congenital dislocation of the radial head may be familial, especially on the paternal side. It is sometimes associated with chondro-osteodystrophy.

A congenitally dislocated radial head is usually irreducible either manually or surgically because of adaptive changes in the soft tissues and the absence of normal surfaces for articulation with the ulna and humerus. Consequently open reduction of the dislocation and reconstruction of the annular ligament in childhood are inadvisable. Any disability is usually caused by restriction of rotation of the forearm, and in children physical therapy to improve this motion is the only treatment indicated. Any resection

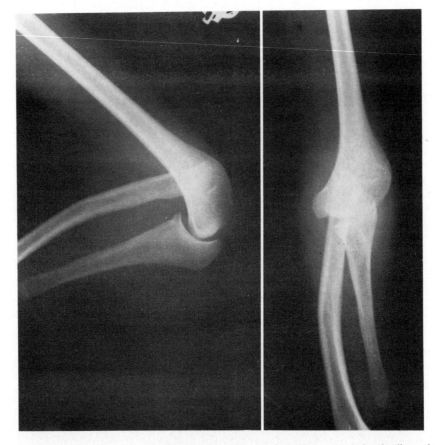

Fig. 63-10. Congenital dislocation of radial head. Head is dislocated anteriorly, and shafts of radius and ulna are abnormal (see text).

of the radial head should be postponed until growth is complete, but even then it may not improve motion because of the contractures of the soft tissues. The technique for resection of the radial head is described on p. 688.

CONGENITAL PSEUDARTHROSIS OF CLAVICLE

Congenital pseudarthrosis of the clavicle is a rare anomaly (Fig. 63-11). Several theories concerning its cause have been proposed. One is that since the clavicle develops in two separate masses by medial and lateral ossification centers, pseudarthrosis could be explained by failure of ossification of the precartilaginous bridge that would normally connect the two ossification centers. Another is that the lesion may be caused by direct pressure from the subclavian artery on the immature clavicle on the right. In one review, congenital pseudarthrosis of the clavicle was found to occur almost invariably on the right side. In a series of 60 unilateral lesions, 59 were on the right, and in the one patient with a pseudarthrosis on the left, dextrocardia was found.

Pseudarthrosis of the clavicle is present at birth and is usually in the middle third of the clavicle.

Congenital pseudarthrosis of the clavicle requires treatment not because of hypermobility of the shoulder girdle but usually because it is unsightly. Spontaneous union is

unknown, and consequently any desired union requires open reduction and bone grafting. Most surgeons agree that the ideal time for grafting is between the ages of 3 and 5 years. However, it can be carried out at any age though the older the patient is the more difficult is the grafting. Simple resection of the prominent ends of the bone has resulted in pain, prominence of the ends during movements of the shoulder, and asymmetry of the shoulder girdles.

Union is easier to obtain in congenital pseudarthrosis of the clavicle than in that of the tibia. Almost any type of bone grafting suitable for traumatic nonunion of the clavicle has been satisfactory in pseudarthrosis (Fig. 63-12).

We recommend treating congenital pseudarthrosis of the clavicle by open reduction and internal fixation with plate and screws and autogenous iliac bone grafting (Fig. 63-13).

TECHNIQUE. Make a transverse 3-inch (7.5 cm) incision centered over the body of the clavicle, approximately a fingerbreadth above the superior border of the bone. Carry sharp dissection through the subcutaneous tissue to expose the clavicle, both medially and laterally and in the central third in the area of the pseudarthrosis. Expose the bone subperiosteally, taking care to protect the underlying neurovascular structures. Debride the site of the pseudarthrosis of all fibrous and cartilaginous tissue down to normal bone

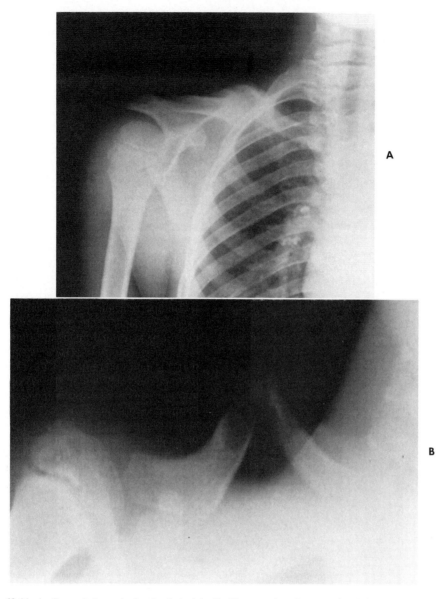

Fig. 63-11. A, Congenital pseudarthrosis of clavicle. **B,** Close-up view demonstrating defect in middle third of clavicle.

both medially and laterally. Bend a four-hole plate (either semitubular or dynamic compression) to fit the contours of the bone. Then fix the plate to the clavicle in the usual manner. Obtain autogenous iliac grafts and place them on the superior, inferior, and posterior aspects of the pseudarthrosis. Close the wound in layers and the skin with subcuticular sutures.

AFTERTREATMENT. A collar and cuff are worn for 3 to 6 weeks. The plate may be removed at 6 to 18 months when roentgenographic union is present.

CONGENITAL PSEUDARTHROSIS OF RADIUS

Congenital pseudarthrosis of the radius is extremely rare. In 1974 Sprague and Brown reported one patient in whom the lesion was associated with neurofibromatosis, and in 1977 Masihuz-Zaman reported a similar patient. In 1975 Greenberg and Schwartz reported a pseudarthrosis apparently not associated with this disease. In patients with neurofibromatosis the pseudarthrosis developed from a cyst in the radius, and each patient either had skin manifestations of neurofibromatosis or had a strong family history of the disease.

In each instance reported, pseudarthrosis of the radius occurred in the distal third of the bone, and the distal fragment was quite short. Since the lesion is near the distal radial epiphysis, the ends of the bone are attenuated, and the ulna is relatively long, the treatment of choice is dual onlay bone grafting as recommended by Boyd for congen-

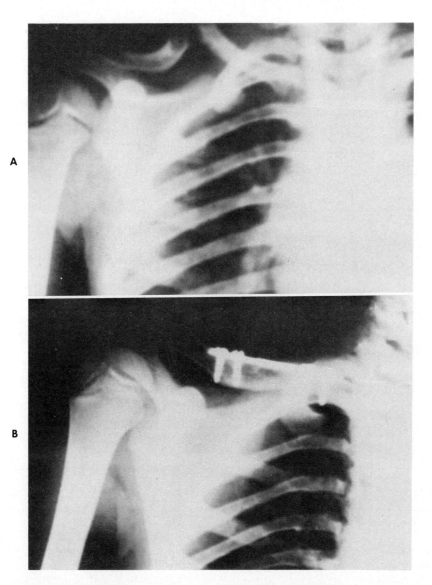

Fig. 63-12. Congenital pseudarthrosis of clavicle. **A,** Before surgery. **B,** Union after open reduction, resection of ends of fragments, application of plate and screws, and insertion of bone chips from resected ends.

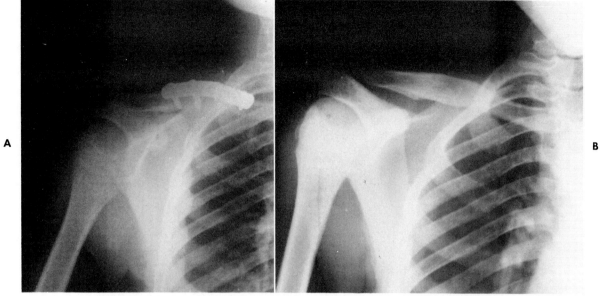

Fig. 63-13. Congenital pseudarthrosis of clavicle. **A,** After open reduction and internal fixation with plate and bone grafting. **B,** Union is solid 1-year after plate removal.

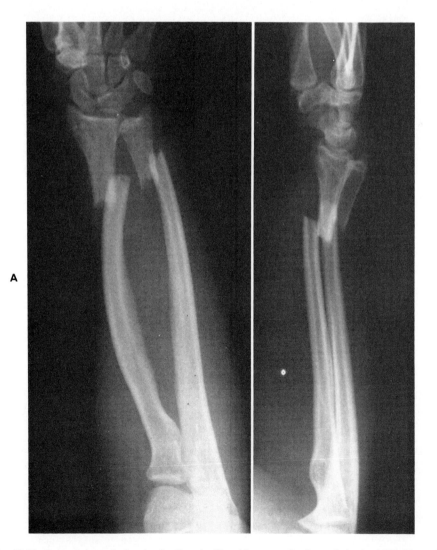

Fig. 63-14. Congenital pseudarthrosis of radius. **A,** Closed fractures of radius and ulna in child with manifestations of neurofibromatosis. *Continued.*

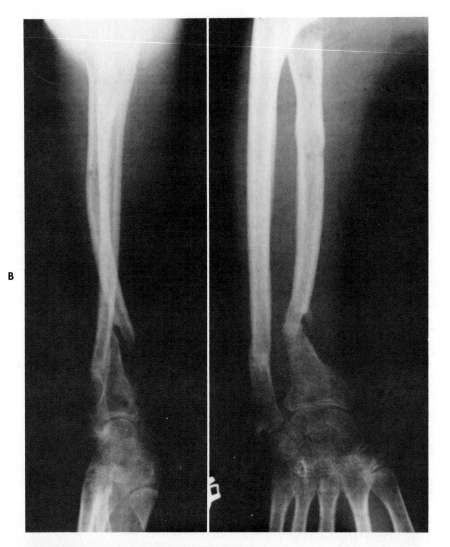

Fig. 63-14, cont'd. B, After 10 weeks of immobilization; ulna has healed but radius has pseudarthrosis with tapering of ends of fragments.

ital pseudarthrosis of the tibia (p. 1816). This operation restores length, provides a vise-like grip on the osteoporotic distal fragment, increases the size of the distal end of the proximal fragment, and usually results in satisfactory union.

We have treated a pseudarthrosis of the radius following fracture in a child with obvious neurofibromatosis and a positive family history of the disease. Roentgenographically the fracture resembled a congenital pseudarthrosis of the clavicle. It failed to unite and was treated by dual onlay bone grafting (Fig. 63-14).

CONGENITAL PSEUDARTHROSIS OF ULNA

Congenital pseudarthrosis of the ulna in neurofibromatosis is extremely rare. Five patients with a solitary ulnar pseudarthrosis have been reported, and one patient had involvement of both bones of the distal forearm. One pseudarthrosis of the ulna occurred through a localized lytic lesion similar to Type 2 congenital pseudarthrosis of the tibia (p. 1813), and all the others showed sclerotic tapering of the ends of the bones characteristic of Type 1. We have treated two patients with neurofibromatosis and congenital pseudarthrosis of the ulna. The ununited ulna produces angulation of the radius, shortening of the forearm, and dislocation of the radial head (Fig. 63-15).

Bone grafting of congenital pseudarthrosis of the ulna has usually failed, but because significant bowing of the radius develops in the very young child, early surgery is indicated. When the pseudarthrosis has developed through a cystic lesion, early curettage of the cyst, internal fixation of the bone, and bone grafting are usually successful. In established pseudarthrosis with tapering of the ends of the bone, the distal ulna should be excised early to relieve its tethering effect on the radius; then the forearm is fitted with a suitable brace. If the radial head dislocates, it should be excised and a synostosis produced between the radius and ulna (Fig. 63-15). Osteotomy of the distal radius to correct bowing may also be indicated.

C

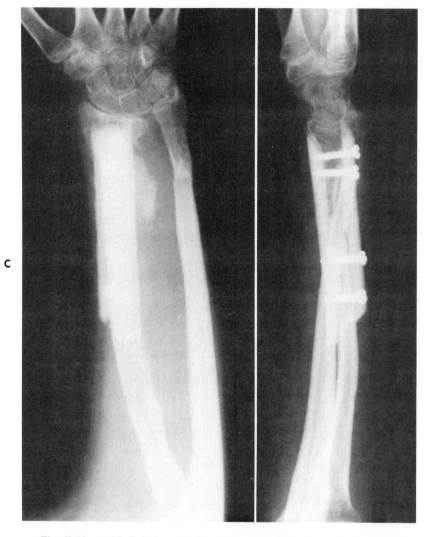

Fig. 63-14, cont'd. C, Union of radius after treatment by dual onlay bone grafting.

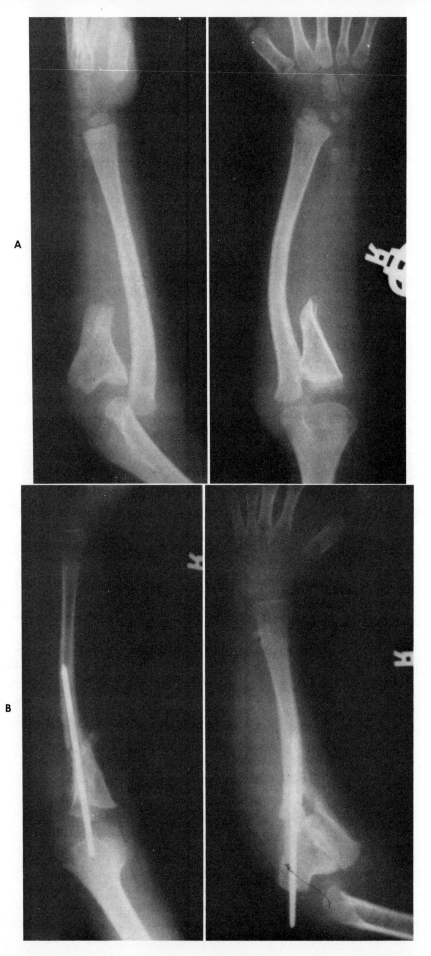

Fig. 63-15. Congenital pseudarthrosis of ulna with dislocation of radial head. **A,** Before surgery. **B,** After excision of radial head, creation of synostosis between proximal radius and ulna, and fixtion with medullary nail.

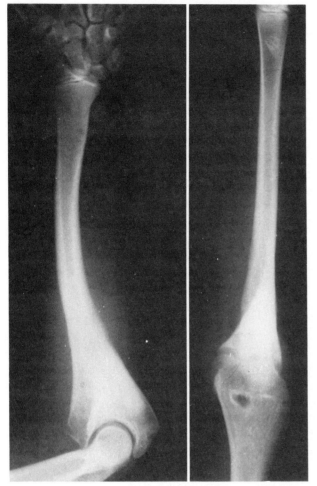

Fig. 63-15, cont'd. C, Final appearance of one-bone forearm.

NEUROVASCULAR COMPRESSION SYNDROME OF SUPERIOR THORACIC OUTLET

The neurovascular compression syndrome of the superior thoracic outlet is ill defined. It results from pressure on the brachial plexus or on the subclavian artery or vein as it courses through the neck and the superior thoracic outlet toward the axilla. The syndrome may be caused by a cervical rib or its fibrous anterior attachment, by hypertrophy or spasm of the scalenus anterior, by an abnormal droop of the shoulder girdle that drags the neurovascular structures downward at the outlet, by spasm of the scalenus medius secondary to trauma or abnormal posture, by edema of the structures bounding the outlet secondary to a direct blow on the shoulder, by anomalies of the first rib, by fractures of the first rib or clavicle, by abnormal tension on the pectoralis minor, or by osteoarthritis at the first costovertebral joint.

Neurovascular compression syndrome of the superior thoracic outlet must be differentiated from the subclavian steal syndrome. In the latter syndrome one of the subclavian vessels is blocked proximal to the origin of the vertebral artery (Fig. 63-16, *B*), resulting in the transfer of blood from the vertebral artery on the contralateral side through the basilar artery to the vertebral artery on the ip-

silateral side. This results in a steal of blood from the cerebral circulation, and neurologic symptoms then develop. It may be confused with the thoracic outlet syndrome because neurologic symptoms in the arm might be caused by increased exercise of the arm. However, the thoracic outlet syndrome is rarely accompanied by symptoms of central nervous system anoxia. Furthermore, the symptoms of subclavian steal syndrome are rarely initiated by any changes in position of the head. The diagnosis is made by subclavian arteriography in which the contrast medium flows superiorly in one vertebral artery into the basilar artery and then inferiorly in the vertebral artery on the opposite side into the subclavian artery.

Since the causes of pressure on the subclavian artery or vein or on the brachial plexus vary much in kind and severity, signs and symptoms of the syndrome vary in like manner. They may be sensory, motor, vascular, or all three, and they may consist of one or more of the following: (1) pain in the supraclavicular region that extends distally along the medial border of the forearm to the hand and fingers, more commonly to the little and ring fingers; (2) paresthesia initiated or aggravated by sudden motions of the shoulder or neck that produce traction on the brachial plexus or the subclavian vessels; (3) atrophy of the interosseus muscles of the hand and thus weakness of the hand; (4) coolness and pallor of the forearm and hand and a decrease in strength of the radial pulse, especially while tilting the chin and turning the head to the affected side (Adson's sign), while exerting downward traction on the extended arm, or while the arm is at the side with the patient holding his breath in deep inspiration; and (5) venous distention caused by pressure on or thrombosis of the subclavian vein.

The syndrome occurs more commonly in people of middle age whose muscle tone is poor, in women more often than in men, and more often on the right side than on the left. Its signs and symptoms may be difficult to differentiate from those of a degenerated or protruded intervertebral disc in the lower cervical spine, of cervical spondylosis, of tumors in the apex of the lung, of pressure or traction on the ulnar nerve at the elbow, or of carpal tunnel syndrome. In addition to routine roentgenograms of the neck, shoulder, and chest, myelograms of the cervical spine, arteriograms or venograms of the subclavian vessels, and electromyography of the muscles of the involved forearm and hand are useful in diagnosis. The combined use of arteriograms and venograms has in many patients indicated the location and type of the offending lesion and has sometimes demonstrated several coexisting lesions. During arteriography and venography the patient should have roentgenograms made in several different positions while traction is exerted on the arm. The arteriography may be performed with the patient sitting or standing to simulate the normal tension on the thoracic outlet. Furthermore, ulnar nerve conduction velocity values have been helpful in deciding which patients are likely to respond to conservative treatment and which are likely to require surgery. When the ulnar nerve conduction velocity is measured from the supraclavicular fossa to the wrist; those patients with a velocity of 60 mm/second are considered more likely to be improved by conservative treatment;

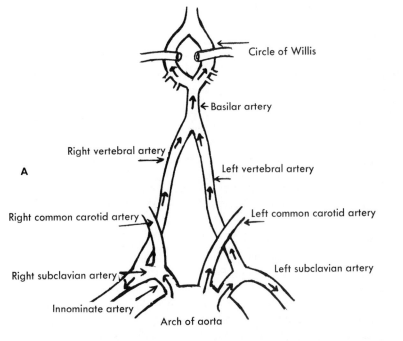

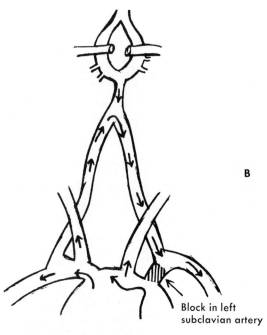

A

B

Circle of Willis

Basilar artery

Right vertebral artery

Left vertebral artery

Right common carotid artery

Left common carotid artery

Right subclavian artery

Left subclavian artery

Innominate artery

Arch of aorta

Block in left subclavian artery

Fig. 63-16. Subclavian steal syndrome. **A,** Normal circulation in various arteries. **B,** Left subclavian artery has been blocked proximal to origin of vertebral artery, resulting in transfer of blood from right vertebral artery through basilar artery to left vertebral artery. (From Heath, R.D.: J. Bone Joint Surg. **54-A:**1033, 1972.)

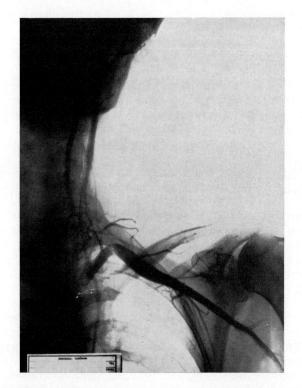

Fig. 63-17. Arteriogram showing compression of subclavian artery by anterior fibrous attachment of cervical rib. (Courtesy Dr. Hector S. Howard.)

most patients in whom the velocity is below 60 mm/second will require surgery.

Treatment

If symptoms are mild, instructing the patient to change postural attitudes, especially while sleeping, and to improve the tone of the neck and shoulder muscles by exercise is usually sufficient. But if symptoms are severe, especially if vascular obstruction can be demonstrated (Fig. 63-17), then the brachial plexus and subclavian vessels should be decompressed by resecting the offending structure, that is, a cervical rib and its anterior fibrous attachment, a part of the scalenus anterior or scalenus medius, or all or part of the first rib. Removal of the entire first rib appears to be a common factor in satisfactory surgery regardless of whether a cervical rib with an anterior fibrous attachment is present. Removing the first rib releases both the scalenus anterior and scalenus medius, and an adequate outlet is thus established. Partial resection of the first rib probably results in a greater rate of recurrence of symptoms than does resection of the entire rib. A technique that permits good exposure to the region and resection of all or part of the offending structure is necessary. In almost every instance the first rib is a factor, and resection of all or part of it is often included in the operation.

SUPRACLAVICULAR TECHNIQUE (BRANNON AND WICKSTROM). Begin the incision 2 cm superior to the sternoclavicular joint and extend it posteriorly and slightly superiorly for 7 to 9 cm (Fig. 63-18, *A*). Retract the sternocleidomastoid muscle medially and divide and ligate the external jugular vein and the transverse scapular and transverse cervical arteries that lie anterior to the scalenus anterior. Directly su-

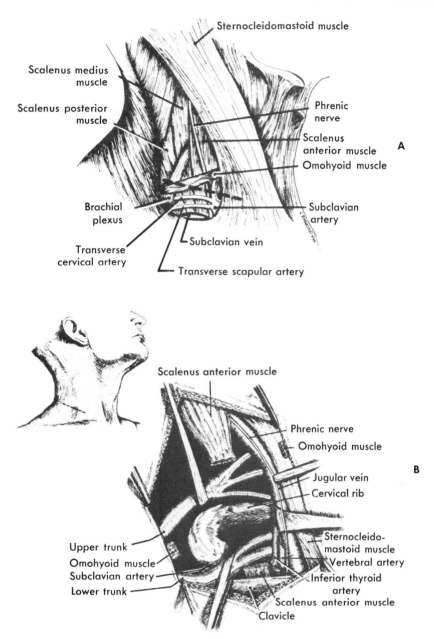

Fig. 63-18. Supraclavicular technique of Brannon and Wickstrom for neurovascular compression syndromes of superior thoracic outlet. **A,** Incision and underlying structures in neck. **B,** Part of scalenus anterior has been resected. Cervical rib is to be resected next (see text). *Inset,* Incision. (Modified from Brannon, E.W., Jr., and Wickstrom, J.: Clin. Orthop. **51:**65, 1967.)

perior to these vessels either retract or divide the inferior belly of the omohyoid muscle as it crosses the scalenus anterior. Next isolate and retract medially the phrenic nerve that descends inferiorly along the anterior border of the scalenus anterior. Then proximal to its inferior attachment divide the scalenus anterior and resect a part of it (Fig. 63-18, *B*). Identify and protect the subclavian artery posterior to the scalenus anterior. Next identify and retract medially the internal jugular vein, the carotid sheath, the carotid artery, and the vagus nerve. Look for a cervical rib extending laterally from the seventh cervical vertebra and traversing anterioly between the scalenus anterior and scalenus medius and crossed by the brachial plexus. If such a rib is found, gently retract the components of the brachial plexus, expose the rib subperiosteally, and with a rongeur resect it. Then carefully inspect the trunks of the brachial plexus to be sure they are free of any fibrous bands. Secure meticulous hemostasis. Close the skin, apply a light pressure dressing, and support the arm in a sling.

• • •

For resecting the first rib, Roos described a transaxillary approach that, according to him, is easier, faster, and safer. In this approach blood loss is less, no muscles are divided, the offending rib and other structures can be completely resected, and proximal exposure is better, permitting easier control of any injured major vessel. Furthermore, discomfort in the shoulder after surgery is minimal. The wound is simply and quickly closed, and the resulting axillary scar is small and inconspicuous.

TECHNIQUE (ROOS). Place the patient in the straight lateral position with the involved shoulder upward. Tilt the thorax posteriorly 60 degrees, supporting it on a sandbag. Prepare the entire limb from the fingertips proximally to include half of the chest. Drape the surgical field to allow free manipulation of the extremity during the operation. Then abduct the arm fully. In the inferior fourth of the axilla and in a normal skin line, make a transverse curved inci-sion convex distally 6 to 10 cm long overlying the third rib (Fig. 63-19, *A*). Deepen the incision directly toward the thorax in the plane of loose areolar tissue that lies on the thorax and the serratus anterior muscle. The lateral thoracic artery and the thoracoepigastric vein cross the line of dissection vertically in the midaxillary line; divide and ligate these structures. As the serratus anterior muscle is reached, develop a plane of dissection in the aerolar tissue by finger dissection up to the first rib. This plane should lie deep to the nodes and vessels of the axilla and to the axillary fat pad. Take care not to injure the intercostobrachial cutaneous nerve that is encountered in the middle of the field, coming from the second intercostal space. One of the complications of this approach is an uncomfortable paresthesia from trauma or ischemia of this nerve. Just lateral to the edge of the first rib and coursing vertically in the middle of the dissection are the superior thoracic artery

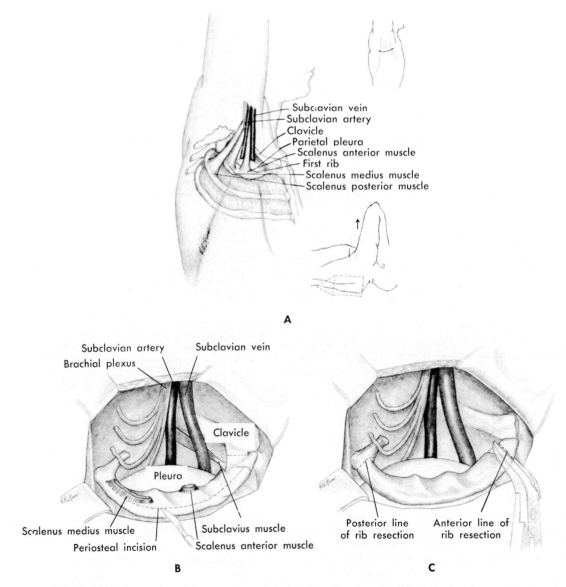

Subclavian vein
Subclavian artery
Clavicle
Parietal pleura
Scalenus anterior muscle
First rib
Scalenus medius muscle
Scalenus posterior muscle

A

Subclavian artery   Subclavian vein
Brachial plexus

Clavicle

Pleura

Scalenus medius muscle   Subclavius muscle
Periosteal incision   Scalenus anterior muscle

B

Posterior line   Anterior line of
of rib resection   rib resection

C

Fig. 63-19. Roos transaxillary approach for resecting first rib in neurovascular compression syndromes of superior thoracic outlet (see text). (Modified from Roos, D.B.: Ann. Surg. **163**:355, 1966.)

and vein that pass into the first intercostal space; clamp, divide, and ligate these structures. By blunt dissection with a fingertip expose the first rib. Now with the shoulder and elbow flexed 90 degrees have an assistant exert traction on the limb directly toward the ceiling. This opens the thoracic outlet and exposes all important structures as they exit over the first rib. These are the large, blue subclavian vein anteriorly, a small ribbon of serratus anterior muscle inserting on the medial edge of the first rib at the scalene tubercle, the pulsating subclavian artery, which is pink and the size of a pencil and is immediately posterior to the scalenus anterior, the T1 root of the brachial plexus immediately posterior to the artery, and the large scalenus medius posterior to the plexus (Fig. 63-19, *A*). During the dissection keep the limb elevated as just described except to lower it occasionally to temporarily relieve tension on the muscles and the brachial plexus. Now check the adequacy of the thoracic outlet by placing a finger on each side of the scalenus anterior superior to the first rib while the shoulder is depressed distally and is abducted and externally rotated 90 degrees (fingertip pinch test). If the surgeon's finger is pinched severely, the diagnosis of costoclavicular compression of the neurovascular structures made before surgery is correct. Next dissect free the taut band of the subclavius tendon that attaches to the first rib anteriorly deep to the head of the clavicle (Fig. 63-19, *B*); divide it under direct vision, taking care not to injure the subclavian vein, which lies medial and posterior to it. With finger dissection free the scalenus anterior and divide it at its insertion on the first rib. The division of this muscle must be exactly on the rib to avoid injuring the phrenic nerve lying 2 to 3 cm above the rib. Avoid opening the superior part of the pleura that rises proximal to the first rib and touches the inner septum of the scalenus anterior. With a periosteal elevator push the scalenus medius and any remaining medial fibers of the scalenus anterior from the superior surface of the posterior third of the rib. Leave intact the periosteum of the rib to minimize scarring after surgery. Now divide the first rib posteriorly 1 cm from the transverse process (Fig. 63-19, *C*). Be careful to protect the root of T1 at this point; it should be clearly visible at all times. After the posterior end of the rib is divided, avulse the anterior end from its costal cartilage; then divide it with rib shears as close to the sternum as possible, leaving a smooth stump. Resect any cervical rib as far posteriorly as the transverse process and any fibrous band attached to it. If necessary a thoracic sympathectomy can be performed through the same incision, and if the subclavian vein is found to be thrombosed, a thrombectomy of this vein can be done as well. Inspect the pleura by irrigating it with saline solution while the lung is forcibly expanded. If no pneumothorax is seen, flood the operative field with saline solution to displace air from the area. If a pneumothorax is found, insert a catheter in the pleural opening and attach it to suction during closure of the wound. Again flood the area with saline solution during forced expansion of the lung and immediately bring the shoulder down to the relaxed position while the fascia is closed. Do not repair any muscles. Close the skin with a subcuticular suture, and during this closure remove any suction tube.

AFTERTREATMENT. The wound is dressed with a plastic spray to seal it. No tape is applied to the axilla. The patient is allowed to shower 1 to 2 days after surgery.

Clagett has recommended a posterior thoracotomy approach for resection of the first rib, and some surgeons prefer it to the supraclavicular or transaxillary approach. A disadvantage to this posterior approach is that any injuries to the major vessels cannot be repaired through it and a second incision must be made anteriorly.

REFERENCES
Congenital pseudarthroses of clavicle, radius, and ulna

Aegerter, E.E.: The possible relationship of neurofibromatosis, congenital pseudarthrosis, and fibrous dysplasia, J. Bone Joint Surg. 32-A:618, 1950.

Alldred, A.J.: Congenital pseudarthrosis of the clavicle, J. Bone Joint Surg. 45-B:312, 1963.

Baldwin, D.M., and Weiner, D.S.: Congenital bowing and intraosseous neurofibroma of the ulna: a case report, J. Bone Joint Surg. 56-A:803, 1974.

Boyd, H.B.: Congenital pseudarthrosis: treatment by dual bone grafts, J. Bone Joint Surg. 23:497, 1941.

Boyd, H.B., and Fox, K.W.: Congenital pseudarthrosis: follow-up study after massive bone-grafting, J. Bone Joint Surg. 30-A:274, 1948.

Compere, E.L.: Localized osteitis fibrosa in the new-born and congenital pseudarthrosis, J. Bone Joint Surg. 18:513, 1936.

Garth, W.P., Jr., and Canale, S.T.: Congenital pseudarthroses of the ulna associated with neurofibromatosis: a report of two cases and review of the literature, Staff meeting report, Campbell Clinic, Memphis, 1977.

Gibson, D.A. and Carroll, N.: Congenital pseudarthrosis of the clavicle, J. Bone Joint Surg. 52-B:629, 1970.

Green, W.T., and Rudo, N.: Pseudarthrosis and neurofibromatosis, Arch. Surg. 46:639, 1943.

Greenberg, L.A., and Schwartz, A.: Congenital pseudarthrosis of the distal radius, South. Med. J. 68:1053, 1975.

Herman, S.: Congenital bilateral pseudarthrosis of the clavicles, Clin. Orthop. 91:162, 1973.

Lloyd-Roberts, G.C., Apley, A.G., and Owen, R.: Reflections upon the aetiology of congenital pseudarthrosis of the clavicle: with a note on cranio-cleido dysostosis, J. Bone Joint Surg. 57-B:24, 1975.

Masihuz-Zaman: Pseudoarthrosis of the radius associated with neurofibromatosis: a case report, J. Bone Joint Surg. 59-A:977, 1977.

McFarland, B.: Congenital deformities of the spine and limbs. In Platt, H., editor: Modern trends in orthopaedics, New York, 1950, Paul B. Hoeber, Inc.

Milgram, J.E.: Impaling (telescoping) operation for pseudarthrosis of long bones in childhood, Bull. Hosp. Joint Dis. 17:152, 1956.

Moore, B.H.: Some orthopaedic relationships of neurofibromatosis, J. Bone Joint Surg. 23:109, 1941.

Moore, J.R.: Delayed autogenous bone graft in the treatment of congenital pseudarthrosis, J. Bone Joint Surg. 31-A:23, 1949.

Morris, H.D.: Amputation as a tool in managing congenital deformities. Movie presented at The Russell A. Hibbs Society, April 1961, New Orleans.

Owen, R.: Congenital pseudarthrosis of the clavicle, J. Bone Joint Surg. 52-B:644, 1970.

Richin, P.F., Kranik, A., Van Herpe, L., and Suffecool, S.L.: Congenital pseudarthrosis of both bones of the forearm: a case report, J. Bone Joint Surg. 58-A:1032, 1976.

Sofield, H.A., and Millar, E.A.: Fragmentation, realignment, and intramedullary rod fixation of deformities of the long bones in children: a ten-year appraisal, J. Bone Joint Surg. 41-A:1371, 1959.

Sprague, B.L., and Brown, G.A.: Congenital pseudarthrosis of the radius, J. Bone Joint Surg. 56-A:191, 1974.

Wall, J.J.: Congenital pseudarthrosis of the clavicle, J. Bone Joint Surg. 52-A:1003, 1970.

Congenital torticollis or wryneck

Armstrong, D., Pickrell, K., Fetter, B., and Pitts, W.: Torticollis: an analysis of 271 cases, Plast. Reconstr. Surg. 35:14, 1965.

Brown J.B., and McDowell, F.: Wry-neck facial distortion prevented by resection of fibrosed sternomastoid muscle in infancy and childhood, Ann. Surg. 131:721, 1950.

Canale, S.T., Griffin, D.W., and Hubbard, C.N.: Congenital muscular torticollis: a long-term follow-up, J. Bone Joint Surg. **64-A:** 1982.

Chandler, F.A.: Muscular torticollis, J. Bone Joint Surg. **30-A:**566, 1948.

Chandler, F.A., and Altenberg, A.: "Congenital" muscular torticollis, JAMA **125:**476, 1944.

Coventry, M.B., and Harris, L.: Congenital muscular torticollis in infancy: some observations regarding treatment, J. Bone Joint Surg. **41-A:**815, 1959.

Feil, A.: Seventeenth report of progress in orthopedic surgery. (Abstracted from Presse Med. **29:**515, 1921.)

Ferkel, R.D., Westin, G.W., Dawson, E.G., and Oppenheim, W.L.: Muscular torticollis: a modified surgical approach, J. Bone Joint Surg. **65-A:**894, 1983.

Hummer, C.D., Jr., and MacEwen, G.D.: The coexistence of torticollis and congenital dysplasia of the hip, J. Bone Joint Surg. **54-A:**1255, 1972.

Kaplan, E.B.: Anatomical pitfalls in the surgical treatment of torticollis, Bull. Hosp. Joint Dis. **15:**154, 1954.

Ling. C.M.: The influence of age on the results of open sternomastoid tenotomy in muscular torticollis, Clin. Orthop. **116:**142, 1976.

Meyerding, H.W.: Cogenital torticollis, J. Orthop. Surg. **3:**91. 1921.

Mickelson, M.R., Cooper, R.R., and Ponseti, I.V.: Ultrastructure of the sternocleidomastoid muscle in muscular torticollis, Clin. Orthop. **110:**11, 1975.

Congenital elevation of scapula

Bonola, A.: Surgical treatment of the Klippel-Feil syndrome, J. Bone Joint Surg. **38-B:**440, 1956.

Cavendish, M.E.: Congenital elevation of the scapula, J. Bone Joint Surg. **54-B:**395. 1972.

Chung, S.M.K., and Farahvar, H.: Surgery of the clavicle in Sprengel's deformity, Clin. Orhtop. **116:**138, 1976.

Chung, S.M.K., and Nissenbaum, M.M.: Congenital and developmental defects of the shoulder, Orthop. Clin. North Am. **6:**381, 1975.

Green, W.T.: The surgical correction of congenital elevation of the scapula (Sprengel's deformity), J. Bone Joint Surg. **39-A:**1439, 1957.

Green, W.T.: The surgical correction of congenital elevation of the scapula. Personal communication, 1962.

Green, W.T.: Sprengel's deformity: congenital elevation of the scapula. In American Academy of Orthopaedic Surgeons: Instructional course lectures, vol. 21, St. Louis, 1972, The C.V. Mosby Co.

Greville, N.R., and Coventry, M.B.: Congenital high scapula (Sprengel's) deformity, Mayo Clin. Proc. **31:**465, 1956.

Halley D.K., and Eyring, E.J.: Congenital elevation of the scapula in a family, Clin. Orthop. **97:**31, 1973.

Horwitz, A.E.: Congenital elevation of the scapula—Sprengel's deformity, Am. J. Orthop. Surg. **6:**260, 1908.

Huc, G.: De l'adaptation de la ceinture scapulaire au thorax; essai d'anatomie de physiologie, de pathologie et de therapeutique, Paris, 1924, no. 403, Viellemard Imp.

Inclan, A.: Congenital elevation of the scapula or Sprengel's deformity: two clinical cases treated with Ober's operation, Cir. Ortop. Traum. Habana **15:**1, 1949.

Jeannopoulos, C.L.: Congenital elevation of the scapula, J. Bone Joint Surg. **34-A:**883, 1952.

Jeannopoulos, C.L.: Observations on congenital elevation of the scapula, Clin. Orthop. **20:**132, 1961.

Koenig, F.: Eine neue Operation des angeborenen Schulterblatthochstandes, Beitr. Klin. Chir. **94:** 1914. (Cited in Lange, M.: Orthopädisch-chirurgische Operationslehre, München, 1951, J.F. Bergmann.)

Lange, M.: Orthopädisch-chirurgische Operationslehre, München, 1951, J.F. Bergmann.

McClure, J.G., and Raney, R.B.: Anomalies of the scapula, Clin. Orthop. **110:**22, 1975.

McFarland, B.: Congenital deformities of the spine and limbs, In Platt, H., editor: Modern trends in orthopaedics, New York, 1950, Paul B. Hoeber, Inc.

Robinson, R.A., Braun, R.M., Mack, P., and Zadek, R.: The surgical importance of the clavicular component of Sprengels' deformity (abstract), J. Bone Joint Surg. **49-A**1481, 1967.

Schrock, R.D.: Congenital elevation of the scapula, J. Bone Joint Surg. **8:**207, 1926.

Schrock. R.D.: Congenital elevation of the scapula, Nelson's new loose leaf surgery, vol. 3, New York, 1935, Thomas Nelson & Sons.

Smith, A.D.: Congenital elevation of the scapula, Arch. Surg. **42:**529, 1941.

Whitman, A.: Congenital elevation of scapula and paralysis of serratus magnus muscle, JAMA **99:**1332, 1932.

Woodward, J.W.: Congenital elevation of the scapula: correction by release and transplantation of muscle origins: a preliminary report, J. Bone Joint Surg. **43-A:**219, 1961.

Congenital radioulnar synostosis and congenital dislocation of radial head

Almquist, E.E., Gordon, L.H., and Blue, A.I.: Congenital dislocation of the head of the radius, J. Bone Joint Surg. **51-A:**1118, 1969.

Cohn, B.N.E.: Congenital bilateral radio-ulnar synostosis, J. Bone Joint Surg. **14:**404, 1932.

Dawson, H.G.W.: A congenital deformity of the forearm and its operative treatment, Br. Med. J. **2:**833, 1912.

Exarhou, E.I., and Antoniou, N.K.: Congenital dislocation of the head of the radius, Acta Orthop. Scand. **41:**551, 1970.

Fahlstrom, S.: Radio-ulnar synostosis: historical review and case report, J. Bone Joint Surg. **14:**395, 1932.

Gibson, A.: A critical consideration of congenital radio-ulnar synostosis, with special reference to treatment, J. Bone Joint Surg. **5:**299, 1923.

Hansen, O.H., and Andersen, N.O.: Congenital radio-ulnar synostosis: report of 37 cases, Acta Orthop. Scand. **41:**225, 1970.

Keats, S.: Congenital bilateral dislocation of head of the radius in a seven-year-old child, Orthop. Rev. **3:**33, August 1974.

McFarland, B.: Congenital dislocation of the head of the radius, Br. J. Surg. **24:**41, 1936.

Milch, H.: So-called dislocation of the lower end of the ulna, Ann. Surg. **116:**282, 1942.

White, J.R.A.: Congenital dislocation of the head of the radius, Br. J. Surg. **30:**377, 1943.

Wilkie, D.P.D.: Congenital radio-ulnar synostosis, Br. J. Surg. **1:**366, 1913-1914.

PART XVI

Nervous System Disorders

CHAPTER 64

Peripheral nerve injuries

Phillip E. Wright

Many peripheral nerve injuries are seen during armed conflicts. Because of the disabilities caused by such injuries, much attention is given to the initial treatment and later to reconstruction and rehabilitation after injury. During World War I the Peripheral Nerve Registry was established for the continuing study of nerve injuries. Later evaluations were not carried out and the early research was ignored. Between the two world wars there was little research in peripheral nerve injuries, and good surgical treatment of such injuries was available in only a few hospitals. During World War II neurosurgical centers for the army were established in the United States by Dr. R. Glen Spurling and in England by Mr. H.J. Seddon. Dr. Barnes Woodhall established a Peripheral Nerve Registry under the direction of the Surgeon General of the United States Army. The diligent work of these surgeons culminated in the publication in 1954 of the British Medical Research Council's Special Report, *Peripheral Nerve Injuries,* edited by Seddon, and in the United States in 1956 of the Veterans Administration Medical Monograph, *Peripheral Nerve Regeneration,* edited by Woodhall and Beebe. Valuable contributions were made later by numerous workers in both basic and clinical research. Noteworthy are the works of Sir Sydney Sunderland, recorded to a great extent in *Nerves and Nerve Injuries,* and of Sir Herbert Seddon, summarized in his *Surgical Disorders of the Peripheral Nerves.* The reader is also referred to the more recent excellent works of Omer and Spinner.

In this chapter the diagnosis and treatment of peripheral nerve injuries are described as simply and as practically as possible. The details of surgical technique and aftertreatment are included in the discussion of each nerve. For de-

2783

tails of embryology, microscopic anatomy, and physiology the reader is referred to other works. The appropriate reconstructive operations are described in other sections of this book, and cross-references are provided.

ANATOMY OF SPINAL NERVES

Each segmental spinal nerve is formed at or near its intervertebral foramen by the union of its dorsal or sensory root with its ventral or motor root. In most of the thoracic segments these mixed spinal nerves retain their autonomy and supply one intercostal segment both dermatomal and myotomal. In virtually all other segments of the spinal axis the spinal nerves join with others to form a plexus that innervates a limb or a special body segment that no longer retains the primitive myomeric pattern.

Thirty-one mixed spinal nerves leave their respective foramina on each side of the spine to innervate the homolateral trunk and extremities: eight cervical, twelve thoracic, five lumbar, five sacral, and one coccygeal.

Components of mixed spinal nerves

A typical mixed spinal nerve has three distinct components as follows (Fig. 64-1).

MOTOR

Several rootlets leave the anterolateral sulcus of the spinal cord and unite to form each motor root. The fibers traversing these roots arise from the anterior horn cells and innervate the skeletal muscles.

SENSORY

The sensory fibers arise from pain, thermal, tactile, and stretch receptors. Cell bodies for these fibers are located within the dorsal root ganglia with axons entering the posterolateral sulcus of the cord by way of several rootlets. The fibers conveying joint or position sensibility and some tactile fibers turn cephalad in the dorsal columns and do not synapse before reaching the gracile and cuneate nuclei at the cervicomedullary junction. Pain and temperature fibers synapse in the substantia gelatinosa and cross to ascend in the dorsal spinothalamic tract. Tactile fibers enter,

synapse, and cross to ascend in the ventral spinothalamic tract.

SYMPATHETIC

The sympathetic component of all 31 mixed spinal nerves leaves the spinal cord along only 14 motor roots. The cells of origin are in the intermediolateral cell column that extends throughout the thoracic and upper lumbar cord segments. The fibers exit from the cord with the 12 thoracic and first 2 lumbar motor roots, enter the respective mixed spinal nerve, and then promptly emerge from it as white rami. The white rami pass anteriorly to the corresponding sympathetic ganglion. Synapse may occur within the ganglion with which the ramus is associated, and postganglionic fibers then pass back to the mixed spinal nerve as a gray ramus. More often, however, the fibers entering the ganglion by way of the white rami pass for variable distances up or down the paravertebral chain to synapse at higher or lower levels. The postganglionic fibers then pass along gray rami to cervical, lower lumbar, or sacrococcygeal mixed spinal nerves having no white rami. Sweat glands, blood vessels, and erector pili are thus innervated too in a segmental pattern.

Gross anatomy

Mixed spinal nerves, having left the intervertebral foramina, receive their sympathetic component and promptly branch into anterior and posterior primary rami. The posterior primary rami are directed posteriorly and supply the paraspinal musculature and the skin along the posterior aspect of the trunk, the neck, and the head. The upper three cervical posterior rami are larger than their corresponding anterior rami, supplying relatively large areas of the scalp posteriorly and the musculature about the craniocervical junction. With these exceptions, posterior primary rami are small and the major part of each spinal nerve continues laterally in an anterior primary ramus either to enter a plexus or to become an intercostal nerve.

Anterior primary rami of all the cervical, the first thoracic, and all the lumbosacral nerves join in the formation of plexuses. Alteration of the metameric pattern results

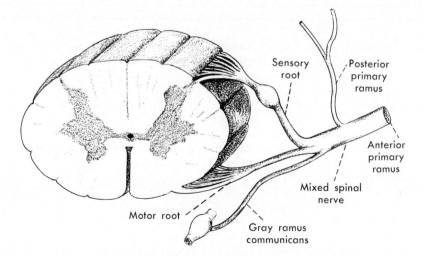

Fig. 64-1. Components of mixed spinal nerve.

from the migration of dermatomes and myotomes into the limb buds. The upper four cervical anterior rami form the cervical plexus, and the lower four cervical and first thoracic anterior rami form the brachial plexus. The first three and a part of the fourth lumbar anterior rami form the lumbar plexus. The sacral anterior rami along with the fifth lumbar and a part of the fourth join to form the lumbosacral plexus. The enlargement and prolongation of the limb bud rather markedly alter the myotomal pattern, resulting in the union of some myotomes and the division or partial extended migration of others. The fibers, then, of any one mixed spinal nerve may be distributed through several peripheral nerves. By the same token any one peripheral nerve may contain fibers from several spinal nerves.

The area of skin supplied by the fibers of a single spinal root is called a dermatome. Segmental dermatomal patterns (Fig. 64-2) are well preserved in the thoracic region but not in the limbs. Migration of the limb buds accounts for the displacement of midcervical dermatomes along the lateral aspect of the arm and radial aspect of the forearm and of the lower cervical and upper thoracic dermatomes along the medial aspect of the arm and the ulnar aspect of the forearm. Lumbar and sacral dermatomal alignment along the various aspects of the lower extremity is similarly explained. The line separating the more rostral segmental dermatomes from the more caudal ones is called the axial line and may be followed into the spinal axis.

Foerster's *remaining sensibility* dermatomes outlined by the *isolation* method of Sherrington depict the areas of maximal supply as large. These areas were determined by section of several roots above and below the root in question with retained sensibility outlined as the *maximal zone*

of that dermatome. Normally there is extensive overlap between adjacent dermatomes. The area of hypesthesia or hypalgesia resulting from the section of a single nerve or root is called the *intermediate zone*. A relatively small area of complete anesthesia may or may not be evident after section of a peripheral nerve or a root, and this area is called the *autonomous zone* of the nerve or root. More often the overlap is so extensive that no autonomous root zone can be delineated.

Microscopic anatomy

Each nerve fiber, or axon, with a diameter greater than 1μ has a myelin sheath of variable thickness (Fig. 64-3). The axon is a direct extension of a dorsal root ganglion cell, an anterior horn cell, or it represents a postganglionic fiber arising in the regional sympathetic ganglion and entering the mixed spinal nerve through the gray ramus. Each axon is encircled by its Schwann cell sheath (Fig. 64-4). In the unmyelinated or sparsely myelinated fibers the Schwann cell alone acts as a sheath and encloses minimal amounts of myelin. In the more heavily myelinated fibers the Schwann cell by rotation forms a multilaminated structure that encloses a myelin sheath. The axon with its Schwann cell and myelin sheath is in turn surrounded by a veil of delicate fibrous tissue called the *endoneurium*. Visualized longitudinally the endoneurium forms a tube encircling individually the Schwann cell sheaths that cluster together to form a funiculus. Each funiculus or separate group of sheathed axons is in turn surrounded by a denser layer of *perineurium*. The entire group of funiculi with their surrounding perineurium is encased as a mixed spinal or peripheral nerve in a denser *epineurium*.

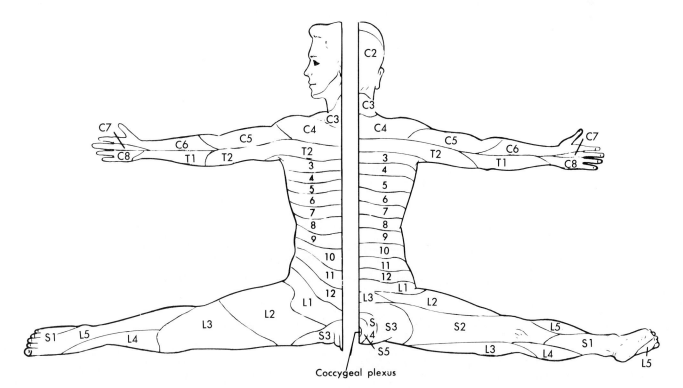

Fig. 64-2. Dermatomal patterns.

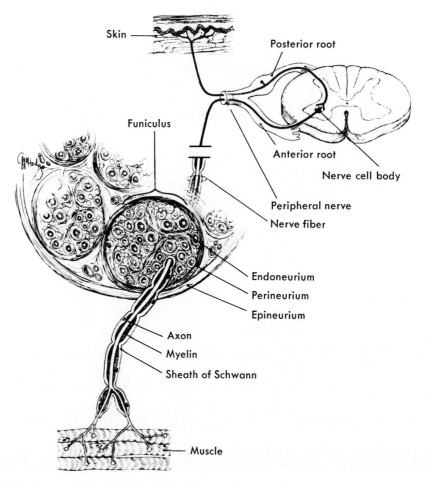

Fig. 64-3. Anatomy of nerve cell, showing cell body and nerve fiber, or axon, with its component parts. (From Grabb, W.C.: Orthop. Clin. North Am. **1**:419, 1970.)

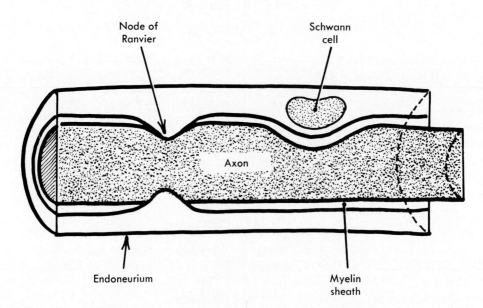

Fig. 64-4. Basic anatomy of myelinated nerve fiber. (From Urbaniak, J.R., and Warren, F.H.: Application of microsurgical techniques in the care of the injured peripheral nerve. In American Academy of Orthopaedic Surgeons: Symposium on microsurgery, St. Louis, 1979, The C.V. Mosby Co.)

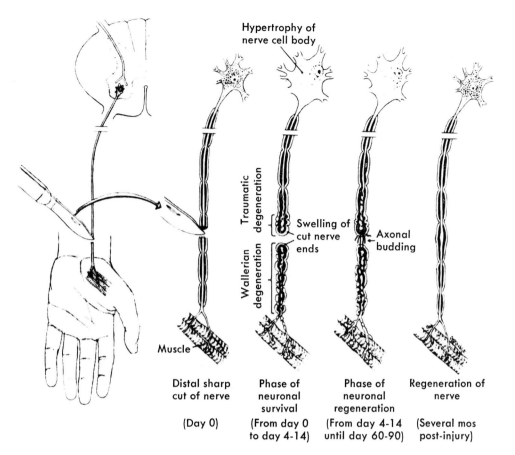

Fig. 64-5. Physiologic changes in regeneration of peripheral motor nerve axon after division with sharp object (see text). (From Grabb, W.C.: Orthop. Clin. North Am. **1**:419, 1970.)

NEURONAL DEGENERATION AND REGENERATION

Any part of a neuron detached from its soma degenerates and is destroyed by phagocytosis. This process of degeneration distal to a point of injury is called secondary or wallerian (1852) degeneration (Fig. 64-5). The reaction proximal to the point of detachment is called primary or retrograde degeneration. The time required for degeneration varies somewhat between sensory and motor segments and is also related to the size and myelinization of the fiber.

During the first three days after injury definite morphologic changes become apparent in the axon. Response to faradic stimulation can be obtained for periods varying from 18 to 72 hours. After 2 or 3 days the distal segment becomes fragmented, and with subsequent fluid loss the fragments begin to shrink and to assume a more oval or globular appearance. A concomitant fragmentation and shrinkage of the myelin sheath parallels the axonal degenerative change. By the seventh day macrophages have reached the area in greater numbers, and clearing of the axonal debris is virtually complete after 15 to 30 days. Schwann cell division by mitosis is evident by the seventh day, the cells increasing in number to fill the area previously filled by the axon and myelin sheath.

The primary retrograde degeneration proceeds for at least a segment or more, depending on the degree of prox-

imal insult. The changes in the parent cell body vary to some degree with the type of cell and the nearness of the injury to the cell body. The more proximal the site of injury, the more pronounced will be the changes. Chromatolysis with swelling of the cytoplasm and eccentric placement of the nucleus is commonly evident. This reaction within the cell body is easily evident by the seventh day, and death or evidence of beginning recovery is apparent after 4 to 6 weeks. With recovery the edema begins to subside, the nucleus migrates toward the center of the cell, and Nissl substance begins to reaccumulate.

Distal to the point of injury or to the proximal extent of retrograde degeneration, there is then an endoneurial tube filled with Schwann cells to accept regenerating sprouts from the axonal stump. If the endoneurial tube with its contained Schwann cells has been uninterrupted by the injury, the sprouts may readily pass along their former courses, and after regeneration the surviving cells innervate their previous end organs. If, however, the injury has been severe enough to interrupt the endoneurial tube with its contained Schwann cells, then sprouts that may number as many as 100 from any one axonal stump may migrate aimlessly throughout the damaged area into the epineurial, perineurial, or adjacent regions to form a stump neuroma or neuroma in continuity. Other migrating axonal sprouts barred from their endoneurial tube by scar tissue might enter empty endoneurial tubes of other injured funiculi and regenerate to myotomal or dermatomal areas other than their own.

Lesser injuries without disruption of the endoneurial and Schwann cell sheaths are associated with excellent or acceptable anatomic regeneration. Conversely, more extensive injuries with complete disruption of the entire nerve, with wide separation of the ends of the nerve, and with the regenerating fibers obstructed by extensive scar tissue are associated with little or no return of function.

CLASSIFICATION OF NERVE INJURIES

The classification of nerve injuries proposed by Seddon (1943) was generally accepted but rarely used. He divided such injuries into three groups as follows.

1. *Neurapraxia,* designating minor contusion or compression of a peripheral nerve with preservation of the axis-cylinder but with possibly minor edema or breakdown of a localized segment of myelin sheath. Thus transmission of impulses is physiologically interrupted for a time, but recovery is complete in a few days or weeks.

2. *Axonotmesis,* designating more significant injury with breakdown of the axon and distal wallerian degeneration but with preservation of the Schwann cell and endoneurial tubes. Spontaneous regeneration with good functional recovery can be expected.

3. *Neurotmesis,* designating a more severe injury with complete anatomic severance of the nerve or extensive avulsing or crushing injury. The axon and the Schwann cell and endoneurial tubes are completely disrupted. The perineurium and epineurium are also disrupted to varying degrees. Segments of the latter two may bridge the gap if complete severance is not apparent. In this group significant spontaneous recovery cannot be expected.

A more useful classification was described by Sunderland in 1951. This classification is more readily applicable clinically, each degree of injury suggesting a greater anatomic disruption with its correspondingly altered prognosis. In this classification peripheral nerve injuries are arranged in ascending order of severity from the first to the fifth degree. Anatomically the various degrees represent differences in loss or disruption of (1) conduction in the axon, (2) the continuity of the axon, (3) the endoneurial tube and its contents, (4) the funiculus and its contents, and (5) the entire nerve trunk.

In *first-degree* injury conduction along the axon is physiologically interrupted at the site of injury, but the axon is not actually disrupted. No wallerian degeneration occurs, and recovery is spontaneous and is usually complete within a few days or weeks. This injury coincides with the neurapraxia of Seddon. The loss of function is variable. Usually motor function is more profoundly affected than is sensory function. Sensory modalities are affected in order of decreasing frequency as follows: proprioception, touch, temperature, and pain; sympathetic fibers are the most resistant to this type of injury. If sensory modalities are markedly affected, paresthesias may be present for several days. If disturbed at all, sympathetic function often returns promptly; the modalities of pain and temperature are also commonly preserved or return promptly. Proprioception and motor function are usually the last to return. Electrical excitability of the nerve distal to the site of injury is pre-

served. A characteristic of this injury is the simultaneous return of motor function in the proximal and distal musculature; this would never occur in injuries with wallerian degeneration in which the "motor march" is evident because of progressive regeneration or reinnervation of the more proximal motor units earlier in the course of recovery. In most instances the final result is complete restoration of function.

In *second-degree* injury disruption of the axon is evident, with wallerian degeneration distal to the point of injury, and degeneration proximally for one or more nodal segments. However, the integrity of the endoneurial tube is maintained, and the Schwann cell sheath within this tube is also maintained, filling it to provide a perfect anatomic course for regeneration. The advancement of the axonal stump is confined within the endoneurial tube, and reinnervation is accomplished in the normal anatomic pattern. Any permanent deficit is related to the number of neural somas that die, such death being more common in injuries at the more proximal levels. Clinically the neurologic deficit is complete with loss of motor, sensory, and sympathetic function. Motor reinnervation is accomplished in a progressive manner from proximal to distal in the order in which nerve branches leave the parent trunk. Commonly the Tinel sign can be followed along the course of the nerve, tracing the progression of regeneration. Usually good functional return is achieved.

In *third-degree* injury the axons, the Schwann cell sheaths, the endoneurial tubes, and the internal funiculi are all disrupted, but the perineurium is preserved. The result then is disorganization resulting from disruption of the endoneurial tubes. Intrafunicular fibrosis can obstruct certain tubes and divert sprouts to paths other than their own. Commonly fusiform swelling is apparent in one or more funiculi resulting in a neuroma in continuity. Variable degrees of regeneration and return of function can be anticipated; at times aberrant regeneration is evident because of competition among the various sprouts for the available endoneurial tubes. Clinically the neurologic loss is complete in most instances, and because of the additional time required for the regenerating axon tips to penetrate the fibrous barrier, the duration of loss is more prolonged than in second-degree injury. Returning motor function is evident from proximal to distal but with varying degrees of permanent motor or sensory deficit. In this injury the Tinel sign is less accurate as a guide of the quality of recovery.

In *fourth-degree* injury the funiculi and endoneurium are disrupted, but some of the epineurium and possibly also some of the perineurium are preserved so that complete severance of the entire trunk does not occur. Retrograde degeneration is more severe following this degree of injury, and the mortality among neuronal soma is higher, sometimes resulting in a significant reduction in the number of surviving axons. Often the axonal sprouts are confronted with an extensive gap or with dense fibrous tissue and with few available endoneurial tubes for which they can compete. Axonal sprouts exit through defects in the perineurium and epineurium and wander about in the surrounding tissues. Prognosis for significant return of useful function is uniformly poor without surgery.

In *fifth-degree* injury division or loss of continuity of the nerve trunk is complete with a variable distance between the neural stumps. Often this type of injury occurs in a compound fracture wound and is commonly associated with sepsis, extensive scarring, and a marked gap between the neural stumps. The likelihood of any significant bridging by axonal sprouts is remote, and the possibility of any significant functional return without appropriate surgery is equally remote.

Mixed injuries occur in which a nerve trunk is partially severed and the remaining part of the trunk sustains fourth-, third-, second-, or rarely even first-degree injury.

To avoid unnecessary delay before any indicated surgical reconstruction of the nerve is carried out, determining the degree of injury is important. Of equal importance is avoiding unnecessary exploration in first-, second-, and a significant percentage of third-degree injuries.

EFFECTS OF PERIPHERAL NERVE INJURIES
Motor

When a peripheral nerve is severed at a given level, all motor function of the nerve distal to that level is abolished. All muscles supplied by branches of the nerve distal to that level are paralyzed and become atonic. Significant electromyographic changes are not apparent for 8 to 14 days, at which time transient fibrillation potentials on needle insertion may become apparent. Spontaneous fibrillations may become evident after 2 to 4 weeks, which time also coincides with the onset of atrophic change within the muscle fibers. Atrophy of muscle bulk progresses rather rapidly to some 50% to 70% at the end of about 2 months (Sunderland, 1952). Then atrophy continues at a much slower rate, and the connective tissue component of the muscles increases somewhat. Striations and motor end-plate configurations are retained for longer than 12 months whereas the empty endoneurial tubes shrink to about one third their normal diameter (Sunderland and Bradley, 1950). Complete disruption and replacement of muscle fibers may not become complete until after 3 years. Several methods are used in evaluating motor return following peripheral nerve injuries. They involve assessment of muscle strength against gravity and against graded resistance. The use of pinch meters, grip meters, and evaluation of endurance, speed of movement, and individual muscle function help to document the progress of motor return.

The British Medical Research Council established the following system for assessing the return of muscle function after peripheral nerve injuries: in M_0 no contraction has returned; in M_1 perceptible contraction in proximal muscles has returned; in M_2 perceptible contraction in both proximal and distal muscles has returned; in M_3 all important muscles act against resistance; in M_4 all synergic and independent movements are possible; and in M_5 recovery is complete.

Sensory

Sensory loss usually follows a definite anatomic pattern, although the factor of overlap from adjacent nerves may confuse the inexperienced. After severance of a peripheral nerve only a small area of complete sensory loss is found. This area is supplied exclusively by the severed nerve and is called the *autonomous zone* or *isolated zone* of supply for that nerve. A somewhat larger area of tactile and thermal anesthesia is readily delineated and corresponds more closely to the gross anatomic distribution of the nerve (Fig. 64-6); this larger area is known as the *intermediate zone*. When a nerve is intact and the adjacent nerves are blocked or sectioned, there is an area of sensibility that exceeds the gross anatomic distribution of the nerve; this area is known as the *maximal zone*.

That the autonomous zone becomes smaller during the first few days or weeks after injury, long before regeneration is possible, has long been recognized. Livingston believes this is caused by ingrowth of adjacent nerves, but resumption of or increase in function in anastomotic branches from adjacent nerves is a more plausible explanation. This decrease in the area of sensory loss might be interpreted by the inexperienced surgeon as evidence of regeneration or of incomplete injury and thus be responsible for needless delay in exploration of the nerve.

Dellon, Curtis, and Edgerton reported their experience with 12 patients with injuries to the median and ulnar nerves. They described a method in which constant touch, moving touch, and a graded vibratory stimulus (tuning fork) were used to evaluate recovery from upper-extremity peripheral nerve injuries. They found that the perception of pinprick was the first to return. The next perceptions to return were those of a 30-cycles/second vibratory stimulus followed by moving touch. The perception of constant touch and finally the perception of a 256-cycles/second vibratory stimulus were the last to return. They inferred that the early return of pain perception resulted from the faster regeneration of the small-diameter pain fibers. The larger-diameter touch fibers regenerated more slowly. That the appreciation of moving touch mediated by quickly adapting fibers and pacinian corpuscles returned sooner than that of constant touch mediated by slowly adapting fibers and Merkel's disks was explained by differential maturation of the respective receptors rather than by the diameter of the fibers alone. The system of evaluating by moving touch, constant touch, vibratory stimulus, pinprick, and the Weber two-point discrimination was proposed as a method for screening patients to determine specific exercises for reeducation of constant-touch perception. The evaluation of sensory return following peripheral nerve injuries is important regardless of the site of the injury. This is especially true in the upper extremity where sensibility in the hand is extremely important.

The clinical evaluation of sensory return is also done using other methods such as pinprick appreciation and von Frey hairs. The British Medical Research Council established the following six-level grading scale for sensory return: in S_0 there is absence of sensibility in the autonomous area, in S_1 there is recovery of deep cutaneous pain within the autonomous area, in S_2 there is return of some superficial cutaneous pain and tactile sensibility within the autonomous area of the nerve, in S_3 there is return of superficial cutaneous pain and tactile sensibility throughout the autonomous area with disappearance of overreaction, in S_{3+} there is some recovery of two-point discrimination within the autonomous area, and in S_4 there is complete recovery.

Moberg has emphasized the limitations of the traditional methods of correlating touch and pain as well as cold and warmth with the eventual function of the hand following peripheral nerve injury. In his evaluation, tests with the

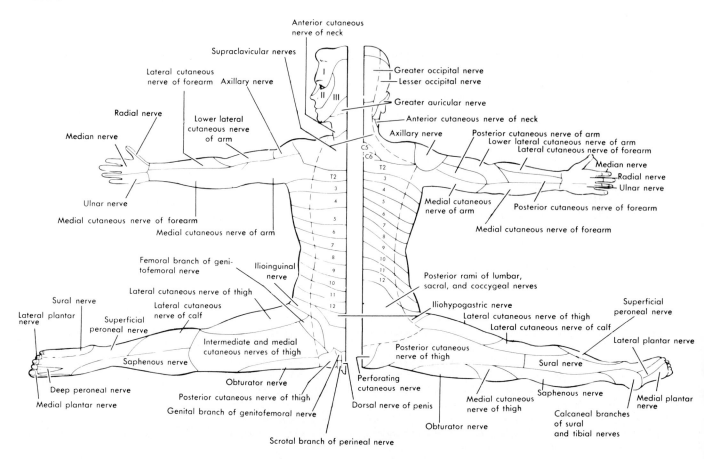

Fig. 64-6. Cutaneous distribution of peripheral nerves.

pinpricks and cotton wool were discarded in favor of the Weber two-point discrimination test, the picking-up test, and the triketohydrindene hydrate (Ninhydrin) printing test.

Leonard described four children who experienced surprisingly satisfactory return of sensation after documented, untreated transection of digital nerves. This observation has been explained on the basis of adaptability of the sensory cortex, maturation of nerves, nerve overlap, and nerve budding. Terzis, using single–fascicle electrophysiologic recording techniques, studied the reinnervation of free skin grafts in rabbits. She found that early reinnervation occurred with ingrowth of fibers that conducted impulses at slow velocities corresponding to unmyelinated sensory fibers. Later, with maturation of the skin grafts, reinnervation was characterized electrically by the ingrowth of fibers having shorter latencies and faster conduction velocities, consistent with an increasing number of myelinated fibers. Such techniques should have future clinical application in the restoration of sensibility after reconstructive operations and in the management of peripheral nerve injuries.

Reflex

Complete severance of a peripheral nerve abolishes all reflex activity transmitted by that nerve. This is true in severance of either the afferent or efferent arc. Commonly, however, reflex activity is abolished in partial nerve injuries when neither arc is completely interrupted and thus is not a reliable guide to the severity of injury.

Autonomic

Interruption of a peripheral nerve is followed by loss of sweating and of pilomotor response and by vasomotor paralysis in the autonomous zone. The area of anhydrosis usually corresponds to but may be slightly larger than the sensory deficit. This area may be easily outlined by the starch-iodine test, by the triketohydrindene hydrate (Ninhydrin) printing test popularized by Aschan and Moberg, or by instruments for determining skin resistance (Richter dermometer). Another objective test described by O'Riain and by Leukens is the wrinkle test. When normal skin is immersed in water for a time, wrinkling occurs. Denervated skin does not wrinkle under these circumstances. As reinnervation occurs, wrinkling of the skin returns. If the injury is incomplete and especially if it is associated with causalgia, sweating may be excessive and may involve areas beyond the intermediate zone of the nerve. Vasodilatation occurs in complete lesions, and the area affected is at first warmer and pinker than the rest of the limb. After 2 to 3 weeks, however, the affected area becomes colder than the adjacent normal areas, and the skin may be pale, cyanotic, or mottled in an area often extending beyond the maximal zone of the injured nerve. Trophic changes occur commonly and are most evident in the hands and feet. The skin becomes thin and glistening and, when subjected to trauma that ordinarily does little harm, breaks down to form ulcers that heal slowly. The fingernails become distorted, often ridged or brittle, and may be lost entirely.

Osteoporosis often follows peripheral nerve injuries. It is more likely to be pronounced in incomplete lesions associated with pain. Incomplete lesions of the median nerve seem to be more often associated with osteoporosis, with changes occurring in the distal phalanges of the thumb and index and long fingers. Partial ankylosis from fibrosis of the periarticular structures may also develop. These changes are similar to atrophy of disuse but are much more severe.

Causalgia

Causalgia was first described by Mitchell, Morehouse, and Keen in 1864. This description is quite specific, and if it is heeded, considerable confusion will be avoided. Causalgia is a clinical syndrome associated with a lesion of a peripheral nerve that contains sensory fibers and is characterized by pain in the affected extremity, usually in the hand or foot. It occurs as a complication in about 3% of major nerve injuries. It is most often associated with incomplete lesions of the median and sciatic nerves, primarily the tibial part of the latter. These two nerves account for about 60% of the cases collected by Shumacker (1948); the rest of the cases involved primarily the nerves of the upper extremity. However, almost every major nerve in both the upper and lower extremity as well as the face has been implicated in isolated reports. Various theories as to the cause of causalgia have been proposed, including short-circuiting effects at the area of injury, permitting irritation of sensory afferent fibers by the efferent sympathetic impulses, periarteritis involving the vessels about the injured neural segments, and abnormal feedback into the internuncial centers of the spinal cord (Gerard, 1951). Lankford has made a detailed study of the historical aspects, etiologic theories, clinical manifestations, and methods of managing this difficult disorder. Because of the apparent involvement of the sympathetic nervous system in this disorder, he recommends the term reflex sympathetic dystrophy be used instead of causalgia. His work is recommended for study by anyone treating patients with causalgia states.

The syndrome is one of excruciating burning pain often described as having a superimposed throbbing, aching, bursting pressure, knifelike stabbing, twisting, or crushing component. In many instances (in about one third of patients reported by Rasmussen and Freedman, 1946) pain begins immediately after injury; it usually begins sometime during the first week. The pain is usually located in an area corresponding to the cutaneous distribution of the nerve but is not necessarily limited to this area. Another characteristic of the pain, one usually necessary for a positive diagnosis, is accentuation by stimuli to such emotions as surprise and anger and by other disturbances in the patient's environment. Some of the factors that aggravate or relieve the pain are so fantastic as to be hardly credible and may lead the patient to unjustified psychiatric consultation. For example, some patients keep the injured extremity wrapped in a wet towel because moisture relieves the pain; others keep the normal hand moist because to touch an object with a normal dry hand causes severe pain in the injured extremity. Examining some patients is impossible unless the examiner's own hands are moistened. Some patients put water in their shoes to avoid increasing the pain when they walk, even though the lesion is in the upper extremity. Some cannot sleep on sheets or pillowcases and prefer instead to sleep on a rough blanket. To touch, feel, or even hear the name of a slick object such as paper or a sheet will cause severe increase in pain in some patients. In many instances light touch, heat, or minor movements of the trunk and extremity will increase existing pain. Some patients insist the pain seems less severe on cool, damp days or at night and is more readily relieved by a drink of whiskey than by morphine.

After having seen a patient with severe causalgia one is not likely to forget the picture of a pain-racked patient guarding the affected extremity with extreme care. The skin of the affected part may show evidence of vasodilatation early after injury, and this may or may not be replaced later by vasoconstriction. Thus the skin of the affected part may be dark red, dry, glossy, and atrophied or cold, mottled, and moist. The skin may be devoid of hair, or, on the contrary, may have an abnormal growth of hair (Mayfield and Devine, 1945). As noted, causalgia is thought to occur most often in incomplete lesions of peripheral nerves, although the syndrome reportedly has followed complete lesions. Furthermore, sepsis, pressure injuries, systemic viral infections, and spinal cord concussion in which no direct injury to the extremity was detectable have reportedly been followed by causalgia. Accurate evaluation of the completeness of the nerve lesion is commonly impossible because of the extreme pain caused by handling the affected limb. Lankford has classified the various clinical types of reflex sympathetic dystrophy as follows:

1. Minor causalgia
2. Minor traumatic dystrophy
3. Shoulder-hand syndrome
4. Major traumatic dystrophy
5. Major causalgia

Echlin, Owens, and Wells attempted to separate so-called major causalgia from minor causalgia. The latter term was coined by Homans and de Takats and referred to the same thing as "reflex dystrophy of the extremities" or "causalgic states." Minor causalgia or causalgic states include conditions such as Sudeck's atrophy and painful osteoporosis. In them the pain is much less severe, and they should rarely be mistaken for true causalgia. They occasionally respond to the same treatment as causalgia; however, Omer et al., Kleinert et al., Buker et al., and Wirth and Rutherford have reported successful treatment of vaious causalgic states by intensive physical therapy, oral medications, perineural infiltration of nerves with local anesthetics, sympathetic ganglion blocks with local anesthetics, and thoracic and lumbar sympathectomies. In a study of 17,500 operations carried out over a period of 5 years,

Kleinert et al. found 506 patients with posttraumatic causalgic states or reflex dystrophy. Twenty-five percent of these followed operations for crushing injuries, and another 25% followed elective operations on the upper extremity, including carpal tunnel release and palmar fasciotomies; the remaining 50% developed after such injuries as sprains and contusions and after other elective operations.

When causalgia is severe, the diagnosis is usually clear and is easily confirmed by local anesthetic block of the second and third sympathetic ganglia if the pain is in the hand or of the second or third lumbar sympathetic ganglion if the pain is in the foot. Rarely will other neurologic conditions be confused with true causalgia.

Many mild or moderate causalgias subside spontaneously after a few months. Occasionally, especially in the early stages of the disease, a series of several sympathetic blocks with a local anesthetic will relieve the pain either completely or enough to make it tolerable. If, however, the pain returns to the level present before injection and is severe, sympathectomy may be necessary.

Preganglionic sympathectomy, consisting of section of the sympathetic chain distal to the third thoracic ganglion and division of the rami between the second and third ganglia and their respective intercostal nerves, will usually relieve the pain in the upper extremity. Excision of the second and third lumbar sympathetic ganglia and chain through a high transverse abdominal incision will usually relieve pain in the lower extremity; occasionally a more extensive sympathectomy is necessary (Mayfield).

ETIOLOGY OF PERIPHERAL NERVE INJURIES

Peripheral nerves may be injured by metabolic or collagen diseases, malignancies, endogenous or exogenous toxins, or thermal, chemical, or mechanical trauma. Only injuries caused by mechanical trauma are considered here. Every patient having injured a limb or limb girdle should be evaluated for possible musculoskeletal, vascular, and peripheral nerve damage (Table 64-1). During times of war 14% to 18% of extremity injuries include injury to peripheral nerves. Omer in his report on Vietnam war casualties found that 22% of the patients with injuries to the

upper extremity had associated injuries to major peripheral nerves. Comparable figure for injuries incurred in civilian life are not available. Lacerating or penetrating wounds caused by sharp objects or weapons accounted for about 40% of the noncombat peripheral nerve injuries reported by Lyons and Woodhall.

Bone or joint injury was associated with about 40% of 3656 peripheral nerve lesions followed by the Veterans Administration and National Research Council. Of the lesions reported by Lyons and Woodhall, 21% were associated with enough bone or joint injury to make combined orthopaedic and neurosurgical care necessary. *Primary* injury of a peripheral nerve results from the same trauma that injures a bone or joint. In some instances, however, the neural injury is caused by displaced osseous fragments, by stretching, or by manipulation rather than by the initial injuring force. *Secondary* injury results from involvement of the nerve by infection, scar, callus, or vascular complications. These complications may be hematoma, arteriovenous fistula, ischemia, or aneurysm.

The *radial nerve* is the one most commonly injured. Fourteen percent of humeral shaft fractures are said to be complicated by injury of this nerve. Thirty-three percent of radial nerve injuries are associated with fracture of the middle third of the humerus, 50% with fracture of the distal third of the humerus, 7% with supracondylar fracture of the humerus, and 7% with dislocation of the radial head.

The *ulnar nerve* is injured in about 30% of patients with combined skeletal and neural injury involving the upper extremity. This injury is most commonly associated with fractures about the medial humeral epicondyle but is often secondary to the formation of callus about the elbow.

The *median nerve* is injured in only about 15% of combined skeletal and neural injuries of the upper extremity. It is injured most commonly in dislocation of the elbow or secondarily in the carpal tunnel after injury of the wrist or distal forearm.

The *peroneal nerve* is injured most commonly at the fibular neck in fracture of the tibia and fibula or dislocation of the knee.

Branches of the *lumbosacral plexus* are injured in less than 3% of pelvic fractures; it is reportedly injured in 10% to 13% of the posterior dislocations of the hip. The *tibial nerve* may be injured in fractures of the proximal tibia and injuries about the ankle.

Peripheral nerve injuries should be carefully excluded in every patient with an acute extremity injury. Equal diligence should be applied in evaluation after surgery, manipulation, casting, and recovery from skeletal injury to detect secondary neural injury.

CLINICAL DIAGNOSIS OF NERVE INJURIES

Immediately after a severe injury to an extremity, recognition of a peripheral nerve injury is not always easy. Pain is often so severe that cooperation by the patient is limited at best. Here the preservation of life and limb is always the first objective. However, when possible, some simple tests should be made to detect injuries of major nerves of the extremity. In the upper extremity, for instance, loss of pain perception in the tip of the little finger

Table 64-1. Frequency of specific nerve involvement associated with long bone fractures based on 300 cases reported by Spurling

Extremity	Bone	Nerve	%
Upper, 74%	Humerus	Radial	70
		Median	8
		Ulnar	22
	Radius and/or ulna	Radial	35
		Median	24
		Ulnar	41
Lower, 20%	Femur	Complete sciatic	60
		Tibial component	20
		Peroneal component	20
	Tibia and/or fibula	Tibial	7
		Peroneal	70
		Both nerves	23

indicates ulnar nerve injury. Loss of pain perception in the tip of the index finger indicates median nerve injury, and inability to extend the thumb in the hitchhiker's sign usually indicates radial nerve injury though the extensor tendons may be severed and render this test invalid. Similarly, in the lower extremity loss of pain perception in the sole of the foot usually indicates sciatic or tibial nerve injury, whereas inability to extend the great toe or the foot indicates peroneal or sciatic nerve injury. As with the radial nerve, injury to the tendons or muscle bellies may render these tests useless. However, they may be carried out quickly and usually serve as effective screening procedures.

In evaluating peripheral nerve lesions, a precise knowledge of the course of the nerve, of the level of origin of its motor branches, and of the muscles that these branches supply is essential. Knowledge of the more common anatomic variations in nerve supply is extremely helpful. Furthermore, one must be familiar with the various zones of sensation as well as with the areas in which sweating may be diminished or absent and in which skin resistance may be increased. Evaluation of motor loss is highly important.

This can be accurate only if one can palpate or see the tendon or muscle belly under consideration. If one relies on analysis of movement alone as an indication of intact nerve supply, errors will be made because of substitution and trick movement. For example, opposition of the thumb to the little finger can be accomplished by many patients even though the nerve supply to the opponens pollicis is completely severed and the muscle is paralyzed. In addition, the wrist may be partially extended, even when the muscles supplied by the radial nerve are completely paralyzed, by simple flexion of the fingers, and the elbow can be forcefully flexed, even when the musculocutaneous nerve is completely severed and the biceps paralyzed by substitution of the brachioradialis. Palpation of the opponens pollicis, extensor tendons of the wrist, and biceps tendon or muscle prevents such deceptions. Some muscles cannot be tested by palpation or sight. They include the lumbricals, the short adductor of the thumb, and the interossei except for the first dorsal. There are enough muscles supplied by each nerve that can be so tested as to allow an accurate diagnosis in most instances. The muscles that may be examined accurately and easily are enumerated in the discussion of each nerve. To make a clinical assessment of the strength of the muscles is helpful. A scale recommended by Highet has been widely accepted. According to that scale the following designations are assigned: 0 for total paralysis, 1 for muscle flicker, 2 for muscle contraction, 3 for muscle contraction against gravity, 4 for muscle contraction against gravity and resistance, and 5 for normal muscle contraction as compared with the opposite side.

Diagnostic tests

ELECTROMYOGRAPHY

Immediately after section of a peripheral nerve the electromyogram will demonstrate normal insertion activity (Fig. 64-7). There will be no muscle response following stimulation of the nerve proximal to the site of injury. During the interval between 5 and 10 days after section, early denervation changes may be seen. Within 5 to 14 days positive sharp waves consistent with denervation are seen (Fig. 64-8). Within 12 days denervation fibrillation potentials may be seen. No motor unit potentials are evident during attempted volitional contraction of the muscle, confirming the clinical finding of paralysis involving the

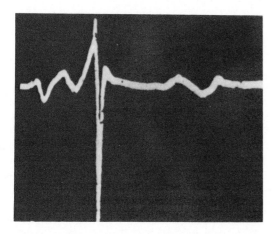

Fig. 64-7. Electromyogram demonstrating normal insertion activity. (From Pierce, D.S.: Clin. Orthop. **107:**25, 1975.)

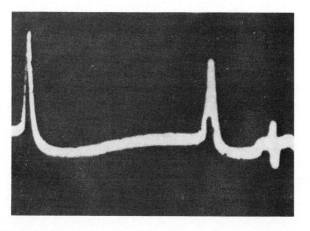

Fig. 64-8. Electromyogram demonstrating positive sharp wave consistent with denervation. (From Pierce, D.S.: Clin. Orthop. **107:**25, 1975.)

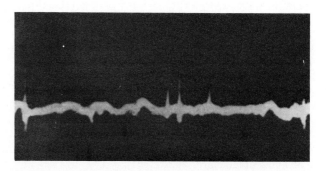

Fig. 64-9. Electromyogram demonstrating spontaneous denervation fibrillation potentials. (From Pierce, D.S.: Clin. Orthop. **107:**25, 1975.)

muscle being tested. Electromyography immediately after injury is valuable to demonstrate residual innervation or retained motor unit potentials during atempted volitional contraction that could be so minimal as to be undetected clinically. Retained motor unit potentials found under these circumstances suggest that complete interruption of the supplying nerve did not result from the injury. In such a situation anomalous innervation must be excluded.

As wallerian degeneration progresses, fibrillation may be detected on electrode insertion at 7 to 14 days. Fifteen to 30 days after complete interruption of its motor supply, spontaneous fibrillation potentials of the muscle will be evident (Fig. 64-9). If denervation fibrillation potentials have not appeared by the end of the second week, this may be considered a good prognostic sign. Fibrillations of denervation will last indefinitely until the muscle has become either reinnervated or fibrotic. Denervation potentials may increase transiently and then progressively decrease as reinnervation progresses.

Evidence of reinnervation is judged to be present when highly polyphasic motor unit potentials are detected on attempts at volitional activity. Initially these may be of low amplitude with diphasic or triphasic configurations of short duration. With progression of reinnervation, these become more numerous and of higher amplitude and eventually become more normal in configuration.

As regeneration progresses along the course of a peripheral nerve, the muscles innervated by the more proximal branches will reveal evidence of electrical reinnervation, whereas those more distally served will retain only fibrillation or denervation activity.

The electromyogram merely indicates that the muscle is or is not innervated but gives no specific indication as to the level of injury to its nerve. Each muscle served by a peripheral nerve should be evaluated; the most proximal level of paralysis gives an excellent indication of the level of injury. In injuries occurring as high as a nerve root at or near its foramen of exit, additional denervation potentials will be detectable in the erector spinae muscles, which are innervated by the posterior primary ramus of the root. By careful evaluation at various levels about the proximal and distal areas of the limb a reasonably definite determination can be made as to what part of a plexus is injured, and frequently a definite level of injury can be established.

Denervation fibrillations do not in any sense determine whether the nerve has sustained a second-, third-, fourth-, or fifth-degree injury. By the same token, reinnervation potentials may be evident after regeneration of only a few motor fibers, and thus the presence of reinnervation potentials does not necessarily indicate that good return of volitional motor function will occurr.

NERVE CONDUCTION STUDIES

Stimulation of a peripheral nerve by an electrode placed on the skin overlying the nerve will readily evoke a response from the muscle or muscles innervated by that nerve. This response can be seen, palpated, or measured electromyographically.

Immediately after section of a peripheral nerve, stimulation distal to the point of injury will still elicit an essentially normal response. Such a response can be obtained for 18 to 72 hours after injury or until wallerian degeneration reaches a point that conduction along the degenerating nerve is no longer possible. This failure of response after about 3 days is the earliest evidence of the severity of an injury and excludes from further consideration the first-degree or neurapraxia type of injury.

Finding a slowed conduction time at a specific point along the course of a peripheral nerve is often valuable in confirming a clinical diagnosis of compression neuropathy as opposed to other possible causes of nerve damage. This is especially valuable in compression neuropathies of the ulnar nerve at the level of the medial humeral epicondyle and of the median nerve within the carpal tunnel.

The techniques of both peripheral nerve stimulation studies and electromyography are exceedingly useful in separating hysterical or functional problems and malingering from organic illness that they might mimic.

TINEL SIGN

The Tinel sign is elicited by gentle percussion by a finger or percussion hammer along the course of an injured nerve. A transient tingling sensation should be experienced by the patient in the distribution of the injured nerve rather than at the area percussed, and the sensation should persist for several seconds following stimulation. A positive Tinel sign is presumptive evidence that regenerating axonal sprouts that have not obtained complete myelinization are progressing along the endoneurial tube. With progressive regeneration, the positive response fades proximally presumably because of progressive myelinization along the more proximal part of the regenerated segment. Distal progression of the response along the course of the nerve in question can be measured, and the rate of this progression has been used by some to establish prognosis or suggest the need for exploration. But the ease with which the sign may be elicited has been used as quantitative evaluation by others for the same purposes. The presence of such a sign alone with its progressive distal migration is certainly encouraging. Electrodiagnostic techniques for the evaluation of nerve-evoked potentials as well as electromyograms in the office and operating room provide sophisticated means for evaluating the progress of nerve regeneration as well as the assessment of neuromas in continuity. The work of Kline et al. in evaluating whole nerves and the reports of Terzis and of Williams and Terzis in assessing single fasciculi are recommended. It must be recalled that a few regenerating sensory fibers can result in a positive Tinel's sign; thus the presence of such a sign cannot be construed as absolute evidence that any motor fibers are regenerating or even that significant sensory return is necessarily to be expected.

SWEAT TEST

Sympathetic fibers within a peripheral nerve are among the most resistant to mechanical trauma. The presence of sweating within the autonomous zone of an injured peripheral nerve reassures the examiner to a degree, suggesting that complete interruption of the nerve has not occurred. Preservation of sweating can be determined very simply, as pointed out by Kahn, by observing beads of sweat through the +20 lens of an ophthalmoscope. The time-honored sweat test (iodine starch test) consists of dusting the extremity with quinizarin powder. Sweating is induced by various means. The powder remains dry and light gray throughout the denervated area and assumes a deep purple color throughout the area of normal sweating. The triketohydrindene hydrate (Ninhydrin) print test as recommended by Aschan and Moberg is another method of assessing sweat patterns in the hand.

SKIN RESISTANCE TEST

The skin resistance test is another method of evaluating autonomic interruption; in it a Richter dermometer is used. The autonomous zone with absence of sweating demonstrates an increased resistance to the passage of electric current. The adjacent innervated areas have a normal resistance, and further decreased resistance in these areas can be elicited by high external temperatures that will not affect the denervated area. The area outlined by the Richter dermometer roughly approximates the autonomous zone of the nerve in question.

ELECTRICAL STIMULATION

Electrical stimulation through the intact skin has been used in one form or another by many investigators and clinicians for a long time. Faradic stimulation is often of little value because normally innervated muscles may fail to respond to this current. Additionally, if response to faradic stimulation is still present after 3 weeks, then the muscles in most instances are capable of voluntary contraction and no additional information is obtained by the study. Galvanic stimulation is useful in determining chronaxy and the strength-duration curve. These determinations frequently give early evidence of denervation after nerve injury and are useful in following the evolution of reinnervation, which is less readily assessed by other methods.

EARLY MANAGEMENT OF NERVE INJURIES

As in any other injury, initial management of the patient with peripheral nerve damage should begin with careful assessment of the vital functions. When indicated, appropriate actions to prevent cardiopulmonary failure and shock should be taken and systemic antibiotics and tetanus prophylaxis should be provided. Once the extent of any injury to the major viscera has been determined and appropriate resuscitative measures have been started, the injury to the peripheral nerve should be evaluated and the specific nerve deficit should be carefully assessed.

An open wound in which a peripheral nerve has been injured should be thoroughly cleansed and debrided of any foreign material and necrotic tissue, using local, regional, or general anesthesia. If the wound is clean and sharply incised, if the condition of the patient is satisfactory, and if a repair can be carried out in a quiet and unhurried setting with adequate personnel and equipment, immediate primary repair of the nerve is preferred. On the other hand, if the general medical condition of the patient does not permit adequate repair or if circumstances otherwise cause an undue delay, we prefer to perform the neurorrhaphy during the first 3 to 7 days after injury; in this instance the wound first is covered with a sterile dressing and is observed for evidence of sepsis.

When open wounds are caused by blasting, abrading, or crushing agents and when contamination with foreign material is severe, the wound is thoroughly cleansed and debrided and a sterile dressing is applied. If the ends of the nerve can be identified, they are marked with sutures such as those of stainless steel that can be easily identified later. In the absence of a significant nerve gap, loose end-to-end apposition prevents retraction of the nerve segments and makes later repair easier. In the presence of a segmental gap in the nerve, suturing the ends to the soft tissues prevents their retraction. Soft tissue coverage of the wound consistent with the management of the injured part is carried out, and the nerve is repaired at a later date when the soft tissues have healed, usually between 3 and 6 weeks after injury.

A closed injury in which a peripheral nerve has been damaged requires careful assessment of residual function and documentation of discrete deficits. After the initial pain has subsided, and the wound has healed, early active motion of all joints of the involved extremity should be started. When necessary, gentle passive exercises that avoid disrupting nerves and tendons may be instituted. All joints of the extremity must be kept supple, and soft tissue contractures must be avoided. Exercises help keep the soft tissues of the extremity in a better physiologic state so that when the nerve has regenerated, rehabilitation is easier. The specific effects of electrical stimulation of muscles remain unclear. Regardless of the details of the treatment program the patient must become actively involved in it to prevent contractures and to strengthen muscles with intact innervation. Similarly an extremity with a peripheral nerve injury should not be immobilized indefinitely. Dynamic and static splinting to support joints and to prevent contractures should be used intermittently.

When closed fractures are complicated by peripheral nerve deficits, to await reinnervation seems reasonable, and early surgical exploration is usually avoided. Then the progress of return of function in the injured extremity is evaluated with periodic electromyograms, nerve conduction velocities, and frequent clinical evaluation. Conversely, if the nerve deficit follows manipulation or casting of a closed fracture in the absence of a prior nerve deficit, early exploration of the nerve is favored.

General considerations of treatment

FACTORS THAT INFLUENCE REGENERATION AFTER NEURORRHAPHY

Few worthwhile reports have been published on the results of neurorrhaphy and the factors that influence them, first because few people have had access to a large enough group of patients to make evaluations statistically significant and second because reports have only rarely been based on sound criteria of regeneration. Valuable reports have been compiled from studies of such injuries incurred in World War II and later conflicts. As a result of these studies, the influence of many factors on regeneration after nerve suture is now better understood.

Rarely should a fracture interfere with nerve repair. In the usual situation, a nerve may be explored if the fracture requires open reduction. In many open injuries, the nature of the wound may be such that early repair of the nerve cannot be done satisfactorily. Every effort should be made by repeated debridement of necrotic material to promote rapid healing of any open wounds without sepsis. Nerves may be successfully repaired during a second debridement, followed by closure and healing. Associated vascular injury may adversely affect nerve regeneration because of tissue ischemia.

Several important factors that seem to influence nerve regeneration are (1) the age of the patient, (2) the gap between the nerve ends, (3) the delay between the time of injury and repair, (4) the level of injury, (5) the condition of the nerve ends, and (6) the experience and techniques of the surgeon. The first five of these are discussed here.

Age. Age undoubtedly influences the rate and degree of nerve regeneration. All other factors being equal, neurorrhaphies are more successful in children than in adults and are more likely to fail in elderly patients; why this is true has not been completely explained. We do not know precisely what results can be expected in either of the extremes of age, for practically all significant studies have dealt with military personnel whose average age was from 18 to 30 years. Omer, in reviewing peripheral nerve injuries in upper extremities incurred in Vietnam, found the most successful results after neurorrhaphy in patients less than 20 years old. The work of Onne suggests a close correlation between the age at the time of neurorrhaphy and the two-point discrimination obtained after median and ulnar nerve repairs. Most of his patients between the ages of 20 and 40 years were found to have two-point discrimination values in the range of 30 mm. During the teens the values did not exceed 15 mm, and in patients 10 years old or younger the values, with one exception, were less than 10 mm. However, he observed that following digital nerve repair the final two-point discrimination was not as closely related to age. Kankaanpää; and Bakalim in studying sensory recovery after 137 peripheral neurorrhaphies in 96 patients found that a higher percentage of those less than 20 years old at the time of repair had two-point discrimination of less than 6 mm than did those over 20.

Gap between nerve ends. The nature of the injury is the most important factor in determining the defect remaining between the nerve ends after any neuromas and gliomas are resected. When a nerve is severed by a sharp instrument, such as a razor or knife, damage is slight both proximally and distally, and although the nerve ends do inevitably retract, the gap can usually be overcome easily. Conversely, when a nerve is severed by a high-velocity missile, proximal and distal nerve damage is extensive. Ultimately both ends must be widely resected to expose normal funiculi, producing a larger gap. The gap is further increased, of course, if part of the nerve is carried away by a missile, as in shrapnel injuries. Methods of closing troublesome gaps include (1) nerve mobilization, (2) nerve transposition, (3) joint flexion, (4) nerve grafts, and (5) bone shortening. The greater the defect, the more dissimilar is the funicular pattern of the two ends because of the constantly changing arrangement of fibers within the nerve as it progresses distally. Agreement is widespread that excessive tension on a neurorrhaphy harms nerve regeneration. Brooks advises nerve grafting if, after the nerve is mobilized, the gap cannot be closed by flexing the main joint of the limb 90 degrees. Sunderland cautions against excessive tension on the line of suture after surgery to avoid excessive fibrosis. He advises a combination of transplantation, transposition, and mobilization of the nerve to close gaps. Millesi after experimental and clinical observations concluded that tension at the line of suture is the most important factor influencing the results of neurorrhaphy. He advises intrafascicular nerve grafting to close the large gaps. Nicholson and Seddon as well as Sakellarides observed that the upper limit of a gap beyond which results will deteriorate is approximately 2.5 cm. The observations of Kirklin, Murphey, and Berkson in 1949 that recovery will be slightly better when the gap is relatively small remain valid (Fig. 64-10).

Delay between time of injury and repair. Delay of neurorrhaphy affects motor recovery more profoundly than sensory recovery (Fig. 64-11). Scarff has suggested that this is related to the survival time of denervated striated muscle. Bowden and Gutmann reported that human muscle develops irreversible changes that can be demonstrated 3 years after injury. Sunderland reported that satisfactory reinnervation of human muscle can occur after denervation of up to 12 months. The observations of patients with peripheral nerve injuries during World War II revealed that for every delay of 6 days between injury and repair there is a variable loss of potential recovery that averages about 1% of maximum performance; after 3 months this loss increases rapidly. In addition, return of function in distal muscles is poor when suture is late. The influence of delay on sensory return is unclear; in the Veterans Administration study little influence could be found, and useful sensation returned in a few patients when suture was performed as late as 2 years after injury. Thus the critical limit of delay beyond which sensation will not return is unknown. However, the British found early suture important in reducing the number of painful paresthesias and in regaining a useful degree of sensation. Kankaanpää and Bakalim studied sensory return after 137 neurorrhaphies and found that if carried out within 3 months after injury, the results were usually better after secondary repair than after primary. Twenty-one percent of the 85 primary repairs and 38% of the 52 secondary repairs regained two-point discrimination of 6 mm or less. The difference in return of sensation was most marked in digital nerve repairs. No difference in return between the primary and secondary repairs was noted in the nerve injuries at the wrist or in the forearm. The experimental work of Ducker et al. reveals a consistent timetable for intracellular metabolic events following nerve injury. They found that between 3 and 6 weeks the degenerative and reparative changes within the nerve cell body and the proximal and distal nerve trunks were well established. Kleinert et al. have reported their clinical impression that a delayed primary repair carried out between 7 and 18 days after injury is best for return of satisfactory function. In Omer's study 70% of successful repairs of lacerated nerves in the upper extremity had been carried out within 6 weeks after injury and all successful repairs within 3 months. Our practice is to perform neurorrhaphies in clean, sharp wounds immediately or during the first 5 to 7 days. In the presence of extensive soft tissue contusion, laceration, crushing, or contamination, a delay of 3 to 6 weeks is preferred.

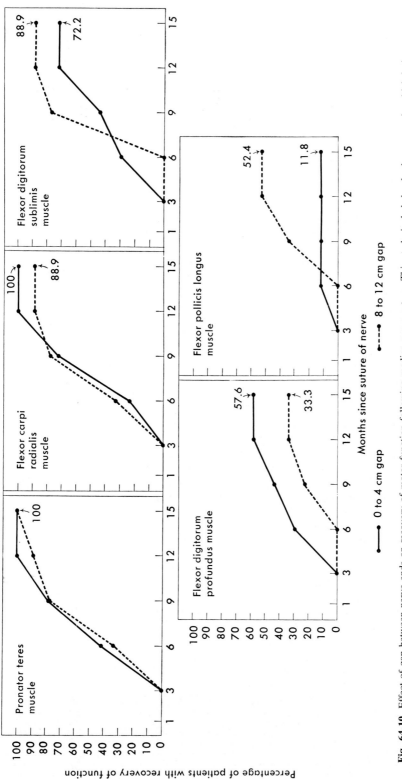

Fig. 64-10. Effect of gap between nerve ends on recovery of motor function following median nerve suture. This study included only those cases in which lesion was located from 0 to 15 cm proximal to medial epicondyle and in which nerve suture was performed within 6 months after injury. (Modified from Kirklin, J.W., Murphey, F., and Berkson, J.: Surg. Gynecol. Obstet. **88:**719, 1949.)

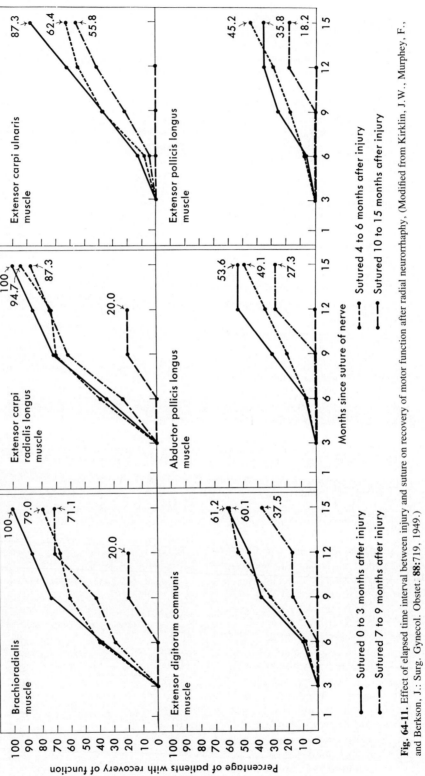

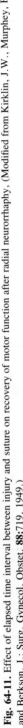

Fig. 64-11. Effect of elapsed time interval between injury and suture on recovery of motor function after radial neurorrhaphy. (Modified from Kirklin, J.W., Murphey, F., and Berkson, J.: Surg. Gynecol. Obstet. **88:**719, 1949.)

Level of injury. The more proximal the injury the more incomplete is the overall return of motor and sensory function, especially in the more distal structures. Sunderland observed that conditions are more favorable for recovery in the more proximal muscles because (1) the neurons that innervate the distal portions of the limb are more severely affected by retrograde changes following proximal injury, (2) a greater proportion of the cross-sectional area of the nerve trunk is occupied by fibers to the proximal muscles, and (3) the potential for disorientation of regrowing axons and for axon loss during regeneration is greater for the distal muscles than for those more proximally situated after a proximal injury. Boswick et al., in a review of 81 patients with 102 peripheral nerve injuries, found that of those injuries below the elbow 87% regained protective sensation and 14% regained normal two-point discrimination. Sakellarides found that after closed peripheral nerve injuries above the elbow return of function was delayed when compared with such injuries below the elbow. Of those patients treated surgically, 143 were followed for 12 months or more after neurorrhaphy. Recovery of good clinical function was found in 13 (27%) of 48 lesions above the elbow and in 37 (39%) of 95 lesions below this joint. Except for parts of the brachial plexus, useful function will at times return regardless of the level of injury if the critical limit of delay has not passed.

Condition of nerve ends. Sunderland has stressed the importance of the condition of the nerve ends at the time of neurorrhaphy. He suggested that meticulous handling of the nerve ends, asepsis, care with nerve mobilization, preservation of neural blood supply, avoidance of tension, and the provision of a suitable bed with minimal scar all exert favorable influences on nerve regeneration. Distal stump shrinkage has been found maximal at about 4 months, leaving the distal fascicular cross-sectional area diminished to 30% to 40% of normal size. Intraneural plexus formation and fascicular dispersal make accurate fascicular alignment and appropriate axonal regeneration more difficult. Edshage demonstrated that a neurorrhaphy with a satisfactory external appearance is no guarantee of optimal internal fascicular alignment. Fascicular malalignment was found commonly in his specimens taken from human nerve repairs. He has used, in addition to a special miter box for nerve trimming, a variety of special knives and scissors designed to assure satisfactory fascicular identification during neurorrhaphy. It is generally agreed that the nerve ends should be prepared in such a way that a satisfactory fascicular pattern is apparent in both the proximal and distal stumps. No scar, foreign material, or necrotic tissue should be allowed to remain about the ends to interfere with axonal regeneration. Sometimes resection of the nerve ends so that satisfactory fasciculi are exposed will leave a gap that cannot be closed by end-to-end repair. As noted previously, clinical and experimental, evidence indicates that excessive tension on the neurorrhaphy both at the time of repair and when an acutely flexed limb is later mobilized causes excessive intraneural fibrosis. These findings and the promising results achieved after the interfascicular nerve grafting technique advocated by Millesi and by Millesi, Meissl, and Berger suggest that such a technique is preferable to repair of nerves under too much tension or with limbs in acutely flexed or awkward positions.

Cuffs at neurorrhaphy. During World War II tantalum cuffs were wrapped around nerve repairs, but they made no significant statistical difference in the results. Since that time other substances have been used without definite benefit. In experimental settings, Kline and Hayes, Ducker and Hayes, and others have reported their experiences with Silastic cuffing of neurorrhaphies. Reports of clinical results using these techniques are insufficient to allow assessment of their effectiveness. We have had no experience with them.

General considerations for surgery
INDICATIONS

In the presence of a traumatic peripheral nerve deficit exploration of the nerve is indicated as follows:

1. When a sharp injury has obviously divided a nerve, early exploration is indicated for diagnostic, therapeutic, and prognostic purposes. Neurorrhaphy may be carried out at the time of exploration or may be delayed.

2. When abrading, avulsing, or blasting wounds have rendered the condition of the nerve unknown, exploration is required for identification of the nerve injury and for marking the ends of the nerve with sutures for later repair.

3. When a nerve deficit follows blunt or closed trauma and no clinical or electrical evidence of regeneration has occurred after an appropriate time, exploration of the nerve is indicated. This is also true when a nerve deficit complicates a closed fracture. In this instance it has been our practice to observe the patient for evidence of nerve regeneration for an appropriate time, depending on the nerve and its level of muscle innervation. Then if regeneration has not occurred, we favor exploration. In situations in which a nerve has been intact before closed reduction and casting of a fracture but a significant deficit is found immediately after, we explore the nerve as soon as feasible.

4. When a nerve deficit follows a penetrating wound such as that caused by a low-velocity gunshot, the part is observed for evidence of nerve regeneration for an appropriate time. Then if evidence of regeneration is absent, exploration is indicated.

Conversely, delay in exploration of a nerve injury is indicated if progressive regeneration is evidenced by improvement in sensation, motor power, and electrodiagnostic tests and by progression of the Tinel sign.

TIME OF SURGERY

It has been the time-honored policy to advise primary suture when possible. This is logical when one considers what happens to the distal end of the nerve, motor end plates, sensory nerve endings, muscles, joints, and other tissues of the denervated extremity. The controversy concerning whether primary or secondary nerve repair is better remains unsolved. Primary repair carried out in the first 6 to 8 hours or delayed primary repair carried out in the first 7 to 18 days is appropriate when the injury is caused by a sharp object, the wound is clean, and there are no other major complicating injuries. Ideally such repairs should be performed by an experienced surgeon in an institution where adequate equipment and personnel are available. The development of magnification devices, new instruments, and new techniques and the modification of a variety of small instruments for use in nerve surgery have improved the technique of early repair. Primary repair should shorten the time of denervation of the end organs, and fascicular alignment should be improved because minimal excision of the nerve ends is required. But in regard to war wounds Seddon has stated, ''The delayed operation converts the suture from a procedure carried out under restriction into one in which the surgeon is free to do as he wishes. At Oxford [England], all the primary sutures compare unfavorably with early secondary suture, and if I had the misfortune to suffer a nerve injury myself, I would prefer the secondary operation.''*

Once the diagnosis of division of a peripheral nerve has been made, if conditions are suitable and repair is indicated, one should not delay repair in anticipation of spontaneous regeneration. Only if the patient's life or limb is seriously endangered should the operation be long postponed. A fracture is not a contraindication for operation. Operation before the fracture becomes united may be advantageous for two reasons: (1) if bone shortening is necessary, resection of an ununited or partially united fracture is a much less formidable procedure than resection of a fully united bone; and (2) restriction of joint motion is minimal if the nerve is repaired soon after the injury; later motion will be more limited, perhaps so severely as to prevent flexing the joint enough to overcome a gap between the nerve ends.

INSTRUMENTS AND EQUIPMENT

A nerve stimulator should be available for all peripheral nerve procedures; many satisfactory permanent and disposable ones are available commercially. A stimulator is indispensable in the investigation of partially severed nerves and of neuromas in continuity and in locating and thus preserving nerve branches given off proximal to or at the lesion that are still functioning but are encased in scar tissue. Kline in 1968 described in vivo recording of nerve action potentials across neuromas or areas of injury in exposed peripheral nerves to assist the surgeon in deciding whether neurorrhaphy is desirable. Terzis, Hakstian, and Grabb individually have described their experiences with intraoperative recordings of potentials from nerve trunks and individual fasciculi. These techniques require sensitive and sophisticated recording and monitoring equipment, as well as trained technicians. For details of these monitoring techniques, the reader is referred to the references at the end of this chapter. Despite the technical difficulties involved in these methods, we have found intraoperative recording to be helpful when assessing partial nerve lesions and neuromas in continuity. Landi et al. found intraoperative somatosensory evoked potentials and nerve action

potentials useful in surgical planning and in predicting the outcome in 15 patients with brachial plexus injuries. Instruments for handling and dissecting delicate tissues are always essential. Nerve surgery in the extremities is also made easier by the use of a pneumatic tourniquet, suction apparatus, and electrocautery. Gelfoam and thrombin are useful for controlling the bleeding from the cut ends of nerves. For suture material we prefer 8-0, 9-0, and 10-0 monofilament nylon. The tensile strength, easy handling qualities, and minimal tissue reaction of nylon make it the most desirable suture material now available for neurorrhaphy. In our experience most epineurial repairs are best done with 8-0 or 9-0 nylon. For perineurial or epiperineurial repair 9-0 or 10-0 monofilament nylon is preferable.

ANESTHESIA

Peripheral nerve operations may be carried out with the patient under general, regional, or local anesthesia for the upper extremities or general, spinal, or local anesthesia for the lower extremities. Local anesthesia has the advantage of allowing one to evaluate the passage of sensory impulses through the injured nerve. However, if evaluation is to be accurate, little if any anesthetic agent should be injected around the nerve, and consequently the procedure is painful. Furthermore, there is always the possibility that the agent will infiltrate the tissues around the nerve and interfere with motor response to stimulation. As a rule we prefer general anesthesia in the upper extremities and neck and general or spinal anesthesia in the lower extremities.

PREPARATION AND DRAPING

Since the exact length of an incision can rarely be predicted, it is mandatory that the entire extremity and its environs be prepared. For an operation on the upper extremity the axilla, shoulder, neck, and chest should be included in the field of preparation; for any on the lower extremity the buttock and the area up to the iliac crest posteriorly should be included.

After preparation of the entire field the proposed incision is marked on the extremity and is crosshatched with washable ink before any of the landmarks are covered. It is a good policy to mark the incision along the course of the nerve in the entire prepared area. The extremity is then encased in a sterile stockinette so that it may be moved freely over the sterile drapes. If it is desirable to watch the movement of the muscles in the hand when the nerve is stimulated, the hand may be left exposed and bare.

Technique of nerve repair

In no type of surgery is the incision more important. Every incision should extend well proximal and distal to the lesion and when possible should follow the course of the nerve. An incision should never cross the flexor creases of the skin at a right angle. Short incisions are probably the cause of more futile nerve operations than any other single factor except the surgeon's inexperience. One should never hesitate to extend an incision great distances, for example, even from the axilla to the wrist to overcome a large defect in the ulnar or median nerve.

A tourniquet is generally helpful and is not usually con-

---

*From Seddon, H.J.: Practical value of peripheral nerve repair, Proc. R. Soc. Med. **42**:427, 1949.

traindicated. If used, as in surgery of the hand, it should be loosened and deflated at hourly intervals for periods of 5 to 10 minutes or longer to obtain hemostasis and to allow temporary resumption of circulation.

It is essential that the injured nerve is exposed first proximal to and then distal to the lesion before approaching the site of injury. Dissection and exposure are thus made simpler, and there is less chance of damaging the nerve and any branches remaining in the scar. The nerve should then be stimulated proximal to and distal to the lesion, and the response should be recorded. When a nerve is dissected from scar tissue, it should be repeatedly stimulated to locate any branches that might still be functioning. Before the nerve is mobilized completely, sutures are placed in the epineurium proximal to and distal to the lesion for orientation so that if neurorrhaphy is necessary the ends may be joined without rotation. Also, inspection of the external surface of the nerve may allow alignment of the longitudinal epineurial vessels; this too may aid in appropriate rotation of the nerve ends.

Handling of the nerve during mobilization is made easier by the use of moist umbilical tape or pieces of rubber tissue drains. Thread should never be used for this purpose because it is more likely to damage the nerve. Any part of the nerve not being operated on at the moment should be covered with moist sponges.

If the nerve has not been completely severed or if a neuroma in continuity is present, it may be difficult to decide whether neurolysis, partial neurorrhaphy, or complete neurorrhaphy will be best. The surgeon may need to call on all of the experience at his command to arrive at the wisest decision. Stimulation proximal to the injury for motor response distal to it is a sine qua non. If local anesthesia is used, stimulation distal to the lesion may give some idea of whether a significant number of sensory fibers have escaped injury or have regenerated, but sensory response is far less reliable than motor response. If a pneumatic tourniquet is used, it should be deflated to allow the muscles and nerves to recover from ischemia so that stimulation of the nerve to elicit motor response will have more validity. Examination at the site of injury may assist one in determining what course to pursue. The neuroma may be injected with saline solution, and if the solution passes up and down the nerve trunk with little difficulty, the neuroma should probably be left alone. This, however, can be misleading, and unless both motor and sensory response to stimulation are good, endoneural exploration is advisable.

ENDONEUROLYSIS

When an endoneural exploration is undertaken, it should be borne in mind that neurolysis or partial or complete neurorrhaphy may be necessary, and one should preserve intact as much of the epineurium and normal nerve as possible.

The epineurium is incised longitudinally proximal to the lesion, beginning not more than 0.5 cm from the level of gross changes in the nerve as determined by palpation. The incision is not extended more proximal to this point unless necessary, since the epineurium may become frayed, and if neurorrhaphy becomes necessary, more of the nerve may have to be sacrificed. For the same reason the distal end

of the incision is limited. The flaps of epineurium on each side may be retracted laterally by nylon sutures and are undermined widely. Then the funiculi are separated if possible with a pointed or diamond-bladed knife, using sharp or blunt dissection as necessary. Spring-loaded microscissors are also helpful in this dissection. If most of the funiculi are intact and can be separated and traced through the neuroma, nothing further should be done. On the other hand, if stimulation fails to elicit a response and few if any intact funiculi can be found, resecting the neuroma and neurorrhaphy are probably indicated. The use of magnifying loupes or the operating microscope is essential when doing intraneural dissection to avoid injury to intact nerve tissue (Chapter 21).

PARTIAL NEURORRHAPHY

Partial severance of the larger nerves, such as the sciatic nerve and the cords and trunks of the brachial plexus, is common. In such an injury partial neurorrhaphy is best. It is occasionally necessary and justifiable in smaller nerves but is never quite as satisfactory technically as is complete neurorrhaphy. The decision to perform partial neurorrhaphy is likewise often difficult. It should be made only after the most careful investigation of the lesion. If one half of the nerve, particularly a large one, is disrupted, partial neurorrhaphy is advisable. However, if the motor response to stimulation is good, it would obviously be unwise in some nerves such as the peroneal or ulnar to risk injury of good motor funiculi in an attempt to restore sensation to a small area on the dorsum of the foot or to the little finger. If most of the funiculi in smaller nerves are severed and if stimulation cannot demonstrate important function in the few that remain, complete neurorrhaphy is probably better. Suture of a few funiculi is usually impractical.

Once the decision has been made to perform partial neurorrhaphy (Fig. 64-12), the incision is extended longitudinally in the epineurium both proximally and distally several centimeters, as necessary. Then the intact funiculi are dissected out for the same distance. The ends of the injured part of the nerve are resected to normal tissue. At the cut ends an end-to-end neurorrhaphy is performed. If the epineurium is inadequate for placement of epineurial sutures, then epiperineurial or perineurial (fascicular) su-

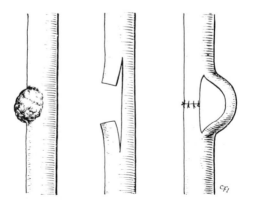

Fig. 64-12. Technique of partial neurorrhaphy.

tures will suffice. The proximal and distal dissection should be extensive enough to prevent kinking of the loop of intact nerve.

NEURORRHAPHY AND NERVE GRAFTING

When a nerve has been completely severed and when conditions as already outlined are appropriate, neurorrhaphy after sufficient resection of the proximal and distal ends of the nerve is indicated. Sometimes a considerable gap will remain after excision of any glioma and neuroma, and selecting a method for overcoming the gap is difficult. Regardless of the technique used, there is general agreement that nerve repair under tension is detrimental to satisfactory regeneration. Extension of the incision both proximally and distally may be helpful in permitting adequate dissection for closure of the gap.

METHODS OF CLOSING GAPS BETWEEN NERVE ENDS

There are several methods of closing gaps between nerve ends without appreciable damage to the nerve itself. The ones most often used are mobilization of the nerve ends and positioning of the extremity. Other methods include nerve transplantation, bone resection, bulb suture, nerve grafting, and nerve crossing (pedicle grafting).

Mobilization. Most small gaps may be closed by mobilizing the nerve ends for a few centimeters both proximal and distal to the point of injury. Large gaps require extensive dissection of the nerve from its adjacent tissues. Although the exact distance that any given nerve may be mobilized without damaging its circulation is unknown, care should be taken to avoid excessive stripping of the small vessels to the nerve. Fortunately a nerve seems to suffer little if mobilized from the axilla to the wrist so long as its branches are not sacrificed. A larger gap may be closed distal to the point of emergence of most of its branches than proximal to that point. For example, a gap of 12 cm in the median nerve distal to its branches into the muscles of the forearm is easily closed, but closing one so large proximal to the elbow is nearly impossible. The branches must be dealt with carefully by intraneural dissection up the nerve trunk, usually with the back of a pointed scalpel blade but occasionally with sharp dissection. At times a small branch as it enters the nerve merges with a funiculus and cannot be dissected out. It should be sacrificed rather than damaging the funiculus. Occasionally branches of some importance may be sacrificed if, after all justifiable means have been tried, they still prevent the ends from coming together. One should weigh carefully the importance of the branch against the probable result of the neurorrhaphy. For example, the branch of the radial nerve to the brachioradialis muscle commonly prevents one from closing a gap proximal to the point where this branch emerges from the nerve, but if the biceps brachii is functioning, this branch may be sacrificed without much loss of function. Excessive tension must be avoided at all times.

Positioning of extremity. Relaxing nerves by flexing various joints and occasionally by other maneuvers, such as abducting, adducting, rotating, and elevating the extremity, is as important as mobilization in closing large gaps in nerves. Through use of both methods long gaps may be

closed in nearly all of the peripheral nerves, and many unsatisfactory neurorrhaphies result from failure to make the most of their possibilities. When joints that are excessively flexed or awkwardly positioned are mobilized later, tension on the neurorrhaphy may be too great and may cause intraneural fibrosis that will compromise axonal regeneration. Consequently a joint should never be flexed forcibly to obtain end-to-end suture. It is a reasonable policy to flex the knee and elbow no more than 90 degrees. Flexion of the wrist more than 40 degrees is also probably unwise. After the wound has healed sufficiently, the joint can be extended about 10 degrees per week until motion is regained. Flexing joints is most important in repairing gaps in the long nerves of the extremities. External rotation and abduction are helpful when repairing radial and axillary nerves as is elevation of the shoulder girdle in brachial plexus injuries. Rarely extension of a joint may be helpful, as in extension of the hip in sciatic injuries.

Transplantation. The anatomic course of some nerves may be changed to shorten the distance between severed ends. This is particularly true of the ulnar nerve at the elbow. The median nerve may also be transplanted anterior to the pronator teres if the lesion is distal to its branches to the long flexor muscles of the forearm, and the tibial nerve may be placed superficial to the soleus or gastrocnemius in the leg if the lesion is distal to its branches to the calf muscles. Most surgeons recommend transplantation of the proximal end of the radial nerve anterior to the humerus and deep to the biceps to obtain needed length. Considerable length may be gained in most patients by the simpler maneuver of externally rotating the arm, provided of course the mobilization has been carried into the axilla and that the branches of the radial nerve to the triceps muscle have been dissected well up the nerve.

Bone resection. In civilian injuries bone resection should almost never be necessary to accomplish neurorrhaphy. Even in war wounds it was rarely employed, usually when the joints of the extremity had become so stiff from immobilization because of fracture or injudicious use of casts that flexion was limited. Intact long bones and most bones in children should rarely if ever be shortened to aid in nerve repair. Bone resection is of particular value in the upper arm for closing large gaps in the ulnar, radial, or median nerves when the humerus has already been fractured. In such patients if early delayed suture is carried out before the fracture has healed, shortening the bone if necessary is not difficult. After the fracture has healed, however, osteotomy is more difficult. It is rarely worthwhile, to shorten the femur in injuries of the sciatic nerve unless this bone has already been fractured; shortening of the bone may then he helpful. Both bones of the forearm or leg in the absence of a fracture should never be shortened.

Nerve stretching and bulb suture. Stretching of the nerve at operation by more than gentle traction is condemned. Gentle traction sufficient to bring the ends together under slight tension seemingly does not hinder regeneration.

Stretching of nerves by bulb suture (neuroma to glioma) with the joints acutely flexed followed by progressive extension of the joints and later by end-to-end neurorrhaphy during a second operation has been proposed in the past.

This method of overcoming gaps should be avoided because excessive fibrosis results, making later neurorrhaphy difficult or impossible and the prospects for successful axon regeneration poor. Furthermore, two operations are required.

Nerve grafting. The usefulness of nerve grafting remains controversial. After the early optimistic reports by Brooks and by Seddon, few additional clinical reports appeared to support the widespread use of nerve grafting techniques. Although reports of the use of irradiated nerve homografts in animals suggest that they are beneficial, clinical substantiation has been insufficient to recommend their general use. The most notable recent contributions to nerve grafting techniques have been made by Millesi et al. of Vienna, Austria. In animal experiments they observed that the connective tissue proliferation and scarring between nerve ends were directly related to tension on the line of suture. They also observed that if the gap in the nerve exceeded 4% of the free length of the nerve, then the tension required to close the gap rose sharply compared with shorter gaps. In addition, they found that regenerating axons pass more easily through two lines of suture in 5 mm nerve grafts than through a single line of suture at neurorrhaphy made under excessive tension. They also noted that connective tissue proliferation occurred in the epineurium, perineurium, and endoneurium with the epineurium producing most of the scarring. From their clinical experience Millesi et al. reported good results using an interfascicular nerve autografting technique to close gaps without undue tension. In the upper extremity especially good results were achieved in repairing injuries to the digital, median, ulnar, and radial nerves. The technique has also been used with encouraging results in the brachial plexus and in nerve injuries in the lower extremities. We have used this method, and although our experience is not as extensive as that of Millesi and others, we believe it is promising. Useful sensory return does occur, and reinnervation of proximal forearm musculature has been seen. Reinnervation of hand intrinsic musculature is unpredictable in our experience. The technique is described later. Taylor and Ham have further increased our knowledge of nerve grafting by transferring an autogenous superficial radial nerve graft to repair a segmental defect in a contralateral median nerve; the graft was revascularized by microvascular anastomosis. Improvement in sensation after surgery was reported. This technique, however, should be tried only by those surgeons who have had sufficient training and experience in microvascular techniques (p. 509) and have facilities to support such an effort.

Nerve crossing (pedicle grafting). Nerve-crossing operations in the extremities are rarely wise or possible. When a combined median and ulnar lesion is so great that the gap cannot be closed in either nerve in any other way, the ulnar nerve may be sectioned again in the upper arm, creating a segment long enough to bridge the gap between the two ends of the median nerve. The proximal end of the median nerve is then sutured to the proximal end of the free segment of the ulnar nerve. At a second operation 6 weeks later the distal end of the free segment of the ulnar nerve is sutured to the distal end of the median nerve. This procedure has been advised in situations such as nerve injury caused by massive ischemic necrosis of the forearm, but in light of current knowledge other nerve grafting techniques seem more appropriate in these situations.

TECHNIQUES OF NEURORRHAPHY

Fibrin clot, micropore tape, collagen tubulization techniques, adhesives, and many varieties of sutures and suture techniques have been proposed for neurorrhaphy. Neurorrhaphy by suture with nonreactive and nonabsorbable materials such as stainless steel and monofilament nylon have widest application and acceptance. The use of magnification, appropriate small instruments, and meticulous technique is essential. Experimental evidence is conflicting concerning the relative merits of epineurial and perineurial (fascicular) neurorrhaphy techniques. Clinical evidence to support the use of one technique instead of the other is meager and inconclusive. The technique selected by the individual surgeon will depend on his training and experience. Our preference is epiperineurial repair at the periphery of the nerve combined with perineurial (fascicular) neurorrhaphy for large fascicles within the nerve. Sunderland points out that funicular (fascicular) repair cannot be accurately done in every instance because (1) funicular patterns at nerve ends match exactly only after clean transection, (2) numbers of funiculi at nerve ends may not correspond, and (3) any discrepancies in funiculi within the nerve would require excessive intraneural suture material. He suggests that funicular repair might be practical when (1) funicular groups are large enough to take sutures that will maintain funicular apposition, (2) nerve ends demonstrate a funicular pattern that would predispose to wasteful regeneration of axons if epineurial repair were done, and (3) each funicular group is made up of nerve fibers to a particular branch occupying a constant position at the nerve ends. The latter arrangement can be seen in the median and ulnar nerves at and above the wrist and the radial nerve at and just proximal to the elbow. He recommends suturing groups of funiculi in such situations.

TECHNIQUE OF EPINEURIAL NEURORRHAPHY. After exposing and dissecting the ends of the nerves, determine that any remaining gap can be closed by end-to-end repair without excessive tension. Resect the glioma and neuroma with a sharp razor blade or a diamond-bladed knife against a sterile wooden tongue depressor in a nerve miter box or with sharp nerve scissors. Make serial cuts about 1 mm apart in the end of the nerve until normal-appearing fasciculi are exposed; this is best determined by use of the operating microscope. When doubt remains concerning the amount of any remaining scar in the nerve end, frozen histologic sections of the nerve will be helpful. Have permanent histologic sections made for later review to help in determining the prognosis. If the distal end contains glioma or if more than one third of the proximal end consists of neuroma, carry out additional trimming as required. Control excessive bleeding with thrombin or Gelfoam.

If positioning of the extremity is required to relieve tension, use an assistant at this point. Sometimes a traction or sling suture of 7-0 or 8-0 nylon passed through the nerve may be required. Our preference in such a situation is the gentle placement of a straight stainless steel Keith or Bunnell needle transversely through each of the nerve stumps with the nerve ends approximated, transfixing the nerve to the adjacent soft tissues. Next determine appropriate rotational alignment by observing the orientation of surface vessels and the appearance and location of fasciculi within the nerve. Epineurial orientation sutures placed 1 cm from each cut edge are also helpful. Now place a piece of plastic or rubber glove material beneath the nerve for visual contrast and less cumbersome handling of sutures. For this repair 8-0 or 9-0 monofilament nylon is usually sufficient. Place the first suture in the posterior or deep surface of the nerve in the epineurium and leave the suture long to make later rotation of the nerve easier. Now place the next three sutures in the remaining three quadrants of the nerve and leave them long, too. Determine as accurately as possible that no kinking or deviation of the fasciculi has occurred. Now place sufficient interrupted sutures of 8-0 or 9-0 nylon to produce a satisfactory neurorrhaphy (Fig. 64-13). Rotate the nerve with the quadrant sutures to be sure of satisfactory posterior surface repair. Next about 1 cm from each end of the repair place a 5-0 stainless steel suture in the epineurium to be used as roentgenographic markers. Because of the position of the extremity it is sometimes helpful to close parts of the wound before completing the neurorrhaphy. When appropriate this may be done even before beginning the repair. Finally remove the sling suture or steel needles from the nerve ends and close the remaining parts of the wound.

TECHNIQUE OF PERINEURIAL (FASCICULAR) NEURORRHAPHY. To perform perineurial (fascicular) neurorrhaphy the surgeon must be proficient in the use of the operating microscope (p. 509) and must also be able to handle the delicate No. 10-0 suture with ease and speed. Expose the nerve injury and resect the ends of the nerve as described for epineurial neurorrhaphy (p. 2803). Place the nerve ends in proper rotation. Next using magnification attempt to identify corresponding groups of fasciculi in the proximal and distal nerve stumps. It is helpful at this point to diagram the arrangement of the fascicular groups on sterile paper from glove or suture packages. Transfix the nerve ends to the soft tissues with stainless steel straight needles. Now incise the epineurium longitudinally both proximally and distally to expose the fasciculi, approximate them individually with interrupted 9-0 or 10-0 nylon sutures (Fig. 64-14). Where the nerve is composed of multiple small fasciculi, approximate several fasciculi as a group. After the fasciculi have been matched and approximated, close the epineurium with interrupted nylon sutures, or if the neurorrhaphy is secure and there is no tension on the repair, omit the epineurial closure to decrease the amount of fibrosis after surgery.

TECHNIQUE OF EPIPERINEURIAL NEURORRHAPHY. Expose and resect the ends of the nerve as described for epineurial repair (p. 2803). Avoid excessive dissection of the epineurium. Place the nerve ends in proper rotation and transfix them with straight stainless steel needles to the surrounding soft tissues. Next attempt to identify the major fasciculi and groups of large and small fasciculi. Now begin the repair on the posterior (deep) surface of the nerve. If possible place the first No. 9-0 or 10-0 nylon suture

through the epineurium of the nerve and then through the perineurium of the largest fasciculus in one cut surface and carry it to the other cut surface, placing it through the perineurium of the matching fasciculus and out through the epineurium. Continue in this manner from the deep surface of the nerve toward the superficial surface. Meanwhile in the central part of the nerve approximate the appropriate

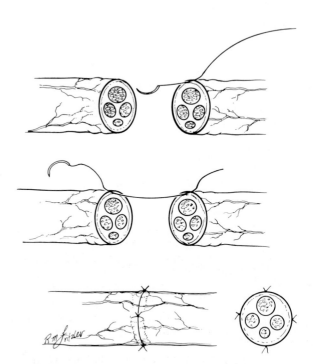

Fig. 64-13. Epineurial neurorrhaphy (see text).

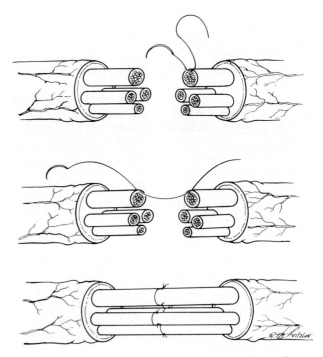

Fig. 64-14. Perineurial (fascicular) neurorrhaphy (see text).

fasciculi with interrupted single perineurial sutures of No. 10-0 nylon. Then continue with the epineurial and perineurial repair to the superficial surface of the nerve (Fig. 64-15). Next insert steel marking sutures in the epineurium of both nerve segments and remove the straight needles. With this technique rotating the nerve to complete the repair of the deep surface is usually unnecessary because the repair proceeds from the deep surface to the superficial. When the repair has been completed, close the wound in the routine manner.

TECHNIQUE OF INTERFASCICULAR NERVE GRAFTING (MILLESI, MODIFIED). Keep the extremity in the extended position so that the graft will not be under tension after surgery. Expose the nerve as for neurorrhaphy (p. 2803). Beginning in normal-appearing tissue, dissect and expose the proximal and distal stumps. Incise the epineurium on the stumps in areas where the nerve appears normal. Next excise a circumferential cuff of epineurium from each stump. Using the operating microscope carry out intraneural dissection in the normal part of the nerve, working toward the neuroma and glioma in the proximal and distal ends respectively. Attempt to identify large fasciculi and groups of smaller fasciculi. Ensure hemostasis by coagulating the smaller vascular branches with bipolar microcoagulating forceps. As intraneural fibrosis is encountered, transect each fasciculus or group of fasciculi individually at the level where the fibrosis begins. When this dissection has been completed, the fasciculi and groups should be transected at different levels depending on the extent of scarring. From four to six fasciculi or fascicular groups, all of different lengths, now should be present in each end of the stump. At this point deflate the tourniquet and compress the wound with saline-moistened packs. Next draw a sketch of each nerve stump and attempt to identify the corresponding fasciculi and groups of fasciculi in each. The more proximal the lesion the less well-defined are the fas-

cicular groups. Use clinical judgment in matching the fasciculi and the fascicular groups in the ends of the stumps. Now by measuring the gaps remaining between the fasciculi and fascicular groups at each end of the nerve, estimate the length of nerve graft needed. Each major fasciculus or group will require a segment of graft; the graft should be 10% to 15% longer than the combined gaps to be filled. Nerves that may be used as donors are the sural, the saphenous, the lateral cutaneous of the thigh, the lateral and medial cutaneous of the forearm, the posterior cutaneous of the forearm, the superficial branch of the radial, the dorsal branch of the ulnar, and the intercostals. We prefer the sural nerve for most situations. A level for transection should be selected to allow the proximal end of the donor nerve to retract beneath fascia or muscles and thus avoid as much as possible the formation of a painful neuroma.

If the sural nerve is to be used, expose it through a short transverse incision posterior to the lateral malleolus. Now separate the nerve from the small saphenous vein that lies just anterior to it. Determine the course of the nerve in the calf by applying traction to the nerve. Next along the course of the nerve make additional transverse incisions to allow further dissection. If long segments of nerve are to be harvested, a single longitudinal incision is used (Fig. 64-16). This will minimize the potential harm caused by traction on the donor nerve during a difficult dissection. Although scissors or nerve strippers can be used during this part of the procedure, take considerable care to avoid injuring the nerve graft. Transect the nerve so that its proximal end retracts beneath the fascia in the proximal calf. Close the incisions in the calf and keep the graft moist with saline during the rest of the operation. Next dissect any excess fat from the ends of the graft and section the graft so that shorter grafts of appropriate lengths can be placed between the ends of corresponding fasciculi or fascicular groups. Using the operating microscope place each graft between the corresponding fasciculi and secure the epineurium of each end to the perineurium of the fasciculus or fascicular group with a single suture of No. 10-0 monofilament nylon (Fig. 64-17). If the extremity has been positioned in extension and if the grafts are placed without tension, the single sutures are sufficient. Obtain meticulous hemostasis and close the wound. Avoid suction drainage tubes.

The same technique may be used for a nerve lesion in continuity or for repair of an unsuccessful primary neurorrhaphy.

AFTERTREATMENT. After neurorrhaphy or nerve grafting the extremity is immobilized in a plaster splint or cast. A posterior molded plaster splint is usually satisfactory for the arm unless the shoulder girdle must be immobilized; a Velpeau dressing reinforced with plaster is then essential. After neurorrhaphy in the lower extremity a spica cast may be needed. The use of a long leg cast alone frequently results in separation of the line of suture.

The wound should not be dressed until the seventh to tenth day. The sutures are then removed. In removing the splint or cast, extreme care is necessary to avoid tension on the line of suture.

Opinions differ widely as to when extension of the joints

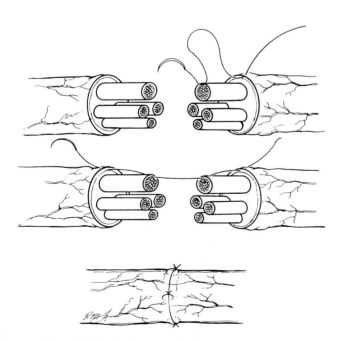

Fig. 64-15. Details of epiperineurial neurorrhaphy (see text).

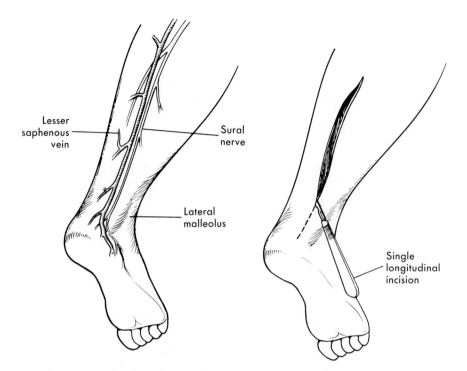

Fig. 64-16. Sural nerve graft. If long nerve grafts are required, use single longitudinal incision to minimize traction injury to nerve graft.

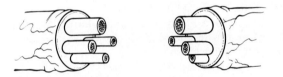

Nerve grafts placed between nerve ends

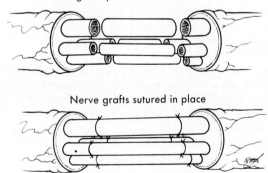

Nerve grafts sutured in place

Fig. 64-17. Interfascicular nerve grafting (see text).

may be safely begun after end-to-end repairs. It is our policy in the upper extremity to retain the plaster splint for 4 weeks and then to replace it with a metal splint that can be extended gradually over a period of 2 or 3 weeks. In the lower extremity, especially when the peroneal or sciatic nerve has been sutured, we keep the patient in the spica cast for at least 6 weeks, then apply a long leg brace that controls extension of the knee, and allow 4 weeks or more, depending on the tension on the line of suture, for

complete extension of the knee. Roentgenograms may be made monthly for the first 3 months to determine the integrity of the line of suture. Physical therapy is essential to recovery of function of the extremity.

After interfascicular grafting, the joints should be immobilized no longer than 10 days. Then the plaster cast or splint is removed, and active exercises of all joints are begun. The progress of regeneration is determined by the advance of the Tinel sign. As this sign progresses along the graft, it may temporarily stop at the distal repair. However, it will usually resume progress eventually. If it does not progress after 3 to 4 months, blockage at the distal line of suture is assumed, and resection of this area followed by repair is indicated.

RESULTS OF OPERATION

The results of such procedures as neurolysis and partial neurorrhaphy cannot be accurately determined. We know, however, that neurorrhaphy is never followed by full return of motor and sensory function. Rarely full return is approached after suture of the radial nerve and occasionally after suture of the median nerve in children. Yet a useful degree of recovery will often occur when the factors that influence recovery are favorable (p. 2795). The degree of recovery will vary from nerve to nerve and with the relative extent of damage to the motor and sensory components within each nerve. It must also be understood that recovery of function of the limb as a whole is not necessarily proportionate to neurologic recovery. For example, a patient may recover fairly good neurologic function; yet, because of other defects in the limb, its overall functional recovery may be unsatisfactory.

Since it is helpful to know what result can be expected after suture of any given nerve, a statement is made at the end of the discussion of each nerve when this information is available.

Practical functional considerations

Injury to a nerve is often associated with such severe trauma to the neighboring bone and soft tissues that the loss of sensation and motor power resulting from the nerve injury is less important than the bone and soft tissue injuries. In the lower extremity, where proper weight-bearing alignment is essential, any disabling deformity of bone must be corrected, and endurance and stability must be restored. In the upper extremity movement and sensation are more important than strength and endurance, but a useful hand depends on the position and stability of the wrist, elbow, and shoulder; the hand is useless if it cannot be maintained in a position of function. Loss of sensation is of major importance in some parts of the body, for example, in the median nerve distribution in the hand and the tibial nerve distribution in the foot. For the little finger to be completely anesthetic is often more disabling than is an amputation of it.

Prolonged immobilization of a part while awaiting nerve regeneration after suture allows fibrosis of both the paralyzed and normal muscles and stiffness of joints. If the prognosis for return of nerve function after suture is doubtful, rigid splinting of joints is not justified, especially if it must be in a poor functional position. For example, prolonged flexion of the knee to maintain an end-to-end suture of a nerve usually results in at least a slight flexion deformity, disturbing the weight-bearing alignment of the limb and causing fatigue while standing and a limp while walking. One must be practical in managing such problems and remember that the function of the limb as a whole is more important than restoring power to any given group of muscles. Still, any treatment that offers a reasonable chance of decreasing a disability should be carefully considered and if indicated should be undertaken.

CERVICAL PLEXUS

The anterior primary rami of the first four cervical nerves unite to form the cervical plexus. Sensory fibers from the upper two or three segments course through the lesser occipital, greater auricular, and anterior cutaneous nerves of the neck. Sensory fibers from the lower two segments course through the supraclavicular nerves. Muscular branches join in the ansa hypoglossi to innervate the thyrohyoid, geniohyoid, omohyoid, sternothyroid, and sternohyoid muscles. Branches from C3, C4, and C5 unite to form the phrenic nerve. Fibers arising from the lateral aspect of the anterior horns of the upper five cervical segments unite to form the spinal accessory nerve, which ascends into the cranial cavity through the foramen magnum. At that point the nerve is joined by its cranial part, which consists primarily of rootlets destined to pass with the vagus nerve. These rootlets diverge from the spinal accessory nerve after its exit from the jugular foramen and thereafter course with the vagus fibers. The spinal accessory nerve descends in the neck beneath the posterior belly of the digastric muscle, receiving branches from the anterior primary rami of C2, C3, and C4 and branching to innervate the sternocleidomastoid. It then leaves the posterior aspect of this muscle and descends farther to innervate the superior third of the trapezius muscle.

SPINAL ACCESSORY NERVE

The spinal accessory nerve may be injured at any point along its course. Because of its superficial location in the posterior cervical triangle it is especially susceptible to damage from penetrating injuries. It may also be injured during operations such as lymph node biopsy or radical neck dissection. Woodhall has given an accurate description of the symptoms and findings that follow surgical injury to this nerve: the patient complains of generalized weakness in the affected shoulder girdle and arm, inability to abduct the shoulder above 90 degrees, and a sensory disturbance that may vary from a pulling sensation in the region of the scar to aching in the shoulder and arm. The aching may radiate to the medial margin of the scapula and down the arm to the fingers and is sometimes incapacitating. The superior one third of the trapezius muscle on the affected side always atrophies, the shoulder sags, and power to elevate it is weak. The scapula rotates distally and laterally and flares slightly; its inferior angle is closer to the midline than is its superior angle. This position is accentuated when the arm is abducted; the flaring of the inferior angle disappears when the arm is raised anteriorly, in contrast to the usual deformity caused by paralysis of the serratus anterior.

Treatment. If the nerve has been injured by a low-velocity missile and if no vascular or visceral injuries require immediate surgical exploration, simple observation for 3 to 4 weeks may be best. However, if after that time electrodiagnostic examination reveals denervation of the trapezius and if clinical evidence of return of function is absent, exploration of the nerve is indicated. When injury to the nerve is detected during an operation and when circumstances permit, primary repair should be attempted. However, when the injury is not appreciated during an operation or when removal of a segment of the nerve is necessary as part of an operation for malignancy, attempts to repair the nerve or any reconstructive procedure should be delayed 2 to 3 weeks to allow the initial wound to heal. Furthermore, when a segment of the nerve has been removed as part of an operation for malignancy, the condition of the patient or later treatment such as irradiation may prevent additional procedures. When the patient's condition permits, when symptoms warrant additional treatment, and when the gap created by segmental resection of the nerve is too great to close by end-to-end suture, interfascicular grafting (p. 2805) or tendon transfer are the remaining alternatives. If the nerve is to be repaired, the approach described here allows satisfactory exposure for suture or nerve grafting. When the initial wound has healed well, the incision is made across the middle of the posterior triangle, following the skin folds of the neck. Remember that the terminal part of the spinal accessory nerve emerges at the junction of the proximal and middle thirds of the sternocleidomastoid muscle and courses diagonally distally and posteriorly to enter the lateral border of the trapezius muscle at the junction of its middle and distal thirds. The incision should be long enough to permit exact identification of both the distal and proximal parts of the nerve. Care must be taken not to confuse the lesser occipital and greater auricular nerves with the spinal accessory. The proximal part of the nerve should be stimulated. Contraction of the trapezius muscle indicates that the nerve has not been severed. The entire nerve is exposed in the posterior triangle. If scarring is extensive within or about the nerve, a neurolysis is performed. If the nerve has been divided, its ends should be mobilized and sectioned back to good funiculi. An end-to-end suture is performed under little or no tension. Awkward positioning of the head, neck, and shoulders in a cast to allow suturing of the nerve without tension should be avoided. Instead, interfascicular nerve grafting (p. 2805) may be a satisfactory alternative. If the line of suture is not under tension, the shoulder should be immobilized in a Velpeau bandage for 3 to 4 weeks. Gentle active exercises are then started, and normal daily activities are resumed between 6 and 8 weeks after surgery.

Results of suturing spinal accessory nerve. There is no information that is statistically significant on the results of suturing of the spinal accessory nerve. However, the reports of Woodall, of Dunn, of Vastamäki and Solonen, and of Wright suggest that neurolysis or repair when necessary may result in relief of symptoms and return of function. Seddon has emphasized that good results may be expected because the spinal accessory nerve is purely a motor nerve.

BRACHIAL PLEXUS

The brachial plexus is formed by the union of the anterior rami of C5, C6, C7, C8, and T1 (Fig. 64-18); C5 usually receives some fibers from C4 and T1 from T2. Shortly after leaving the intervertebral foramen each root receives its sympathetic component by way of a gray ramus. The cervical roots receive their sympathetic components from one of the lower cervical sympathetic ganglia and the T1 root from its own sympathetic ganglion after contributing a white ramus to it.

The formation of the brachial plexus begins just distal to the scalene muscles. Here the C5 and C6 roots unite to form the upper trunk, the C7 root continues alone to form the middle trunk, and the C8 and T1 roots unite to form the lower trunk. The three trunks thus formed proceed inferolaterally behind the clavicle, and each divides into anterior and posterior divisions. The three posterior divisions unite to form the posterior cord, the anterior divisions of the upper and middle trunks unite to form the lateral cord, and the anterior division of the lower trunk continues alone to form the medial cord. These three cords embrace the axillary artery in the relationships that their names imply.

The surgically important nerves arising from the brachial plexus are described as follows. The long thoracic nerve arises from C5, C6, and C7 immediately after they emerge from the intervertebral foramina. It traverses the neck posterior to the brachial plexus, continues distally along the lateral aspect of the thoracic wall, and innervates the serratus anterior muscle. The dorsal scapular nerve arises from the C5 root just lateral to its contribution to the long thoracic nerve. The dorsal scapular nerve also traverses the neck posterior to the brachial plexus; as it courses to the medial border of the scapula it innervates the levator scapulae, the rhomboideus major, and the rhomboideus minor. These two are the only nerves that leave the roots before their union to form the trunks.

The only surgically significant nerve to arise from a trunk is the suprascapular, which arises from the lateral aspect of the upper trunk well superior to the clavicle. This

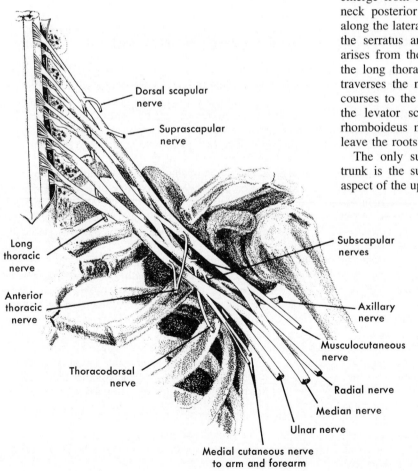

Dorsal scapular nerve

Suprascapular nerve

Long thoracic nerve

Anterior thoracic nerve

Thoracodorsal nerve

Medial cutaneous nerve to arm and forearm

Ulnar nerve

Median nerve

Radial nerve

Musculocutaneous nerve

Axillary nerve

Subscapular nerves

Fig. 64-18. Brachial plexus.

is the first important branch seen when the plexus is explored superior to the clavicle. This nerve proceeds distally, passing through the scapular notch to the posterior aspect of the scapula, where it supplies the supraspinatus muscle and, after proceeding around the lateral border of the scapular spine, supplies the infraspinatus muscle. No branches arise from the divisions of the plexus.

The lateral anterior thoracic nerve arises from the lateral cord and the medial anterior thoracic nerve from the medial cord. These two nerves descend, communicate by an anastomotic loop, and innervate the pectoralis major and minor. The musculocutaneous nerve is the only additional branch of the lateral cord. The remainder of this cord joins the medial cord to form the median nerve.

The medial brachial cutaneous and medial antebrachial cutaneous nerves arise from the medial cord, which then divides into its two main branches, one the ulnar nerve and the other its contribution to the median nerve.

The upper and lower subscapular nerves, which innervate the subscapularis and teres major muscles, arise from the posterior cord. The thoracodorsal nerve, which also arises from the posterior cord, passes distally between the two subscapular nerves to innervate the latissimus dorsi. The last branch of the posterior cord is the axillary nerve, which turns laterally to course around the surgical neck of the humerus; en route it innervates the teres minor, the deltoid, and the skin overlying the deltoid. The posterior cord then continues distally in the arm as the radial nerve.

Injuries of brachial plexus. In military combat penetrating wounds cause most brachial plexus injuries. In civilian life, in addition to injuries related to birth, the plexus may be injured by missiles, stab wounds, traction applied to the plexus during falls, vehicular accidents, or sports activities. Other injuries that may be associated with those of the brachial plexus include fractures of the proximal humerus, the scapula, the ribs, the clavicle, and the transverse processes of the cervical vertebrae and dislocation of the shoulder, the acromioclavicular, and the sternoclavicular joints.

Upper plexus injury (Erb) involves the segments innervated by the C5 and C6 nerve roots with or without dysfunction of the C7 root. Typically the limb is extended at the elbow, flaccid at the side of the trunk, and adducted and internally rotated. Abduction is impossible because of paralysis of the deltoid and supraspinatus muscles, and external rotation is impossible because of paralysis of the infraspinatus and teres minor muscles. Active flexion of the elbow is impossible because of paralysis of the biceps, brachialis, and brachioradialis muscles. Paralysis of the supinator muscle causes pronation deformity of the forearm and inability to supinate the forearm. Sensation is absent over the deltoid muscle and the lateral aspect of the forearm and hand. Injury in which the roots of the upper plexus are avulsed from the spinal cord should always be recognized because surgical repair is impossible. It can be diagnosed by finding segmental motor and sensory deficits involving the C5 and C6 roots with paralysis of the serratus anterior, the levator scapulae, and the rhomboids, indicating that the lesion of the nerve roots is medial to the emergence of the long thoracic and dorsal scapular nerves that supply these muscles. Long tract signs may or may

not be present, depending on whether the spinal cord has been damaged. The diagnosis is often confirmed by demonstrating denervation potentials in the segmental paraspinous musculature innervated by the posterior primary rami. In 1947 Murphey, Hartung, and Kirklin demonstrated that myelography (Fig. 64-19) can be extremely helpful by demonstrating a pseudomeningocele or complete absence of root shadows at the level of the avulsion. Myelography, however, may be inaccurate early after injury because clotted blood may occlude the opening into the pseudomeningocele. Therefore a delay of 6 to 12 weeks is recommended before a myelogram is made. Rorabeck and Harris found that of 34 patients with pseudomeningocele formation, 31 showed no recovery.

The cutaneous axon reflexes have been found useful in differentiating preganglionic intraspinal lesions from postganglionic extraspinal lesions, although they indicate nothing regarding the severity of the lesion. These reflexes are elicited by placing a drop of histamine on the skin along the distribution of the nerve being examined. After the skin is scratched through the drop of histamine, a sequential response consisting of cutaneous vasodilatation, wheal formation, and flare response is normally seen. If the nerve is interrupted proximal to the ganglion, there is anesthesia along its cutaneous course, but the normal axon response will be seen. If the injury is distal to the ganglion, there is also anesthesia along the course of the nerve, and vasodi-

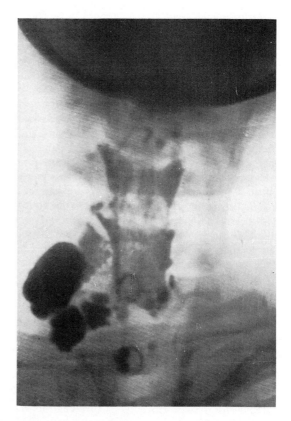

Fig. 64-19. Pantopaque myelogram showing pseudomeningocele produced by avulsion of roots of C7 and C8; C5 and C6, which were also avulsed, did not fill. T1 still functions.

latation and wheal formation are seen, but the flare response is absent; this negative axonal response suggests injury at a site where recovery might be possible after repair. Techniques such as the cold vasodilatation test and sensory nerve velocity studies may assist in differentiating the level of the injury.

In upper plexus injuries when avulsion of the roots can be excluded, exploration is justified and repair is sometimes possible. Of 134 brachial plexus injuries reviewed by Rorabeck and Harris, isolated injuries to the upper trunk had the best prognosis.

Lower plexus injury (Klumpke) can be diagnosed by finding segmental sensory and motor deficits involving C8 and T1 with or without C7 dysfunction. Associated Horner's syndrome should alert the examiner to the possibility of an avulsing injury of the lower plexus, and myelography and electromyographic studies may be necessary to exclude such an injury. In addition to penetrating wounds, many lower plexus injuries are caused by difficult births, falling on the outstretched arm, or trauma from crutches. The primary dysfunction is apparent in the intrinsic musculature of the hand along with paralysis of the wrist and finger flexors. The sensory deficit is along the medial aspect of the arm, forearm, and hand.

Injuries to the upper or lower trunks of the plexus produce essentially the same sensory and motor deficits as do injuries to their respective rami except for preservation of function of the long thoracic and dorsal scapular nerves in the upper trunks and absence of Horner's syndrome in the lower trunks. Isolated injuries of the divisions of the plexus are extremely rare and are usually associated with or mistaken for injuries of the cords or trunks.

Injuries of the cords produce fairly regular patterns of altered function. Injuries of the lateral cord cause motor and sensory deficits in the distribution of the musculocutaneous nerve (paralysis of the biceps) and of the lateral root of the median nerve (paralysis of the flexor carpi radialis and pronator teres). Glenohumeral subluxation may result. This may be prevented by an aggressive program of rehabilitation of the remaining intact musculature. Sensory deficit can be detected over the anterolateral aspect of the forearm in the relatively small autonomous zone of the musculocutaneous nerve. Injuries of the posterior cord cause motor and sensory deficits in the distribution of the following nerves: the subscapular (paralysis of the subscapularis and teres major), the thoracodorsal (paralysis of the latissimus dorsi), the axillary (paralysis of the deltoid and teres minor), and the radial nerve (paralysis of extension of the elbow, wrist, and fingers). The disability consists mainly of inability to internally rotate the shoulder, elevate the limb, and extend the forearm and hand. Sensory loss is most often apparent only in the autonomous zone of the axillary nerve overlying the deltoid muscle. Injuries of the medial cord produce the motor deficit of a combined ulnar and median nerve lesion (except for the flexor carpi radialis and pronator teres) and extensive sensory loss along the medial aspect of the arm and hand.

Indications for surgery. The surgical treatment of brachial plexus injuries has been discussed by Seddon, Brooks, Barnes, Leffert, Narakas, Tracy and Brannon, Berger and Millesi, and others. The importance of careful evaluation and preparation before surgery is emphasized by all. These injuries may be divided for purposes of treatment into two broad categories, open injuries and closed injuries.

Open injuries are usually caused by sharp objects or missiles. When components of the plexus have been cut by sharp objects, when the patient is seen soon after injury, and when the patient's general condition permits, exploration and primary repair may be attempted. Usually, however, injuries to adjacent vessels or to the mediastinal or thoracic viscera must be treated first, and thus repair of the plexus injury must be delayed. In these situations the plexus should be inspected and the injured parts marked with wire sutures to make later evaluation and treatment easier. When the patient is not seen soon after injury but only after the initial management, it is best to await healing of the wound and stabilization of any other injuries. During this waiting period the extremity should be carefully examined, and the neurologic deficits are documented to determine the level of injury and to serve as a baseline for later evaluation. Electromyography 3 to 4 weeks after injury is also helpful in determining the level of the injury. Exploration of the plexus and neurorrhaphy, autogenous interfascicular nerve grafting, or neurolysis are indicated 3 to 6 weeks after injury. Millesi and Lusskin et al. reported limited return of function in small groups of patients treated in this manner. Lusskin et al. found this treatment especially useful in periplexus scar formation with conduction block, in lacerations sufficiently distal to allow repair or grafting, and in neuromas that could be resected, leaving sufficient stumps for grafting or repair. Leffert emphasized the poor prognosis after lower trunk injuries but advised surgical exploration for sharp injuries of the upper and middle trunks.

Sedel reported results of surgical treatment of 63 traumatic brachial plexus palsies, 32 complete and 31 partial. Of the 32 complete palsies, 26 had repair procedures; 21 were improved. Of the 31 partial palsies, 23 had repair procedures; 20 were improved. Results of nerve transfer were disappointing.

Solonen et al. reviewed 52 brachial plexus injuries treated surgically. Grafts were used in 24, neurolyses in 14, direct suture in 2, and intercostal neurotization in 12 avulsions. Good results were seen in 19 patients after fascicular grafting with return of function of the biceps muscle. Neurotization produced function in 4 of 12 patients.

When an open injury has been caused by a low-velocity missile, early exploration is not indicated unless injuries to adjacent vessels or viscera make immediate treatment necessary. In these situations the condition of the patient usually prevents extensive repair or grafting of the plexus. However, the injury should be inspected and its extent documented. These injuries often result in either neurapraxia or lesions in continuity. Consequently a period of observation is indicated because considerable function may return spontaneously. Leffert emphasized the importance of periodic examinations and the establishment of reasonable timetables for recovery. Again electromyograms should be obtained 3 to 4 weeks after injury to aid in determining the extent of denervation. Thereafter periodic examinations are indicated every 4 to 6 weeks. When such examinations during a reasonable period of time reveal the absence of recovery or that any recovery has halted, exploration and neurorrhaphy, grafting, or neurolysis may be beneficial. The timing of exploration is difficult to determine, but 4 to 6 weeks is a reasonable period in which to expect some recovery. Bonney found that in high-velocity injuries involving the whole plexus, severe spasmodic pain and Horner's syndrome were unfavorable prognostic signs.

Closed injuries are most often caused by traction, either with the arm forcibly abducted or with the arm adducted and the neck deviated to the opposite side. Barnes divided them into four groups as follows: (1) injuries at C5 and C6, (2) injuries at C5, C6, and C7, (3) degenerative lesions of the entire plexus, and (4) injuries at C7, C8 and T1 (rare). He found that 11 of 14 patients with C5 and C6 lesions spontaneously regained shoulder abduction and elbow flexion against gravity and some resistance. Eleven of 19 with C5, C6, and C7 lesions spontaneously regained shoulder abduction, elbow flexion, and finger and wrist extension against gravity and some resistance. Of 24 patients with degenerative lesions of the entire plexus, 7 showed no recovery, 10 showed recovery of the C8 and T1 innervated muscles but no upper root recovery, and 7 showed recovery of the C5 and C6 innervated muscles but no lower root recovery. Bonney also reported incomplete recovery from this type of whole plexus injury in 24 patients and found no useful finger or wrist extensor function, although function of the trapezius, the rhomboids, and the serratus anterior muscles returned. Infraclavicular brachial plexus injuries are less common than supraclavicular injuries, and the prognosis after them is better. They are usually associated with fractures or dislocations about the shoulder. Leffert and Seddon found satisfactory results in 31 patients with infraclavicular injuries regardless of which part of the plexus was damaged and stated that surgical treatment for these is rarely necessary. Narakas reported surgical treatment by repair, grafting, or neurolysis in 164 patients with traction injuries and found that 85% of 20 patients with infraclavicular injuries improved after surgery and that only 55% of 58 patients with supraclavicular injuries improved. In treating closed injuries electromyography should be carried out at 3 to 4 weeks as in open injuries. Observation and physical therapy should be continued, and at 6 to 8 weeks additional studies including myelography and axon reflex evaluation may be performed if no return of function is seen. If no return of function has occurred or if any return has ceased and if there is evidence that the lesions are at the postganglionic level, then exploration is justified at 6 to 12 months after injury. Leffert emphasized that exploration assists in determining the extent of postganglionic injury in the absence of preganglionic damage. When the lesion is preganglionic in two or more roots, the prognosis is poor, but if the lower two roots are involved, then exploration is justified to determine the status of the upper roots (Fig. 64-20). Excision of neuromas in continuity, repair or grafting, or neurolysis when indicated has been found beneficial in these injuries. Yeoman and Seddon found that the prognosis in flail arms after whole plexus injuries can be determined by proper investigation within 8 weeks after injury, and when return of function is impossible reconstructive operations should then be started.

COMPREHENSIVE APPROACH TO BRACHIAL PLEXUS. The brachial plexus may be approached either superior or inferior to the clavicle, depending on the site of injury. When a neurorrhaphy is to be carried out near or superior to the clavicle, then osteotomy of this bone may be necessary. However, a nerve graft may be placed posterior to the clavicle without osteotomy. The approach described here exposes the entire plexus, and any appropriate part of it may be used to explore a part of the plexus. A transverse approach to the plexus is not recommended because it is not extensile and thus exposure is restricted.

Begin the incision at the anterior border of the sternocleidomastoid muscle about 4 cm superior to the clavicle. Carry it laterally over the muscle parallel to the clavicle as far as the junction of the lateral and middle thirds of the clavicle and then curve it distally across the clavicle along the anterior border of the deltoid muscle to the anterior pectoral fold. Curve it posteriorly along the natural skin folds of the axilla to the midpoint of the medial aspect of the arm and then curve it again distally parallel with the neurovascular bundle (Fig. 64-21).

Superior to the clavicle, deepen the incision through the subcutaneous tissue and the platysma. Ligate the external jugular vein, retract or divide the omohyoid muscle, and expose the deep fascia. The subclavian vein (Fig. 64-22) is seldom seen because it is several centimeters inferior to this region. Open the deep fascia transversely and clear away the exposed areolar tissue. By retracting or dividing the clavicular head of the sternocleidomastoid muscle, expose the scalenus anterior medially. It is then usually necessary to divide and ligate the transverse cervical artery, which crosses the scalenus anterior superficial to the phrenic nerve. The phrenic nerve crosses this muscle from lateral to medial; identify and retract it medially. All the rami of the brachial plexus should now be visible as they emerge from deep to the lateral border of the scalenus anterior to form the upper, middle, and lower trunks of the plexus. If a fuller view of the rami is needed, divide the scalenus anterior transversely so that the subclavian artery is visible inferior to and the rami of the brachial plexus just superior to the point of division.

To see or to mobilize the parts of the plexus that lie deep to or inferior to the clavicle, deepen that part of the incision that crosses the junction of the lateral and middle thirds of the clavicle. Divide the fascia distally in the cleft identified by the cephalic vein between the pectoralis major and the deltoid muscle. Sever the tendon of the pectoralis major about 1 cm proximal to its insertion on the humerus, retract the muscle medially, identify the clavipectoral fascia, and incise it longitudinally. Then divide the tendon of the pectoralis minor, mark it with a suture, and retract it. After exposing the clavicle from superiorly and inferiorly, divide it with a Gigli saw (if necessary, part of the bone may be resected later) and separate the divided ends. Sever the subclavius muscle and ligate and divide the cephalic vein. Now incise longitudinally the deep fascia of the arm and that which encases the neurovascular bundle until the entire brachial plexus is visible.

The relationships of the various parts of the brachial plexus to each other and to the vessels are described in standard texts on anatomy and need not be discussed at

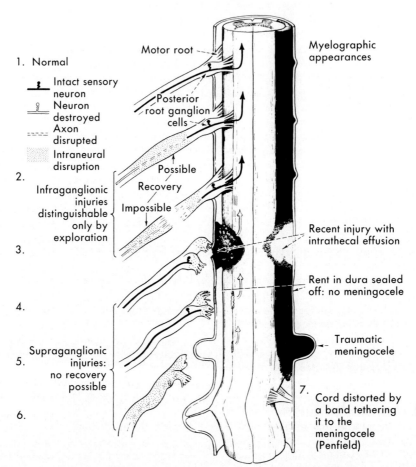

Types of injury suffered by roots of the brachial plexus

Myelographic appearances

1. Normal

Motor root

⌐●─┐ Intact sensory neuron

⌐◖─┐ Neuron destroyed

----- Axon disrupted

░░░ Intraneural disruption

Posterior root ganglion cells

2.

Infraganglionic injuries distinguishable only by exploration

Possible

Recovery

Impossible

3.

Recent injury with intrathecal effusion

4.

Rent in dura sealed off: no meningocele

Supraganglionic injuries: no recovery possible

5.

Traumatic meningocele

6.

7. Cord distorted by a band tethering it to the meningocele (Penfield)

Fig. 64-20. Types of injuries suffered by roots of brachial plexus. Spinal cord is viewed from posteriorly. On *left* are shown types of injuries and prognosis in each at postganglionic (infraganglionic) and preganglionic (supraganglionic) levels. On *right* are shown myelographic appearances for various injuries *1,* Normal nerve root. *2,* An injury in continuity distal to posterior root ganglion. All axons degenerate; axon reflex tests are negative, and there is no nerve conduction. Some recovery is possible if regenerating axons can penetrate intraneural scar. *3,* The same, but there has been disruption of the nerve. Repair is impossible because of extensive intraneural damage; *2* and *3* are distinguishable only by exploration in the posterior triangle of the neck. *4,* Recent supraganglionic lesion. Nerve root has been torn out of the cord, and there is an intrathecal effusion that shows as a filling defect in the myelogram. Posterior root ganglion cell bodies are intact. Whereas their central connections degenerate (there is no way of demonstrating this) their peripheral axons are intact, as can be shown by axon reflex tests and by nerve conduction. *5,* Same, but rent in dura matter has healed and myelographic appearance is normal. *6,* If rent in dura does not heal, a saccular protrusion forms a traumatic meningocele, easily visible in the myelogram. Nerve root here is shown as having suffered extensive interstitial damage, sufficient to destroy posterior root ganglion cells. Axon reflex tests and nerve conduction would therefore be negative, suggesting infraganglionic lesion—but for myelographic demonstration of meningocele. *7,* Rare distortion of spinal cord, late consequence of supraganglionic rupture of nerve root. (From Seddon, H.: Surgical disorders of the peripheral nerves, Edinburgh, 1972, Churchill Livingstone.)

length here. Some matters, however, need special emphasis.

When proceeding distally along the proximal part of the arm, one usually finds first the medial antebrachial cutaneous nerve crossing the large axillary vein. *Do not mistake this nerve for the ulnar nerve.* The ulnar nerve is nearby and is easily exposed by mobilizing and retracting the vein laterally. By retracting the same vein *medially,* the axillary artery is brought into view. Retracting this artery medially exposes the median nerve well on the lateral aspect of the bundle; retracting *laterally* the axillary artery, axillary vein, and ulnar nerve, one can easily identify the radial nerve, which lies well posterior to all other structures in the bundle. As the axillary artery is followed proximally, it is found to lie posterior to the point where the median nerve is formed from branches of the medial and lateral cords. Proximal to that point and posterior to the

pectoralis minor tendon, the axillary artery separates the medial and lateral cords and lies directly anterior to the posterior cord.

It is also wise to recall that the point of emergence of the musculocutaneous nerve from the lateral cord varies: usually it is deep to the tendon of the pectoralis minor, but it may be much more distal. Sometimes several branches emerge from the lateral cord to form this nerve. The axillary nerve usually emerges from the posterior cord a little more proximally than does the musculocutaneous nerve from the lateral cord and then winds posteriorly through the quadrangular space.

METHODS OF CLOSING GAPS. Extensive defects in the more proximal elements of the brachial plexus—its nerve roots, trunks, and divisions—and those on its lateral side are difficult to close because of the limitation of mobilization imposed on the surgeon by the various branches it gives off, including the suprascapular, the anterior thoracic, the subscapular, and the axillary nerves. Nevertheless, a gap of 5 to 6 cm can be closed with either autogenous nerve grafts or maneuvers that position the shoulder so that tension on an end-to-end repair is minimized. If positioning is selcted as the method, the plexus and the branches are first mobilized as far as possible. Then as much as 2.5 cm of the clavicle is resected, allowing the shoulder to collapse toward the body. The neck is bent sharply to the involved side, and the shoulder girdle is elevated. Finally the arm is adducted, the elbow is flexed, and the arm is brought across the chest. Often all sutures must be placed in the nerve ends but not tied, the clavicular osteotomy must be fixed, preferably with a plate and screws, and the wound must be closed except at the actual point of neurorrhaphy before the extremity can be positioned and the neurorrhaphy completed by tying the sutures. If such extreme positions of the head and extremity are required to allow closure of the gap, a cast incorporating the arm and extending

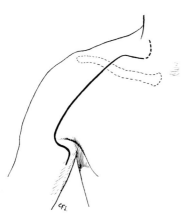

Fig. 64-21. Incision for approach to brachial plexus (see text).

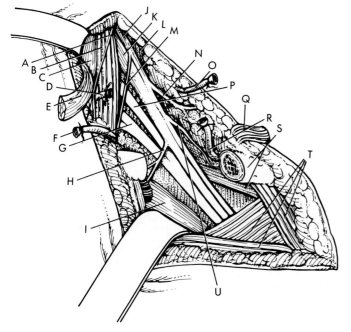

Fig. 64-22. Exposure of brachial plexus with section of clavicle. *A,* Phrenic nerve; *B,* scalenus anterior; *C,* internal jugular vein; *D,* transverse cervical artery; *E,* omohyoid muscle; *F,* suprascapular artery; *G,* eighth cervical and first dorsal roots; *H,* muscular branch; *I,* subclavian vein; *J,* fifth root; *K,* sixth root; *L,* scalenus medius muscle; *M* nerve to subclavian muscle; *N,* suprascapular nerve; *O,* transverse cervical artery; *P,* seventh root; *Q,* omohyoid muscle; *R,* suprascapular artery; *S,* clavicle and subclavius muscle; *T,* pectoralis major, pectoralis minor, and deltoid muscles; *U,* anterior thoracic nerve (Redrawn from Stookey, B.: Surgical and mechanical treatment of peripheral nerves, Philadelphia, 1922, W.B. Saunders Co.)

from the head to both iliac crests is necessary to prevent disruption of the line of suture.

In the region of the cords the closure of gaps is somewhat easier. Mobilization of the major nerves to the elbow or distal to it, if necessary, elevation of the shoulder girdle, flexion of the elbow, flexion of the shoulder, and adduction of the arm across the chest allow considerable length to be gained. Gaps as long as 10 cm, except in the posterior cord, can be closed in this manner. Rarely is it necessary to extend the incision superior to the clavicle, and sacrifice of a portion of the clavicle is not necessary here. Immobilization after surgery may require a shoulder spica cast with the shoulder flexed and adducted, or a Velpeau bandage reinforced with plaster may suffice.

AFTERTREATMENT. At 10 days the skin sutures are removed through a window in the cast, and if metal marking sutures were placed in the nerve ends, a roentgenogram is made to determine the integrity of the line of suture. At 6 to 8 weeks, depending on the tension on the line of suture, the cast is removed, and another roentgenogram is made. An abduction humeral splint is applied, and the shoulder gradually is adducted and the elbow extended during a period of 2 to 3 weeks; then physical therapy and active movement of the shoulder and other joints may be started. Subsequently braces should not be worn during the day except to prevent a joint from extending too rapidly. Occupational therapy is extremely important as soon as active motion is possible.

When an interfascicular grafting technique is used, the aftertreatment is different. A Velpeau bandage is applied for immobilization. Any drains left in the wound are removed at 36 to 48 hours. The sutures are removed at 10 to 14 days, and the Velpeau dressing is removed at 3 to 4 weeks. Active pendulum exercises are started at 4 weeks and gentle abduction exercises at 6. Significant return of function may require 3 to 5 years. During this time physical therapy to prevent contractures of joints and muscles is essential. Vocational rehabilitation is equally important. Whether electrical stimulation of denervated muscles is beneficial is not known for certain.

Results of treatment. As is true in all peripheral nerve injuries, many variables influence the results after injuries to the brachial plexus. Consequently dogmatic statements concerning the prognosis after the various injuries are difficult to prove. Since the time of publications describing the results of treatment of plexus injuries incurred during World War II, the experience of later surgeons has increased our knowledge of the prognosis after different methods of treatment.

Some brachial plexus injuries, usually those that are closed, may be treated without surgery with the expectation of relatively good results. Barnes found that 13 patients with plexus injuries but without electromyographic evidence of degenerative changes at 3 weeks recovered rapidly and completely. Of 33 upper plexus injuries, 22 spontaneously regained significant function of the muscles of the shoulder, elbow, and wrist. Of 26 lower plexus injuries, 18 regained some proximal muscle function. Brooks found that spontaneous recovery was good in lesions of the roots of C5 and C6 or of the upper trunk, fair in lesions of the posterior cord, and poor in those of C8 and T1 or the medial cord. According to Leffert and Sed-

don, the prognosis is remarkably good in infraclavicular plexus injuries. They found these injuries commonly associated with closed fractures or dislocations about the shoulder. All of their 14 patients regained almost normal strength in the muscles proximal to the hand. Some function returned in the median- and ulnar-innervated intrinsic muscles of the hand, and useful sensation returned. In a later study of 92 infraclavicular injuries Seddon found almost normal recovery in 42 and some recovery in 31. Narakas reported that of 248 injuries that were considered not serious or injuries in which early signs of recovery had occurred, the result was good or fair in 98.4%. Of 17 for whom surgery was considered but was rejected because of early recovery, the result was good or fair in 86.7%.

Until recently, with occasional exceptions, the surgical treatment of brachial plexus injuries was viewed with pessimism. The Veterans Administration monograph of 1956, *Peripheral Nerve Regeneration,* edited by Woodhall and Beebe, reported the results of the surgical treatment of a few such injuries incurred during World War II. Usually the results were better after repair in the upper plexus than in the lower. Suture of C5 and C6 nerve roots or of the upper trunk resulted in the return of significant muscle power in 10 of 14 patients. Brooks reported the results of exploration of 54 of 170 open plexus injuries treated in the British Peripheral Nerve Injuries Centers during World War II. Neurorrhaphies were carried out in 11 injuries, but only after upper trunk repairs was recovery satisfactory.

In the past the use of nerve grafts for brachial plexus injuries offered little hope of benefit. Sunderland proposed, however, that advancements in nerve grafting techniques might improve the prognosis after severe stretching injuries. Seddon in 1947 reported incomplete recovery of one of three patients treated with autogenous cable grafts for traction injuries. In 1955 Brooks reported incomplete return of function in three of six patients treated with nerve grafting. In 1973 Lusskin et al. reported the results of 20 patients treated by exploration of the plexus following trauma; 19 had some degree of paralysis. The proximal muscles were significantly reinnervated in the two patients treated with autogenous nerve grafts. When the transection was distal enough or when a nontransmitting neuroma in continuity could be resected leaving stumps long enough, they recommended autogenous grafting. Millesi, using the interfascicular autogenous nerve grafting technique, reported return of M-3 or better power (Highet) in 38 (70%) of 54 patients with injuries to various components of the plexus. Narakas used a similar grafting technique in 164 patients with traction injuries of the plexus and obtained good or fair results in 61%. He concluded that repair of brachial plexus injuries with grafts offers a chance for useful return of function for lesions in the following locations: (1) in the upper or middle trunk or in the cords posterior and inferior to the clavicle, (2) at the origin of the nerves leaving the plexus, (3) in the extraforaminal region with rupture of any two of C5, C6, or C7 spinal nerves but with no more than one avulsion and without injury to C8 and T1 and the median and ulnar nerves, and (4) in the upper plexus with partial lesions but without root avulsion when plexus repair is combined with tendon transfers to restore hand function.

In some situations neurorrhaphy may be the treatment of choice. Usually lesions of the C5 and C6 nerve roots, the upper trunk, and the lateral cord proximal to the origin of the musculocutaneous nerve may be treated with some success by neurorrhaphy, while lesions of other elements of the brachial plexus do not respond as well. It is unusual for intrinsic muscle function of the hand to return when C8 and T1 roots have been repaired. This does not mean that useful function may not be recovered when other elements of the plexus are repaired in children or when such surgery is carried out early in young adults.

Neurolysis is indicated in some injuries of the plexus. However, the results of this type of treatment have varied. Of 17 patients treated by neurolysis and reported by Lusskin et al., 13 were significantly improved. In their opinion neurolysis is beneficial in periplexus scarring, and they found in some instances that recovery was rapid. Narakas reported 47.6% good and fair results and 52.4% poor results among 21 patients treated by neurolysis.

The limited experiences of Narakas and of Millesi et al. with neurotization of distal stumps of avulsed nerve roots with intercostal nerves suggest that this might prove a useful alternative to other types of surgery, especially if the return of only one function is needed.

The results of the surgical treatment of pain after brachial plexus injuries have been unpredictable. Narakas reported improvement after exploration in 18 patients and no change in 10. Lusskin et al. reported no relief in three patients, one of whom was treated by silicone capping and two by neurolysis. Rhizotomy or some other type of treatment appears more appropriate.

BRACHIAL PLEXUS COMPRESSION SYNDROME

The neurovascular structures passing from the thorax may be compressed by the pectoralis minor at its coracoid attachment. The symptoms of aching pain in the arm and shoulder referred to the anterior chest and periscapular area may be reproduced by abduction of the arm or by pressure in the region of the coracoid process. Roentgenograms of the cervical spine, the chest, and the shoulder, angiography, and electromyography may help in diagnosis. Conservative measures consisting of heat and postural exercises are usually effective in relieving symptoms, but occasionally surgical release of the pectoralis minor may be necessary for relief of persistent pain.

The neurovascular compression syndrome of the superior thoracic outlet is discussed in Chapter 63.

SUPRASCAPULAR NERVE

Arising from the upper trunk of the brachial plexus, the suprascapular nerve lies in the posterior triangle of the neck near the posterior belly of the omohyoid muscle. It courses across the posterior triangle, passing under the belly of the omohyoid muscle and the anterior border of the trapezius to the scapular notch. It traverses the scapular notch, passing below the superior transverse ligament (transverse scapular ligament) and enters the supraspinatus fossa, where it sends a motor branch to the supraspinatus muscle and an articular branch to the shoulder joint. It passes around the lateral border of the spine of the scapula (spinoglenoid notch) into the infraspinatus fossa where it sends a muscular branch to the infraspinatus muscle with branches also to the shoulder joint and the scapula.

The nerve may be injured by penetrating trauma in the posterior triangle of the neck, by cancer surgery in the same area, by blunt or penetrating trauma in the supraclavicular region, by fractures of the superolateral portion of the scapula, especially involving the region of the suprascapular notch, following anterior dislocations of the shoulder joint, by entrapment in the suprascapular notch, and by space-occupying lesions such as a ganglion at the spinoglenoid notch.

Examination. Pain in the shoulder and weakness of the shoulder girdle are common complaints. Atrophy of both the supraspinatus and infraspinatus muscles may be seen if the nerve is injured at or proximal to the suprascapular notch. Atrophy of only the infraspinatus muscle suggests entrapment distal to the supraspinatus fossa, as may occur at the spinoglenoid notch.

Electrodiagnostic studies are helpful in confirming the diagnosis.

APPROACH (SWAFFORD AND LICHTMAN). (Fig. 64-23). With the patient prone, make an incision parallel to and about 3 cm superior to the scapular spine. Elevate the trapezius subperiosteally and expose the supraspinatus muscle. Identify the nerve by elevating the supraspinatus muscle, and dissecting superior and inferior to the muscle. Identify the suprascapular notch and release the transverse ligament. It may be necessary to enlarge the notch with a rongeur if it is narrow. Smooth the edges of the notch if it is enlarged. If no definite entrapment is identified in the notch, follow the nerve around the spinoglenoid notch to exclude entrapment in that area, especially if only the infraspinatus muscle is involved. Return of function following release is variable.

Results of suture. There are no conclusive reports regarding results following suture of this nerve.

LONG THORACIC NERVE

The serratus anterior muscle alone is occasionally paralyzed by injury to the long thoracic nerve. Such injuries may result from either sharp or blunt trauma or from traction when the head is forced acutely away from the shoulder or when the shoulder is depressed as when carrying heavy weights. Other causes include exposure to cold, viral infections, and placing patients in the Trendelenburg position with shoulder braces that compress the supraclavicular areas. When the serratus anterior is paralyzed, the patient cannot fully flex the arm above the level of the shoulder anteriorly, and active abduction may also be restricted. When the patient attempts to exert forward pushing movements with the hands, ''winging'' of the scapula occurs and its vertebral border and inferior angle become unduly prominent.

When the nerve has been stretched rather than severed, it is usually enough to immobilize the shoulder girdle in extension with the arm against the chest. Care should be taken to avoid contractures of the shoulder, elbow, and wrist while awaiting recovery. According to Sunderland, the nerve may recover after 3 to 12 months. If paralysis persists or if the nerve has been severed, the prognosis for recovery is poor, and a reconstructive operation may be indicated (see also the discussion of muscle transfers and

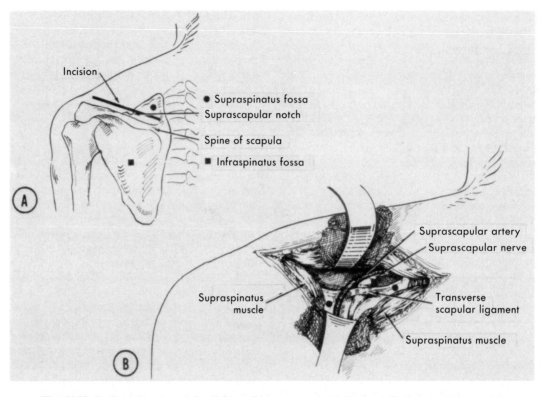

Fig. 64-23. A, Posterior approach for division of transverse scapular ligament. **B,** Suprascapular artery is above and suprascapular nerve is beneath ligament. (From Swafford, A.R., and Lichtman, D.H.: J. Hand Surg. **7:**57, 1982.)

fascial transplants for paralysis of the scapular muscles in Chapter 66). There are no significant reports of results following suture of the long thoracic nerve. For reconstructive operations for paralysis of the long thoracic nerve see p. 3049.

AXILLARY NERVE

The axillary nerve, composed of fibers from C5 and C6, is a branch of the posterior cord of the brachial plexus emerging inferior to the subscapular and thoracodorsal nerves at the level of the humeral head; it then winds around the neck of the humerus, passing through the quadrangular space to supply the deltoid and teres minor muscles. This nerve is commonly injured by fractures or dislocations about the shoulder, penetrating wounds, and direct blows.

Examination. Because a lesion of the axillary nerve sometimes does not cause anesthesia, the diagnosis must rest solely on the presence or absence of function in the deltoid muscle. Usually deltoid paralysis is easily detected by the inability to actively abduct the arm. However, it is well documented that full abduction of the arm is possible in the presence of deltoid paralysis because of the action of the supraspinatus and because of rotation of the scapula. Therefore it is essential to observe and palpate the deltoid muscle for contraction during the examination. Electrical stimulation of the nerve in situ is easily accomplished by inserting the needles along the posterior border of the deltoid.

APPROACH. If the wound is anterior, the axillary nerve is best exposed through the incision used for the more distal parts of the brachial plexus. Although occasionally it may be possible to expose the nerve in the axilla without detaching the pectoralis major tendon, dividing the insertion of this muscle greatly increases exposure. Externally rotate the arm so that the nerve may be followed into the quadrangular space. If the wound is posterior, the nerve may be exposed after it emerges from the quadrangular space through an incision beginning about 5 cm proximal to the posterior axillary fold, extending distally parallel to the posterior border of the deltoid, and ending at a point posterior to the deltoid tuberosity of the humerus. Then separate the posterior border of the deltoid muscle from the infraspinatus, teres minor and major, and triceps muscles. Locate the nerve as it emerges from the quadrangular space; the branch to the teres minor often arises proximal to this point. At varying distances after emerging from the space, sometimes as much as 2.5 cm, the axillary nerve divides into motor branches to the deltoid muscle and sensory branches to the skin. If the nerve is injured in the quadrangular space or if a long gap must be closed, both anterior and posterior incisions will be necessary.

METHODS OF CLOSING GAPS. A gap of 4 to 5 cm can be closed by mobilizing the nerve and the posterior cord of the brachial plexus proximally to the clavicle and by stripping the nerve up the plexus for 3 to 4 cm. Rarely other procedures used for mobilizing the brachial plexus such as resecting part of the clavicle may be indicated to gain more length. As in the brachial plexus, all sutures must be inserted in the nerve ends, and the wound or wounds must be closed as much as possible before neurorrhaphy is completed. Positioning after surgery is the same as that for the brachial plexus.

Millesi et al. reported satisfactory results after interfascicular nerve grafting to close gaps in the axillary nerve.

AFTERTREATMENT. Aftertreatment is as described for the brachial plexus (p. 2814).

Results following axillary nerve injury. If the injury is a closed one, signs of return of function may not be observed for 3 to 12 months. No statistical information is available concerning the results of suturing the axillary nerve.

TENDON AND MUSCLE TRANSFERS FOR PARALYSIS OF DELTOID

These tendon and muscle transfers are discussed in Chapter 66.

MUSCULOCUTANEOUS NERVE

The musculocutaneous nerve, composed of fibers from C5 and C6, is a branch of the lateral cord of the brachial plexus. It is most commonly injured by penetrating injuries but occasionally by anterior dislocation of the shoulder or fractures of the humeral neck. When this nerve is injured in the axilla, the injury is often in conjunction with injuries to other components of the brachial plexus. Complete division of the nerve may be overlooked because the sensory loss may be ill-defined and flexion of the elbow by the brachioradialis may be strong enough to mask biceps paralysis. In these instances it is essential to palpate the biceps while testing its function to identify specific muscle contractions.

Examination. The only muscle supplied by the musculocutaneous nerve that can be examined accurately is the biceps; the brachialis and the coracobrachialis are difficult to palpate. Sensory examination is of no great value because complete anesthesia is rare. Division of this nerve may cause less disability than that of any other major nerve in the body, and for this reason, especially in older patients, suture is occasionally not even indicated.

APPROACH. The incision is the same as for exposing the more distal parts of the brachial plexus (Fig. 64-21). If certain that no other nerves are involved, carry the incision in the proximal part of the arm about 2.5 cm anterior to that shown. Divide the tendon of the pectoralis major and identify the musculocutaneous nerve where it emerges from the lateral cord of the brachial plexus and before it pierces the coracobrachialis muscle. Then follow the nerve through the coracobrachialis muscle and as it passes into the arm, locate it in the plane between the biceps and brachialis muscles. The muscular branches of the nerve to the biceps are given off just after the nerve emerges from the coracobrachialis muscle and those to the brachialis at or just proximal to the level of junction of the middle and distal thirds of the arm. Exposing the nerve distal to this point is not necessary.

METHODS OF CLOSING GAPS. Gaps up to 8 cm may be closed by mobilizing the lateral cord of the brachial plexus proximally into the neck and the musculocutaneous nerve distally to its muscular branches, by adducting the shoulder sharply, and by bringing the arm anteriorly across the chest as for relaxing the brachial plexus. Occasionally one may transplant the musculocutaneous nerve so that it no longer pierces the coracobrachialis but runs across the axilla medial to this muscle between the biceps and brachialis muscles. As in repair of the brachial plexus, all sutures may be inserted in the nerve ends, and the wound is closed except at the site of neurorrhaphy before the sutures are tied. Interfascicular grafting may also be done if the gap is too wide to close by mobilization and limb positioning. After surgery, immobilization is the same as for the brachial plexus.

AFTERTREATMENT. Aftertreatment is as described for the brachial plexus (p. 2814).

Results following injury to musculocutaneous nerve. Signs of recovery of the musculocutaneous nerve may appear at 4 to 9 months after injury. Seddon reported excellent results in five of six nerves treated by secondary repair and satisfactory results in three treated by nerve grafting. According to him, the results of repair by either secondary suture or grafting are excellent.

RADIAL NERVE

The radial nerve, a continuation of the posterior cord of the brachial plexus, consists of fibers from C6, C7, and C8 and sometimes T1. It is primarily a motor nerve and innervates the triceps, the supinators of the forearm, and the extensors of the wrist, fingers, and thumb. This nerve is injured most often by fractures of the shaft of the humerus and gunshot wounds and lacerations of the arm and proximal forearm.

Entrapment syndromes of the radial nerve may develop when the nerve or one of its branches is compressed at some point along its course. Compression of the radial nerve in the arm may be caused by the fibrous arch of the lateral head of the triceps muscle. The posterior interosseous nerve may be compressed by the fibrous arcade of Frohse, fracture-dislocations or dislocations of the elbow, fractures of the forearm, Volkmann's ischemic contracture, neoplasms, enlarged bursae, aneurysms, or rheumatoid synovitis of the elbow. According to Spinner, posterior interosseous nerve entrapment is of two types. In one type all of the muscles supplied by the nerve are completely paralyzed; these include the extensor digitorum communis, extensor indicis proprius, extensor digiti quinti, extensor carpi ulnaris, abductor pollicis longus, and extensor pollicis brevis. In the second type only one or a few of these muscles are paralyzed. Roles and Maudsley have emphasized that entrapment of the posterior interosseous nerve may be a cause of chronic and refractory tennis elbow (p. 2515). Such entrapment may occur at the origin of the extensor carpi radialis brevis, at the arcade of Frohse, or in adhesions about the radial head. Pain in the region of the radial nerve anterior to the elbow, pain on resistance to supination of the forearm, and electrodiagnostic measures aid in differentiating this particular type of tennis elbow. Lotem et al. found that when symptoms and signs of radial nerve entrapment in the arm develop only after muscular effort, spontaneous recovery can be anticipated. However, when entrapment is caused by other conditions, especially in the forearm, surgical exploration and decompression of the nerve are usually beneficial.

Compression of the superficial radial nerve causes pain in the forearm and sensory impairment on the dorsum of the thumb. The nerve may be caught in scar tissue at the wrist after surgery or trauma. Constricting jewelry has also been cited as a potential cause for entrapment here.

After repair of the radial nerve the prognosis for regeneration is more favorable than for any other major nerve in the upper extremity, primarily because it is predominantly a motor nerve and secondarily because the muscles innervated by it are not involved in the finer movements of the fingers and hand.

Examination. The following muscles supplied by the radial nerve can be tested accurately because their bellies or tendons or both can be palpated: the triceps brachii, brachioradialis, extensors carpi radialis, extensor digitorum communis, extensor carpi ulnaris, abductor pollicis longus, and extensor pollicis longus. Injury to this nerve results in inability to extend the elbow or supinate the forearm and in a typical wristdrop. The inexperienced examiner, however, may often be misled by the patient's ability to extend the wrist merely by flexing the fingers. The examiner therefore should be discriminating because analysis of movements may often result in error in evaluating the function of a nerve. The triceps is not seriously affected by injuries of the nerve at the level of the middle of the humerus or distally. In injuries of the nerve at its bifurcation into the deep and superficial branches the brachioradialis and the extensor carpi radialis longus continue to function; thus the arm can be supinated and the wrist can be extended. The nerve is especially susceptible to electrical stimulation in situ just proximal to the elbow; elsewhere this is difficult, and the results are uncertain.

Sensory examination is relatively unimportant, even when the nerve is divided in the axilla, because there is usually no autonomous zone. When present, the autonomous zone is usually over the first dorsal interosseus muscle, between the first and second metacarpals. It is usually too inconsistent to afford more than confirmatory evidence of complete interruption of the nerve proximal to its bifurcation at the elbow.

APPROACH. Expose the radial nerve in the axilla and proximal third of the arm by the usual incision for the distal part of the brachial plexus (Fig. 64-21) and carry this incision distally in the arm a little more posteriorly than is necessary for exposing the ulnar and median nerves. Incise the fascia over the neurovascular bundle and expose the bundle between the triceps posteriorly and the biceps, brachialis, and coracobrachialis anteriorly. Expose and retract laterally the more superficial structures of the bundle—the ulnar nerve, the brachial artery and vein, and the median nerve—thereby exposing the radial nerve and one or two of its branches, first to the long head and then to the medial head of the triceps. Then trace the nerve to the point where it winds around the humerus.

To expose the nerve on the posterior and lateral aspects of the humeral shaft, begin the incision along the posterior border of the distal third of the deltoid between the deltoid and the long head of the triceps. Then curve it distalward along the lateral aspect of the arm, curving at first anteriorly along the medial aspect of the brachioradialis and then, if necessary, laterally at the elbow across the belly of this muscle and the extensor carpi radialis longus. Finally if the deep radial nerve is to be explored, carry the

incision distally on the dorsum of the forearm along the radial side of the extensor digitorum communis.

In the incision proximal to the elbow it is wise to expose the nerve at its most superficial position by incising the fascia between the brachialis and brachioradialis and to identify the nerve at this point by retracting the brachioradialis laterally. The nerve can then be easily exposed proximally by incising the fascia and retracting the lateral head of the triceps laterally to the point where the nerve winds around the humerus. This approach, with minor changes, is shown in Fig. 64-24.

The nerve may then be carefully traced distally to the elbow. Five or 6 cm proximal to the elbow it sends branches to the brachioradialis and then a little more distally to the extensor carpi radialis longus and brevis; at the elbow the nerve divides into the superficial and deep radial (posterior interosseous) nerves. The superficial radial nerve is entirely sensory but should be protected to avoid painful neuromas. The deep radial nerve is injured often, and such an injury is quite disabling. Expose this nerve through the distal part of the incision just described, beginning 8 to 10 cm proximal to the elbow and continuing to the middle of the dorsum of the forearm (Fig. 64-25). Follow the nerve beneath the brachioradialis into the supinator muscle. If the injury is at this point or is more distal, expose the nerve distal to the supinator by incising the fascia between the extensor carpi radialis longus and brevis and the extensor digitorum communis and by developing this plane of cleavage. After exposing the nerve, follow it proximally to the distal border of the supinator where numerous branches are given off. After identifying these, incise the superficial part of the supinator at a right angle to the direction of its fibers to complete the exposure of the entire deep radial nerve.

METHODS OF CLOSING GAPS. Gaps in the radial nerve are closed less easily than those in the ulnar and median nerves. In general, however, the same extensive mobilization and positioning of the extremity enable one to close most of them. In the axilla and in the proximal arm on the medial side proximal to the point of emergence of the branches to the triceps, closing a gap of more than 6 to 7 cm is difficult without sacrificing the branches to the triceps; this is hardly justifiable. Resecting the humerus is rarely feasible at this level. Gaps here are best closed either by mobilizing the nerve and the posterior cord of the brachial plexus proximally to the clavicle and the nerve distally well into the lateral side of the arm or by interfascicular nerve grafting.

In the middle third of the arm, defects of 10 to 12 cm may be closed by mobilizing the nerve from the elbow to the clavicle and widely stripping the branches of the nerve, by flexing the elbow, by externally rotating and strongly adducting the arm across the chest, and finally if necessary by sacrificing the branch to the brachioradialis (if the biceps is functioning). Transplanting the nerve beneath the biceps anterior to the humerus, advocated by most authors on this subject, actually adds variable length and is occasionally worthwhile. In one patient Gore reported mobilization of a proximal branch of the radial nerve to the triceps to suture to the distal end of the nerve with good results. In the presence of a nonunited fracture of the hu-

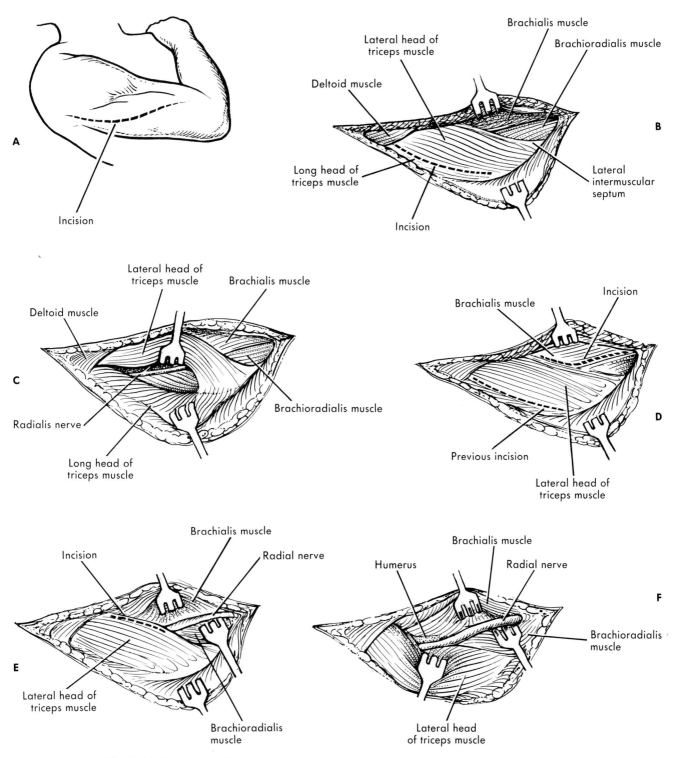

Fig. 64-24. Exposure of radial nerve in middle and distal thirds of arm. **A,** Skin incision begins at posterior margin of deltoid muscle and extends distally in midline and then laterally and anteriorly. It ends at interval between brachioradialis and brachialis. **B** Posterior skin flap has been dissected and retracted; deep fascia is incised in line with skin incision. *Dotted line,* incision in triceps muscle between long and lateral heads. **C,** Radial nerve and accompanying vascular bundle have been exposed by retraction of these two heads of triceps muscle. Radial nerve has been dissected to point at which it passes beneath lateral head of triceps muscle. **D,** Arm is externally rotated a few degrees. Interval between proximal end of brachioradialis and brachialis is to be dissected, exposing radial nerve along anterolateral aspect of humerus. **E,** *Dotted line,* incision through which lateral head of triceps is mobilized from underlying bone, facilitating exposure of radial nerve deep to it. **F,** Exposure. (Modified from Banks, S.W., and Laufman, H.: An atlas of surgical exposures of the extremities, Philadelphia, 1953, W.B. Saunders Co.)

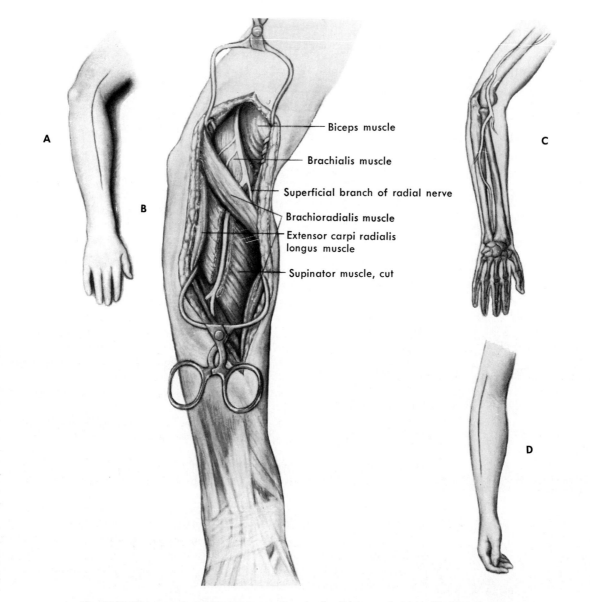

Fig. 64-25. Exposure of posterior interosseous branch of radial nerve. **A,** Line of incision, forearm prone, elbow flexed. **B,** Nerve exposed. **C,** Diagram of course of nerve with arm in position **A. D,** Line of incision, elbow extended. (Modified from Mayer, J.H., Jr., and Mayfield, F.H.: Surg. Gynecol. Obstet. **84**:979, 1947.

merus, 3 to 4 cm of the bone may be resected, but if the procedures just mentioned are used, resecting part of a normal humerus should almost never be necessary to repair the radial nerve. Before such extreme dissection and awkward positioning are attempted, serious consideration should be given to interfascicular nerve grafting.

In the distal third of the arm, at the elbow, and in the forearm, the procedures mentioned here will allow closure of almost any gap up to 10 to 12 cm long.

AFTERTREATMENT. If adducting the arm across the chest has been necessary, immobilization is maintained by a Velpeau bandage reinforced with plaster. Otherwise, as in repair of the ulnar and median nerves, a posterior molded plaster splint is sufficient; the treatment after surgery is the same as for the ulnar nerve (p. 2822). If nerve grafting techniques have been used, the aftercare is as described on p. 2805.

Results of suture of radial nerve. Only motor recovery is important in suture of the radial nerve. Eighty-nine percent of patients with sutures of this nerve will obtain recovery of proximal muscles, 63% will regain useful function of all muscles supplied by the radial nerve, and 36% will regain some fine control of the extensors of the fingers and thumb. Thus when circumstances are most favorable, more than three fourths of these patients recover useful function of all the muscles supplied by this nerve. Millesi reported return of motor power of M-3 (Highet) or better in 17 of 18 radial nerve lesions treated by interfascicular grafting.

Critical limit of delay of suture. Return of motor function should not be expected when suture has been delayed for more than 15 months. Zachary found that return of function in muscles innervated by the posterior interosseous nerve is unlikely if the delay is more than 9 months.

ULNAR NERVE

The ulnar nerve is composed of fibers from C8 and T1 coming from the medial cord of the brachial plexus. It may be divided at any point along its course by missile wounds or lacerations. When it is injured in the upper arm, other nerves or the brachial artery because of their proximity may also be injured. In the middle of the arm the ulnar nerve is relatively protected, but in the distal arm and at the elbow it is often injured by dislocations of the elbow and supracondylar and condylar fractures. An ulnar nerve deficit complicating a fracture or dislocation may be caused by the initial trauma, by repeated manipulations of the osseous injury, or by scar formation developing sometime after injury. The nerve is injured most commonly in the distal forearm and wrist; in these locations it may be injured by gunshot wounds, lacerations, fractures, or dislocations. In civilian life lacerations cause most of the injuries at the wrist.

Traction on the nerve, subluxation or dislocation of the nerve, and entrapment syndromes may also cause ulnar nerve deficits that may require surgical treatment. Tardy ulnar nerve palsy may develop after malunited fractures of the lateral humeral condyle in children, displaced fractures of the medial humeral epicondyle, dislocations of the elbow, and contusions of the nerve. In malunion of the lateral humeral condyle, cubitus valgus develops; in this deformity the ulnar nerve is gradually stretched and may become incompletely paralyzed. Tardy ulnar nerve palsy may also develop in patients who have a shallow ulnar groove on the posterior aspect of the medial humeral epicondyle, hypoplasia of the humeral trochlea, or an inadequate fibrous arch that normally keeps the nerve in the groove, resulting in recurrent subluxation or dislocation of the nerve. Childress found recurrent subluxation or dislocation of the nerve in 16.2% of 2000 elbows. Subluxation is more common than dislocation, and the ulnar nerve is more likely to be injured repeatedly in subluxations. In most patients flexion of the elbow aggravated the symptoms of pain and paresthesias. Entrapment or compression of the ulnar nerve may also occur at the supracondyloid process of the humerus medially, at the arcade of Struthers near the medial intermuscular septum, between the heads of origin of the flexor carpi ulnaris, and at the wrist in Guyon's canal. In other areas the nerve may be compressed by tight fascia or ligaments, neoplasms, rheumatoid synovitis, aneurysms, vascular thromboses, or anomalous muscles.

Examination. Interrupting the ulnar nerve proximal to the elbow is followed by paralysis of the flexor carpi ulnaris, the flexor profundus to the little and ring fingers, the lumbricals of the same fingers, all of the interossei, the adductor of the thumb, and all of the short muscles of the little finger. Occasionally when a nerve is completely divided at this level, the intrinsic muscles of the hand function normally because of anomalous innervation of these muscles by the median nerve. In these instances the fibers that supply the intrinsic muscles may be incorporated in the median nerve down to the middle of the forearm where they leave the median nerve to join the ulnar nerve (Martin-Gruber anastomosis). Complete division of the ulnar nerve at the wrist usually causes paralysis of all ulnar-innervated intrinsic muscles unless there is an anatomic

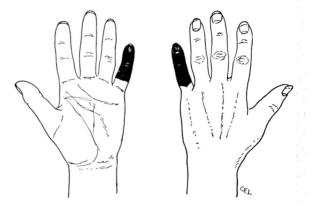

Fig. 64-26. Autonomous zone of ulnar nerve.

variation through which the median and ulnar nerves are connected in the palm (Riche-Cannieu anastomosis). Usually when the nerve is divided at the wrist, only the opponens pollicis, the lateral or superficial head of the flexor pollicis brevis, and the lateral two lumbricals remain functional.

In practice only three muscles—the flexor carpi ulnaris, the abductor digiti quinti, and the first dorsal interosseus muscle—can be tested accurately. The bellies or tendons (or both) of these muscles may be easily palpated or seen. One may be tempted to test other muscles by their well-known functions but would be misled by the occasional patient who can by substituting other muscles perform perfectly the actions of paralyzed muscles.

Atrophy of the muscles supplied by the ulnar nerve and clawing of the little and ring fingers are usually confirmatory evidence of paralysis of the muscles supplied by this nerve. However, if the nerve has been injured proximal to the elbow, clawing of these two fingers may be absent because the flexor digitorum profundus to the ring and little fingers is also denervated. Electrical stimulation of the nerve in situ is easy at the elbow and wrist.

The sensory examination is usually straightforward, although anatomic variations may cause confusing sensory findings. One need examine only the middle and distal phalanges of the little finger, which make up the autonomous zone of the ulnar nerve (Fig 64-26). Complete anesthesia to pinpricks in this area strongly suggests total division of the nerve. If one is in doubt about the sensory examination, skin resistance studies or an iodine starch test will be useful.

APPROACH. In the axilla the ulnar nerve is exposed through the usual more distal brachial plexus incision (p. 2811). To expose the nerve in the upper arm begin the incision over the tendon of the pectoralis major and curve it into the natural folds of the axilla and then distally along the medial aspect of the upper arm. At a point 6 to 8 cm proximal to the elbow curve the incision posteriorly slightly behind the medial epicondyle (Fig. 64-27). To expose the nerve in the forearm continue the incision distally along the ulnar side of the volar aspect of the forearm to the proximal flexor crease of the wrist.

In the axilla and upper arm the nerve lies just medial to the brachial artery, usually beneath the brachial vein. At about the middle of the upper arm the nerve leaves

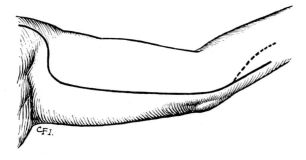

Fig. 64-27. Skin incision for exploration of median and ulnar nerves in upper arm.

the neurovascular bundle, gradually courses posteriorly through the intermuscular septum superficial to the medial head of the triceps muscle, and enters the ulnar groove behind the medial humeral epicondyle. Here the medial antebrachial cutaneous nerve may be confused with the ulnar nerve. In the region of the ulnar groove the ulnar nerve gives off no important branches, although there are articular branches to the elbow joint and one or two branches to the flexor carpi ulnaris. Muscular branches to the medial half of the flexor digitorum profundus and additional branches to the flexor carpi ulnaris are given off distal to the groove.

Trace the nerve into the forearm by freeing the flexor carpi ulnaris at its origin from the humeral epicondyle or by resecting the epicondyle. The nerve courses distally in the forearm on the flexor profundus on the radial side of the belly of the flexor carpi ulnaris. At the junction of the middle and proximal thirds of the forearm the ulnar artery approaches the nerve from its lateral side and accompanies it into the hand. The dorsal cutaneous branch is given off about 5 to 8 cm proximal to the pisiform and winds deep to the tendon of the flexor carpi ulnaris to reach the dorsum of the wrist and hand. The main trunk of the ulnar nerve courses distally lateral to the tendon of the flexor carpi ulnaris and enters the hand where it divides into the superficial and deep branches.

METHODS OF CLOSING GAPS. The ulnar nerve may be sutured at any point along its course. A gap in it can probably be closed more easily than in any other nerve, primarily because the nerve can be transplanted to the antecubital fossa to gain length. If the lesion is distal to the muscular branches in the forearm, gaps of 12 to 15 cm can be closed by mobilizing and transplanting the nerve, flexing the wrist and elbow, intraneural dissection of the motor branches up the nerve, and sacrificing the articular branches. In the upper arm gaps of 8 to 10 cm may be closed by the same methods without sacrificing motor branches to the long flexors. Sacrificing these branches is rarely justified because recovery of motor function will probably be limited to these muscles after suture of the ulnar nerve in the upper arm.

The nerve should be transplanted only after the most painstaking intraneural dissection of the branches to the flexor profundus and flexor carpi ulnaris. In our experience satisfactory results have been achieved by placing the nerve on the fascia of the flexor-pronator group beneath the thick layer of fat in this region. The fat is then sutured to the fascia medial to the nerve to keep the nerve from slipping back posterior to the epicondyle. Or the nerve may be transplanted anteriorly deep to the flexor-pronator muscles by removing their origins from the medial epicondyle, either by dividing the flexor origin in its tendinous portion or by resecting and later reattaching the medial epicondyle; when this technique is used, the ulnar nerve is transplanted anteriorly to a location near the median nerve. The medial intermuscular septum should be divided proximal to the elbow to allow flexion and extension of the joint without kinking or stretching the nerve. As an alternative to awkward positioning and extensive mobilization of the nerve, interfascicular nerve grafting should be considered.

AFTERTREATMENT. If transplanting the nerve and flexing the wrist and elbow have been necessary, a molded posterior plaster splint from the axilla to the metacarpophalangeal joints is necessary. If the lesion is in the forearm and the gap is closed by flexing the wrist alone, the wrist is immobilized in a posterior molded plaster splint from just distal to the elbow to the metacarpophalangeal joints.

The sutures are removed at 7 to 10 days, and the splint is removed 4 weeks later. While wearing the splint, the patient should be encouraged to use the fingers and keep the metacarpophalangeal joints supple. After the splint is removed, the elbow and wrist, if flexed, are gradually extended during a period of 2 to 3 weeks, depending on the tension on the line of suture, by means of an adjustable metal splint. During this time roentgenograms should be made as necessary to determine the integrity of the line of suture. This is indicated by the position of metal clips or wire sutures placed near the ends of the nerves at the time of repair. After the elbow and wrist can be extended, physical therapy is started to help in regaining full motion in the joints. Splints are rarely used after the limb can be extended.

Results of suture of ulnar nerve. Motor recovery is more important than sensory recovery. After suture of the ulnar nerve about half of these patients may be expected to show return of function in the long flexors of the fingers and wrist and some useful function in the interossei and hypothenar intrinsic muscles. Only 5% of the patients may recover independent function of the interossei. Seventy-eight percent may regain useful motor recovery under favorable circumstances, and 16% may show independent finger motion. About half of the patients may be expected to regain useful sensation with return of sensitivity to touch and pain in the autonomous zone but with persistence of overresponse. Thirty percent regain touch and pain sensation without overresponse; under favorable circumstances this type of return may be obtained in half of these patients.

Seddon reported return of motor power of M_3 (Highet) or better in almost half of the 21 primary ulnar neurorrhaphies at the wrist. Combined good and fair motor return was seen in almost 90% of ulnar neurorrhaphies at the wrist, whether primary or secondary. The poorest motor return occurred when the ulnar nerve was repaired in the axilla. Millesi reported return of motor power of M_3 (Highet) or better in 79.5% of 38 patients after interfascicular grafting.

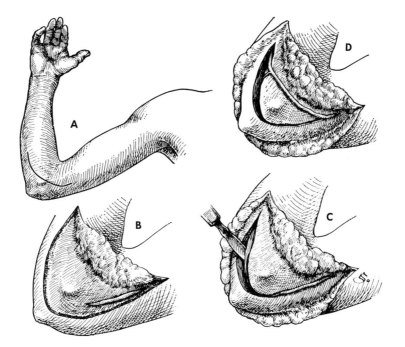

Fig. 64-28. Technique of transplanting ulnar nerve for tardy ulnar nerve palsy. **A,** Skin incision. **B,** and **C,** Exposing and freeing of nerve. It is freed from scar tissue posterior to medial epicondyle and from beneath tendinous arch between humeral and ulnar heads of flexor carpi ulnaris. **D,** Nerve has been transplanted anteriorly.

Critical limit of delay of suture. Useful motor recovery of the ulnar nerve should not be expected if suture is delayed 9 months after injury in high lesions or 15 months in low lesions. Sensory recovery rarely occurs after 9 months in high lesions but has been said to occur as late as 31 months after injury in low lesions. According to Zachary, motor return cannot be expected after a delay of 29 months in lesions above the flexor carpi ulnaris and 18 months in lesions below the branches of the flexor digitorum profundus. Sensory return cannot be expected after a delay of 29 months in lesions above the flexor carpi ulnaris and 31 months below the flexor digitorum profundus.

TARDY ULNAR NERVE PALSY

The treatment for refractory tardy ulnar nerve palsy may require removal of the nerve from its groove, neurolysis if necessary, and anterior transplantation of the nerve to the flexor surface of the elbow.

Craven and Green reported relief of pain and improvement in nerve conduction velocities in 28 of 30 patients with the cubital tunnel syndrome treated by medial epicondylectomy and anterior transposition of the nerve. Jones and Gauntt reported 48% good, 17% fair, and 35% poor results in 22 extremities treated for ulnar nerve compression at the elbow by medial epicondylectomy. Eaton et al. reported improvement in 15 of 16 ulnar neuropathies treated by anterior nerve transposition and construction of a fasciodermal sling from the antebrachial fascia overlying the flexor pronator muscles, based on the medial epicondyle.

Adelaar et al. conducted a prospective study to evaluate release of the cubital tunnel, subcutaneous anterior transposition, and submuscular anterior transposition in 32 patients. They found no significant difference in the results of the three procedures. They recommended careful preoperative evaluation including electromyography.

TECHNIQUE OF TRANSPLANTING ULNAR NERVE. With the arm abducted and externally rotated, make an incision on the posteromedial surface of the elbow beginning 7 cm proximal to the epicondyle, passing distally anterior to the epicondyle, and proceeding farther distally in line with the course of the nerve (Fig. 64-28). Reflect the anterior skin flap to expose the common origin of the flexor muscles. Identify the nerve in its groove posterior to the medial epicondyle and free it of soft tissues. Free the flexor carpi ulnaris from its humeral origin on the epicondyle to further expose the nerve. Identify its branches to the flexor profundus and flexor carpi ulnaris and carefully dissect them intraneurally up the nerve. Dissect any fibrous tissue or callus from the area adjacent to the groove and remove the nerve. Carry out a neurolysis or endoneurolysis as indicated if there is extensive scarring. Now draw the nerve over the epicondyle to the anterior surface of the elbow and place it on the surface of the fascia of the flexor-pronator group beneath the thick fat in this region. Excise the medial intermuscular septum and any other tendinous bands that may constrict or otherwise injure the transplanted nerve. Place a few interrupted sutures through the fascia and subcutaneous fat medial to the nerve to keep the nerve from slipping back posterior to the epicondyle.

As an alternative divide the medial epicondyle, transplant the ulnar nerve anterior to the elbow near the median nerve, and reattach the epicondyle.

AFTERTREATMENT. The elbow is immobilized at a right angle for 3 weeks. Physical therapy is then started and continued to prevent secondary changes in the muscles of the hand. Appropriate splinting is continued until sufficient function has returned to allow the patient to be free of brace or splint.

MEDIAN NERVE

The median nerve, formed by the junction of the lateral and medial cords of the brachial plexus in the axilla, is composed of fibers from C6, C7, C8, and T1 (Fig. 64-29). Median nerve injuries often result in painful neuromas and causalgia. From the sensory standpoint they are more disabling than injuries of the ulnar nerve because they involve the digits used in fine volitional activity.

Median nerve injuries are often caused by lacerations, usually in the forearm or wrist. Sunderland pointed out that in the upper arm the nerve can be injured by relatively superficial lacerations, excessively tight tourniquets, and humeral fractures, and when it is injured near the axilla, the ulnar and musculocutaneous nerves and the brachial artery are also commonly injured. In the arm the median nerve may be compressed by the ligament of Struthers. At the elbow the nerve may be injured in supracondylar fractures and posterior dislocations of the elbow. Rana et al. reported division of the median nerve in a dislocation of the elbow. Pritchard, Linscheid, and Svien reported a 12-year-old boy in whom delayed exploration after dislocation of the elbow revealed an entrapped median nerve; a segment of the nerve was resected, the nerve was repaired, and the result was satisfactory. Median nerve deficits, as seen in the pronator syndrome, may result from compression of the nerve at the pronator teres, the lacertus fibro-

sus, or the fibrous flexor digitorum sublimis arch or from anomalies including a hypertrophic pronator teres, fibrous bands within the pronator teres, the median nerve passing posterior to both heads of the pronator teres, or an accessory tendinous arch of the flexor carpi radialis arising from the ulna. The anterior interosseous nerve may be injured in fractures and lacerations or may be compressed or entrapped by any of the following: the tendinous origins of the flexor digitorum sublimis or the pronator teres, variant muscles such as the palmaris profundus and flexor carpi radialis brevis, accessory muscle slips and tendons from the flexor digitorum sublimis to the flexor pollicis longus, an accessory head of the flexor pollicis longus (Gantzer's muscles), by an aberrant radial artery, by thrombosis of the ulnar collateral vessels, enlargement of the bicipital bursa, or Volkmann's ischemic contracture. For detailed discussions of these particular nerve compressions the reader is referred to the extensive reports by Spinner and to the bibliography.

At the wrist the median nerve may be injured by fractures of the distal radius and by fractures and dislocations of the carpal bones. Wolfe and Eyring reported the unusual occurrence of median nerve entrapment in callus after a fracture of the distal radius; excision of the callus and repair of the nerve were necessary.

Examination. The muscles of the forearm and hand supplied by the median nerve that can be tested with relative accuracy are the pronator teres, flexor carpi radialis, flexor digitorum profundus (index), flexor pollicis longus, flexor digitorum sublimis, and abductor pollicis brevis. Substitution movements caused by action of intact muscles may cause confusion during the examination. The works of Sunderland provide an excellent review of these movements and the methods of recognizing and preventing them. Usually if the forearm can be actively maintained in pronation against resistance, the pronator teres is intact. If the wrist can be actively maintained in flexion and a contracting flexor carpi radialis is palpated, this muscle is intact. Similarly if the interphalangeal joint of the thumb can be maintained in flexion against resistance with the wrist in the neutral position and the thumb adducted, the flexor pollicis longus is functioning. The flexor digitorum sublimis to each finger is examined separately while the remaining fingers are held in full passive extension (Fig. 5-3). Although opposition of the thumb may be difficult to confirm, if the thumb can be actively maintained in palmar abduction and a contracting abductor pollicis brevis is palpated, this muscle is functioning. The lumbricals cannot be discretely tested because they cannot be palpated and because their function may be confused with that of the interosseus muscles.

According to Spinner, the anterior interosseous syndrome may cause varying signs and symptoms. The typical patient has pain in the proximal forearm lasting for several hours and is found to have weakness or paralysis of the flexor pollicis longus, the flexor digitorum profundus to the index and long fingers, and the pronator quadratus. When the patient attempts to pinch, active flexion of the distal phalanx of the index finger is impossible. Variations from these signs and symptoms usually result from atypical patterns of innervation. For example, if all of the flexor

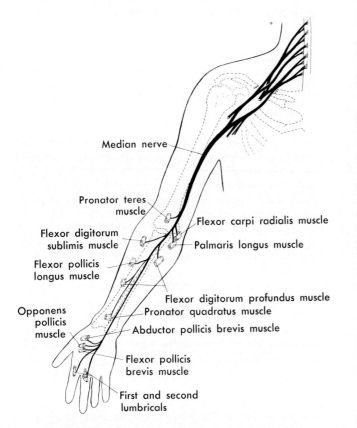

Median nerve

Pronator teres muscle

Flexor carpi radialis muscle

Flexor digitorum sublimis muscle

Palmaris longus muscle

Flexor pollicis longus muscle

Flexor digitorum profundus muscle

Opponens pollicis muscle

Pronator quadratus muscle

Abductor pollicis brevis muscle

Flexor pollicis brevis muscle

First and second lumbricals

Fig. 64-29. Origin, course, and distribution of median nerve.

digitorum profundus muscles are supplied by the anterior interosseous nerve, then all of these muscles are weak or paralyzed. Conversely if innervation overlaps and the ulnar nerve supplies the flexor digitorum profundus to the long finger, this finger is spared. Electromyography, the triketohydrindene hydrate (Ninhydrin) print test, and clinical examination will help to differentiate the syndromes. In well-established lesions atrophy of the forearm flexor mass and of the thenar muscles may be seen.

Variations in the sensory supply of the median nerve may also be confusing, but usually the volar surface of the thumb, of the index and middle fingers, and of the radial half of the ring finger and the dorsal surfaces of the distal phalanges of the index and middle fingers are supplied by the median nerve. The smallest autonomous zone of the median nerve covers the dorsal and volar surfaces of the distal phalanges of the index and middle fingers (Fig. 64-30). The iodine-starch test or triketohydrindene hydrate (Ninhydrin) print test may be helpful in diagnosis. Autonomic changes such as anhydrosis, atrophy of the skin, and narrowing of the digits because of atrophy of the pulp are also valuable signs of sensory deficit.

Operative treatment of the median nerve may be indicated in most of the lesions listed on p. 2824. For the anterior interosseous syndrome Spinner recommends the following plan. If the onset of paralysis has been spontaneous, the initial treatment is nonoperative. Surgical exploration is indicated in the absence of clinical or electromyographic improvement after 12 weeks. If an anterior interosseous nerve injury is caused by a penetrating wound, primary repair is recommended. In irreparable injury to the nerve, tendon transfers are indicated as discussed in Chapter 12. Carpal tunnel syndrome is discussed in Chapter 18.

APPROACH. To expose the median nerve use the same approach as that for the ulnar in the arm and at the elbow and thus avoid crossing the folds of the antecubital fossa (Fig. 64-27).

To expose the median nerve in the forearm continue the incision from the medial epicondyle onto the volar aspect of the forearm and then distally over the course of the nerve. In approaching the wrist curve it toward the radial side (or if exploration of both the median and ulnar nerves is indicated, toward the ulnar side). As the flexor creases

of the wrist are reached, return the incision along one of them to the middle of the wrist. If the nerve is to be explored distal to the wrist, extend the incision down the thenar crease.

Deepen the incision through the fascia along the course of the nerve. To accomplish this at the elbow undermine the skin flap widely. In the arm retract the brachial artery and vein medially to expose the nerve on the lateral aspect of the neurovascular bundle. At the junction of the middle and distal thirds of the arm the nerve crosses to the medial side of the artery, usually coursing posterior although occasionally anterior to it. The nerve enters the forearm beneath the lacertus fibrosus medial to the artery, then courses between the two heads of the pronator teres, and continues distally in the forearm beneath the flexor sublimis, lying on the flexor profundus. Approaching the wrist the nerve becomes more superficial, lies beneath the tendon of the flexor carpi radialis, and is easily found if approached between this tendon and that of the palmaris longus.

At the elbow expose the nerve by incising the fibers of the lacertus fibrosus at its attachment to the fascia over the pronator-flexor group. Dissect the fascia radially from this group of muscles and incise it distally and radially along the proximal border of the pronator teres and thence distally across this muscle and along the medial side of the flexor carpi radialis. Thus the pronator teres may be widely mobilized and separated from the flexor carpi radialis, permitting easy exposure of the nerve and making closure easier later. Next expose the nerve where it emerges from beneath the fibers of the flexor digitorum sublimis. Trace the nerve proximally by retracting the flexor carpi radialis laterally and the pronator proximally and by separating the fibers of the flexor digitorum sublimis. In this way the nerve may be exposed over its entire course. As an alternative cut the radial origin of the flexor digitorum sublimis in line with the nerve and sever the pronator teres by a Z incision near its insertion (Fig. 64-31).

The median nerve gives off no branches in the upper arm. The branches to the pronator teres and flexor carpi radialis emerge as the nerve courses beneath the lacertus fibrosus. There are usually two branches to the pronator, one to the superficial head, and one to the deep head. There are also several branches to the flexor carpi radialis and palmaris longus, one to the flexor sublimis, and one to the profundus. The anterior interosseous nerve emerges from the posteromedial side of the nerve and supplies the flexor pollicis longus, the radial half of the flexor profundus, and the pronator quadratus. Farther distally several more branches are given off to the flexor digitorum sublimis. No other significant branches are given off until the nerve enters the hand.

When exposure of the anterior interosseous nerve deep to the pronator teres is required or when anterior transplantation of the median nerve is preferred, a method whereby the pronator teres insertion is released and is repaired by Z-plasty or a tongue-in-groove suture after the median nerve has been transplanted is suitable.

METHODS OF CLOSING GAPS. By extensively mobilizing the nerve, stripping back its branches in the main trunk, and flexing the wrist and elbow, one may close a gap of 8 to

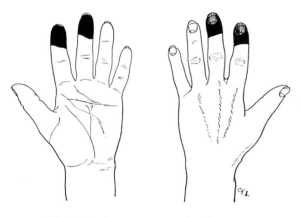

Fig. 64-30. Autonomous zone of median nerve.

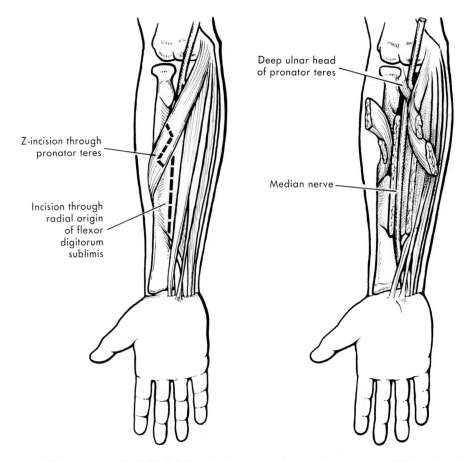

Z-incision through pronator teres

Incision through radial origin of flexor digitorum sublimis

Deep ulnar head of pronator teres

Median nerve

Fig. 64-31. Alternate method of exposing median nerve throughout forearm (see text). (Redrawn from Seddon, H.: Surgical disorders of the peripheral nerves, Edinburgh, 1972, Churchill Livingstone.)

10 cm proximal to the elbow and of 12 to 15 cm distal to the elbow. Transplanting the nerve anterior to the pronator teres allows one to gain more length if the lesion is distal to this muscle. The ease with which the nerve may be transplanted anteriorly depends to some extent on the level at which the branches to the flexor-pronator group emerge. When they emerge distally, transplanting the nerve is much more difficult than when they emerge more proximally. Transplantation is usually necessary in large destructive wounds in the middle of the forearm. In these wounds most of the branches to the flexor sublimis are usually destroyed and therefore need not be considered.

Transplantation is accomplished by stripping the branches to the pronator teres, the flexor carpi radialis, the palmaris longus, and the anterior interosseous nerve intraneurally from the main trunk well proximally in the upper forearm, then by mobilizing the distal end of the nerve all the way to the wrist and beneath the transverse carpal ligament, and then by flexing both the wrist and elbow and suturing the nerve anterior to the flexor-pronator group. Two or 3 cm more in length may be gained by transplantation, thus permitting neurorrhaphy, which could not otherwise be carried out. If too much tension is placed on the nerve, the fascia and lacertus fibrosus must be closed deep to it, and the nerve is left subcutaneous all the way to the wrist. Release of the deep head of the pronator teres and dissection and placement of the flexor carpi radialis deep to the median nerve may make mobilization and transplantation of the nerve to the subcutaneous position easier. To avoid awkward positioning and excessive tension, interfascicular nerve grafting should be considered.

AFTERTREATMENT. Aftertreatment is as described for the ulnar nerve (p. 2822).

Results of suture of median nerve. Motor recovery is extremely important following median nerve repair; however, the hand without median nerve sensory supply is almost useless. Even with the best sensory recovery the patient will probably have difficulty with stereognosis. Under favorable circumstances about half of the patients with median nerve suture will recover sensitivity to pain and touch and some degree of stereognosis. Furthermore, under the same circumstances about 90% of these patients will recover a useful degree of motor function in the long flexors of the forearm. A much smaller number, perhaps one third, will obtain useful recovery in the thenar muscles as well when the lesion is in the upper arm. In more distal lesions about two thirds will attain some useful motor recovery. Seddon reported better than 90% good and fair motor and sensory results after secondary repair of the median nerve in the forearm and wrist in 166 injuries. Of 17

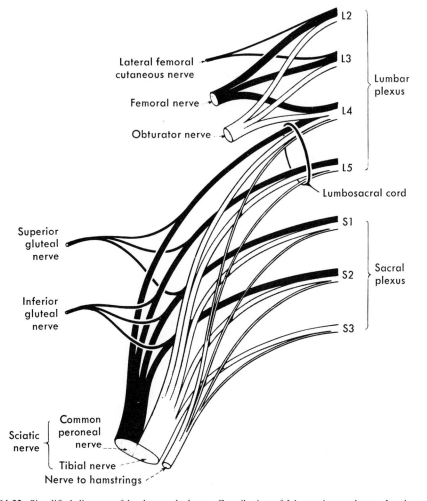

Fig. 64-32. Simplified diagram of lumbosacral plexus. Contribution of L1 root is not shown. Lumbosacral trunk or cord is shown. (From Seddon, H.: Surgical disorders of the peripheral nerves, Edinburgh, 1972, Churchill Livingstone.)

treated by primary repair in the wrist, 14 had good and fair results. After interfascicular grafting of the nerve in 38 patients, Millesi reported 82% with M-3 or better motor recovery and 97.4% with S-3 or better sensory recovery. Simesen et al. treated 24 patients with medial nerve transection using interfascicular grafting techniques; 83% achieved functional motor return (M-3 or higher), and all but one patient obtained protective touch.

Critical limit of delay of suture. Motor recovery in the intrinsic muscles of the hand does not occur if suture is delayed 9 months in high lesions or 12 months in low ones. Useful sensory recovery only rarely occurs after 9 months in high lesions or 12 months in low ones but may occur when suture has been delayed as long as 2 years. Zachary found that useful motor recovery cannot be expected after delays of 9 months in lesions above the pronator teres or 32 months in those below the flexor pollicis longus. For sensory return in adults the critical period of delay appeared to be 12 months in lesions above the pronator teres or 9 months in those below the flexor pollicis longus. Sensory return in children, however, is possible after longer

delays. Inasmuch as sensory recovery is so important, a second operation may be indicated if sensation does not return at the expected time, since this is the only way that sensation can be regained.

LUMBAR PLEXUS

The lumbar plexus is formed by the junction of the anterior primary rami of L1, L2, L3, and L4. White rami leave L1 and L2, less often L3, and rarely L4. All receive gray rami from the sympathetic chain. The L4 nerve makes a significant contribution to the formation of the sacral plexus, joining with the L5 anterior primary ramus to form the lumbosacral trunk (Fig. 64-32). The L4 nerve is frequently called the nervus furcalis because of its contribution to both the lumbar and sacral plexuses.

The L1 anterior primary ramus extends laterally and divides into the iliohypogastric and ilioinguinal nerves. Its only branch leaves the nerve before this division and joins a fasciculus from the L2 nerve root to form the genitofemoral nerve. The L2, L3, and L4 roots divide into anterior and posterior divisions; the anterior divisions of all join to form the obturator nerve, and the posterior divisions of all join to form the femoral nerve. Smaller segments of the posterior divisions of L2 and L3 unite to form the lateral femoral cutaneous nerve. The lumbar nerve roots are occasionally injured by traction in fractures of the pelvis and dislocations of the sacroiliac joints. Myelography, electromyography, and careful physical examination are helpful in evaluating these injuries. Unlike cervical root avulsions, myelographic evidence of dural diverticula does not correlate well with avulsion of lumbar roots. Even though repair of avulsed lumbar roots would seem futile, exploration may be helpful in prognosis. The plexus may also be injured by missile wounds.

The iliohypogastric nerve supplies a small area of skin over the superolateral gluteal region and an area just superior to the pubic bones on the anterior abdominal wall (Fig. 64-6). The ilioinguinal nerve supplies a segmental strip of skin along the inguinal ligament overlying the symphysis pubis and the skin of the upper scrotum, the root and dorsal aspect of the penis, and the medial aspect of the thigh. The genitofemoral nerve traverses the inguinal canal and supplies the cremaster muscle and the skin of the scrotum and adjacent part of the thigh. From a surgical standpoint these three nerves are significant because they may be injured in herniorrhaphy, resulting in persistent neuralgic discomfort that may require surgery.

The lateral femoral cutaneous nerve is formed from the roots of L2 and L3. It courses to the region of the anterosuperior iliac spine to exit between the lateral attachments of the inguinal ligament and the anterosuperior iliac spine and the sartorius muscle. The nerve then becomes superficial, penetrating the fascia lata about 10 cm inferior to the inguinal ligament, and supplies the skin of the lateral aspect of the thigh. Compression of the nerve in the region of the anterosuperior iliac spine by a tight-fitting brace or corset or injury to the nerve along its subcutaneous course often results in hypesthesias and dysesthesias in the area of its cutaneous distribution. This condition, known as meralgia paresthetica, may develop spontaneously. It is often associated with lumbar disc protrusion, impingement of the nerve probably being secondary to abnormal posture or to persistent regional muscle spasm. In most instances spontaneous recovery may be expected. Occasionally symptoms are persistent, but rarely are they sufficiently severe to require decompression and neurolysis at the point of exit of the nerve beneath the inguinal ligament.

The obturator nerve is formed by union of the anterior divisions of the L2, L3, and L4 roots. It descends through the pelvis posterior to the common iliac vessels and exits through the obturator foramen to enter the thigh. Its cutaneous branches supply the medial thigh and occasionally the medial aspect of the knee. Its motor component is divided into anterior and posterior divisons. The anterior division supplies the adductor longus, the gracilis, the adductor brevis, the pectineus, and through articular branches the hip joint. The posterior division supplies the obturator externus, the adductor magnus, occasionally the adductor brevis, and through articular branches the knee joint. The obturator nerve may be compressed against the wall of the pelvis by a mass such as a tumor or a fetus. Because of its relationship to the pubis it may be injured in pelvic fractures or in acutely flexed positions of the hip by being compressed against the pubis. Because of its nearness to the sacroiliac and hip joints, when these joints are diseased or injured, the obturator nerve may be involved too. Obturator neurectomy is sometimes beneficial in relieving adductor spasm of the hip in spastic conditions that cause a scissoring of the lower extremities (see Chapter 65). In significant lesions of the obturator nerve, atrophy of the medial aspect of the thigh, sensory disturbances of the distal medial surface of the thigh and the medial surface of the knee, and weakness or paralysis of adduction of the hip are common findings.

FEMORAL NERVE

The femoral nerve is formed by union of the posterior divisions of the L2, L3, and L4 roots. It passes distally deep to the inguinal ligament, remaining lateral to the femoral artery as it enters the thigh. Just distal to the inguinal ligament it divides into anterior and posterior branches. The anterior branch divides into the intermediate cutaneous and medial cutaneous nerves to supply the anteromedial aspect of the thigh. The motor branches of this part supply the pectineus and sartorius. The posterior branch of the femoral nerve gives off the saphenous nerve, which as the largest cutaneous branch continues distally with the femoral vessels in the subsartorial canal, pierces the fascia along the medial side of the knee to become subcutaneous, and supplies the skin on the anteromedial aspect of the leg distally to the medial malleolus and arch of the foot. The muscular parts of the posterior branch supply the rectus femoris, the vastus lateralis, the vastus medialis, and the vastus intermedius.

The femoral nerve is often injured by penetrating wounds of the lower abdomen (the small intestine may also be injured at the same time). It may also be injured during an operation in this region. Because they are near each other, the iliac artery and femoral nerve may be injured together. Concern over the hemorrhage and the fact that active extension of the knee is rarely lost despite complete division of the femoral nerve cause injury to this nerve to be overlooked as often as injury to the musculocutaneous nerve. Femoral neuropathies may also result from hematomas of the abdominal wall caused by hemophilia, anticoagulant therapy, or trauma. Branches of the femoral nerve may be contused or stretched in pelvic fractures. During operations in which the patient is prone, care must be taken to avoid excessive compression of the nerve.

Examination. Atrophy of the anterior thigh muscles is obvious. The patient is usually able to extend the knee slightly against gravity and can stand and walk, especially on level surfaces, because the gastrocnemius, the tensor fasciae latae, the gracilis, and the gluteus maximus aid in stabilizing the limb. But the patient usually finds it very difficult to go uphill or upstairs. The autonomous zone of supply usually consists of a small area just superior and medial to the patella; the anterior aspect of the thigh and the area supplied by the saphenous nerve show, at most, only varying degrees of hypesthesia. Electrical stimulation with needle electrodes inserted near the femoral nerve is valuable in assessing its function.

APPROACH. Begin the incision 5 cm proximal to the anterosuperior iliac spine and direct it diagonally and distally to the point where the femoral nerve passes beneath the inguinal ligament. This point is usually 2.5 to 3 cm lateral to the femoral artery, which is usually palpable. Next direct the incision medially for about 2.5 cm to avoid crossing the skin flexion creases at a right angle; then continue it distally onto the anterior aspect of the thigh. Proximal to the inguinal ligament deepen the incision through the fascia and the aponeurosis of the external oblique muscle. Open the transversalis fascia and retract the peritoneum medially to expose the iliac fascia. The femoral nerve can then be palpated beneath this thick fascia; split this fascia along the course of the nerve. The nerve can be exposed proximally to the point where it emerges from beneath the lateral edge of the psoas muscle and distally to the point where it passes beneath the inguinal ligament. If necessary, divide the inguinal ligament to expose the nerve as it enters the thigh and at once begins to divide into its motor and sensory branches.

METHODS OF CLOSING GAPS. Gaps of 8 to 10 cm may be closed without too much difficulty. The nerve is mobilized proximally to the point where it emerges from the lateral border of the psoas muscle and distally by freeing the branches of the nerve in the proximal thigh. The hip is flexed acutely, and the nerve is sutured. The inguinal ligament is reconstructed, and the wound is closed like any lower abdominal incision. A hip spica cast is then applied, with the hip acutely flexed.

No significant information is available regarding grafting for defects in the femoral nerve.

AFTERTREATMENT. Aftertreatment is as described for the sciatic nerve (p. 2832).

Results of suture of femoral nerve. No statistically significant information is available about the results of repair of the femoral nerve.

SACRAL PLEXUS

The sacral plexus is formed by the anterior primary rami of L5, S1, S2, and S3 (Fig. 64-32). The anterior primary ramus of L4 contributes a large branch that joins with L5 to form the lumbosacral trunk. A segment of S4 joins a segment of S3 to form the pudendal nerve, which is considered by some to be a part of the sacral plexus, by others to be a separate or pudendal plexus, and by others to be the superior part of the tiny coccygeal plexus. The anterior primary rami converge and split into anterior and posterior divisions. The trunk formed by the posterior divisions gives off the superior and inferior gluteal nerves and then proceeds toward the sciatic notch as the common peroneal part of the sciatic nerve. The trunk formed by the anterior divisions becomes the tibial part of the sciatic nerve and also proceeds toward the notch. Smaller branches that are rarely of concern surgically are given off within the pelvis to the quadratus femoris, obturator internus, superior gemellus, and piriformis. Smaller branches of S1, S2, and S3 unite to form the posterior femoral cutaneous nerve (posterior cutaneous nerve of the thigh). This is a rela-

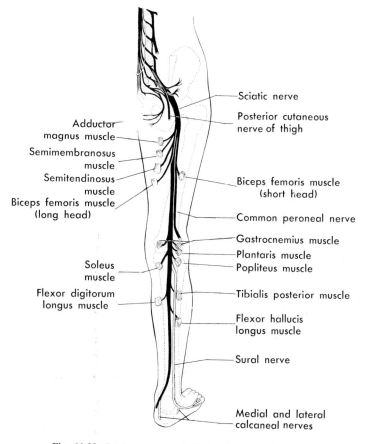

Fig. 64-33. Origin, course, and distribution of sciatic nerve.

tively large nerve that leaves the sciatic notch medial to the sciatic trunk and lies just deep to the deep fascia as it courses distally in the middle of the thigh posteriorly, roughly overlying the sciatic trunk. It is often called the small sciatic nerve. It innervates the skin of the entire posterior aspect of the thigh and the popliteal fossa. The superior gluteal nerve leaves the sciatic notch proximal to the piriformis and supplies the gluteus medius and gluteus minimus, which function as abductors and internal rotators of the hip. The inferior gluteal nerve leaves the sciatic notch with the sciatic nerve and supplies the gluteus maximus, an important extensor of the hip. Paralysis of this muscle results in difficulty in rising from a squatting or sitting position and in ascending steps or a slope. The sacral plexus may be compressed by pelvic neoplasms or during labor and delivery, especially when forceps are used. Sacral fractures and sacroiliac dislocations may also be complicated by injuries of the sacral plexus.

The sciatic nerve is composed of fibers from L4, L5, S1, S2, and S3 (Fig. 64-33). It leaves the pelvis through the sciatic notch, and at this level the large trunk is rather easily separated into its common peroneal part laterally and its tibial part medially. Frequently along the medial side of the trunk a smaller segment, the nerve to the hamstrings, is visible and can be easily dissected from it. Here the sciatic nerve is the largest one in the body, its transverse diameter being 2 to 2.5 cm. It supplies the muscles of the entire leg and foot and the posterior part of the thigh and carries most of the sensory fibers from these same parts. It descends deep to the gluteus maximus to the level of the inferior gluteal fold where it lies in the depression between the ischial tuberosity and the greater trochanter. Then distal to this level it follows a more superficial course to the distal third of the thigh where it divides. While coursing through the posterior thigh, its upper part supplies articular branches to the hip joint. The nerve to the hamstrings, visible along the medial aspect of the trunk, sends branches medially to supply the adductor magnus, semimembranosus, semitendinosus, and the long head of the biceps femoris. A branch leaves the common peroneal part of the trunk laterally to supply the short head of the biceps femoris. Just proximal to the popliteal fossa the sciatic nerve divides into its two large divisions: the common peroneal nerve, which deviates laterally, and the larger tibial nerve, which continues distally in the midline of the limb.

SCIATIC NERVE

The sciatic nerve is analogous in its importance in the lower extremity to the brachial plexus in the upper. It is usually injured by gunshot wounds of the thigh or buttock. Less often it is injured by posterior dislocations and fracture-dislocations of the hip, by intramuscular injections into the buttock, or during operations about the hip joint. When the nerve is injured in dislocations or fracture-dislocations of the hip, the peroneal half of the nerve is injured much more often than is the entire nerve. Compression caused by anatomic variations in the relationship of the nerve to the gluteal and piriformis muscles and to the sciatic notch may cause sciatic pain. In the thigh the nerve is usually injured by penetrating wounds and fractures of the femoral shaft. The semimembranosus and semitendinosus are rarely paralyzed by complete division of the

proximal one third of the sciatic nerve as the result of a gunshot wound and rarely by a dislocation of the hip.

Examination. Of the muscles innervated by the sciatic nerve that can be tested accurately, those supplied by the tibial component include the hamstrings, the gastrosoleus, the tibialis posterior, and the long flexors of the toes; those supplied by the peroneal component include the tibialis anterior and the long extensors of the toes (deep peroneal nerve) and the peroneus longus and the peroneus brevis (superficial peroneal nerve). Testing of the intrinsic muscles of the foot, except the extensor digitorum brevis, is impractical. An extremity in which the sciatic nerve has been divided may develop an equinus deformity of the foot, clawing of the toes, and atrophy of the muscles innervated by the nerve, depending on the level of the injury. Profound weakness of flexion of the knee, inability to dorsiflex the foot or extend the toes, inability to plantar flex and evert the foot, and inability to flex the toes may be seen. When the peroneal part is involved, the sensory loss is primarily over the lateral aspect of the leg and dorsum of the foot. When the tibial nerve is involved, the sensory deficit is primarily over the plantar aspect of the foot. Anesthesia on the plantar surface may result in chronic ulceration. Autonomic disturbances and chronic pain may follow an injury to the sciatic or tibial nerve. The sciatic nerve is difficult to stimulate in situ because it is so deeply located. Stimulation is significant only when it causes contraction or pain. Electromyography is of considerable help in evaluating this nerve.

The autonomous zone of the sciatic nerve (Fig. 64-34), includes the area over the metatarsal heads and over the heel, the lateral and posterior aspects of the sole of the foot, and the dorsum of the foot as far medially as the second metatarsal, as well as a narrow strip up the lateral aspect of the leg. The autonomous zones of the branches of the sciatic nerve—the tibial (branching into the lateral and medial plantar), the common peroneal (branching into the superficial and deep peroneal), and the sural—are smaller and are described later.

As in other nerves, the skin resistance test or iodine starch test is helpful.

In multiple wounds percussing along the course of the nerve to the point where tingling is most pronounced is a fairly accurate method of locating an injury. Exact knowledge of the point of emergence of the various nerve branches is helpful; however, if one attempts to locate an injury by this knowledge alone, one is more likely to err than when using percussion because a branch may be injured after it emerges from the nerve.

If an injury to a branch of the nerve has been caused by external compression as in a poorly fitted cast or an unusual posture as in crossing of the legs, the cause should be corrected. If compression has been of long duration, exploration and neurolysis may be warranted, but the prognosis in these instances is extremely guarded. If a complete division of the sciatic nerve complicates a dislocation or fracture about the hip, exploration of the nerve will assist in determining the extent of injury and whether repair is possible. If complete division of the nerve complicates a femoral shaft fracture or fracture-dislocation about the knee, exploration is also justified early when no signs of recovery are apparent. If a sciatic nerve lesion is caused by a penetrating injury, especially if the wound is proximal in the buttock, early exploration and repair may be worthwhile so that the distal structures are denervated for the shortest possible time.

APPROACH. The sciatic nerve may easily be exposed from its emergence from the sciatic notch to the point of its division into the tibial and peroneal nerves in the popliteal fossa. For injuries near the sciatic notch, begin the incision at the posterosuperior iliac spine and carry it diagonally distally and laterally in the direction of the fibers of the gluteus maximus to a point about 2.5 cm medial to the greater trochanter (Fig. 64-35). Thence curve it medially, distal to the gluteal fold, as far as the midpoint of the fold, and finally distalward along the posterior aspect of the thigh to a point 10 cm proximal to the skin creases of the popliteal fossa. Deepen the proximal part of the incision through the gluteal fascia and separate the fibers of the gluteus maximus muscle as far laterally as the greater trochanter. Then incise the fascia of the thigh longitudinally to the gluteal fold and detach the insertion of the distal fibers of the gluteus maximus from the iliotibial band.

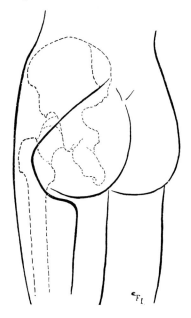

Fig. 64-35. Skin incision for approach to proximal portion of sciatic nerve extends from posterosuperior iliac spine to trochanter and then is curved distally along posterior surface of thigh.

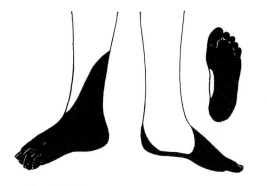

Fig. 64-34. Autonomous zone of sciatic nerve.

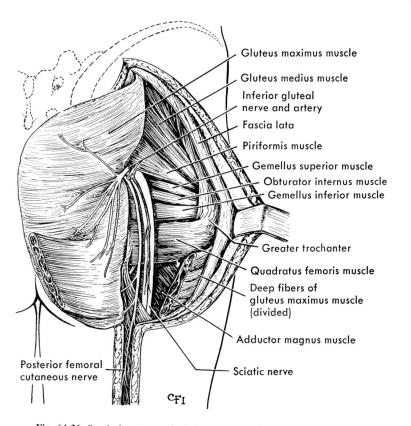

Gluteus maximus muscle

Gluteus medius muscle

Inferior gluteal nerve and artery

Fascia lata

Piriformis muscle

Gemellus superior muscle

Obturator internus muscle

Gemellus inferior muscle

Greater trochanter

Quadratus femoris muscle

Deep fibers of gluteus maximus muscle (divided)

Adductor magnus muscle

Posterior femoral cutaneous nerve

Sciatic nerve

Fig. 64-36. Surgical anatomy of sciatic nerve and related structures in buttock.

Then the muscle with its nerve and blood supply may be reflected medially to expose the nerve as far proximally as the piriformis (Fig. 64-36). Sacrifice the piriformis to expose the nerve as it emerges from the sciatic notch. If better exposure of the nerve within the sciatic notch is necessary, remove with a rongeur a part of the sacrum.

When the injury to the nerve is more distal to the sciatic notch, make the incision over the buttock likewise more distal. When the injury is in the thigh, begin the incision at the gluteal fold and continue it distally along the posterior aspect of the thigh, as just described, to a point 10 cm proximal to the knee. Open the fascia longitudinally in line with the skin incision. Protect the posterior femoral cutaneous nerve, which is just deep to the deep fascia. In the proximal thigh identify the biceps femoris, retract it medially, and identify the sciatic nerve in the depths of the wound. Distally trace the nerve beneath the biceps to its point of bifurcation. For more exposure (Mayfield) curve the distal end of the incision to the lateral aspect of the knee when the peroneal nerve has been injured. Then pass the incision distally along its course around the neck of the fibula. When the tibial nerve has been injured, pass the incision medially and then a few centimeters distally along the medial aspect of the leg. These incisions have two advantages. First, they do not cross the skin folds of the popliteal fossa; consequently contractures and ulcerating scars are less likely. Second, closing the wound is easier with the knee flexed. When the lesion is located in the middle third of the thigh, a posterolateral approach may be preferable.

METHODS OF CLOSING GAPS. Mobilizing the nerve extensively, including its two divisions, flexing the knee, and hyperextending the hip will allow closure of a gap of as much as 15 cm. When the femur has been fractured and the sciatic nerve divided, it is highly important, even in the presence of draining sinuses, to operate on the nerve before the femur has united because, aside from the effect of time on the nerve ends and muscles, the knee may stiffen and it may be impossible to flex it enough to close large defects. Furthermore, resecting a part of the femur may be necessary to help close the gap. When a fracture is present, such a resection may be justified and may be carried out with ease. However, in the absence of a femoral fracture, the bone should not be shortened. Instead, autogeneous interfascicular nerve grafting may be a reasonable alternative, especially in young patients.

AFTERTREATMENT. After any neurorrhaphy of the sciatic nerve the limb should be immobilized in a double spica cast extending from the nipple line to the toes on the affected side and to above the knee on the opposite. On the affected side the knee is flexed and the hip is extended if necessary. The cast is windowed to allow removal of the sutures after about 10 days. At 6 weeks the cast is removed, and a long leg brace with an adjustable knee hinge is applied so that the knee may be extended gradually during the next 6 weeks. Physical therapy and exercises are used to restore function to joints and soft parts. After extension of the knee is complete, an appropriate brace is applied to compensate for paralysis of the leg. When autogenous grafting has been used in repair of the sciatic nerve, the application of a spica cast after surgery is necessary, but maintaining the hip and knee in awkward positions is usually unnecessary; in addition the cast may be removed when the sutures are removed, and motion of the joints may then be started.

Results of suture of sciatic nerve. According to Sunderland, the results of suture of the sciatic nerve are poor, especially in distally innervated muscles because of the extensive retrograde neuronal degeneration, intraneural intermixing of regenerating fibers with loss of fiber localization, and degenerative changes in the distal muscles that must remain denervated for a long time. Usually significant recovery can be expected only in the proximally innervated muscles, especially the hamstring and calf muscles. If sensation returns, it is usually only of a protective nature. Delaria et al. reported 22 sciatic lesions treated surgically. Thirteen required neurolysis only, whereas 9 were treated with nerve grafts. Of those treated by neurolysis, 5 were excellent (''complete'' recovery of muscles), 7 were good, and 1 was poor. Of those treated by grafting, 4 were excellent, 4 were good, and 1 was poor.

Critical limit of delay of suture. Zachary found that useful motor and sensory recovery is not to be anticipated if the sciatic nerve injured high in the thigh or in the buttock is not sutured before 12 to 15 months.

COMMON, SUPERFICIAL, AND DEEP PERONEAL NERVES

The common peroneal nerve, a division of the sciatic, is composed of fibers from L4, L5, S1, and S2. It is injured more often than the tibial nerve even where it is part of the sciatic nerve and is injured by trauma about the knee, including ruptures of the fibular collateral ligament, by fractures and dislocations of the head of the fibula, by casts, and even by crossing the legs. Bony entrapment of the superficial peroneal nerve following fracture and entrapment by the margins of a deep fascial defect during exercise are other reported causes of injury. Release of compressing structures usually relieves the painful symptoms.

The common peroneal nerve is smaller than the tibial after the two nerves separate near the proximal angle of the popliteal fossa. The former nerve deviates laterally in the popliteal fossa, arches around the posterior aspect of the fibular head, encircles the fibular neck, and then divides into the superficial and deep peroneal nerves (Fig. 64-37). The common peroneal nerve itself is relatively short, having only two sensory branches and no motor branches. One sensory branch, the lateral sural cutaneous nerve, supplies the skin along the lateral aspect of the knee and the proximal third of the calf (Fig. 64-6). The other sensory branch, the peroneal anastomotic branch, joins the tibial anastomotic branch to form the sural nerve, which supplies the skin over the posterolateral aspect of the calf and over the lateral malleolus, the lateral aspect of the foot, and the fourth and fifth toes. As already mentioned, at or just inferior to the fibular neck the common peroneal nerve divides into its two branches, the superficial and deep peroneal nerves.

The superficial peroneal nerve continues distally in the leg between the peroneus longus and extensor digitorum longus muscles and the intermuscular septum. Along this

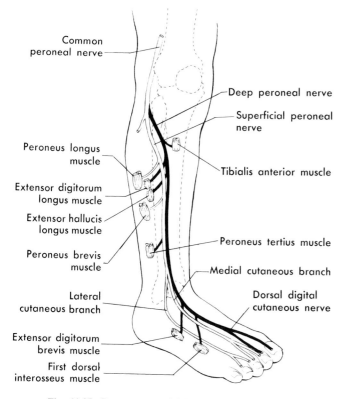

Fig. 64-37. Common, superficial, and deep peroneal nerves.

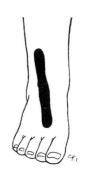

Fig. 64-38. Autonomous zone of peroneal nerve.

route it gives off two motor branches, one each to the peroneus longus and peroneus brevis. It then divides into two cutaneous branches that pierce the deep fascia and course distally to supply the skin on the anterior and lateral aspects of the leg and the dorsum of the foot, with the exception of a small wedge-shaped area in the web between the great and second toes.

The deep peroneal nerve passes obliquely distally on the interosseous membrane beneath the extensor digitorum longus. Along this route it gives off motor branches to the tibialis anterior, extensor digitorum longus, extensor hallucis longus, peroneus tertius, extensor digitorum brevis, and the first dorsal interosseus. Its terminal branch divides into digital cutaneous nerves that supply the web between the great and second toe, the lateral aspect of the dorsum of the great toe, and the medial aspect of the dorsum of the second toe.

Examination. The muscles supplied by the common peroneal nerve that can be tested accurately have been listed previously (see discussion of sciatic nerve). Typically injury of the peroneal nerve results in footdrop, which cannot be overcome or disguised by any supplementary or trick movement. The nerve may be easily stimulated in situ at the head of the fibula. The presence and extent of the autonomous zone of this nerve is extremely variable, but it may have value when present (Fig. 64-38).

APPROACH. The exposure of the peroneal nerve in the distal thigh and popliteal fossa has been described previously (see discussion of sciatic nerve). If the nerve is injured at the head of the fibula or distal to it, begin the incision at

any point proximal to the injury as required; at the head of the fibula, curve it anteriorly over the neck of the fibula and distally along the anterolateral aspect of the leg. Then deepen it proximally through the fascia and identify the nerve on the medial side of the biceps tendon. From here trace the nerve distally as it curves around the neck of the fibula between the origin of the peroneus longus and the bone; just distal to this point it divides into the deep and superficial peroneal nerves. The superficial nerve continues distally in the leg between the peroneus longus and the extensor digitorum longus in the intermuscular septum. The deep nerve passes distally beneath the extensor digitorum longus, whose origin must be freed to expose completely this part of the nerve, from which numerous muscular branches arise; the nerve may then be traced distally beneath the tibialis anterior just lateral to the anterior tibial artery.

METHODS OF CLOSING GAPS. Mobilizing the nerve extensively and flexing the knee allows one to close a gap of as much as 10 to 12 cm in the popliteal fossa. Distal to the neck of the fibula length is hard to get. But even here, mobilizing the nerve in the thigh and the leg, stripping up branches in the leg, and flexing the knee will allow one to close a considerable gap in either division of the common peroneal nerve.

Even though large gaps can be closed, lines of suture in the peroneal nerve are much more likely to separate than are those in other peripheral nerves, even when it is still a part of the sciatic nerve, presumably because it is especially vulnerable to stress between two bony points—the fibula and pelvis—between which no other soft tissue structures effectively protect the nerve from tension. In most patients immobilization in a hip spica cast for 6 weeks after surgery and gradual extension of the knee during the next 6 weeks will prevent such catastrophes. A long leg cast is not enough; the line of suture often separates unless a spica cast is used.

Autogenous interfascicular nerve grafting may prove to be a suitable alternative to the measures described here.

AFTERTREATMENT. Aftertreatment is as described for the sciatic nerve (p. 2832). If autogenous nerve grafting has been used, awkward positioning and prolonged use of casts and braces may not be required.

Results of suture of peroneal nerve. Motor recovery is far more important than sensory recovery because the autonomous zone on the dorsum of the foot is so small. Motor recovery is useful only if it enables the patient to dorsiflex the foot against gravity. Under the most favorable circumstances, that is, after a low lesion with a small gap between the nerve ends and with early suture, 60% to 70% of patients will reach this level of motor recovery. The percentage of success will decrease as circumstances become less favorable but does not reach the point that suture is not worthwhile unless surgery is delayed too long. A second operation to resuture the nerve after initial failure to obtain motor recovery is rarely indicated.

Critical limit of delay of suture. Useful motor function in the peroneal nerve is not to be expected when suture has been delayed 12 months after injury.

Tendon transfer for peroneal nerve paralysis. This operation is discussed on p. 2957.

TIBIAL NERVE

The tibial nerve, composed of fibers from L4, L5, S1, S2, and S3, is the larger and more important of the two divisions of the sciatic nerve. It begins in the distal third of the thigh just proximal to the popliteal fossa as the common peroneal nerve leaves the sciatic nerve to course laterally. It continues distally through the middle of the popliteal fossa and supplies branches to the plantaris, the soleus, the popliteus, and both heads of the gastrocnemius before passing beneath the arch of the soleus (Fig. 64-39). Also given off within the popliteal fossa is the tibial anastomotic branch, which joins the peroneal anastomotic branch to form the sural nerve already described. Deep to the soleus the tibial nerve courses straight distally on the tibialis posterior. It supplies motor branches to the tibialis posterior, flexor hallucis longus, and flexor digitorum longus. In the distal calf it gives off medial calcaneal branches to supply the skin on the medial aspect of the heel. The nerve then passes beneath the laciniate ligament

posterior and inferior to the medial malleolus and divides into the medial and lateral plantar nerves, which innervate the intrinsic muscles and the skin of the plantar surface of the foot much the same as the median and ulnar nerves innervate the hand. Injuries to the tibial nerve are severely disabling because of the large sensory deficit on the plantar surface of the foot. Many such injuries are also associated with causalgia. The effect of a complete tibial nerve lesion on the function of the foot is comparable in importance to that of combined median and ulnar nerve lesions on function of the hand.

In the popliteal fossa the tibial nerve, although protected by a muscular covering, may be injured in dislocations of the knee. In these instances vascular injuries may also be present, and careful evaluation is necessary. Deep to the soleus muscle the tibial nerve is most often injured by penetrating wounds. Suture of the nerve distal to the muscular branches may result in disabling plantar hyperesthesia. It is worthwhile, however, to attempt such repair, especially in children and young adults, to prevent or minimize trophic ulceration on the plantar surface of the foot. Although division of the sural nerve may result in a troublesome neuroma, it rarely causes a severe clinical problem. Compression of this nerve at the lateral aspect of the ankle has been described by Pringle et al. In four patients complaining of pain, paresthesias, dysesthesias, and hypesthesias, relief was achieved by excision of a ganglion or release of a posttraumatic scar. On the medial side of the ankle the tibial nerve may be compressed in the tarsal tunnel between the laciniate ligament and the medial surface of the talus distal to the medial malleolus. Tarsal tunnel syndrome is described on p. 953.

Examination. The muscles supplied by this nerve that may be accurately examined were described in the discussion of the sciatic nerve. The autonomous zone of the tib-

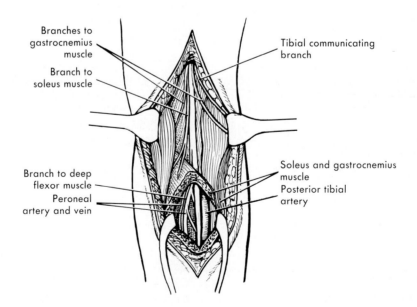

Fig. 64-39. Anatomy of tibial nerve in popliteal space and proximal third of leg (see text for discussion of exposure). (Redrawn from Stookey, B.: Surgical and mechanical treatment of peripheral nerves, Philadelphia, 1922, W.B. Saunders Co.)

ial nerve (including the medial sural cutaneous branch) varies but generally includes the sole of the foot (except the medial border of the instep), the lateral surface of the heel, and the plantar surface of the toes. Because the nerve is deep in the popliteal fossa, stimulating the nerve in this area is not always dependable, and consequently electromyography is indicated. The tibialis posterior, flexor digitorum longus, and flexor hallucis longus are supplied by branches of the tibial nerve after the nerve passes deep to the arch of the soleus muscle. The flexor digitorum longus and flexor hallucis longus may be difficult to test, but the tendon of the flexor hallucis longus may be palpated posterior to the medial malleolus as it passes to cross the medial aspect of the plantar arch. Atrophy of the intrinsic muscles of the foot may allow palpation of the flexor digitorum longus tendons; otherwise this muscle may not be palpable for testing. The autonomous zone of the tibial nerve as it passes deep to the soleus muscle is smaller than that of the nerve as it passes through the popliteal fossa because the sural nerve is excluded. Although electromyography may be necessary for evaluating injury to the tibial nerve beneath the soleus, the nerve may be stimulated with relative ease at the posterior aspect of the medial malleolus.

APPROACH TO TIBIAL NERVE IN POPLITEAL FOSSA. The tibial nerve may be exposed in the popliteal fossa by the incision and the approach described for the sciatic nerve. As usual, avoid crossing the skin folds in the popliteal fossa and if necessary extend the skin incision along the medial side of the hamstring tendons and then distally on the leg just posterior to the medial border of the tibia (Fig. 64-40).

Methods of closing gaps in this part of the nerve, immobilization, and care after surgery are the same as those described for the sciatic nerve.

APPROACH TO TIBIAL NERVE DEEP TO SOLEUS MUSCLE. Explore the tibial nerve deep to the soleus muscle or in the distal third of the leg through a longitudinal incision beginning

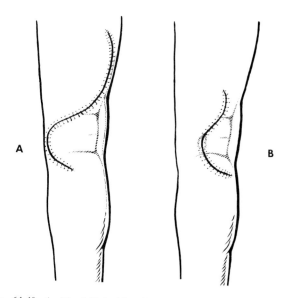

Fig. 64-40. A, Mayfield incision for exposure of nerves in popliteal space. **B,** Ulceration and contracture are likely from incisions across the skin folds.

posterior to the subcutaneous part of the tibia on the medial side of the leg and continuing parallel to the tibia distally to the ankle. Deepen the incision through the superficial fascia and identify and retract laterally the tendo calcaneus. Expose the deep fascia through which the nerve and artery may be easily palpated. Open this fascia longitudinally and identify the nerve lateral to the artery. Distally this part of the nerve may be easily mobilized to the ankle, but proximally it is quite deep beneath the soleus muscle on the tibialis posterior between the flexor hallucis longus laterally and the flexor digitorum longus medially. Proximal to the middle of the leg the origin of the soleus from the tibia interferes with exposure and must be sectioned and reflected laterally to expose the tibial nerve as it comes under the arch of the soleus. Exposing and mobilizing the nerve require great care because of the many vessels with which it is intimately associated. Troublesome bleeding from these vessels may be minimized by using a pneumatic tourniquet and by wide exposure of the nerve in the distal two thirds of the leg.

METHODS OF CLOSING GAPS. Even though the lesion itself can be fully exposed by this approach, one can rarely close a significant gap by mobilizing this part of the nerve alone. Plantar flexing the foot to obtain length may lead to disabling equinus contracture of the ankle and is condemned. Therefore exposing and mobilizing the proximal part of the tibial nerve in the popliteal fossa or even farther proximally as already described are almost always necessary. By connecting the two incisions, the nerve can be exposed and mobilized from the thigh to the ankle. In addition, all muscular branches must be stripped back intraneurally for several centimeters by careful dissection. By flexing the knee to 90 degrees, one may close a gap of 10 to 12 cm. Occasionally more length may be obtained by transplanting the nerve between the soleus and the gastrocnemius or superficial to both of these muscles. This is especially applicable when the distal muscular branches to the flexor hallucis and flexor digitorum longus have been destroyed, although it may be carried out with these branches intact if they are dissected proximally to the popliteal fossa. After one is certain that the defect can be closed but before the nerve is sutured, especially if tension on the line of suture is likely, the incision in the popliteal fossa should be closed because closing the fascia may reduce slightly the length regained.

If the nerve has been transplanted between the soleus and the gastrocnemius or superficial to both, the soleus should also be sutured to its origin before the nerve is sutured. If transplantation has been unnecessary, the soleus is, of course, sutured after neurorrhaphy.

Autogenous interfascicular grafting may prove to be a satisfactory alternative to awkward and sometimes disabling positioning when gaps are to be closed in the tibial nerve.

AFTERTREATMENT. Aftertreatment is as described for the sciatic nerve (p. 2832).

Results of suture of tibial nerve. Both motor and sensory return are extremely important. Even a slight return of pain sensation is valuable because an anesthetic foot tends to develop trophic lesions.

Under favorable circumstances most patients (about

90%) regain fairly strong power in the gastrosoleus group. Slightly fewer regain good function in the other muscles, such as the tibialis posterior, flexor digitorum longus, and flexor hallucis longus. Four fifths of these patients regain some pain perception in the sole of the foot. One fourth develop touch sensation with overresponse, and in one half of these overresponse will disappear. In high lesions regeneration is not nearly as good but is not bad enough to preclude suture of a high sciatic lesion. If the original suture fails to result in regeneration, resuture is rarely worthwhile.

Critical limit of delay of suture. Motor recovery is not to be expected when suture has been delayed 12 months.

REFERENCES

Abbott, L.C.: Reconstructive orthopaedic surgery for disabilities resulting from irreparable injuries to the radial nerve, J. Nerv. Ment. Dis. **99**:466, 1944.

Abbott, L.C., and Saunders, J.B. deC.M.: Injuries of the median nerve in fractures of the lower end of the radius, Surg. Gynecol. Obstet. **57**:507, 1933.

Adelaar, R.S., Foster, W.C., and McDowell, C.: The treatment of the cubital tunnel syndrome, J. Hand Surg. **9-A**:90, 1984.

Aitken, D.R., and Minton, J.P.: Complications associated with mastectomy, Surg. Clin. North Am. **63**:1331, 1983.

Allbritten, F.F., Jr.: The surgical repair of the deep branch of the radial nerve, Surg. Gynecol. Obstet. **82**:305, 1946.

Allbritten, F.F., Jr.: Method for repair of posterior tibial nerve, Am. J. Surg. **73**:588, 1947.

Almquist, E., and Eeg-Olofsson, O.: Sensory-nerve-conduction velocity and two-point discrimination in sutured nerves, J. Bone Joint Surg. **52-A**:791, 1970.

Altman, H., and Trott, R.H.: Muscle transplantation for paralysis of the radial nerve, J. Bone Joint Surg. **28**:440, 1946.

Aschan, W., and Moberg, E.: The ninhydrin finger printing test used to map out partial lesions to hand nerves, Acta Chir. Scand. **123**:365, 1962.

Babcock, J.L., and Wray, J.B.: Analysis of abduction in a shoulder with deltoid paralysis due to axillary nerve injury, Clin. Orthop. **68**:116, 1970.

Baer, R.D., Goka, R.S., and Smith, G.R.: Electrodiagnosis in the entrapment of the intermediate dorsal cutaneous branch of superficial peroneal nerve, Orthop. Rev. **11**:105, 1982.

Bargar, W.L., Marcus, R.E., and Ittleman, F.P.: Late thoracic outlet syndrome secondary to pseudarthrosis of the clavicle, J. Trauma **24**:857, 1984.

Barnes, R.: Traction injuries of the brachial plexus in adults, J. Bone Joint Surg. **31-B**:10, 1949.

Barr, J.S.: Transference of posterior tibial tendon through interosseous membrane for paralytic foot drop. (Personal communication, October 1954.)

Barrington, R.L.: Haemorrhagic femoral neuropathy, Injury **14**:170, 1982.

Bassett, C.A.L., et al.: Peripheral nerve and spinal cord regeneration: factors leading to success of a tubulation technique employing Millipore, Exp. Neurol. **1**:386, 1959.

Bateman, J.E.: Peripheral nerve injuries in the multiply injured patient, Orthop. Clin. North Am. **1**:115, 1970.

Berger, A., and Millesi, H.: Nerve grafting, Clin. Orthop. **133**:49, 1978.

Berkheiser, E.J., and Shapiro, F.: Alar scapula, JAMA **108**:1790, 1937.

Billington, R.W.: Tendon transplantation for musculospiral (radial) nerve injury, J. Bone Joint Surg. **20**:538, 1922.

Boe, S.: The neurovascular island pedicle flap, Acta Orthop. Scand. **50**:67, 1979.

Bonney, G.: The value of axon responses in determining the site of lesion in traction injuries of the brachial plexus, Brain **77**:588, 1954.

Bora, F.W., Jr.: Peripheral nerve repair in cats: the fascicular stitch, J. Bone Joint Surg. **49-A**:659, 1967.

Bora, F.W., Jr.: A comparison of epineurial, perineurial and epiperineurial methods of nerve suture, Clin. Orthop. **133**:91, 1978.

Bora, F.W., Jr., and Osterman, A.L.: Compression neuropathy, Clin. Orthop. **163**:20, 1982.

Bora, F.W., Jr., Pleasure, D.E., and Didizian, N.A.: A study of nerve regeneration and neuroma formation after nerve suture by various techniques, J. Hand Surg. **1**:138, 1976.

Boswick, J.A., Jr., Schneewind, J., and Stromberg, W., Jr.: Evaluation of peripheral nerve repairs below elbow, Arch. Surg. **90**:50, 1965.

Bowden, R.E.M., and Gutmann, E.: Denervation and re-innervation of human voluntary muscle, Brain **67**:273, 1944.

Braun, R.M.: Comparative studies of neurorrhaphy and sutureless peripheral nerve repair, Surg. Gynecol. Obstet. **122**:15, 1966.

Braun, R.M.: Epineurial nerve suture, Clin. Orthop. **163**:50, 1982.

Bristow, W.R.: Injuries of peripheral nerves in two world wars, Br. J. Surg. **34**:333, 1947.

British Medical Research Council (see Medical Research Council).

Brooks, D.M.: Tendon transplantation in the forearm and arthrodesis of the wrist, Proc. R. Soc. Med. **42**:838, 1949.

Brooks, D.M.: Open wounds of the brachial plexus. In Seddon, H.J., editor: Peripheral nerve injuries, London, 1954, Her Majesty's Stationery Office.

Brooks, D.: The place of nerve-grafting in orthopaedic surgery, J. Bone Joint Surg. **37-A**:299, 1955.

Browett, J.P., and Fiddian, N.J.: Delayed median nerve injury due to retained glass fragments: a report of two cases, J. Bone Joint Surg. **67-B**:382, 1985.

Brown, C.: Compressive, invasive referred pain to the shoulder, Clin. Orthop. **173**:55, 1983.

Brown, D.G.: Surgical tape (Micropore) as a substitute for sutures in nerve repair, Tex. Med. **64**:52, 1968.

Brown, P.W.: The time factor in surgery of upper-extremity peripheral nerve injury, Clin. Orthop. **68**:14, 1970.

Bryan, F.S., Miller, L.S., and Panijayanond, P.: Spontaneous paralysis of the posterior interosseous nerve: a case report and review of the literature, Clin. Orthop. **80**:9, 1971.

Bufalini, C., and Pescatori, G.: Posterior cervical electromyography in the diagnosis and prognosis of brachial plexus injuries, J. Bone Joint Surg. **51-B**:627, 1969.

Buker, R.H., et al.: Causalgia and transthoracic sympathectomy, Am. J. Surg. **124**:725, 1972.

Bunnell, S.: Tendon transfers in the hand and forearm, In American Academy of Orthopaedic Surgeons: Instructional course lectures, vol. 6, Ann Arbor, 1949, J.W. Edwards.

Bunnell, S.: Surgery of the hand, ed. 3, Philadelphia, 1956, J.B. Lippincott Co.

Burns, J., and Lister, G.D.: Localized constrictive radial neuropathy in the absence of extrinsic compression: three cases, J. Hand Surg. **9-A**:99, 1984.

Cabaud, H.E., Rodkey, W.G., McCarroll, H.R., Jr., Mutz, S.B., and Niebauer, J.J.: Epineurial and perineurial fascicular nerve repairs: a critical comparison, J. Hand Surg. **1**:131, 1976.

Caldwell, E.H.: Through the operating microscope: improved peripheral nerve repair, Contemp. Surg. **8**:13, May 1976.

Childress, H.M.: Recurrent ulnar-nerve dislocation at the elbow, J. Bone Joint Surg. **38-A**:978, 1956.

Childress, H.M.: Recurrent ulnar-nerve dislocation at the elbow, Clin. Orthop. **108**:168, 1975.

Clark, J.M.P.: Reconstruction of biceps brachii by pectoral muscle transplantation, Br. J. Surg. **34**:180, 1946.

Clark, G.L.: A method of preparation of nerve ends for suturing, Plast. Reconstr. Surg. **34**:233, 1964.

Clein, L.J.: Suprascapular entrapment neuropathy, J. Neurosurg. **43**:337, 1975.

Cozen, L.: Management of foot drop in adults after permanent peroneal nerve loss, Clin. Orthop. **67**:151, 1969.

Craven, P.R., Jr., and Green, D.P.: Cubital tunnel syndrome: treatment by medial epicondylectomy, J. Bone Joint Surg. **62-A**:986, 1980.

Crue, B.L., Pudenz, R.H., and Shelden, H.: Observations on the value of clinical electromyography, J. Bone Joint Surg. **39-A**:492, 1957.

d'Aubigne, R.M.: Treatment of residual paralysis after injury of the main nerves (superior extremity), Proc. R. Soc. Med. **42**:831, 1949.

Davidson, A.J., and Horwitz, M.T.: Late or tardy ulnar-nerve paralysis, J. Bone Joint Surg. **17**:844, 1935.

Davis, L., Martin, J., and Perret, G.: The treatment of injuries of the brachial plexus, Ann. Surg. **125**:647, 1947.

DeAngelis, A.M.: Surgical approach to the tibial nerve below the popliteal fossa, Am. J. Surg. **73**:568, 1947.

Delaria, G., Manupassa, J., Saporiti, E., and Taglioretti, I.: Surgical treatment of lesions of the sciatic nerve, Ital. J. Orthop. Traumatol. **9**:451, 1983.

Dellon, A.L., Curtis, R.M., and Edgerton, M.T.: Evaluating recovery of sensation in the hand following nerve injury, Johns Hopkins Med. J. **130**:235, 1972.

Dellon, A.L.: Reinnervation of denervated Meissner corpuscles: a sequential histologic study in the monkey following fascicular nerve repair, J. Hand Surg. **1**:98, 1976.

Dellon, A.L.: Clinical use of vibratory stimuli to evaluate peripheral nerve injury and compression neuropathy, Plast. Reconstr. Surg. **65**:466, 1980.

Dellon, A.L., and Jabaley, M.E.: Reeducation of sensation in the hand following nerve suture, Clin. Orthop. **163**:75, 1982.

de Takats, G.: Causalgia states in peace and war, JAMA **128**:699, 1945.

Dharapak, C., and Nimberg, G.A.: Posterior interosseous nerve compression: report of a case caused by traumatic aneurysm, Clin. Orthop. **101**:225, 1974.

Drez, D., Jr.: Suprascapular neuropathy in the differential diagnosis of rotator cuff injuries, Am. J. Sports Med. **4**:43, 1976.

Ducker, T.B., and Hayes, G.J.: A comparative study of the technique of nerve repair, Surg. Forum **18**:443, 1967.

Ducker, T.B., and Hayes, G.J.: Experimental improvements in the use of Silastic cuff for peripheral nerve repair, J. Neurosurg. **28**:582, 1968.

Ducker, T.B., Kempe, L.G., and Hayes, G.J.: The metabolic background for peripheral nerve surgery, J. Neurosurg. **30**:270, 1969.

Dunn, A.W.: Trapezius paralysis after minor surgical procedures in the posterior cervical triangle, South. Med. J. **67**:312, 1974.

Eaton, R.G., Crowe, J.F., and Parkes, J.C., III: Anterior transposition of the ulnar nerve using a non-compressing fasciodermal sling, J. Bone Joint Surg. **62-A**:820, 1980.

Echlin, F., Owens, F.M., Jr., and Wells, W.L.: Observations on ''major'' and ''minor'' causalgia, Arch. Neurol. Psychiat. **62**:183, 1949.

Edshage, S.: Peripheral nerve suture: a technique for improved intraneural topography: evaluation of some suture materials, Acta Chir. Scand. Suppl. **331**:1, 1964.

Edshage, S.: Peripheral nerve injuries: diagnosis and treatment, N. Engl. J. Med. **278**:1431, 1968.

Eisen, A.A.: Electromyography and nerve conduction as a diagnostic aid, Orthop. Clin. North Am. **4**:885, 1973.

Erhart, E.A., and Rezze, C.J.: Effect of experimental devascularization on peripheral nerves, Arq. Neuropsiquiatr. **24**:7, 1966.

Escobar, P.L.: Short segment stimulations in ulnar nerve lesions around elbow, Orthop. Rev. **12**:65, 1983.

Feindel, W.: Neurosurgical disorders affecting the hand, Surg. Clin. North Am. **44**:1031, 1964.

Fiddian, N.J., and King, R.J.: The winged scapula, Clin. Orthop. **185**:228, 1984.

Field, J.H.: Peripheral nerve suturing using a nerve miter box to trim the ends, Plast. Reconstr. Surg. **44**:605, 1969.

Finseth, F., Constable, J.D., and Cannon, B.: Interfascicular nerve grafting: early experiences at the Massachusetts General Hospital, Plast. Reconstr. Surg. **56**:492, 1975.

Finsterbush, A., Porat, S., Rousso, M., and Ashur, H.: Prevention of peripheral nerve entrapment following extensive soft tissue injury, using silicone cuffing: an experimental study, Clin. Orthop. **162**:276, 1982.

Fisher, T.R., and McGeoch, C.M.: Severe injuries of the radial nerve treated by sural nerve grafting, Injury **16**:411, 1985.

Foerster, O.: The dermatomes in man, Brain **56**:1, 1933.

Forster, R.S., and Fu, F.H.: Reflex sympathetic dystrophy in children: a case report and review of the literature, Orthopedics **8**:475, 1985.

Freeman, B.S.: Adhesive neural anastomosis, Plast. Reconstr. Surg. **35**:167, 1965.

Friedenberg, Z.B.: Transposition of the biceps brachii for triceps weakness, J. Bone Joint Surg. **36-A**:656, 1954.

Gabrielson, G.J., and Stenström, S.J.: A contribution to peripheral nerve suture technique, Plast. Reconstr. Surg. **38**:68, 1966.

Ganel, A., et al.: Intraoperative nerve fascicle identification using choline acetyltransferase: a preliminary report, Clin. Orthop. **165**:228, 1982.

Ganzhorn, R.W., Hocker, J.R., Horowitz, M., and Switzer, H.E.: Suprascapular nerve entrapment: a case report, J. Bone Joint Surg. **63-A**:492, 1981.

Garcia, G., and McQueen, D.: Bilateral suprascapular-nerve entrapment syndrome: case report and review of the literature, J. Bone Joint Surg. **63-A**:491, 1981.

Gay, J.R., and Love, J.G.: Diagnosis and treatment of tardy paralysis of the ulnar nerve: based on a study of 100 cases, J. Bone Joint Surg. **29**:1087, 1947.

Gelberman, R.H., Szabo, R., Williamson, R.V., and Dimick, M.P.: Sensibility testing in peripheral-nerve compression syndromes, J. Bone Joint Surg. **65-A**:632, 1983.

Gelmers, H.J., and Buys, D.A.: Suprascapular entrapment neuropathy, Acta Neurochir. **38**:121, 1977.

Gerard, R.W.: The physiology of pain: abnormal neuron states in causalgia and related phenomena, Anesthesiology **12**:1, 1951.

Gessini, L., Jandolo, B., and Pietrangeli, A.: Entrapment neuropathies of the median nerve at and above the elbow, Surg. Neurol. **19**:112, 1983.

Gilliatt, R.W.: Physical injury to peripheral nerve: physiologic and electrodiagnostic aspects, Mayo Clin. Proc. **56**:361, 1981.

Goldner, J.L., Nashold, B.S., Jr., and Hendrix, P.C.: Peripheral nerve electrical stimulation, Clin. Orthop. **163**:33, 1982.

Gonza, E.R., and Harris, W.R.: Traumatic winging of the scapula, J. Bone Joint Surg. **61-A**:1230, 1979.

Gore, R.V.: A new method of nerve repair: repair of a lesion of the radial nerve with a branch to the triceps muscle, Br. J. Surg. **65**:352, 1978.

Goto, Y.: Funicular suture: experimental study of nerve autografting by funicular suture, Arch. Jpn. Chir. **36**:478, 1967.

Grabb, W.C.: Management of nerve injuries in the forearm and hand, Orthop. Clin. North Am. **1**:419, 1970.

Grabb, W.C., Bement, S.L., Koepke, G.H., and Green, R.A.: Comparison methods of peripheral nerve suturing in monkeys, Plast. Reconstr. Surg. **46**:31, 1970.

Greenwald, A.G., Schute, P.C., and Shiveley, J.L.: Brachial plexus birth palsy: a 10-year report on the incidence and prognosis, J. Pediatr. Orthop. **4**:689, 1984.

Gregg, J.R., et al.: Serratus anterior paralysis in the young athlete, J. Bone Joint Surg. **61-A**:825, 1979.

Gurdjian, E.S., and Smathers, H.M.: Peripheral nerve injury in fractures and dislocations of long bones, J. Neurosurg. **2**:202, 1945.

Haas, J.: Muskelplastik bei Serratuslähmung, Z. Orthop. **55**:617, 1931.

Haas, S.L.: Serratus anterior paralysis, Orthopaedic Correspondence Club Letter, March 15, 1949.

Hakstian, R.W.: Funicular orientation by direct stimulation: an aid to peripheral nerve repair, J. Bone Joint Surg. **50-A**:1178, 1968.

Hakstian, R.W.: Perineural neurorrhaphy, Orthop. Clin. North Am. **4**:945, 1973.

Hankin, F.M., Jaeger, S.H., and Beddings, A.: Autogenous sural nerve grafts: a harvesting technique, Orthopedics **8**:1160, 1985.

Hargens, A.R., et al.: Peripheral nerve-conduction block by high muscle-compartment pressure, J. Bone Joint Surg. **61-A**:192, 1979.

Hayes, J.M., and Zehr, D.J.: Traumatic muscle avulsion causing winging of the scapula case: a case report, J. Bone Joint Surg. **63-A**:495, 1981.

Haymaker, W., and Woodhall, B.: Peripheral nerve injuries. Principles of diagnosis, ed. 2, Philadelphia, 1953, W.B. Saunders Co.

Henry, A.K.: Extensile exposure applied to limb surgery, Baltimore, 1945, The Williams & Wilkins Co.

Herzmark, M.H.: Traumatic paralysis of the serratus anterior relieved by transplantation of the rhomboidei, J. Bone Joint Surg. **33-A**:235, 1951.

Highet, W.B.: Procaine nerve block in investigation of peripheral nerve injuries, J. Neurol. Psychiatry **5**:101, 1942.

Highet, W.B., and Holmes, W.: Traction injuries to the lateral popliteal nerve and traction injuries to peripheral nerves after suture, Br. J. Surg. **30**:212, 1943.

Hirasawa, Y., Katsumi, Y., and Tokioka, T.: Evaluation of sensibility after sensory reconstruction of the thumb, J. Bone Joint Surg. **67-B**:814, 1985.

Hirasawa, Y., and Sakakida, K.: Sports and peripheral nerve injury, Am. J. Sports Med. **11**:420, 1983.

Hirayama, T., and Takemitsu, Y.: Compression of the suprascapular nerve by a ganglion at the suprascapular notch, Clin. Orthop. **155**:95, 1981.

Homans, J.: Minor causalgia following injuries and wounds, Ann. Surg. **113**:932, 1941.

Hopkins, G.O., Ward, A.B., and Garnett, R.A.F.: Lone axillary nerve lesion due to closed non-dislocating injury of the shoulder, Injury **16:**305, 1985.

Ito, T., Hirotani, H., and Yamamoto, K.: Peripheral nerve repairs by the funicular suture technique, Acta Orthop. Scand. **47:**283, 1976.

Jabaley, M.E.: Nerve stimulation in the awake patient (mimeographed), 1983.

Jabaley, M.E.: Peripheral nerve injuries. In Evarts, C.M.: Surgery of the musculoskeletal system, New York, 1983, Churchill Livingstone.

Jabaley, M.E., Burns, J.E., Orcutt, B.A., and Bryant, W.M.: Comparison of histologic and functional recovery after peripheral nerve repair, J. Hand Surg. **1:**119, 1976.

Jessing, P.: Monteggia lesions and their complicating nerve damage, Acta Orthop. Scand. **46:**601, 1975.

Johnson, E.W., and Olsen, K.J.: Clinical value of motor nerve conduction velocity determination, JAMA **172:**2030, 1960.

Jones, R.: Tendon transplantation in cases of musculospiral injuries not amenable to suture, Am. J. Surg. **35:**333, 1921.

Jones, R.E., and Gauntt, C.: Medial epicondylectomy for ulnar nerve compression syndrome at the elbow, Clin. Orthop. **139:**174, 1979.

Kahn, E.A.: Direct observation of sweating in peripheral nerve injuries, Surg. Gynecol. Obstet. **92:**22, 1951.

Kankaanpää, U., and Bakalim, G.: Peripheral nerve injuries of the upper extremity: sensory return of 137 neurorrhaphies, Acta Orthop. Scand. **47:**41, 1976.

Kendall, J.P., Stokes, I.A.F., O'Hara, J.P., and Dickson, R.A.: Tension and creep phenomena in peripheral nerve, Acta Orthop. Scand. **50:**721, 1979.

Kernohan, J., Levack, B., and Wilson, J.N.: Entrapment of the superficial peroneal nerve: three case reports, J. Bone Joint Surg. **67-B:**60, 1985.

King, T.: The treatment of traumatic ulnar neuritis, Aust. New Zeal. J. Surg. **20:**33, 1950.

King, T., and Morgan, F.P.: Late results of removing the medial humeral epicondyle for traumatic ulnar neuritis, J. Bone Joint Surg. **41-B:**51, 1959.

Kirklin, J.W., Chenoweth, A.I., and Murphey, F.: Causalgia: a review of its characteristics, diagnosis, and treatment, Surgery **21:**321, 1947.

Kirklin, J.W., Murphey, F., and Berkson, J.: Suture of peripheral nerves, Surg. Gynecol. Obstet. **88:**719, 1949.

Kleinert, H.E., and Griffin, J.M.: Technique of nerve anastomosis, Orthop. Clin. North Am. **4:**907, 1973.

Kleinert, H.E., et al.: Post-traumatic sympathetic dystrophy, Orthop. Clin. North Am. **4:**917, 1973.

Kline, D.G.: Early evaluation of peripheral nerve lesions in continuity with a note on nerve recording, Am. Surg. **34:**77, 1968.

Kline, D.G.: Timing for exploration of nerve lesions and evaluation of the neuroma-in-continuity, Clin. Orthop. **163:**42, 1982.

Kline, D.G., Hackett, E.R., and May, P.R.: Evaluation of nerve injuries by evoked potentials and electromyography, J. Neurosurg. **31:**128, 1969.

Kline, D.G., and Hayes, G.J.: The use of a resorbable wrapper for peripheral-nerve repair: experimental studies in chimpanzees, J. Neurosurg. **21:**737, 1964.

Kurze, T.: Microtechniques in neurological surgery, Clin. Neurosurg. **11:**128, 1964.

Landau, W.M.: The duration of neuromuscular function after nerve section in man, J. Neurosurg. **10:**64, 1953.

Landi, A., Copeland, S.A., Wynn Parry, C.B., and Jones, S.J.: The role of somatosensory evoked potentials and nerve conduction studies in the surgical management of brachial plexus injuries, J. Bone Joint Surg. **62-B:**492, 1980.

Lankford, L.L.: Reflex sympathetic dystrophy. In Omer, G., and Spinner, M., editors: Management of peripheral nerve problems, Philadelphia, 1980, W.B. Saunders Co.

Lassmann, G., and Piza, H.: The nerve response after autotransplantation of the rabbit ear, J. Hand Surg. **9-A:**121, 1984.

Lazaro, L., III: Ulnar nerve instability: ulnar nerve injury due to elbow flexion, South. Med. J. **70:**36, 1977.

Leffert, R.D.: Brachial plexus injuries, Orthop. Clin. North Am. **1:**399, 1970.

Leffert, R.D.: Lesions of the brachial plexus, including thoracic outlet syndrome. In American Academy of Orthopaedic Surgeons: Instructional course lectures, vol. 26, St. Louis, 1977, The C.V. Mosby Co.

Leffert, R.D., and Seddon, H.J.: Infraclavicular brachial plexus injuries, J. Bone Joint Surg. **47-B:**9, 1965.

Leonard, M.H.: Return of skin sensation in children without repair of nerves, Clin. Orthop. **95:**273, 1973.

Lerman, B.I., Gornish, L.A., and Bellin, H.J.: Injury of the superficial peroneal nerve, J. Foot Surg. **23:**334, 1984.

Leukens, C.A.: The wrinkle test for nerve loss, Paper presented at the annual meeting, New Mexico Orthopaedic Association, El Paso, Texas, 1974.

Levy, D.M., and Apfelberg, D.B.: Results of anterior transposition for ulnar neuropathy at the elbow, Am. J. Surg. **123:**304, 1972.

Lewis, D., and Miller, E.M.: Peripheral nerve injuries associated with fractures, Ann. Surg. **76:**528, 1922.

Lindstrom, N., and Danielsson, L.: Muscle transposition in serratus anterior paralysis, Acta Orthop. Scand. **32:**369, 1962.

Lipscomb, P.R., and Sanchez, J.J.: Anterior transplantation of the posterior tibial tendon for persistent palsy of the common peroneal nerve, J. Bone Joint Surg. **43-A:**60, 1961.

Livingston, K.E.: A simple method of rapid identification of major peripheral nerve injuries, Lahey Clin. Found. Bull. **5:**118, 1947.

Livingston, K.E., Livingston, W.K., and Andrus, D.: Nerve end separation following suture: resection of the neck of the fibula in suture of the peroneal nerve, J. Neurosurg. **4:**16, 1947.

Livingston, W.K.: Evidence of active invasion of denervated areas by sensory fibers from neighboring nerves in man, J. Neurosurg. **4:**140, 1947.

Lotem, M., et al.: Radial palsy following muscular effort: a nerve compression syndrome possibly related to a fibrous arch of the lateral head of the triceps, J. Bone Joint Surg. **53-B:**500, 1971.

Lowdon, I.M.R.: Superficial peroneal nerve entrapment: a case report, J. Bone Joint Surg. **67-B:**58, 1985.

Lusskin, R., Campbell, J.B., and Thompson, W.A.L.: Post-traumatic lesions of the brachial plexus: treatment by transclavicular exploration and neurolysis or autograft reconstruction, J. Bone Joint Surg. **55-A:**1159, 1973.

Lyons, W.R., and Woodhall, B.: Atlas of peripheral nerve injuries, Philadelphia, 1949, W.B. Saunders Co.

Mackenzie, I.G., and Woods, C.G.: Causes of failure after repair of the median nerve, J. Bone Joint Surg. **43-B:**465, 1961.

Mackinnon, S.E., et al.: Peripheral nerve injection injury with steroid agents, Plast. Reconstr. Surg. **69:**482, 1982.

Madden, J.W., and Peacock, E.E., Jr.: Some thoughts on repair of peripheral nerves, South. Med. J. **64:**17, 1971.

Marshall, S.C., and Murray, W.R.: Deep radial nerve palsy associated with rheumatoid arthritis, Clin. Orthop. **103:**157, 1974.

Matson, D.D., Early neurolysis in the treatment of injury of the peripheral nerves due to faulty injections of antibiotics, N. Engl. J. Med. **242:**973, 1950.

Mayer, J.H., Jr., and Mayfield, F.H.: Surgery of the posterior interosseous branch of the radial nerve; analysis of 58 cases, Surg. Gynecol. Obstet. **84:**979, 1947.

Mayfield, F.H.: Incision for exposure of peroneal nerve at knee, Bull. U.S. Army Med. Dept. **4:**167, 1945.

Mayfield, F.H., and Devine, J.W.: Causalgia, Surg. Gynecol. Obstet. **80:**631, 1945.

McAuliffe, T.B., Fiddian, N.J., and Browett, J.P.: Entrapment neuropathy of the superficial peroneal nerve: a bilateral case, J. Bone Joint Surg. **67-B:**62, 1985.

Medical Research Council, War Memorandum No. 7: Aids to the investigation of peripheral nerve injuries, ed. 2, London, 1943, His Majesty's Stationery Office.

Medical Research Council, Special Report Series No. 282: Peripheral nerve injuries (Seddon, H.J., editor), London, 1954, Her Majesty's Stationery Office.

Michon, J., and Moberg, E., editors: Traumatic nerve lesions of the upper limb, New York, 1975, Churchill Livingstone.

Millender, L.H., Nalebuff, E.A., and Holdsworth, D.E.: Posterior interosseous-nerve syndrome secondary to rheumatoid synovitis, J. Bone Joint Surg. **55-A:**753, 1973.

Millesi, H.: Microsurgery of peripheral nerves, Hand **5:**157, 1973.

Millesi, H.: Treatment of nerve lesions by fascicular free nerve grafts. In Michon, J., and Moberg, E., editors: Traumatic nerve lesions of the upper limb, Edinburgh, 1975, Churchill Livingstone.

Millesi, H.: Interfascicular grafts for repair of peripheral nerves of the upper extremity, Orthop. Clin. North Am. **8:**387, 1977.

Millesi, H.: Surgical management of brachial plexus injuries, J. Hand Surg. **2**:367, 1977.

Millesi, H., Meissl, G., and Berger, A.: The interfascicular nerve-grafting of the median and ulnar nerves, J. Bone Joint Surg. **54-A**:727, 1972.

Mino, D.E., and Hughes, E.C., Jr.: Bony entrapment of the superficial peroneal nerve, Clin. Orthop. **185**:203, 1984.

Mitchell, S.W., Morehouse, G.R., and Keen, W.W.: Gunshot wounds and other injuries of the nerves, Philadelphia, 1864, J.B. Lippincott Co.

Moberg, E.: Criticism and study of methods for examining sensibility in the hand, Neurology **12**:8, 1962.

Moberg, E.: Aspects of sensation in reconstructive surgery of the upper extremity, J. Bone Joint Surg. **46-A**:817, 1964.

Moberg, E.: Evaluation and management of nerve injuries in the hand, Surg. Clin. North Am. **44**:1019, 1964.

Moldaver, J.: Tourniquet paralysis syndrome, Arch. Surg. **68**:136, 1954.

Moneim, M.S.: Interfascicular nerve grafting, Clin. Orthop. **163**:65, 1982.

Mukherjee, S.R.: Tensile strength of nerves during healing, Br. J. Surg. **41**:192, 1953.

Murphey, F., Hartung, W., and Kirklin, J.W.: Myelographic demonstration of avulsing injury of the brachial plexus, Am. J. Roentgenol. **58**:102, 1947.

Murphey, F., Kirklin, J.W., and Finlayson, A.I.: Anomalous innervation of the intrinsic muscles of the hand, Surg. Gynecol. Obstet. **83**:15, 1946.

Naffziger, H.C., and Norcross, N.C.: The surgical approach to lesions of the upper sciatic nerve and the posterior aspect of the hip joint, Surgery **12**:929, 1942.

Narakas, A.: Surgical treatment of traction injuries of the brachial plexus, Clin. Orthop. **133**:71, 1978.

Nashold, B.S., Jr., Goldner, J.L., Mullen, J.B., and Bright, D.S.: Long-term pain control by direct peripheral-nerve stimulation, J. Bone Joint Surg. **64-A**:1, 1982.

Nicholson, O.R., and Seddon, H.J.: Nerve repair in civil practice: results of treatment of median and ulnar nerve lesions, Br. Med. J. **2**:1065, 1957.

Ober, F.R.: Tendon transplantation in the lower extremity, N. Engl. J. Med. **209**:52, 1933.

Oh, S.J.: Electromyographic studies in peripheral nerve injuries, South. Med. J. **69**:177, 1976.

O'Malley, G.M., Lambdin, C.S., and McCleary, G.S.: Tarsal tunnel syndrome: a case report and review of the literature, Orthopedics **8**:758, 1985.

Omer, G.E., Jr.: Injuries to nerves of the upper extremity, J. Bone Joint Surg. **56-A**:1615, 1974.

Omer, G.E., Jr.: Reconstructive procedures for extremities with peripheral nerve defects, Clin. Orthop. **163**:80, 1982.

Omer, G.E., Jr.: Results of untreated peripheral nerve injuries, Clin. Orthop. **163**:15, 1982.

Omer, G.E., Jr.: Management of peripheral nerve problems. In American Academy of Orthopaedic Surgeons: Instructional course lectures, vol. 33, St. Louis, 1984, The C.V. Mosby Co.

Omer, G.E., and Spinner, M.: Peripheral nerve testing and suture techniques. In American Academy of Orthopaedic Surgeons: Instructional course lectures, vol. 24, St. Louis, 1975, The C.V. Mosby Co.

Omer, G.E., Jr., and Thomas, S.R.: Treatment of causalgia: a review of seventy cases at Brooke General Hospital, Tex. Med. **67**:93, 1971.

Onne, L.: Recovery of sensibility and sudomotor activity in hand after nerve suture, Acta Chir. Scand. Suppl. **300**:1, 1962.

Orgel, M.G.: Experimental studies with clinical application to peripheral nerve injury: a review of the past decade, Clin. Orthop. **163**:98, 1982.

O'Riain, S.: New and simple test of nerve function in hand, Br. Med. J. **3**:615, 1973.

Packer, J.W., Foster, R.R., Garcia, A., and Grantham, S.A.: The humeral fracture with radial nerve palsy: is exploration warranted? Clin. Orthop. **88**:34, 1972.

Parisien, S., and Kaplan, J.: A case of recurrent symptomatic dislocation of the ulnar nerve at the elbow, Orthopedics **5**:1323, 1982.

Parry, C.B.W.: Electrodiagnosis, J. Bone Joint Surg. **43-B**:222, 1961.

Pierce, D.S.: Electrodiagnosis in orthopedic surgery, Clin. Orthop. **107**:25, 1975.

Platt, H.: The operative treatment of traumatic ulnar neuritis at the elbow, Surg. Gynecol. Obstet. **47**:822, 1928.

Pollard, C., Jr., and Grantham, E.G.: Peripheral nerve surgery: incisions for exposures of peripheral nerves, Am. J. Surg. **86**:61, 1953.

Popelka, S., and Vainio, K.: Entrapment of the posterior interosseous branch of the radial nerve in rheumatoid arthritis, Acta Orthop. Scand. **45**:370, 1974.

Poppen, N.K., McCarroll, H.R., Jr., Doyle, J.R., and Niebauer, J.J.: Recovery of sensibility after suture of digital nerves, J. Hand Surg. **4**:212, 1979.

Pringle, R.M., Protheroe, K., and Mukherjee, S.K.: Entrapment neuropathy of the sural nerve, J. Bone Joint Surg. **56-B**:465, 1974.

Pritchard, D.J., Linscheid, R.L., and Svien, H.J.: Intraarticular median nerve entrapment with dislocation of the elbow, Clin. Orthop. **90**:100, 1973.

Raji, A.M.: An experimental study of the effects of pulsed electromagnetic field (diapulse) on nerve repair, J. Hand Surg. **9-B**:105, 1984.

Raji, A.R.M., and Bowden, R.E.M.: Effects of high-peak pulsed electromagnetic field on the degeneration and regeneration of the common peroneal nerve in rats, J. Bone Joint Surg. **65-B**:478, 1983.

Rana, N.A., et al.: Complete lesion of the median nerve associated with dislocation of the elbow joint, Acta Orthop. Scand. **45**:365, 1974.

Rapp, I.H.: Serratus anterior paralysis treated by transplantation of the pectoralis minor, J. Bone Joint Surg. **36-A**:852, 1954.

Rappaport, N.H., Clark, G.L., and Bora, W.F., Jr.: Median nerve entrapment about the elbow, Adv. Orthop. **8**:270, 1985.

Rask, M.R.: Suprascapular nerve entrapment: a report of two cases treated with suprascapular notch resection, Clin. Orthop. **123**:73, 1977.

Rask, M.R.: Anterior interosseous nerve entrapment (Kiloh-Nevin syndrome): report of seven cases, Clin. Orthop. **142**:176, 1979.

Rasmussen, T.B., and Freedman, H.: Treatment of causalgia: an analysis of 100 cases, J. Neurosurg. **3**:165, 1946.

Rayner, C.R.: The split sternomastoid muscle flap: a method to improve the bed for brachial plexus grafts, J. Hand Surg. **9-B**:113, 1984.

Richmond, J.C., and Southmayd, W.W.: Superficial anterior transposition of the ulnar nerve at the elbow for ulnar neuritis, Clin. Orthop. **164**:42, 1982.

Riley, D.A., and Lang, D.H.: Carbonic anhydrase activity of human peripheral nerves: a possible histochemical aid to nerve repair, J. Hand Surg. **9-A**:112, 1984.

Richter, C.P.: Instructions for using cutaneous resistance recorder, or "dermometer" on peripheral nerve injuries, sympathectomies and paravertebral block, J. Neurosurg. **3**:181, 1946.

Rockett, F.X.: Observations on the "burner": traumatic cervical radiculopathy, Clin. Orthop. **164**:18, 1982.

Roles, N.C., and Maudsley, R.H.: Radial tunnel syndrome: resistant tennis elbow as a nerve entrapment, J. Bone Joint Surg. **54-B**:499, 1972.

Rorabeck, C.H., and Harris, W.R.: Factors affecting the prognosis of brachial plexus injuries, J. Bone Joint Surg. **63-B**:404, 1981.

Sakellarides, H.: A follow-up study of 172 peripheral nerve injuries in the upper extremity in civilians, J. Bone Joint Surg. **44-A**:140, 1962.

Salisbury, R.E., and Dingeldein, G.P.: Peripheral nerve complications following burn injury, Clin. Orthop. **163**:92, 1982.

Scarff, J.E.: Peripheral nerve injuries: principles of treatment, Med. Clin. North Am. **42**:611, 1958.

Scuderi, C.: Tendon transplants for irreparable radial nerve paralysis, Industr. Med. **23**:258, 1954.

Seddon, H.J.: Three types of nerve injury, Brain **66**:237, 1943.

Seddon, H.J.: The use of autogenous grafts for the repair of large gaps in peripheral nerves, Br. J. Surg. **35**:151, 1947.

Seddon, H.J.: The practical value of peripheral nerve repair, Proc. R. Soc. Med. **42**:427, 1949.

Seddon, H.J.: Transplantation of pectoralis major for paralysis of the flexors of the elbow, Proc. R. Soc. Med. **42**:837, 1949.

Seddon, H.J.: Reconstructive surgery of the upper extremity. In Poliomyelitis, Second International Poliomyelitis Congress, Philadelphia, 1952, J.B. Lippincott Co.

Seddon, H.J.: Nerve grafting, J. Bone Joint Surg. **45-B**:447, 1963.

Seddon, H.J.: Nerve injuries, Univ. Mich. Med. Center J. **31**:4, 1965.

Seddon, H.J.: Surgical disorders of the peripheral nerves, Edinburgh, 1972, Churchill Livingstone.

Seddon, H.J., et al.: Rate of regeneration of peripheral nerves in man, J. Physiol. **102**:191, 1943.

Sedel, L.: The results of surgical repair of brachial plexus injuries, J. Bone Joint Surg. **64-B**:54, 1982.

Shumacker, H.B., Jr.: Causalgia. III. A general discussion, Surgery **24**:485, 1948.

Silver, D.: Thoracic outlet syndrome, Hosp. Phys., October, 1983, p. 42.

Simesen, K., Haase, J., and Bjerre, P.: Interfascicular transplantation in medial nerve injuries, Acta Orthop. Scand. **51**:243, 1980.

Skurja, M., Jr., and Monlux, J.H.: Case studies: the suprascapular nerve and shoulder dysfunction, J. Orthop. Sports Phys. Ther. **6**:254, 1985.

Smith, J.W.: Microsurgery of peripheral nerves, Plast. Reconstr. Surg. **33**:317, 1964.

Smith, J.W.: Factors influencing nerve repair: II. Collateral circulation of peripheral nerves, Arch. Surg. **93**:433, 1966.

Snyder, C.C., et al.: Intraneural neurorrhaphy: a preliminary clinical and histological evaluation, Ann. Surg. **167**:691, 1968.

Solheim, L.F., and Roaas, A.: Compression of the suprascapular nerve after fracture of the scapular notch, Acta Orthop. Scand. **49**:338, 1979.

Solonen, K.A., Telaranta, T., and Ryöppy, S.: Early reconstruction of birth injuries of the brachial plexus, J. Pediatr. Orthop. **1**:367, 1981.

Solonen, K.A., Vastamäki, M., and Ström, B.: Surgery of the brachial plexus, Acta Orthop. Scand. **55**:436, 1984.

Spinner, M.: The anterior interosseous-nerve syndrome: with special attention to its variations, J. Bone Joint Surg. **52-A**:84, 1970.

Spinner, M.: Injuries to the major branches of peripheral nerves of the forearm, Philadelphia, 1978, W.B. Saunders Co.

Spinner, M., and Schreiber, S.N.: Anterior interosseous-nerve paralysis as a complication of supracondylar fractures of the humerus in children, J. Bone Joint Surg. **51-A**:1584, 1969.

Spinner, M., and Spencer, P.S.: Nerve compression lesions of the upper extremity: a clinical and experimental review, Clin. Orthop. **104**:46, 1974.

Spurling, R.G.: Early treatment of combined bone and nerve lesions, Bull. U.S. Army Med. Dept. **4**:444, 1945.

Spurling, R.G., Lyons, W.R., Whitcomb, B.B., and Woodhall, B.: The failure of whole fresh homogenous nerve grafts in man, J. Neurosurg. **2**:79, 1945.

Spurling, R.G., and Woodhall, B.: Experiences with early nerve surgery in peripheral nerve injuries, Ann. Surg. **123**:731, 1946.

Stein, F., Grabias, S.L., and Deffer, P.A.: Nerve injuries complicating Monteggia lesions, J. Bone Joint Surg. **53-A**:1432, 1971.

Stookey, B.: The technic of nerve suture, JAMA p. 1380, May 15, 1920.

Stookey, B.: Surgical and mechanical treatment of peripheral nerves, Philadelphia, 1922, W.B. Saunders Co.

Strange, F.G. St. C.: An operation for nerve pedicle grafting: preliminary communication, Br. J. Surg. **34**:423, 1947.

Sunderland, S.: A classification of peripheral nerve injuries producing loss of function, Brain **74**:491, 1951.

Sunderland, S.: Factors influencing the course of regeneration and the quality of the recovery after nerve suture, Brain **75**:19, 1952.

Sunderland, S.: Funicular suture and funicular exclusion in the repair of severed nerves, Br. J. Surg. **40**:580, 1953.

Sunderland, S.: Nerves and nerve injuries, Baltimore, 1968, The Williams & Wilkins Co.

Sunderland, S., and Bradley, K.C.: Endoneurial tube shrinkage in the distal segment of a severed nerve, J. Comp. Neurol. **93**:411, 1950.

Swafford, A.R., and Lichtman, D.H.: Suprascapular nerve entrapment—case report, J. Hand Surg. **7**:57, 1982.

Swift, T.R.: Involvement of peripheral nerves in radical neck dissection, Am. J. Surg. **119**:694, 1970.

Szabo, R.M., and Gelberman, R.H.: Peripheral nerve compression: etiology, critical pressure threshold, and clinical assessment, Orthopedics **7**:1461, 1984.

Szabo, R.M., et al.: Vibratory sensory testing in acute peripheral nerve compression, J. Hand. Surg. **9-A**:104, 1984.

Takebe, K., Kanbara, Y., Mizuno, K., and Hirohata, K.: Tardy ulnar nerve palsy associated with the isolated dislocation of the head of the radius, Clin. Orthop. **167**:260, 1982.

Tanabu, S., Yamauchi, Y., and Fukushima, M.: Hypoplasia of the trochlea of the humerus as a cause of ulnar-nerve palsy: report of two cases, J. Bone Joint Surg. **67-A**:151, 1985.

Taylor, G.I.: Nerve grafting with simultaneous microvascular reconstruction, Clin. Orthop. **133**:56, 1978.

Taylor, G.I., and Ham, F.J.: The free vascularized nerve graft: a further experiment and clinical application of microvascular techniques, Plast. Reconstr. Surg. **57**:413, 1976.

Taylor, P.E.: Traumatic intradural avulsion of the nerve roots of the brachial plexus, Brain **85**:579, 1962.

Tenny, J.R., and Lewis, R.C.: Digital nerve-grafting for traumatic defects: use of the lateral antebrachial cutaneous nerve J. Bone Joint Surg. **66-A**:1375, 1984.

Terzis, J.K.: Functional aspects of reinnervations of free skin grafts, Plast. Reconstr. Surg. **58**:142, 1976.

Terzis, J.K.: Sensory mapping, Clin. Plast. Surg. **3**:59, 1976.

Terzis, J., Faibisoff, B., and Williams, B.: The nerve gap: suture under tension vs. graft, Plast. Reconstr. Surg. **56**:166, 1975.

Terzis, J.K., and Strauch, B.: Microsurgery of the peripheral nerve: a physiological approach, Clin. Orthop. **133**:39, 1978.

Thompson, R.C., Jr., Schneider, W., and Kennedy, T.: Entrapment neuropathy of the inferior branch of the suprascapular nerve by ganglia, Clin. Orthop. **166**:185, 1982.

Tracy, J.F., and Brannon, E.W.: Management of brachial-plexus injuries (traction type), J. Bone Joint Surg. **40-A**:1031, 1958.

Trail, A.I.: Delayed repair of the ulnar nerve, J. Hand Surg. **10-B**:345, 1985.

Tsuge, K., Ikuta, Y., and Sakaue, M.: A new technique for nerve suture: the anchoring funicular suture, Plast. Reconstr. Surg. **56**:496, 1975.

Urbaniak, J.R.: Fascicular nerve suture, Clin. Orthop. **163**:57, 1982.

Van Beek, A., and Kleinert, H.E.: Practical microneurorrhaphy, Orthop. Clin. North Am. **8**:377, 1977.

Vandeput, J., Tanner, J.C., and Huypens, L.: Electro-physiological orientation of the cut ends in primary peripheral nerve repair, Plast. Reconstr. Surg. **44**:378, 1969.

Vastamäki, M., and Solonen, K.A.: Accessory nerve injury, Acta Orthop. Scand. **55**:296, 1984.

Ventura, R., et al.: Experimental suture of the peripheral nerves with "fibrin glue," Ital. J. Orthop. Traumatol. **6**:407, 1980.

Waisbrod, H., Panhans, Ch., Hansen, D., and Gerbershagen, H.U.: Direct nerve stimulation for painful peripheral neuropathies, J. Bone Joint Surg. **67-B**:470, 1985.

Watson-Jones, R.: Primary nerve lesions in injuries of the elbow and wrist, J. Bone Joint Surg. **12**:121, 1930.

Weaver, H.L.: Isolated suprascapular nerve lesions, Injury **15**:117, 1983.

Weeks, P.M.: Radial, median, and ulnar nerve dysfunction associated with a congenital constricting band of the arm, Plast. Reconstr. Surg. **69**:333, 1982.

Weiss, P.: Nerve reunion with sleeves of frozen-dried artery in rabbits, cats and monkeys, Proc. Soc. Exp. Biol. Med. **54**:274, 1943.

Werner, C.-O., Ohlin, P., and Elmquist, D.: Pressures recorded in ulnar neuropathy, Acta Orthop. Scand. **56**:404, 1985.

Whitcomb, B.B.: Separation of suture sites as cause of failure in regeneration of peripheral nerves, J. Neurosurg. **3**:399, 1946.

Whitman, A.: Congenital elevation of scapula and paralysis of serratus magnus muscle, JAMA **99**:1332, 1932.

Wiggins, C.E.: Pronator syndrome, South Med. J. **75**:240, 1982.

Wilgis, E.F.S.: Techniques for diagnosis of peripheral nerve loss, Clin. Orthop. **163**:8, 1982.

Wilgis, E.F.S., and Maxwell, G.P.: Distal digital nerve grafts: clinical and anatomical studies, J. Hand Surg. **4**:439, 1979.

Williams, H.B., and Terzis, J.K.: Single fascicular recordings: an intra-operative diagnostic tool for the management of peripheral nerve lesions, Plast. Reconstr. Surg. **57**:562, 1976.

Wirth, F.P., Jr., and Rutherford, R.B.: A civilian experience with causalgia, Arch. Surg. **100**:633, 1970.

Wise, A.J., Jr., et al.: A comparative analysis of macro- and microsurgical neurorrhaphy technics, Am. J. Surg. **117**:566, 1969.

Wolfe, J.S., and Eyring, E.J.: Median-nerve entrapment within a greenstick fracture: a case report, J. Bone Joint Surg. **56-A**:1270, 1974.

Woodhall, B.: Peripheral nerve injuries: II. Basic data from the peripheral nerve registry concerning 7,050 nerve sutures and 67 nerve grafts, J. Neurosurg. **4**:146, 1947.

Woodhall, B.: The surgical repair of acute peripheral nerve injury, Surg. Clin. North Am. **31**:1369, 1951.

Woodhall, B.: Trapezius paralysis following minor surgical procedures in the posterior cervical triangle, Ann. Surg. **136**:375, 1952.

Woodhall, B., and Beebe, G.W., editors: Peripheral nerve regeneration: a follow-up study of 3,656 World War II injuries, Veterans Administration Medical Monograph, Washington, D.C., 1956, U.S. Government Printing Office.

Woodhall, B., and Lyons, W.R.: Peripheral nerve injuries: I. The results of ''early'' nerve suture: a preliminary report, Surgery **19:**757, 1946.

Worth, R.M., Kettelkamp, D.B., Defalque, R.J., and Duane, K.U.: Saphenous nerve entrapment: a cause of medial knee pain, Am. J. Sports Med. **12:**80, 1984.

Wright, T.A.: Accessory spinal nerve injury, Clin. Orthop. **108:**15, 1975.

Yeoman, P.M.: Cervical myelography in traction injuries of the brachial plexus, J. Bone Joint Surg. **50-B:**253, 1968.

Yeoman, P.M., and Seddon, H.J.: Brachial plexus injuries: treatment of the flail arm, J. Bone Joint Surg. **43-B:**493, 1961.

Yiannikas, C., and Shahani, B.T.: Special review: painful sequelae of injuries to peripheral nerves, Am. J. Phys. Med. **63:**53, 1984.

Young, L., Wray, R.C., and Weeks, P.M.: A randomized prospective comparison of fascicular and epineural digital nerve repairs, Plast. Reconstr. Surg. **68:**89, 1981.

Zachary, R.B., and Holmes, W.: Primary suture of nerves, Surg. Gynecol. Obstet. **82:**632, 1946.

Zachary, R.B.: Results of nerve suture. In Seddon, H.J., editor: Peripheral nerve injuries, London, 1954, Her Majesty's Stationery Office.

Zalis, A.W., Rodriquez, A.A., Oester, Y.T., and Mains, D.B.: Evaluation of nerve regeneration by means of nerve evoked potentials, J. Bone Joint Surg. **54-A:**1246, 1972.

Zoltan, J.D.: Injury to the suprascapular nerve associated with anterior dislocation of the shoulder: case report and review of the literature, J. Trauma **19:**203, 1979.

CHAPTER 65

Cerebral palsy

Fred P. Sage

This chapter discusses cerebral palsy that occurrs prenatally and perinatally, acquired cerebral palsy in children, and the treatment of adult patients recovering from a cerebrovascular accident, or stroke.

Cerebral palsy is defined as a disorder of movement and posture caused by a nonprogressive defect or lesion in the immature brain. Although lesions that occur in the upper cervical cord just below the decussation of the pyramids do not technically fit the definition, they can be treated like cerebral palsy.

The cerebral palsied population is the largest group of pediatric patients with neuromuscular disorders in the United States. The occurrence of cerebral palsy in various countries and localities ranges from 0.6 to 5.9 patients per 1000 live births, varying according to the amount and type of prenatal care, socioeconomic conditions of the parents, the environment, and the type of obstetric and pediatric care the mother and the child receive. In the United States, there are approximately 25,000 new patients with cerebral palsy each year and approximately 400,000 children afflicted with cerebral palsy at any given time.

It has been speculated that neonatal intensive care units are saving more children with birth injuries or prenatal defects than previously, thereby increasing the cerebral palsied population. Reports are available to support and to refute this premise. Certainly, the distribution of the clinical presentation of the various types of involvement appears to have shifted now that so many children with birth weight of less than 1500 g are being saved. The incidence of prematurity has long been related to the incidence of spastic paraplegia or diplegia.

Cerebral palsy is divided into the following four types according to clinical presentation: spastic, dyskinetic, ataxic, and mixed. Patients with dyskinetic cerebral palsy are further subdivided into the following five groups, characterized by the type of abnormal posture or movement: athetosis, tremor, dystonia, choreiform, and rigidity. Spastic paralysis occurs in at least 65% of patients with cerebral palsy. Patients with dyskinetic cerebral palsy are the next largest group, making up about 25% of the total number. Ataxia without other movement abnormalities is the rarest form, and patients so afflicted make up less than 3%

2843

of the total. The mixed group has been found to account for an increasing number of patients, probably greater than 10%, as we become more skillful in the detection of the various clinical types of abnormal movement and posture. As the immature brain develops, occasionally the clinical manifestations of the type of movement or posture disorder change.

The lesions in the brain causing abnormality in movement or posture occur primarily in the following four areas: the cerebral cortex (spastic paralysis), the midbrain or base of the brain (dyskinesia), the cerebellum (ataxia), and widespread brain involvement (rigidity and mixed). Locating the causative lesion in the brain is easier now than in the past. Cerebral blood flow studies, computed tomography, and magnetic resonance imaging done in the neonatal intensive care unit can pinpoint the exact geographic location of the brain insult and at times define the type of insult as well. In the past, pneumoencephalography, ventriculography, and electrophysiologic localization with multiple channel electroencephalograms were not always accurate and the exact location and type of brain lesion could only be pinpointed at autopsy.

ETIOLOGY

The lesion responsible for cerebral palsy may have its origin in the prenatal, natal, or postnatal period. The prenatal period is from conception until the onset of labor, the natal period is from the onset of labor until the actual time of delivery, and the postnatal period is from the time of delivery until brain maturation at 2½ to 3 years when myelinzation occurs, or up to 8 years in some opinions. Some investigators have defined perinatal as the period between the onset of labor and 7 days after birth when stability with the outside environment has taken place.

Most lesions that cause cerebral palsy occur in the perinatal period, but increasing evidence shows that prenatal causes occur more often than suspected. Perlstein kept extensive records on all cerebral palsied patients who attended his clinic. He found that 30% of lesions were caused by prenatal factors, 60% by natal factors, and 10% by postnatal factors. Blumel, Eggers, and Evans found postnatal causes to account for 7% of the 110 lesions in their study. In 1981 O'Reilly and Walentynowicz reported 1503 patients who were followed between 1947 and 1980 and for whom adequate etiologic data were available. They found that 38.5% of lesions had a prenatal cause, 46.3% occurred during the natal period, and 15.2% occurred postnatally. They also found that the number of patients seen in each decade since 1950 had gradually decreased. They attributed this to the decreased birth rate in the United States since 1950, as well as to the improvements in obstetric and perinatal care since that time.

Of 142 children with cerebral palsy born during the 1970s, Holm found 50% of the lesions to have a prenatal cause, 33% occurred in the natal period, 10% occurred postnatally, and 7% had a mixed origin. A similar high incidence of prenatal causes was found in a recent study in Sweden.

O'Reilly and Walentynowicz reported a steady increase in the percentage of patients who had spasticity, especially paraplegia and quadriplegia. In their study, they found a drastic decrease in the incidence of athetosis, from 10.8% between 1930 and 1949 to 3.6% between 1970 and 1979. They attributed this to the marked decrease in patients with erythroblastosis fetalis and to the decrease in instances of perinatal anoxia. Bleck also noted that the incidence of cerebral palsy has definitely decreased.

Prenatal causes

One cause of cerebral palsy in the prenatal period is a congenital brain defect. This is common in children whose mothers had rubella (German measles) or viral infections in early pregnancy. These patients usually have other congenital anomalies, such as cataracts, congenital heart defects, deafness, and mental retardation. Erythroblastosis fetalis was formerly a common prenatal cause, as was fetal anoxia, but fetal monitoring now routinely performed in most obstetric centers has decreased significantly the incidence of these conditions. Anoxia in the prenatal period may result from various causes, such as abruptio placentae, placental infarction, maternal pneumonia, or cardiorespiratory disease. Chemical dependency on alcohol or drugs in the mother has been shown to increase the incidence of cerebral palsy. Maternal metabolic disturbances, such as diabetes mellitus and thyroid abnormalities, likewise contribute to prenatal cerebral palsy. Cerebral palsy in an older sibling would also indicate a probable congenital origin rather than a lesion of perinatal origin, as would congenital hydrocephalus and microcephaly. Genetically inherited errors in metabolism may result in motor disabilities as well as cause numerous other defects.

Natal causes

Natal causes are usually trauma or anoxia incurring during labor, often caused by dystocia and delay in delivery. Such traumatic injuries can result in intracranial hemorrhage. Rupture of the great vein of Galen causes spastic paraplegia or quadriplegia. Spastic hemiplegia can be caused by localized trauma such as impingement of the head on the sacral promontory in dystocia. A fetal stroke during periods of maternal eclampsia may cause hemiplegia. Delay in delivery, as in breech or other abnormal presentations, may cause anoxia, as may fetal tracheobronchial tree aspiration or maternal asphyxia from any cause, such as anesthetic complications or oversedation.

Prematurity is by far the most common natal cause. Low birth weight (below 2268 g) and cerebral palsy have long been known to be causally related. The premature infant's brain is immature and susceptible to anoxia, and the respiratory tree is also underdeveloped and may be unable to assimilate oxygen in the tracheobronchial-alveolar tree. With anoxia there is respiratory depression, which may lead to further anoxia and more widespread brain damage. The second twin often suffers anoxia because of a delay in being delivered; in addition, twins are often born prematurely. The blood vessels in the premature infant are fragile and subject to rupture, especially during sudden pressure changes, such as in precipitous labor.

Postnatal causes

The most common causes of cerebral palsy in the postnatal period are encephalitis, meningitis, trauma, vascular accidents, and anoxia. During the acute stage of encephalitis, the motor deficit may progress with increasing involvement. In the postacute stage it may also increase as the brain undergoes scarring. During these periods the motor deficit may change in its clinical presentation, but the lesion will ultimately become stable, as will the motor deficit, unless the infection recurs. With increasing infection control measures, such as immunization, organism-specific antibiotics, and other chemotherapeutic measures, cerebral palsy resulting from infections is decreasing.

Traumatic head injuries, mainly from motor vehicular accidents and child abuse, account for a significant number of cerebral palsied children in the postnatal period. Anoxia from near drowning, fibrocystic disease, and other assorted lesion mainly result in disorders of movement that are often choreiform or athetoid. Cerebral palsy resulting from trauma or associated hemorrhage is usually spastic. Patients with neurologic disorders from anoxia and trauma tend to improve with time, often for a year or more after the injury. In an excellent study of brain-traumatized children, Brink and Hoffer related the prognosis for recovery directly to the level and length of unconsciousness after the initial insult. Deep coma for longer than 1 week results in a poor prognosis for any significant recovery.

Removal of brain tumors may result in a motor deficit, but after the immediate postoperative period any remaining motor injury can be expected to be nonprogressive. Postnatal cerebral palsy from toxins such as lead, either inhaled or ingested, are seldom seen but do occur.

CLINICAL TYPES

The location of the lesion in the brain determines the clinical type of cerebral palsy. A lesion in the cerebral cortex generally causes spasticity or lack of voluntary initiation of motion. Most insults are not neatly confined to an area of the brain supplying one muscle, as in the lower motor neuron pareses. The area involved is geographically larger, and the entire portion of the body supplied by that area of the brain is involved. This is why whole extremities are involved to some degree, instead of a single muscle as in poliomyelitis. If a single muscle shows predominant involvement, spasticity must be suspected in other muscles in that area. For example, hamstring spasticity will usually be accompanied by some quadriceps spasticity, and this antagonistic spasticity must be recognized and evaluated before deciding on the appropriate therapy. Motor deficits are usually evaluated in individual muscles, but in cerebral palsy this is inappropriate. Brodmann's areas 4 and 6 in the brain are the beginning of the pyramidal tracts; lesions in this region are called pyramidal tract disease and commonly cause spasticity.

The degree of functional deficit may be increased by the lack of facilitation and the inhibition of movement resulting from the brain's failure to interpret proprioceptive impulses and stretch information from the muscle spindles inside the muscles. This results in a lack of coordinated movement between agonistic and antagonistic muscles and the presence of stretch reflexes in the muscles.

Spasticity, a state of increased tension in the muscle when it is passively lengthened, is caused by an exaggeration of the normal muscle stretch reflex. An exaggerated stretch reflex is pathognomonic of spasticity. In an exaggerated stretch reflex, resistance is felt to sudden passive movement of the muscle, followed by relaxation of the muscle to a certain point. The degree of functional impairment caused by spasticity may be affected by the lack of balance between facilitation and inhibition in the centers of the midbrain and brainstem, but defects in the motor cortex of the cerebral hemispheres are the primary cause of the spasticity.

If the insult to the brain is near the vertex in both hemispheres, then both legs will be involved; if the insult extends deeper into the brain, then the arms are involved as well. An insult localized to one side of the cerebral cortex results in involvement of only one side of the body, and a hemiplegia develops on the side opposite the lesion in the brain. Increased spasticity causes hypercontractility of the muscles when stretched. Deep tendon reflexes in the spastic muscles are hyperactive, and clonus of the muscle may be present, indicating an increased response to stretch.

Lesions in the base of the brain usually result in dyskinesia, or movement disorders with retained primitive reflexes. Impulses may be released that result in many types of involuntary movement disorders. The motions may be rapid or slow, constant or intermittent, or appear only during voluntary effort. Athetoid cerebral palsy is the most common type of dyskinetic cerebral palsy; other types are rarely seen except in widespread brain damage, which can cause rigidities.

Because the lesion causing dyskinesia is in the base of the brain or in the midbrain, total body involvement generally results. It is unusual to see a movement disorder confined to one extremity. Facial muscles and the muscles that control speech are commonly involved in these patients, and the constant grimacing, drooling, and difficulty with speech may lead one to believe that these patients are mentally retarded, but in fact many have normal intelligence.

Dyskinesia is a disorder of motion and tone in the muscles. The motion is irregular and uncontrollable and is usually accentuated by voluntary effort. Primitive reflexes are retained longer in a dyskinetic child than in a normal child. Chorea, athetosis, and dystonia are similar; the difference is in the amount of tone present. The motion is slower in athetosis than in choreiform movements, but more tension is present in the muscles. In dystonia tension in the muscles in the affected area is marked. Tension predominates over movement, so abnormal postural manifestations may inhibit abnormal movements.

Many patients with athetosis show increased tension in their muscles, and this may be mistaken for spasticity. The increased tension may be caused by voluntary efforts to control the involuntary motion or by emotional overlay. Tension mimicking spasticity may be removed from the muscle by repeated, rapid, passive stretching and relaxation of the muscle (shaking the tension out). Spasticity and the exaggerated stretch reflex cannot be shaken out.

A tremor is a small, pendular, repetitive movement that usually follows encephalitis and is rarely congenital.

Rigidity is usually caused by diffuse lesions of the brain, which may follow prolonged anoxia after birth or multiple punctuate hemorrhages caused by venous stasis in the brain. This type of cerebral palsy is characterized by a loss of elasticity of the muscles and a "lead-pipe" response to passive flexion or extension of the joints. When trying to stretch the muscles, the examiner elicits a stiffness from beginning to end of the attempted passive motion. The passive motion may trigger an exaggerated stretch reflex, however, so that rigidity in the muscles may be intermittent. Because the brain is diffusely damaged in these children, the incidence of mental impairment is relatively high, and these children do not respond well to treatment programs.

Lesions in the cerebellum cause a loss of kinesthetic sense; orientation in space is lost from the failure to correctly interpret incoming stimuli. This causes ataxia, or a loss in the sense of balance and position in space. Most cerebellar insults are congenital. They cause not only loss of position sense, but usually hypotonic muscles and hypermobile joints as well. Often nystagmus is present, and motion sickness may occur when trying to fix the eyes on small objects, such as when reading. Ataxia usually improves with time, as the patient learns from experience to voluntarily control balance. This is one type of cerebral palsy that seems to show spontaneous improvement.

The mixed type of cerebral palsy may result from damage in more than one area, but usually not from diffuse damage. A lesion in the midbrain may cause athetosis whereas a concomitant lesion in the cerebellum causes spasticity. Along with spastic diplegia, balance and righting reactions are often lost. Retention of primitive reflex patterns and righting reactions also leads to ataxia.

Geographic classification

To properly describe the cerebral palsied patient, the geographic area involved by the motor or postural deficit must be described. This is done by assigning names to the different patterns of paresis.

Monoplegia. Only one extremity, either upper or lower, is affected. This is an extremely uncommon type of paresis, and the examiner must carefully evaluate the other extremities before making this designation.

Hemiplegia. Both extremities on the same side are affected. The arm is usually worse than the leg in the cerebral palsied patient, and these patients are usually spastic.

Paraplegia. This pattern is often associated with prematurity; as neonatal care improves, a greater percentage of the cerebral palsied population falls into this category. In this pattern, both lower extremities are affected, usually about equally so, unless a hydrocephalus or a congenital defect in an asymmetric location is present. These patients are usually spastic.

Triplegia. Three of the four extremities are affected. These patients are most often spastic, but may be dyskinetic. This is also an extremely unusual distribution, and one should carefully evaluate the unaffected extremity before classifying a patient as a triplegic.

Quadriplegia. All four extremities are involved by the brain insult. These patients are usually subdivided further to indicate whether the upper or lower extremities are more involved. They may have either spasticity or dyskinesia or a mixed type of involvement.

Diplegia. All four extremities are affected, but the upper extremities are less affected than the lower extremities.

Double hemiplegia. All four extremities are affected, but the lower extremities are less involved than the upper extremities (as in a hemiplegia). These deficits are usually spastic. This is an uncommon pattern of involvement.

Tetraplegia. All four extremities are equally involved. This type is usually spastic.

Total body involvement. The trunk, head, and neck are affected, as well as all four extremities. These patients are mainly dyskinetic and primarily athetoid. They retain primitive reflexes that interfere with head control in relation to the extremities, and their sense of balance may be severely impaired.

In a review of 3800 patients with cerebral palsy, Perlstein found that the geographic distribution of the 2490 patients with spasticity was hemiplegia 50%, quadriplegia 25%, paraplegia and diplegia 21%, triplegia 3.1%, and monoplegia 0.3%. O'Reilly and Walentynowicz found a different distribution in the 1503 patients that they reported in 1980 (Table 65-1). We have found hemiplegia and diplegia to be by far the most common patterns in the patients affected by spasticity. The quadriplegic or totally involved patient is seen less often, and most often has dyskinesia, which is almost always athetoid.

Tone and severity

Cerebral palsy may also be classified in other terms to give a better clinical picture of the patient. These terms concern the tonicity of the muscles and the severity of the impairment.

Muscles may be hypertonic, hypotonic, or normal in tone. Tone is variable and may change with time. Children with athetoid cerebral palsy are hypotonic at birth, but usually become hypertonic as they grow older. On the other hand, children with ataxia are hypotonic at birth and

Table 65-1. Diagnostic distribution of cerebral palsy

	Total patient group (%)	Known etiology group (%)		Total patient group (%)	Known etiology group (%)
Spastic	62.8	63.8	Athetosis	11.7	10.4
Monoplegia	3.0	3.3	Ataxia	4.9	4.6
Hemiplegia	26.0	26.2	Rigidity	7.2	7.1
Paraplegia	15.7	15.5	Atonia	1.1	1.3
Triplegia	4.5	5.0	Tremor	0.3	0.2
Quadriplegia	13.5	13.8	Mixed	12.0	12.6

From O'Reilly, D.E., and Walentynowicz, J.E.: Etiological factors in cerebral palsy: an historical review, Dev. Med. Child Neurol. **23:**633, 1980.

usually remain so. Changes in spatial orientation and in emotional stability cause decreased or increased tone in many patients. Thus, although tone may be used in the classification of a patient's condition, it is subject to change.

The severity of the impairment may be mild, moderate, or severe. A mildly affected patient is ambulatory and independent in the activities of daily living. These patients make up about 25% of the cerebral palsied population. Although orthopaedic treatment may not be required, occupational therapy in fine motor skills, special education, and speech therapy may be indicated. A cerebral palsied child with moderate involvement needs help in the activities of daily living and ambulation, or has difficulty in speech or other functional disabilities. These make up about 50% of all patients. A severely involved patient is fully incapacitated and is usually bedridden or confined to a wheelchair. Because mobility may never be improved, treatment is aimed at functional improvement in other activities rather than attempted ambulation.

Associated handicapping conditions

Almost all patients with a motor or postural deficit have some other handicapping condition, and often the motor deficit is not the most severe impairment. From a functional standpoint, the most severe impairment may be secondary to some other deficit, such as the inability to communicate, deafness, blindness, learning disabilities, or sensory loss. Between 50% and 60% of patients with spastic hemiplegia have a sensory deficit in the affected hand. Homan's studies have demonstrated that the greatest loss is in two-point discrimination, stereognosis, position sense, or tactile sense. If this sensory deficit is significant in the upper extremity, the hand is of little value.

Tablan found that 82% of the cerebral palsied population had problems with speech, 19% were mentally retarded, 15% had some element of deafness, 34% had visual defects, and 13.6% had perceptual problems. In 1961 Henderson reported that 25% of his cerebral palsied patients had seizures. Perlstein and Barnett found that seizures occur in approximately 40% of the children with cerebral palsy, but in only 0.5% of the general population. Seizures are more common in more severely involved children, such as those with spasticity and rigidity, than in children with athetosis.

Emotional problems add to these handicapping conditions. The attitudes of the parents, the siblings, the community, and the treatment team are all important. The child's self-image plays an important role especially during adolescence when he is unable to keep up with his peers. As young adulthood is reached, concerns about employment, self-care, sexual gratification, marriage, and child-bearing all cause anxiety and may lead to emotional instability.

Hoffer states that "the two most crucial abilities for any human being are the ability to think and the ability to communicate." Communication is of prime importance if one has cognitive ability. As the experienced pediatric orthopaedic surgeon can attest, some type of communication aid can often lead to the discovery of a normal cognitive ability in a child thought to be mentally retarded. In the absence of speech, some alternative for communication must be found so that cognitive abilities can function. As orthopaedic surgeons, we have in the past placed too much emphasis on the ability to walk and to do so in a more normal manner, rather than on the habilitation of the child as a whole. Many cerebral palsied adults on consumer symposia have been explicit in telling us this.

TREATMENT

There is no cure for cerebral palsy. The initial insult to the brain in the newborn may heal to some extent, but the residual defect will remain the same throughout life. The brain lesion that causes the deficit in voluntary muscle control and posture, balance abnormalities, and disorders in tone remains constant. With proper management, we can decrease the functional impairment in many children, but the child will never be normal. Treatment techniques that claim the production of normalcy as their goal should be received with suspicion.

The aim of management in cerebral palsy is to increase the patient's assets as much as possible and minimize his defects. We strive to increase his emotional maturity, physical independence, cognitive abilities, and speech or communication, and to create a socioeconomic independence, as well as create or improve his sense of self-worth. All of these may be idealistic goals, but we can temper them with a realistic appraisal of the patient's assorted abilities.

Adults with cerebral palsy have given us the following order of preference in improving their quality of life: (1) education and communication, (2) activities of daily living, (3) mobility, and (4) ambulation. Too much emphasis has been placed on gait and its refinement. If we had spent as much effort in improving the educational and communicative levels of our patients, it would have been more to their advantage.

Regardless of their mental capacity, almost all patients can be taught something about self-care, mobility, and communication. The severity of the physical impairment is paralleled by impaired cognitive abilities in about 50% of patients. About 70% of children with athetoid cerebral palsy have an IQ above 70, and about 12% have an IQ above 100. A number of totally involved spastic children are found to be quite bright if given the ability to communicate at their cognitive levels. The mental capacity of the individual patient is crucial because it establishes what is normal for him and therefore what the goal of treatment is for him. A patient who has 75% normal intelligence is functioning at his normal level when he acquires motor, social, and other skills at 75% of the usual normal rate. A specific motor defect, as is present in cerebral palsy, imposes an additional handicap that further retards the rate of acquiring new motor skills.

Mental deficiency alone does not make treatment inadvisable. Treatment, including surgery, may be indicated to correct a deformity in an ambulatory patient and make him more socially acceptable, to help a wheelchair patient sit better, transfer, or walk, to help a bedridden patient sit with more stability, or to improve his nursing care and hygiene. Treatment may be indicated to make life fuller and more enjoyable for the patient and for those around him. However, each problem must be faced realistically, each goal must be identified, and a method of treatment must be used for each goal that is consistent with the expected benefits.

Ingram, Withers, and Speltz in a study of hospitalized children receiving intensive inpatient rehabilitation treatment (physical, occupational, and speech therapy, and special education) demonstrated that 50% of the children with an IQ below 70 benefited more than would be expected from normal maturation. Their test involved an extensive evaluation of motor and social skills and is described in a later section (see below and p. 2852).

Numerous tests have been devised to predict the probable improvement resulting from treatment in the cerebral palsied patient and to measure that improvement or the lack of it. We have not developed a standardized method to evaluate treatment adequately. The variables in this group of patients are so numerous that to establish a group of controls is practically impossible. Also it may be inhumane to withhold a promising treatment program from a group of patients so that they may act as controls. Almost all studies are retrospective ones and relate to the ability to perform certain functions that would occur in the process of normal development. We measure motor milestones by the date at which certain activities appear or fail to appear with regard to chronologic age, such as the presence of primitive reflex patterns, sitting, crawling, creeping, cruising, standing, speaking, walking, and social adjustment. A number of proven tests that measure these normal milestones are available, and we use them to compare a handicapped child's achievements to those of normal children. Some of the tests currently in use are the Gesell Developmental Scales, the Bayley Scales of Infant Development, the Denver Developmental Screening Test, and the Milani-Comparetti Motor Development Test.

Primitive reflex patterns of motor activity that are outgrown as the normal nervous system matures are demonstrated in children with cerebral palsy for longer periods of time after birth, and some remain permanently. Furthermore, some cerebrocortical reactions needed for standing and walking in the normal child may develop fully, late, or not at all in the child with cerebral palsy. Other reflex patterns, on which integrated and skillful function of the motor system seems to be built, may be delayed or may never appear. In a child with cerebral palsy, these and other patterns of primitive motor activity should be sought. First, they can be used to determine the patient's neurologic age and, by comparing this age with the chronologic age, a neurologic quotient can be established that may significantly influence treatment and the prognosis for improvement. Second, the continued presence of the primitive reflex patterns contributes much to the development of deformities.

Johnson, Zuck, and Wingate and Ingram, Withers, and Speltz developed tests that measure the rate at which motor and social skills are acquired by patients with cerebral palsy. By regular and repeated testing they were able to assess the extent of the handicap and whether it was being influenced by the treatment program and to make tentative predictions concerning the future development of the patient. Ingram, Withers, and Speltz found that when the motor quotient (motor age times 100, divided by the chronologic age) was 15 or less, independent walking was

unlikely, but when it was 25 or more, walking could be expected. Beals, using a test of motor performance similar to that described by Ingram, Withers, and Speltz, studied 93 spastic paraplegic or diplegic patients followed to the age of 7 years or older. In an attempt to determine the severity of the handicap in a given patient, he developed a "severity index," which is a statement of the motor age in months at the chronologic age of 3 years. Using this index, Beals attempted to predict the ultimate motor performance of the individual patient and thus to establish realistic goals in treatment.

Paine observed that the presence of tonic neck reflexes is usually incompatible with independent standing balance and with the ability to make alternating movements of the lower extremities necessary for walking. In his experience, if a child learns to sit alone before the age of 2 years, usually he will learn to walk independently. If a child learns to sit alone between the ages of 2 and 4 years, the likelihood of his learning to stand and walk independently is about 50%. If a child has not learned to sit alone before the age of 4 years, rarely will he learn to stand or walk without support. Finally, if a child has not learned to walk before the age of 8 years and if he does not have severe contractures that would otherwise prevent walking, it is unlikely he will ever learn to walk.

Bleck studied the incidence and persistence of certain pathologic reflexes in children with cerebral palsy, and developed certain prognostic signs based on the presence or absence of a few important infantile reflexes. A favorable sign in prognosis for walking is sitting by the age of 2 years. Poor prognostic signs for walking are (1) an impossible asymmetric tonic neck reflex (Fig. 65-1, A); (2) a persistent Moro reflex (Fig. 65-1, B) (a loud noise or a sudden jerk of the table causes the upper limbs to extend away from the side of the body and then to come together in an embracing pattern); (3) a strong extensor thrust on vertical suspension (Fig. 65-1, C) (when the child is held upright by the armpits, the lower extremities stiffen out straight); (4) a persistent neck-righting reflex (Fig. 65-1, D) (when the head is turned, the shoulder, trunk, pelvis, and lower limbs follow the turned head); and (5) absence of the normal parachute reaction (Fig. 65-1, E) after 11 months (when the child is lifted horizontally by the waist and suddenly lowered to the table, normally the arms and hands extend to the table as though to protect from the fall). In Bleck's experience, spastic hemiplegics usually walked by 21 months; most children with cerebral palsy who will walk at all will walk by the age of 7 years.

Bleck has also analyzed pathologic reflexes in children 1 to 8 years old. The reflexes recorded in the study were symmetric tonic neck reflex (Fig. 65-1, F), neck-righting reflex, foot placement reflex, asymmetric tonic neck reflex, Moro reflex, parachute reflex, and positive supporting reaction. Figure 65-2 shows the incidence of these various reflexes in children with cerebral palsy who have not walked by age 8 years. The supporting reaction reflex is positive in practically all children who do not walk, the parachute reflex is absent in seven-eighths of them, and the Moro and asymmetric tonic reflexes are present in three-fourths of children who do not walk by age 8 years. The persistence of these infantile automatisms indicates

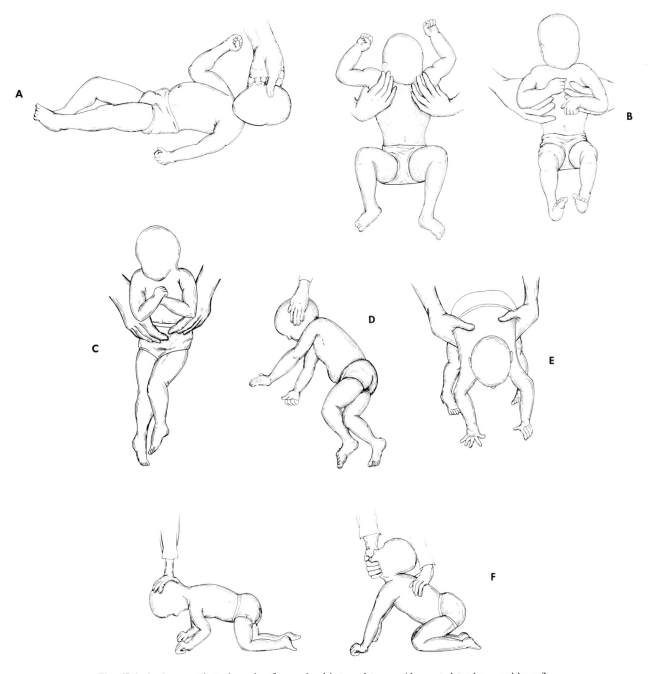

Fig. 65-1. A, Asymmetric tonic neck reflex: as head is turned to one side, contralateral arm and knee flex. **B,** Moro reflex: as neck is suddenly extended, upper limbs extend away from body and then come together in embracing pattern. **C,** Extensor thrust reflex: as child is held upright by armpits, lower extremities stiffen out straight. **D,** Neck-righting reflex: as head is turned, shoulders, trunk, pelvis, and lower extremities follow turned head. **E,** Parachute reaction: as child is suspended at waist and suddenly lowered forward toward table, arms and hands extend to table in a protective manner. **F,** Symmetric tonic neck reflex: as neck is flexed, arms flex and legs extend. Opposite occurs as neck is extended.

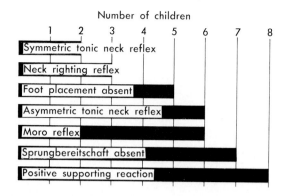

Number of children

Fig. 65-2. Incidence of pathologic reflexes in children with cerebral palsy who have not walked by age 8 years (see text). (Courtesy Dr. E.E. Bleck; from Goldner, J.L.: In American Academy of Orthopaedic Surgeons: Instructional course lectures, vol. 20, St. Louis, 1971, The C.V. Mosby Co.)

extensive, severe brain damage and a poor prognosis for ambulation, self-help, and the performance of activites of daily living.

Training program

The training program for a child with cerebral palsy should be directed toward developing (1) speech or communication, (2) self-help, (3) locomotion or mobility, and (4) education. Bobath and Köng (1966) have both emphasized that the earlier the training program is begun, the better. The earlier the diagnosis of a motor or postural deficit is made, the earlier the training can be started. The experience of movement plays an important part is a child's motor, cognitive, social, and emotional development.

The responsibility for an early diagnosis is placed on the pediatrician, and children ''at risk'' must be carefully evaluated. All patients who have been treated in a neonatal intensive care unit for prematurity, perinatal anoxia, or perinatal seizures, and all patients who have an ''at risk'' mother should be followed closely to detect any early abnormalities. Treatment should begin preferably by 3 months of age, when feeding and handling problems or abnormal muscle tone become apparent. During the first 2 years of life there is said to be a plasticity of the developing central nervous system (Bobath, 1967), and this plasticity may be molded by appropriate sensorimotor stimuli in the early years. Early treatment programs strongly involve the parents and teachers in the so-called intervention technique.

Early treatment may use one of several techniques. The most popular types of programs are briefly summarized, but the choice of the program used will probably depend on the knowledge and training of the treating developmental therapists (physical and occupational therapists specifically trained in developmental therapies). Early treatment methods are molded into a developmental training program that continues into later life.

Harris has summarized the following four types of intervention therapy for young patients: (1) the neurodevelopmental approach, (2) the sensorimotor treatment approach, (3) the proprioceptive neuromuscular facilitation approach, and (4) the neuromuscular reflex treatment approach.

The neurodevelopmental approach was developed by Carl and Berta Bobath and has gained worldwide popularity. The aim is to achieve normal muscle tone, movement patterns, and posture by appropriate sensory stimuli. The child is trained by being placed in positions that inhibit abnormal muscle tone and reflex patterns and that favor automatic movements rather than the performance of conscious voluntary movements. Automatic reactions are the prerequisites of voluntary movement by which sitting, standing, and walking are achieved.

The sensorimotor stimulation technique is based on the neurologic concepts of Rood. Different types of sensory stimuli are used to inhibit unwanted abnormal patterns of movement and to encourage more normal patterns. The therapeutic program follows a normal developmental sequence and is based on the blending and interacting of phasic muscle activity for movement and mobility responses with the tonic muscle groups to provide postures and positions. This is achieved by various sensory stimuli such as stretch, vibration, joint compression, lateral resistance to improve posture, and subcutaneous stimuli, such as brushing and icing of muscles to lower the threshold of muscle responses. These techniques are described in detail by Stockmeyer.

Proprioceptive neuromuscular facilitation is a technique developed by Knott and Voss. Motor learning by this method involves movement patterns rather than the use of individual muscle groups. These movement patterns are based on a developmental sequence and involve patterns that are spiral or diagonal. Resistance is used to stimulate other parts of the body, thereby encouraging stronger muscle action. Auditory stimulation, proprioception, and tactile stimulation (in the form of touch, stretch, and pressure), are used to improve posture, muscle tone, and movement.

Fay developed a neuromuscular reflex treatment program before 1950 that attempts to teach motion as it developed in an evolutionary pattern. Patterns of movement are emphasized before complex integrated movement is sought. Passive exercises and total patterns are used to affect sensory feedback, and reflex responses are used to develop coordinated movement and tone. After the basic reflex patterns are established, active exercises are used. The patterns used progress from the prone to the quadriped position, to the plantigrade position, and then to the erect posture.

The early intervention techniques may be used in other handicapping conditions, such as those with an element of mental retardation, because all are based on primitive reflex activity, either its use or its inhibition.

There are some questions concerning the value of early intervention: how much is good for the child, how much is bad for the child, and what is the effect on the whole family unit? Denhoff reviewed the status of the infant stimulation or enrichment programs after 15 years of use in this country. Any treatment program must first establish, through proper evaluation of the patient, long-term goals that are appropriate. Short-term goals to be achieved are then set to advance to the long-term ones.

Early intervention techniques are practiced in the home with the parents as the primary caregivers. The child must first establish his relationship with the family, and the family must establish its relationship with the child. A strong family bond in the home of a handicapped child is a much-needed asset. Periodic visits for evaluation clarify the techniques and measure the progress as goals are achieved. Thus the treatment program is updated periodically for the caregiver.

Available training facilities should be used appropriately according to the patient's potential and should not be overprescribed when little if any potential for improvement is present. Physical therapy is not a panacea to be prescribed indiscriminately for all patients. The waste of time and effort in the absence of potential for improvement is intolerable. Unfortunately, it does occur as a response to parental or caretaker pressure.

There are other techniques for treatment of the cerebral palsied child. Some are based on Phelps' teaching and are applied according to each child's clinical type of involvement.

Spastic paralysis is characterized by the presence of an exaggerated stretch reflex. Because of this reflex, a spastic muscle when stretched will contract as much as possible. Passive stretching of a spastic muscle in an infant is of course not met with as much resistance as in an older child, and if treatment is begun early, contractures can often be prevented. Gross movements of the arms and legs and the value of relaxation can be taught early; the more complicated fundamental movements can then be taught later. Muscles are educated by encouraging the child to repeat the fundamental movements; the intact parts of the brain are thus gradually trained to perform the functions of the parts that have been damaged.

The older child with spastic paralysis is helped by active exercises to strengthen the weak antagonists. Passive exercises should be avoided if possible, but when they are necessary, the stretch reflex should be excited as little as possible. Simple conditioning exercises are indicated first; skilled movements are postponed until later. The muscles are first taught to move through accurate ranges of motion at properly regulated speeds. As training progresses, coordination is sought. This is manifested by improvement in the rhythm, speed, and accuracy of movements. Training is continued in voluntary motion that overcomes the stretch reflex and increases the child's ability to carry out a given motion without being hindered by this reflex.

Because any affected extremity has a combination of spastic, normal, weak, and paralyzed muscles and therefore muscle imbalance, contractures are likely to develop. Every effort should be made, of course, to prevent these contractures. The most common is contracture of the triceps surae, resulting in equinus deformity. This muscle group should therefore be stretched repeatedly to gain the full range of dorsiflexion of the ankle (with the knee and hip extended) and to maintain it. A brace should be worn at night to prevent the foot from resting in equinus position and to maintain the position gained. A brace with a single round caliper (a rod), a right-angled stop, and a T-strap is the most efficient; the rod may be increasingly bent from time to time to dorsiflex the ankle and gradually stretch the triceps surae. The brace must be worn every night until growth of the long bones is complete, usually at age 14 to 15 years.

Heat-molded, plastic ankle-foot orthoses are presently being used more often than braces. They are more comfortable and lighter in weight, may be worn inside the shoes, and are easily made. For the most part, they cannot be adjusted to accommodate for growth and must be periodically replaced.

Braces are also used to enable the patient to stand and thus to gain balance as well as strength; and when standing, of course, he can use his arms more easily and can see better what goes on about him.

Athetosis is characterized by constant involuntary motions (which disappear during relaxation or sleep), but the fundamental ability of the patient to move muscles normally is unimpaired. It is also characterized by voluntary tension of entire extremities because the patient constantly tries to overcome the involuntary motions. This tension eventually becomes habitual and produces findings suggestive of spasticity. Still another characteristic is the placing of parts in distorted positions. All available muscles are used to produce a given position, and when an attempt is made either by braces or surgery to interfere with this position and to correct the distortion, other muscles may produce the same position or a similar one.

Repetitive exercises are an unsuccessful treatment for athetosis. Rather, the patient should be trained in voluntary and conscious relaxation by the Jacobson technique. After involuntary motions have been abolished, purposeful and coordinated ones are taught. Any contractures are treated with braces or, if severe enough, with surgery. Braces may also be used to control involuntary motions.

In *ataxia* the kinesthetic sense is disturbed or lost, and consequently balance and coordination are impaired. The training program should include measures to improve muscle tone, to develop sitting and standing balance, to teach walking, to improve the gait, and to improve eye-to-hand skills. Muscle tone is improved by physical therapy. Sitting balance is taught first, then standing balance, and finally walking. To improve the gait, various schemes are used to narrow the width of its base, to improve the placement of the feet, and to increase the patient's sense of security. Short braces to prevent extension of the ankle beyond the neutral position are often required. The shoes should have rubber soles and heels because they grip the floor better. Eye-to-hand skill is usually hard for the patient to develop because of his characteristic difficulty in fixing his eyes on objects close by. Surgery is almost never indicated. Bioelectric feedback training is especially effective in the ataxic patient.

The training program for *rigidity* is similar to that for spastic paralysis, but because of the more severe damage to the brain, it is less effective.

For *tremors* medication is often useful in controlling involuntary movements. The training program is similar to that for athetosis.

An orthopaedic surgeon seldom sees cerebral palsied children before 12 months of age unless he directs a training or treatment center that receives referrals from a neonatal intensive care unit or from pediatricians. Thus the orthopaedic surgeon is seldom involved in the care of infants with cerebral palsy. Once abnormal postural and movement patterns appear, especially if there is an inability to stand or walk, the orthopaedic surgeon is consulted. Treatment depends first on a provisional prognosis and

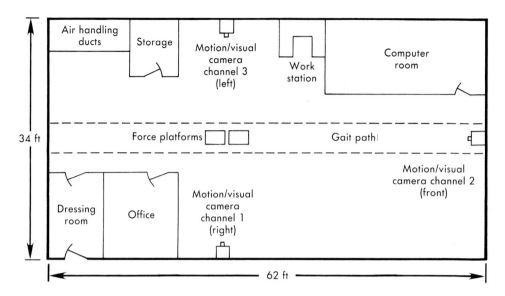

Fig. 65-3. Typical floor plan of gait laboratory with adequate space for ease in working. (Redrawn from Gage, J.R.: Bull. Hosp. Jt. Dis. Orthop. Inst. **43**:148, 1983.)

then on more accurate prognoses arrived at by various tests. To measure both the level and the progress of development in patients with neuromuscular disorders such as cerebral palsy, three tests have been devised.

The first test was designed by Johnson, Zuck, and Wingate to measure the level and progress of motor development alone. It uses artificial situations and mechanical devices; each item in the test is given a value, and the motor ages of the upper and of the lower extremities are determined by adding the values of the items successfully completed. The motor age of the upper extremities is then divided by the chronologic age to arrive at an upper motor quotient; in the same way a lower motor quotient is derived for the lower extremities. These two quotients provide an index of motor handicap. Progress of motor development in terms of months is then correlated with such variables as the type of palsy, the IQ, and the type and duration of treatment.

The second test was designed by Ingram, Withers, and Speltz to measure the level and progress of both motor and social development. After much consultation with Gesell and Ilg and with Zuck, Johnson, and Wingate, a system of age zones was adopted, a series of activities to be performed by patients in each age zone was listed, and a scale of development of both motor and social behavior was devised. The test is principally based on the developmental schedules outlined by Gesell and Amatruda. It yields both a motor age and a social age. The motor age obtained indicates basic motor skills of the upper and lower extremities and is roughly in the province of physical therapy; the social age obtained indicates ability to operate in society and to perform necessary acts of daily living and is in the province of occupational therapy. Both of these tests attempt to satisfy a need for an objective test of the progress of a patient under a given training program.

The third test was designed by Beals and, as already mentioned, is similar to that developed by Ingram, Withers, and Speltz. The "severity index" measured by his test

seems to be valuable chiefly in children who have been observed repeatedly before the age of 3 years.

The prognostic signs of Bleck to forecast the ability to walk (p. 2848) is another useful guide.

As a general rule, all hemiplegics will walk. Most diplegics will walk, although some may require assistance, and a large number of quadriplegics and patients with total body involvement will never walk; most of these patients can at least be propped sitters. Thus our goals for hemiplegics are to make the foot plantigrade and to correct the alignment of the involved leg and thus the spine. In the diplegic patient our aim is for better general alignment and stride in the lower extremities, along with leveling of the pelvis to help prevent scoliosis. In the severe quadriplegic our aim may be to modify posture in the legs and feet to aid in wheelchair transfers or simply to aid in daily hygiene. In the bedridden patient alterations in bed posture may be necessary, as well as measures to improve hygiene.

The alignment of the spine is most often linked to the position of the pelvis and lower extremities. Scoliosis appears often enough (40%) that measures to recognize and prevent its occurrence should always be taken.

In the ambulatory patient gait should always be analyzed preoperatively and postoperatively. Static testing of muscles, bones, and joints should be done first, but never solely relied on. Gait analysis may be simple, such as merely watching the patient's posture, gait, stride, foot placement, and extremity and spine alignment while walking. Video taped recordings of gait analysis are invaluable in preoperative and postoperative evaluations; they are also a great teaching aid.

Kinetic or dynamic electromyography has improved to the point that it is beneficial in the preoperative and postoperative assessment of both the upper and lower extremities, especially so in problem patients. It is no longer a simple research tool (Fig. 65-3). In its simplest form, it consists of a measured gait path or track, a timing instru-

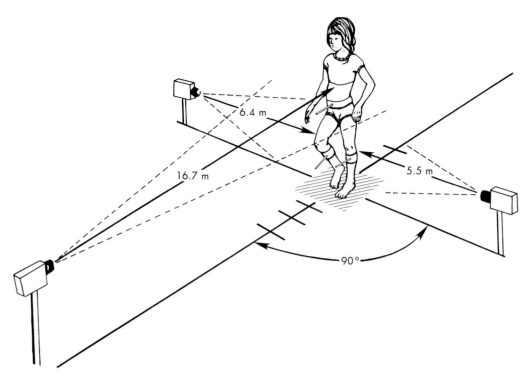

Fig. 65-4. The child's gait is recorded from three directions as he strikes a force plate in the floor. (Redrawn from Sutherland, D.H., et al.: J. Bone Joint Surg. **62-A:**336, 1980.)

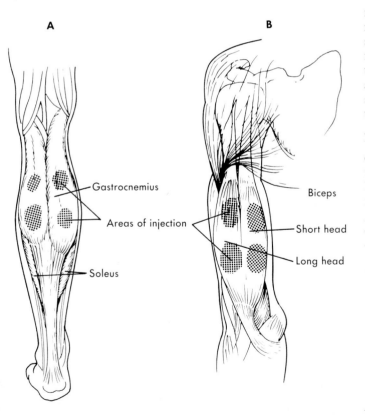

Fig. 65-5. Sites of injection of 45% alcohol solution in calf muscles, **A,** and biceps, **B,** to temporarily weaken muscles. (Redrawn from Carpenter, E.B., and Seitz, D.C.: Dev. Med. Child Neurol. **22:**497, 1980.)

ment, recording cameras in the frontal and lateral planes, multichannel EMG using skin or needle electrodes, foot switches to record foot reactions, and a device to simultaneously record the foot reactions, time, and the tracings on the oscilloscope of the muscle activity. In this way muscle activity may be coordinated with the phases of stance and swing in the gait pattern. Force plates may be added so that the force transmitted through the foot to the force plate gives information about vertical and horizontal loading as well as torque on the extremity (Fig. 65-4). Other peripherals may be added to record ankle, knee, hip, and pelvic flexion, extension, and rotation during the gait cycle. Telemetry is needed to transmit the information to the recording device so that the patient is not encumbered by dangling or trailing wires. All of these may then be computerized to generate graphic reproductions of the gait cycle for easier study and analysis.

Kinesthetic electromyography can also be used to evaluate phasic activity in the upper extremities. Gait analysis in the evaluation of the cerebral palsied patient has been reported extensively by Sutherland, Perry, and Hoffer, Simon et al., and Gage et al.

Another useful tool in the preoperative evaluation is the temporary weakening of the spastic muscles by the injection of alcohol into them at selected sites (Fig. 65-5). This weakening of the muscles shows the permanent improvement that may be expected after surgery. The alcohol injection occasionally results in a permanent alteration of muscle dynamics so that surgery is no longer necessary.

It must be remembered that the lesion causing the alteration of the normal pattern of muscle control is a brain lesion; the patterns of control are determined in the brain, and we may merely alter the peripheral display of these patterns by our treatment.

Indications for surgery

Surgery is most often indicated in patients with *spastic* cerebral palsy and less often in those with dyskinesia.

Its chief role is to help correct local physical defects that interfere with the patient's rehabilitation, but it can also help to correct those that interfere with nursing care. The nonsurgical treatment of patients with cerebral palsy has been emphasized too much in recent years, and thus the help that surgery can bring has often been overlooked. Statistical reports support the thesis that well-performed surgical procedures on properly selected patients yield good results, provided that treatment after surgery is carefully managed. Indeed, a program for treating cerebral palsy that fails to make orthopaedic procedures available to its patients deprives them of one of its most effective aids. However, no surgery should be performed until the patient has been thoroughly evaluated.

Although necessary surgery is justifiably delayed to permit a thorough evaluation of the patient, it should not be delayed too long. Early surgery may shorten the months or years required for physical therapy or sometimes may even eliminate the need for it. It may also make later treatment by bracing and physical therapy more effective than otherwise. The benefits of early surgery may not always be maintained throughout the period of growth, and surgery may become necessary again later; even so, years of physical therapy may be avoided by a carefully planned series of operations.

During the course of conservative treatment, surgery is often necessary because progress has become arrested or because a new deformity or some other complication has developed. Usually surgery is only an incident in the total treatment of a patient with cerebral palsy. But surgery is an important incident, and both the indications for it and the proper time for it should be decided by the group of medical attendants responsible for the care of the specific patient. Much of the success of the operation depends on the quality of care after surgery because few operations used in treating cerebral palsy are definitive. Clear provision must therefore be made for informed aftercare and other treatment for as long as necessary.

Surgery is indicated less often in *athetosis*. Spastic paralysis affects individual muscles, but athetosis is characterized by the placing of parts in distorted positions by any muscles capable of doing so. Consequently, if athetoid muscles or groups of muscles responsible for a given distorted position are transferred or otherwise operated on, the athetosis may shift to other muscles of similar function to produce the same distorted position or a similar one; for example, the finger flexors may become affected after athetoid wrist flexors have been transferred to the dorsum of the wrist. Fortunately, when athetosis has been so shifted, the distorting muscles are usually weaker and are thus less harmful functionally and cosmetically; consequently, surgery is occasionally indicated, even though the athetosis may be expected to shift. Surgery may also be indicated for postural contractures, such as equinus deformities of the ankles and flexion contractures of the knees and hips,

that result from prolonged sitting or lying in poor position before walking is learned; bracing and walking must be postponed until these contractures have been corrected, usually by surgery.

In *rigidity,* the brain is so severely damaged that surgery is rarely indicated except to correct major deformities.

Operations useful in cerebral palsy

Surgery may be useful in cerebral palsy (1) to correct deformity, whether static, dynamic, or both, (2) to balance muscle power, or (3) to stabilize uncontrollable joints.

Static deformities are corrected chiefly by lengthening tendons, by capsulotomies, fasciotomies, and osteotomies such as of the tarsal bones for varus or valgus deformity, or of the tibia, femur, or forearm bones for angular or rotary deformity. Dynamic deformities are corrected, at least partially, by lengthening musculotendinous units (which also weakens the units) or by tenotomy of tendons such as the tibialis posterior, psoas, hamstring, hip adductor, and soleus muscles, or by tenotomy or myotomy of some muscles of the forearm and hand.

Balancing the muscle power acting on a joint is difficult in cerebral palsy. Some of the obstacles to satisfactory function after tendon transfers in patients with this affection are (1) the impairment in voluntary control of muscles, (2) the slowness of voluntary movements, (3) the lowered threshold to stretch reflexes, (4) the frequency of associated sensory deficits, (5) the frequency with which antagonistic muscle groups exhibit synchronous electric activity without regard to the function being undertaken (dysphasic activity), (6) the fact that voluntary contraction of a spastic muscle begins simultaneously throughout the muscle, in contrast to a normal muscle in which different parts contract at different times, and (7) the fact that coordinated and skillful use of a muscle, already difficult enough for the cerebral palsied patient to learn when the muscle is in its normal location and serving its normal function, is even more difficult to learn when the function of the muscle has been changed or even reversed after surgery (that he has difficulty in learning to integrate the transferred muscle into patterns of normal and reflex activity is easily understood). For these and other reasons most tendon transfers in cerebral palsy lack the highly coordinated function of most tendon transfers seen in poliomyelitis or peripheral nerve injury. Often their chief functions are to remove a dynamic but deforming force and to serve as a motorized tenodesis.

Rerouting a muscle to alter its function has limited popularity. Once a spastic muscle is transferred, it still retains its spasticity. The muscle may be weakened, but it is still spastic. For example, if the spastic tibialis posterior muscle is rerouted anteriorly through the interosseous membrane to the dorsum of the foot, it is changed from a spastic invertor and plantar flexor to a spastic dorsiflexor. The phasic activity of the muscle can be easily sorted out for decision making by kinetic electromyography.

Neurectomy of some of the motor branches of nerves to a particular muscle is based on the idea that by resecting some of the branches that innervate a spastic muscle its strength may be decreased so that its power equals that of its antagonist; in practice, however, muscle balance is rarely if ever attained. To minimize errors in indications for neurectomy, Barnett has temporarily paralyzed the branches considered for neurectomy by exposing and crushing them. While the branches are regenerating, the effects of the contemplated neurectomy can be accurately evaluated, and if the desired results have been obtained, neurectomy is indicated. To obtain a more transient paralysis of the branches considered for neurectomy, they may be infiltrated with procaine; the immediate effects of such a paralysis are apparent, but the permanent effects and the patient's ability to learn new patterns of motor activity usually cannot be evaluated in such a short time.

Uncontrollable joints may be stabilized by operations that continue to be among the most satisfactory in orthopaedic surgery. In cerebral palsy, triple arthodesis is useful in stabilizing the unbalanced foot, and the Grice extraarticular arthrodesis of the subtalar joint (p. 2963) is valuable in correcting equinovalgus deformity; when indicated, arthrodesis of the wrist is satisfactory.

Treatment after surgery. If the patient is to receive the maximum benefit from a given operation and if this benefit is to be retained for future use, continued attention to the many details in the period immediately after surgery is extremely important. Recurrence of a deformity after satisfactory correction is often caused by inadequate treatment after surgery. Treatment should continue until the patient is skeletally mature.

FOOT

In cerebral palsy, spastic paralysis may cause one or more of the following deformities of the foot: (1) equinus, (2) valgus, (3) varus, (4) talipes calcaneus, (5) clawing of the toes, and (6) adduction deformity of the forefoot.

Equinus deformity

Equinus deformity in spastic paralysis is caused by one of the following mechanisms:
1. Spastic triceps surae versus spastic dorsiflexors
2. Spastic triceps surae versus normal dorsiflexors
3. Spastic triceps surae versus weak dorsiflexors
4. Normal triceps surae versus weak dorsiflexors
5. Weak triceps surae versus weak dorsiflexors

Regardless of its cause, equinus deformity in spastic paralysis should be treated by the simplest technique, conservative or surgical, that is capable of correcting it. Conservative treatment is often sufficient, especially in children, but sometimes the deformity is so severe that surgery is obviously indicated, and months of conservative treatment would only be a waste of time. In any event, the method of treatment must be appropriate to the deformity. If not effective in correcting the deformity within a reasonable time, it should be abandoned in favor of a different course of treatment.

In a *young child* the deformity can usually be corrected conservatively by stretching the triceps surae both manually and by using a brace. The most satisfactory brace is the single-caliper brace with a round rod, this rod at first being bent to accommodate the deformity. As the deformity gradually decreases, the rod is bent from time to time to help stretch the triceps surae. When the deformity is mild, this brace is worn only at night. When the deformity

is severe enough to prevent the foot from being placed properly on the floor in walking, another brace of the same type is also worn during the day. The heel of the shoe is elevated so that the stretch reflex is not excited.

Since the development of heat-molded plastic, most braces or orthoses are now made of this material rather than metal. The development of these improved appliances has led to a change in terminology: *orthosis* is now preferred over *brace*. A particular orthosis is described by the initials of the joints that it stabilizes. For example, an orthosis that stabilizes the ankle and foot is called an AFO (ankle-foot orthosis); one that also stabilizes the knee is called a KAFO (knee-ankle-foot orthosis); if the hip is included in the orthosis, it is known as an HKAFO. These abbreviations are useful to describe the basic orthoses. Heat-treated plastic orthoses are actually more comfortable, lighter, less noisy, and more cosmetically acceptable because they can be worn inside the shoes. Their effectiveness can be easily evaluated since the foot, ankle, and leg can be easily viewed while in the orthosis. When heated, they may be molded into different shapes to place the foot in more dorsiflexion as heel cord length is gained.

After the deformity has been corrected enough to allow dorsiflexion to the neutral position, the daytime brace or AFO is omitted. One is still worn at night and it is appropriately bent at the ankle, usually at intervals of 8 to 10 weeks, until full dorsiflexion is possible. This position is then maintained by an orthosis at night until growth of the long bones is complete. Unless a brace or orthosis is worn at night until skeletal maturity, the deformity usually recurs, just as it may recur after surgery unless a brace is worn. The deformity tends to recur during growth because the tibia grows in length faster than the triceps surae, making the muscle group act like a bowstring. That the foot usually rests in an equinus position at night is also a factor. It must always be remembered when treating crippled children, especially those with cerebral palsy, that muscle imbalance combined with habitually faulty body posture and growth almost always results in deformity.

When the deformity is severe or fails to yield to stretching and to the use of a brace or orthosis as just outlined, it can usually be corrected promptly by using wedging plaster casts similar to those described by Kite for treating congenital clubfoot. After the deformity has been completely corrected, the ankle is immobilized in full dorsiflexion in a cast for about 3 weeks. The cast is then removed, and an AFO is worn at night.

When conservative treatment has failed, or when deformity is so severe that conservative treatment would be ineffective, surgery is indicated.

In *older children* and *adults* conservative treatment may be sufficient, but surgical correction is necessary more often than in young children.

Care must be taken when surgically correcting an equinus deformity. Overcorrection leads to a calcaneus deformity that is difficult to brace against, interferes more with gait, and is difficult to correct surgically.

Ankle equinus may be secondary to knee flexion, and any dynamic knee flexion deformity must be evaluated as a possible cause of the equinus. If placing the knee in a cylinder cast in extension causes the ankle equinus to disappear, then lengthening the tendo calcaneus will not correct the knee flexion deformity. A dynamic EMG will reveal a decrease in activity in the triceps surae as the knee is passively extended. Equinus is preferred to calcaneus; the ''jump'' position of flexed hips and knees and equinus ankles is better handled than the crouched position of flexed hips and knees and calcaneus feet that lowers the buttocks closer to the walking surface and affords no push-off in walking.

Ankle clonus can be treated by lengthening the tendo calcaneus if there is a fixed equinus contracture. If the equinus is dynamic, a partial neurectomy of the motor nerves to the gastrocnemius or soleus muscles or merely advancing the insertion of the tendo calcaneus anteriorly on the calcaneus may be performed.

SURGICAL CORRECTION OF EQUINUS DEFORMITY

Surgery is indicated in equinus deformity when conservative treatment has failed or when the deformity is so severe that conservative treatment would be ineffective. Because the contracture tends to recur until growth is complete, the status of the length of the tendo calcaneus must be continuously monitored until growth is complete.

The following five types of operations, listed in order of preference, are useful for correcting an equinus deformity, depending on whether it is dynamic or fixed: (1) lengthening the tendo calcaneus (TAL), (2) lengthening the tendon of the gastrocnemius alone, (3) releasing the heads of origin of the gastrocnemius from the femur, (4) advancing the insertion of the tendo calcaneus anteriorly on the calcaneus (heel cord advancement, HCA), and (5) partial tibial nerve neurectomy, at times combined with recession of the heads of origin of the gastrocnemius.

The proper operation can be selected by determining the mechanism responsible for the equinus deformity. The amount of lengthening required must be determined to prevent overlengthening the tendo calcaneus which would cause an undesirable calcaneus gait. There is no mathematic method for determining the amount of lengthening required, but two methods have recently been proposed to prevent overlengthening. Gaines and Ford divided their patients into three groups according to the severity of the spasticity and the strength and degree of voluntary control of the ankle plantar flexors and dorsiflexors. After the tendon had been divided by a Z-plasty procedure, the knee was fully extended and the passive excursion of the proximal gastrocsoleus muscle group was determined by pulling it down with a Kocher clamp. It was allowed to retract proximally one half of this distance, and the distal end of the tendo calcaneus was then sutured to the proximal end by absorbable sutures in a side-to-side fashion. The ankle was placed in a neutral position in the mildly involved patients; it was placed in 10 degrees of dorsiflexion in those in the moderate group, and in 20 degrees of dorsiflexion in the most severe group. Of 43 patients, there were none with a postoperative calcaneus gait, and only three had recurrent equinus gait.

Garbarino and Clancy reported a method of geometric analysis to determine the amount to lengthen the tendo calcaneus (Fig. 65-6). They also did the lengthening through an open incision and with a Z-plasty procedure. With the

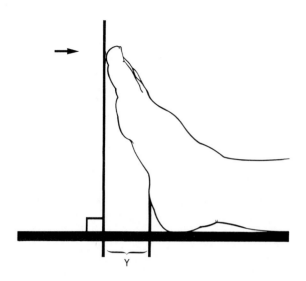

Fig. 65-6. Geometric formula for tendo calcaneus lengthening. Tendo calcaneus is lengthened one-half of distance Y (see text). (Redrawn from Garbarino, J.L., and Clancy, M.: J. Pediatr. Orthop. **5:**573, 1985.)

patient relaxed or lightly anesthetized, a straight edge was placed under the head of the first metatarsal and perpendicular to the long axis of the tibia. The distance from the straight edge to the heel pad was halved, and the tendo calcaneus was lengthened this amount. In their review of 26 such operations, there were no patients with iatrogenic calcaneus gait, and none with recurrent equinus in a 6-month follow-up period.

Either of these methods may be used to determine at surgery how much to lengthen the tendon, but postoperative care and a long follow-up are always necessary.

OPERATIONS THAT RELEASE TRICEPS SURAE

In 1924 Silfverskiöld made an important contribution to the analysis and treatment of spastic equinus contracture by distinguishing two significant types of this deformity: (1) those that cannot be corrected regardless of the position of the knee, and (2) those that cannot be corrected when the knee is fully extended, but that can be passively corrected when the knee is flexed.

The *first type* of deformity is caused by contracture of both the gastrocnemius and soleus. For this type Silfverskiöld lengthened the tendo calcaneus; this operation is appropriate for the mechanics of the structures concerned. In spastic paralysis, the tendon should be lengthened only enough to allow dorsiflexion of the ankle to the neutral position.

According to Silfverskiöld, the *second type* of deformity is caused chiefly by contracture of the gastrocnemius muscle, because when this muscle is relaxed by passively flexing the knee the deformity disappears. By transplanting the heads of origin of the gastrocnemius muscle to a level distal to the knee, he transformed a muscle that crossed two joints into a muscle that crosses only one. The gastrocnemius thus becomes, as it were, a second soleus. In some instances he also resected appropriate branches of the tibial nerve to the gastrocnemius, to make its motor action still weaker. He left the soleus undisturbed so that it could function during push-off in walking. According to Silver and Simon equinus deformity in cerebral palsy, especially in children, is almost always caused by contracture of the gastrocnemius muscle alone; only 4 children in their series of 70 who had surgery to correct equinus deformity required lengthening of the tendo calcaneus because of contracture of both the gastrocnemius and soleus.

Perry et al. have reported a clinical and electromyographic study of the triceps surae in a group of 17 patients with cerebral palsy before and after surgery. They used the Silfverskiöld test already described, and a positive test indicated a contracture of the gastrocnemius muscle alone. By the use of electromyography, during gait and during the time of clinical examination, electromyographic activity of the gastrocnemius muscle could be separated from that of the soleus. If isolated gastrocnemius phase distortion or clonus or both were found, a gastrocnemius recession was performed. If combined soleus and gastrocnemius distortion or clonus was found, the tendo calcaneus was lengthened.

Before surgery, plantar flexion tension against gentle pressure was greatest in all patients when the knees were extended. During a vigorous stretch to a point of discomfort, only eight patients demonstrated more than 15 degrees of difference in the dorsiflexion arc of the foot with change in the knee position. During surgery with the patients under general anesthesia, no significant differences in the dorsiflexion arc with changes in knee position were noted, even in these eight patients. Consequently none of this group of patients had contractures, only a tonic neurologic imbalance. Also before surgery all patients had a distortion of the phasic activity of the triceps surae muscles; that is, the gastrocnemius or soleus muscle or both were active in the swing phase as well as in the stance phase. In normal people even in stance, the soleus becomes active after a delay of about 10% of the stance phase of the gait cycle and the gastrocnemius usually waits a bit longer, averaging a 17% delay. Therefore any initiation of triceps surae activity during swing phase is a sign of abnormal muscle action. In most patients the electromyogram after surgery revealed diminished activity of the gastrocnemius, the soleus, or both in the swing phase.

Electromyographic recordings of the triceps surae during the quick stretch test demonstrated in some patients a neurologic mechanism that simultaneously activates both the soleus and the gastrocnemius, and patients with this primitive synergy have increased tone in both muscles whatever the position of the knee. In this situation, correction of the equinus deformity requires lengthening of the tendo calcaneus rather than the gastrocnemius alone to decrease the hyperreaction of both muscles.

During the Silfverskiöld test in an awake child, it cannot always be determined whether the test is positive because of gastrocnemius spasticity (or contracture) or because of the primitive extensor reflex in which both the soleus and the gastrocnemius are activated by the quick stretch. If electromyography is not available, the child can be examined under anesthesia and the findings can be compared with those elicited when the child is fully awake. During anesthesia deep enough to eliminate all reflexes, the simple mechanical status of the muscles can be determined, that is, which of the two muscles is contracted. The surgeon can determine whether the deformity is primarily dynamic or is caused by a contracture. Then the proper choice between lengthening the tendo calcaneus and releasing the gastrocnemius can be made in the operating room. It must be remembered, however, that a contracture causes a spastic muscle to respond to stretch sooner than otherwise and that this mechanism apparently accounts for the differential findings shown only by gait electromyography, which can demonstrate whether the patient exhibits the primitive extensor reflex or whether the contracted gastrocnemius is responding early during walking.

In practice, we always lengthen the tendo calcaneus for an equinus deformity. We no longer do gastrocnemius recessions or lengthen only the gastrocnemius portion of the tendo calcaneus.

OPEN LENGTHENING OF TENDO CALCANEUS

Based on his observation that the tendo calcaneus rotates about 90 degrees on its longitudinal axis between insertion and origin, in 1942 White described his method of lengthening the tendo calcaneus. The rotation of the tendon fibers is from medial to lateral when viewed from the posterior aspect.

TECHNIQUE (WHITE). Using a posteromedial incision, expose the tendo calcaneus from its insertion onto the calcaneus proximally for 10 cm. Near its insertion onto the calcaneus, divide the anterior two thirds of the tendon. Apply a moderate force in dorsiflexion to the foot, and then divide the medial two thirds of the tendon 5 to 8 cm proximal to the site of the distal division. Forcefully dorsiflex the foot to lengthen the tendon (it slides on itself). Suturing the tendon is usually unnecessary, but may be done when its continuity is doubtful. This method provides a smooth posterior surface of the tendon inferiorly where little subcutaneous fat is present between it and the skin. Close the tendon sheath and skin and apply a long leg cast with the knee extended and the ankle in neutral dorsiflexion.

When heel varus accompanies the equinus, the two incisions may be altered to give a lateral insertion of the tendo calcaneus into the bone (Fig. 65-7).

AFTERTREATMENT. The patient is allowed to bear weight in the long leg cast the day after surgery. The cast is left in place with the knee in full extension for 3 weeks, then a short leg cast is worn for an additional 3 weeks. This cast is then removed and an AFO is fitted with the ankle in neutral dorsiflexion (right angle) for night use until longitudinal bone growth is complete. See also the after treatment for the Hauser technique (p. 2858).

TECHNIQUE (HAUSER). Expose the tendon through a posteromedial incision. Incise two thirds of the tendon transversely at a level 8 to 12 cm proximal to its insertion by inserting a tenotome transversely into the tendon so that its flat surface faces anteroposteriorly, and so that two thirds of the tendon is posterior to the blade. Turn the tenotome blade posteriorly and cut through the tendon to its posterior surface. Then incise the tendon 1.2 cm proximal to its insertion on the calcaneus as follows. Insert a curved tenotome anterior to the medial two thirds of the tendon and

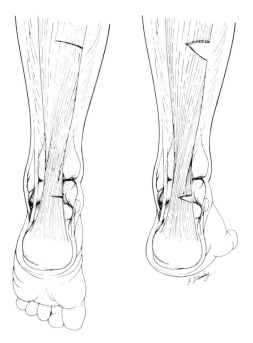

Fig. 65-7. Modification of White technique to effect more lateral insertion of tendo calcaneus onto calcaneus. Distal cut in tendon is made through its medial half, and proximal cut is made through posteromedial half of tendon. (Redrawn from Tachdjian, M.O.: Pediatric orthopaedics, Philadelphia, 1972, W.B. Saunders Co.)

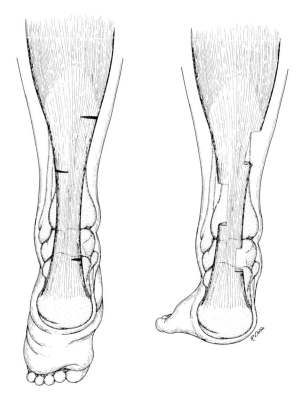

Fig. 65-8. Incisions for percutaneous tendo calcaneus lengthening. Cut ends slide on themselves with forceful dorsiflexion of foot. (From Hsu, J.D., and Hsu, C.L.: In Jahss, M.H. (editor): Disorders of the foot, Philadelphia, 1982, W.B. Saunders Co.)

draw it posteromedially to partially divide the tendon at this point. Dorsiflex the foot and the tendon will slide on itself and lengthen. It is beneficial to incise the slender tendon of the plantaris as it lies alongside the medial aspect of the tendo calcaneus. A concerted effort should be made to repair the defects in the tendon sheath after the tendon has been lengthened to prevent the skin from adhering to the tendon by scar.

AFTERTREATMENT. A cast is applied from midthigh to toes with the knee in full extension and the ankle in neutral dorsiflexion, making certain that the skin along the incision does not blanch when the foot is in neutral dorsiflexion. If it does blanch, it may slough in the postoperative period and cause massive scarring. If the skin blanches in these circumstances, allow the foot to fall into a little equinus before applying the cast. The foot can be brought up to neutral dorsiflexion at the first cast change. The long leg cast is removed at 6 weeks and then an AFO is used as a brace and as a night splint for as long as necessary to prevent recurrence of the equinus.

Often a daytime orthosis will not be needed after lengthening because the dorsiflexor strength is then adequate to overcome the equinus thrust of the spastic triceps surae.

PERCUTANEOUS LENGTHENING OF TENDO CALCANEUS

TECHNIQUE. With the patient prone and the leg prepared from a level above the knee to include the toes, extend the knee and dorsiflex the ankle to tense the tendo calcaneus so that it is subcutaneous, easily outlined, and away from the neurovascular structures anteriorly. Make three partial

tenotomies in the tendo calcaneus (Fig. 65-8). Make the first medial just at the insertion of the tendon onto the calcaneus; cut through one half of the width of the tendon. Make the second tenotomy proximally and medially just below the musculotendinous junction. Make the third laterally through half the width of the tendon midway between the two medial cuts. Dorsiflex the ankle to the desired angle. The incisions do not require closure, only a sterile dressing and a long leg cast with the knee in extension. The two incisions are on the medial side if the heel is in varus as it usually is. If the heel is in valgus, then two incisions are placed laterally and one medially in between.

AFTERTREATMENT. The aftertreatment is the same as described for open lengthening of the tendo calcaneus (p. 2857).

SEMIOPEN SLIDING TENOTOMY OF TENDO CALCANEUS

The small incisions used for this procedure cause little scarring, which decreases the postoperative morbidity and is preferred from a cosmetic standpoint. If equinus recurs, no extensive scarring is present in the skin and subcutaneous tissues or in the tendon itself.

TECHNIQUE. With the patient prone and the leg prepared from above the knee to include the toes, extend the knee fully and dorsiflex the ankle to tense the tendo calcaneus subcutaneously. Make two longitudinal incisions, each 2

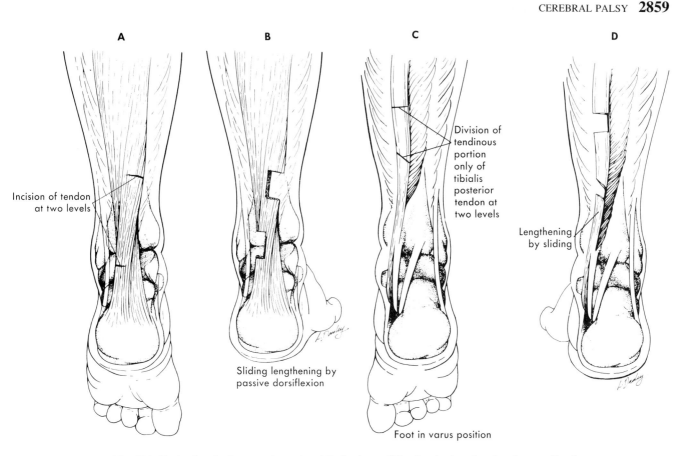

Fig. 65-9. Tendon lengthening procedures. **A** and **B**, Semiopen sliding lengthening of tendo calcaneus. **C** and **D**, Sliding lengthening of tibialis posterior tendon.

cm long, centered over the tendo calcaneus, one at the level of its insertion onto the calcaneus and the other just below the musculotendinous junction (Fig. 65-9). Deepen the lower incision down to the tendon and incise the tendon sheath. Cut the lateral half of the tendon just above its insertion. Deepen the proximal incision down to the tendon sheath and incise it. Under direct view tenotomize the tendon of the plantaris and the posteromedial half of the tendo calcaneus.

Dorsiflex the ankle and the cut portions of the tendon will slide on themselves to the desired length. Close the incision with absorbable subcuticular sutures. Because the skin incisions are made vertically, there is no tendency for them to gap open as the skin is tensed by dorsiflexing the ankle. Apply a sterile dressing and a long leg cast.

AFTERTREATMENT. The aftertreatment is the same as described for open lengthening of the tendo calcaneus (p. 2857).

• • •

Open lengthening is required in recurrent equinus because the normal rotation of the tendon fibers is no longer present and a sliding tenotomy cannot be done easily.

Posterior capsulotomy of the ankle is rarely needed in the cerebral palsied patient. Since some ability to dorsiflex the ankle is usually retained, the posterior capsule does not usually become tight. However, in equinus of long dura-

tion that is allowed to persist into adulthood, the posterior ankle capsule may be contracted and in such instances posterior capsulotomy of the talotibial joint may be necessary to allow adequate ankle dorsiflexion.

LENGTHENING OF GASTROCNEMIUS MUSCLE

The rest of this section discusses the type of deformity described by Silfverskiöld, in which the gastrocnemius muscle is the chief cause of equinus.

In 1942 Green and McDermott reported 15 instances in which they had lengthened the origin of the gastrocnemius muscle to correct equinus deformity in spastic paralysis. According to Banks and Green, this operation is used chiefly for patients with mild deformity and in conjunction with lengthening of the hamstring tendons for flexion contracture of the knee. They do not consider it a valuable operation when equinus deformity alone must be corrected.

In 1950 Strayer described an operation in which the aponeurotic tendon of the gastrocnemius is divided transversely near its junction with that of the soleus, the foot is dorsiflexed to the neutral position, and the retracted proximal part of the tendon is sutured to the underlying soleus. He concluded that the operation is helpful because it alters the proprioceptive impulses received from the extremity, and these impulses in turn modify the stretch reflexes. In 1958 he reviewed his results in 23 patients and rated them as good or excellent in 16. The operation described by Strayer is similar in principle to that of Vulpius in which the aponeurotic tendon of the gastrocnemius is divided and its distal part is allowed to retract distally but is not sutured to the soleus.

Sharrard and Bernstein in 1972 compared lengthening of the tendo calcaneus with gastrocnemius recession using the Strayer technique to correct equinus deformity in cerebral palsy. The tendo calcaneus was lengthened in 77 limbs, and in 18, or 23%, the deformity recurred and surgery was again required. Gastrocnemius recession was performed on 53 limbs, and the deformity recurred enough in 8, or 15%, to require another operation. They concluded that either operation is satisfactory, but that gastrocnemius recession is usually better in paraplegia and lengthening of the tendo calcaneus is better in hemiplegia.

In 1954 Baker reported performing a procedure similar to the Silfverskiöld operation but without partial neurectomy of the tibial nerve. According to Calandriello, Scaglietti has also used a technique similar to that of Silfverskiöld.

In 1959 Silver and Simon reported their experience with that operation of Silfverskiöld that combines transplantation of the heads of origin of the gastrocnemius with neurectomy of some branches of the tibial nerve. They had performed it 110 times, and only five times did the equinus deformity recur. According to them, these five failures were each the result of weakness of the dorsiflexor muscles of the foot that was not properly evaluated before surgery.

In 1966 Bassett and Baker reported their experiences with the three basic operations used to treat equinus deformity: neurectomy of branches of the tibial nerve, distal transplantation of the heads of origin of the gastrocnemius (gastrocnemius recession), and lengthening the aponeurotic tendon of the gastrocnemius. Of 85 extremities treated by neurectomy, the deformity recurred in 26%; of 62 treated by gastrocnemius recession, it recurred in 16%; and of 447 treated by lengthening the aponeurotic tendon of the gastrocnemius using Baker's "tongue-in-groove" modification of the Vulpius operation, it recurred in only 4%. According to them, when the deformity recurred, usually it had been incompletely corrected or care after surgery had been inadequate.

Craig and van Vuren have used metal markers and roentgenograms made before, during, and after lengthening of the tendo calcaneus to demonstrate that the gastrocnemius cannot be sufficiently released by division of this tendon alone. In their opinion, to ensure relaxation of the gastrocnemius muscle, the operation of choice is a combination of gastrocnemius recession by the method of Strayer and lengthening of the tendo calcaneus to correct any deformity that may be caused by the shortened soleus. In 1976 they reported 100 limbs treated by this method and followed for an average of 6 years after surgery; equinus deformity recurred in 9%, and a calcaneus deformity developed in 3%, resulting in insufficient push-off during walking. Their criterion for recurrence was inability to actively dorsiflex the foot above the neutral position with the knee extended.

This combined operation was developed because, in their opinion, the flat tendon and muscle belly of the gastrocnemius muscle are invariably adherent to the underlying soleus and therefore can retract only as far as the belly of the soleus retracts. Because the origin of the soleus extends halfway down the tibia and fibula, this muscle cannot retract further proximally than the middle of the leg; proximal to this point the spastic gastrocnemius still exerts its pull on the underlying structures. To substantiate this opinion, they attached a metal marker to the tendon of the gastrocnemius proximal to the soleus aponeurosis. The foot was then passively forced into maximal dorsiflexion with the knee extended and a roentgenogram was made. Then the tendo calcaneus was lengthened, the foot was again forced into dorsiflexion with the knee extended, and a second roentgenogram was made, revealing that the marker had not moved much proximally as a result of the tendon lengthening. A gastrocnemius recession by the method of Strayer was performed, and only then did the marker move proximally to any marked degree on passive dorsiflexion of the foot with the knee extended. According to Craig and van Vuren, reduction of spasm in the gastrocnemius is especially indicated when some of the equinus deformity is caused by a persistence of the positive support reflex or by the hyperactive stretch reflex.

For equinus deformity in spastic paralysis in which the chief cause is contracture of or increased electrical activity within the gastrocnemius alone, one of the techniques described here (or a modification of one) is recommended; the choice of technique depends on the preference of the surgeon and on the findings in the specific patient. Considering the electromyographic findings before and after surgery by Perry et al. that tendon lengthening diminishes electrical activity within a muscle unit and in the absence of any electromyographic findings to support partial neurectomy, we doubt that such neurectomy is indicated at the time the affected tendon is lengthened.

TECHNIQUE (SILFVERSKIÖLD; SILVER AND SIMON). With the patient under general anesthesia, place him prone on the operating table and apply a pneumatic tourniquet. Make a transverse incision in the popliteal fossa parallel with the skin creases, beginning at a point 1 cm lateral to the biceps femoris tendon and ending at a point 1 cm medial to the semitendinosus tendon. Deepen the incision transversely through the deep fascia and expose the two heads of origin of the gastrocnemius muscle. If neurectomy is to be done, identify the tibial nerve and isolate its motor branches to the heads of origin of the gastrocnemius; one or two branches emerge from each side of the nerve and course obliquely distalward to the medial or lateral head. Pinch these branches gently to identify them. Then resect a small segment from enough of these branches to interrupt half or more of this innervation (Fig. 65-10, A); take great care to avoid injuring the popliteal vein, which lies immediately deep to the tibial nerve.

Now with a curved clamp elevate each head of the gastrocnemius muscle and free it from the posterior aspect of the femoral condyle by dividing it transversely near its attachment to the bone (Fig. 65-10, B and C); take care to avoid injuring the peroneal nerve, which courses near the lateral head. Then by dissecting bluntly with a gauze

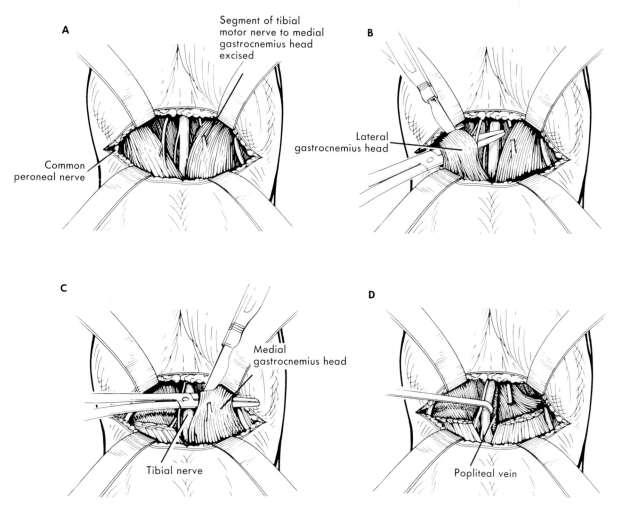

A

Segment of tibial
motor nerve to medial
gastrocnemius head
excised

Common
peroneal nerve

B

Lateral
gastrocnemius head

C

Medial
gastrocnemius head

Tibial nerve

D

Popliteal vein

Fig. 65-10. Technique of Silfverskiöld as described by Silver and Simon. **A,** Segment has been resected from nerve to medial head of gastrocnemius. **B,** Lateral head of gastrocnemius is isolated leaving its nerve intact. **C,** Medial head of gastrocnemius is isolated and divided. **D,** Both heads have been divided and have retracted distally. (Redrawn from Silver, C.M., and Simon, S.D.: J. Bone Joint Surg. **41-A:**1021, 1959.)

sponge, elevate the two heads of the muscle until they are free to a level distal to the knee joint (Fig. 65-10, *D*). Close the wound routinely.

AFTERTREATMENT. A long leg cast is applied, with the ankle dorsiflexed 10 degrees and the knee fully extended. A window is cut from the cast over the apex of the heel to prevent pressure sores. After 6 weeks the cast is removed, and rehabilitation is begun.

TECHNIQUE (VULPIUS, COMPERE). Make a posterior longitudinal incision 7.5 cm long over the middle of the calf. Identify the medial sural cutaneous nerve and retract it. Then expose the aponeurotic tendon of the gastrocnemius and make an inverted V-shaped incision through it (Fig. 65-11). Force the ankle into slight dorsiflexion and thus separate the segments of the tendon. If the aponeurosis of the soleus is also contracted, divide it but do not disturb the soleus muscle itself.

AFTERTREATMENT. A cast is applied from the groin to the toes, with the knee fully extended and the ankle in either slight dorsiflexion or in the neutral position. At 6 weeks the cast is removed, and a single-caliper brace that holds the ankle in the same position is fitted; it is worn at night until growth is complete.

Baker modified the Vulpius technique by lengthening the aponeurotic tendon of the gastrocnemius in a "tongue-in-groove" fashion (Fig. 65-12).

• • •

TECHNIQUE (STRAYER). With the patient prone and with a tourniquet inflated, make a posterior longitudinal incision 10 to 15 cm long over the middle of the calf (Fig. 65-13). Identify and retract the medial sural cutaneous nerve. Deepen the incision through the fascia to expose the gastrocnemius muscle; by blunt dissecton separate this muscle from the underlying soleus distally to where its aponeurotic tendon joins that of the soleus to form the tendo calcaneus. Insert a probe or clamp deep to the gastrocnemius and sever its tendon. Then dorsiflex the foot; a gap 2 to

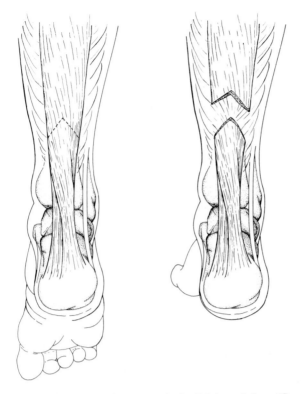

Fig. 65-11. Lengthening of gastrocnemius by Vulpius technique. (Courtesy Drs. E.L. Compere and W.T. Schnute.)

2.5 cm wide will appear between the segments of severed tendon. Then dissect the two muscle bellies from their medial and lateral attachments to the deep fascia proximally into the popliteal fossa and pass a finger from side to side beneath the muscle to completely separate the gastrocnemius from the soleus. This allows the gastrocnemius to retract farther proximally. Then suture the proximal part of the aponeurotic tendon to the underlying soleus with fine interrupted silk sutures at a level at least 2.5 cm more proximal than its original attachment. Close the wound with subcuticular catgut sutures so that the sutures need not be removed.

AFTERTREATMENT. Bilateral casts are applied from the groin to the toes with the knees in extension and the ankles in the neutral position. If needed, spreader bars may be attached to the casts both at the knees and at the feet to keep the hips abducted. Intensive exercises are carried out to develop the gluteal muscles. At 4 weeks the casts are removed but are used as night splints thereafter until the muscles have regained their tone.

ADVANCEMENT OF INSERTION OF TENDO CALCANEUS

Because equinus deformity recurs rather frequently after lengthening of the tendo calcaneus in children, Pierrot and Murphy devised a different surgical method consisting of anterior advancement of the insertion of the tendo calcaneus. By transferring the insertion of the tendon anteriorly to the dorsum of the calcaneus just posterior to the subtalar joint, the effective leverage of the triceps surae is decreased; further, because the resting length of the triceps

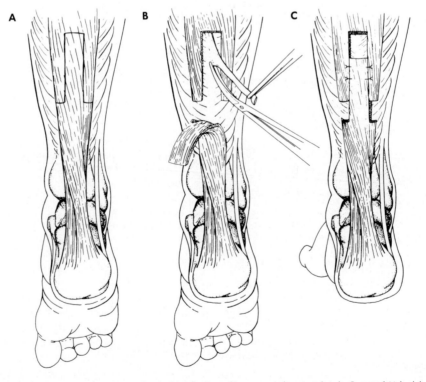

Fig. 65-12. Baker technique of aponeurotic lengthening of gastrocnemius muscle. **A,** Inverted-U incision is made through aponeurosis. **B,** Central aponeurosis of soleus is dissected free. **C,** After ankle is dorsiflexed sliding end of tendon is sutured distally.

surae is not changed, the final result should not be affected by growth. In the resting position the fulcrum for function of the triceps surae is at the center of the ankle joint, and anterior transfer of the tendo calcaneus weakens the muscle by 48% (Fig. 65-14, *A*); during push-off, however, the fulcrum is transferred to the head of the first metatarsal, and push-off is weakened by only 15% (Fig. 65-14, *B*).

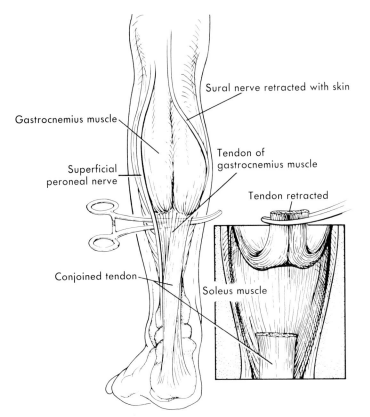

Fig. 65-13. Lengthening of gastrocnemius by Strayer technique (see text). (Redrawn from Strayer, L.M., Jr.: J. Bone Joint Surg. **32-A**:671, 1950.)

Thus theoretically equinus deformity is lessened but push-off is not greatly weakened. In contrast, lengthening of the tendo calcaneus weakens the action of the triceps surae equally during rest and during push-off by lengthening the muscle itself. In a series of 22 extremities treated by lengthening the tendo calcaneus poor results were obtained in 10 as compared with a series of 32 treated by advancement of the tendo calcaneus in which the results were poor in only 8.

In 1975 Throop et al. reported their experience in 95 advancements of the tendo calcaneus in 48 patients. The time from surgery to study was only 1 to 4 years, but the improvement in these patients was encouraging. Using the criteria of Pierrot and Murphy, the result was excellent in 17.7% (heel-toe gait, good push-off, and no hyperextension of the knee), good in 72.2% (flat-footed strike with or without push-off, no hyperextension of the knee), and poor in 10.1% (toe-heel gait, recurrence of equinus deformity, or calcaneus gait). By addition of the excellent and good results, 89.9% were satisfactory. Their indication for the procedure was the presence of a dynamic equinus deformity with no more than 15 degrees of fixed equinus deformity in a predominantly spastic foot. They did not advance the tendon anterior to the flexor hallucis longus tendon, but this did not affect the results. They found that in time a small slip of tendon reattached itself to the point of original insertion on the calcaneus while the main bulk of the tendon remained in the advanced location.

We have found the operation most useful in treating a child with little or no fixed equinus deformity but with either severe clonus or severe extensor thrust while walking. Any fixed equinus deformity should be corrected by wedging plaster casts before surgery.

TECHNIQUE (PIERROT AND MURPHY). Make a longitudinal posteromedial incision 7.5 to 10 cm long, exposing the distal 7.5 cm of the tendo calcaneus. Detach the tendon from the tuberosity of the calcaneus as far distally as possible to preserve length (Fig. 65-15, *A*). Take care not to injure the epiphysis of the calcaneus. Then place a pullout

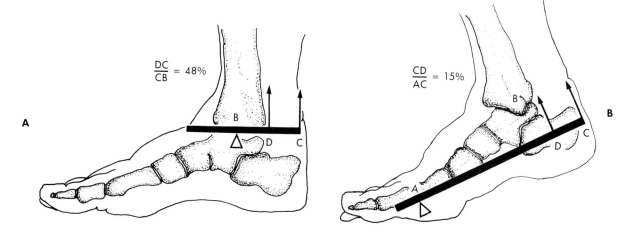

Fig. 65-14. Advancement of insertion of tendo calcaneus. **A,** In resting position power of triceps surae is reduced 48% when tendo calcaneus is advanced from *C* to *D*. **B,** During push-off power of triceps surae is reduced only 15% when tendo calcaneus is so advanced. (Redrawn from Pierrot, A.H., and Murphy, O.B.: Orthop. Clin. North Am. **5**:117, 1974.)

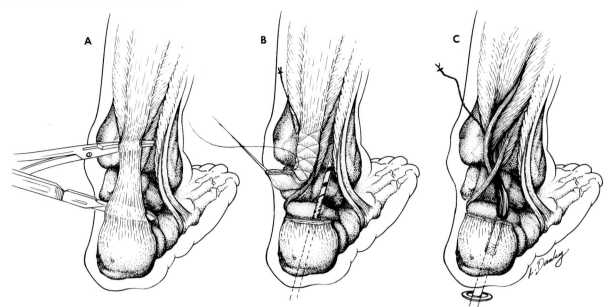

Fig. 65-15. Pierrot and Murphy technique of advancement of insertion of tendo calcaneus. **A,** Tendon is detached from calcaneus as far distally as possible. **B,** Pull-out wire suture is placed in tendon and hole is drilled in calcaneus. **C,** Tendon is routed anterior to flexor hallucis longus tendon and is anchored in calcaneus with pull-out wire over padded button on heel pad.

wire suture in the tendon (Fig. 65-15, *B*) and expose the dorsal surface of the calcaneus and the musculotendinous junction of the flexor hallucis longus muscle. Next drill a hole 0.6 cm in diameter from the superior aspect of the calcaneus just posterior to the subtalar joint to the infero-medial aspect of the bone in the non-weight-bearing part of the foot. Then route the pull-out wire and tendo calcaneus anterior to the flexor hallucis longus, pass the wire through the hole, and tie it over a plastic heelplate on the plantar surface of the foot with the foot in 15 degrees of plantar flexion (Fig. 65-15, *C*). The tendon will often return to its original insertion if not routed anterior to the flexor hallucis longus. Next close the fat pad over the flexor hallucis longus and tendo calcaneus. Close the wound in layers and apply a long leg cast with the foot in 15 degrees of plantar flexion.

AFTERTREATMENT. The cast, pull-out wires, and sutures are removed in 6 weeks and physical therapy is begun to restore ankle motion. Full motion is usually regained after an additional 1 or 2 months.

NEURECTOMY OF BRANCHES OF TIBIAL NERVE

Occasionally neurectomy of branches of the tibial nerve to the gastrocnemius or soleus or both, or advancement of the insertion of the tendo calcaneus may correct equinus deformity caused only by spasm of one or both muscles, but neurectomy alone is unsuccessful when the triceps surae is contracted.

Troublesome clonus on weight bearing, however, can usually be reduced by neurectomy, as in Phelps' method described here. Before surgery, the surgeon should determine which muscle, the gastrocnemius or the soleus, is the cause of clonus: when clonus is caused chiefly by the gastrocnemius, it disappears or decreases when the knee is flexed because the muscle takes origin proximal to the knee and flexion relaxes it; when clonus is caused chiefly by the soleus, changes in position of the knee do not affect it because the soleus takes origin distal to the knee. Even when clonus is severe, lengthening of the tendo calcaneus at the time of neurectomy is inadvisable because after neurectomy the lengthening might be unnecessary. Usually resecting only one or two branches of the tibial nerve is sufficient to relieve clonus.

When the equinus deformity persisted after release of the patellar retinacula and transfer of the hamstring tendons to the femoral condyles, Eggers carried out neurectomy of the branches of the tibial nerve to the soleus alone. Lengthening the tendo calcaneus was then rarely necessary. This neurectomy is described in the second technique here.

TECHNIQUE (PHELPS). Anesthesia should not be deep enough to obliterate the stretch reflex. Make a transverse incision 7.5 cm long over the distal part of the popliteal fossa; this incision follows the flexion creases of the skin and is preferable to a longitudinal one because the scar does not tend to hypertrophy. Divide the fascia to expose the tibial nerve, which lies superficial to the vessels. Do not disturb the first branch of the nerve; it is purely sensory. The next two branches, one emerging from the medial side and the other from the lateral side of the nerve, course to the medial and lateral heads of the gastrocnemius muscle and are easily found and identified (Fig. 65-16). They enter the muscle close to the origin of its heads; the branch to the medial head divides into three twigs just before it disappears into the muscle and the branch to the lateral head divides into two. Just distal to where these two branches emerge, a single branch emerges from the posterior surface of the tibial nerve and divides into two

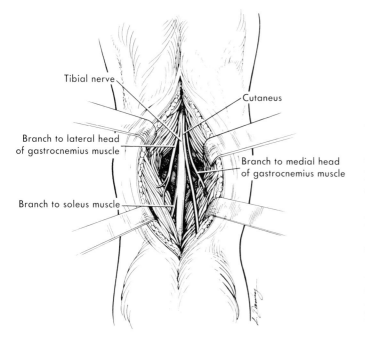

Fig. 65-16. Exposure of tibial nerve and its branches for neurectomy. Most proximal and superficial branch to emerge is cutaneous one; next are medial and lateral branches to heads of gastrocnemius and soleus. Branch to tibialis posterior emerges at more distal level as nerve disappears beneath soleus. (Curved longitudinal skin incision that does not cross flexion crease at right angle, or transverse one, is preferred to one shown here.)

twigs, one to each head of the soleus muscle; further distally another branch that enters the medial head of the soleus emerges from the tibial nerve deep to the soleus. Stimulate each branch either by an electric current or by gently pressing it with a smooth forceps. While the branches are being stimulated an assistant gently dorsiflexes the foot; thus the branch or branches chiefly responsible for the clonus or spasticity can be identified. Then decide which branches should be sacrificed, divide them where they emerge from the trunk, and avulse them from the muscle by winding each separately around a clamp.

When the decision has been made before surgery to resect only branches to the gastrocnemius, identifying branches to other muscles is unnecessary. Occasionally, however, when spasticity of the long toe flexors is disabling, branches of the tibial nerve to these muscles should be identified and resected.

AFTERTREATMENT. If only neurectomy has been carried out, a pressure dressing is usually sufficient immobilization. Exercises to reeducate the dorsiflexors are begun promptly after surgery, and walking is allowed as soon as the wound has healed.

TECHNIQUE (EGGERS). With the patient prone, begin the incision at a point just posterior to the neck of the fibula and continue it distally about 10 cm. Identify and protect the peroneal nerve. Locate and develop the interval between the gastrocnemius and soleus muscles; now retract the gastrocnemius posteriorly to expose the posterior surface of the soleus muscle in the floor of the wound. A triangular mass of fat is seen proximally and medially; in it courses

the main branch to the soleus muscle, usually accompanied by a small vein. Trace the nerve into the soleus, where it usually terminates in two branches. After the nerve has been identified by stimulation, resect a segment from each of these two branches.

AFTERTREATMENT. Aftertreatment is the same as described for the Phelps technique.

Varus or valgus deformity

In cerebral palsy, varus or valgus deformity is most often accompanied by equinus, either of the forefoot or the hindfoot. Both neurologic and biomechanical forces may cause these deformities. The position of the extremity above the ankle has a direct and indirect influence on the position of the foot; for example, a diplegic patient with internally rotated and adducted hips and flexed knees may develop external tibial torsion that causes the foot to assume a valgus position. If the gastrocsoleus is spastic, there will be equinovalgus, that is, an equinus heel with the foot abducted or in valgus at the midtarsal joint. A patient with hemiplegia usually has an internally rotated thigh, but the knee usually comes into extension in the stance phase of gait causing the foot to be internally rotated and to assume a varus posture. Neurologic deformities are usually caused by retained primitive reflex patterns, inappropriate phasic activity of muscles during the gait cycle, loss of voluntary control of muscle activity, mass reflexes to stimuli of any type (labyrinthian, visual, auditory, or sensory), and an imbalance of agonist versus antagonist muscle activity.

In a study of 230 children, Bennett et al. found that in hemiplegia the foot deformity was equinus or equinovarus, and in diplegia or quadriplegia the foot deformity was valgus in 64% and varus in 36%.

Initially the deformity is dynamic and can be corrected and often controlled by some physiotherapeutic or orthotic means. If left uncorrected, an uncontrolled dynamic deformity, however, will become fixed in the muscles, tendons, ligaments, and joint capsules and in the growing child will lead to bony deformities. Dynamic, static, and bony deformities require different approaches for proper treatment. The aim of treatment for dynamic deformities is to balance the muscles by lengthening or transferring a muscle-tendon complex. Static deformities also require muscle-tendon lengthening or transferring, but may also require ligamentous or capsular releases about the joint. Bony deformities require realignment of the bones by osteotomy or arthrodesis. Dynamic muscle balance must be established once the bones have been realigned. Otherwise the deformity will recur or the foot will remain poorly functional.

Varus deformity is more easily corrected surgically and is more functionally disabling in walking and standing. Valgus deformity is more difficult to correct surgically and is less functionally disabling. Consequently, surgery is done more often and more successfully for varus deformities than for valgus deformities.

Surgery is indicated to improve function when standing and walking, to aid in fitting the patient with shoes, to correct deformity when an orthosis will not hold it corrected, and to allow the extremity to be used without the impairment of an orthosis. When an orthosis is holding the deformity corrected and when other deformities in the same extremity require the continued use of an orthosis even after a surgical correction, then surgery would be useless.

VARUS DEFORMITY

This deformity is most often accompanied by equinus. One must be sure that varus is not secondary to internal femoral or tibial torsion. Root has observed that when a child with a varus foot stands on his toes, the varus is accentuated by an overactive tibialis posterior muscle. Dynamic gait studies may show that the tibialis posterior tendon is active in the swing phase or it may be active continuously. In any event, in true varus or equinovarus of the foot the tibialis posterior tendon is usually the offending structure. The other invertor muscles and weakness of the evertor muscles, whether actual or relative, may contribute to the deformity. Triceps surae spasticity or contracture adds considerably to the functional varus impairment.

Operations on the invertor muscles of the foot include lengthening the tibialis posterior tendon, rerouting it from behind to in front of the medial malleolus, transferring its insertion through the interosseous membrane into the dorsum of the foot, and transferring part of it behind the tibia into the peroneus brevis. All of these tend to weaken its evertor action.

Hoffer, Reiswig, Garrett, and Perry studied ambulatory electromyograms in patients with spastic varus hindfoot deformities and found inappropriate hyperactivity of the tibialis anterior tendon in some. For the patients with abnormal electromyograms they devised a new procedure to correct deformity called the split tibialis anterior tendon transfer. It has been used extensively in adults with cerebrovascular accidents, and the results of 21 procedures performed in children with spastic cerebral palsy were reported. In 15 feet fixed deformities required lengthening the tendo calcaneus, lengthening the tibialis posterior tendon, or releasing the medial hindfoot. In six feet the deformity was dynamic, flexible, and correctable, and in these the split tibialis anterior transfer was performed as an isolated procedure. In only one instance was the procedure unsuccessful. In the remainder the split tendons worked with equal force in their spastic pattern as noted before surgery. In all of these patients, electromyograms before surgery revealed the tibialis anterior to be overactive and nonphasic; after surgery the gait electromyograms were often slightly modified but not dramatically so. When the gait electromyogram before surgery shows the tibialis anterior tendon to be neither overactive nor nonphasic but there is phase reversal in the tibialis posterior muscle, then transfer of the tibialis posterior is recommended.

LENGTHENING OF TIBIALIS POSTERIOR TENDON

The tibialis posterior tendon may be lengthened by a Z-plasty procedure, a step cut procedure, or a sliding lengthening at its musculotendinous junction. If the tendon is lengthened by a step cut or Z-plasty procedure, it may bind down behind the medial malleolus in its tendon sheath and with growth act as a tether and cause the deformity to recur. In recurrent deformity, a previously lengthened ten-

don is less suitable for transfer because it is scarred and may be attenuated. Majestro, Ruda, and Frost described a modified lengthening of this muscle at its musculotendinous junction that is a more desirable procedure. If the deformity recurs, the tendon is more easily transferred because it will not have developed any intratendinous scarring. Majestro et al. reported only a 6% recurrence rate after this procedure. Intratendinous lengthening of the tibialis posterior tendon can be combined with an open tendo calcaneus lengthening through the same incision.

Z-PLASTY LENGTHENING OF TIBIALIS POSTERIOR TENDON

TECHNIQUE. Incise the skin longitudinally just above and posterior to the medial malleolus for a distance of 8 cm. By sharp dissection, divide the subcutaneous fat directly behind the medial border of the tibia down to the tendon sheath of the tibialis posterior tendon. Incise the tendon sheath directly over the tendon for 6 to 8 cm. Incise the tendon in its middle at the lower end of the incision and cut the lateral one half of the tendon; then incise the tendon in a proximal direction in line with its fibers for about 6 cm. At this proximal level, incise the tendon transversely medially to sever the medial one half of the tendon. Place the foot in the neutral position with regard to varus and neutral dorsiflexion. While holding the foot corrected, overlap the ends of the tendon and suture them together with nonabsorbable sutures. Repair the incision in the tendon sheath with small absorbable sutures. Close the subcutaneous tissue and skin with absorbable sutures and apply a short leg cast with the foot in the neutral or a slightly overcorrected position.

AFTERTREATMENT. Protected weight bearing is allowed for 3 weeks, and then full weight bearing in a short leg cast is allowed for an additional 3 weeks. When the cast is removed at 6 weeks, the foot is placed in an AFO to hold it in the corrected position. Daytime use of the AFO may be discontinued at 3 months. Protection of the foot in the corrected position with the AFO at night should be continued until skeletal growth of the limb is complete.

STEP CUT LENGTHENING OF TIBIALIS POSTERIOR TENDON

TECHNIQUE. Expose the tendon sheath as described above, but do not incise it over its length. Just above the medial malleolus, incise the lateral one half of the tendon sheath and the tendon. Move 6 to 8 cm proximally from this level and incise the medial one half of the tendon sheath and tendon. Dorsiflex the foot to the neutral position and forcibly correct the hindfoot and midfoot varus. The incised tendon should slide on itself within the sheath. Do not close the tendon sheath or suture the tendon. Close the subcutaneous tissues and skin in a routine fashion. Hold the foot and ankle in the corrected or a slightly overcorrected position and apply a short leg cast.

AFTERTREATMENT. The aftertreatment is the same as described for Z-plasty lengthening of the tibialis posterior tendon.

INTRAMUSCULAR LENGTHENING OF TIBIALIS POSTERIOR TENDON

TECHNIQUE (MAJESTRO, RUDA, AND FROST). With the patient supine and the pneumatic tourniquet inflated, make a longitudinal incision 3 cm long over the posteromedial corner of the tibia centered at the junction of the middle and distal thirds of the leg. Incise the deep fascia at this corner of the bone, identify the flexor digitorum longus, and retract it posteriorly. Now identify the musculotendinous junction of the tibialis posterior by placing a hemostat beneath it and by observing its action when inverting the foot without flexing the toes. Next pass a curved hemostat beneath the tendinous part of the tibialis posterior, isolate this part from the muscle fibers that envelop it, and divide the tendon fibers completely, leaving the muscle fibers intact and allowing the tendon ends to retract freely within the muscle. Close the wound and apply a soft dressing.

AFTERTREATMENT. No cast is applied, and walking is allowed the day of surgery. The use of orthoses after surgery is not recommended until the final effect of the operation on motor balance of the foot during walking and running has been determined, usually at 2 months.

• • •

Baker and Hill have noted that when a spastic tibialis posterior muscle causes varus and internal rotational deformities of the foot, rerouting its tendon anterior to the medial malleolus improves alignment immediately. This was true in 34 feet in which the operation was used.

Bisla, Louis, and Albano reported anterior rerouting of the tibialis posterior tendon as described by Baker and Hill in 21 feet of 16 patients with cerebral palsy. In 5 the involvement was mild, in 10 moderate, and in 1 severe. On clinical evaluation after surgery 4 were improved and in 14 there was no significant change. Varus or equinus deformity was not completely corrected in a single patient, and in 3 the equinovarus deformity increased significantly, requiring additional surgery. Examination both clinically and by electromyograms revealed neither voluntary nor involuntary action in the rerouted tendon.

A tendon so rerouted still acts as an invertor, although it is somewhat weakened. In our experience anterior rerouting has not corrected the dynamic imbalance, and we no longer use the procedure.

REROUTING INSERTION OF TIBIALIS POSTERIOR TENDON TO DORSUM OF FOOT THROUGH INTEROSSEOUS MEMBRANE

This operation has proved to be useful because it allows the tibialis posterior tendon to assist in dorsiflexion and removes a dynamic invertor and plantar flexor force. Bisla et al., Williams, Gritzka et al., and Root have all reported 80% or more excellent or good results after this procedure. On the other hand, Turner and Cooper found only 21% of their results were excellent or good, and in 71% of their patients the result was poor. Root states that failures of this operation are caused by the following four factors: (1) unrecognized fixed varus deformity that cannot be corrected by a tendon transfer alone, and thus the varus attitude persists; (2) simultaneous tendo calcaneus lengthening, which can lead to a calcaneus deformity; (3) transplanting the tendon too far laterally, which may lead to excessive valgus; and (4) insecure insertion of the tendon into the bone, which allows it to detach. Although originally we were enthusiastic about this procedure, 13 of 20 feet so treated

have subsequently required a triple arthrodesis to correct heel and midfoot valgus. For this reason, we prefer one of the tendon-splitting transfer procedures to correct dynamic varus of the hindfoot or midfoot.

TECHNIQUE. This technique is described on p. 2957.

SPLIT TENDON TRANSFERS FOR VARUS DEFORMITY

In 1977 Kaufer reported treating varus deformities of the foot by split tendon transfer. The procedure was performed 30 times, 20 in adults with deformities after stroke or central nervous system trauma and 10 in patients with spastic cerebral palsy with varus deformities. Split tendon transfers for valgus deformity produced inconsistent results and were abandoned.

Any significant fixed deformity should be corrected before or during the transfer procedure. The split transfer functions reliably as a control mechanism only if the strongest deforming muscle is selected. The strongest deforming muscle is usually apparent in a varus deformity. When the tibialis posterior muscle is the principal deforming force, its tendon is prominent subcutaneously through the distal part of its course and, in addition to the adduction of the forefoot and varus of the heel, the metatarsals are in plantar flexion. When the tibialis anterior muscle is at fault, in addition to the varus deformity of the heel, adduction of the forefoot, and prominence of the tibialis anterior tendon in the subcutaneous tissues, the forefoot is supinated more and the metatarsals are in less plantar flexion.

If the tibialis posterior is the deforming structure, the plantar half of its tendon is detached from its insertion, is split proximally to the musculotendinous junction, is rerouted posterior to the tibia, and is then sutured to the peroneus brevis tendon. The tension is adjusted so that the foot rests in a neutral position when it dangles. If the tibialis anterior muscle is the major deforming force, its tendon is split to the musculotendinous junction and the lateral half is rerouted to the lateral border of the foot and is then sutured to the tendon of the peroneus brevis or is fixed in the cuboid. Again the tension should be sufficient to allow the foot to rest in a neutral position when it dangles.

Of the first 30 feet in which this procedure was done by Kaufer, the postural deformity was corrected in 29. In one foot the deformity partially persisted, presumably as a result of failure of the tendon suture. In no instance did the deformity reverse, and all patients have been free of braces since surgery. Furthermore, the deformity has not tended to recur after an average of more than 5 years.

In 1985 Kling, Kaufer, and Hensinger reported excellent or good results in 34 of 37 cerebral palsied patients who had undergone this operation, 26 of whom had reached skeletal maturity. In no instance did a calcaneus deformity result. Green, Griffin, and Shiavi have likewise reported good results. In our experience it has been a worthwhile procedure when combined with a tendo calcaneus lengthening, although our experience with it does not cover as long a time as those cited previously. It has never resulted in a calcaneus deformity or recurrence of the varus, although the patient must be watched closely until skeletal maturity for recurrent equinus.

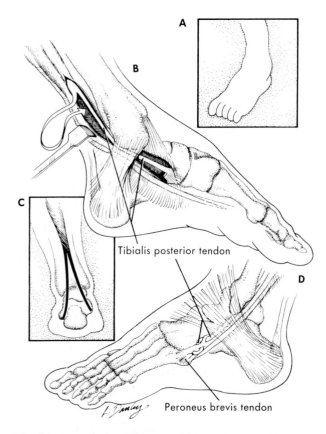

Fig. 65-17. Kaufer split transfer of tibialis posterior tendon for varus deformity. **A,** Foot is in varus position. **B,** Tibialis posterior tendon has been split, one half is freed distally, and flexor tendons of toes and neurovascular bundle are retracted posteriorly. **C** and **D,** Freed half of tendon is passed from medial to lateral behind tibia and sutured to peroneus brevis tendon near its insertion. (Courtesy Dr. H. Kaufer.)

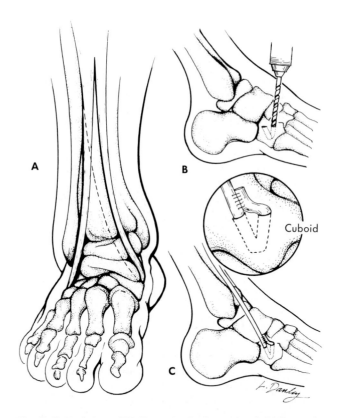

Fig. 65-18. Technique of Hoffer et al. of split transfer of tibialis anterior tendon for varus deformity. **A,** After transfer. **B,** Two holes are drilled in cuboid at converging angles to create tunnel in bone. **C,** One half of tibialis anterior tendon is passed through tunnel and sutured. Route of lateral one half of tibialis anterior tendon is shown. Transfer completed. (Redrawn from Hoffer, M.M., et al.: Orthop. Clin. North Am. **5:**31, 1974.)

SPLIT TRANSFER OF TIBIALIS POSTERIOR TENDON

TECHNIQUE (KAUFER). Begin a curvilinear incision at the tuberosity of the navicular and extend it inferiorly and posteriorly to the medial malleolus and then proximally to the posterior midline over the tendo calcaneus. Deepen the incision through the skin and subcutaneous tissue and expose the tibialis posterior tendon sheath and the neurovascular bundle. Completely excise the tendon sheath over the tibialis posterior tendon except for a band 1 cm wide at the tip of the medial malleolus. Split the tibialis posterior tendon longitudinally into dorsal and plantar halves by a stab wound through it just distal to the medial malleolus. Introduce hemostats and split the tendon into two halves in the direction of its fibers proximally to the musculotendinous junction and distally to the tuberosity of the navicular. Continue the split beyond the tuberosity by sharp dissection, identify that part of the tendon that extends into the sole of the foot, divide this part, and withdraw it into the proximal part of the wound. Next carry out any necessary lengthening of the tendo calcaneus through the same incision. By blunt dissection separate the flexor tendons of the toes and the neurovascular bundle from the posterior aspect of the tibia and retract them posteriorly (Fig. 65-17,

B). Retract further laterally so that the fascia forming the peroneal muscle compartment can be seen in the depths of the wound. Excise a large window from this fascia and reposition the foot for access to its lateral side. Now make an incision from the tip of the lateral malleolus to the base of the fifth metatarsal and expose the peroneal tendons. Identify the peroneus brevis tendon and pass a tendon carrier proximally within its sheath posterior to the lateral malleolus. Reposition the foot, identify the tendon carrier within the peroneal muscle compartment, and bring it out through the window in the peroneal fascia and into the medial incision. Insert the freed half of the tibialis posterior tendon into the carrier and draw it through the peroneal muscle compartment and through the peroneal tendon sheath posterior to the lateral malleolus and bring it out through the lateral incision next to the peroneus brevis tendon. Now close the medial wound. Place the foot in the corrected position with the forefoot abducted and pronated, and suture the freed half of the tendon to the peroneus brevis tendon near its insertion and under tension so that the foot dangles in a neutral position (Fig. 65-17, *C* and *D*). Close the wound and apply a long leg plaster cast, holding the foot in the corrected position.

AFTERTREATMENT. At 2 months the cast is removed and a short leg walking cast is applied and worn for 2 more months. Then all external support is discontinued.

SPLIT TRANSFER OF TIBIALIS ANTERIOR TENDON

Hoffer et al. use this procedure when tibialis anterior hyperactivity causes a varus hindfoot and when the deformity is dynamic and correctable. Gait analysis by electromyography will confirm the hyperactivity of the tibialis anterior muscle in such patients.

We have used this procedure extensively and have found it appropriate when there is varus in the swing phase of gait with a clinically apparent functioning tibialis anterior muscle-tendon unit. If equinus is also present, lengthening the tendo calcaneus and the tibialis posterior tendon may be necessary.

TECHNIQUE (HOFFER ET AL.). With the patient supine and the tourniquet inflated, make the first longitudinal incision on the dorsomedial aspect of the foot over the first cuneiform. Identify the tibialis anterior tendon at its insertion, split it, and insert an umbilical tape. Then make a second longitudinal incision over the anterolateral aspect of the ankle, identify the tibialis anterior tendon, and draw the umbilical tape into this second incision splitting the tendon further. Then release the lateral half of the tendon distally, tag it, and bring it into the second incision. Now make a third short longitudinal incision over the dorsum of the cuboid. Pass the lateral half of the tendon subcutaneously into the third incision. Using a $\frac{7}{64}$-inch (2.73 mm) drill, make two holes in the cuboid at converging angles (Fig. 65-18, *B*). Then use a small curet to join the depths of the holes, making a tunnel. Take care to preserve a roof of bone. Pass the slip of tendon through the tunnel and suture it on itself with the ankle in slight dorsiflexion (Fig. 65-18, *C*).

AFTERTREATMENT. A long leg cast is applied. After 2 weeks weight bearing in the cast is permitted. At 6 weeks the cast is discarded and a weight-bearing orthosis is applied. A splint is used at night. At 6 months bracing is discontinued if possible.

• • •

For equinovarus deformity of the foot Tohen, Carmona, and Barrera have transferred the extensor hallucis longus and tibialis anterior tendons to the dorsum of the foot at either its center or lateral side. In 14 feet in which the deformity could be manually reduced, the tendons were transferred to the proximal end of the second metatarsal, and in six in which the deformity could not be so reduced, they were transferred to the base of the fifth metatarsal. In addition to eliminating a dynamically deforming force, the newly created extensor responds to the abnormal Babinski reflex and to the triple flexion response as an active dorsiflexor of the ankle. In all feet the deformity was corrected and the transfer functioned actively after completion of an exercise program. In six feet the tendo calcaneus was lengthened at the time of tendon transfer, in three a triple arthrodesis was carried out at the time of transfer, and in one foot a triple arthrodesis and lengthening of the tendo calcaneus were performed and the tendons were transferred later.

ANTERIOR TRANSFER OF TIBIALIS POSTERIOR TENDON

This technique is described on p. 2958.

TRANSFER OF EXTENSOR HALLUCIS LONGUS AND TIBIALIS ANTERIOR TENDONS

TECHNIQUE (TOHEN ET AL.). Make a longitudinal incision slightly curved laterally extending from the base of the first metatarsal proximally to the proximal phalanx of the great toe distally. Identify the tibialis anterior and extensor hallucis longus tendons. Free the insertion of the tibialis anterior tendon, then divide the extensor hallucis longus tendon and suture its remaining distal end to the extensor hallucis brevis tendon. Next make a longitudinal incision 5 cm long proximal to the cruciate ligament of the ankle and lateral to the tibial crest. Through this incision locate the two tendons to be transferred and draw them into the wound. Then make three small incisions in the tibialis anterior tendon and weave the extensor hallucis longus tendon through them; sew the end of the tibialis anterior tendon to the extensor hallucis longus tendon while both are held under equal tension. Then pass this newly created conjoined tendon subcutaneously to the base of the second or fifth metatarsal (depending on the deformity as already mentioned) and anchor it either subperiosteally or by the method of Cole (see Fig. 1-8). Close the wound and apply a long leg cast.

AFTERTREATMENT. At 5 weeks the cast is removed. The muscles of the transfer are then reeducated by stimulating the sole of the foot so that they contract, and by having the patient actively flex the hip while in a sitting position, so that dorsiflexion of the foot is produced synergistically. At 6 or 7 weeks walking is resumed in a short leg brace that eliminates plantar flexion, and when the muscles of the transfer function well, the brace is discarded.

• • •

In any of these procedures, the flexor hallucis longus and the flexor digitorum communis may be so shortened as to require lengthening. These muscles will rarely prevent passive correction of the deformity, but will draw the toes into marked plantar flexion once the hindfoot and forefoot are corrected, making weight bearing painful.

OSTEOTOMY OF CALCANEUS

Once the heel becomes fixed in varus, a corrective procedure on the bone is required, combined with a muscle-balancing soft tissue procedure. Osteotomy of the calcaneus as advocated by Dwyer will correct the varus of the heel and does not impair mobility in the subtalar or midtarsal joints as does a triple arthrodesis.

Silver et al. reported a series of patients in whom an osteotomy of the calcaneus had been made for varus or valgus deformities of the foot in cerebral palsy. The operation is basically a modification of the Dwyer osteotomy (Fig. 65-19). It had been carried out on 27 feet in 20 children whose ages ranged from 2½ to 13 years and who had been observed for 2 to 5½ years after surgery. Twenty open-wedge osteotomies had been made to correct valgus deformity, and they had been held open by autoclaved homogenous tibial grafts; in 14 the result was excellent, in 4

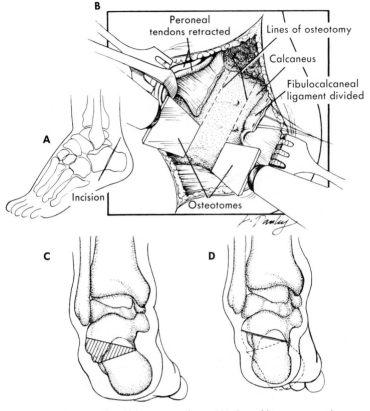

Fig. 65-19. Dwyer closing wedge osteotomy of calcaneus for varus heel. **A,** Lateral skin incision is made inferior and parallel to peroneal tendons. **B,** Wedge of bone is resected with its base laterally. **C,** Wedge of bone is tapered medially. **D,** Calcaneus is closed after bone is removed and varus deformity is corrected to slight valgus.

a mild valgus deformity persisted, and in 2 a varus deformity was produced. Seven closing wedge osteotomies had been made through a lateral approach to correct varus deformity and the fragments had been fixed by staples; in 6 the result was excellent and in 1 a valgus deformity was produced. In 11 of the 27 operations, procedures on the soft structures had been carried out at the same time. Silver et al. recommended that the minimum age for this osteotomy be 3 years, and that in children 9 years old or older a triple arthrodesis be performed.

We do not recommend opening wedge osteotomies of the calcaneus. The skin laterally and medially along the bone is only slightly mobile, and opening wedges put too much tension on the suture line and tend to cause incisional skin sloughs. Furthermore, the medial calcaneal nerves may be stretched by an opening wedge osteotomy made from the medial side, causing painful neuromas. For these reasons, we do only closing wedge resection osteotomies on the calcaneus. For varus deformities the incision is lateral and the base of the wedge of bone removed is lateral.

OSTEOTOMY OF CALCANEUS FOR VARUS DEFORMITY

TECHNIQUE (DWYER). Expose the lateral aspect of the foot through a curved incision parallel and about 1 cm posterior and inferior to the peroneus longus tendon. Retract the superior wound edge until the tendon sheath of the peroneus longus is exposed. Strip the periosteum from the superior, lateral, and inferior surfaces of the calcaneus posterior to this tendon. Remove a wedge of bone from the calcaneus just inferior and posterior to the tendon and parallel with it (Fig. 65-19, *B*). Make the base of the wedge 8 to 12 mm wide as needed for correction of the deformity and taper the wedge medially to but not through the medial cortex of the calcaneus (Fig. 65-19, *C*). Manually break the medial cortex and close the gap in the bone. Bring the bony surfaces snugly together by pressing the foot into dorsiflexion against the pull of the tendo calcaneus (Fig. 65-19, *D*). Failure to close the gap in the calcaneus indicates that a small piece of bone has been left behind at the apex of the wedge and should be removed. Now be certain that the varus deformity has been corrected and that the heel is in the neutral or a slightly varus position. Close the wound and apply a cast from the toes to the tibial tuberosity.

AFTERTREATMENT. Walking may be permitted as soon as soft tissue healing is secure. Cast immobilization is continued until the osteotomy is solid, usually no longer than 8 weeks.

VALGUS DEFORMITY

Hindfoot valgus deformity is more common in cerebral palsy than varus deformity and is more difficult to correct.

Fortunately, it requires correction less often than varus deformity because the skin along the medial border of the foot is better protected from the underlying bone than it is laterally, and skin breakdown and painful callus formation occur less often than in varus deformity.

In cerebral palsy, valgus deformity may be caused by overpull of the peroneal and other evertor muscles and weakness, either relative or actual, of the invertor muscles. But Bassett and Baker and Keats and Kouten have pointed out that the primary deforming factor in valgus deformity is most often contracture of the triceps surae. The contracted mechanism acts like a bowstring on the calcaneus and thus blocks normal dorsiflexion at the ankle joint. The desired dorsiflexion must then occur at the midtarsal joint, and as a part of this dorsiflexion the calcaneus usually rolls into eversion, removing the sustentaculum tali from its normal supporting position beneath the head of the talus. The forefoot abducts at the midtarsal joint, and the talus drops into a more medial and vertical position than normally. A standing lateral roentgenogram of the foot will indicate that the talus is in fact oriented vertically and standing on its head. The first step in correcting this deformity is to release the contracted triceps surae.

Treatment of the valgus foot should at first be conservative with an orthosis or a shoe insert such as the UCB. If this approach is unsuccessful and the tendo calcaneus is tight, causing the foot to break in the midtarsal joint, then a tendo calcaneus lengthening is indicated. Tight or spastic peroneus brevis and longus muscles may contribute to the deformity and their tendons may require lengthening to correct the deformity. However, if the peroneal tendons are lengthened an opposite varus deformity may develop. Several operations have been suggested to alter the effect of the peroneal muscles on the valgus foot, but these have not gained much popularity. Most of the operations have been recommended after intensive gait analysis and should not be undertaken without a strong scientific indication such as an electromyographic gait analysis. The peroneal tendons may be transferred to the midline dorsally, to the calcaneus, or to the tibialis posterior tendon. Perry and Hoffer have transferred the peroneus longus or peroneus brevis posteromedially into the tibialis posterior tendon if either or both are active during the stance phase only. Little has been written about peroneal muscle-tendon surgery, probably because of its tendency to produce a varus deformity.

Much has been written about the role of the Grice subtalar extraarticular arthrodesis for valgus deformity in cerebral palsy since Grice reported it in 1952. Keats and Kouten reported a series of 63 Grice operations for planovalgus deformity. To correct the equinus position of the talus and the lateral displacement of the calcaneus, they recommended opening the capsule of the talonavicular joint and, using a bone hook, reducing the head of the talus into its normal position over the sustentaculum tali before the bone grafts are locked in place. They also recommended homogenous bank bone for grafts, and in the 53 feet in which it was used, it caused no complications. The result was satisfactory in 61 feet in patients whose ages ranged from 2 to 8 years.

In 1974 Engstrom, Erikson, and Hjelmstedt studied the results of the Grice subtalar arthrodesis in 27 feet of patients with cerebral palsy. In 9 the grafts failed to unite, and they were either fully or partially absorbed in 6. In 4 abduction deformity of between 15 and 30 degrees persisted, the foot was unstable, and weight bearing was unsatisfactory. They again emphasized the importance of correcting any existing deformity either before or during surgery, the use of strong autogenous bone for grafting, and the use of internal fixation to maintain the position until union has occurred.

Tohen et al. and others have reported their unsuccessful experience with the classic Grice procedure in a large number of patients. Despite this, the Grice subtalar extraarticular arthrodesis seems to have become the procedure of choice for stabilizing the planovalgus foot in cerebral palsy, especially between the ages of 4 and 9 years. It should be preceded or accompanied by operations that correct deformity of the soft structures and that attempt to balance muscle power. The bone grafts should be so placed that they lie at a right angle to the axis of motion of the subtalar joint and, as seen in a lateral roentgenogram of the foot, parallel to the weight-bearing axis of the leg, ankle, and foot. The dislocation of the head of the talus from the sustentaculum tali should be reduced before the grafts are inserted. Some surgeons recommend the use of homogenous bank bone as grafts, but we prefer autogenous bone. Finally the extremity must be immobilized until fusion is solid. We use a long leg cast for 8 weeks, followed by a short leg walking cast for 4 more weeks.

Several modifications of the extraarticular subtalar fusion have appeared since Grice originally reported his procedure. Most are aimed at better retention of the calcaneus beneath the talus by some means, such as the use of a fibular graft or a perpendicular cancellous screw across the joint, because postoperative loss of position and nonunion have been among the complications. Other modifications include the use of other types of grafts and the donor areas from which they are obtained. A well-done extraarticular subtalar fusion has established itself as a useful procedure in the treatment of the cerebral palsied valgus foot.

Baker and Hill described a different osteotomy of the calcaneus for correcting valgus deformities of the foot. It is a horizontal osteotomy made immediately beneath the posterior articular facet (Fig. 65-20). Its purpose is to correct the valgus inclination of this articular surface caused by prolonged weight bearing with the foot in the deformed position. Forty-one such osteotomies were followed after surgery for an average of over 2 years. In 31 feet the osteotomy was the only operation performed on the bones; in 21 the result was satisfactory, in 2 a mild to moderate varus deformity was produced, and in 8 a mild valgus deformity persisted. In 10 feet the osteotomy was combined with the Grice extraarticular subtalar arthrodesis; in 5 the result was excellent, in 4 some valgus deformity persisted, and in 1 foot a varus deformity was produced.

We have had no experience with the Baker-Hill osteotomy, since the Grice procedure or its modifications have proved satisfactory in most instances.

EXTRAARTICULAR ARTHRODESIS OF SUBTALAR JOINT FOR EQUINOVALGUS DEFORMITY

TECHNIQUE FOR THE TECHNIQUE FOR EXTRAARTICULAR AR-THRODESIS OF SUBTALAR JOINT FOR EQUINOVALGUS DEFORMITY (GRICE AND GREEN). See p. 2963.

MODIFICATIONS OF GRICE EXTRAARTICULAR SUBTALAR ARTHRODESIS

TECHNIQUE (BATCHELOR AS REPORTED BY BROWN). Inflate a midthigh tourniquet and make a small vertical incision over the dorsum of the head and neck of the talus. Expose

the neck of the talus and invert the calcaneus to the corrected position beneath it. Next drive an awl through the neck of the talus inferiorly, posteriorly, and a little laterally, then through the inferior surface of the talar neck, across the subtalar joint, and into the calcaneus for 2 to 3 cm. Invert and evert the foot with the awl in place to be sure the subtalar joint is stable.

Expose the middle third of the ipsilateral fibula through a straight lateral incision, remove subperiosteally a full-thickness segment of the bone 5 cm long, and trim the narrow end to a point. Enlarge the awl track with a 9 to 12 mm diameter burr to accommodate the fibular graft. Drive the point of the graft into the track made in the talus and calcaneus, across the subtalar joint, and into the calcaneus (Fig. 65-21). Close all wounds, deflate the tourniquet, and apply a below-knee cast.

AFTERTREATMENT. A walking cast is applied at 2 weeks and is worn for an additional 6 weeks.

Gross has reported a pseudarthrosis rate of 41% in 34 feet in which this procedure was done.

TECHNIQUE (DENNYSON AND FULFORD). Obliquely incise the skin in line with the skin creases over the sinus tarsi be-

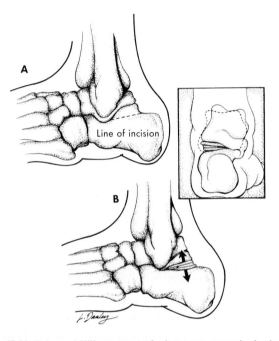

Fig. 65-20. Baker and Hill osteotomy of calcaneus to correct heel valgus. **A,** *Broken line,* site of horizontal osteotomy made from lateral side; medial cortex is left intact to act as hinge. **B** and *Inset,* Osteotomy is opened enough laterally to place calcaneus in neutral position and is held open by homogenous bone grafts. (Redrawn from Baker, L.D., and Hill, L.M.: J. Bone Joint Surg. **46-A:**1, 1964.)

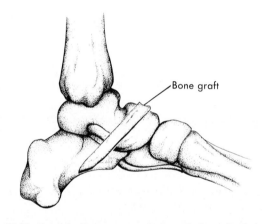

Fig. 65-21. Batchelor-Brown extraarticular subtalar arthrodesis using segment of fibula placed in neck of talus across subtalar joint and into calcaneus.

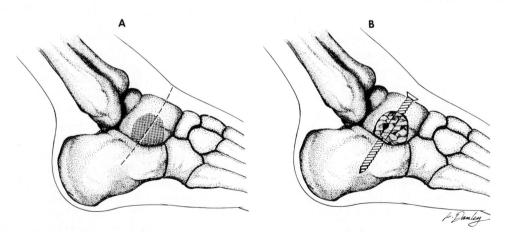

Fig. 65-22. Dennyson and Fulford technique of extraarticular subtalar arthrodesis using screw and cancellous bone chips. **A,** Skin incision and bone area curetted from lateral side of talus and calcaneus. **B,** Placement of iliac bone chips in side of talus and calcaneus after screw has been inserted across subtalar joint with heel in corrected position. (Redrawn from Dennyson, W.G., and Fulford, G.E.: J. Bone Joint Surg. **58-B:**507, 1976.)

ginning proximally at the middle of the ankle and proceeding distally to the peroneal tendons (Fig. 65-22, *A*). Incise and reflect as one flap the subcutaneous fat and the origins of the extensor brevis muscles. By sharp dissection excise the fat from the sinus tarsi down to bone proximally and distally. With a small gouge remove cortical bone from the apex of the sinus tarsi to expose cancellous bone on both the talar neck and the superior surface of the calcaneus. Do not remove the cortical bone from the outer part of the sinus tarsi where a transfixion screw is to pass.

Dorsally expose the small depression just behind the neck of the talus through a small separate skin incision and by blunt dissection between the neurovascular bundle and the tendons of the extensor digitorum longus. Hold the calcaneus in the corrected position and pass an awl from on top of the talus, through the talus, across the subtalar joint, and through the calcaneus. Direct the awl posteriorly, inferiorly, and slightly laterally so that it passes through cortical bone of the talus above and below, and of the calcaneus above and inferolaterally. Use the awl to determine the desired length of a screw needed for fixation, and insert a screw in the hole. Remove chips of cancellous bone from the iliac crest and pack them into the sinus tarsi and against the bone that has been denuded on the talus and calcaneus (Fig. 65-22, *B*). Replace the extensor digitorum brevis and close the skin. Apply a short leg cast over padding. Mold it well around the heel and leave it in place for 6 to 8 weeks.

Barrasso, Wile, and Gage have modified this technique by using a Kirschner wire extending from the talus into the calcaneus as a guide for screw placement and as a holding device during screw insertion. They also do not decorticate the bone in the sinus tarsi until the screw has been placed across the subtalar joint.

Guttman has modified the subtalar extraarticular arthrodesis by placing a dowel of iliac bone in a cylindrical bed cut from the subtalar joint after the foot has been placed in the corrected position (Fig. 65-23).

Others have recommended the use of a dowel bone graft taken from the calcaneus posterior to the peroneal tendons and placed in the subtalar joint. This eliminates the need for a second incision to harvest bone from the ilium, but

it adds the possibility of fracture occurring in the calcaneus through the donor site.

Calcaneus deformity

Talipes calcaneus in spastic paralysis is usually secondary to excessive or repeated lengthening of the tendo calcaneus either alone or in conjunction with neurectomy of branches of the tibial nerve. However, it may also develop as a primary deformity when the dorsiflexors of the foot are spastic and the triceps surae is weak. Surgical correction of talipes calcaneus in spastic paralysis, whatever its cause, is usually unsatisfactory. If the dorsiflexors of the foot are spastic, the toe extensors can be partially denervated and the tibialis anterior tendon can be transferred to the tendo calcaneus, which is shortened at the same time. If this does not restore muscle balance, the peroneus longus and tibialis posterior tendons can both be inserted into the tendo calcaneus to further strengthen plantar flexion. The treatment of this condition in most instances is prevention by avoiding inappropriate lengthening or denervating procedures on the gastrocsoleus muscle group.

CRESCENTIC OSTEOTOMY OF CALCANEUS

Occasionally talipes calcaneus is purely in the hindfoot and is accompanied by a cavus deformity in the midfoot. In such instances, Samilson has recommended a crescentic osteotomy of the calcaneus to lengthen the foot and elevate the base of the heel.

TECHNIQUE (SAMILSON). Inflate a midthigh tourniquet and incise the skin laterally over the calcaneus posterior to the subtalar joint and overlying the posterior tuberosity of the calcaneus. The peroneal tendons should lie anterior to the incision, and the incision should parallel them. Expose the lateral side of the calcaneus, protect the peroneal tendons, and then perform a plantar fasciotomy from the lateral surface of the foot. Make a crescentic osteotomy in the calcaneus with a motor saw using a curved blade or with a large curved osteotome (Fig. 65-24, *A*). Free the posterior tuberosity of the calcaneus and then shift it proximally and posteriorly in the line of the osteotomy to correct the calcaneocavus deformity (Fig. 65-24, *B*). Secure the fragments with a staple or a Kirschner wire and apply a short leg cast.

AFTERTREATMENT. The cast and staple or Kirschner wire are removed 6 weeks after surgery and full weight bearing is allowed.

Cavus deformity

Talipes cavus deformity is uncommon in cerebral palsy. It may occur as a hindfoot cavus in which the calcaneus is in a calcaneus position, or as a forefoot cavus in which the apex of the angulation is at the midtarsal joints or distally. Hindfoot cavus is best treated by the crescentic osteotomy of the calcaneus combined with a plantar release as recommended by Samilson (see above). Forefoot cavus may respond to an extensive plantar release and preoperative wedging casts. In adolescents and adults, correction may require osteotomies as described in the chapter on progressive neuromuscular deformities (Chapter 67).

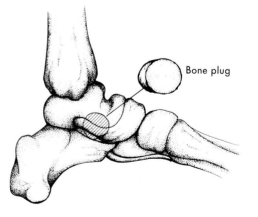

Fig. 65-23. Guttmann technique of subtalar extraarticular arthrodesis with dowel of bone from ilium. (Redrawn from Guttmann, G.: J. Pediatr. Orthop. **1:**219, 1981.)

• • •

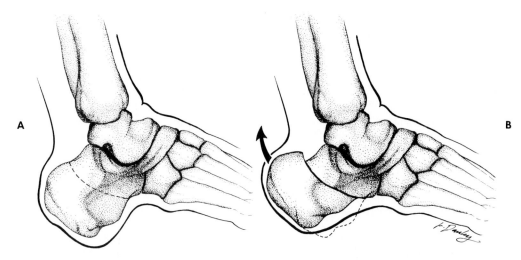

Fig. 65-24. Samilson technique of crescentric osteotomy of calcaneus. **A,** Line of osteotomy. **B,** Displacement of posterior fragment of calcaneus posterosuperiorly. (Redrawn from Samilson, R.L.: Crescentric osteotomy of the os calcis for calcaneocavus feet. In Bateman, J.E., editor: Foot science, Philadelphia, 1976, W.B. Saunders Co.)

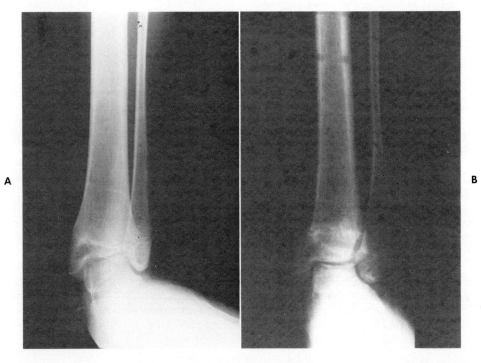

Fig. 65-25. A, Standing anteroposterior view of ankle demonstrating valgus deformity of ankle joint. **B,** Alignment of the ankle achieved by supramalleolar osteotomy.

After skeletal maturity, all residual deformities in the ankle, hindfoot, and midfoot can be corrected by a triple arthrodesis with appropriate wedge resections (see Chapter 66, p. 2935). Before undertaking a triple arthrodesis in the cerebral palsied child, standing anteroposterior roentgenograms of the ankle should always be made. What often appears to be a valgus of the heel is in fact valgus of the ankle mortise and should be corrected by supramalleolar osteotomy and realigning the ankle, rather than creating a secondary compensatory deformity in the subtalar joint (Fig. 65-25). Any external tibial torsion should be recognized before a triple arthrodesis is done, for if the ankle joint is externally rotated, the foot will continue to appear to be in valgus and abduction after the triple arthrodesis.

Adduction deformity of forefoot

Bleck has noted in 10 patients with spastic paralysis an adduction deformity of the forefoot caused by spasticity of the abductor hallucis muscle that appeared after the triceps surae had been lengthened. The abductor hallucis becomes more active after this lengthening because a substitute pattern of muscle function develops. When the great toe is passively adducted at the metatarsophalangeal joint, the tight abductor hallucis tendon is palpable. To be sure this muscle is deforming, it may be paralyzed by infiltrating it with procaine as a diagnostic procedure. An alternative method of making certain the abductor hallucis is the deforming force is to passively abduct the forefoot while holding the heel stable and the foot plantigrade and take a roentgenogram in the anteroposterior plane. If forefoot adduction can be passively corrected, Bleck recommends resecting a segment of the muscle and its tendon. Nine patients were observed for more than 2½ years after this operation was performed bilaterally; in 2 feet a hallux valgus deformity developed, but in the other 16 the adduction deformity did not increase and function and appearance of the feet were satisfactory.

TECHNIQUE (BLECK). Make a longitudinal incision 4 cm long over the medial aspect of the first metatarsal neck and curve it distally to the dorsomedial aspect of the proximal phalanx of the great toe. Expose and identify the abductor hallucis muscle and tendon, and resect a segment of muscle and tendon 2.5 cm long. If the medial part of the capsule of the metatarsophalangeal joint is tight, do a partial capsulectomy. Close the wound, pad the medial border of the forefoot and great toe, and apply a boot cast molded to force the forefoot in abduction.

AFTERTREATMENT. At 6 weeks the cast is removed and physical therapy is started.

Forefoot adduction in an older child that cannot be corrected passively should be treated by osteotomies of the bases of all five metatarsals (see p. 2635) and metatarsal realignment and internal fixation with Kirschner wires until union has occurred. In the younger child, this condition can be treated by tarsometatarsal capsulotomies and metatarsal realignment (see p. 2633). Both of these procedures should be accompanied by release of the abductor hallucis as described by Bleck.

HALLUX VALGUS

Hallux valgus deformity is usually secondary to equinovalgus in the foot, valgus in the heel, or external torsion of the tibia. As the foot pronates, the hallux is forced passively into abduction and hallux valgus results. The tendon of the extensor hallucis longus then subluxates into the space between the first and second metatarsals, and in this position acts as an active adductor on the hallux. When the foot everts, the origin of the adductor hallucis arising from the peroneal tendon sheath is moved laterally and distally, thereby furthering its deforming influence on the hallux.

Correction of the equinovalgus, heel valgus, or external tibial torsion should precede any bunion procedure. If the hindfoot deformity is allowed to remain, recurrence of the hallux valgus is almost certain after any soft tissue procedure on the hallux, especially if arthrodesis of the metatarsophalangeal joint is not performed.

Correction of the hallux valgus may require fusion of the metatarsophalangeal joint by the McKeever method (see p. 886). A combined bony and soft tissue procedure may be preferred. We do a soft tissue realignment medially and laterally at the metatarsophalangeal joint with transfer of the adductor hallucis into the neck of the first metatarsal, plicating the medial capsule and performing an osteotomy of either the base or head of the first metatarsal along with realignment of the extensor hallucis longus, lengthening it when needed. Realignment of the first metatarsal and hallux must be stabilized temporarily with Kirschner wires until the soft tissue is stable or the osteotomies have healed. The spastic toe muscles may cause recurrence of the deformity.

Operations for hallux valgus are described on p. 879.

Claw toes

Claw toe deformity is common in adolescents or adults with cerebral palsy. Although neurectomy of the lateral plantar nerve has been recommended for these deformities, we prefer to treat claw toes by metatarsophalangeal joint capsulotomies and proximal interphalangeal joint resections or fusions using Kirschner wire fixation until the bone and soft tissues are stable.

Operations for claw toes are described on p. 2938.

KNEE

Deformities and disabilities of the knee in cerebral palsy are difficult to evaluate and treat. Pelvic, hip, knee, ankle, and foot deformities are interrelated. Deformities in the pelvis or the ankle and foot can cause deformities in the knee, and deformities in the knee may cause deformities in the pelvis, hip, or ankle. A number of muscles that cross the extensor and flexor sides of the hip and muscles that arise above the knee joint and that cause equinus or calcaneus deformities in the ankle can also cause deformities in the knee. These ''two joint'' muscles—the rectus femoris anteriorly, the gracilis, semitendinosus, and semimembranosus posteriorly (the medial hamstrings), and the biceps femoris (the lateral hamstrings)—all directly affect the position of the knee as well as the position of the hip. The gastrocnemius muscle originates above the knee joint and extends to the ankle joint; therefore, it affects knee and ankle motion and position. A person who walks with his knees flexed does not necessarily have hamstrings that are tight or spastic. A person may walk with the knees in recurvatum, but this does not mean that the quadriceps is overactive because this condition may be caused by an equinus contracture of the ankle or weakened hamstrings.

The patient must be studied carefully while walking, and the examiner should look not only at the knee but also at the hip and ankle. Some of the tendons attached to the muscles are subcutaneous, and their activity can often be determined by a good clinical examination. This assessment should be accompanied by recorded studies of the patient's gait. A videotape camera and recorder should be available to anyone who treats cerebral palsied patients.

Kinetic electromyography provides another means of assessing the influence of hip and knee muscles on gait. It is a useful tool for evaluating which muscles are active and in which part of the gait cycle they are most influential. Electromyography is not necessary in the clinical evaluation of all patients, but it is certainly an excellent tool in the evaluation of the problem patient.

In 1969 Sutherland et al. reported a clinical and electromyographic study of seven children with spastic cerebral palsy with internal rotation gait characterized by flexion of the knee, internal rotation and flexion of the hip, and hamstring spasticity. They noted the multiple and widespread deformities that often occur in the lower extremities in children with cerebral palsy caused by contracture, spasticity, unequal muscle pull, and bony deformity. They also noted that it is impossible by visual means alone to record and analyze the many abnormalities of gait. Consequently they studied these children using combined electromyograms and motion pictures of gait made with special equipment that superimposed electromyograms on motion pictures in which it was possible to view the patient simultaneously in the sagittal and coronal planes. This method made possible a frame-by-frame analysis of the timing of contraction of muscles and a positive correlation with the observed movements during gait. In this group of patients increased internal rotation at the hip appeared to occur just before heelstrike and to continue through most of the stance phase; this rather striking internal rotation was observed consistently in patients with spastic muscles about the hip, a characteristic not seen during normal gait. These investigators demonstrated that the iliopsoas, the tensor fasciae latae, and the sartorius failed to contract during the movements of greatest internal rotation. On the contrary, the hamstring muscles, especially the medial ones, consistently contracted in definite synchrony with the internal rotation movement, and the most consistent finding was an abnormal prolongation of the time of their contraction that extended well into the stance phase. The medial hamstrings appeared to be spastic more consistently than did the biceps femoris.

The operations carried out on this group of patients were based on the clinical findings of hamstring tightness and spasticity, electromyographic confirmation of increased hamstring activity with prolongation of contraction, and positive correlation of the abnormal internal rotation movement of the extremity with hamstring contraction. The operation began with division of the semimembranosus and semitendinosus at their insertions and of the gracilis if the hip adductors had not already been released. This combined muscle unit was mobilized, transferred laterally deep to the tibial and common peroneal nerves and superficial to the popliteal artery and vein, passed through a window deep to the lateral intermuscular septum, and sutured to itself; thus these muscles were converted to external rotators and their action as knee flexors was eliminated. Clinical, electromyographic, and photographic studies of the patients after these operations revealed satisfactory results in six out of seven.

In 1976 Perry et al. studied 23 ambulatory children with spastic diplegic cerebral palsy who walked with flexion of the hip and knee and internal rotation of the hip. They had previously based their indications for surgery on a clinical examination that included observations of the gait and the performance of certain "stretch tests" originally designed to distinguish specific muscle tightness and spasticity. The patients in this study were evaluated by electromyography during gait and stretch tests before and after surgery. Eight muscles were studied electromyographically: the rectus femoris, the gluteus maximus, the gluteus medius, the lateral hamstrings, the medial hamstrings, the gracilis, the adductor longus, and the iliacus. They assumed that iliacus activity was similar to that of the psoas, that of the tensor fasciae latae was similar to that of the gluteus medius during gait and to the hip flexors during stretch, and that of the vastus muscles was similar to that of the rectus femoris during gait. The following stretch tests were performed while electromyographic recordings were made: straight leg raising, hip flexion with knees flexed, adductor stretch with hips and knees flexed, the Thomas test for hip flexion deformity, external rotation of the extended hip, external rotation of the flexed hip, extension of the knee with the hip flexed and abducted (the Phelps-Baker gracilis test), and prone flexion of the knee with the hip extended (the prone rectus test of Duncan or Ely). None of these eight stretch tests were found to be specific for any one muscle electromyographically. The one most nearly specific was the straight leg raising test, which caused activity almost exclusively in the hamstrings; frequently the gracilis also showed increased activity. Most of the tests produced marked activity in muscles that the tests were designed to exclude from stretching; thus no test distinguished between the medial hamstrings and the gracilis. Activity in the iliopsoas and rectus femoris muscles was also similar, and the adductors were markedly sensitive to the gracilis, the Thomas, and the adductor stretch tests.

The clinical and electromyographic indications for the operations performed were as follows. When a fixed flexion contracture of the hip was present, the psoas tendon was detached and sutured to the anterior capsule of the joint. When fixed adduction contracture of the hip was present, the adductor longus and brevis were released and the released portions were sutured to the adductor magnus; no obturator neurectomies were performed. When fixed anteversion of the femoral neck exceeded 45 degrees, derotational trochanteric osteotomy of the femur was performed. When anteversion and coxa valga produced subluxation of the hip, varus derotational osteotomy was performed. When the gracilis was contracted, it was released either proximally or distally, depending on whether adductor or hamstring surgery was carried out at the same time. When the medial hamstrings required release, the semitendinosus and semimembranosus were lengthened. When obvious fixed deformities were absent but the posture and gait suggested marked muscle imbalance as occurred in seven patients, gait electromyograms helped to select the appropriate operations; prolonged and inappropriate activity in a muscle during the gait cycle was the indication for each procedure used in treating these dynamic deformities.

In 1975 Sutherland, Larsen, and Mann studied eight patients with cerebral palsy and contracture of the rectus femoris muscle. They considered this muscle contracted if, with the patient supine and with the hip fully extended, the knee could not be passively flexed past 90 degrees or if, with the patient prone, passive flexion of the knee caused the pelvis to rise from the examining table (positive prone rectus or Ely test). All eight patients fulfilled these criteria. The patients were examined for range of motion of the joints, strength of the muscles, and neurologic abnormalities, and phasic activity electromyograms were made before and after surgery along with two-plane gait photographs. After release of the rectus femoris, lack of improvement in two of the eight patients appeared to be caused by faulty indications for surgery. The improvement in the remaining six patients was apparently produced by improvement in flexion of the knee and especially in the initiation of this movement. In the opinion of these investigators the indications for rectus release are precise and relatively uncommon. Many patients with spastic cerebral palsy have a positive rectus test. In the absence of objective, dynamic functional abnormalities, surgery should not be considered. A prolonged stance phase with slow, labored, and insufficient flexion of the knee is the most important objective sign of rectus overactivity; this should be confirmed by electromyography.

Evans has also reviewed the findings in the most common gait posture assumed by children with spastic cerebral palsy. In this gait, as already described, the hips and knees are flexed, the thighs are usually adducted and internally rotated, and the ankles are either plantar flexed or dorsiflexed. This gait may be caused by flexion contracture at either the hip or the knee, a strong plantar thrust at the ankle, or a combination of these. He notes an interaction of the rectus femoris and the hamstrings in which flexion of the hip imposes a stretch on the hamstrings, which in turn flex the knee. Contracture or spasticity of the hamstrings exaggerates this mechanism in that the hamstrings are, in effect, too short to allow simultaneous extension of the knee and flexion of the hip. Similarly the rectus femoris cannot allow flexion of the knee and extension of the hip. Thus the presence of flexion of the knee without contracture of the joint may be a result of deformity at the hip or ankle and may be relieved by surgical correction of any flexion contracture of the hip or equinus deformity. Evans also points out that an isolated adduction contracture of the hip may cause flexion of the knee because of gracilis spasticity or contracture and that the scissors gait makes flexion of the knee easier. Therefore adductor tenotomy alone may relieve moderate flexion deformity of the knee as well as moderate internal rotation deformity of the hip. Transposition of the tendons of origin of the adductors to the ischial tuberosity, according to Evans, results in excellent correction of adduction and internal rotation of the thigh; flexion of the hip and knee if not relieved immediately are likely to decrease progressively. This operation will not, however, correct severe flexion deformities of the knee. He further points out that the aim of any surgery on the hamstrings should not be to obtain full extension of the knee; rather it should be to obtain a balance of power in flexion and extension of the joint. Any operation that lengthens the hamstrings will increase the lumbar lordosis because it decreases the posterior stabilizing effect of the hamstrings on the pelvis; it will also decrease the power of flexion of the knee and may cause genu recurvatum. Surgery on the hamstrings should not be performed in the presence of fixed equinus deformity or a strong plantar thrust because then genu recurvatum will almost certainly result. Likewise, if the knees are straightened surgically in the presence of a flexion deformity of the hip, the patient will be unable to stand erect without severely increasing the lumbar lordosis, and he will frequently lean forward and require crutches for support. Evaluation of the strength and spasticity of the quadriceps is important and only that surgery necessary to obtain active extension of the knee should be performed; but obtaining full extension of the knee surgically is unnecessary. When contractures and deformities are present at the hip, knee, and ankle, simultaneous surgical correction at all three levels is technically feasible and is indicated. We agree with Evans that advancement of the patella is rarely indicated; if the overpull resulting from spasticity and contracture of the hamstrings is released, the quadriceps usually regains enough power for full extension of the knee. Because of the functional interrelationship of the rectus femoris and hamstrings, when attempting to produce a freer swing of the knee, Evans now frequently releases the rectus femoris when surgery is performed on the hamstrings; this is especially true in those patients with moderate or severe involvement regardless of the findings on stretch testing.

Banks and Green, on the other hand, point out the importance of the adductors in producing internal rotation and adduction of the hips and flexion of the knees. According to them, adductor myotomy, including the adductor longus, the adductor brevis, and the gracilis, and neurectomy of the anterior branch of the obturator nerve correct not only flexion and adduction of the hip but also flexion of the knee in two of every three patients. Fixed flexion contractures of the knee caused by significant hamstring spasticity and contracture require operations on the hamstrings after the role of the adductors in producing the contracture of the knee has been identified and corrected.

As Chandler pointed out in 1933, when a patient has walked for a long time with the knees in flexion, elongation of the patellar tendon may develop (the patella, of course, then comes to lie at a more proximal level on the femoral condyles than normal). The extensor mechanism of the knee is then unable to completely extend the joint actively even after flexion contracture or significant muscle imbalance has been corrected. Chandler transplanted the tibial tuberosity distally to enable the extensor mechanism to function more normally. But damage to the proximal tibial epiphyseal plate is often incurred during this operation, causing a disturbance in growth that results in genu recurvatum. It is therefore no longer performed unless the epiphysis has already fused. Chandler later plicated the patellar tendon to shorten it (Fig. 65-26); this operation does not endanger the epiphyseal plate and is as satisfactory as transplanting the tibial tuberosity. Each of these operations effects a patellar advancement, and both with their modifications are described here. But we agree with Evans that they are rarely indicated.

Eggers has found that when the patellar tendon elongates, the patellar retinacula fail to do so (Fig. 65-27, A). These retinacula are attached chiefly to the sides of the patella and to the proximal end of the tibia on its anteromedial and anterolateral sides. Thus when the patellar tendon has become elongated, the quadriceps must exert its force on the tibia through the retinacula rather than through the patellar tendon. Division of the patellar retinacula enables the quadriceps to extend the knee completely (Fig. 65-27, B), just as does transplanting the tibial tuberosity distally (Fig. 65-27, C) or the patellar tendon distally (Fig.

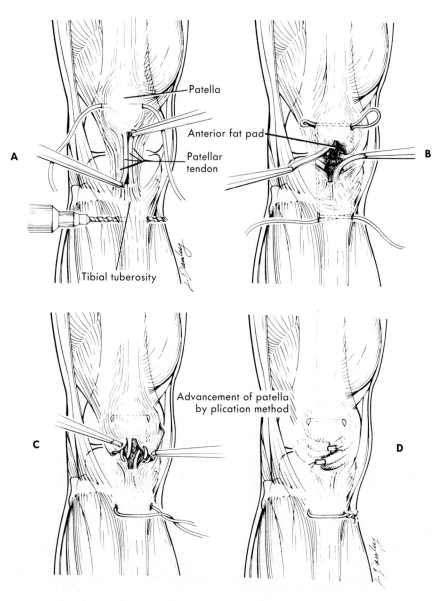

Patella

Anterior fat pad

Patellar tendon

Tibial tuberosity

A

B

Advancement of patella by plication method

C

D

Fig. 65-26. Chandler technique of patellar advancement by plication of patellar tendon (see text). (Modified from Lewis: Practice of surgery, Hagerstown, Md., 1947, W.F. Prior Co., Inc.)

65-28) or plicating the patellar tendon (Fig. 65-27, *D*). It is a simple operation, convalescence from it is brief, and complications after it are rare. Eggers considers that division of the retinacula and transfer of the hamstring tendons to the femoral condyles (p. 2884) are interdependent operations. In an excellent review of surgery of the lower extremities in cerebral palsy, Evans recommends division of the retinacula if when the hip is extended the knee cannot be actively extended beyond 20 degrees of flexion or when active extension of the knee is significantly less than passive extension.

Imbalance between the flexors and extensors of the knee is difficult to treat. A difference of not more than one grade in strength is necessary for satisfactory reciprocal flexion and extension of the joint. When the imbalance was caused by spasticity of the hamstring muscles, Silver-

skiöld transferred their origins from the ischium to the posterior subtrochanteric aspect of the femur. Seymour and Sharrard released their origins from the ischium. They recommended this operation (1) when fixed flexion deformity of the knee is absent, (2) when the stride is short and the pelvis rotates at the end of each step, (3) when straight leg raising is limited to 30 degrees or less, and (4) when sitting upright is impossible if the knees are extended but not if they are flexed. In their nine patients, the length of the stride was doubled after surgery, walking was easier, and rotation of the pelvis was lessened; in all patients straight leg raising was possible to at least 65 degrees and in two thirds to 85 degrees or more.

In 1974 Drummond, Rogala, Templeton, and Cruess reported the results of complete release of the hamstring muscles from the ischium in 50 extremities of 25 patients.

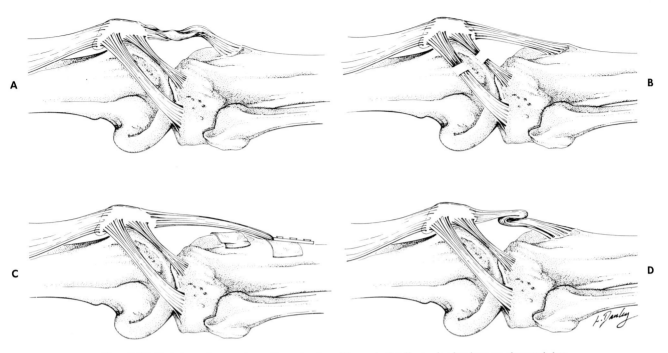

Fig. 65-27. Techniques for restoring active extension of knee. **A,** Patellar tendon has become elongated, but retinacula have not. Thus, retinacula limit proximal excursion of patella and prevent complete active extension of knee. **B,** Eggers divides retinacula to allow quadriceps to extend completely. **C,** Bosworth transplants tibial tuberosity distally to allow quadriceps to extend knee completely. **D,** Chandler plicates patellar tendon to allow quadriceps to extend knee completely. (**A** and **B,** after Eggers.)

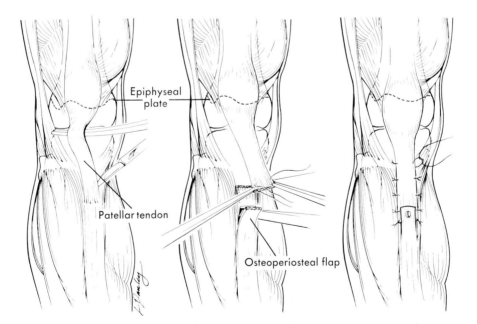

Fig. 65-28. Baker technique of patellar advancement (see text). (Modified from Roberts, W.M., and Adams, J.P.: J. Bone Joint Surg. **35-A:**958, 1953.)

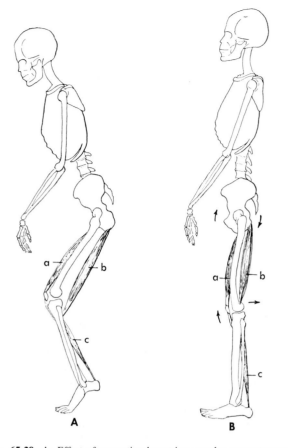

Fig. 65-29. A, Effect of overactive hamstring muscles on posture and gait. Crouched position caused by hip and knee flexion. **B,** Effect of hamstring tenodesis. Since hamstring muscles no longer flex knees, quadriceps extensor group can now extend knee joints. If retinacula are contracted, these are divided. Transplanted hamstrings can now rotate pelvis and extend hips. End result is erect stance, with heels in improved walking position. *a,* Quadriceps femoris muscles; *b,* hamstring muscles; *c,* soleus muscle. (From Eggers, G.W.N.: J. Bone Joint Surg. **34-A:**827 1952.)

The spastic flexion deformity of the knee was corrected sufficiently. In most instances posture was corrected, gait was improved, and a longer stride was possible. However a significant increase in lumbar lordosis developed in four patients and genu recurvatum developed in seven. As a result of this study, they are now performing a limited proximal hamstring release in a few carefully selected patients whose flexion deformity of the hip is less than 25 degrees and whose abdominal muscles are not weak.

Eggers recommended a converse operation: he transferred the insertion of the hamstrings to the posterior supracondylar aspect of the femur. Besides eliminating the function of the hamstrings in flexing the knee, this operation also improved their function in extending the hip; thus it reduced both the primary flexed position of the hip and the secondary flexed position of the knee (Fig. 65-29). According to Evans and to Evans and Julian, the original Eggers operation in which all of the hamstrings are transferred proximal to the knee often causes genu recurvatum, weakness in flexion of the knee, and increased lumbar lor-

dosis; consequently it is no longer used. The operation most often used consists of tenotomy of the gracilis with resection of 5 cm or more of its tendon, lengthening the semimembranosus by dividing its aponeurosis, and lengthening or transferring the semitendinosus to the lateral femoral condyle; if this procedure allows sufficient passive extension of the knee, the biceps femoris is left intact.

According to Keats and Kambin, lengthening the biceps is usually unnecessary. Pollock and English reported 54 operations on 31 patients in which some type of hamstring transfer had been performed; the biceps femoris had been transferred 49 times, the semitendinosus 45 times, the semimembranosus 19 times, and the gracilis 7 times. They also advise leaving at least one hamstring intact to assist in flexing the knee; however, it may be lengthened if necessary. Twenty-one patients were improved after surgery. Patients with severe flexion deformities of the hip before surgery improved less than those without. Moderate flexion deformities of the hip that averaged 30 degrees before surgery averaged only 15 degrees after.

Reimers, in a prospective study of 60 patients with cerebral palsy and flexion deformity of the knee caused by contracture of the hamstrings, reported 112 operations on these muscles performed by three different techniques. As a result of this study, transposition of the hamstrings by the Eggers' method was abandoned because of unsatisfactory results. Lengthening the hamstrings proximally at or near the ischial tuberosity when the fixed flexion deformity of the knee does not exceed 5 degrees has become the standard operation. Lengthening the medial hamstrings distally is used when fixed flexion deformity of the knee exceeds 5 degrees; the gracilis and the biceps tendon are divided and not sutured, and the other hamstrings are lengthened by Z-plasty incisions. In every instance the hamstring operation has been preceded by operations to correct flexion contracture of the hip or equinus deformity of the ankle.

Knee flexion deformity

Flexion, by far the most common knee deformity, may be caused by tight hamstring muscles, weak quadriceps muscle, or a combination of both. It may be secondary to hip flexion deformities in which the hip flexors are spastic, the hip extensors are weak, or a combination of the two. It may be secondary to equinus of the ankles, or the so-called jump position, in which the hips are flexed, the knees are flexed, and the ankles are in equinus. It may also be secondary to a weak triceps, in which the tendo calcaneus or another portion of the triceps surae has been overlengthened, or in which spastic ankle dorsiflexors overpull the ankles into calcaneus. If the ankles are in calcaneus, the knees must flex to get the forefeet on the ground.

To find the cause of knee flexion, the muscles must be assessed to determine whether the joint itself is contracted or whether the deformity is caused by spasticity. If possible, the strength of the muscles should be assessed, though this is difficult in the cerebral palsied patient. Remember that cerebral palsy is an upper motor neuron lesion and is caused by a lesion in the brain. The brain is geographically affected and the body is regionally affected. Nerves to one

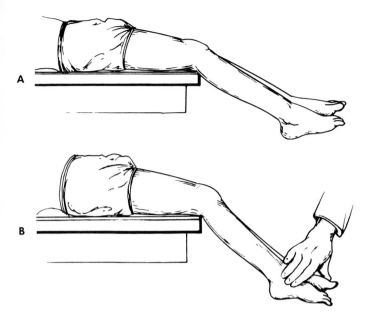

Fig. 65-30. Testing for quadriceps strength. **A,** With hips extended, knees are allowed to flex off end of table. **B,** Patient voluntarily extends knees from flexed position against resistance. (Redrawn from Evans, E.B.: American Academy of Orthopaedic Surgeons: Instructional course lectures, vol. 20, St. Louis, 1971, The C.V. Mosby Co.)

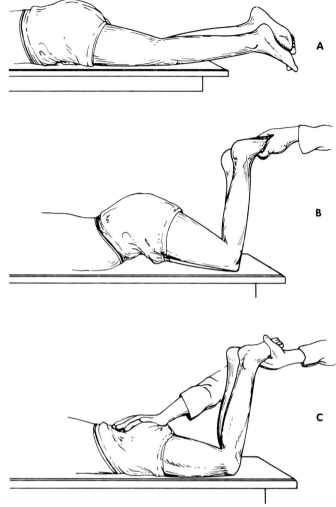

Fig. 65-31. Prone rectus test. **A,** Patient is prone and knees are extended. **B,** Flexing knees causes buttocks to rise from table. **C,** Spasticity in rectus is overcome by downward pressure on buttocks. (Redrawn from Evans, E.B.: American Academy of Orthopaedic Surgeons: Instructional course lectures, vol. 20, St. Louis, 1971, The C.V. Mosby Co.)

specific muscle are not affected, but rather nerves to a group of muscles. If the hamstring muscles are spastic, then the quadriceps will probably be spastic too, perhaps to a lesser degree. The same is true for the gastrocnemius, the dorsiflexors of the foot, and the flexors and extensors and the abductors and adductors of the hip. It is not unusual to correct a knee flexion deformity by transferring or lengthening a hamstring and then have a spastic rectus femoris pull the knee into hyperextension because spasticity in the rectus femoris was not detected before the hamstring muscles were altered. An extended knee in the swing phase of gait tremendously hampers propulsion. If a person has flexed hips and extended knees, he may have difficulty even bending his knees enough to get up on a curbing or to climb steps. To effect this elevation, he must hike up his pelvis and abduct his hips.

Testing hip flexion and extension, as well as adduction and abduction, is discussed later. The strength of the quadriceps muscle, whether it is under voluntary control, and whether it has functional strength is best checked with the patient supine and his feet off the end of the table. Extend the hips and allow the knees to flex passively (Fig. 65-30, *A*), then ask the patient to voluntarily extend his knees against resistance (Fig. 65-30, *B*). An opinion can then be formed as to how strong the quadriceps is. To determine if the rectus femoris muscle is spastic, turn the patient prone and do the prone rectus test (Ely test) (Fig. 65-31). With the patient prone and the knees extended, flex the knees. If the rectus is spastic, the hips will flex and the buttocks will rise off the table when the rectus is thus stretched. It is best to do this test one side at a time to determine the relative spasticity in each rectus femoris.

The hamstring spasticity and contracture test is done with the patient prone and then supine (Fig. 65-32). With the patient prone, extend the hips as much as possible and exert gentle pressure on the calves. The angle that the femur and the tibia make after the spasticity is overcome is the degree of absolute contracture of the soft tissues behind the knee. Next place the patient supine to test hamstring spasticity. Stabilize the opposite knee in as much extension as possible, and then raise the leg that is to be examined with the knee straight. If knee extension is limited as the hip is flexed, then either the medial or lateral hamstrings are tight. The patient can also be examined for medial hamstring spasticity in the prone position with the knees flexed and feet off the table. This relaxes the hamstrings proximally and allows the hip to be abducted if there is no contracture of the adductor muscles. Extend the knees and if extension is not possible then, unless the hip is adducted, the gracilis and medial hamstrings are tight. This may also be done with the patient supine and the hips and knees flexed (Fig. 65-33). To test for gastrocnemius contracture, the amount of equinus in the ankle is measured with the knee fully extended and then with the knee flexed (Fig. 65-34). If the ankle can be dorsiflexed more with the knee flexed than with it extended, there is gastrocnemius contracture or spasticity.

An absolute contracture of about 10 degrees is compatible with walking without flexing the hips and knees excessively. Contracture beyond 10 degrees should be corrected, usually by changing the strength of the hamstring muscles.

Weakened hamstrings are the major cause of recurvatum in the knees. Thus, only partial lengthening of the hamstring tendons is indicated in most instances. It is our practice to selectively lengthen the gracilis and semitendinosus muscles with a Z-plasty procedure and to partially lengthen the semimembranosus by merely sectioning the fascia as it surrounds the muscle. If the biceps femoris is determined to be tight, then it is lengthened by incising its fascia circumferentially.

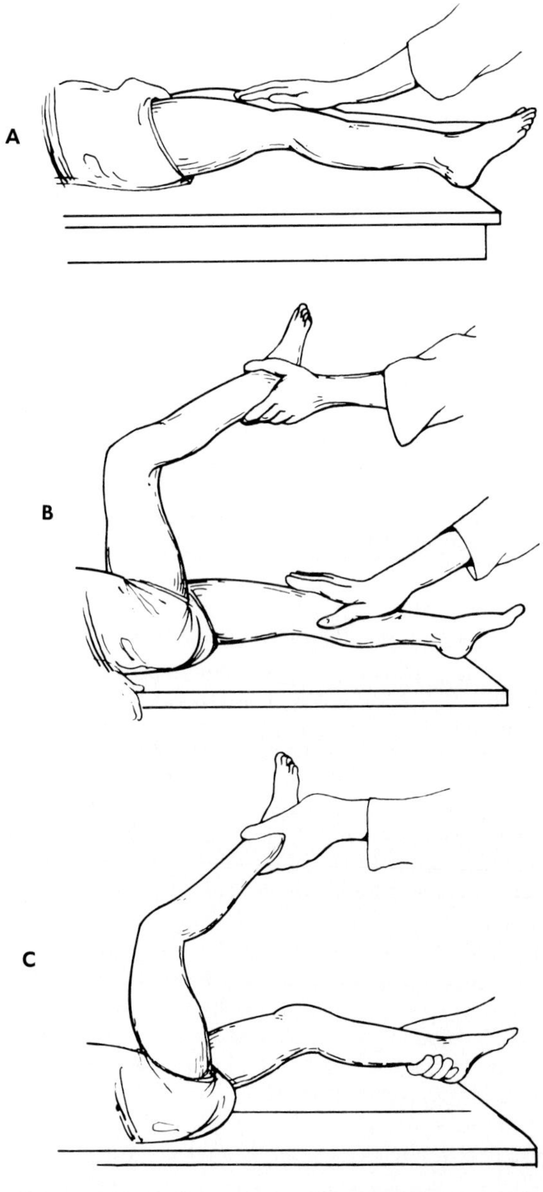

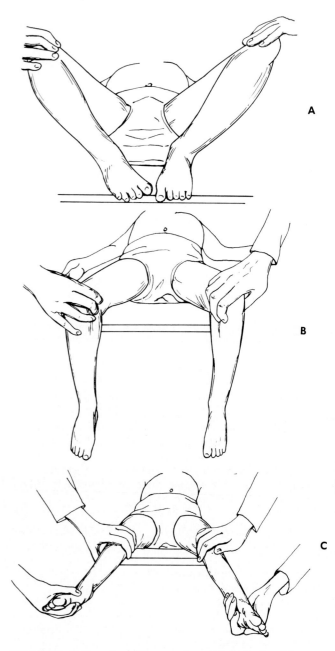

Fig. 65-32. Testing for hamstring spasticity and contracture. **A,** Patient is supine with hips extended. Pressure is exerted over knees forcing them into extension. Flexion remaining in knees is absolute knee flexion contracture. **B,** Knee on side to be tested is flexed while opposite knee is stabilized in extension. **C,** Attempted flexion of hip results in more flexion of knee. (Redrawn from Evans, E.B.: American Academy of Orthopaedic Surgeons: Instructional course lectures, vol. 20, St. Louis, 1971, The C.V. Mosby Co.)

Fig. 65-33. Testing for adductor and medial hamstring tightness. **A,** Thighs abduct well with hips and knees flexed indicating no adductor contracture. **B,** With hips extended and knees flexed hips abduct well. **C,** With hips extended, bringing knees into extension causes thighs to adduct, indicating medial hamstring spasticity. (Redrawn from Evans, E.B.: American Academy of Orthopaedic Surgeons: Instructional course lectures, vol. 20, St. Louis, 1971, The C.V. Mosby Co.)

Some authors recommend transferring a portion of the hamstrings to the supracondylar area. Sutherland and his group transfer the semimembranosus and semitendinosus muscles into the periosteum along the lateral side of the femur. Baker recommended semitendinosus transfer to the lateral femoral condyle. In our experience, transferring the hamstring tendons laterally has been no more effective than fractionally lengthening them.

Proximal hamstring lengthenings or releases have not

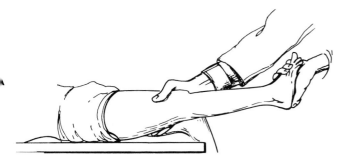

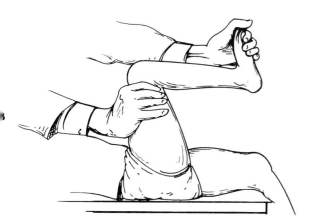

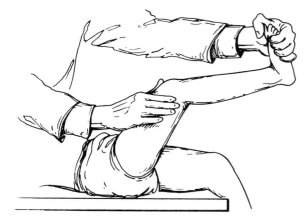

Fig. 65-34. Testing for gastrocnemius contracture and spasticity. **A,** With knee extended equinus in ankle is noted. **B,** With knee flexed ankle is easily dorsiflexed indicating no soleus contracture. **C,** As knee is extended ankle dorsiflexion is resisted by tight or spastic gastrocnemius muscles. (Redrawn from Evans, E.B.: American Academy of Orthopaedic Surgeons: Instructional course lectures, vol. 20, St. Louis, 1971, The C.V. Mosby Co.)

been satisfactory in our experience. Little correction of knee flexion has been obtained, and increased hip flexion and lumbar lordosis have developed, although stride length was improved. It is possible that we used this procedure in patients who had too much uncorrected hip flexion.

Hamstring tenotomies are rarely if ever indicated except in patients with flexion contractures of the knees that interfere with the use of a wheelchair. If a percutaneous hamstring tenotomy is done, the lateral incision should be large enough to make sure the peroneal nerve is not mistaken for a tendon.

In a hamstring contracture of long duration, soft tissue releases may not allow full knee extension, or a full release may compromise the nerves and vessels behind the knee. If further alignment of the leg in extension is necessary, it may be obtained by a corrective supracondylar osteotomy. Grant, Small, and Lehman have advised that supracondylar osteotomy be performed if fixed knee flexion exceeds 15 to 20 degrees. They have developed a geometric osteotomy to correct the flexion attitude about the knees that leaves relatively even surfaces anteroposteriorly at the osteotomy site.

OPERATIONS TO CORRECT KNEE FLEXION
PATELLAR ADVANCEMENT

Patellar advancement is designed to enable the quadriceps to completely extend the knee on weight bearing. We believe the elongation of the patellar tendon is usually caused by spasticity and contracture of the hamstring muscles. After correction of the hamstring imbalance, with or without retinacular release, the quadriceps usually gains enough strength to fully extend the knee actively against gravity; thus patellar advancement is rarely indicated. If strength is insufficient 6 to 12 months after correction of the hamstring muscle imbalance, patellar advancement may be indicated (1) when the patellar tendon has become elongated, the patella thus lying at a more proximal level than normal, (2) when the knee can be completely extended passively, and (3) when the knee cannot be actively extended beyond a position of 10 to 20 degrees flexion. Before patellar advancement any flexion contracture should be corrected by the use of wedging casts when the deformity is mild or, when it is moderate or severe, by posterior capsulotomy and lengthening of the hamstrings or by supracondylar osteotomy.

Transplanting the tibial tuberosity as originally described by Chandler is contraindicated until growth is complete because it is likely to damage the proximal tibial epiphyseal plate.

Chandler later devised a technique of patellar advancement in which surgery is limited to the soft tissues, and thus injury of the proximal tibial epiphyseal plate is prevented. The patella is held in its normal position by plicating the patellar tendon.

McCarroll and Baker have each also devised a technique of patellar advancement that avoids injuring the epiphyseal plate. The patellar tendon is freed at its insertion, and its distal end is transplanted distally and is fastened beneath an osteoperiosteal flap (Fig. 65-28).

TECHNIQUE (CHANDLER). Expose the patellar tendon through a curved bayonet-shaped incision. Begin the incision just lateral to and 2.5 cm proximal to the proximal border of the patella and continue it distally and medially across the distal part of the patellar tendon to a point about 2.5 cm distal to the tibial tuberosity. Undermine the skin edges as needed. Now drill a hole transversely through the center of the patella and pass a wire through it (Fig. 65-26, *A*). Then drill a second hole transversely through the tibial crest just distal to the tibial tuberosity. Insert a short, curved cannula beneath the aponeurosis at the lateral end of the hole in the tibia and force it proximally to emerge at the lateral end of the hole in the patella. Then feed the wire distally through the lumen of the cannula to the hole in the tibia and withdraw the cannula. Repeat this procedure on the medial side. Then pass both ends of the wire through the hole in the tibia (Fig. 65-26, *B*). Now incise the patellar tendon in the midline (Fig. 65-26, *A* and *B*) and cut narrow strips from its free margin, leaving one strip attached to the patella and the other to the tibia. Then draw the wire taut enough to bring the patella distally to its normal position and twist it on itself. Thread the strips of tendon on a heavy fascia needle and use them to plicate the patellar tendon (Fig. 65-26, *C* and *D*); add interrupted silk sutures.

Occasionally the quadriceps is so contracted that dividing the proximal tendon of the rectus femoris at its pelvic origin is necessary before the patella can be drawn distally to its proper place.

AFTERTREATMENT. A posterior splint is worn for several days, and then active motion is begun. The wire will break if left in place; it should be removed at 8 weeks.

Burns, instead of inserting a wire as just described, inserts a Kirschner wire through the patella and incorporates it in a long leg cast. The patella is thus held in position, but the patellar tendon is relieved of undue tension during healing.

RELEASE OF PATELLAR RETINACULA

TECHNIQUE (EGGERS). Make anteromedial and anterolateral curved incisions about 7.5 cm long as shown in Figs. 65-35, *a*, and 65-36, *a*. Begin them distally 1 cm lateral or medial to the patellar tendon at a point midway between the patella and the tibial tuberosity and extend them first proximally and then posteriorly to end at a point just anterior to the femoral attachment of the respective collateral ligaments. Deepen the incisions. The fascial retinacula are exposed by the distal part of each incision; divide them parallel with the patellar tendon and patella. The muscular retinacula are exposed by the proximal part of each incision; divide them in line with the incisions. Do not incise the capsule of the knee joint. Close the subcutaneous tissue and skin with interrupted sutures. The hamstring tendons may be transferred to the femoral condyles at the same time if desired.

AFTERTREATMENT. A long leg cast is applied with the knee in extension and is worn for 3 weeks.

TRANSFER OF HAMSTRING TENDONS TO FEMORAL CONDYLES

As already indicated, the Eggers transfer is often followed by weakness of the knee in flexion, increased lumbar lordosis, and genu recurvatum. According to Evans, it is now used only in skeletally mature patients who have severe flexion deformity of the knee and weakness of the quadriceps. It is generally agreed that to prevent excessive weakness in flexion of the knee, at least one hamstring should not be transferred and this hamstring should be the biceps femoris or semimembranosus, or both. The operation used most often consists of tenotomy or proximal transfer of the gracilis, proximal transfer of the semitendinosus, and lengthening of the semimembranosus and biceps femoris.

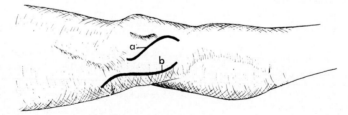

Fig. 65-35. Medial incisions for, *a,* division of patellar retinacula and, *b,* hamstring transplantation. (From Eggers, G.W.N.: J. Bone Joint Surg. **34-A**:827, 1952.)

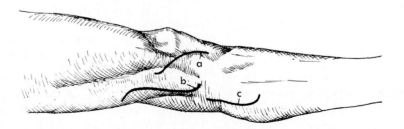

Fig. 65-36. Lateral incisions for, *a,* division of patellar retinacula, *b,* release of biceps femoris and transplantation to femoral condyle, and *c,* soleus neurectomy. (From Eggers, G.W.N.: J. Bone Joint Surg. **34-A**:827, 1952.)

TECHNIQUE (EGGERS). Make a curvilinear incision (Fig. 65-36, b) 7.5 cm long over the biceps femoris tendon: curve the distal end of the incision anteriorly just proximal to the head of the fibula. Isolate and gently retract the peroneal nerve and expose the biceps tendon. Now divide the tendon transversely just proximal to its insertion on the fibula and embed it subperiosteally in a groove in the posterolateral margin of the lateral femoral condyle. Anchor it firmly to the periosteum and adjacent lateral intermuscular septum with interrupted silk sutures (Fig. 65-37).

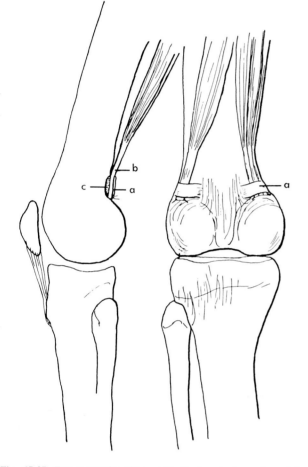

Fig. 65-37. Eggers transfer of hamstring tendons to femoral condyles. Tendons, b, are anchored in grooves, c, beneath periosteum, a. Tendons are sutured to periosteum and adjacent fibrous tissue. (From Eggers, G.W.N.: J. Bone Joint Surg. **34-A:**827, 1952.)

Make a similar medial incision (Fig. 65-35, b). Identify and isolate the semimembranosus, semitendinosus, and gracilis tendons and divide them just proximal to their insertions. Embed them in the medial intermuscular septum and periosteum at the posteromedial aspect of the medial femoral condyle as described for the biceps tendon.

The patellar retinacula may be released at the same time if desired.

AFTERTREATMENT. Aftertreatment is as described for release of patellar retinacula (p. 2884).

MODIFIED EGGERS PROCEDURE AS ADVOCATED BY EVANS

See Table 65-2.

FRACTIONAL LENGTHENING OF HAMSTRING TENDONS

In 1942 Green and McDermott reported fractionally lengthening the hamstring tendons and other tendons about the knee in spastic flexion deformities. Some modification of their original operation is now used by most surgeons to modify spastic knee flexion when indicated.

TECHNIQUE (TACHDJIAN). Place the patient prone and inflate a midthigh tourniquet; then make a midline longitudinal incision beginning just above the popliteal crease and extend it 7 to 10 cm proximally (Fig. 65-38, A). Divide the subcutaneous tissue and deep fascia in line with the skin incision. Protect the posterior femoral cutaneous nerve in the proximal part of the wound. Next identify the hamstring tendons by blunt dissection. Divide the tendon sheaths of each longitudinally, and tag them with silk sutures. Expose the tendon of the biceps femoris laterally and isolate it from the peroneal nerve lying along its medial side. Pass a blunt instrument deep to the biceps tendon, incise its tendinous portion transversely at two levels 3 cm apart and leave the muscle fibers intact (Fig. 65-38, B). The tendon lengthens over the muscle fibers as the hip is flexed and the knee is extended (Fig. 65-38, C). Next, isolate the semimembranosus tendon medially. Incise its tendon sheath and mark it as above. Divide its tendinous fibers on its deep side at two levels as in the biceps femoris (Fig. 65-38, D). Extend the knee and flex the hip and the tendinous parts will slide on the muscle. Expose the semitendinosus tendon and divide the distal part of the tendon obliquely up to its muscle fibers. Incise the tendon transversely above and lengthen it in a similar manner, or perform a Z-plasty procedure to lengthen the tendon (Fig. 65-38, E). Close all tendon sheaths meticulously, but do not close the deep fascia (Fig. 65-38, F). After the tourniquet

Table 65-2. Suggested surgery for hamstring weakness

Condition	Suggested surgery
Full active knee extension in recumbency	No hamstring surgery
Active recumbent knee extension to within 5 to 10 degrees of full extension with good quadriceps power	Semitendinosus lengthening or transfer, usually with gracilis tenotomy; occasionally, because of operative testing, aponeurotic lengthening of semimembranosus or biceps
An absolute contracture of greater than 10 degrees but less than 20 degrees	Usually requires gracilis tenotomy, semitendinosus lengthening or transferring, and semimembranosus or biceps lengthening; much depends on quadriceps strength
An absolute contracture of 20 degrees or more and a measurable contracture of 45 degrees or more with the hip at 90 degrees	May require lengthening or transferring all hamstrings and releasing retinaculum, again depending on quadriceps strength

Modified from Evans, B.: American Academy of Orthopaedic Surgeons: Instructional course lectures, vol. 20, St. Louis, 1971, The C.V. Mosby Co.

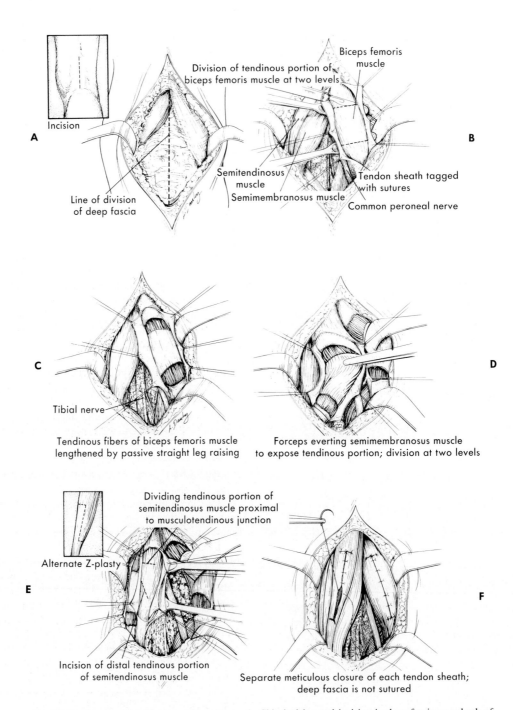

Fig. 65-38. Fractional lengthening of hamstrings. **A,** Skin incision and incision in deep fascia over back of knee. **B,** Incisions in tendon of biceps femoris in lateral compartment after opening and retracting its tendon sheath, protecting peroneal nerve medially. **C,** Tendon of biceps femoris lengthens as knee is extended and hip is flexed. **D,** Division of tendon of semimembranosus in similar fashion. **E,** Semitendinosus is lengthened by Z-plasty, as seen in inset, or by step-cuts in its tendon at multiple levels. **F,** Tendon sheaths of biceps femoris and semimembranosus are sutured before closure of wound. (Redrawn from Tachjdian, M.O.: Pediatric orthopaedics, Philadelphia, 1972, W.B. Saunders Co.)

is deflated, secure all bleeding points and close the subcutaneous tissues and skin. Apply a long leg cast with the knee in extension.

AFTERTREATMENT. Straight leg raising exercises are performed 15 times once a day while the cast is on to stretch the hamstring tendons. At 3 to 4 weeks, a new long leg cast is applied and bivalved so that active and passive exercises to alter knee flexion and strengthen knee extension may be started. The patient is allowed to walk with crutches and the cast is discontinued when a functional range of motion and muscle control of the knees are acquired.

LATERAL TRANSFER OF MEDIAL HAMSTRINGS FOR INTERNAL ROTATIONAL DEFORMITY OF HIP

Baker and Hill described an operation in which the semitendinosus tendon is transferred laterally to the anterior surface of the lateral femoral condyle for internal rotational deformity of the hip (Fig. 65-39). They first used it in an athetoid patient with a dynamic deformity. But it has also been found to be useful when the tendon has been divided in treating flexion deformity of the knee. The tendon is passed through a subcutaneous tunnel from the posteromedial aspect of the middle of the thigh to the anterior aspect of the lateral femoral condyle, where it is anchored opposite the superior pole of the patella.

Sutherland et al. used a technique of simultaneous electromyographic and photographic studies before and after

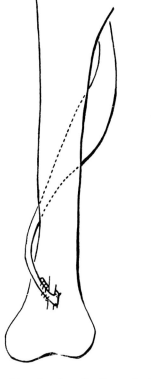

Fig. 65-39. Baker lateral transfer of semitendinosus for internal rotation deformity of hip (see text). (From Baker, L.D., and Hill, L.M.: J. Bone Joint Surg. **46-A:**1, 1964.)

surgery to record the timing of contraction of muscles, which coincided with the abnormal internal rotational movement at the hip. As a result of these studies, they transferred the semimembranosus and semitendinosus, and also the gracilis if the adductors had not been previously released, to the lateral aspect of the femur and anchored them to the lateral intermuscular septum.

TECHNIQUE (SUTHERLAND ET AL.). With the patient prone, inflate a pneumatic tourniquet high on the thigh and make an S-shaped incision on the posterior aspect of the knee. Begin the incision proximally on the lateral aspect of the popliteal space over the biceps femoris tendon and extend it distally 7.5 cm, then medially across the popliteal space in the flexor crease, and then again distally for 5 cm over the insertion of the semitendinosus muscle (Fig. 65-40, A). Mobilize the proximal flap. Pass a clamp beneath the semitendinosus and semimembranosus tendons and divide them near their insertions. If the adductors have not been previously released, identify the gracilis tendon, free it proximally, and divide it near its insertion. Next gently mobilize the tibial and common peroneal nerves and develop the interval deep to the nerves but superficial to the femoral artery and vein and extend it down to the lateral intermuscular septum (Fig. 65-40, B). Next incise the lateral intermuscular septum at its attachment to the periosteum of the femur just proximal to the lateral femoral condyle (Fig. 65-40, C). Gently tease the fibers of the vastus lateralis muscle away from the anterior surface of the intermuscular septum, pass the tendons through the incision in the septum, loop them around the septum, and suture them to themselves with interrupted nonabsorbable sutures (Fig. 65-40, D). Sometimes the semimembranosus alone is passed through the septum and the semitendinosus is sutured to it. The tendons must not be fixed under too much tension since Perry et al. have pointed out that this may cause inappropriate electrical activity in the transfer after surgery. Close the wound in layers and apply a long leg cast.

AFTERTREATMENT. At 4 weeks the cast is removed and a walking cylinder cast is applied. At 6 weeks this cast is removed and physical therapy is started.

EXTENSION OSTEOTOMY OF LOWER FEMUR

When release of soft tissue contractures fails to result in full extension of the knee, or when the deformity is so severe that the neurovascular structures may be damaged if soft tissues are released too vigorously, an extension osteotomy of the lower femur in the supracondylar area to realign the femur with the tibia may be indicated.

Grant, Small, and Lehman believe that a true flexion contracture of more than 15 to 20 degrees warrants a corrective extension osteotomy with or without femoral shortening. They have devised a geometric osteotomy that does not require preoperative cutouts or measurements to align the femur with the tibia. However, the operation is not recommended for children with significant growth remaining.

Geometric supracondylar extension osteotomy

TECHNIQUE (GRANT, SMALL, AND LEHMAN). Without using a tourniquet, expose the lateral side of the femur by a straight lateral approach. Reflect the vastus lateralis ante-

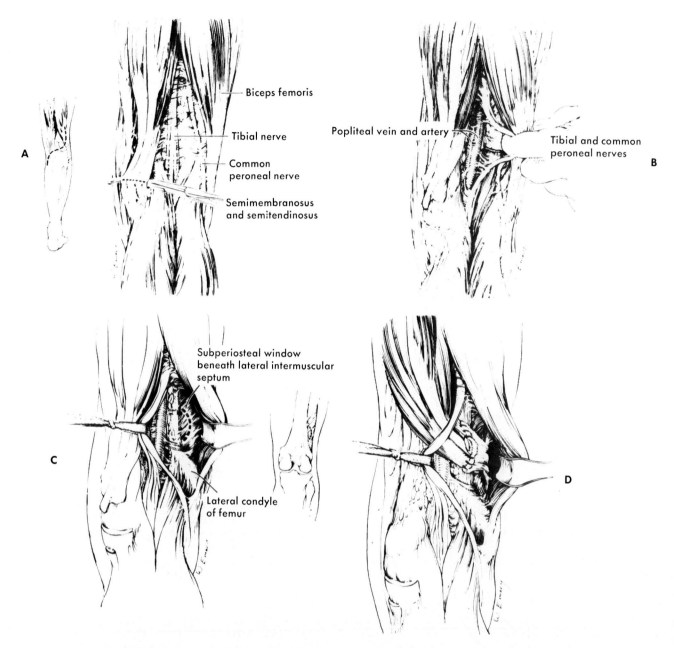

Fig. 65-40. Technique of Sutherland et al. for lateral transfer of medial hamstrings. **A,** *Inset,* skin incision. Semitendinosus and semimembranosus tendons are divided. **B,** Tibial and common peroneal nerves are mobilized, and lateral intermuscular septum is exposed. **C,** Septum is incised at attachment to periosteum. **D,** Divided tendons are passed through incision in septum, are looped around septum, and are sutured to themselves. (From Sutherland, D.H., et al.: J. Bone Joint Surg. **51-A:**1070, 1969.)

riorly off the linea aspera and intermuscular septum. Then expose the supracondylar area of the femur laterally, anteriorly, and medially by subperiosteal stripping distally to the articular surface of the patellofemoral joint. Avoid the epiphyseal plate in skeletally immature patients. Extend the knee maximally and select a point just above the femoral articular cartilage on the anterolateral edge of the femur. At this level score with an osteotome the lateral edge of the femur perpendicular to a line in the long axis of the tibia (Fig. 65-41, *A*). Proximally, where this scored line

intersects the posterolateral edge of the femur, score the lateral surface of the femur anteriorly to form a line perpendicular to the long axis of the femur. The distance between these two points on the anterolateral margin of the femur is the width of the wedge of bone to be removed. Convert the triangular wedge of bone so marked into an isosceles triangle. Outline this triangle on the lateral, anterior, and medial surfaces of the femur, and remove this triangular wedge of bone with a bone saw or an osteotome. If the correction is enough to damage the neurovascular

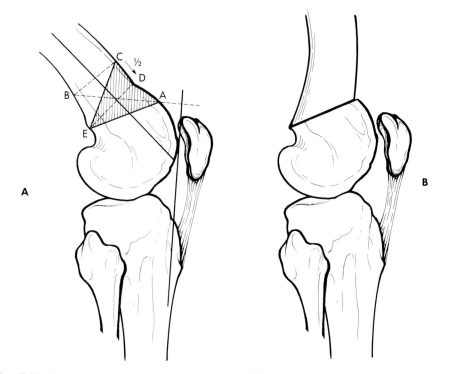

Fig. 65-41. Supracondylar geometric extension osteotomy of femur. **A,** With knee maximally extended score line *BA* on femur perpendicular to longitudinal axis of tibia. Score line *BC* perpendicular to longitudinal axis of femur, starting posteriorly at point *B*. Convert triangle so formed into isosceles triangle by *D* projecting line from anterior to posterior on femur *E*, beginning one half distance from *A* to *C*. Correct *AE* and *CE*. Point *E* is apex of triangle, *(ACE)* to be removed. **B,** After wedge has been removed, close and fix femur. (Redrawn from Grant, A.D., Small, R.D., and Lehman, W.B.: Bull. Hosp. Jt. Dis. Orthop. Inst. **42:**30, 1982.)

supply to the leg, merely shorten the proximal femoral fragment by cutting parallel to its cut edge. Close the wedge and fix the osteotomy by any appropriate method (Fig. 65-41, *B*). Grant et al. prefer the AO condylar plate.

AFTERTREATMENT. Aftertreatment is the same as for any other supracondylar osteotomy.

Recurvatum of knee

Recurvatum may be primarily the result of quadriceps spasticity or quadriceps spasticity that is greater than any spasticity of the hamstrings. It may be secondary to hamstring weakness when the hamstrings have been lengthened too much or transferred or by weakness of the gastrocnemius muscle when its proximal heads have been recessed. Recurvatum may also be secondary to equinus of the ankle; if a patient tries to put his foot on the ground with the ankle in equinus, then the knee must go into recurvatum if his heel is to touch the surface.

To test for quadriceps spasticity the prone rectus test (Ely test) is used. The same test may also be done with the patient sitting. If the rectus femoris is tight, it is lengthened at the hip. We prefer to lengthen it at the Y-bifurcation where it divides into the direct and oblique heads.

To determine if recurvatum of the knee is secondary to equinus of the ankle, a short leg cast or ankle orthosis is applied with the ankle in neutral dorsiflexion. If the knee goes into recurvatum with the foot plantigrade, then the

recurvatum is secondary to either weakened hamstrings or a spastic quadriceps. If the ankle will not dorsiflex to neutral (right angle), the heel can be built up to accommodate for the equinus. If the knee goes into recurvatum as this built-up heel touches the floor, then equinus is not the cause of the recurvatum. If equinus is the cause, cast correction or surgery to correct it is indicated.

Recurvatum of the knee secondary to overlengthening or transferring the hamstrings is difficult to treat. Even if replanting the tendons is technically possible, the hamstrings will not regain normal strength because they will have been weakened by the previous surgery. Evans has recommended that significant recurvatum of this nature be treated with bilateral long leg braces with a pelvic band. He recommends locking the knees at 20 degrees to prevent full extension and ankle stops at 5 degrees above a right angle. When hip control is achieved, he removes the pelvic band but retains the long leg braces for months or years until a satisfactory knee stance is achieved. He advises against flexion osteotomy for recurvatum.

Knee valgus

Knee valgus is usually caused by a hip adduction deformity, which is coupled with internal rotation and flexion. Usually the valgus looks worse than it actually is, because it is a combination of flexion and internal rotation that accentuates the appearance of valgus. Correction of the spastic hip adduction and internal rotational deformity is indicated. Either the hip adductors, the medial hamstrings, or the iliopsoas causes the deformity. The cause must be determined and corrected surgically, but in such patients the knee does not require surgery.

A tight iliotibial band may also cause knee valgus. It is easily tested by positioning the patient on the contralateral side and having him flex the knee nearest the table up onto his abdomen. With the knee flexed, the hip being tested is flexed and abducted, then is moved from the position of flexion to extension, and then is adducted. If the hip will not adduct without flexing, then the iliotibial band is tight and can be palpated subcutaneously along the distal third of the thigh. The tight band should be resected by a Yount procedure (p. 2987).

Severe valgus deformities of the ankle can cause structural knee valgus. It is rarely severe enough to warrant any surgery at the knee, but if it is, then a supracondylar varus osteotomy may be performed. This deformity is more common in myelodysplasia than in cerebral palsy.

Patella alta

Patella alta causes chondromalacia. The patella rides above the femoral condyles and the patellar tendon is lengthened (Fig. 65-42). This may be caused primarily by quadriceps spasticity or it may be secondary to a marked knee flexion deformity of long duration. Plication of the patellar tendon is the procedure of choice for patella alta. Transplantation of the bony insertion of the patellar tendon distally is contraindicated because this condition usually occurs in growing children with open proximal tibial epiphyses and damage to the front of the epiphysis can result in recurvatum of the knee. In severe flexion deformity of the knee with elongation of the patellar tendon, correction of the flexion deformity is all that is needed. Usually an operation on the patella is unnecessary because the quadriceps lag will disappear with time.

Subluxation or dislocation of patella

Subluxation or dislocation of the patella can result from a valgus knee deformity. It may also be caused by flexion, adduction, and internal rotation contracture of the hip causing the quadriceps muscle to pull the patella laterally. If the patella becomes chronically dislocated, then it should be reduced surgically because the knee cannot be adequately extended with a dislocated patella. Transferring the patellar tendon insertion (p. 2177) by a soft tissue procedure is the preferred treatment. Lateral patellar retinacular release alone may suffice, but in chronic dislocation or subluxation it probably will not. Reefing the quadriceps tendon medially with a Campbell sling or transferring half of the patellar tendon medially into the upper tibia is the preferred method of alignment, along with releasing the patellar retinaculum. If a valgus knee deformity is the cause of the patellar subluxation, then a varus supracondylar osteotomy of the femur is needed (p. 2983).

RECESSION OF RECTUS FEMORIS AT HIP

TECHNIQUE (SAGE). Place the patient supine with a small elevation under the buttocks. Through the lower end of an

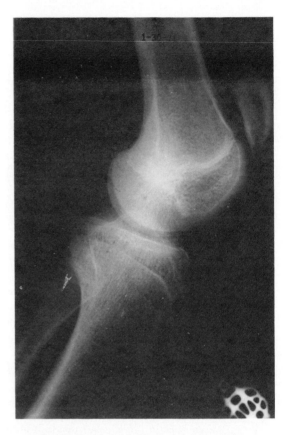

Fig. 65-42. Patella alta in cerebral palsied patient.

iliofemoral approach (p. 59) divide the fascia of the anterior thigh at the anterosuperior iliac spine, taking care not to injure the lateral femoral cutaneous nerve in this area. At the anterosuperior spine, separate the origin of the sartorius and the anterior border of the tensor fasciae latae. Retract the sartorius medially and the tensor fasicae latae laterally, and elevate the latter muscle about 5 cm off the anterior edge of the outer iliac wing. Locate the straight head of the rectus femoris at its attachment to the anteroinferior iliac spine, lying between the medial border of the tensor fasicae latae and lateral to the iliacus (Fig. 65-43, A). Expose its straight head distally until the Y-bifurcation into the straight and reflected heads is found. By sharp and blunt dissection clear the reflected head toward its origin proximally on the superior hip capsule. Free its attachment from the capsule and mark it with a suture. Follow the reflected head back to the Y-bifurcation, and split it longitudinally along the course of its fibers distally toward the musculotendinous junction for at least 3 cm. Turn the scalpel anteriorly at this point and cut the attachment of the straight head from the remainder of the muscle and tendon, leaving it attached at the anteroinferior iliac spine (Fig. 65-43, B). Then extend the hip and flex the knee and suture the distal end of the straight head to the proximal end of the reflected head (Fig. 65-43, C). This effectively lengthens the tendon 5 cm but leaves it still attached to the anteroinferior iliac spine. Close the wound routinely.

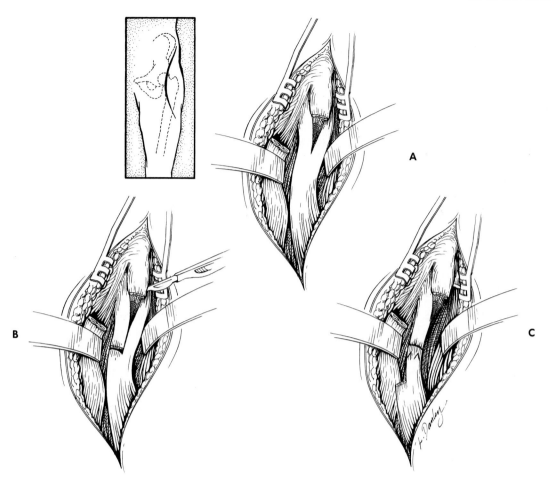

Fig. 65-43. Recession of origin of rectus femoris at hip. **A,** Y-bifurcate tendon of the proximal end of rectus femoris is found between iliacus muscle and tensor fasciae latae after sartorius has been released and retracted. **B,** The straight head of rectus femoris is incised from its muscle as far distally as possible leaving it attached to anteroinferior iliac spine above. Reflected head is then incised from hip capsule as far proximally as possible. **C,** Distal end of straight head is sutured to proximal end of reflected head, thus lengthening tendinous attachment proximally.

HIP

Deformities of the hip in cerebral palsy are the second most common deformities encountered. They are caused by imbalance of muscle power, retained primitive reflexes, habitually faulty posture, absence of weight-bearing stimulation on bone, and growth. If the imbalance in muscle power is marked and if the faulty postural habits are allowed to continue, adaptive changes develop in the soft tissues and bones. Congenital anteversion of the femoral neck fails to correct spontaneously and even increases, and valgus deformity of the femoral neck caused by muscle imbalance and prolonged absence of weight bearing gradually increases. The hip may eventually subluxate or dislocate. According to Baker, Dodelin, and Bassett, every cerebral palsied patient with appreciable involvement of the lower limbs should be considered to have abnormal hips until proved otherwise.

Sharrard states that if hemiplegic spastic patients and other patients with nonspastic varieties of cerebral palsy are excluded, then 92% of the remaining patients will show some degree of hip deformity, especially spastic, diplegic, triplegic, and quadriplegic patients.

Baker et al. in a study of the pathogenesis, incidence, and treatment of structural changes in 258 hips of 129 patients with cerebral palsy found only 55 hips they considered entirely normal. There was valgus deformity of the femoral neck in 197, increase in obliquity of the acetabular roof in 160, subluxation in 42, and dislocation in 31; varus deformity of the neck was found in only 6. They noted that valgus deformity of the neck was found by Banks in 179 of 180 hips of patients with cerebral palsy. They believe that the strong overpull of the spastic muscles weakens and gradually overcomes the abductor muscles; this causes a decrease in stimulation and thus in growth of the greater trochanter and, in turn, a failure in development of the normal varus inclination of the femoral neck. They also believe that if balanced muscle power about the hip can be established and normal alignment of the femur can be restored, later deformity of the hip may be prevented;

precisely how and when these can be accomplished is the problem.

Therefore each patient should be examined both clinically and roentgenographically and the examination should be repeated every 6 months to make sure the hips are not subluxating or dislocating or becoming dysplastic.

It is important that the deformity of flexion and internal rotation be distinguished from adduction deformity, although they frequently coexist. Each may cause a scissors gait, but the treatment of each is different. The flexion–internal rotational deformity is usually caused by spastic internal rotators acting against weak external rotators; often spasticity of the tensor fasciae latae is a major cause. The habitually faulty postures in this deformity are assumed while sitting on the floor: the hips are flexed 90 degrees and fully rotated internally, the knees are flexed more than 90 degrees, and the legs and feet are externally rotated and positioned alongside the greater trochanters (the "reversed tailor position"). Often the cerebral palsied child habitually sits in this position because it increases stability while sitting by broadening the base. This favors development of excessive internal torsion of the femur (anteversion of the femoral neck), external torsion of the tibia, and planovalgus deformity of the foot. This habit should be corrected as soon as possible. True adduction deformity is caused by spastic adductors acting against normal, less spastic, or weak abductors; the limbs are pulled together and do not rotate internally when forcibly separated by the examiner.

The relationships of flexion of the hip, with or without internal rotation, flexion of the knee, and plantar flexion of the ankle, usually referred to as the "crouched position" have been discussed many times by Silfverskiöld, Bleck, Roosth, Samilson, Evans, Reimers, Sharrard, and others.

A patient with flexion deformities of the hips must flex the knees, overload the forefeet, and extend the lumbar spine to place the center of gravity over the weight-bearing surface. Likewise, a patient with fixed flexion deformities of the knees must flex the hips to place the center of gravity over the weight-bearing surface (Fig. 65-44, *A*). Furthermore, a patient with plantar flexion deformities of the ankles may flex the knees, hips, and lumbar spine for the same reason (Fig. 65-44, *B*). The decisions concerning whether the deformities are dynamic or fixed and which joint should be treated first and in what manner are controversial. For instance, if there are fixed plantar flexion deformities of the ankle and fixed flexion deformities of the hip and knee, and the deformity of the knee is corrected without correcting the deformities of the hip and ankle, genu recurvatum will probably develop, and because the posterior support of the hip has been decreased, increased flexion of the hip and increased lumbar lordosis will also probably develop. Therefore it is important to determine among the hip, knee, and ankle which joints are affected and the degree of any fixed deformities.

An isolated fixed deformity in any of the three joints that significantly interferes with the patient's activities can be corrected. When flexion contractures of the hip and knee coexist, the patient will, of course, stand with flexion of the hip and knee, overloaded forefoot, and increased lumbar lordosis. The patient will sit with the lumbar spine flexed because of the downward pull of the contracted hamstrings and will walk with a short stride, rotating the pelvis as the extremity is swung forward. When the fixed flexion deformity of the hip is from 15 to 30 degrees, most surgeons now recommend psoas recession and resection of the rectus femoris. When the deformity is greater than 30 degrees, a more extensive anterior release is necessary, in-

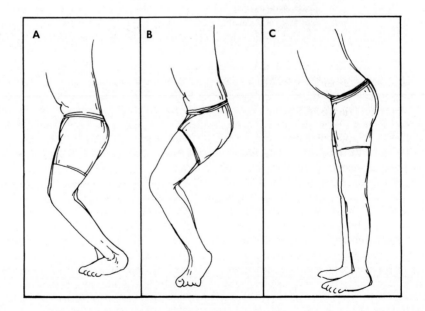

Fig. 65-44. Typical deformities of lower extremities and spine with flexed hip posture. **A,** Crouch posture. **B,** Jump posture. **C,** Extended lumbar spine with flexed hips and normal knees and ankles. (Redrawn from Bleck, E.E.: American Academy of Orthopaedic Surgeons: Instructional course lectures, vol. 20, St. Louis, 1971, The C.V. Mosby Co.)

cluding the sartorius, tensor fasciae latae, and the anterior fibers of the gluteus medius and minimus; this operation results in decreased flexion deformity of the hip, weakness of the flexors of the hip, decreased lumbar lordosis, posterior tilting of the pelvis, and a relative lengthening of the hamstrings. If after surgery, significant flexion deformity of the knee persists, the hamstrings should be lengthened. When flexion contracture of the knee and plantar flexion deformity of the ankle coexist, the patient will, of course, stand with flexion of the hip and knee and equinus deformity of the foot. He will still sit with the lumbar spine flexed and will walk with a short stride, rotating the pelvis forward. In this instance the flexors of the knee and the tendo calcaneus should be lengthened at the same time. When flexion contractures of the hip and knee and contracture of the triceps surae coexist, the patient again will walk with increased lumbar lordosis, flexion of the hip and knee, equinus deformity of the foot, and a short stride with rotation of the pelvis anteriorly; he will sit with his lumbar spine flexed as though he were sitting on the sacrum. In this instance release of the contracted muscles beginning at the hip and followed soon by release at the knee and ankle is indicated.

The extent of surgery necessary to correct flexion deformity of the hip is also controversial. Bleck recommends recession of the psoas muscle and insertion of its tendon and the iliacus muscle fibers into the anterior capsule of the hip near the base of the femoral neck. He recommends this operation for children with flexion deformity of the hip of more than 15 degrees; the optimum age for surgery is from 7 to 9 years. The operation is also recommended in children with any one of the following three gait patterns: (1) flexed and internally rotated hips and flexed knees (spastic hamstrings), (2) flexed and internally rotated hips and hyperextended knees (spastic quadriceps), and (3) flexed and internally rotated hips and normal knees. Bleck performed additional surgery on these patients depending on the analysis of the gait pattern and examination before surgery. In patients who walked with a scissors gait or had limited abduction of the hip to 15 degrees or less, adductor longus myotomy and neurectomy of the anterior branch of the obturator nerve were performed. In those who walked with hyperextended knees, the rectus femoris was released at its origin. In those who walked with flexed-knee gait patterns, the semitendinosus tendon was transferred to the medial femoral condyle and the semimembranosus was lengthened. Any contracture of the triceps surae was treated by lengthening the tendo calcaneus. The mean correction of the flexion deformity of the hip was 20 degrees; after surgery passive internal rotation of the hip gradually decreased and passive external rotation gradually increased. Subluxations of the hips in three nonambulatory patients were reduced.

According to Roosth, on the other hand, muscles that span two joints, namely the tensor fasciae latae, the rectus femoris, and the sartorius muscles, and also the anterior fibers of the gluteus medius and minimus cause the flexion deformity of the hip, and release of these flexors of the hip at an early age without disturbing the psoas will eliminate the "crouch posture" and improve gait. At surgery he sequentially divided the different flexors of the hip and observed the flexion contracture after each muscle had been divided. He established to his satisfaction that the muscles just mentioned caused the flexion contracture. When all of these muscles were sectioned, the deformity of the hip was relieved, but when all were not sectioned a flexion contracture of 15 degrees or less remained. Of 23 children with internal rotational deformity of the limbs before surgery, only one could not correct this deformity actively when examined after surgery. The flexion deformity of the knee disappeared after correction of the flexion deformity of the hip, and according to Roosth, hamstring transfer after release of the hip flexors is necessary only in children with fixed flexion contracture of the knee and in those with no fixed flexion contracture but who still lack satisfactory extension of the knee when walking or standing. When full active extension of the knee is possible despite spasticity, hamstring surgery is unnecessary. Any uncorrected equinus deformity will usually cause genu recurvatum and in this instance lengthening the tendo calcaneus is indicated.

Perry and Hoffer, and Sutherland, Simon, Gage, and others have used kinetic electromyography and gait analysis to assess hip muscle dynamics and joint positions in cerebral palsied patients. Hoffer used kinetic electromyography in patients who had a flexed hip posture to differentiate between rectus femoris and iliopsoas hyperactivity. In the internally rotated, adducted gait, electromyograms have been used to differentiate between medial hamstring, gracilis, and adductor hyperactivity. Bleck used them in addition to determine the activity of the gluteus medius when considering whether to transfer them. He studied kinetic electromyograms about the hip in 25 patients with spastic hip muscle patterns. In all patients dysphasic activity was present in the adductors during the stance and swing phases of gait. In most patients the gluteus medius fired in phase, but its activity was prolonged. Kinetic electromyograms of 11 patients showed the iliacus to be phasic in five and dysphasic in six. He also studied the sartorius, rectus femoris, and the tensor fasciae latae—all hip flexors. The rectus was almost uniformly dysphasic. In hip extension deformity, the hamstrings were found to be the offending muscles more often than the gluteus maximus. Gait analysis has come to play a major role in decision making concerning the dynamics of hip deformities.

The hip may become dislocated when its adductors, flexors, and internal rotators are all severely spastic or rigid. The dislocation may be unilateral or bilateral, one hip may be dislocated and the opposite hip subluxated, or one hip may be dislocated and the opposite hip may present a combined abduction and external rotational deformity.

Tachdjian and Minear, in a careful study of 590 patients with cerebral palsy, found dislocation or subluxation of the hip in 25, an incidence of 4.2%. They note that Mathews, Jones, and Sperling reported an incidence of 2.5% and Gherlinzoni and Pais of 4.6%. Tachdjian and Minear believe that dislocation of the hip in cerebral palsy is preventable and therefore that each child with spastic paralysis of the lower extremities should be watched carefully for the development of subluxation or dislocation. Their results show that the following measures are valuable and effective; tenotomy of the spastic adductors, closed reduction of any dislocation or subluxation, immobilization in abduction during convalescence, and strengthening of the abductors either by active exercises of if they are not under cerebral control by automatic reflex.

Samilson et al. found dislocated or subluxated hips in 28% of a population of severely involved cerebral palsied patients. The patients of Pollock and Sharrard had a 23% incidence of dislocation or subluxation.

Bleck found dislocation of the hip only in patients unable to walk, and this has been the experience of many investigators. In dislocation, Bleck recommends adductor tenotomy and iliopsoas recession. In addition to the soft tissue surgery, he recommends varus derotational osteotomy of the femur in children after the age of 5 years. In acetabular dysplasia, he recommends a Pemberton innominate osteotomy up to the age of 10 years. After the age of 10 years, in addition to soft tissue surgery, he recommends a femoral shortening derotational osteotomy and a Chiari acetabular reconstruction. In older patients in whom the femoral articular surface is unsatisfactory, he recommends a hip fusion or femoral head and neck resection and capsular interpositional arthroplasty for the painful hip.

All agree that the best treatment for dislocation of the hip in spastic paralysis is prophylactic. This requires a constant awareness that dislocation may develop. Only by such awareness can dislocation be prevented by appropriate measures or at least be diagnosed early when treatment is most effective.

Surgery for hip deformities

ADDUCTION DEFORMITY

Adduction is the most common deformity of the hip. It causes a scissoring gait and subluxation and dislocation of the hip itself. If an adduction deformity is fixed at 20 degrees or less, obturator neurectomy and adductor tenotomy are indicated. Before obturator neurectomy it may be helpful at first to paralyze the adductor muscles temporarily by infiltrating the branches of the nerve with lidocaine. Then the strength of the abductors can be more accurately determined, and the result of neurectomy can be more accurately predicted. Adductor tenotomy and neurectomy of the anterior branch of the obturator nerve are indicated, as is discussed later, in spastic subluxation of the hip and as a preliminary measure in spastic dislocation of the joint. They may also be useful in improving hygiene or the sitting position of a patient who cannot walk.

Intrapelvic obturator neurectomy should not be done. After this type of neurectomy some adductor power remains because the femoral nerve supplies the pectineus and the sciatic nerve supplies that part of the adductor magnus that takes origin from the ischial tuberosity; power may be insufficient, however, especially when the abductors are strong, and an abduction deformity may develop. It is usually better to begin with neurectomy of the anterior branch of the obturator nerve alone; if necessary, the posterior branch may be treated similarly later.

Phelps pointed out that sometimes the gracilis muscle is a major cause of adduction deformity of the hip, especially when there is also a flexion deformity of the knee. Because the gracilis is the only adductor muscle that spans both joints, extending both joints simultaneously will make the adduction deformity more severe. Phelps has developed the best test to detect contracture of the gracilis. The patient is placed prone, knees flexed and hips abducted as far as possible. Each knee is then gradually extended; if the gracilis is shortened, the hip will then adduct. Dividing the gracilis alone at its musculotendinous junction often corrects the contracture. Baker, Dodelin, and Bassett have pointed out that tightness of the medial hamstrings is also important in causing adduction deformity; they modified Phelps' gracilis test to include these muscles (Fig. 65-45). Keats noted improvement in 35 of 38 children with adduction deformity caused by cerebral palsy after tenotomy of the gracilis as well as of the adductors (combined with neurectomy of the anterior branch of the obturator nerve). Perry et al. conducted electromyographic studies of eight muscles acting on the hip and knee while conducting various stretch tests intended to indicate specific muscle tightness, including the Phelps' test. None of the tests were specific for any one muscle electromyographically; no test distinguished between the medial hamstrings and the gracilis. Consequently the only way to isolate the medial hamstrings from the gracilis is by kinetic electromyography.

Banks and Green made a statistical study of patients treated for adduction deformity. For 157 hips treated by adductor tenotomy and neurectomy of the anterior branch of the obturator nerve, they classified the results as fair, good, or excellent in 81% and as poor in only 19%. In some of the patients the abductor muscles were weak, but in no patient was the gait made worse by operation. Their study did not substantiate the idea that such surgery should be deferred until growth is complete; most of their patients were operated on in childhood, and they found no correlation between the result and the age of the patient. In a few severely handicapped patients with severe fixed adduction deformities of the hips, the purpose of surgery was simply to improve nursing care.

In the treatment of an adduction deformity by intrapelvic obturator neurectomy or neurectomy of both branches of the obturator nerve, an abduction deformity, as already mentioned, may result and the patient may be unable to adduct the hip. This is especially true when adductor tenotomy has also been performed. In two patients with spastic paralysis in whom this abduction deformity had developed, Pollock transferred the origin of the hamstrings to the inferior ramus of the pubis and the insertion of the hamstrings to the distal femur in such a way as to make them forceful adductors of the hip. The results were satisfactory in both patients.

Flexion–internal rotational deformity was once frequently corrected by the Durham operation, in which the gluteus medius and minimus muscles are released by dividing their tendons and, if it is tight, leaving the tensor fasciae latae unsutured. But this operation should not be used because it weakens the power of abduction. Rather the deformity can be corrected by one or more of several procedures, depending on the severity of the deformity and on whether it can be corrected passively.

When the deformity is mild to moderate and is present only when the limb is used (is not fixed), it can often be corrected by lateral transfer of the medial hamstrings or the Soutter operation (p. 2989), followed by immobilization in external rotation. Barr has advocated instead an operation similar to that of Legg in which the origin of the tensor fasciae latae, instead of being stripped from the ilium and allowed to retract distally, is transplanted posteriorly on the ilium to convert the muscle into an external rotator and abductor. Steele has recommended an anterior and inferior transfer of the insertions of the gluteus medius

and minimus for dynamically internally rotated thighs when no other contractures exist. Bleck recommends iliopsoas recession when the hip is flexed and internally rotated during walking and when passive external rotation of the hip is impossible if the joint is extended but is possible to 15 to 20 degrees if the joint is passively flexed to 90 degrees. He advises that the operation be carried out before the age of 10 years.

Transfer of the origins of the adductor muscles of the

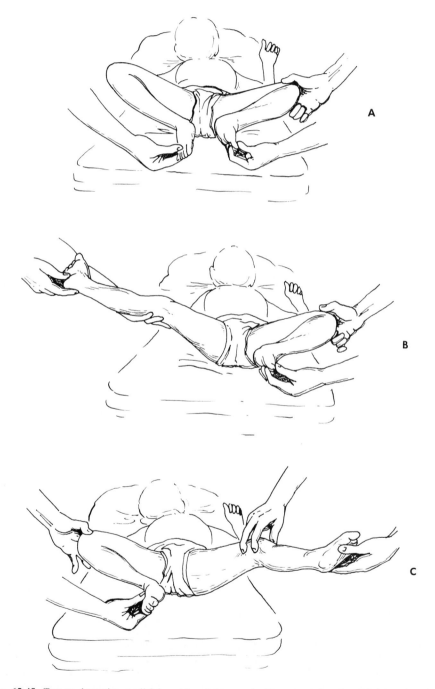

Fig. 65-45. Test to determine medial hamstring tightness. **A,** Hips are abducted and knees are flexed to exclude adductor tightness. **B** and **C,** Knee is extended and tightness of medial hamstrings is determined by palpation. (Redrawn from Baker, L.D., Dodelin, R., and Bassett, F.H., III: J. Bone Joint Surg. **44-A:**1331, 1962.)

hip to the ischial tuberosity was first described in 1966 by Nickel, Perry, Garrett, and Feiwell in treating paralytic dislocation of the hip. More recently Stephenson and Donovan, Griffin et al., and Couch et al. have found it useful in treating flexion, adduction, and internal rotational deformities in children with cerebral palsy. It consists of transferring the origin of the adductor longus and gracilis posteriorly to the ischium and releasing the origins of the adductor brevis and the anterior part of the adductor magnus. After surgery usually the width of the gait is increased, abduction of the hips improves, internal rotation of the lower limbs disappears, and some patients unable to walk before surgery are able to do so. Furthermore, in most patients flexion deformity of the knee and equinus deformity of the ankle decrease. Aftercare is easy because prolonged use of abduction splints at night to prevent recurrence of deformity is unnecessary.

When the deformity is present constantly and cannot be corrected passively (is fixed), it is caused by contracture of the internal rotators and of the soft tissue structures about the hip itself and by internal femoral torsion. In older patients structural changes of the acetabulum may also have developed. This deformity cannot be corrected by releasing the soft tissues alone; rather, the rotational component of the deformity can be corrected only by rotational osteotomy of the femur, preferably at the subtrochanteric level (Chapter 62). Any disabling flexion component can be corrected as described later. When the osteotomy is being planned, the patient should be examined while supine or sitting, the leg hanging over the edge of the table and the knee flexed 90 degrees; both the range of rotation and the arc of rotation of the hip should be carefully noted. With this information available, the amount of correction desired can be determined. After surgery the range of internal rotation should equal that of external rotation. For example, if the hip can be rotated internally 90 degrees and externally only to the neutral position, then at osteotomy the distal fragment should be rotated externally 45 degrees. (We prefer to measure the internal femoral torsion or anteversion of the femoral neck by the technique of Magilligan, p. 2725.) When a subtrochanteric osteotomy is carried out, the fragments should be fixed with a blade plate, and the hip should be immobilized in a spica cast after surgery. When a supracondylar osteotomy is carried out, a Kirschner wire is passed through the femur just proximal to the osteotomy; the wire holds the proximal fragment in full internal rotation while the distal fragment is externally rotated enough to correct the deformity.

For *flexion deformity* of the hip of more than 15 degrees in patients who must walk with crutches and are less than 11 years old, Bleck recommends iliopsoas recession. Any other indicated operations such as adductor tenotomy and neurectomy of the anterior branch of the obturator nerve may be carried out at the same time. Keats and Morgese recommend iliopsoas tenotomy when excessive lumbar lordosis does not respond to stretching of the hip flexors. They describe an approach to the lesser trochanter and the iliopsoas tendon similar to that of Ludloff (Fig. 2-53). According to them, the best time for this tenotomy is between the ages of 8 and 11 years. They described the preliminary results of 34 operations on 17 patients as "gratifying," but the extent of flexor weakness after surgery and detailed information about the ability to walk were not reported.

Transfer of the iliac crest (p. 2987) is rarely necessary. However, when a flexion deformity is severe, the Soutter operation and the following additional measures are indicated. The fascia lata is divided transversely, and the intermuscular septa about the anterior aspect of the hip are released. In some instances dividing the adductor longus is necessary before complete extension is possible. The anterior branch of the obturator nerve is resected when adduction deformity is also disabling. Rarely dividing the anterior part of the joint capsule and tenotomy of the psoas are required. Long leg casts that hold the knees and ankles in the neutral position are applied. Immediately after surgery, pillows are placed beneath the buttocks to keep the hips extended. At 3 to 6 weeks the casts are removed and long leg braces are fitted.

A fixed adduction deformity or an early subluxation of the hip is corrected by neurectomy of the anterior branch of the obturator nerve, tenotomy of the contracted adductors or gracilis, or both, and immobilization in abduction for 6 weeks. Then a program of exercises to strengthen the abductors is begun and walking is eventually started. Bleck recommends a varus subtrochanteric osteotomy for patients 9 years old or older when roentgenograms show that half or more of the femoral head is out of the acetabulum; for younger patients with less severe subluxation he recommends operations that release the soft tissues.

In 1975 Sharrard, Allen, Heaney, and Prendiville compared the clinical and roentgenographic status of hips in two groups of children with cerebral palsy with adduction and flexion deformities of the hips and imbalance of muscle power about these joints. The first group had been treated without surgery, and in that group 11% of the hips had become dislocated, 28% had become subluxated, 46% had become dysplastic, and 15% had remained normal. The second group had been treated by surgery to correct the deformity of the hip and to balance the power of the muscles about the joint, and in that group no hip had become dislocated, 13% had become subluxated, 35% had become dysplastic, and 52% had remained normal. In the second group surgery was carried out if the range of abduction was less than 45 degrees, if early dysplastic changes such as a break in Shenton's line were present, or if the hip was dysplastic or subluxated. A dysplastic hip was one in which more than two thirds of the femoral head was covered by the acetabulum, but Shenton's line was clearly interrupted or the acetabulum or femoral head was abnormal. A subluxated hip was one in which less than two thirds of the femoral head was covered by the acetabulum. Surgery to prevent subluxation or dislocation was based on the concept that these abnormalities are caused by strong flexors and adductors of the hip in the presence of weak abductors and extensors. The aim of surgery was to lengthen and weaken the short adductor and flexor muscles by adductor tenotomy and myotomy and, if necessary, by lengthening of the psoas tendon. When the adductor muscles were more than two grades stronger than the abductors, the adductors were further weakened by dividing the anterior branch of the obturator nerve. Only one operation was needed in 101 hips (75%), two in 28 hips (21%), and three or more in 5 hips (4%). These investigators concluded that early subluxation is an urgent indication for surgical treatment and that the need for surgery is independent of age, severity of involvement, or neurologic maturity of the child.

Samilson et al. in 1972 reported a study of dislocation and subluxation of the hip in cerebral palsy. Of 1013 severely involved patients who were neurologically and developmentally immature, the hips dislocated or subluxated in 274. The severity of their handicaps was indicated by the fact that 62% of the patients required total bed care, 15% could sit up if propped, 12% were independent sitters, 11% were able to walk some, and only 1% were able to walk independently. Scoliosis was present in 124 patients, predominantly long thoracolumbar C curves. Fixed pelvic obliquity was present in 122 patients. The mean age at which the hip dislocated was 7 years. In dislocation of the hip the average angle between the femoral shaft and neck was 160.8 degrees, and in subluxation the average angle was 154 degrees. Anteversion of the femoral neck averaged 69 degrees in 142 patients. When arthrograms of the hip showed one third or more of the femoral head to be uncovered by the acetabulum, the hip was considered subluxated, and when the femoral head lay completely outside the acetabulum, the hip was considered dislocated. The retention of neonatal reflexes was considered an important cause of deformity of the hip. For example, asymmetric incurvatum reflexes (Galant's sign) result in positioning of the hips ''windblown'' into the concavity of any long thoracolumbar C curve. Other reflexes considered important were symmetric and asymmetric tonic neck reflexes, crossed extension responses, and positive supporting reactions, and these were frequently found in the patients studied. Shallowness of the acetabulum was rarely seen and is explained by the fact that the mean age at the time of dislocation was only 7 years. Thus according to these investigators, acetabuloplasty in spastic dislocation of the hip is rarely indicated.

Samilson et al. observed that skeletal traction was tolerated poorly, if at all, and was ineffective in maintaining reduction of a dislocated hip. Based on their experience with this group of patients, they now recommend for subluxated hips a percutaneous adductor tenotomy, release of the iliopsoas and rectus femoris, osteotomy of the femur to correct anteversion of the femoral neck, coxa valga, and when necessary flexion deformity of the proximal femur, and closed reduction of the hip. Tenotomy of the gracilis was added if this muscle was thought to be contributing to deformity. For dislocated hips, in addition to the operations just mentioned, they frequently found it necessary to remove a segment of the femur at the level of the lesser trochanter between 2 and 5 cm long as a wedge based medially to obtain reduction, varus positioning, and derotation. The decision to remove a segment was made at the time of attempted reduction of the hip: if reduction was difficult, removing the segment made it easy. Any osteotomy was fixed, preferably in 90 to 100 degrees of varus position, using a bent plate and six screws. The younger the child, the greater was the varus position in which the osteotomy was fixed. The hip was immobilized in a one

and one-half spica cast for 10 weeks after surgery. When bilateral operations were required, the second side was operated on 6 weeks after the first. The goals of surgery and how often they were attained were as follows: (1) to improve perineal care, 156 of 202, (2) to prevent progression of subluxation or dislocation, 42 of 64, (3) to increase the status of activity, 4 of 32, (4) to reduce a dislocation and maintain the reduction, 19 of 26, (5) to reduce pain, 4 of 6, (6) to improve sitting balance, 2 of 3, and (7) to reduce the incidence of fractures, 2 of 3. The most common complication after surgery was fracture of the femur, which occurred in 40 patients. Twelve of 46 hips in which subtrochanteric varus derotational osteotomies were performed in combination with appropriate soft tissue releases and reduction of the hip, either closed or open, redislocated; in these the angle between the femoral shaft and neck exceeded 100 degrees. When the angle was between 90 degrees and 100 degrees, no hips redislocated. In a separate group of children not included in this study, 152 hips without subluxation or dislocation but with comparable degrees of coxa valga, increased anteversion of the femoral neck, and adduction contracture were treated by soft tissue releases and varus derotational osteotomies; at an average of 4 years after surgery frank dislocation developed in only 13. In another group of 156 untreated children without subluxation or dislocation of the hip and with the same deformities, surgery was not permitted by the parents or was contraindicated from a medical standpoint, and in all the hips dislocated or subluxated. Therefore appropriate soft tissue releases combined with varus derotational osteotomy are effective in preventing dislocation and subluxation in a hip with an adduction contracture and anteversion of the femoral neck.

An old dislocation in which severe adaptive osseous changes have developed, such as coxa valga, anteversion of the femoral neck, and insufficiency of the acetabulum, is treated as follows. If the patient is so disabled otherwise by cerebral palsy that walking is impracticable, no treatment is indicated except for relief of pain. If walking is practicable, then the surgeon, the patient, and the patient's family must choose between (1) arthrodesis of the hip, (2) osteotomy of the femur to correct its angular and torsional deformities and osteotomy of the pelvis to correct the insufficiency of the acetabulum, (3) pelvic support osteotomy of the femur, or (4) no surgical treatment at all. The operations just listed are indeed major ones; furthermore, after any of them the morbidity is considerable, complications are likely, and the result may be unsatisfactory.

ILIOPSOAS RECESSION

As already mentioned, Bleck recommends iliopsoas recession when the hip internally rotates during walking and when passive external rotation of the hip is impossible if the joint is extended but is possible to 15 to 20 degrees if the joint is passively flexed to 90 degrees.

At the time of iliopsoas recession other operations may be indicated depending on the analysis of the gait pattern before surgery. If adductor spasm interferes with walking and if the hips cannot be passively abducted past 20 degrees, then adductor tenotomy and neurectomy of the anterior branch of the obturator nerve are indicated. If the

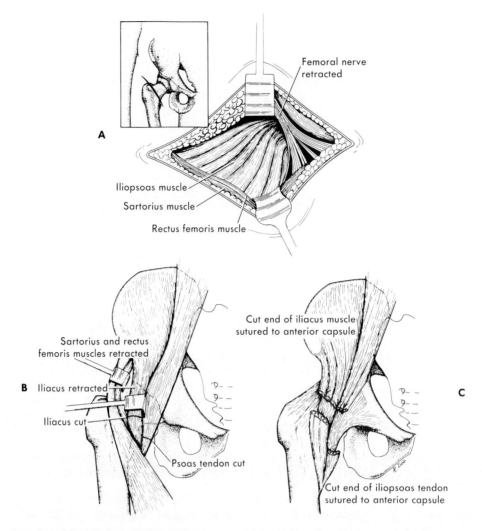

Fig. 65-46. Bleck iliopsoas recession. **A,** *Inset,* Skin incision. Sartorius muscle is retracted laterally and femoral nerve is separated from iliacus muscle. **B,** Iliacus muscle and psoas tendon are divided. **C,** Psoas tendon and iliacus fibers are transferred superiorly and are sutured to anterior capsule. (From Bleck, E.E.: J. Bone Joint Surg. **53-A:**1468, 1971.)

child walks with the knees hyperextended, then release of the rectus femoris is indicated. If the child walks with the knees flexed and has not previously had surgery on the hamstrings, lengthening or transferring the medial hamstrings may be indicated. If the foot is fixed in equinus deformity, lengthening the tendo calcaneus or gastrocnemius is indicated.

TECHNIQUE (BLECK). Make an anterior iliofemoral incision beginning 1.5 cm distal to the anterosuperior iliac spine and coursing obliquely distally and medially for 10 to 15 cm, depending on the size of the patient (Fig. 65-46, A). Next identify the sartorius muscle and retract it laterally. Then identify the femoral nerve and the medial and lateral borders of the iliacus muscle and separate the nerve from the muscle. The iliacus muscle fibers overlap the broad psoas tendon that hugs the anteromedial aspect of the capsule of the hip. Now divide the iliacus muscle transversely as far distally as possible and the psoas tendon at its attachment to the lesser trochanter (Fig. 65-46, B).

Transfer the psoas tendon superiorly and suture it to the anterior capsule of the hip joint near the base of the femoral neck. Then suture the iliacus fibers to the capsule (Fig. 65-46, C).

AFTERTREATMENT. Immobilization in a cast is unnecessary. Bedrest, either prone or supine, is continued for 3 weeks.

OBTURATOR NEURECTOMY AND ADDUCTOR TENOTOMY

We agree with Banks and Green that obturator neurectomy and adductor tenotomy are indicated for severe scissors gait caused by adduction contracture of the hip in a child who retains a fundamental sense of balance. They are also indicated in a patient whose hip has either already become dislocated or is so subluxated that dislocation seems imminent.

The power of adduction is not entirely destroyed even by neurectomy of both branches of the obturator nerve because a small branch of the sciatic nerve supplies a part of the adductor magnus muscle and because the pectineus muscle supplied by the femoral nerve is preserved.

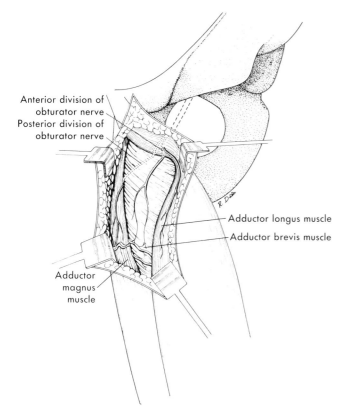

Anterior division of
obturator nerve
Posterior division of
obturator nerve

Adductor longus muscle

Adductor brevis muscle

Adductor
magnus
muscle

Fig. 65-47. Extrapelvic neurectomy of obturator nerves. Exposure of anterior and posterior divisions of obturator nerve; vessels on surfaces of adductor brevis and magnus muscles serve as guides. Note two branches of anterior division. When adductor spasm is mild, only anterior division is resected; when moderate or severe, both anterior and posterior divisions are resected.

Veleanu, Rosianu, and Ionescu have described an improved approach for obturator neurectomy with or without adductor tenotomy. We have had no experience with this approach, but it seems to have merit.

TECHNIQUE. Beginning at the pubis make a longitudinal incision 5 cm long on the medial aspect of the thigh in line with the adductor longus muscle (Fig. 65-47). Separate this muscle from the adductor brevis. Now locate the anterior branch of the obturator nerve on the superior surface of the adductor brevis and resect it. Then, if indicated, resect the posterior branch after retracting the adductor brevis anteriorly and finding the branch between the adductors brevis and magnus. If an adduction contracture is present, divide the tendinous origins of the appropriate adductor muscles through the proximal end of the incision.

TECHNIQUE (VELEANU, ROSIANU, AND IONESCU). Mark the position of the pubic spine and inguinal ligament with a skin pencil. Then starting at the pubic spine make an incision in the skin 6 or 7 cm long parallel to the inguinal ligament and 0.5 cm distal to it. Incise the subcutaneous tissue and the cribiform fascia and retract the linguinal ligament proximally. Then cut from the superior pubic ramus the insertion of the pectineus muscle covered by its fascia close to the periosteum. Reflect the underlying periosteum inferiorly toward the obturator foramen. Palpate the fora-

men beneath the detached periosteum and at the middle of the line of incision divide the periosteum vertically just inferior to the superior pubic ramus. The obturator nerve then appears in the wound wrapped in a layer of fat. At this level the anterior and posterior branches of the nerve are only a few millimeters apart. Dissect each branch free and identify each by stimulation; then resect as indicated either the anterior branch or both branches. The adductor tendons can be easily approached in the medial part of the incision and can be divided if necessary. Suture the cribiform fascia and skin.

TRANSFER OF ADDUCTOR ORIGINS TO ISCHIUM

Transferring the adductor origins to the ischium was first described by Nickel, Perry, Garrett, and Feiwell for treating paralytic dislocation of the hip. It consists of transferring the origins of the adductor longus and gracilis posteriorly to the ischium and releasing the origins of the adductor brevis and anterior part of the adductor magnus. Couch, DeRosa, and Throop studied the results of this operation in 32 patients with spastic cerebral palsy whose gait was characterized by flexion, adduction, and internal rotation of the hips and flexion of the knees. The following are the results in the 32 patients studied: (1) the width of the base of gait was increased in 26 of 28 patients from an average before surgery of 13 cm to an average after surgery of 24 cm; (2) combined abduction of the flexed hips increased in all patients from an average of 50 degrees before surgery to an average of 110 degrees after surgery; (3) internal rotation at the knees while walking was present before surgery in 24 patients and after surgery in only 5; (4) toe-in gait was present in 22 patients before surgery and in only 8 after surgery; (5) walking was impossible in 12 patients before surgery, and all 12 were walking after surgery; (6) the parents of 31 of the 32 patients stated that the operation had been beneficial to the child; and (7) movies made before and after surgery in 28 patients were available, and in all patients the gait and other functional abilities were improved. In 28 patients on whom sufficient data were available, the result was excellent in 16, good in 11, and poor in only 1. The results were better in younger children, and the operation is recommended for patients who can walk or almost do so. The operation is not intended to replace the traditional adductor myotomy and obturator neurectomy used in preventing subluxation of the hip.

In 1971 Stephenson and Donovan reported their use of transfer of the adductor origins in cerebral palsy. They had used it for 10 years and considered it better than other types of operations involving the adductor muscles. It was effective in treating flexion, adduction, and internal rotation deformities of the hip. It was also effective in some patients by simply making nursing care easier. Eighty-seven patients were studied after surgery. None were made worse by the operation, and in none did an abduction contracture develop. In 83% the gait was improved or the patient walked for the first time after surgery. Thus the result was good or fair in 83% and poor in 17%. As in all other orthopaedic operations, patients with spastic cerebral palsy obtained better results than those with athetosis. In addition to a decrease in the hip deformities, flexion deformities of the knee and equinus deformities of the ankle also decreased.

In 1977 Griffin, Wheelhouse, and Shiavi reported a study of five cerebral palsied patients with spasticity of the adductors and limited abduction of the hip treated by transfer of the adductor origins. Each patient was studied before and after surgery by physical examination and by videotape recordings and electromyographic analysis of gait. All patients could walk or almost do so, had voluntary control of the gluteus medius, and were intelligent enough to cooperate in the treatment program after surgery. Those who walked did so with the hip adducted and internally rotated on the affected side. After surgery the most consistent finding was a prolongation of stance phase activity in the transferred muscle. In all patients the gait was improved and endurance was increased, and all were classified as community walkers. In the opinion of these investigators, patients treated by this operation walk with a narrower base, with more security, with less trunk shift, with longer single support phase and stance, and with more endurance than patients similarly involved but treated by adductor myotomy or obturator neurectomy or both. Further, the management after surgery is easier because there is less need for prolonged use of abduction splints at night to prevent recurrence of deformity.

In 1981 Root and Spero reported the results of a 10-year study comparing adductor transfer (gracilis, adductor longus, and adductor brevis) to the ischium with adductor myotomy and anterior branch obturator neurectomy. They concluded that adductor transfers provided greater pelvic stability, reduced hip instability, and decreased hip flexion contracture more consistently than adductor myotomy and obturator neurectomy.

Reimers and Poulson compared a similar group of patients using the two operations and found no significant difference in the results. For this reason, they abandoned the adductor transfer operation because it was technically more difficult and was more stressful to the child.

Goldner has reported equally good results with recessing the adductor longus and brevis and the gracilis from their pelvic attachment to the fasia and intermuscular septum around the adductor magnus without obturator neurectomy. Patients with adductor recessions had decreased adduction, a realigned pelvis without obliquity, improved gait, and no apparent loss of strength.

When several adductor muscles have been transferred, a gait with excessive abduction sometimes occurs. Reimers and Poulson believe that the functional advantages of the adductor transfer are only of theoretical value.

ADDUCTOR TRANSFER

TECHNIQUE (COUCH, DEROSA, AND THROOP). Place the patient in the lithotomy position with the buttocks resting at the end of the operating table. Position the legs in pelvic stirrups and, with adhesive tape 3 inches (7.5 cm) wide placed just proximal to the knees and attached to the uprights of the pelvic stirrup, hold the knees and thighs abducted as much as the contracted tissues permit. Carefully prepare the entire perineum, the buttocks, the lower abdomen, and the proximal thighs and drape the operative field, using paper draping from a gynecologic pack. Sit

between the patient's legs. Now begin an incision just superior to the tendon of adductor longus and extend it posteriorly in a straight line to the ischial tuberosity, paralleling as closely as possible the borders of the inferior pubic ramus and the ischium. After the skin and subcutaneous tissues have been divided, use self-retaining retractors to increase the exposure. Identify the adductor longus tendon, tag it with a suture, and sever it from its origin on the pubic ramus with the cutting electrocautery. Next, also with the electrocautery, release the origins of the adductor brevis, gracilis, and anterior part of the adductor magnus next to the bone. End this dissection at the shiny fascia of the obturator externus. Now extend and slightly adduct the hip to allow the adductor longus tendon to reach the ischial tuberosity. Make an incision in the apophysis of the ischial tuberosity and push the adductor brevis, the adductor magnus, and the gracilis posteriorly toward the tuberosity, rolling them under the tendon of the adductor longus. Then free the adductor longus distally in the thigh, place it in a straight line, and secure it with several nonabsorbable sutures to the apophysis of the ischium. Now thoroughly irrigate the wound and close it. Place the child in long leg braces with a pelvic band.

AFTERTREATMENT. The child is kept in long leg braces with a pelvic band for 4 weeks. During the first 2 weeks the hip and knee locks are released occasionally for comfort and to allow the child to flex the hips about 45 degrees while eating. During the second week active and passive exercises of the hips and knees in the braces are begun. Four weeks after surgery the braces are discarded and intensive physical therapy is started.

TECHNIQUE (ROOT). Incise the medial thigh 1 cm lateral and parallel to the groin crease, over the adductor longus, and carry the incision posteriorly for a distance of 6 cm. Dissect the fasica overlying the adductor longus to expose the insertion of the adductor longus and pectineus on the pubic ramus. Locate the interval between these muscles and identify and protect the branches of the obturator nerve. Using electrocautery, incise along the pubic ramus the origin of the gracilis, adductor longus, and adductor brevis. Strip the tendons from their insertion at the pubic ramus subperiosteally while preserving the thick fibrous periosteal origin of these muscles. Free the remainder of the adductor brevis muscular attachments by blunt dissection. With a clamp, grasp the freed periosteal attachments of the tendons and hold them alongside the ischial tuberosity while suturing them to the tuberosity with nonabsorbable sutures, the most distal part of insertion being on the anteroinferior aspect of the ischial tuberosity. Obtain meticulous hemostasis with the electrocautery. Close the wound in a standard manner and apply a double spica cast.

AFTERTREATMENT. The spica cast is left on for 3 weeks and then removed to begin mobilization exercises.

FLEXION-INTERNAL ROTATIONAL DEFORMITY
GLUTEUS MEDIUS AND MINIMUS ADVANCEMENT
FOR CORRECTION OF INTERNAL ROTATIONAL GAIT

In 1980 Steel reported 42 hips in 26 patients in whom the gluteal muscles were advanced anteriorly and distally. All walked preoperatively with a toe-in gait. All were between the ages of 5 and 16 years and 16 had simultaneous bilateral operations. In follow-up periods varying from 3 to 11 years all patients walked with their lower extremities in neutral or outward rotation. There was no loss in abductor strength in 90% of the patients, and in 10% of the younger ones who were followed to skeletal maturity the angle of femoral anteversion was significantly reduced. The operation converts the gluteus minimus and medius from internal rotators of the thighs to external rotators.

TECHNIQUE (STEEL). Place the patient supine and drape both lower extremities from the lower ribcage to the toes. Make the skin incision proximal to the greater trochanter where the distal muscle bellies of the gluteus medius and minimus can be exposed. Begin it at the anterior border of the gluteus maximus and the posterior border of the gluteus medius and carry it anteriorly to the greater trochanter: then extend it posteriorly and distally to the posterior border of the femur 5 cm below the greater trochanter (Fig. 65-48, A). Incise the fascia lata between the gluteus maximus and tensor fasciae latae in a bloodless interval. Extend the incision in the fascia lata 5 cm distal to the trochanter. Abduct the leg to relax the fascia lata and retract it anteriorly. This exposes the insertion of the gluteus medius and minimus into the greater trochanter. Free these two muscles on all sides, but maintain their blood supply.

Strip the attachment of the gluteus minimus from the superior part of the capsule of the hip joint. With an osteotome remove the conjoined tendinous insertion of these two muscles and a thin wafer of bone from the greater trochanter (Fig. 65-48, B), being sure to stay distal to the greater trochanteric epiphysis. Expose and reflect for a short distance inferiorly the origin of the vastus lateralis from the intertrochanteric line (Fig. 65-48, C). Roughen the exposed femoral surface with a gouge to accept the wafer of bone that is attached to the tendon ends. Position the hip in 10 degrees less than the maximum abduction and external rotation the hip joint will permit. Place the wafer of bone and tendinous structures anteroinferiorly on the femur, and internally fix them with pins, screws, or staples. Replace and suture the origin of the vastus lateralis over the newly positioned wafer of bone (Fig. 65-48, D). Close the fascia lata and the remainder of the wound in a standard manner and apply a double spica cast.

AFTERTREATMENT. The spica cast is removed 6 weeks after surgery, and walking and exercises are begun.

VARUS DEROTATIONAL OSTEOTOMY

In the presence of excessive anteversion and valgus deformity of the femur and a hip that is either subluxated or

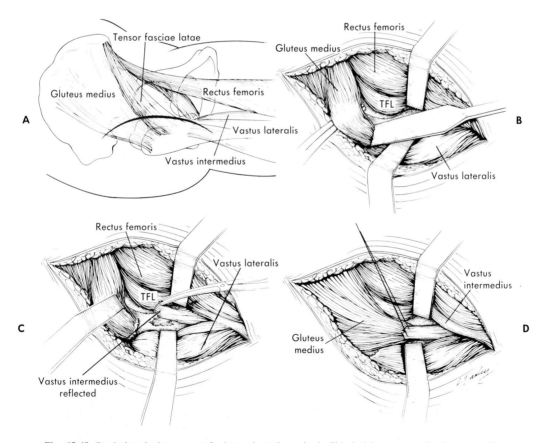

Fig. 65-48. Steel gluteal advancement for internal rotation gait. **A,** Skin incision exposes distal muscle bellies of gluteus medius and minimus. **B,** Conjoined tendinous insertion of muscles is removed with a thin wafer of bone from greater trochanter. **C,** Origin of vastus lateralis is reflected a short distance inferior to greater trochanter. **D,** Insertion of gluteus medius and minimus is advanced inferiorly and anteriorly and vastus lateralis is replaced over it. (Redrawn from Steel, H.H.: J. Bone Joint Surg. **62-A:**919, 1980.)

dislocated, a varus derotational osteotomy may be required in addition to soft tissue corrective surgery to keep the hip reduced and stable (Fig. 65-49). It is usually required in a child more than 6 years old and in whom 80 to 90 degrees of internal rotation of the femur is possible and only 15 degrees or less of external rotation when the hips are extended. This is best determined by examination with the patient prone. The corrective osteotomy can usually be made when any soft tissue correction is performed. It is best done at the level of the lesser trochanter through either a straight lateral or posterior approach. In 1980 Root and Siegal reported 100 hips operated on through a posterior approach with the patient prone. The approach was relatively bloodless, and the image intensifier allowed easy viewing of the femur. Union occurred in 99% of the patients. However, this approach cannot be used when an open reduction of the hip is anticipated.

TECHNIQUE (ROOT AND SIEGAL). Place the patient prone on a table suitable for the image intensifier or anteroposterior roentgenograms. Drape the buttocks and lower extremities free in the sterile field. Make an incision 15 cm long over the greater trochanter beginning proximally in line with the fibers of the gluteus maximus and extending distally from the greater trochanter in line with the posterolateral border of the femur (Fig. 65-50, A and B). Deepen the incision through the fascia lata and gluteus maximus to expose the superior part of the posterior and posterolateral surfaces of the femur, including the greater trochanter. Using an electrocautery, detach the origin of the vastus lateralis from the proximal femur by a transverse cut at the base of the greater trochanter and a longitudinal cut along the linea aspera (Fig. 65-50, C). Reflect the vastus lateralis anteriorly from the lateral surface of the femur subperiosteally. At the level of the proximal edge of the lesser trochanter, use an electrocautery to cut proximally through the tendinous and muscular attachment of the quadratus femoris and reflect it from the back of the femur medially and distally. This allows palpation of the inferior surface of the

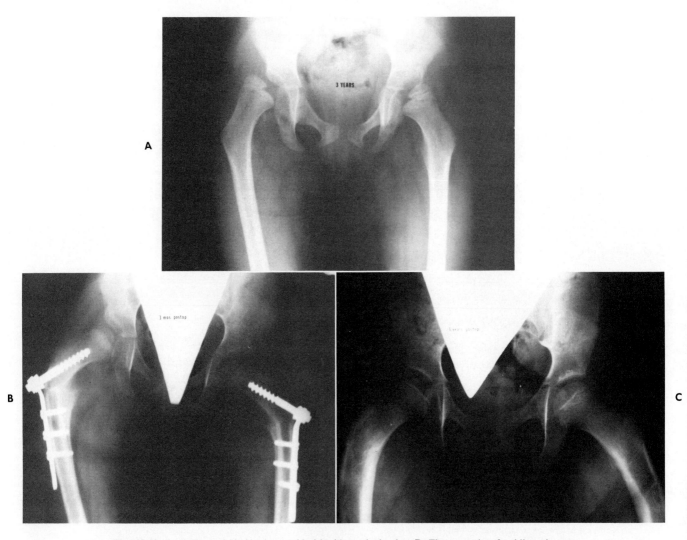

Fig. 65-49. A, Subluxated hips in 4-year-old girl with cerebral palsy. **B,** Three months after bilateral varus and derotational osteotomies combined with adductor releases and psoas tenotomies. **C,** Four years after surgery.

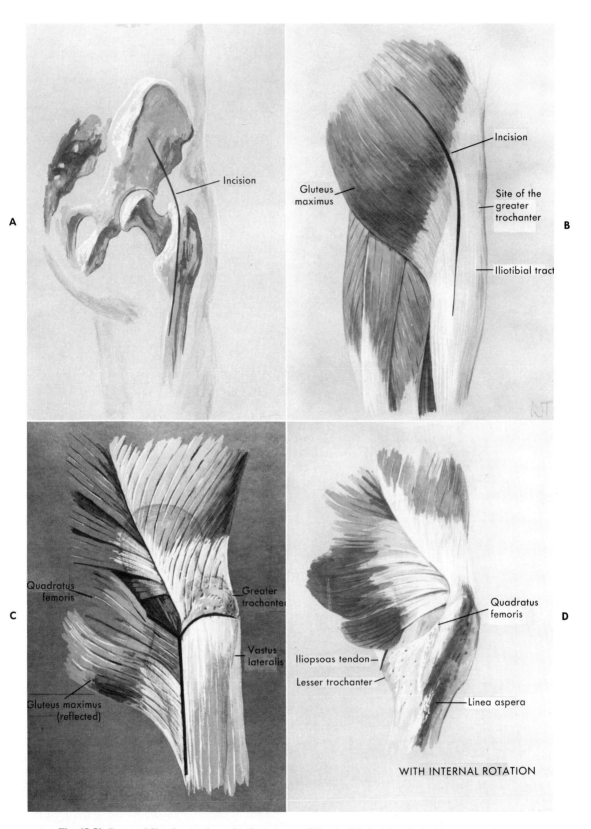

Fig. 65-50. Root and Siegal varus derotational osteotomy of hip. **A,** Skin incision. **B,** Incision through gluteus maximus and fascia lata (iliotibial tract). **C,** Greater trochanter, quadratus femoris, origin of vastus lateralis, tendinous attachment of gluteus maximus, and linea aspera are identified. **D,** Osteotomy site is exposed in area of lesser trochanter; psoas tendon may be released if necessary.

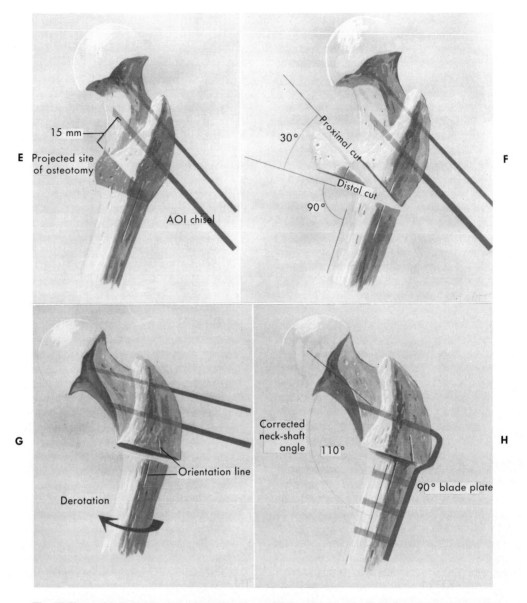

Fig. 65-50, cont'd. E, Guide wire and chisel are inserted in parallel position. Shaded area represents wedge to be excised; scored line is for reference for later rotation. **F,** Location of osteotomy planes; proximal osteotomy is 15 mm distal to chisel. **G,** Rotation is accomplished by external rotation of femur. **H,** Osteotomy is fixed with AO plate and screws. (**A, C,** and **I** courtesy Dr. Leon Root; **B, D, E, F,** and **G** from Root, L., and Siegal T.: J. Bone Joint Surg. **62-A:**571, 1980.)

neck of the femur and identification of the lesser trochanter (Fig. 65-50, *D*). Isolate the iliopsoas tendon and free it from the lesser trochanter. The area of bone to be osteotomized is thus completely exposed. Perform an osteotomy at the level of the lesser trochanter (Fig. 65-50, *E*). Remove the wedge of bone calculated by preoperative measurements (Fig. 65-50, *F*) and place the neck-shaft angle at 100 to 110 degrees in patients younger than 8 years old. In older patients the neck-shaft angle should be at 115 to 120 degrees.

Locate the proper level of the two osteotomy cuts by using a guide wire in the neck of the femur for orientation

(Fig. 65-50, *E*). It should be placed in the trochanter and upper femoral neck parallel with the intended proximal osteotomy cut. With the guide wire in proper position, insert an osteotome parallel with the guide wire and at the expected site of blade plate insertion into the subtrochanteric area of the femur. Verify the position of the osteotomy with the image intensifier or plain roentgenograms. Use the electrocautery to score a line in the bone posteriorly in line with the femoral shaft (vertically) as a later guide to rotational alignment (Fig. 65-50, *G*). Make the first osteotomy cut 1.5 to 2 cm below the level of the osteotome in the femoral neck and parallel with it, but not into the femoral

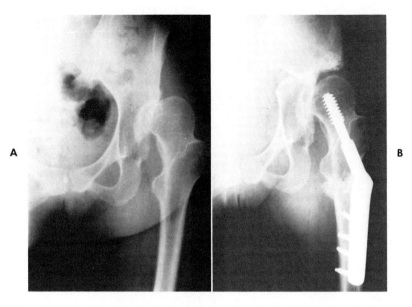

Fig. 65-51. A, Painful subluxed hip in 40-year old athetoid cerebral palsied patient. **B,** Hip is no longer painful after femoral shortening and Chiari osteotomy.

neck. Make the second osteotomy cut distally at a right angle to the shaft of the femur and remove a medially based bone wedge of previously determined width to allow the proper varus position of the neck of the femur. This wedge should include all or part of the lesser trochanter. The distal osteotomy should go to but not through the lateral cortex of the femur. Clamp the distal femur to the plate portion of the blade plate with a bone-holding forceps. This closes the open wedge-shaped space where the bone was removed. Check for proper position of the blade plate and the osteotomy with the image intensifier or roentgenograms. Release the bone clamp from the blade plate and derotate the femur to correct anteversion, using the previously scored longitudinal line on the posterior surface of the femur as a reference (Fig. 65-50, *H*). When corrective rotation has been made, again clamp the blade plate to the distal fragment for stability. Check for correction of anteversion by flexing the knee and rotating the hip. Approximately 15 to 20 degrees of internal rotation at the hip should be preserved. After proper rotation of the distal fragment has been determined, fix the blade plate to this fragment with screws and close the wound in a standard manner. Apply a hip spica cast.

AFTERTREATMENT. The spica cast is usually removed 3 weeks after surgery but may be used longer if the fixation is questionable.

DISLOCATION

Dislocated or subluxated hips become painful in many patients and it cannot be predicted which will be painful and which will not. In a young child with a subluxation or dislocation, we believe that an aggressive approach should be taken to reduce a dislocation, relieve pain, improve perineal hygiene, improve balance when sitting and standing, and help prevent pelvic obliquity. In a young child who has the potential for remodeling the acetabulum, a procedure need not be done on this side of the joint. After the age of 8 years, an operation on the ilium is indicated to correct or decrease the acetabular dysplasia and prevent redislocation. We prefer a Chiari osteotomy (Fig. 65-51) or a triple innominate osteotomy as described by Steele (p. 2739) with a minor modification, or Sutherland and Greenfield (p. 2741) along with derotational and varus osteotomies and adductor or flexor releases (Fig. 65-52). In patients who walk with assistance, we use the triple innominate rather than the Chiari osteotomy. However, as our experience with Chiari's procedure has increased, we have used it more often. Acetabuloplasty, as described by Pemberton (p. 2738), or innominate osteotomy (p. 2733), as described by Salter, has been unsatisfactory in this group of patients.

We have modified the Steele triple innominate osteotomy by dividing the pubic and ischial rami near the symphysis pubis with a rongeur through the same incision at the time an open adductor release is done (Fig. 65-53). This requires little added exposure and it is technically much easier than Steele's approach to these bones. The iliac osteotomy is performed as in a Salter procedure and the redirected acetabulum is stabilized by pin fixation in the ilium and cast immobilization.

Drummond et al. believe that a dislocated hip is not usually disabling in a patient who is neurologically immature, extremely intellectually impaired, bedridden, and institutionalized. In 1974 they established the following four criteria for open reduction of a dislocated hip: first, the patient had to be moderately mature neurologically and have moderate intelligence; second, the patient should have walking ability or at least have sitting potential; third, pelvic obliquity should have been corrected; and fourth, the dislocation ideally should be unilateral. In a 1979 study that included some of these same authors, Moreau et al. reviewed 88 hips in institutionalized adult cerebral palsied

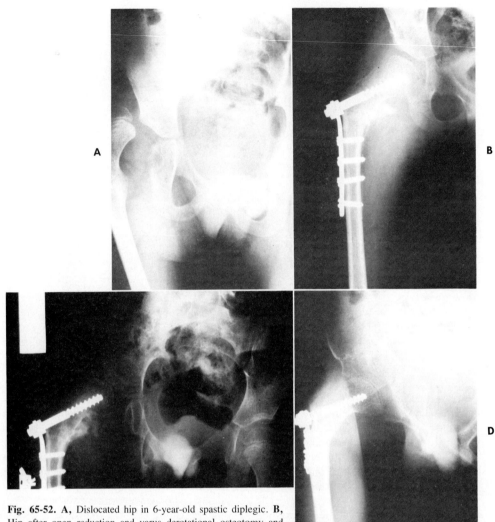

Fig. 65-52. A, Dislocated hip in 6-year-old spastic diplegic. **B,** Hip after open reduction and varus derotational osteotomy and adductor and flexor releases. **C,** Four months later hip has subluxed from inadequate acetabulum. **D,** Hip is reduced after open reduction and triple innominate osteotomy.

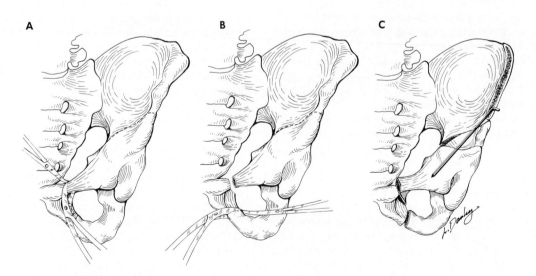

Fig. 65-53. Modification of triple innominate osteotomy through adductor and iliofemoral approach. **A** and **B,** After subperiosteal stripping of adductors from pubic and ischial rami of symphysis, pubic bone is rongeured free of its attachment to symphysis. **C,** Innominate osteotomy is done and acetabulum is rotated over femoral head.

patients (average age, 26.5 years). Forty-one of the 88 patients had unstable hips. In 24 patients the hips were dislocated and in 9 they were subluxated. Pain was present in 11 of the patients who had dislocations. One third of the patients with hip subluxation or dislocation had problems with perineal care, and in 14 of these pelvic obliquity and scoliosis were present. It was their conclusion that dislocation and subluxation should be prevented, but that surgery for a dislocated hip should be reserved for the neurologically mature patient and those patients with athetosis. They combined adductor release or varus derotational osteotomy of the femur with a femoral shortening if needed and open reduction of the hip, as well as iliopsoas muscle release. A Chiari osteotomy was performed 2 or 3 weeks later followed by immobilization in a hip spica cast for 2 months.

In their review of 274 subluxated or dislocated hips in institutionalized patients, Samilson et al. found that the mean age for dislocation was 7 years, and this has been the experience of others. They also found that pain from the dislocation was uncommon, occurring in only 6 patients, whereas perineal care was the primary indication for surgical treatment in 202 patients. They concluded that the proper treatment of subluxation was percutaneous adductor tenotomy (at times including the gracilis), open release of the iliopsoas and the rectus femoris, varus and derotational osteotomy of the femur to correct coxa valga and anteversion, and closed reduction of the hip. In patients with dislocations needing surgery, they performed the soft tissue releases as above, a varus derotational osteotomy of the femur combined with femoral shortening of 2 to 5 cm, and an open reduction of the hip with plication of any redundant capsule.

Arthrodesis of the hip or total hip arthroplasty has been successful in a small number of skeletally mature patients with hip pain. Root recommends that the hip be arthrodesed in 45 degrees of flexion, 15 degrees of abduction, and neutral rotation. This procedure should be limited to the patient with total body involvement who has pain both when sitting and when lying. Total hip arthroplasty should be reserved for the adult ambulatory patient or the minimally involved patient with a painful subluxation or dislocation, because success with this procedure requires good motor function about the hip.

Modified Girdlestone procedures (see p. 687) and resection arthroplasties of the proximal femur with capsular interposition have been somewhat successful and are probably preferred over arthrodesis. Although these procedures are no longer favored because of recurrent deformity, recurrent pain, and ectopic bone formation, they still have merit. In 1984, Kalen and Gamble reviewed 18 hips in 15 patients who had proximal femoral resection arthroplasty at a mean age of 17.5 years with an average follow-up of 4.7 years. All patients were nonambulatory preoperatively, severely retarded, and totally dependent for all activities. In each patient, nursing hygiene and care was made easier by the operation. Of the 10 patients with preoperative pain, 8 were improved by the procedure, and sitting and supine posture was improved in 8 of the 9 patients. Although some complications occurred, all nursing goals were achieved and most of the patients were free of pain.

PELVIC OBLIQUITY, HIP DISLOCATION, AND SCOLIOSIS

In 1979 Drummond et al. stated that pelvic obliquity in cerebral palsy was caused by a combination of scoliosis and contractures about the hip. In their review of 88 institutionalized adult patients, they found an incidence of hip dislocation that resulted in pelvic obliquity in 15% of patients. However they concluded that a pelvic obliquity should be corrected before a paralytic hip deformity for although the hip problem might be resolved surgically, a remaining pelvic obliquity would probably cause recurrence of the hip deformity. In their opinion pelvic obliquity was usually caused by scoliosis.

Scoliosis is seen in about 7% of ambulatory cerebral palsied patients and in 35% of those who are not ambulatory. The more common type of scoliosis is a long, gentle, C-shaped curve extending down into the pelvis, which with time becomes fixed, producing a fixed pelvic obliquity. Often a dislocated hip is also present. Drummond et al. reported that a thoracic lumbar spinal orthosis (TLSO) can control some curvatures and halt their progression for a period of time, but when use of such an orthosis was discontinued the curvature in the spine recurred. They recommended corrective surgery and noted that often the fusion mass had to extend into the sacrum.

The treatment of paralytic scoliosis is discussed on p. 3224.

When studying the relationship of scoliosis, pelvic obliquity, and dislocated hips, Lonstein and Beck reviewed 500 children treated by the Cerebral Palsy Spine Service at the Gillette Children's Hospital. They found no correlation between the frequency of dislocated hips, either bilateral or unilateral, and pelvic obliquity. All degrees of pelvic obliquity were found in children whose hips were both not dislocated or were both dislocated. Furthermore, the frequency of hip dislocation on the same side as the elevated pelvis had no direct correlation with the degree of the pelvic obliquity. They also found that the convexity of a lumbar or thoracolumbar curve occurred on the side opposite the high side of the pelvis, but that in "windswept" hips there was no correlation between the direction of the windswept hips and the direction of the pelvic obliquity. Thus they concluded that hip dislocation and subluxation are the result of muscle imbalance about the hip and that pelvic obliquity and scoliosis are related to muscle imbalance of the trunk and independent of the position of the hips.

Other than the inability to think and comprehend and the inability to communicate, two of the most disabling conditions in cerebral palsy are dislocated hips and scoliosis. The first is preventable and the second is manageable, and both are handled more easily the earlier they are detected. Awareness and vigilance in their detection is of great importance.

UPPER EXTREMITY

In cerebral palsy, upper extremity paralysis is often accompanied by sensory deficits, particularly in proprioception, sterognosis, barognosis, and light touch. There is seldom normal sensation in the hand of the paralyzed extremity. In many instances this sensory loss causes the patient to totally disregard the hand, and there appears to be a direct relationship between the use of the hand and its sensitivity or lack of it. When a patient uses an involved extremity to play, grasp, eat, or assist the opposite hand it is functionally useful and may be improved by surgery. In an extremity that has been isolated from use by the patient, reconstructive surgery has seldom been of any benefit except to improve cosmesis and hand hygiene.

For a hand to function in grasp, release, pinch, and transfer activities, it must be able to reach the object to be handled. The hand may be so restrained by lack of motion at the shoulder and elbow that its maximum functional capacity cannot be used. If the hand is functional or can be made functional by surgical reconstruction, then surgery on the shoulder, elbow, and forearm may be justified.

In spastic paralysis the most common deformities are those of position: flexion of the fingers, flexion of the thumb with or without adduction, flexion of the wrist, pronation of the forearm, flexion of the elbow, and adduction and internal rotation of the shoulder.

The results of surgery on the upper extremity, in which the goal is functional mobility, are poor when compared with those of the lower extremity, in which the goal is painless stability. Although operations often fail and their results are usually only fair to good, the possibility of improving the part, either cosmetically or functionally, makes surgery sometimes indicated.

Operations on the upper extremities are designed primarily to place the arm and forearm in a functional position and to enable the patient to extend the fingers and wrist while retaining active flexion of the fingers.

Not only should the motor and sensory evaluation of the extremity be considered when making a decision, but also the intellectual level and age of the patient. More postoperative training is required after surgery of the upper extremities than of the lower extremities, and for this reason age and cognition are of primary importance. Kinetic electromyographic evaluation is extremely useful when evaluating the upper extremity. Hoffer et al. have shown that phasic activity in the muscle is unchanged after transfer surgery, so no benefit is derived in transferring a muscle whose phasic ability preoperatively is less than that desired postoperatively. Operations to weaken a severely spastic muscle or to transfer one to assist as a tenodesis are the exceptions.

Shoulder

Contracture of the shoulder or spasticity of the muscles that control it usually is not disabling enough to justify surgery. Any deformity is usually one of adduction and internal rotation. When surgery is indicated, neurectomy of motor nerves to the involved muscles is impracticable because the nerves are not easily accessible. For this reason the only useful operations to correct the deformity are (1) the operation of Fairbank modified by Sever or procedures similar to those performed for obstetric paralysis (p. 3045) and (2) rotational osteotomy of the humerus made at the level of the deltoid tubercle.

Elbow

In an extremity in which the hand is functional or has been made so by surgery, an elbow flexion contracture inhibits its use by restricting the ability to reach forward. In the nonfunctional extremity, a flexion contracture at the elbow may cause skin breakdown in the antecubital fossa, which may be painful and result in poor skin hygiene. In such instances, release of an elbow flexion contracture may be justified.

Although we have released flexion contractures, we do not attempt to obtain full extension in the elbow. The brachial artery and the median nerve have become shortened by the constant elbow flexion, and an effort to obtain full extension may result in neurovascular injury. During the operation, we locate and isolate the radial nerve, the brachial artery, and the median nerve on either side of the brachialis muscle before the dissection is continued.

In 1979 Mital reported the results of 50 anterior elbow releases in which there were no neurovascular complications and no recurrences of the deformity. Other operations that improve forearm supination and hand function by releasing the flexor-pronator muscle origins from the medial capsule result in a mild amount of elbow extension as well.

RELEASE OF ELBOW FLEXION CONTRACTURE

Mital's indications for this operation are a fixed elbow flexion contracture of 45 degrees or more or a functional flexion attitude of the elbow of 110 degrees (10 degrees above a right angle) that interferes with the ability to reach forward with a functional forearm and hand.

TECHNIQUE (MITAL). With the patient supine, the arm fully draped, and with or without a tourniquet, approach the intercubital space through a gently curving, S-shaped incision over the flexor crease. If needed, ligate the veins that cross the region transversely. Dissect the soft tissue and deep fascia to the muscle belly of the biceps proximally, and then follow it distally to its tendon and the lacertus fibrosis. Isolate the lacertus fibrosis and excise it (Fig. 65-54, *A*). Identify and protect the lateral antebrachial cutaneous nerve as it enters the area between the biceps and the brachialis laterally. Retract the nerve laterally, then flex the elbow partially, and free the biceps tendon down to its insertion on the tuberosity of the proximal radius. Divide the biceps tendon for a Z-plasty lengthening (Fig. 65-54, *B*). The musculofascial surface of the brachialis muscle can then be seen under it. The radial nerve lies lateral to the brachialis muscle, and the brachial artery and the median nerve lie medial to it. Identify and protect these structures. Extend the elbow maximally and circumferentially incise the aponeurotic tendinous fibers of the brachialis muscle at its distal end at one or two levels (Fig. 65-54, *C*). Then maximally extend the elbow and if necessary perform an anterior elbow capsulotomy. Allow the tourniquet to deflate and secure hemostasis. Then extend the elbow and repair the previously divided biceps tendon (Fig. 65-54, *D*). Assure the integrity of the brachial artery and the median nerve. Close only the subcutaneous tissue and skin, and immobilize the arm in a well-padded cast with the elbow maximally but not forcefully extended and the forearm fully supinated. Bivalve the cast and reapply it with straps at the operating table.

AFTERTREATMENT. The arm is elevated over the head for 48 hours and finger motion is encouraged. The bivalved cast is loosened if any swelling occurs. At 4 days the

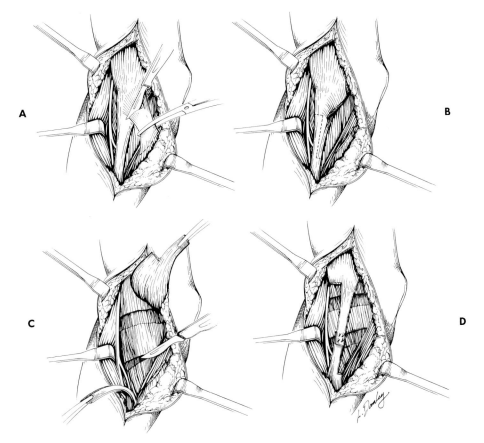

Fig. 65-54. Mital elbow flexion release. **A,** Lacertus fibrosus is severed through incision in antecubital space. **B,** Tendon of insertion of biceps muscle is lengthened by Z-plasty. **C,** Fascia covering brachialis muscle anteriorly is cut at two levels. **D,** Z-plasty in biceps tendon is sutured after elbow is extended.

dressing is changed and at 5 days flexion-extension exercises out of the cast are begun. For 6 weeks after surgery the arm is replaced in the cast when the exercise period is completed. Pronation-supination exercises are added to the routine three weeks after surgery. The bivalved cast is continued at night for 6 months. Maximum elbow motion is usually obtained from 3 to 5 months after the operation.

Forearm, wrist, and hand

Deformities of the forearm, wrist, and hand are considered in the discussion of the cerebral palsied hand, Chapter 13.

Fractures in cerebral palsy

McIvor and Samilson studied 134 fractures in 92 patients with cerebral palsy. One hundred and thirty-one fractures healed, but about one half healed in malposition. Refracture occurred 19 times and decubitus ulcers 17 times. According to them, treatment must be individualized because the usual methods are not appropriate in paraplegia. Skin traction often causes ulceration, Steinmann pins or Kirschner wires may cause infection, and plaster casts may cause decubitus ulcers. For these reasons molded plaster splints that can be removed frequently for inspection of the skin are recommended when feasible in the particular fracture.

POSTNATAL CEREBRAL PALSY

To this point in the chapter the diagnosis and treatment of the traditional types of cerebral palsy in children, developing in the prenatal, perinatal, and early postnatal periods have been discussed. Here the causes and treatment of cerebral palsy developing in the later postnatal period in both children and adults are considered.

Children

The chief neuromuscular manifestations of postnatal cerebral palsy in children are spasticity and paralysis of muscles. Hoffer et al. and later Hoffer and Brink reported the experience of the staff of Rancho Los Amigos Hospital in postnatal or acquired cerebral palsy in children. The most common cause of palsy was traumatic head injury; less common ones were near-fatal anoxia, hydrocephalus, cerebrovascular accidents, sclerosing brain syndromes, slowly growing inaccessible brain tumors, and meningitis or encephalitis. As might be expected, these children had many significant medical problems, including convulsive disorders, hypertension, visual difficulties, and behavioral disorders.

As already mentioned, the most common cause of cerebral palsy in this group was head injury, which occurred in 221 children. The prognosis for independence in self-care and walking was found to be directly related to the duration and depth of the coma and not to the age of the child. Coma was defined in five levels, ranging from level 1, those children normal in terms of cognition and recorded daily events, to level 5, those in deep unresponsive coma. The children were also grouped in categories related to their independence in self-care and walking, ranging from group A, those who were totally independent in self-care and were community ambulators, to group C, those who were totally dependent and were nonambulatory. This classification was necessary to evaluate the patients accurately and to record their progress during treatment.

In the acute phase, the first 7 to 10 days after a head injury, the orthopaedist must accurately evaluate the skeletal injuries and properly treat them. They should be treated as though the patient is certain to make a complete neurologic recovery; in other words, the skeletal injury should be treated as if there were no head injury. In a review by Garland and Rhoades of 90 head-injured patients, 60 patients sustained a total of 97 skeletal injuries, and of those 12 had major skeletal fractures that were initially unrecognized. These authors recommended that all comatose patients who experienced a high velocity accident have anteroposterior and lateral roentgenograms of the cervical, thoracic, and lumbar spines, an anteroposterior roentgenogram of the pelvis that includes both hips, and anteroposterior and lateral roentgenograms of both knees. No comatose patient should be treated on the assumption that he will not recover, for if he recovers and the fractures have not been treated satisfactorily, their treatment becomes more complicated and the results less certain.

During the recovery or subacute phase, lasting from 10 days to 1½ years after injury, the neurologic status was found to be changeable and unpredictable and consequently definitive operations should not be carried out until at least 1 year after injury. In patients admitted during the first year, any deformed joints of the limbs were treated in serial plaster casts that were changed weekly and were used until after the deformity had been corrected. After the fully corrected position had been maintained for 2 or 3 weeks, the casts were bivalved and used as night splints. Shoulder and hip contractures were treated by stretching exercises. Occasionally the musculocutaneous, median, and ulnar nerves were blocked by local anesthesia to distinguish between fixed flexion contractures and spasticity. When the deformity could be corrected after blocking of a nerve, the limb was placed in a plaster cast in the desired position, and the cast was usually tolerated well. Open blocking of peripheral nerves was also occasionally used; 2 to 5 ml of a 3% to 5% solution of phenol were injected into the motor nerve under direct vision using a tuberculin syringe and a 26-gauge needle. The injection was continued until the nerve ballooned slightly and until stimulation of the nerve proximal to the site of injection showed that nerve transmission was blocked. Such an injection can be expectd to decrease spasticity significantly for about 6 months. During this time a treatment program to strengthen the antagonistic muscles can be started, and if it is ineffective, suitable transfers can be carried out to improve muscle balance. The most common orthopaedic operations performed in these children were tenotomies,

tendon transfers, osteotomies, tendon lengthenings, and advancement of muscle origins, all of which were borrowed from the established treatment of traditional cerebral palsy. The results of these operations were similar to those in cerebral palsy, but the number of children involved was too few for precise evaluation.

Children with anoxic brain damage and neuromuscular disabilities were much more severely involved than those with head injuries. Very few who had been in deep coma for longer than a week developed any useful function. One of their major problems was early dislocation of the hip, and this can be prevented by early soft tissue releases.

Children with progressive cerebral disease such as sclerosing syndromes, inaccessible brain tumors, and hydrocephalus and those after meningitis or encephalitis required few orthopaedic operations. Many were aided by braces, but some eventually required surgery to correct deformities in the lower extremities.

Adults (stroke patients)

Much has been written in recent years about the orthopaedic evaluation and treatment of patients after cerebrovascular accidents, or strokes. Among those making significant contributions are Braun, Caldwell, Hoffer, McCollough, McKeever, Mooney, Nickel, Roper, Waters, and Tracy.

LOWER EXTREMITY

Of patients who have had a stroke, 65% to 75% recover enough function in their lower extremities to permit them to walk. This is because the lower extremity does not depend as much on sensation for its function as does the upper extremity and the activities necessary for walking are gross motor functions that are enhanced by primitive postural reflexes in the weight-bearing position. Most patients with residual hemiparesis require the use of an external support and a brace, at least initially, to become independently ambulatory.

After stroke orthotic management of the lower extremity begins in the early phases of recovery when prevention of contracture is the chief aim of treatment. This treatment extends through the period of motor recovery and gait training to the time when the neurologic deficit becomes stationary and a definitive brace is required. In the early phase the paralysis is usually flaccid and deformities result from poor positioning. Equinus deformity should be prevented by appropriate splinting, and frequently repeated range-of-motion exercises of all the joints of the extremity are indicated. The prevention of deformity of the lower extremities is greatly assisted by the patient's standing and walking as soon as his medical condition permits. Motor recovery usually occurs during the first 3 or 4 months, and the quality of gait may change considerably during this time. To become a functional ambulator, the patient must obtain adequate spontaneous improvement to allow voluntary control of the hip and knee. A brace for the ankle and foot is usually required, but any brace necessary to stabilize the knee is difficult to apply and manage and significantly interferes with walking. When maximum motor recovery has been obtained and the gait pattern has been stabilized, usually within 4 to 6 months, the patient should be fitted with a definitive brace. It must be the most functional, comfortable, and cosmetically acceptable one available that will control the gait defect.

Perry et al. have contributed much to the understanding of neurophysiology in both normal people and patients with stroke. They list seven neurologic sources of motion. Two of these are sophisticated components of normal function (selected control and habitual control); five are forms of primitive control that are normally subliminated into a preparatory background, but in the spastic patient they are exposed as overt sources of motion (locomotor pattern, verticality, limb synergy, fast stretch, and slow stretch).

Selected control is the normal ability to move one joint independently of another, to contract an isolated muscle, or to select a desired combination of motions. How fast, strong, or continuous a motion is can also be controlled, and this is a cortical function. *Habitual control* is the normal automatic performance of a learned skill such as walking and probably arises from the basal ganglia. Primitive *locomotor patterns* are mass movements of flexion or extension. The patient can initiate or terminate the movements but cannot otherwise modify them. If the knee is extended, the ankle also is automatically plantar flexed and the hip is extended. The opposite movements occur in knee flexion. This voluntary motion is preserved after a loss of cortical control and presumably is controlled by the midbrain. Control of *verticality* is a vestibular function and is an antigravity mechanism. When the body is erect, the extensor muscles have more tone than when it is supine, and standing creates a more intense stimulus than does sitting. In the upper extremity the flexor muscles respond in this manner. Primitive *limb synergy* is the result of a multisegmental spinal cord reflex, tying the action of the extensor muscles to the posture of the limb. Thus when the knee is extended, the tone of both the soleus and the gastrocnemius is greatly increased, making them much more sensitive to stretch than when the knee is flexed. Likewise the tone in antagonistic muscles may be inhibited. It is this activity that confuses the results in the Silfverskiöld test used to differentiate contracture of the gastrocnemius from that of the soleus. The *fast stretch*, the stretch reflex characterized by the familiar clonic response, is caused by an intermittent burst of muscle activity. It is initiated by the velocity sensors in the muscle spindles. The *slow stretch* reflex is characterized by rigidity, a clinical term for continuous muscle reaction to stretch and often misinterpreted as joint contracture; however, when the patient is anesthetized and the muscles are relaxed, the deformity disappears. It is caused by the length-change sensors in the muscle spindles.

In addition to these motor problems the stroke patient frequently has impaired sensation. Impaired proprioception is especially important, and this causes a delay or hesitancy in making a voluntary motor response. The duration of this delay indicates the time it takes to process the central nervous system signals, and if the delay is too great, walking will not be a realistic goal.

Perry et al. also point out the importance of gait analysis and various standing tests, including double limb support, hemiparetic single limb stance, and hemiparetic limb flex-

ion; the results of gait analysis and these various tests determine whether the patient can expect to walk and whether orthopaedic operations might be expected to decrease the handicap. Further information is also gained from kinesiologic electromyography, and some decisions for surgery cannot be made without this new aid.

Surgery should be deferred until at least 6 months after the stroke. Most patients make rapid spontaneous recovery during the first 6 to 8 weeks. They then strengthen these gains and learn to live with their disability. Progress in control of the limb occurs, and this is a contribution that surgery cannot make. By 6 to 9 months after the stroke the patient will have obtained the maximum spontaneous improvement and must come to realize the permanence of the limitations. The results of surgery must be carefully and thoroughly explained to avoid unrealistic expectations after surgery. Although improvement in a single deficit may be expected, restoration of normal function in the extremity is impossible.

FOOT

Talipes equinovarus is the most common foot deformity in the stroke patient. Other deformities can occur, such as equinus without varus, varus of the forefoot, dropfoot without spasticity in the triceps surae, occasionally planovalgus, and often in-curling of the toes.

Talipes equinus. The goal of surgery is to correct talipes equinus in the midswing and midstance phases while preserving heel lift support in the terminal stance phase and accepting a flat-footed contact with the floor. The recommended operation is a closed subcutaneous triple hemisection of the tendo calcaneus. The distal cut is made medially proximal to the insertion of the tendon, the next is made 2.5 cm proximal to the first through the lateral half of the tendon, and the final one is made 2.5 cm proximal to the second through the medial half of the tendon. After surgery the foot is immobilized in a cast in a slightly equinus position so that walking does not stretch the tendon further. Walking in the cast is started immediately and the cast is removed at 4 weeks.

Isolated contracture of the gastrocnemius muscle may be suspected when the plantar flexion deformity is mild and clonus in the soleus muscle is absent. It may be demonstrated by a nerve block and the traditional Silfverskiöld test. In these patients gait electromyography shows pre-stance action in the gastrocnemius but not in the soleus.

Talipes equinovarus. Talipes equinovarus is usually seen in stroke patients and can result from either dorsiflexor-evertor insufficiency or excess activity in their antagonists. The goal of surgery should be to render the patient free of brace or to improve walking in a brace when proprioception is defective or the dorsiflexor muscles are inadequate. In the presence of moderate action of the tibialis anterior without assistance of the toe extensors, the equinus deformity is corrected by rebalancing the foot to eliminate the varus deformity. The tibialis anterior, the tibialis posterior, the soleus, the flexor hallucis longus, and the flexor digitorum longus, despite their swing phase and stance phase action, can be active well into the other phase and are often active continuously. Furthermore, they can also be inactive. Therefore varus deformtiy in either the swing or

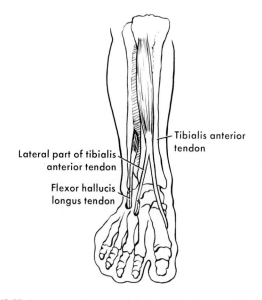

Fig. 65-55. Technique of Perry et al. to correct equinovarus deformity in stroke patients. Lateral three fourths of tibialis anterior tendon and flexor hallucis longus tendon are transferred to third cuneiform. Flexor digitorum longus is released (see text). (From Perry, J., and Waters, R.L.: In American Academy of Orthopaedic Surgeons: Instructional course lectures, vol. 24, St. Louis, 1975, The C.V. Mosby Co.)

stance phase can be caused by any of these muscles. Based on surgical experience and on the new techniques of gait electromyography, Perry el al. recommend the following operation to correct equinovarus deformity. Three fourths of the tibialis anterior tendon is transferrred laterally to the third cuneiform, the flexor hallucis longus tendon is transferred anteriorly to the same area, the flexor digitorum longus tendon is released, and the tibialis posterior tendon is not disturbed (Fig. 65-55).

TECHNIQUE (PERRY ET AL.). Identify and expose the insertion of the tibialis anterior tendon. Separate and detach the lateral three fourths of the tendon from the medial one fourth. Bring the detached part out through an incision made just proximal to the ankle and route it subcutaneously to the dorsal surface of the third cuneiform. Here expose the cuneiform, drill converging holes into the bone, and use a curet to construct a tunnel. Loop the free part of the tendon through this tunnel to be anchored later. Then in the arch of the foot release the plantar flexors of the toes. Next through a posterior incision identify the flexor hallucis longus tendon at its tunnel, detach it, and pass it anteriorly through a large window made in the interosseous membrane. Insert this tendon through the tunnel in the third cuneiform in the direction opposite to that of the tibialis anterior. Lengthen the tendo calcaneus as just described. With the ankle in neutral position and the foot slightly everted, sew the two tendons to themselves as loops and to each other. The flexor digitorum longus may be transferred instead of the flexor hallucis longus if the toe flexors are active in the swing phase of gait.

AFTERTREATMENT. Because the tendo calcaneus has been lengthened at the same time, a cast is applied with the foot in slight plantar flexion. A 6 weeks the cast is removed and the foot is protected by a locked ankle brace for an additional 6 months. Because muscles in a hemiplegic pull

with marked vigor or none at all, several months are necessary for the scar to mature enough not to yield under tension.

• • •

In 1976 Tracy reported satisfactory results in 32 of 35 adult hemiplegics with talipes equinovarus. He used an operation originally described by Mooney et al. consisting of triple hemisection of the tendo calcaneus, open Z-plasty lengthening and suturing of the tibialis posterior tendon just proximal to the medial malleolus, transfer of one half of the tibialis anterior tendon to the third cuneiform, and transverse division of the flexor digitorum brevis and flexor digitorum longus tendons at the base of each toe. All patients who could satisfactorily dorsiflex the foot after surgery had been able to contract the tibialis anterior selectively at will or had some activity in the muscle before surgery.

Varus. The tibialis anterior muscle is usually the deforming force in forefoot varus. A split tibialis anterior transfer (p. 2869) is the procedure of choice for this condition, although it will not correct a fixed hindfoot varus.

AFTERTREATMENT. A short leg walking cast is worn for 6 weeks, then an AFO is used when walking to protect the muscle transfer for an additional 4 to 5 months.

Planovalgus. If a pes planus preceded the stroke, a planovalgus deformity may occur after the stroke. Spasticity of the triceps surae pulls the calcaneus laterally, and the peroneals may be hyperactive with no function occurring in the tibialis posterior tendon during stance.

If walking is impeded by pain, then surgical correction is indicated. As in equinus deformity, the treatment is to lengthen the tendo calcaneus, with a triple level hemitenotomy. The distal hemisection in the tendo calcaneus is performed in the lateral one half of the tendon, however, so as to decrease the valgus placement or thrust of the tendon on the calcaneus.

If the peroneals are hyperactive during the stance phase, the peroneus brevis may be transferred medially into the tibialis posterior tendon to support the medial border of the foot.

A triple arthrodesis may ultimately be required if an AFO does not control the deformity.

Toe flexion. Toe flexion occurs at the metatarsophalangeal joint and is different from the clawtoe deformity seen in most neurologic disorders in which extensors are hyperactive. Toe curling or toe flexion in the stroke patient occurs from overactivity of the long toe flexors. If all toes are involved, the flexor digitorum longus and the flexor hallucis longus may be tenotomized through a plantar incision along the medial border of the foot, reflecting the abductor hallucis plantarward and locating the tendons between the first and third layers of the plantar surface of the foot. An alternative is to merely tenotomize the toe flexors at the plantar surface of the metatarsophalangeal joints of all toes.

KNEE

Flexion contractures of the knee, like other deformities in the stroke patient, are better prevented than treated. Although the hamstrings are important extensors of the hip, occasionally a patient with a flexion contracture of the knee and good power in the gluteus maximus and quadriceps muscles will benefit from releasing the hamstrings or transferring the medial hamstrings.

Deficient flexion of the knee during the swing phase, producing a stiff knee gait, is usually caused by increased electric activity in the rectus femoris during the swing phase. Release of the rectus femoris from the patella by excision of its distal segment can result in 15 to 20 degrees of flexion of the knee during the swing phase.

HIP

The scissors gait caused by adductor spasticity is the only disability about the hip now treated surgically. To determine whether the adductors are necessary in flexion of the hip in a given patient, obturator nerve block using a local anesthetic is advisable. If the patient is unable to walk with the obturator nerve blocked, then surgery will be of no benefit. On the other hand, if the gait is improved temporarily, a neurectomy of the anterior branch of the obturator nerve is recommended. If the effect of the local anesthetic is prolonged, the nerve block may be repeated once or twice and occasionally the results will be permanent.

Surgical release of a flexion contracture of the hip is rarely indicated in stroke patients because the decrease in the power of active flexion of the hip may make the patient unable to walk. When gait electromyography shows continuous activity in the flexors of the hip and in the medial hamstrings, then releasing the iliopsoas, tenotomy of the adductor longus, and transferring the medial hamstrings to the femur will sometimes allow the limb to assume an upright position.

UPPER EXTREMITY

The prognosis for recovering normal function in the upper extremity in stroke patients is poor, and approximately one third are left with a permanently functionless limb. The most important reason for this is that the patterns of neuromuscular activity in the normally functioning upper extremity are highly sophisticated and complex and are modified by multiple sophisticated sensory impulses. Permanent impairment in motor and sensory function in the upper extremity is incurable, and permanent impairment of function is to be expected. Thus rehabilitation of the arm and hand consists primarily of training the patient to accomplish the activities of daily living as a one-handed person. In those who show sufficient neurologic recovery additional training for development of assistive function is indicated.

The orthopaedic surgeon may release contractures, weaken spastic muscles that cause imbalance and deformity, and transfer functioning muscle units to attempt to restore some balance in the extremity. These operations may also relieve persistent pain, which causes immobility and lack of participation in other areas of the rehabilitation program.

SHOULDER

Some stroke patients complain of pain localized precisely to the shoulder and specifically to the adductor and internal rotator groups of muscles. In others a hemicorporal type of diffuse discomfort is present and is untreatable by present methods. Patients with the first type of pain develop progressively decreasing ranges of motion in the joint despite intensive conservative treatment. They also have an exaggerated stretch reflex on rapid external rotation of the shoulder, abduction of less than 45 degrees, and internal rotation of less than 15 degrees. Surgery is recommended only for those patients who will have an exercise program available to them after surgery, for those who will participate in it fully, and for those who have a reasonable potential for rehabilitation. Braun et al. reviewed their initial experience with the operation described here and noted complete relief of pain and significant improvement in motion in 10 of the first 13 patients in whom it was used. Of 12 control patients with similar symptoms not treated by surgery, none had spontaneous resolution of the painful contracture of the joint.

TECHNIQUE (BRAUN ET AL.). Make an anterior deltopectoral approach to the shoulder (p. 77). Identify the subscapularis tendon and cauterize the vascular bundle at its distal edge. Excise this broad tendon, but preserve the anterior capsule of the shoulder joint. Palpate the tendon of the pectoralis major and, with scissors passed distally along the humerus, cut its tendinous insertion.

AFTERTREATMENT. A sling is worn on the arm. A program of assisted range-of-motion exercises is begun within the first few days after surgery and reciprocal pulley exercises within the first 5 days. It is important to supervise the patient's participation in the exercises.

ELBOW

Fixed flexion of the elbow causes a serious impairment of function of the upper extremity. Anterior release in the antecubital fossa, however, is a major operation and may be followed by serious complications. Sometimes a fixed flexion deformity can be prevented by an open injection of phenol into the musculocutaneous nerve carried out with minimal added dissection at the time the shoulder is released. This injection will usually allow the patient 6 months in which to develop adequate extensor muscles before motor power returns to the flexor muscles of the elbow supplied by this nerve.

Any necessary release is carried out through an S-shaped incision over the anterior aspect of the elbow. The neurovascular bundle is isolated and protected throughout the operation. The biceps tendon is lengthened in a step-cut manner. The fascia over the brachialis muscle is divided and, if necessary, the brachialis itself is divided at its musculotendinous junction, the flexor-pronator origin is divided, the brachioradialis fascia is released, the capsule of the elbow joint is divided, the ulnar nerve is transplanted anteriorly, and the wound is closed over a drain. This operation is rarely carried out because the results of it are so uncertain.

Phenol nerve block

Braun, Hoffer, Mooney, McKeever, and Roper reported the results of injection of phenol into motor nerves in 24 adults and 10 children with spastic hemiplegia. The nerves were exposed surgically. That the correct nerve had been exposed was confirmed by a nerve stimulator, and the nerve was injected intraneurally with 3% to 5% phenol solution beneath the neural sheath and into the substance of the nerve. The volume of solution injected ranged from 2 to 5 ml within a 2 cm segment of the nerve. The injection was continued until electrical stimulation proximal to the site of injection revealed that the nerve had in fact been blocked. Such blocks in 18 patients initially resulted in improvement in 17, but review later revealed that 11 of these good results disappeared in 6 months. In two patients the deformity recurred in 1 year, and in only 2 patients did the good results last longer than 1 year. In these latter two some selective control of the antagonistic muscles was present before the injection. In four patients phenol block of the spastic flexor-pronator muscles was combined with transfer of the flexor carpi ulnaris tendon to the extensor carpi radialis brevis. Relaxation of the excessive flexor tone was seen during the 3 months required for strengthening of the the transfer. These investigators concluded that open intraneural phenol nerve blocks can be expected to decrease muscle tone for about 6 months. During this time other treatment programs to prevent contractures or to strengthen and train weakened or transferred muscles can be carried out. A few patients showed prolonged benefits, and most of these had selective muscle control of their spastic muscles before the nerves were blocked.

Functional electric stimulation in stroke patients

Functional electric stimulation is a product of modern electronic rehabilitation engineering whereby function is restored in paralyzed muscles by electrical stimulation. The aim is to have functional muscle control occur during the stimulation, but occasionally a carryover occurs and the muscle comes under voluntary control even during periods without electrical stimulation. Functional electrical stimulation (FES) theoretically depends on one stimulation, such as heel lift, being transmitted through an antenna to an electric implant, which then fires another signal to the nerve supply to the muscles, such as the peroneal nerve, to perform a function, such as dorsiflexion of the foot. The device needs to be small and cosmetically acceptable, and activity of the stimulator should be partly under voluntary control; otherwise too much stimulation or erroneous stimulation may occur. Although development of FES is still in its infancy, it is being used in the upper and lower extremities, around the foot and ankle to suppress spasticity, to correct scoliosis, for electrophrenic respiration, and in bladder control. There remains a need for external control of motor unit graduation, for synergistic acitivity with other muscles, and for some proprioceptive kinesthetic feedback. This will come as reseach progresses.

REFERENCES
General

Allen, M.C.: The appearance of selected primitive reflexes in a population of very low birthweight premature infants. Presented at the Annual Meeting of the American Academy of Cerebral Palsy and Developmental Medicine, Washington, D.C., October 24-27, 1984.

Arvidsson, J., and Eksmyr, R.: Cerebral palsy and perinatal deaths in geographical defined populations with different perinatal services, Dev. Med. Child Neurol. **26:**709, 1984.

Baker, L.D., and Bassett, F.H.: Surgery in the rehabilitation of cerebral palsied patients (abstract), J. Bone Joint Surg. **51-A:**1040, 1969.

Banks, H.H.: Cerebral palsy. In Lovell, W.W., and Winter, R.B., (editors): Pediatric orthopaedics, ed. 1, vol. 1, Philadelphia, 1978, J.B. Lippincott Co.

Barrnett, H.E.: Orthopedic surgery in cerebral palsy, JAMA **150:**1396, 1952.

Bax, M.C.O.: Terminology and classification of cerebral palsy, Dev. Med. Child Neurol. **6:**295, 1964.

Bayley, N.: Bayley scales of mental and motor development, New York, 1969, The Psychological Corp.

Beals, R.K.: Spastic paraplegia and diplegia: an evaluation of non-surgical and surgical factors influencing the prognosis for ambulation. J. Bone Joint Surg. **48-A:**827, 1966.

Bennett, F.C., et al.: Spastic diplegia in premature infants: etiological and diagnostic considerations, Am. J. Dis. Child. **135:**732, 1981.

Bennett, F.C., Crowe, T., Deitz J., and TeKolste, K.: Childhood motor skills of premature infants. Presented at the Annual Meeting of the American Academy of Cerebral Palsy and Developmental Medicine, Washington, D.C., October 24-27, 1984.

Biasini, F.J., and Mindingall, A.: Developmental outcome of very low birthweight children, Orthop. Trans. **8:**115, 1984.

Bleck, E.E.: Locomotor prognosis in cerebral palsy, Dev. Med. Child Neurol. **17:**18, 1975.

Bleck, E.E.: Cerebral palsy. In Bleck, E.E., and Nagel, D.A., editors: Physically handicapped children: a medical atlas for teachers, New York, 1975, Grune & Stratton, Inc.

Bleck, E.E.: Orthopaedic management of cerebral palsy, Philadelphia, 1979, W.B. Saunders.

Bleck, E.E., (editor): Physically handicapped children—a medical atlas for teachers, ed. 2, New York, 1982, Grune & Stratton, Inc.

Bleck, E.E.: Where have all the CP children gone?—the needs of adults, Dev. Med. Child Neurol. **26:**674, 1984.

Blumel J., Eggers, G.W.N., and Evans, E.B.: Genetic, metabolic, and clinical study on one hundred cerebral palsied patients, JAMA, **174:**860, 1960.

Bobath, B.: Abnormal postural reflex activity caused by brain lesions, ed. 2, New York, 1976, William Heinman Publishers.

Bobath, B., and Bobath, K.: Motor development in the different types of cerebral palsy, New York, 1978, William Heinman Publishers.

Bobath, K.: The motor deficit in patients with cerebral palsy, Clin. Develop. Med. No. 23, London, 1966, Spastics International Medical Publications in association with William Heinemann Medical Books Ltd.

Bost, F.C., Ashley, R.K., and Kelley, W.J.: Role of the orthopedic surgeon in treatment of cerebral palsy, JAMA, **160:**256, 1956.

Bozynski, M.E.A., et al.: Two-year follow-up of 1,200 gram and less premature infants: long-term sequelae of intracranial hemorrhage (abstract), Orthop. Trans. **8:**115, 1984.

Brink, J.D., and Hoffer, M.M.: Rehabilitation of brain injured children, Orthop. Clin. North Am. **9:**451, 1978.

Butler, C.: Effects of powered mobility on self-initiative behavior of very young, locomotor-disabled children. Presented at the Annual Meeting of the American Academy of Cerebral Palsy and Developmental Medicine, Washington, D.C., October 24-27, 1984.

Campos da Paz, A., Nomura, A.M., Braga, L.W., and Burnett, S.M.: Cerebral palsy: a retrospective study. Presented at the Annual Meeting of the Pediatric Orthopaedic Society, Vancouver, Canada, 1984.

Capute, A.J., Shapiro, B.K., and Palmer, F.B.: Spectrum of developmental disabilities, Orthop. Clin. North Am. **12:**3, 1981.

Capute, A., et al.: Primitive reflex profile, Baltimore, 1978, University Park Press.

Capute, A., and Palmer, F.: A pediatric overview of the spectrum of developmental disabilities, J. Dev. Behav. Pediatr. **1:**66, 1980.

Carlson, W., Carpenter, B., and Wenger, D.: Myoneural blocks for preoperative planning in cerebral palsy surgery. Presented at the Annual Meeting of the American Academy for Cerebral Palsy and Developmental Medicine, Chicago, 1983.

Carlson, W., Carpenter, B., and Wenger, D.: Myoneural blocks for preoperative planning in cerebral palsy surgery (abstract), Orthop. Trans. **8:**111, 1984.

Cech, D., and Gallagher, R.J.: Infant motor assessment: Bayley scales of infant development as compared to the Chicago Infant Neuromotor Assessment. Presented at the Annual Meeting of the American Academy of Cerebral Palsy and Developmental Medicine, Washington, D.C., October 24-27, 1984.

Cliff, G., and Nymann: Mothers can help, El Paso, 1974, El Paso Rehabilitation Center.

Connolly, B., and Russell, F.: Interdisciplinary early intervention program, Phys. Ther. **56:**155, 1976.

Craig, C.L., Sosnoff, F., and Zimbler, S.: Seating in cerebral palsy: a possible advance. Presented at the Annual Meeting of the Pediatric Orthopaedic Society, Vancouver, Canada, 1984.

Crothers, B., and Paine, R.: The natural history of cerebral palsy, Cambridge, 1959, Harvard University Press.

Crothers, B., and Paine, R.: The natural history of cerebral palsy, Cambridge, 1959, Harvard University Press.

Cruickshank, W.M. (editor): Cerebral palsy: a developmental disability, ed. 3, Syracuse, New York, 1976, Syracuse University Press.

Dale, A., and Stanley, F.J.: An epidemiological study of cerebral palsy in Western Australia, 1956-1975. II: Spastic cerebral palsy and perinatal factors, Dev. Med. Child. Neurol. **22**:13, 1980.

Davies, P.A., and Tizard, J.P.M.: Very low birthweight and subsequent neurological deficit, Dev. Med. Child Neurol. **17**:3, 1975.

Denhoff, E.: Current status of infant stimulation or enrichment programs for children with developmental disabilities, Pediatrics **67**:32, 1981.

Denhoff, E., and Holden, R.H.: Early diagnosis of cerebral palsy by assessment of upper extremities, Clin. Orthop. **46**:37, 1966.

Denhoff, E., Holden, R.H., and Silver, M.L.: Prognostic studies in children with cerebral palsy, JAMA **161**:781, 1956.

Dierdorf, S.F., et al.: Effect of succinylcholine on plasma potassium in children with cerebral palsy, Anesthesiology **62**:88, 1985.

Drennan, J.C.: Orthopaedic management of neuromuscular disorders, Philadelphia, 1983, J.B. Lippincott Co.

Elliman, A.M., Bryan, E.M., Elliman, A.D., Palmer, P., and Dubowitz, L.: Denver developmental screening test and preterm infants, Arch. Dis. Child. **60**:20, 1985.

Evans, P., Agassiz, C.D.S., Pritchard, F.E., and Nissen, J.J.: Symposium on cerebral palsy, Proc. R. Soc. Med. **44**:82, 1951.

Fay, T.: Neurophysiocal aspects of therapy in cerebral palsy, Arch. Phys. Med. **29**:327, 1948.

Florentino, M.: Reflex testing: methods for evaluating C.N.S. development, Springfield, Ill., 1979, Charles C Thomas.

Florentino, M.: A basis for sensorimotor development: normal and abnormal, Springfield, Ill. 1981, Charles C Thomas.

Frankenburg, W.K., and Dodds, J.B.: Denver developmental screening test, J. Pediatr. **71**:181, 1967.

Gage, J.R.: Orthopaedic aspects of cerebral palsy. Presented at American Academy for Cerebral Palsy and Developmental Medicine Symposium, Growing Up With Cerebral Palsy, Wilmington, Delaware, April 19-20, 1985.

Gage J.R.: Deformities of the knee and foot. Presented at American Academy for Cerebral Palsy and Developmental Medicine Symposium, Growing Up With Cerebral Palsy, Wilmington, Delaware, April 19-20, 1985.

Gage, J.R., Fabian, D., Hicks, R. and Tashman, S.: Pre- and postoperative gait analysis in patients with spastic diplegia: a preliminary report, J. Pediatr. Orthop. **4**:715, 1984.

Georgieff, M., Hoffman-Williamson, M., Spungen, L., Borian, F., and Bernbaum, J.: Abnormal muscle tone as an indicator of later development in preterm infants (abstract), Orthop. Trans. **8**:108 1984.

Gesell, A., and Amatruda, C.: Developmental diagnosis, ed. 2, New York, 1947, Harper & Row.

Gesell, A., and Amatruda, C.S.: Developmental diagnosis: normal and abnormal child development: clinical methods and pediatric applications, ed. 2, New York, 1947, Paul B. Hoeber, Inc.

Gesell, A., and Ilg, F.L.: Infant and child in the culture of today, New York, 1943, Harper & Brothers.

Goldner, J.L.: Cerebral palsy: Part I. General principles. In American Academy of Orthopaedic Surgeons: Instructional course lectures, vol. 20, St. Louis, 1971, The C.V. Mosby Co.

Green, W.T., and McDermott, L.J.: Operative treatment of cerebral palsy of spastic type, JAMA **118**:434, 1942.

Hagberg, B., Hagberg, G., and Olow, I.: The changing panorama of cerebral palsy in Sweden, 1954-1970. 1: Analysis of the general changes, Acta Paediatr. Scand. **64**:187, 1975.

Hagberg, B., Hagberg, G., and Olow, I.: Gains and hazards of intensive neonatal care: an analysis from Swedish cerebral palsy epidemiology, Dev. Med. Child. Neurol. **24**:13, 1982.

Hagberg, B., Hagberg, G., and Olow, I.: The changing panaroma of cerebral palsy in Sweden, 1954-70. II: Analysis of the various syndromes, Acta Paediatr. Scand. **64**:193, 1975.

Hagberg, B., Hagberg, G., and Olow, I.: The changing panaroma of cerebral palsy in Sweden, 1954-70, III: The importance of fetal deprivation of supply, Acta Paediatr. Scand. **65**:403, 1976.

Harris, S.: The school-aged child. Physical therapy: developmental vs. functional goals. Presented at American Academy for Cerebral Palsy and Developmental Medicine Symposium, Growing Up With Cerebral Palsy, Wilmington, Delaware, April 19-20, 1985.

Harris, S.R., and Tada, W.L.: Providing developmental therapy services. In Garwood, S.G., and Fewell, R.R.: Educating handicapped infants: issues in development and intervention, Rockville, M, 1983, Aspen Systems Corp.

Henderson, J.L.: Cerebral palsy in childhood and adolescence: a medical, psychological, and social study, Edinburgh, 1961, E & S Livingston, Ltd.

Hensinger, R.N., Fraser, B., Machello, J., and Taylor, S.: Head and neck control in the severely involved cerebral palsy patient. Presented at the Annual Meeting of the Pediatric Orthopaedic Society, Vancouver, Canada, 1984.

Heyman, C.H.: The surgical treatment of spastic paralysis. In Lewis practice of surgery, vol. 3, Hagerstown, Md., 1945, W.F. Prior Co., Inc.

Hoffer, M.M.: Basic considerations and classifications of cerebral palsy, American Academy of Orthopaedic Surgeons: Instructional course lectures, vol. 25, 1976, The C.V. Mosby Co.

Hoffer, M., and Brink, J.: Orthopedic management of acquired cerebral spasticity in childhood, Clin. Orthop. **110**:224, 1975.

Hoffer, M.M., and Bullock, M.: The functional and social significance of orthopedic rehabilitation of mentally retarded patients with cerebral palsy, Orthop. Clin. North Am. **12**:185, 1981.

Hoffer, M.M., and Koffman, M.: Cerebral palsy: the first three years, Clin. Orthop. **151**:222, 1980.

Hoffer, M.M.,, et al.: The orthopaedic management of brain-injured children, J. Bone Joint Surg. **53-A**:567, 1971.

Hoffman-Williamson, M., et al.: Comparable development progress in infants of birthweights less than 1000 grams and 1001-1500 grams (abstract), Orthop. Trans. **8**:115, 1984.

Holm, V.A.: The causes of cerebral palsy: a contemporary perspective, JAMA **247**:1473, 1982.

Ingram, A.J., Withers, E., and Speltz, E.: Role of intensive physical and occupational therapy in the treatment of cerebral palsy: testing and results, Arch. Phys. Med. **40**:429, 1959.

Johnson, M.K.: The use of motor age test in the evaluation of cerebral palsy patients. In American Academy of Orthopaedic Surgeons: Instructional course lectures, vol. 9 Ann Arbor, 1952, J.W. Edwards.

Johnson, M.K., Zuck, F.N., and Wingate, K.: The motor age test: measurement of motor handicaps in children with neuromuscular disorders such as cerebral palsy, J. Bone Joint Surg. **33-A**:698, 1951.

Johnston, R.B.: Development disorders: assessment, treatment, education, Austin, Texas, 1976, Pro-Ed.

Jones, M.H., and Ogg, H.L.: The use of sensory modalities in the training of infantile cerebral palsied patients. Clin. Orthop. **46**:63, 1966.

Kenney, W.E.: The importance of sensori-perceptuo-gnosia in the examination, the understanding, and the management of cerebral palsy, Clin. Orthop. **46**:45, 1966.

Kiely, M., Lubin, R.A., and Kiely, J.L.: Descriptive epidemiology of cerebral palsy, Pub. Health Rev. **12**:79, 1984.

Kling, T.F., Hensinger, R.N., and Taylor, S.R.: Transparent spinal orthosis for the neurologically handicapped child. Presented at the Annual Meeting of the American Academy for Cerebral Palsy and Developmental Medicine, Washington, D.C., 1984.

Knoblock, H., and Passamanick, B. editors: Gessell and Amatruda's developmental diagnosis, ed. 3, Scranton, Harper & Row.

Knott, M., and Voss, D.E.: Proprioceptive neuromuscular facilitation, New York, 1956, Hoeber-Harper.

Kong, E.: Very early treatment of cerebral palsy, Dev. Med. Child Neurol. **8**:198, 1966.

Levy, H.B.: Square pegs, round holes (The learning disabled child in the classroom and at home), Boston, 1973, Little, Brown & Co.

Lindsey, R.W, and Drennan, J.C.: Management of foot and knee deformities in the mentally retarded, Orthop. Clin. North Am. **12**:107, 1981.

Lipper, E.G.,, Voorhies, T., Ross, G., Auld, P.A.M., and Vanucci, R.: Early neurological predictors of one year outcome in birth asphyxiated infants. Presented at the Annual Meeting of the American Academy of Cerebral Palsy and Developmental Medicine, Washington, D.C., October 24-27, 1984.

Little, W.J.: The classic: deformities of the human frame, Clin. Orthop. **131:**3, 1978.

Lord, J.: Cerebral palsy: a clinical approach, Arch. Phys. Med. Rehabil. **65:**542, 1984.

Mann, R.: Biomechanics in cerebral palsy, Foot Ankle, **4:**114, 1983.

Marquis, P.J., Ruis, N.A., Lundy, M.S., and Dillard, R.G.: Primitive reflexes and early motor development in very low birth weight (VLBW) infants (abstract), Orthop. Trans. **8:**108, 1984.

Masland, R.L.: Spastic diplegia after short gestation, Dev. Med. Child Neurol. **12:**127, 1970.

McCarroll, H.R.: Surgical treatment of spastic paralysis. In American Academy of Orthopaedic Surgeons: Instructional course lectures, vol. 6, Ann Arbor, 1949. J.W. Edwards.

McCarroll, H.R., and Schwartzmann, J.P.: Spastic paralysis and allied disorders, J. Bone Joint Surg. **25:**745, 1943.

McIvor, W., and Samilson, R.L.: Fracture in patients with cerebral palsy, J. Bone Joint Surg. **48-A:**858, 1966.

Milani-Comparetti, A., and Gidoni, E.A.: Routine developmental examination in normal and retarded children, Dev. Med. Child Neurol. **9:**631, 1967.

Nelson, M.N., Bozynski, M.E.A., Genaze, D., Rosati-Skertich, C., and O'Donnell, K.J.: Comparative evaluation of motor development of 1,200 grams (or less) infants during the first postnatal year using the Bayley scales versus the Milani-Comparetti (abstract), Orthop. Trans. **8:**108, 1984.

Nissen, K.I.: Orthopaedic operations in congenital spastic paralysis, Proc. R. Soc. Med. **44:**87, 1951.

Norlin, R., and Tkaczuk, H.: One-session surgery for correction of lower extremity deformities in children with cerebral palsy, J. Pediatr. Orthop. **5:**208, 1985.

O'Neill, D.L., and Harris, S.R.: Developing goals and objectives for handicapped children, Phys. Ther. **62:**295, 1982.

O'Reilly, D.E., and Walentynowicz, J.E.: Etiological factors in cerebral palsy: an historical review, Dev. Med. Child Neurol. **23:**633, 1981.

Ough, J.L., Garland, D.E., Jordan, C., and Waters, R.L.: Treatment of spastic joint contractures in mentally disabled adults, Orthop. Clin. North Am. **12:**143, 1981.

Paine, R.S.: Cerebral palsy: symptoms and signs of diagnostic and prognostic significance. In Adams, J.P., editor: Current practice in orthopaedic surgery, vol. 3, St. Louis, 1966, The C.V. Mosby Co.

Pearson, D.T.: Psychological needs of the handicapped. Presented at American Academy for Cerebral Palsy and Developmental Medicine Symposium, Growing Up With Cerebral Palsy, Wilmington, Delaware, April 19-20, 1985.

Pearson, P.H.: The results of treatment: the horns of our dilemma, Dev Med. Child Neurol. **24:**417, 1982.

Pearson, P.H., and Williams, C.E. (editors): Physical therapy services in the developmental disabilities, Springfield, Ill., 1972, Charles C Thomas.

Pearson, P., and Williams, C.E.: Physical therapy services in the developmental disabilites, Springfield, Ill., 1980, Charles C Thomas.

Perlstein, M.A., and Barnett, H.E.: Nature and recognition of cerebral palsy in infancy, JAMA **148:**1389, 1952.

Perlstein, M: Personal communication, 1958.

Perlstein, M.A., and Hood, P.N.: Etiology of postneonatally acquired cerebral palsy, JAMA **188:**850, 1964.

Perlstein, M.: The clinical significance of kernicterus. In Swinyard, C., editor: Kernicterus and its importance in cerebral palsy, Springfield, Ill., 1957, Charles C Thomas

Perry, J., Simon, S., and Sutherland, D.: Gait analysis: an evaluation of measurement systems and their applications. Presented at the American Academy for Cerebral Palsy and Developmental Medicine Annual Meeting, Washington, D.C., October 24-27, 1984.

Perry, J., et al.: Electromyography before and after surgery for hip deformity in children with cerebral palsy: a comparison of clinical and electromyographic findings, J. Bone Joint Surg. **58-A:**201, 1976.

Phelps, W.M.: Treatment of paralytic disorders exclusive of poliomyelitis. In Bancroft, F.W., and Marble, J.C.:Surgical treatment of the motor-skeletal system, Philadelphia, 1951, J.B. Lippincott Co.

Phelps, W.M.: Complications of orthopaedic surgery in the treatment of cerebral palsy, Clin. Orthop. **53:**39, 1967.

Rang, M., Douglas, G., Bennet, G.C. and Koreska, J.: Seating for children with cerebral palsy, J. Pediatr. Orthop. **1:**279, 1982.

Rang, M., Silver, R., and de la Garza, J.: Cerebral palsy. In Lovell, W.W., and Winter, R.B., editors: Pediatric orthopaedic, ed. 2, vol. 1, Philadelphia, 1986.

Reimers, J.: Static and dynamic problems in spastic cerebral palsy, J. Bone Joint Surg. **55-B:**822, 1973.

Robinault, I.: Sex, society and the disabled, Scranton, P, 1978, Harper & Row.

Rood, M.S.: Neurophysiological reactions as a basis for physical therapy, Phys. Ther. Rev. **34:**444, 1954.

Roseberg, L.K., Blackman, J, and Sustik, J.: Assessment of motor dysfunction in infants: a computer-videodisc program (abstract), Orthop. Trans. **8:**102, 1984.

Rosenbaum, P.L.: Early diagnosis of developmental delay. Presented at American Academy for Cerebral Palsy and Developmental Medicine Symposium, Growing Up With Cerebral Palsy, Wilmington, Delaware, April 19-20, 1985.

Royle, N.D.: Treatment of spastic paralysis by sympathetic ramisection, Proc. R. Soc. Med. (orthopedic sect.) **20:**63, 1927.

Royle, N.D.: The clinical results following the operation of sympathetic ramisection, Br. Med. J. **2:**628, 1930.

Rutter, M., Graham, P., and Yule, W.: A neuropsychiatric study in childhood, London, 1970, Heinemann.

Sabel, K.G,. Olegard, R.,, and Victorin, L.: Remaining sequelae with modern perinatal care, Pediatrics **57:**652, 1976.

Samilson, R.L.: Orthopaedic aspects of cerebral palsy, Clin. Dev. Med., **52/53:**183, 1975.

Samilson, R.L.: Orthopaedic aspects of cerebral palsy, Philadelphia, 1975, J.B. Lippincott Co.

Samilson, R.L.: Current concepts of surgical management of deformities of the lower extremities in cerebral palsy, Clin. Orthop. **158:**99, 1981.

Samilson, R.L., and Dillin, L.: Postural impositions on the foot and ankle from trunk, pelvis, hip, and knee in cerebral palsy, Foot Ankle **4:**120, 1983.

Scherzer, A.L., Mike, V., and Ilson, J.: Physical therapy as a determinant of change in cerebral palsied infants, Pediatrics **58:**47, 1976.

Scherzer, A.L., and Mike, V.: Cerebral palsy and the low birthweight child, Am. J. Dis. Child. **128:**199, 1974.

Schlesinger, E.R., Allaway, N.C., and Peltin, S.: Survivorship in cerebral palsy, Am. J. Pub. Health **49:**343, 1959.

Scrutton, D., and Gilbertson, M.: The physiotherapist's role in the treatment of cerebral palsy. In Samilson, R., editor: Orthopedic aspects of cerebral palsy, Philadelphia, 1975, J.B. Lippincott Co.

Scrutton, D., and Gilbertson, M.: The physiotherapist's role in the treatment of cerebral palsy. In Samilson, R., editor: Orthopedic aspects of cerebral palsy, Philadelphia, 1975, J.B. Lippincott Co.

Shapiro, B., Accardo, P., and Capute, A.: Factors affecting walking in a profoundly retarded population, Dev. Med. Child Neurol. **21:**369, 1979.

Sherk, H.H.: Indications for orthopedic surgery in the mentally retarded patient, Clin. Orthop. **90:**174, 1973.

Snell, E.E.: Physical therapy. In Cruickshank, W.M., editor: Cerebral palsy: a developmental disability, ed. 3, Syracuse, New York, 1976, Syracuse University Press.

Stanley, F.J.: An epidemiological study of cerebral palsy in Western Australia, 1956-1975. I: Changes in total cerebral palsy incidence and associated factors, Dev. Med. Child Neurol.**21:**701, 1979.

Steindler, A.: Orthopedic operations, Springfield, Ill., 1940, Charles C Thomas, Publisher.

Steindler, A.: Post-graduate lectures on orthopedic diagnosis and indications, vol. 2, Springfield, Ill., 1951, Charles C Thomas, Publisher.

Stockmeyer, S.A.: A sensorimotor approach to treatment. In Pearson, P.H., and Williams, C. editors : Physical therapy services in the developmental disabilities, Springfield, Ill., 1972, Charles C Thomas.

Tablan, D.J.: Clinical analysis of the brain injured child: an analysis of 333 cases in the Phillipines. In Samilson, R.L., editor: Orthopedic aspects of cerebral palsy, Philadelphia, 1975, J.B. Lippincott.

Tachdjian, M.O.: The neuromuscular system. In Tachdjian, M.O.: Pediatric orthopaedics, vol. 1, Philadelphia, 1972, W.B. Saunders.

Tachdjian, M.O.: Affections of brain and spinal cord. In Tachdjian, M.O.: Pediatric orthopaedics, Philadelphia, 1972, J.B. Lippincott Co.

Tachdjian, M.O., and Minear, W.L.: Sensory disturbances in the hands of children with cerebral palsy, J. Bone Joint Surg. **40-A:**85, 1958.

Taft, L.T.: Intervention programs for infants with cerebral palsy: a clinician's view. In Brown, C.E., editor: Infants at risk: assessment and intervention, 1981, Johnson & Johnson Baby Products.

Taylor, S., and Kling, T.F., Jr.: An improved system of orthotic management in neuromuscular disease. Presented at the Annual Meeting of the American Academy for Cerebral Palsy and Developmental Medicine, Chicago, 1983.

Taylor, S., and Kling, T.F., Jr.: An improved system of orthotic management in neuromuscular disease (abstract), Orthop. Trans. **8:**105, 1984.

Thompson, G.H., Rubin, I.L., and Bilenker, R.M., editors: Comprehensive management of cerebral palsy, New York, 1983, Grune and Stratton.

Thibodeau, A.A., Wagner, L.C., and Carr, F.J., Jr.: The evaluation of surgical procedures on bones, muscles and peripheral nerves in spastic paralysis , Am. J. Surg. **43:**821, 1939.

Turnbull, A., and Turnbull, H.R., III: Parents speak out: a view from the other side of the two-way mirror, Columbus, Ohio, 1978, Charles E. Merrill Publishing Co.

Twitchell, T.E.: The nature of the gait disorder in infantile cerebral palsy, Clin. Orthop. **36:**111, 1964.

Twitchell, T.E.: Sensation and the motor deficit in cerebral palsy, Clin. Orthop. **46:**55, 1966.

Vining, E.P., Accardo, P.J., Rubenstein, J.E., Farrell, S.E., and Roizen, N.J.: Cerebral palsy: a pediatric developmentalist's overview, Am. J.. Dis. Child. **130:**643, 1976.

Vulpius, O., and Stoffel, A.: Orthopädische Operationslehre, ed. 2, Stuttgart, 1920, Ferdinand Enke.

Waters, R.L., et al.: Stiff-legged gait in hemiplegia: surgical correction, J. Bone Joint Surg. **61-A:**927, 1979.

Waters, R.L., Perry, J., and Garland, D.: Surgical correction of gait abnormalities following stroke, Clin. Orthop. **131:**54, 1978.

Westin, G.W., and Dye, S.: Conservative management of cerebral palsy in the growing child, Foot Ankle **4:**160, 1983.

Williams, S.F., Ferguson-Pell, M., and Cochran, G.V.B.: Characterization and treatment patterns of 122 spastic diplegic patients. Presented at the Annual Meeting of the American Academy of Cerebral Palsy and Developmental Medicine, Washington, D.C., October 24-27, 1984.

Winters, T.F., and Gage, J.R.: Gait patterns in spastic hemiplegia secondary to cerebral palsy. Presented at the American Academy for Cerebral Palsy and Developmental Medicine Annual Meeting, Washington, D.C., October 21-27, 1984.

Yale Clinic of Child Development: The first five years of life: a guide to the study of the preschool child, New York, 1940, Harper & Brothers.

Zimbler, S., Craig, C., Harris, J., Sohn, R., and Rosenberg, G.: Orthotic management of severe scoliosis in spastic neuromuscular disease: results of treatment. Presented at the Annual Meeting of the American Academy for Cerebral Palsy and Developmental Medicine, Washington, D.C., 1984.

Zuck, F.N., and Johnson, M.K.: Progress of cerebral palsy patient under in-patient circumstances, In American Academy of Orthopaedic Surgeons: Instructional course lectures, vol. 9, Ann Arbor, 1952, J. W. Edwards.

Lower Extremity

Close, J.R., and Todd, F.N.: The phasic activity of the muscles of the lower extremity and the effect of tendon transfer, J. Bone Joint Surg. **41-A:**189, 1959.

Gage, J.R.: Development disorders of gait. Presented at American Academy for Cerebral Palsy and Developmental Medicine Symposium, Growing Up With Cerebral Palsy, Wilmington, Delaware, April 19-20, 1985.

Green, N.E.: The knee, ankle and foot in cerebral palsy. Presented at the Annual Meeting of the American Academy of Orthopaedic Surgeons, Las Vegas, 1985

Lindsey, R.W. and Drennan, J.C.: Management of foot and knee deformities in the mentally retarded, Orthop. Clin. North Am. **12:**107, 1981.

Norlin, R., and Tkaczuk, H.: One-session surgery for correction of lower extremity deformities in children with cerebral palsy, J. Pediatr. Orthop. **5:**208, 1985.

Perry, J., et al.: Electromyography before and after surgery for hip deformity in children with cerebral palsy: a comparison of clinical and electromyographic findings, J. Bone Joint Surg. **58-A:**201, 1976.

Samilson, R.L.: Current concepts of surgical management of deformities of the lower extremities in cerebral palsy, Clin. Orthop. **138:**99, 1981.

Samilson, R.L., and Dillin, L.: Postural impositions on the foot and ankle from trunk, pelvis, hip, and knee in cerebral palsy, Foot Ankle **4:**120, 1983.

Simon, S.R., et al.: Genu recurvatum in spastic cerebral palsy, J. Bone Joint Surg. **60-A:**882, 1978.

Tachdjian, M.O.: Affections of brain and spinal cord, In Tachdjian, M.O.: Pediatric orthopaedics, Philadelphia, 1972, W.B. Saunders.

Winters, T.F., and Gage, J.R.: Gait patterns in spastic hemiplegia secondary to cerebral palsy. Presented at the Annual Meeting of the Pediatric Orthopaedic Society, Vancouver, Canada, 1984.

Lower Extremity—Foot and Ankle

Adelaar, R.S., et al.: A long term study of triple arthrodesis in children, Orthop. Clin. North Am. **7:**895, 1976.

Baker, L.D.: A rational approach to the surgical needs of the cerebral palsy patient, J. Bone Joint Surg. **38-A:**313, 1956.

Baker, L.D.: Triceps surae syndrome in cerebral palsy, Arch. Surg. **68:**216, 1954.

Baker, L.D., and Hill, L.M.: Foot alignment in the cerebral palsy patient, J. Bone Joint Surg. **46-A:**1, 1964.

Banks, H.H.: Equinus and cerebral palsy: its management, Foot Ankle **4:**149, 1983.

Banks, H.H., and Grun, W.T.: The correction of equinus deformity in cerebral palsy, J. Bone Joint Surg. **40-A:** 1359, 1958

Barrasso, J.A., Wile, P.B., and Gage, J.R.: Extraarticular subtalar arthrodesis with internal fixation, J. Pediatr. Orthop. **4:**555, 1984.

Bassett, F.H., III, and Baker, L.D.: Equinus deformity in cerebral palsy. In Adams, J.P., editor: Current practice in orthopaedic surgery, vol. 3, St. Louis, 1966, The C.V. Mosby Co.

Baumann, J.U., and Zumstein, M.: Experience with a plastic ankle-foot orthosis for prevention of muscle contracture. Presented at the American Academy for Cerebral Palsy and Developmental Medicine Annual Meeting, Washington, D.C., October 24-27, 1984.

Bennett, G.C., Rang, M., and Jones, D.: Varus and valgus deformities of the foot in cerebral palsy, Dev. Med. Child Neurol. **24:**499, 1982.

Bernau, A.: Long-term results following Lambrinudi arthrodesis, J. Bone Joint Surg. **59-A:**473, 1977.

Bisla, R.S., Louis, H.J., and Albano, P.: Transfer of tibialis posterior tendon in cerebral palsy, J. Bone Joint Surg. **58-A:**497, 1976.

Bleck, E.E.: Spastic abductor hallucis, Dev. Med. Child Neurol. **9:**602, 1967.

Bleck, E.E.: Forefoot problems in cerebral palsy: diagnosis and management, Foot Ankle **4:**188, 1984.

Bleck, E.E., and Rinsky, L.A.: Decision making in surgical treatment of paralytic deformities of the foot with gait electromyograms (abstract), Orthop. Trans. **9:**90, 1985.

Boss, J.A., Gugenheim, J.J., and Tullos, H.S.: Dennyson-Fulford subtalar arthrodesis in fifty feet (abstract), Orthop. Trans. **8:**63, 1984.

Brown, A.: A simple method of fusion of the subtalar joint in children, J. Bone Joint Surg. **50-B:**369, 1968.

Bowser, B.L., Dimitrijevic, M.M., Erdmann, M., and Solis, I.S.: Effects of neuromuscular stimulation on passive ankle dorsiflexion in children with cerebral palsy: preliminary report (abstract), Orthop. Trans. **9:**98, 1985.

Burman, M.S.: Spastic intrinsic-muscle imbalance of the foot, J. Bone Joint Surg. **20:**145, 1938.

Calandriello, B.: The detachment of gastrocnemius muscles in the treatment of spastic equinus foot, Bull. Hosp. Joint Dis. **20:**48, 1959.

Carpenter, E.B.: Role of nerve blocks in the foot and ankle in cerebral palsy: therapeutic and diagnostic, Foot Ankle **4:**164, 1983.

Carpenter, E.B., and Mikhail, M.: The use of intramuscular alcohol as a diagnostic and therapeutic aid in cerebral palsy (abstract), Dev. Med. Child Neurol. **14:**113, 1972.

Coleman, S.S.: Complex foot deformities in children, Philadelphia, 1983, Lea & Febiger.

Compere, E.L.: Personal communication, 1946.

Craig, J.J., and van Vuren, J.: The importance of gastrocnemius recession in the correction of equinus deformity in cerebral palsy, J. Bone Joint Surg. **58-B:**84, 1976.

Dennyson, W.G., and Fulford, G.E.: Subtalar arthrodesis by cancellous grafts and metallic internal fixation, J. Bone Joint Surg. **58-B:**507, 1976.

Duncan, J.W., and Lovell, W.W.: Hoke triple arthrodesis, J. Bone Joint Surg. **60-A:**795, 1978.

Duncan, W.R., and Mott, D.H.: Foot reflexes and the use of the "inhibitive cast," Foot Ankle **4:**145, 1983.

Eilert, R.E.: Cavus foot in cerebral palsy, Foot Ankle **4:**185, 1984.

Engström, A., Erikson, U., and Hjelmstedt, A.: The results of extra-articular subtalar arthrodesis according to the Green-Grice method in cerebral palsy, Acta Orthop. Scand. **45:**945, 1974.

Gaines, R.W., and Ford, T.D.: A systematic approach to the amount of Achilles tendon lengthening in cerebral palsy, J. Pediatr. Orthop. **4:**448, 1984.

Garbarino, J.L., and Clancy, M.: A geometric method of calculating tendo Achilles lengthening, J. Pediatr. Orthop. **5:**573, 1985.

Green, W.T., and Grice, D.S.: The surgical correction of the paralytic foot. In American Academy of Orthopaedic Surgeons: Instructional course lectures, vol. 9, Ann Arbor, 1952, J.W. Edwards.

Green, W.T., and McDermott, L.J.: Operative treatment of cerebral palsy of the spastic type, JAMA **118:**434, 1942.

Green, N.E., Griffin, P.P., and Shiavi, R.: Split posterior tibial-tendon transfer in cerebral palsy, J. Bone Joint Surg. **65-A:**748, 1983.

Grice, D.S.: An extra-articular arthrodesis of the subastragular joint for correction of paralytic flat feet in children, J. Bone Joint Surg. **34-A:**927, 1952.

Grice, D.S.: Further experience with extra-articular arthrodesis of the subtalar joint, J. Bone Joint Surg. **36-A:**246, 1955.

Grice, D.S.: The role of subtalar fusion in the treatment of valgus deformities of the feet. In American Academy of Orthopaedic Surgeons: Instructional course lectures, vol. 16, St. Louis, 1959, The C.V. Mosby Co.

Gritzka, T.L., Staheli, L.T., and Duncan, W.R.: Posterior tibial tendon transfer through the interosseous membrane to correct equinovarus deformity in cerebral palsy: an initial experience, Clin. Orthop. **89:**201, 1972.

Gross, R.H.: A clinical study of the Batchelor subtalar arthrodesis, J. Bone Joint Surg. **58-A:**343, 1976.

Guttman, G.: Modificaton of the Grice-Green subtalar arthrodesis in children, J. Pediatr. Orthop. **1:**219, 1981.

Hauser, E.D.: Diseases of the foot, Philadelphia, 1939, W.B. Saunders.

Hoffer, M.M., and Perry, J.: Pathodynamics of gait alterations in cerebral palsy and the significance of kinetic electromyography in evaluating foot and ankle problems, Foot Ankle **4:**128, 1983.

Hoffer, M.M., Reiswig, J.A., Garrett, A.M. and Perry, J.: The split anterior tibial tendon transfer in the treatment of spastic varus hindfoot of childhood, Orthop. Clin. North Am. **5:**31, 1974.

Jahss, M.H.: Evaluation of the cavus foot for orthopedic treatment, Clin. Orthop. **181:**52, 1983.

Jahss, M.H.: Disorders of the foot, Philadelphia, 1982, W.B. Saunders Co.

Kasser, J.R., and MacEwen, G.D.: Examination of the cerebral palsy patient with foot and ankle problems, Foot Ankle **4:**135, 1983.

Kaufer, H.: Personal communication, 1977.

Keats, S., and Kouten, J.: Early surgical correction of the planovalgus foot in cerebral palsy: extra-articular arthrodesis of the subtalar joint, Clin. Orthop. **61:**223, 1968.

Kennan, M.A., Creighton, J., Garland, D.E., and Moore, T.A.: Surgical correction of spastic equinovarus deformity in the adult (abstract), Orthop. Trans. **8:**195, 1984.

Kilfoyle, R.M. and Bryne, D.P.A.: Nonexcision triple arthrodesis of the foot, Orthop. Clin. North Am. **7:**941, 1976.

King, H.A., and Staheli, L.T.: Torsional problems in cerebral palsy, Foot Ankle **4:**180, 1984.

Kling, T.F., Jr., and Hensinger, R.N.: The results of split posterior tibial tendon transfer in children with cerebral palsy (abstract), Orthop. Trans. **8:**102, 1984.

Kling, T.F., Jr., Kaufer, H. and Hensinger, R.N.: Split posterior tibial-tendon transfer in children with cerebral spastic paralysis and equinovarus deformity, J. Bone Joint Surg. **67-A:**186, 1985.

Majestro, T.C., Ruda, R., and Frost, H.M.: Intramuscular lengthening of the posterior tibialis muscle, Clin. Orthop. **79:**59, 1971.

Menelaus, M.B., and Ross, E.R.S.: The management of curly and hammer toes by flexor tenotomy. Presented at the Annual Meeting of the Pediatric Orthopaedic Society, Vancouver, Canada, 1984.

Miller, G.M., Hsu, J.D., Hoffer, M.M. and Rentfro, R.: Posterior tibial tendon transfer: a review of the literature and analysis of 74 procedures, J. Pediatr. Orthop. **2:**363, 1982.

Mortens, J., Moller, H., and Salmonsen, L.: Early stabilizing operation for spastic talipes equino-valgus by Grice's extraarticular osteoplastic subtalar arthrodesis, Acta. Orthop. Scand. **32:**485, 1962.

Muburak, S.J., and Katz, M.M.: Hereditary tendo-Achilles contractures. Presented at the Annual Meeting of the Pediatric Orthopaedic Society, Vancouver, Canada, 1984.

O'Reilly, D.E., and Carter, E.E.: Surgical treatment of equinus in cerebral palsy. Presented at the American Academy for Cerebral Palsy and Developmental Medicine Annual Meeting, Washington, D.C., October 24-27, 1984.

Perry, J., Hoffer, M.M., Giovani, P., Antonelli, D., and Greenberg, R.: Gait analysis of the triceps surae in cerebral palsy: a preoperative and postoperative clinical and electromyographic study, J. Bone Joint Surg. **56-A:**511, 1974.

Pierrot, A.H., and Murphy, O.B.: Heel cord advancement: a new approach to the spastic equinus deformity, Orthop. Clin. North Am. **5:**117, 1974.

Root, L.: Varus and valgus foot in cerebral palsy and its management, Foot Ankle **4:**174, 1984.

Rosenthal, R.K.: The use of orthotics in foot and ankle problems in cerebral palsy, Foot Ankle **4:**195, 1984.

Ruda, R., and Frost, H.M.: Cerebral palsy. Spastic varus and forefoot adductus, treated by intramuscular posterior tibial tendon lengthening, Clin. Orthop. **79:**61, 1971.

Ryerson, E.W.: Arthrodesing operations on the feet, J. Bone Joint Surg. **5:**453, 1923.

Samilson, R.L.: Crescentric osteotomy of the os calcis for calcaneocavus feet. In Bateman, J.E., editor: Foot science, Philadelphia, 1976, W.B. Saunders.

Schneider, M., and Balon, K.: Deformity of the foot following anterior transfer of the posterior tibial tendon and lengthening of the Achilles tendon for spastic equinovarus, Clin. Orthop. **125:**113, 1977.

Seymour, R., and Evans, D.K.: A modification of the Grice subtalar arthrodesis, J. Bone Joint Surg. **50-B:**372, 1968.

Sharrard, W.J.W., and Bernstein, S.: Equinus deformity in cerebral palsy: a comparison between elongation of the tendo calcaneus and gastrocnemius recession, J. Bone Joint Surg. **54-B:**272, 1972.

Sharrard, W.J.W., and Smith, T.W.D.: Tenodesis of flexor hallucis longus for paralytic clawing of the hallux in childhood, J. Bone Joint Surg. **58-B:**224, 1976.

Silfverskiöld, N.: Reduction of the uncrossed two-joint muscles of the leg to one-joint muscles in spastic conditions. Acta Chir. Scand. **56:**315, 1923-1924.

Silver, C.M., and Simon, S.D.: Gastrocnemius muscle recession (Silfverskiöld operation) for spastic equinus deformity in cerebral palsy, J. Bone Joint Surg. **41-A:**1021, 1959.

Silver, C.M., Simon, S.D., Spindell, E., Litchman, H.M., and Scala, M.: Calcaneal osteotomy for valgus and varus deformities of the foot in cerebral palsy: a preliminary report on twenty-seven operations, J. Bone Joint Surg. **49-A:**232, 1967.

Simon, S.R., Fernandez, O., Rosenthal, R.K., and Griffin, P.: The effect of heel cord lengthening and solid ankle foot orthosis on the gait of patients with cerebral palsy. Presented at the Annual Meeting of the American Academy for Cerebral Palsy and Developmental Medicine, Washington, D.C., 1984.

Skinner, S.R., and Lester, D.K.: Dynamic EMG findings in valgus hindfoot deformity in spastic cerebral palsy (abstract), Orthop. Trans. **9:**91, 1985.

Skinner, S.R., and Lester, D.K.: Gait EMG evaluation of long toe flexors in spastic cerebral palsy (abstract), Orthop. Trans. **8:**268, 1984.

Stöffel, A.: The treatment of spastic contracture, Am. J. Orthop. Surg. **10:**611, 1912-1913.

Strayer, L.M., Jr.: Recession of the gastrocnemius: an operation to relieve spastic contracture of the calf muscles, J. Bone Joint Surg. **32-A:**671, 1950.

Strayer, L.M., Jr.: Gastrocnemius recession: five-year report of cases, J. Bone Joint Surg. **40-A:**1019, 1958.

Throop, F.B., DeRosa, G.P., Reeck, C., and Waterman, S.: Correction of equinus in cerebral palsy by the Murphy procedure of tendo calcaneus advancement: a preliminary communication, Dev. Med. Child Neurol. **17:**182, 1975.

Tohen, Z.A., Carmona, P.J., and Barrera, J.R.: The utilization of abnormal reflexes in the treatment of spastic foot deformities: a preliminary report, Clin. Orthop. **47:**77, 1966.

Trumble, T., Banta, J.V., Raycroft, J., and Curtis, B.H.: Talectomy for equinovarus deformity in myelodysplasia. Presented at the American Academy for Cerebral Palsy and Developmental Medicine Annual Meeting, Washington, D.C., October 24-27, 1984.

Turner, J.W., and Cooper, R.R.: Posterior transposition of tibialis anterior through the interosseous membrane, Clin. Orthop. **79:**71, 1971.

Turner, J.W., and Cooper, R.R.: Anterior transfer of the tibialis posterior through the interosseous membrane, Clin. Orthop. **83:**241, 1972.

White, J.W.: Torsion of the Achilles tendon: its surgical significance, Arch. Surg. **46:**784, 1943.

Wilcox, P.G., and Weiner, D.S.: The Akron midtarsal dome osteotomy: preliminary review of a new surgical procedure for treatment of rigid pes cavus. Presented at the American Academy for Cerebral Palsy and Developmental Medicine Annual Meeting, Washington, D.C., October 24-27, 1984.

Wilcox, P., and Weiner, D.S.: The Akron dome osteotomy: preliminary review of a new surgical procedure for the treatment of rigid pes cavus. Presented at the Annual Meeting of the Pediatric Orthopaedic Society, Vancouver, Canada, 1984.

Williams, P.F., and Menelaus, M.B.: Triple arthrodesis by inlay grafting: a method suitable for the undeformed or valgus foot, J. Bone Joint Surg. **59-B:**333, 1977.

Williams, P.F.: Restoration of muscle balance of the foot by transfer of the tibialis posterior, J. Bone Joint Surg. **58-B:**217, 1976.

Lower extremity—knee

Baker, L.D.: A rational approach to the surgical needs of the cerebral palsy patient, J. Bone Joint Surg. **38-A:**313, 1956.

Chandler, F.A.: Reestablishment of normal leverage of the patella in knee flexion deformity in spastic paralysis, Surg. Gynecol. Obstet. **57:**523, 1933.

Chandler, F.A.: Patellar advancement operation: a revised technic, J. Int. Surg. **3:**433, 1940.

Cleveland, M., and Bosworth, D.M.: Surgical correction of flexion deformity of knees due to spastic paralysis, Surg. Gynecol. Obstet. **63:**659, 1936.

Drummond, D.S., Rogala, E., Templeton, J., and Cruess, R.: Proximal hamstring release for knee flexion and crouched posture in cerebral palsy, J. Bone Joint Surg. **56-A:**1598, 1974.

Eggers, G.W.N.: Surgical division of the patellar retinacula to improve extension of the knee joint in cerebral spastic paralysis, J. Bone Joint Surg. **32-A:**80, 1950.

Eggers, G.W.N.: Transplantation of hamstring tendons to femoral condyles in order to improve hip extension and to decrease knee flexion in cerebral spastic paralysis, J. Bone Joint Surg. **34-A:**827, 1952.

Evans, E.B.: The status of surgery of the lower extremities in cerebral palsy, Clin. Orthop. **47:**127, 1966.

Evans, E.B.: Cerebral palsy: Part III. Knee flexion deformity in cerebral palsy. In American Academy of Orthopaedic Surgeons: Instructional Course Lectures, vol. 20, St. Louis, 1971, The C.V. Mosby Co.

Evans, E.B., and Julian, J.D.: Modifications of the hamstring transfer. Dev. Med. Child. Neurol. **8:**539, 1966.

Gage, J.R.: Deformities of the knee and foot. Presented at American Academy for Cerebral Palsy and Developmental Medicine Symposium, Growing Up With Cerebral Palsy, Wilmington, Delaware, April 19-20, 1985.

Gherlinzoni, G., and Pais, C.: Trattamento della lussazione patologica dell'anca; indicazioni, tecnica e resultati lontani, Chir. Organi. Mov. **34:**335, 1950.

Grant, A.D., Small, R.D., and Lehman, W.B.: Correction of flexion deformity of the knee by supracondylar osteotomy, Bull. Hosp. Jt. Dis. **42:**28, 1982.

Herndon, C.H.: Tendon transplantation at the knee and foot: In American Academy of Orthopaedic Surgeons: Instructional course lectures, vol. 18, St. Louis, 1961, The C.V. Mosby Co.

Hoyt, W.A., Jr., Davis, W.M., and Schulze, K.W.: Reconstruction of the quadriceps mechanism by vastus medialis transposition in selected cases of patellar luxation: a preliminary report (abstract), J. Bone Joint Surg. **51-A:**1040, 1969.

Keats, S., and Kambin, P.: An evaluation of surgery for the correction of knee-flexion contracture in children with cerebral spastic paralysis, J. Bone Joint Surg. **44-A:**1146, 1962.

Lloyd-Roberts, G.C., Jackson, A.M., and Albert, J.S.: Avulsion of the distal pole of the patella in cerebral palsy. A cause of deteriorating gait, J. Bone Joint Surg. **67-B:**252, 1985.

McCarroll, H.R.: Surgical treatment of spastic paralysis. In American Academy of Orthopaedic Surgeons: Instructional course lectures, vol. 6, Ann Arbor, 1949, J.W. Edwards.

Perry, J., et al.: Electromyography before and after surgery for hip deformity in children with cerebral palsy, J. Bone Joint Surg. **58-A:**201, 1976.

Pollock, G.A., and English, T.A.: Transplantation of the hamstring muscles in cerebral palsy, J. Bone Joint Surg. **49-B:**80, 1967.

Reimers, J.: Contracture of the hamstrings in spastic cerebral palsy: a study of three methods of operative correction, J. Bone Joint Surg. **56-B:**102, 1974.

Roberts, W.M., and Adams, J.P.: The patellar-advancement operation in cerebral palsy, J. Bone Joint Surg. **35-A:**958, 1953.

Seymour, N., and Sharrard, W.J.: Bilateral proximal release of the hamstrings in cerebral palsy, J. Bone Joint Surg. **50-B:**274, 1968.

Sullivan, R.C., Gehringer, K.M., and Harris,G.F.: A computer assisted survey of results of medial hamstring surgery in children with cerebral palsy. Presented at the Annual Meeting of the American Academy for Cerebral Palsy and Developmental Medicine, Chicago, 1983.

Sutherland, D.H., et al.: Clinical and electromyographic study of seven spastic children with internal rotation gait, J. Bone Joint Surg. **51-A:**1070, 1969.

Sutherland, D.H., Larsen, L.J, and Mann, R.: Rectus femoris release in selected patients with cerebral palsy: a preliminary report, Dev. Med. Child Neurol. **17:**26, 1975.

Lower extremity—hip

Anthonsen, W.: Treatment of hip flexion contracture in cerebral palsy patients, Acta Orthop. Scand. **37:**387, 1966.

Baciu, C.C.: Translocation du muscle petit fessier dans la hanche spastique: a propos de onze cas, Ann. Chir. **38:**435, 1984.

Baker, L.D., Dodelin, R., and Bassett, F.H., III: Pathological changes in the hip in cerebral palsy: incidence, pathogenesis, and treatment: a preliminary report, J. Bone Joint Surg. **44-A:**1331, 1962.

Banks, H.H., and Green, W.T.: Adductor myotomy and obturator neurectomy for the correction of adduction contracture of the hip in cerebral palsy, J. Bone Joint Surg. **42-A:**111,1960.

Barr, J.S.: Muscle transplantation for combined flexion-internal rotation deformity of the thigh in spastic paralysis, Arch. Surg. **46:**605, 1943.

Beals, R.K.: Developmental changes in the femur and acetabulum in spastic paraplegia and diplegia, Dev. Med. Child Neurol. **11:**303, 1969.

Bell, M.: Proximal hamstring release: anterior approach (abstract), J. Bone Joint Surg. **55-B:**661, 1973.

Bleck, E.E.: Cerebral palsy: Part IV, Hip deformities in cerebral palsy, In American Academy of Orthopaedic Surgeons: Instructional course lectures, vol. 20, St. Louis, 1971, The C.V. Mosby Co.

Bleck, E.E.: Postural and gait abnormalities caused by hip-flexion deformity in spastic cerebral palsy: treatment by iliopsoas recession, J. Bone Joint Surg. **53-A:**1468, 1971.

Bleck, E.E.: Management of hip deformities in cerebral palsy. In Adams, J.P., editor: Current practice in orthopaedic surgery, vol. 3, St. Louis, 1966, The C.V. Mosby Co.

Bleck, E.E.: The hip in cerebral palsy, Orthop. Clin. North Am. **11:**79, 1980.

Bunnell, W.P., and Goncalves, J.: Varus derotational osteotomy of the hip in cerebral palsy. Presented at the American Academy for Cerebral Palsy and Developmental Medicine Annual Meeting, Washington, D.C., October 24-27, 1984.

Castle, M.E., and Schneider, C.: Proximal femoral resection interposition arthroplasty, J. Bone Joint Surg. **60-A:**1051, 1978.

Chiari, K.: Medial displacement osteotomy of the pelvis, Clin. Orthop. **98:**55, 1974.

Cote, P.S., and Drennan, J.C.: The role of proximal femoral derotational osteotomy in pediatric acetabular dysplasia. Presented at the Annual Meeting of the American Academy of Orthopaedic Surgeons, Las Vegas, 1985.

Couch, W.H. Jr., De Rosa, G.P., and Throop, F.B.: Thigh adductor transfer for spastic cerebral palsy, Dev. Med. Child Neurol. **19:**343, 1977.

Cristofaro, R.L., Taddonio, R.F., and Gelb, R.: The effect of correction of spinal deformity and pelvic obliquity on hip stability in neuromuscular disease. Presented at the Annual Meeting of the American Academy for Cerebral Palsy and Developmental Medicine, Washington, D.C., 1984.

Drummond, D.S., Rogala, E.J., Cruess, R., and Moreau, M.: The paralytic hip and pelvic obliquity in cerebral palsy and myelomeningocele, American Academy of Orthopaedic Surgeons: Instructional course lectures, vol. 28, St. Louis, 1979, The C.V. Mosby Co.

Durham, H.A.: A procedure for the correction of internal rotation of the thigh in spastic paralysis, J. Bone Joint Surg. **20:**339, 1938.

Eilert, R.E., and MacEwen, G.D.: Varus derotational osteotomy of the femur in cerebral palsy, Clin. Orthop. **125:**168, 1977.

Evans, E.B., and Julian, J.D.: Modifications of the hamstring transfer, Dev. Med. Child Neurol. **8:**539, 1966.

Fulford, G.E., and Brown, J.K.: Position as a cause of deformity in children with cerebral palsy, Dev. Med. Child Neurol. **18:**305, 1976.

Gage, J.R.: Gait analysis for decision making in cerebral palsy, Bull. Hosp. Jt. Dis. **43:**147, 1983.

Gherlinzoni, C., and Pais, C.: Trattamento della lussazione patalogia dell'anca: indicazioni, technica e resultati lontani, Chir. Organ. Mov. **34:**335, 1950.

Goldner, J.L.: Hip adductor transfer compared with adductor tenotomy in cerebral palsy (letter), J. Bone Joint Surg. **63-A:**1498, 1981.

Griffin, P.P., Wheelhouse, W.W., and Shiavi, R.: Adductor transfer for adductor spasticity: clinical and electromyographic gait analysis, Dev. Med. Child Neurol. **19:**783, 1977.

Gross, M.S., Ibrahim, K., Wehner, J., and Dvonch, V.: Combined surgical procedure for treatment of hip dislocation in cerebral palsy (abstract), Orthop. Trans. **8:**113, 1984.

Gross, M.S., Ibrahim, K., Wehner, J., and Dvonch, V.: Combined surgical procedure for treatment of hip dislocation in cerebral palsy. Presented at the Annual Meeting of the American Academy for Cerebral Palsy and Developmental Medicine, Chicago, 1983.

Gurd, A.R.: Surgical correction of myodesis of the hip in cerebral palsy (abstract), Orthop. Trans. **8:**112, 1984.

Gurd, A.R.: Surgical correction of myodesis of the hip in cerebral palsy. Presented at the Annual Meeting of the American Academy for Cerebral Palsy and Developmental Medicine, Chicago, 1983.

Handelsman, J.E.: The Chiari pelvic sliding osteotomy, Orthop. Clin. North Am. **11:**105, 1980.

Hill, L.M., Bassett, F.H., III, and Baker, L.D.: Correction of adduction, flexion and internal rotation deformities of the hip in cerebral palsy, Dev. Med. Child Neurol. **8:**406, 1966.

Hiroshima, K., and Ono, K.: Correlation between muscle shortening and derangement of the hip joint in children with spastic cerebral palsy, Clin. Orthop. **144:**186, 1979.

Hoffer, M.M., Abraham, E. and Nickel, V.L.: Salvage surgery at the hip to improve sitting posture of mentally retarded, severely disabled children with cerebral palsy, Dev. Med. Child Neurol. **14:**51, 1972.

Hoffer, M.M., Prietto, C. and Koffman, M.: Supracondylar derotational osteotomy of the femur for internal rotation of the thigh in the cerebral palsied child, J. Bone Joint Surg. **63-A:**389, 1981.

Horstmann, H.M., and Rosabal, O.G.: Varus derotation osteotomy. Presented at the Annual Meeting of the American Academy for Cerebral Palsy and Developmental Medicine, Chicago, 1983.

Horstmann, H.M. and Rosabal, O.G.: Varus derotation osteotomy (abstract), Orthop. Trans. **8:**113, 1984.

Howard, C.B., McKibbin, B., Williams, L.A., and Mackie, I.: Factors affecting the incidence of hip dislocation in cerebral palsy, J. Bone Joint Surg. **67-B:**530, 1985.

Houkom, J., et al.: Treatment of acquired hip dysplasia in cerebral palsy. Presented at the Annual Meeting of the Pediatric Orthopaedic Society, Vancouver, Canada, 1984.

Huang, S., and Eilert, R.E.: Important radiographic signs for decision making in surgery of the hip in cerebral palsy. Presented at the American Academy for Cerebral Palsy and Developmental Medicine Annual Meeting, Washington, D.C., October 24-27, 1984.

Jones, G.B.: Paralytic dislocation of the hip, J. Bone Joint Surg. **36-B:**375, 1954.

Jones, G.B.: Paralytic dislocations of the hip, J. Bone Joint Surg. **44-B:**573, 1962.

Kaga, C.S., and Huurman, W.W.: Supracondylar detoration osteotomy of the femur for femoral anteversion (abstract), Orthop. Trans. **8:**82, 1984.

Kalen, V., and Gamble, J.G.: Resection arthroplasty of the hip in paralytic disorders, Dev. Med. Child Neurol. **26:**341, 1984.

Kalen, V., and Bleck, E.E.: Prevention of spastic paralytic subluxation and dislocation of the hip (abstract), Orthop. Trans. **8:**112, 1984.

Kalen, V., and Gamble, J.G.: Resection arthroplasty of the hip in paralytic dislocations (abstract), Orthop. Trans. **8:**113, 1984.

Keats, S.: Combined adductor-gracilis tenotomy and selective obturator-nerve resection for the correction of adduction deformity of the hip in children with cerebral palsy, J. Bone Joint Surg. **39-A:**1087, 1957.

Keats, S.: Surgery of the extremities in treatment of cerebral palsy, JAMA **174:**1266, 1960.

Keats, S., and Morgese, A.N.: A simple anteromedial approach to the lesser trochanter of the femur for the release of the iliopsoas tendon, J. Bone Joint Surg. **49-A:**632, 1967.

Kling, T.F., Jr.: Adductor release with and without obturator neurectomy in children with cerebral palsy. Presented at the Annual Meeting of the American Academy for Cerebral Palsy and Developmental Medicine, Chicago, 1983.

Kling, T.F. Jr.: Adductor release with and without obturator neurectomy in children with cerebral palsy (abstract), Orthop. Trans. **8:**112, 1984.

Koffman M.: Proximal femoral resection or total hip replacement in severely disabled cerebral-spastic patients, Orthop. Clin. North Am. **12:**91, 1981.

Legg, A.T.: Transplantation of tensor fasciae femoris in cases of weakened gluteus medius, New Engl. J. Med. **209:**61, 1933.

Letts, M., Shapiro, L., Mulder, K., and Klassen, O.: The windblown hip syndrome in total body cerebral palsy, J. Pediatr. Orthop. **4:**55, 1984.

Lonstein, J.E., and Beck, K.: Hip dislocation and subluxation in cerebral palsy. Presented at the Annual Meeting of the American Academy for Cerebral Palsy and Developmental Medicine, Chicago, 1983.

Lonstein, J.E., and Beck, K.: Hip dislocation and subluxation in cerebral palsy. Presented at the American Academy for Cerebral Palsy and Developmental Medicine Annual Meeting, Washington, D.C., October 24-27, 1984.

Lonstein, J.B., and Beck, K.: Hip dislocation and subluxation in cerebral palsy. Presented at the Annual Meeting of the Pediatric Orthopaedic Society, Vancouver, Canada, 1984.

Ludloff, K.: Zur blutigen Einrenkung der angeborenen Huftluxation, Ziet. Orthop. Chir. **22:**272, 1908.

Magilligan, D.J.: Calculation of the angle of anterversion by means of horizontal lateral roentgenography, J. Bone Joint Surg. **38-A:**1231, 1956.

Majestro, T.C., and Frost, H.M.: Cerebral palsy: spastic internal femoral torsion, Clin. Orthop. **79:**44, 1971.

Majestro, T.C., and Frost, H.M.: Posterior transposition of the origins of the anatomic internal rotators of the hip, Clin. Orthop. **79:**57, 1971.

Markee, J.E., et al.: Two-joint muscles of the thigh, J. Bone Joint Surg. **37-A:**125, 1955.

Mathews, S.S., Jones, M.H., and Sperling, S.C.: Hip derangements seen in cerebral palsied children, Am. J. Phys. Med. **32:**213, 1953.

McCarroll, H.R.: Early management of congenital dislocation of the hip. In American Academy of Orthopaedic Surgeons: Instructional course lectures, vol. 2, Ann Arbor, 1948, J.W. Edwards.

Moreau, M., Drummond, D.S., Rogala, E., Ashworth, A., and Porter, T.: Natural history of the dislocated hip in spastic cerebral palsy, Dev. Med. Child Neurol. **21:**749, 1979.

Nickel, V.L., Perry, J., Garrett, A., and Feiwell, E.N.: Paralytic dislocation of the hip, J. Bone Joint Surg. **48-A:**1021, 1966.

Pemberton, P.A.: Pericapsular osteotomy of the ilium in the treatment of congenital dislocation and subluxation of the hip, J. Bone Joint Surg. **47-A:**65, 1965.

Perry, J.: Kinesiology of lower extremity bracing, Clin. Orthop. **102:**18, 1974.

Perry, J., and Hoffer, M.M.: Preoperative and postoperative dynamic electromyography as an aid in planning tendon transfers in children with cerebral palsy, J. Bone Joint Surg. **59-A:**531, 1977.

Phelps, W.M.: Personal communication, 1947.

Phelps, W.M.: Prevention of acquired dislocation of the hip in cerebral palsy, J. Bone Joint Surg. **41-A:**440, 1959.

Pillard, D., Benoit, S., and Taussig, G.: Résection élargie de l'éxtremitié supérieure du fémur chez l'enfant infirme moteur d'origine cérébrale (extensive excision of the upper end of the femur in cerebral palsy), Rev. Chir. Orthop. **70:**623, 1984.

Pollock, G.A.: Treatment of adductor paralysis by hamstring transposition, J. Bone Joint Surg. **40-B:**534, 1958.

Pollock, G.A.: Surgical treatment of cerebral palsy, J. Bone Joint Surg. **44-B:**68, 1962.

Pollack, G.A., and Sharrard, W.J.W.: Orthopaedic surgery in the treatment of cerebral palsy, London, 1958, Churchill.

Ray, R.L., and Ehrlich, M.G.: Lateral hamstring transfer and gait improvement in the cerebral palsy patient, J. Bone Joint Surg. **61-A:**719, 1979.

Reimers, J.: The stability of the hip in children, Acta Orthop. Scand. (suppl.) **184,** 1980.

Reimers, J., and Poulsen, S.: Adductor transfer versus tenotomy for stability of the hip in spastic cerebral palsy, J. Pediatr. Orthop. **4:**52, 1984.

Roach, J.W., Herring, J.A., and Norris, E.N.: Treatment of acquired hip dysplasia in cerebral palsy. Presented at the Annual Meeting of the Pediatric Orthopaedic Society, Vancouver, Canada, 1984.

Roosth, H.P.: Flexion deformity of the hip and knee in spastic cerebral palsy: treatment by early release of spastic hip-flexor muscles: technique and results in thirty-seven cases, J. Bone Joint Surg. **53-A:**1489, 1971.

Root, L.: The hip in cerebral palsy. Presented at American Academy for Cerebral Palsy and Developmental Medicine Symposium, Growing Up With Cerebral Palsy, Wilmington, Delaware, April 19-20, 1985.

Root, L., and Bourman, S.N.: Combined pelvic osteotomy with open reduction and femoral shortening for dislocated hips. Presented at the American Academy for Cerebral Palsy and Developmental Medicine Annual Meeting, Washington, D.C., October 24-27, 1984.

Root, L., and Siegal, T.: Osteotomy of the hip in children: posterior approach, J. Bone Joint Surg. **62-A:**571, 1980.

Root, L., and Spero, C.R.: Hip adductor transfer compared with adductor tenotomy in cerebral palsy, J. Bone Joint Surg. **63-A:**767, 1981.

Root, L., and Washington, R.: Pathological changes in the femoral head in cerebral palsy (abstract), Orthop. Trans. **8:**111, 1984.

Root, L., and Washington, R.: Pathological changes in the femoral head in cerebral palsy. Presented at the Annual Meeting of the American Academy for Cerebral Palsy and Developmental Medicine, Chicago, 1983.

Rosenthal, R.K.: Soft tissue procedures about the hip in spastic cerebral palsy. Presented at the Annual Meeting of the American Academy for Cerebral Palsy and Developmental Medicine, Chicago, 1983.

Samilson, R.L.: Orthopedic surgery of the hips and spine in retarded cerebral palsy patients, Orthop. Clin. North Am. **12:**83, 1981.

Salter, R.B.: Innominate osteotomy in the treatment of congenital dislocation and subluxation of the hip, J. Bone Joint Surg. **43-B:**518, 1961.

Salter, R.B., and De Castro, A.: The role of iliopsoas recession in the management of spastic hip flexion deformity (abstract), J. Bone Joint Surg. **55-B:**661, 1973.

Samilson, R.L., Carson, J.J., James, P., and Raney, F.L., Jr.: Results and complications of adductor tenotomy and obturator neurectomy in cerebral palsy, Clin. Orthop. **54:**61, 1967.

Samilson, R.L., Trace, P., Aamoth, G., and Green, W.M.: Dislocation and subluxation of the hip in cerebral palsy: pathogenesis, natural history, and management, J. Bone Joint Surg. **54-A:**863, 1972.

Seger, B.M., and Dickson, J.H.: Chiari osteotomy in the treatment of hip dysplasia: indications and long-term follow-up (abstract), Orthop. Trans. **8:**62, 1984.

Sharps, C.H., Clancy, M., and Steel, H.H.: A long-term retroprospective study of proximal hamstring release for hamstring contracture in cerebral palsy, J. Pediatr. Orthop. **4:**443, 1984.

Sharrard, W.J.W.: The hip in cerebral palsy. In Samilson, R.L.: Orthopaedic aspects of cerebral palsy, Philadelphia, 1975, J.B. Lippincott Co.

Sharrard, W.J.W., Allen, J.M.H., Heaney, S.H., and Prendiville, G.R.G.: Surgical prophylaxis of subluxation and dislocation of the hip in cerebral palsy, J. Bone Joint Surg. **57-B:**160, 1975.

Silberstein, C.E.: The place of innominate osteotomy (Salter) in the management of hip problems in cerebral palsy (abstract), Dev. Med. Child Neurol. **13:**247, 1971.

Silfverskiöld, N.: Reduction of the uncrossed two-joint muscles of the leg to one-joint muscles in spastic conditions, Acta Chir. Scand. **56:**315, 1923-24.

Soutter, R.: A new operation for hip contractures in poliomyelitis, Boston Med. Surg. J. **170:**380, 1914.

Steel, H.H.: Triple osteotomy of the innominate bone, J. Bone Joint Surg. **55-A:**343, 1973.

Steel, H.H.: Gluteus medius and minimus insertion advancement for correction of internal rotation gait in spastic cerebral palsy, J. Bone Joint Surg. **62-A:**919, 1980.

Stein, G.A., Hoffer, M.M., and Koffman, M.: Long-term follow-up of proximal femoral varus derotation osteotomy for hip dislocations in cerebrospastic children. Presented at the Annual Meeting of the American Academy of Orthopaedic Surgeons, Las Vegas, 1985.

Stephenson, C.G., and Donovan, M.M.: Transfer of hip adductor origins to the ischium in spastic cerebral palsy, Dev. Med. Child Neurol, **13:**247, 1971.

Stephenson, C.T., and Donovan, M.M.: Transfer of hip adductor origins to the ischium in spastic cerebral palsy (abstract), J. Bone Joint Surg. **51-A:**1040, 1969.

Stephenson, C.T., Griffith, B., Donovan, M.M., and Franklin, T.: The adductor transfer and iliopsoas release in the cerebral palsy hip (abstract), Orthop. Trans. **6:**94, 1982.

Sussman, M.D.: Adductor and iliopsoas release: results after early mobilization (abstract), Orthop. Trans. **8:**112, 1984.

Sussman, M.D.: Adductor and iliopsoas release: results after early mobilization. Presented at the Annual Meeting of the American Academy for Cerebral Palsy and Developmental Medicine, Chicago, 1983.

Sussman, M.E.: Myositis ossification in young children following adductor and iliopsoas release. Presented at the Annual Meeting of the Pediatric Orthopaedic Society, Vancouver, Canada, 1984.

Sutherland, D.H.: Gait analysis in cerebral palsy, Dev. Med. Child Neurol. **20:**807, 1978.

Sutherland, D.H., Olshen, R., Cooper, L., and Woo, S.K.: The development of mature gait, J. Bone Joint Surg. **62-A:**336, 1980.

Tachdjian, M.O., and Minear, W.L.: Hip dislocation in cerebral palsy, J. Bone Joint Surg. **38-A:**1358, 1956.

Tylkowski, C.M., Rosenthal, R.K., and Simon, S.R.: Proximal femoral osteotomy in cerebral palsy, Clin. Orthop. **151:**183, 1980.

Uematsu, A., Bailey, H.L., Winter, W.G.R., and Brower, T.D.: Results of posterior iliopsoas transfer for hip instability caused by cerebral palsy, Clin. Orthop. **126:**183, 1977.

Vanden Brink, K.D., Beck, K.O., and Comfort, T.H.: Management of the hip in young children with severe cerebral palsy: a surgical dilemma. Presented at the Annual Meeting of the Pediatric Orthopaedic Society, Vancouver, Canada, 1984.

Veleanu, C., Rosianu, I., and Ionescu, L.: An improved approach for obturator neurectomy for cerebral spastic paralysis. J. Bone Joint Surg. **52-A:**1693, 1970.

Vidal, J., et al.: The success and limitations of adductor tenotomy in dysplasia of the hip in cerebral palsy (abstract), Orthop. Trans. **8:**34, 1984.

Weinert, C., Jr., and Ireland, M.L.: Abduction osteotomy for the severely contracted hip in spastic quadriplegia: a new technique with rigid fixation using the compression hip screw system. Presented at the Annual Meeting of the American Academy for Cerebral Palsy and Developmental Medicine, Washington, D.C., 1984.

Wenger, D.R., and Carrell, T.: Chiari osteotomy and the migrating acetabulum: modifications to improve hip stability. Presented at the Annual Meeting of the Pediatric Orthopaedic Society, Vancouver, Canada, 1984.

Wheeler, M.E., and Weinstein, S.L.: Adductor tenotomy-obturator neurectomy, J. Pediatr. Orthop. **4:**48, 1984.

Zuckerman, J.D., Staheli, L.T., and McLaughlin, J.F.: Acetabular augmentation for progressive hip subluxation in cerebral palsy, J. Pediatr. Orthop. **4:**436, 1984.

Upper extremities

Craig, C.L., Ruby, L.K., Sosnoff, F., and Zimbler, S.Z.: The upper extremity in Duchenne dystrophy: an unsolved problem. Presented at the Annual Meeting of the American Academy for Cerebral Palsy and Developmental Medicine, Washington, D.C., 1984.

Filler, B.C., Stark, H.H., and Boyes, J.H.: Capsulodesis of the metacarpophalangeal joint of the thumb with cerebral palsy, J. Bone Joint Surg. **58-A:**667, 1976.

Goldner, J.L.: Upper extremity surgical procedures for patients with cerebral palsy, In American Academy of Orthopaedic Surgeons: Instructional course lectures, vol 28, St. Louis, 1979, The C.V. Mosby Co.

Goldner, J.L: Upper extremity reconstructive surgery in cerebral palsy or similar conditions. In American Academy of Orthopaedic Surgeons: Instructional course lectures, vol. 18, St. Louis, 1961, The C.V. Mosby Co.

Hoffer, M.M., Perry, J., and Melkonian, G.J.: Dynamic electromyography and decision-making for surgery in the upper extremity of patients with cerebral palsy, J. Hand Surg. **4:**424, 1979.

Hoffer, M.M., Perry, J., Garcia, M., and Bullock, D.: Adduction contracture of the thumb in cerebral palsy: a preoperative electromyographic study, J. Bone Joint Surg. **65-A:**755, 1983.

House, J.H., Gwathmey, F.W., and Fidler, M.O.: A dynamic approach to the thumb-in-palm deformity in cerebral palsy: evaluation and results in fifty-six patients, J. Bone Joint Surg. **63-A:**216, 1981.

Inglis, A.E., and Cooper, W.: Release of the flexor-pronator origin for flexion deformities of the hand and wrist in spastic paralysis: a study of eighteen cases, J. Bone Joint Surg. **48-A:**847, 1966.

Manske, P.R.: Extensor pollicis longus re-routing for treatment of spastic thumb in palm deformity (abstract), Orthop. Trans. **8:**95, 1984.

Mital, M.A.: Flexion contractures and involuntary flexor bias in the upper extremities at elbows: its surgical management (abstract), J. Bone Joint Surg. **57-A:**1031, 1975.

Mital, M.A.: Lengthening of the elbow flexors in cerebral palsy, J. Bone Joint Surg. **61-A:**515, 1979.

Mital, M.A., and Sakellarides, H.T.: Surgery of the upper extremity in the retarded individual with spastic cerebral palsy, Orthop. Clin. North Am. **12:**127, 1981.

Mowery, C.A., Gelberman, R., and Roades, C.E.: Upper extremity tendon transfers in cerebral palsy: an electromyographic and functional analysis. Presented at the American Academy for Cerebral Palsy and Developmental Medicine Annual Meeting, Washington, D.C., October 24-27, 1984.

Mowery, C.A., Gelberman, R.H., and Rhoades, C.E.: Upper extremity tendon transfers in cerebral palsy: electromyographic and functional analysis, J. Pediatr. Orthop. **5:**69, 1985.

Ober, F.R.: Transplantation to improve the function of the shoulder joint and extensor function of the elbow joint. In American Academy of Orthopaedic Surgeons: Instructional course lectures, Ann Arbor, 1944, J.W. Edwards.

Omer, G.E.: Proximal row carpectomy with muscle transfers for spastic paralysis of the wrist (abstract), Orthop. Trans. **1:**191, 1977.

Patella, V., and Martucci, G.: Transposition of the pronator radii teres muscle to the radial extensors of the wrist in infantile cerebral paralysis: an improved operative technique, Ital. J. Orthop. Traumatol. **6:**61, 1980.

Patella, V., Franchin, B., Moretti, B., and Mori, F.: Arthrodesis of the wrist with mini-fixators in infantile cerebral palsy, Ital. J. Orthop. Traumatol. **10:**75, 1984.

Pletcher, D.F.-J., Hoffer, M.M., and Koffman, D.M.: Nontraumatic dislocation of the radial head in cerebral palsy, J. Bone Joint Surg. **58-A:**104, 1976.

Sakellarides, H.T.: The management of the unbalanced wrist in cerebral palsy. Presented at the American Academy for Cerebral Palsy and Developmental Medicine Annual Meeting, Washington, D.C., October 24-27, 1984.

Sakellarides, H.T., Mital, M.A., and Lenzi, W.D.: Treatment of pronation contractures of the forearm in cerebral palsy by changing the insertion of the pronator radii teres, J. Bone Joint Surg. **63-A:**645, 1981.

Sakellarides, H.T., Matza, R.A., and Mital, A.: The surgical treatment of the different types of thumb-in-palm deformities in cerebral palsy (abstract), Dev. Med. Child Neurol. **21:**116, 1979.

Sakellarides, H.T., Mital, M.A., and Matza, R.A.: The surgical treatment of the different types of "thumb-in-palm" deformities seen in cerebral palsy (abstract), Orthop. Trans. **4:**9, 1980.

Samilson, R.L., and Morris, J.M.: Surgical improvement of the cerebral-palsied upper limb: Electromyographic studies and results of 128 operations, J. Bone Joint Surg. **46-A:**1203, 1964.

Skoff, H., and Woodbury, D.F.: Current concepts review: management of the upper extremity in cerebral palsy, J. Bone Joint Surg. **67-A:**500, 1985.

Tachdjian, M.O.: Affections of brain and spinal cord. In Pediatric Orthopaedics, Philadelphia, 1972, W.B. Saunders.

Thometz, J.G., and Tachdjian, M.O.: Results of the flexor carpi ulnaris transfer in cerebral palsy. Presented at the Annual Meeting of the American Academy for Cerebral Palsy and Developmental Medicine, Washington, D.C., 1984.

Spine

Akbarnia, B.A.: Spinal deformity in patients with cerebral palsy. Presented at the Annual Meeting of the American Academy for Cerebral Palsy and Developmental Medicine, Chicago, 1983.

Akbarnia, B.A.: Spinal deformity in patients with cerebral palsy (abstract), Orthop. Trans. **8:**116, 1984.

Akbarnia, B.A., Winter, R.B., Moe, J.H., Bradford, D.S., and Lonstein, J.E.: Operative treatment of spine deformity in cerebral palsy (abstract), Orthop. Trans. **1:**140, 1977.

Allen, B.A., Jr., and Ferguson, R.L.: L-rod instrumentation for scoliosis in cerebral palsy, J. Pediatr. Orthop **2:**87, 1982.

Baumann, U.: Indications for Harrington's spine instrumentation for scoliosis in cerebral palsy. In Chapchal, G., editor: Operative treatment of scoliosis, Stuttgart, 1973, Thieme.

Beck, K.O., Lonstein, J.E., and Carlson, J.M.: Functional evaluation of the sitting support orthosis for cerebral palsy (abstract), Orthop. Trans. **4:**34, 1980.

Bonnett, C., Brown, J.C., and Grow, T.: Thoracolumbar scoliosis in cerebral palsy, J. Bone Joint Surg. **58-A:**328, 1976.

Bonnett, C., Brown, J.C., and Brooks, H.L.: Anterior spine fusion with Dwyer instrumentation for lumbar scoliosis in cerebral palsy: a preliminary report (abstract), J. Bone Joint Surg. **55-A:**425, 1973.

Bunnell, W.P., and MacEwen, G.D.: Non-operative treatment of scoliosis in cerebral palsy: preliminary report on the use of a plastic jacket, Dev. Med. Child. Neurol. **19:**45, 1977.

Bunnell, W.P.: Spinal deformities in cerebral palsy. Presented at American Academy for Cerebral Palsy and Developmental Medicine Symposium, Growing Up With Cerebral Palsy, Wilmington, Delaware, April 19-20, 1985.

Charney, E.B., McMorrow, M., Bruce, D.A., and Sherk, H.H.: Assessment of spinal deformities in children with myelomeningocele (abstract), Orthop. Trans. **8:**116, 1984.

Cristofaro, R.L., Taddonio, R.F., and Gelb, R.: Stability in neuromuscular disease. Presented at the American Academy for Cerebral Palsy and Developmental Medicine Annual Meeting, Washington, D.C., October 24-27, 1984.

Fulford, G.E., and Brown, J.K.: Position as a cause of deformity in children with cerebral palsy, Dev. Med. Child Neurol. **18:**305, 1976.

Horstmann, H.M., and Boyer, B.: Progression of scoliosis in cerebral palsy patients after skeletal maturity. Presented at the Annual Meeting of the American Academy for Cerebral Palsy and Developmental Medicine, Chicago, 1983.

Horstmann, H.M., and Boyer, B.: Progression of scoliosis in cerebral palsy after skeletal maturity (abstract), Orthop. Trans. **8:**116, 1984.

Kalen, V., Bleck, E.E., and Rinsky, L.A.: Preliminary results of Luque instrumentation in neuromuscular scoliosis. Presented at the Annual Meeting of the American Academy for Cerebral Palsy and Developmental Medicine, Washington, D.C., 1984.

Lonstein, J.E., and Akbarnia, B.A.: Operative treatment of spinal deformities in patients with cerebral palsy or mental retardation: an analysis of one hundred and seven cases, J. Bone Joint Surg. **65-A:**43, 1983.

Lonstein, J.E., Winter, R.B., Moe, J.H., and Bradford, D.S.:A combined anterior and posterior approach for the operative treatment of cerebral palsy spine deformity (abstract), Orthop. Trans. **2:**230, 1978.

Lonstein, J.E.: Deformities of the spine in cerebral palsy, Orthop. Rev. **10:**33, 1981.

Madigan, R.R., and Wallace, S.L.: Scoliosis in the institutionalized cerebral palsy population, Spine **6:**583, 1981.

Mital, M.A., Belkin, S.C., and Sullivan, M.A.: An approach to head, neck and trunk stabilization and control in cerebral palsy by use of the Milwaukee brace, Dev. Med. Child Neurol. **18:**198, 1976.

Mubarak, S.J., Kurz, L., Schultz, P., and Park, S.M.: Correlating scoliosis and pulmonary function in Duchenne muscular dystrophy (abstract), Orthop. Trans. **8:**116, 1984.

Rinsky, L., Bleck, E., and Gamble, J.: The "growing" segmental spinal instrumentation technique in young children with progressive spinal deformity. Presented at the Annual Meeting of the American Academy for Cerebral Palsy and Developmental Medicine, Washington, D.C., 1984.

Robson, P.: The prevalance of scoliosis in adolescents and young adults with cerebral palsy, Dev. Med. Child Neurol. **10:**447, 1968.

Rosenthal, R.K., Levine, D.B., and McCarver, C.L.: The occurrence of scoliosis in cerebral palsy, Dev. Med. Child Neurol. **16:**664, 1974.

Samilson, R.L.: Orthopedic surgery of the hips and spine in retarded cerebral patients, Orthop. Clin. North Am. **12:**83, 1981.

Shufflebarger, H.L., Price, C.T., and Riddick, M.F.: L-rod instrumentation and spinal fusion: the Florida experience (abstract), Orthop. Trans. **8:**43, 1984.

Stanitski, C.L., et al.: Surgical correction of spinal deformity in cerebral palsy, Spine **7:**563, 1982.

Thompson, G.H., Wilber, R.G., Shaffer, J.W., and Nash, C.L.: Segmental spinal instrumentation in spinal deformities (abstract), Orthop. Trans. **8:**82, 1984.

Adult stroke patient

Bloch, R., and Bayer, N.: Prognosis in stroke, Clin. Orthop. **131:**10, 1978.

Braun, R.M., Hoffer, M.M., Mooney, V., McKeever, J., and Roper, B.: Phenol nerve block in the treatment of acquired spastic hemiplegia in the upper limb, J. Bone Joint Surg. **55-A:**580, 1973.

Braun, R.M., et al.: Surgical treatment of the painful shoulder contracture in the stroke patient. J. Bone Joint Surg. **53-A:**1307, 1971.

Caldwell, C., and Braun, R.M.: Spasticity in the upper extremity, Clin. Orthop. **104:**80, 1974.

Casey, J.M., Moore, M.L., and Nickel, V.L.: Spasticity: what to do when it becomes harmful, J. Musculoskel. Med., October 1985, p. 29.

Garland, D.E., and Rhoades, M.E.: Orthopedic management of brain-injured adults, Part II, Clin. Orthop. **131:**111, 1978.

Hoffer, M.M., and Brink, J.: Orthopedic management of acquired cerebrospasticity in childhood, Clin. Orthop. **110:**244, 1975.

McCollough, N.C., III: Orthopaedic evaluation and treatment of the stroke patient. Part I. Incidence and functional prognosis of hemiplegia. In American Academy of Orthopaedic Surgeons: Instructional course lectures, vol. 24, St. Louis, 1975, C.V. Mosby Co.

McCollough, N.C., III: Orthopaedic evaluation and treatment of the stroke patient. Part II. Lower extremity management. Orthotic management. In American Academy of Orthopaedic Surgeons: Instructional course lectures, vol. 24, St. Louis, 1975, C.V. Mosby Co.

McCollough, N.C., III: Orthopaedic evaluation and treatment of the stroke patient: Part III. Upper extremity management: evaluation and management. In American Academy of Orthopaedic Surgeons: Instructional course lectures, vol 24, St. Louis, 1975, The C.V. Mosby Co.

McCollough, N.C., III: Orthothic management in adult hemiplegia, Clin. Orthop. **131:**38, 1978.

Mooney, V., Perry, J., and Nickel, V.L.: Surgical and non-surgical orthopaedic care of stroke, J. Bone Joint Surg. **49-A:**989, 1967.

Perry, J.: Orthopaedic evaluation and treatment of the stroke patient: Part II. Lower extremity management: examination: a neurologic basis for treatment. In American Academy of Orthopaedic Surgeons: Instructional course lectures, vol. 24, St. Louis, 1975, The C.V. Mosby Co.

Perry, J., and Waters, R.L.: Orthopaedic evaluation and treatment of the stroke patient. Part II. Lower extremity management. Surgery. In American Academy of Orthopaedic Surgeons: Instructional course lectures, vol. 24, St. Louis, 1975, C.V. Mosby Co.

Perry, J., and Waters, R.L.: Orthopaedic evaluation and treatment of the stroke patient. Part III. Upper extremity management. Surgery. In American Academy of Orthopaedic Surgeons: Instructional course lectures, vol. 24, St. Louis, 1975, C.V. Mosby Co.

Perry, J., Waters, R.L., and Perrin, T.: Electromyographic analysis of equinovarus following stroke, Clin. Orthop. **131:**47, 1978.

Perry, J., Giovan, P., Harris, L.J., Montgomery, J., and Azaria, M.: The determinants of muscle action in the hemiparetic lower extremity (and their effect on the examination procedure), Clin. Orthop. **131:**71, 1978.

Savinelli, R., Timm, M., Montgomery, J., and Wilson, D.J.: Therapy evaluation and management of patients with hemiplegia, Clin. Orthop. **131:**15, 1978.

Solomonow, M.: Restoration of movement by electrical stimulation: a contemporary view of the basic problems, Orthopedics **7:**245, 1984.

Tracy, H.W.: Operative treatment of the plantar-flexed inverted foot in adult hemiplegia, J. Bone Joint Surg. **58-A:**1142, 1976.

Vodovnik, L., Kralj, A., Stanic, U., Acimovic, R., and Gros, H.: Recent applications of functional electrical stimulation to stroke patients in Ljubljana, Clin. Orthop. **131:**64, 1978.

Waters, R.L.: Upper extremity surgery in stroke patients, Clin. Orthop. **131:**30, 1978.

Waters, R.L.: Stroke rehabilitation (editoral comment), Clin. Orthop. **131:**2, 1978.

Waters, R.L., Perry, J., and Garland, D.: Surgical correction of gait abnormalities following stroke, Clin. Orthop. **131:**54, 1978.

Waters, R.L., Frazier, J., Garland, D.E., Jordan, C., and Perry, J.: Electromyographic gait analysis before and after operative treatment for hemiplegic equinus and equinovarus deformity, J. Bone Joint Surg. **64-A:**284, 1982.

Waters, R.L., Garland, D.E., Perry, J., Habig, T., and Slabaugh, P.: Stiff-legged gait in hemiplegia: surgical correction, J. Bone Joint Surg. **61-A:**927, 1979.

CHAPTER 66

Paralytic disorders

Alvin J. Ingram

The following paralytic disorders will be discussed in this chapter: anterior poliomyelitis, spina bifida occulta and myelomeningocele, arthrogryposis multiplex congenita or congenital muscular contractures, obstetric paralysis, and paralysis caused by peripheral nerve injuries. Although some disorders have their origin before birth and some afterward, their associated deformities are primarily caused by muscle imbalance resulting from a neurologic lesion of the lower motor neurons, and if the imbalance continues throughout the growth period, the deformities are likely to increase in severity.

Only recently have neurologic lesions been identified as the cause of the deformities present at birth in spina bifida occulta, lumbar and sacral agenesis, and arthrogryposis multiplex congenita (AMC), or multiple congenital contractures (MCC). This relationship of cause and effect makes it important that the deformity and its cause be recognized early, the deformity corrected, and balanced muscle power established to prevent either recurrence or reversal of the deformity with growth.

Although the same surgical procedures may be indicated in any of the paralytic disorders included in this chapter, we have attempted to indicate the difference in patient management and in philosophy for each specific etiologic group as it is discussed.

Poliomyelitis

Since the introduction and extensive use of the poliomyelitis vaccine, the incidence of acute anterior poliomyelitis in the Western world has dropped dramatically. At present it is a disease affecting children under the age of 5 years in developing tropical and subtropical countries and unimmunized persons in other temperate climates.

Prevention of the disease is required if it is to be eliminated, and this can be achieved by administration of at least two and preferably three doses of Sabin's oral polio vaccine containing all three types of attenuated virus. Intensive immunization campaigns are necessary, and all babies and children should be immunized from age 3 months onward. Paradoxically, as the hygiene of a primitive community improves, poliomyelitis epidemics become more likely. Since the poliomyelitis virus is endemic and is transmitted by fecal contamination, infants thus receive passive immunity from their mothers and, on ingestion of the virus, develop subclinical, nonparalytic disease with resulting active immunity. When public hygiene improves, infections are sustained after passive immunity has been lost, and paralytic poliomyelitis results. Epidemics of paralytic poliomyelitis in developing countries of the tropics have increased in the recent past; thus nationwide immunization campaigns should be mounted promptly and must be repeated periodically and regularly if future epidemics are to be prevented.

After 14 years of treating crippled persons in Uganda, Huckstep recently published a valuable monograph on the management of poliomyelitis in developing countries. He estimated that of Uganda's population of 10 million there were 90,000 with some residual poliomyelitis effects and 30,000 with severe paralysis. The number of untreated paralyzed individuals in Nigeria was estimated at 200,000 to 300,000, in Africa well over 1 million, and in the developing nations of the world several million. These unfortunate people are impoverished, untreated, uneducated, and neglected and, although possessing a normal mentality, spend their lives without the awareness or the hope that the services of a competent orthopaedic surgeon could correct or minimize their deformities and make them erect and ambulatory so that with proper education they could become productive citizens in their own societies.

Our hope is that this chapter will serve as a reference

for surgeons who have been trained in the developed nations since poliomyelitis became extinct and now find themselves treating paralyzed patients either in a temporary or a permanent setting.

In recent years, many individuals have observed that a significant number of adults who suffered acute poliomyelitis during past prevaccine epidemics develop symptoms of renewed pain, fatigue, and muscle weakness in previously unaffected muscles as well as affected ones, and increased functional impairment some 30 to 35 years after the acute illness. Four factors are strongly associated with these aftereffects: being over 10 years of age at onset, having paralytic involvement in four extremities during the acute stage, requiring a mechanical ventilator, and having been hospitalized at onset. The exact cause of these symptoms presently is not clear. Some suspect that they result from the reactivation of an old virus or the activation of a new one, but as yet no scientific evidence supports this hypothesis. Others reason that affected patients lost a significant portion of their muscular mass, strength, and muscular reserve during the acute disease. Therefore the asymptomatic decline in muscular strength that normal people experience with aging, diminished physical activity, and weight gain produces symptoms and increased functional impairment in postpoliomyelitis patients because of the chronic limitation of functional reserve imposed by their original illness.

Another theory is that anterior horn cells that survive the acute infection are perennially and abnormally overloaded and may die prematurely.

Whatever the cause, the symptoms are real and have been reported in 20% to 80% of surviving patients. These patients will likely consult orthopaedic surgeons in their search for relief.

PREOPERATIVE CONSIDERATIONS

During the convalescent stage of poliomyelitis, which begins after the acute febile illness and ends 16 to 24 months later, orthopaedic operations are usually not indicated, although sometimes one is necessary to prevent or correct a deformity that could not otherwise be prevented or corrected and that would interfere with rehabilitation during the next stage. It is during the residual stage of the disease, which begins after the convalescent stage and continues for life, that orthopaedic surgery makes its greatest contribution to the rehabilitation of the patient: preventing or correcting deformities, reestablishing muscle power, stabilizing flail joints, and eliminating the need for such external supports as braces and corsets.

Before treatment is begun, a carefully planned program of rehabilitation is outlined; its ultimate aim is to help the patient become a self-sufficient citizen. Cooperation is desirable with physical and occupational therapists; vocational and social guidance is valuable. The surgeon's role is primarily to help the patient become physically self-sufficient, but to do this requires appraising the affected part in relation to the patient as a human being with all his present and future potentials. The individual procedures chosen must not be random but must be coordinated steps in a complex program.

The patient as a whole must be evaluated before undertaking a surgical program, and especially the surgeon must decide whether the proposed surgical program can be expected to render the patient ambulatory and whether ambulation will benefit the patient socially. For instance, if both lower limbs are moderately or severely paralyzed along with weakness of one of both upper extremities, especially the triceps, the patient will be unable to walk with crutches or with calipers. If both lower limbs and the trunk are weak, both arms must be strong to permit walking.

Generally speaking, every child with a reasonable expectation of walking after surgery should undergo such surgery, since the emotional and social benefits of walking in a handicapped child are great. On the other hand, older patients with severe deformities requiring extensive surgery usually are subject to greater technical difficulties, a higher incidence of complications, longer and more difficult rehabilitation periods, and less dramatic emotional and social benefits. In fact, a wheelchair is often preferable to crutches and long leg braces in severely paralyzed adults. Sometimes, especially in developing countries, the patient who can crawl rapidly and earn his living on the ground prefers this status to slow and labored walking with crutches and long leg braces.

PREVENTION AND CORRECTION OF DEFORMITY

A skeletal deformity may be caused by any one or a combination of any of the following factors: muscle imbalance, unrelieved muscle spasm, habitually faulty posture, dynamics of activity, and growth. To prevent deformity is of course the happiest outcome of any patient's program. It requires close observation by the orthopaedist at regular frequent intervals and close cooperation from the patient and attendants until growth is complete. The skillful use of braces, plaster casts, and dynamic splinting techniques is important. Repeated accurate evaluations of muscle power should be made, for even when deformity is absent on first examination, gross imbalances of muscle power may be discovered that if left untreated would lead to deformity with growth.

Sometimes even with expert treatment, deformity may be impossible to prevent. For example, when poliomyelitis strikes early in childhood and leaves a severe imbalance between the opposing muscle groups of the leg and foot, shortening and other deformities of the foot may develop despite treatment. When seen early, a deformity can often be corrected by conservative means, and appropriate measures can be taken to prevent its recurrence. But when it cannot be prevented and cannot be corrected by conservative means, surgery is indicated.

Although several factors must be considered in timing the procedures properly, the age of the patient is the most important. Some progressive deformities such as scoliosis and pelvic obliquity require early definitive treatment, since when they are neglected, their influence may damage much of the body. An arthrodesis should usually be deferred until the patient is so near skeletal maturity that growth of the part will not be impeded or injured; this is especially important in considering arthrodesis of the tarsus. Arthrodesis of other joints such as the shoulder and knee should often be postponed until the patient's social and occupational status can be clarified. In transferring tendons to eliminate a dynamic force, or to supplement the power of a partially or completely paralyzed muscle group, or both, to await skeletal maturity is usually unnecessary, but operation should if possible be deferred until the child is old enough to cooperate in muscle reeducation. Although inequality of leg length may be present or may be anticipated on first examination of a small child, procedures to equalize leg length must be carefully planned and coordinated with skeletal maturation.

REESTABLISHMENT OF MUSCLE POWER
Tendon transfer

Tendon transference (or transfer) is sometimes incorrectly called tendon transplantation (or transplant). Transplantation refers to excision of all or part of a tendon to use elsewhere as a free transplant; a transfer shifts a tendinous insertion from its normal attachment to another location so that its muscle may be substituted for a paralyzed muscle in the same region. Many have been responsible for making tendon transfers practical—in Europe, Nicoladoni, Velpeau, Helferich, Salvia, Lange, Vulpius, and Codivilla, and in the United States, Parrish, Goldthwait, Mayer, and Milliken. Hundreds of variations of the pioneer procedures have been devised; we give here only those that have proved most efficient and make no attempt to establish priority.

In selecting a tendon for transfer, the following factors must be carefully considered.

1. The muscle to be transferred must be strong enough to do reasonably well what the paralyzed muscle did or to supplement the power of a partially paralyzed muscle. If weakened itself by paralysis or when its normal power is insufficient, the expected action may be impossible, or the muscle may function for a short time and then because of overstretching lose its power. A muscle to be transferred should have a rating of good or better. It must be remembered that a transferred muscle loses at least one grade in power after transfer.

2. For efficiency the freed end of the transferred tendon should be attached close to the insertion of the paralyzed tendon and should be routed in a comparatively direct line between its origin and new insertion.

3. The transferred tendon should be retained in its own sheath or should be inserted into the sheath of another tendon; otherwise it should be passed through tissues such as fat that will allow it to glide. Routing a tendon through tunnels in fascia, bone, or an interosseous membrane is not usually wise because scar tissue and adhesions will rapidly form.

4. The nerve and blood supply to the transferred muscle must not be impaired or traumatized in making the transfer.

5. The joint on which the muscle is to act must be in a satisfactory position; all contracted structures must be released before the tendon transfer. A transferred muscle cannot be expected to correct a deformity—satisfactory function across a reasonably normal joint is enough to expect of it.

6. The transferred tendon must be securely attached to bone under tension slightly greater than normal. If tension is insufficient, then energy will be used in taking up slack

in the musculotendinous unit rather than in producing the desired function.

7. Agonists are preferable to antagonists.

8. The tendon to be transferred should have, when possible, a range of excursion similar to the one it is reinforcing or replacing.

In a study of 300 tendon transfers, mostly in the lower extremity, Peabody examined 215 patients from 3 to 10 years after surgery and found a strong functioning transfer in 90%. From this study he found that the extent to which the disability or deformity is dynamic (positive) or static (negative) must be determined. The calcaneus foot is an example of a dynamic deformity; an almost flail planovalgus foot without invertor power is a static deformity. When the deformity is dynamic, arthrodesis alone, regardless of its extent, will not prevent its recurrence in a growing child. On the other hand, when a deformity is static, it will usually not recur after fusion or blocking procedures. Frequently both dynamic and static elements are present—for example, in a planovalgus deformity with strong peroneal muscles—and if the dynamic element is overlooked, an arthrodesis may be ineffective. When a deformity is dynamic, as Peabody stated, redistribution of muscle power is imperative and tendon transfers may often, without arthrodesis, restore both balance and function, especially in adults. Transfers are not limited to any age group; in young children even when complete stabilization is not obtained by redistribution of muscle power alone, deformity becomes easily preventable by using minimal support after transfers until the patient is old enough for arthrodesis. Sometimes the redistribution of muscle power may be combined with fusion at a single operation. When a deformity is mainly static, tendon transfers alone will never suffice, and fusion is necessary. But, also in contrast with dynamic deformities, a static one may be controlled mechanically without transfers until arthrodesis is feasible.

Close and Todd studied with continuous oscillographic records the phasic activity of muscles of the lower extremity and the effect of tendon transfer; they found the patterns of electrical activity exhibited by the muscles to be quite consistent. In normal people the anterior muscles of the leg are predominantly swing-phase muscles and the posterior muscles, or flexors, are stance-phase muscles; in the thigh the quadriceps is characteristically a stance-phase muscle and the hamstrings are basically swing-phase muscles. In general, phasic transfers retain their preoperative phasic activities; they also seem to regain their preoperative duration of contraction and electrical intensity. Many muscles transferred from stance-phase to swing-phase functions or vice versa (called nonphasic transfers) retain their preoperative phasic activity and thus fail to assume the action of the muscles for which they are substituted. Some nonphasic transfers are capable of phasic conversion. Some of the factors that seemed to influence phasic conversion are as follows:

1. Training a nonphasic muscle to assume the proper phase of the walking cycle seems essential after some transfers but unnecessary after others. When the tibialis anterior is transferred to the calcaneus, it undergoes phasic conversion only after several months of intensive reeducation. The only patients who had phasic conversion after

transfer of the hamstrings to the patella were "extensively trained by the physical therapist." On the other hand, the one patient in whom phasic conversion occurred after transfer of the peroneus longus to the dorsum of the foot received little or no instruction; many others after the same operation were extensively instructed for several years but never developed swing-phase activity. Phasic conversion of the peroneus brevis after transfer to the dorsum of the foot seemed to be spontaneous.

2. The mixing of swing-phase and stance-phase transfers dooms the nonphasic transfer to failure of phasic conversion unless the latter transfer is made as a separate procedure.

3. Phasic conversion is not related to the time from onset of the disease to transfer.

4. Bracing or splinting after surgery, so helpful in maintaining physiologic length and vigor of the muscles, seems to have no effect on phasic conversion.

According to Mann, the ideal muscle for tendon transfer would have the same phasic activity as the paralyzed muscle, would be of about the same size in cross section and of equal strength, and could be placed in proper relationship to the axis of the joint to allow maximum mechanical effectiveness. Unfortunately not all of these criteria can be met in every instance.

Muscle transplantation

Schottstaedt, Larsen, and Bost have described (1955 and 1950) techniques for complete transplantation of a muscle to replace the power of a paralyzed muscle. In these procedures both the origin and insertion of a muscle are detached, and the muscle, along with its neurovascular pedicle, is transplanted to a completely new location so that it will perform a more important function. They also set down (1958) the following basic principles of muscle transplantation:

1. The muscle chosen for transplantation must be large enough and strong enough to accomplish the task proposed for it. "If it is ineffective in its normal position it can be expected to be even less effective in a new location."*

2. The musculotendinous unit must be transplanted so that it works in a straight line; occasionally a freely gliding pulley system is effective, but usually pulleys increase the friction of the system and thus are doomed to failure.

3. A muscle essential to body mechanics should never be transplanted without making sufficient provision for its loss from its normal position; for example, when wrist extensors are substituted for finger flexors, the wrist should be fused. The procedure is contraindicated when such a provision cannot be made.

4. The transplanted muscle must be securely attached in its new location. When possible it should be attached to bone, although in the upper extremity where forces are not so great as in the lower, it may be successfully attached to tendon or to dense unyielding fascia.

5. Each transplantation requires specific care and fixation after surgery; each demands specific immobilization before function can be safely resumed.

6. The musculotendinous unit must be placed under sufficient tension, usually "about 80% of the elasticity of the muscle with the joint in the corrected position. It should be noted that this is quite snug or tight."*

7. A muscle chosen for transplantation should have a length of fiber that permits a desirable range of motion in its new location. This length is directly proportional to the range of excursion of the muscle in its normal location.

8. "The neurovascular bundle must not be damaged by kinking or by stretching."* Occasionally injury to a nerve from stretching is temporary, and complete or partial recovery occurs in 3 or 4 months; when injury to the nerve has been severe, however, or when the arteriovenous system is seriously impaired, the transplanted muscle will not function.

9. A muscle should never be expected to perform two separate functions; one half of a muscle cannot continue a previous function and the other half perform a new and separate function.

These authors describe the following techniques in detail: transplantation of the pectoralis major to restore elbow flexion, to replace the sternocleidomastoid and associated neck flexors, or to replace the anterior part of the deltoid; transplantation of the latissimus dorsi to restore elbow flexion or extension or to replace the rhomboids; and transplantation of the sternocleidomastoid to reinforce the rotators of the scapula, to replace the masseter, or to replace the facial muscles. Since these procedures are rarely indicated, we refer the reader to their well-prepared and well-illustrated articles for the details of surgical technique.

STABILIZATION OF RELAXED OR FLAIL JOINTS

A relaxed or flail joint is stabilized by partially or completely restricting its normal range of motion or by eliminating an abnormal motion. Although a properly constructed brace may work fairly well, it is less desirable than a reconstructive operation that will not only eliminate the need for a brace but will also improve function.

Stabilization has been attempted by tenodesis, fixation of ligaments, and construction of artificial check ligaments from fascia lata or silk. With few exceptions these procedures have been discarded for two reasons: (1) even when such a stabilization seems successful, a deformity in the opposite direction may occur if the soft tissue or artificial ligament does not stretch with growth and (2) although the artificial check ligament fashioned from a tendon or fascia lata may be satisfactory for a few months or years, it may then overstretch and lose its function, especially in the lower extremity. Stabilization by operation on bone is usually much more permanent and efficient. Tenodeses that use flexor or extensor tendons to stabilize joints of the fingers (Chapters 5 and 12) are notable exceptions, as are tenodeses of the peroneus longus or tendo calcaneus in paralytic calcaneus deformity; results are satisfactory here because the pull of gravity and body weight is usually not enough to overstretch the tendons.

---

*From Schottstaedt, E.R., Larsen, L.J., and Bost, F.C.: The surgical reconstruction of the upper extremity paralyzed by poliomyelitis, J. Bone Joint Surg. **40-A:**633, 1958.

The bone operations designed to stabilize joints are of two types: bone blocks and arthrodeses. Usually, a bone block preserves some useful motion; an arthrodesis completely fixes the joint in one functional position. Since the lower extremities are designed primarily to support the weight of the body, whether standing or walking, it is important that their joints be stable and their muscles powerful. When the control of one or more joints of the foot and ankle is lost because of paralysis, stabilization may be required. In the upper extremity, on the other hand, reach, grasp, pinch, and release require more mobility than stability and more dexterity than power. Thus an operation to limit or obliterate motion in a joint of an upper extremity should be performed only after careful study of its local advantages and disadvantages and of its general effect on the patient, especially in normal daily activity. Arthrodesis of the shoulder is useful for some patients but has certain objections, cosmetic and functional, that must be weighed. Arthrodesis of the elbow is rarely if ever indicated in poliomyelitis. Arthrodesis of the wrist, although useful for some patients, may in others increase their disability. For example, a patient who must use a wheelchair or crutches, if his wrist is fused in the ''optimum'' position (for grasp and pinch), may be unable to lift himself from the chair or to manipulate crutches because he cannot shift his body weight to the palm of his hand with the wrist extended. Arthrodesis of the joints of the fingers and thumb, rarely indicated in poliomyelitis, is discussed in detail in Chapter 10.

FOOT AND ANKLE

Since the foot and ankle are the most dependent parts of the body and are subjected to greater strain than other parts, they are especially susceptible to deformity from paralysis. After tendon transfers and stabilization are discussed, these deformities will be discussed under the following headings: claw toes, cavus deformity and claw foot, dorsal bunion, talipes equinus, talipes equinovarus, talipes cavovarus, talipes equinovalgus, and talipes calcaneus. When the paralysis is of short duration, these dynamic deformities are not fixed and may be evident only on contracture of unopposed muscles or on weight bearing; later as a result of muscle imbalance, habitually faulty posture, growth, and abnormal weight-bearing alignment, a permanent deformity is established from contracture of the soft tissues and from distortion of the normal contour of the bones.

Tendon transfers

The results of tendon transfers are better in patients over 10 years old; surgical stabilization of the joints of the feet is also associated with fewer complications and failures if the procedure can be delayed until skeletal maturity. A child under age 10 or 11 years must be examined regularly, and should a deformity appear, it must be corrected before irreversible secondary skeletal changes develop. If the deformity recurs or persists despite conservative measures, as is characteristic of talipes calcaneocavus, it must be corrected surgically, and appropriate tendons must be transferred to prevent recurrence. In these instances the parents must be told that foot stabilization will be necessary when the bones are more mature.

Tendon transfers about the foot and ankle after age 10 or 11 years are usually supplemented by stabilizing procedures to correct fixed deformities, to establish enough lateral stability for weight bearing, and to compensate in part for the loss of power in the abductor-evertor and adductor-invertor muscles. In addition, when tendons are transferred to the dorsum of the foot to be used for active dorsiflexion, a bone block operation to limit plantar flexion may be necessary to prevent overstretching of the transferred tendons. When tendon transfers and bone stabilization are combined at the same operation, the latter is done first. When there is any significant imbalance, the transfer of even a single tendon should usually be preceded or accompanied by foot stabilizations; to balance the muscle power about the foot accurately with tendon transfers alone is impossible in a child because even the slightest imbalance, when combined with a long period of growth, usually results in significant deformity. This is not true in the adult; when the onset of paralysis is after skeletal maturity, significant deformity is rare. After foot stabilization only plantar flexion and dorsiflexion remain, and since these are ankle motions, to preserve or restore muscle power on the medial and lateral sides of the ankle is unnecessary.

Transfer of a tendon is usually preferable to excision not only to preserve function, but also to prevent further atrophy of the leg. When the paralysis is severe enough to require stabilization, there is usually some weakness of either the dorsiflexor or plantar flexor muscles, and invertor or evertor muscles should be transferred either to the midline of the foot anteriorly or into the calcaneus and tendo calcaneus posteriorly as the case may be. In the rare instance when a muscle function is discarded, 7 to 10 cm of its tendon should be excised to prevent reunion of the tendon ends by fibrous tissue.

After foot stabilization and tendon transfers, any deformities of the leg, such as excessive tibial torsion, knock-knee, or bowlegs, should be corrected, since otherwise they might cause recurrence of the foot deformity.

Peabody classified paralysis of the muscles of the foot and ankle as follows: (1) limited extensor-invertor insufficiency, (2) gross extensor-invertor insufficiency, (3) evertor insufficiency, and (4) triceps surae insufficiency. He offered the following suggestions as to treatment.

LIMITED EXTENSOR-INVERTOR INSUFFICIENCY

Severe weakness or paralysis of the tibialis anterior muscle produces a slowly progressive deformity—equinus and cavus or varying degrees of planovalgus. Muscle power is redistributed by transferring the extensor hallucis longus tendon to the base of the first metatarsal; plantar fasciotomy is usually the only other operative procedure needed. When the foot is severely relaxed or when the valgus deformity is fixed, the tendon transfer is combined with triple arthrodesis. The equinus deformity can usually be corrected by stretching before operation; otherwise, lengthening of the tendo calcaneus is necessary.

When the peroneus tertius muscle is functioning, it may be transferred along with the extensor hallucis longus to the base of the first metatarsal, thus reinforcing the latter muscle.

GROSS EXTENSOR-INVERTOR INSUFFICIENCY

TYPE A

Weakness or paralysis of the tibialis anterior muscle and the extensor muscles of the toes in the presence of a relatively normal tibialis posterior muscle produces a paralytic equinus or equinovalgus deformity. Muscle power is redistributed by transfer of the peroneus longus tendon to the dorsum of the foot; the tendon is not passed through the sheath of the tibialis anterior to its insertion, since this might reverse the invertor-evertor imbalance and leave the foot unstable in a varus position. Rather, the tendon is usually inserted on the dorsum of the first cuneiform. When the structural changes of the soft tissues and bone prevent satisfactory alignment, triple arthrodesis may be combined with the tendon transfer.

In the weakness or paralysis described here we prefer transferring the peroneus brevis tendon to the distal tarsus. When the power of the tibialis posterior balances that of the peroneus longus, then the tendon is transferred to the midline of the foot, but when the tibialis posterior is the stronger of the two, the tendon is transferred in line with the fourth ray, and conversely when the peroneus longus is the stronger, the tendon is transferred in line with the first or second ray. We also prefer to stabilize the foot by triple arthrodesis.

TYPE B

Severe paralysis of both tibial muscles and of the toe extensor muscles characterizes this type. Transfer of both peroneal muscles to the dorsum of the foot should result in good function. For a severe deformity of long standing the Hoke arthrodesis may be added to the tendon transfers.

EVERTOR INSUFFICIENCY

For paralysis of the peroneal muscles, the extensor hallucis longus or tibialis anterior muscle is transferred to the lateral side of the foot. When the impairment is slight to moderate, the extensor hallucis longus tendon is transferred to the base of the fifth metatarsal; when it is gross, the tibialis anterior tendon is transferred to the cuboid and the extensor hallucis longus to the first metatarsal. When the peroneal muscles are completely paralyzed and the tibialis posterior muscle is normal, varus imbalance is less likely if the tibialis posterior tendon is transferred to the anterolateral aspect of the foot. For a varus deformity of long standing a triple arthrodesis is combined with the tendon transfers.

Transfer of the tibialis anterior tendon to the lateral side of the foot is one of the most effective transfers available. Where the tendon should be anchored is determined by any balance or imbalance in power between the tibialis posterior and peroneus longus muscles as already described for gross extensor-invertor insufficiency. Rather than resecting the tibialis posterior tendon, we prefer transferring it anteriorly through the interosseous membrane to the distal tarsus. This transfer is beneficial because it not only removes the dynamic deforming force of the muscle but also

produces at least a motorized tenodesis; however, the patient may learn to use the transfer in the swing phase in walking and then the operation becomes even more beneficial. According to Turner and Cooper, this operation is effective when other plantar flexors are satisfactory.

For paralysis of the peroneal muscles we now prefer the split anterior tibial tendon transfer as described by Hoffer et al., originally used in the treatment of patients with cerebral palsy in which the tibialis anterior tendon is overactive. One half of the tendon, or slightly more in severe cases, can be detached distally, brought out to the midline of the lower leg near the musculotendinous junction, split proximally nearly to the musculotendinous junction, rerouted deep to the transverse crural ligament, and securely fixed to the insertion of the peroneus brevis tendon with the foot in the slightly overcorrected position.

TRICEPS SURAE INSUFFICIENCY

According to Peabody, redistribution of muscle power in the early residual stage of paralysis (2 to 3 years) will prevent a progressive calcaneus or calcaneocavus deformity. In his experience the only operation that will restore heel-and-toe gait and the ability to stand on tiptoe is posterior transfer of the tendon of the tibialis anterior through the interosseous membrane into the calcaneus; he also thinks that function would perhaps be more completely restored by the additional transfer of the extensor hallucis longus tendon to the dorsum of the foot, provided that the muscle is competent. For a calcaneovalgus deformity the peroneal tendons are attached to the calcaneus; for a calcaneovarus deformity both the tibialis posterior and flexor hallucis longus tendons are transferred. A calcaneocavus deformity in which both the invertors and evertors are strong is corrected by transfer of the peroneal and tibialis posterior tendons to the calcaneus. When a deformity is of long duration, correction of the distorted bones by triple arthrodesis is also necessary.

• • •

In summary, Peabody made the following recommendations: (1) for early weakness of the triceps surae group only, without bone deformities, posterior transfer of the tibialis anterior without arthrodesis; (2) for early lateral imbalance, transfer of the acting invertors or evertors; (3) for old lateral imbalance associated with bone deformities, supplementary resections and arthrodesis of the tarsal joints combined with transfer of the acting invertors or evertors; and (4) for old weakness of the triceps surae group only, a combination of tarsal reconstruction and posterior transfer of the peroneus longus and tibialis posterior tendons. Excepting the tarsal reconstruction and posterior transfer of the tibialis anterior tendon, these procedures may be done at a single operation.

Reidy, Broderick, and Barr reported a study of 125 tendon transfers about the foot and ankle performed at the Massachusetts General Hospital from 1920 through 1949. About one third of the transfers were rated as failures, one third as fair, and one third as good to excellent. Transfers performed before age 11 years were frequently unsuccessful; in 60% of the patients in this age group reoperations were necessary. In properly selected patients tendon transfers improved the result of arthrodesis by reinforcing the power of dorsiflexion or plantar flexion. Anterior transfers to reinforce dorsiflexion were generally more successful than posterior transfers to reinforce plantar flexion.

Kuhlmann and Bell, in a study of 395 tendon transfers in the lower extremities performed between 1914 and 1949, found that in about 40% of the anterior transfers of the peroneus longus tendon some muscle power was lost in the process of transfer; on the other hand, when the tibialis anterior and the extensor hallucis longus tendons were transferred to the dorsum of the foot, power was rarely lost. They further noted that the results of tendon transfers depend as much on the strength and function of the neighboring tendons as on the strength of the transferred tendons; although the extensor hallucis longus muscle was not strong enough to substitute for the action of the paralyzed tibialis anterior, yet when it was reinforced by a functioning peroneus longus muscle, the substitution was satisfactory. Tendon transfer into the calcaneus was reasonably effective when combined with a tarsal arthrodesis; although the push-off in the gait of many patients was improved, none were able to rise up actively on tiptoe and bear full weight on the involved foot alone. Removing a deforming muscle force by transfer was important in controlling a progressive deformity, especially in children.

Stabilization of joints of foot and ankle

The object of foot stabilization for paralysis about the leg and foot is to reduce the number of joints the weakened or even paralyzed muscles must attempt to control. Excellent discussions of the evolution and history of foot stabilization have been presented by Hart, by Hallgrimsson, and by Schwartz.

Albert in 1878 first attempted to stablize a paralytic equinus foot by curetting the articular surfaces of the ankle joint to fuse it; with the same object in view, von Lesser in 1879 resected the joint between the lateral malleolus and the talus. The first arthrodesis of the ankle was done at the Hospital for Ruptured and Crippled in 1894. However, Whitman must be given credit for placing the principles of foot stabilization on a sound basis. In 1901 he reported his method of talectomy for paralytic talipes calcaneus and pointed out the importance of posterior displacement of the foot when the triceps surae is weak. He found that arthrodesis of the ankle alone is of little value in the presence of lateral distortion; in such patients the operation must also include the subtalar and midtarsal joints. Nierny of Germany in 1905 also performed a subtalar arthrodesis for lateral instability. In 1913 G.G. Davis of Philadelphia described a method of ''horizontal transverse section'' of the foot with posterior displacement. Davis must be given credit for popularizing foot stabilization. However, his method does not permit much posterior displacement of the foot; other procedures have since been developed that permit more such displacement and also better correction of other deformities.

Hoke in 1921 and Dunn in 1922 first suggested removing bone from between the cuneiform bones and the body of the talus to produce posterior displacement of the foot. Hoke's method combined subtalar arthrodesis with resec-

tion, reshaping, and reimplantation of the head and neck of the talus and posterior displacement of the foot. In the method described by Dunn the foot is displaced posteriorly by excising the navicular and part of the head and neck of the talus; the amount of displacement is determined by the amount of bone removed. Actual shortening of the foot is slight. Both Dunn and Hoke advised balancing the foot by tendon transfers when necessary. Hoke also emphasized the need for correcting any tibial torsion or knock-knee deformity.

In 1923 Ryerson recognized that if the entire physiologic unit involved in lateral deformities of the foot is to be stabilized, the calcaneocuboid joint should also be fused. His technique of triple arthrodesis is rational, since lateral movements of the foot are functions of both the subtalar and talonavicular joints. After fusion of the calcaneocuboid joint, deformity is less likely to recur, and a severe varus or valgus deformity can be better corrected.

Steindler in 1923 presented a method of pantalar arthrodesis to stabilize the flail ankle. Goldthwait had already described a method of arthrodesis that denuded the ankle and subtalar joints but not the talonavicular joint; Sir Robert Jones had also described an arthrodesis of the same joints but done in two stages. Steindler did not originally include fusion in the calcaneocuboid joint; he added this later.

Many modifications of these basic methods of foot stabilization and related procedures have been devised. Most seek partial limitation of ankle motion. Chief among those still in use are the posterior bone block of Campbell and the stabilization described by Lambrinudi, both of which limit plantar flexion. These are described on pp. 2952 and 2955.

Foot stabilization is indicated only when a deformity of the foot is accompanied by lateral stability of the talus in the ankle mortise. When this stability is questionable, anteroposterior roentgenograms of the ankle should be made with the foot in extreme varus and in extreme valgus position; any lateral instability can be detected by comparing these films. When the talus is unstable, ankle fusion as well as foot stabilization may be indicated. Failure to recognize instability of the ankle before surgery will mean an unstable ankle after surgery and perhaps an unstable foot as well; the deformity may even recur after satisfactory foot stabilization.

Knowing that anterior subluxation of the ankle often follows stabilization of the foot for paralytic equinus deformity, Flint and MacKenzie studied 60 feet with this deformity that had not been treated surgically; they found such subluxation in 43%. They recommend that before surgery lateral roentgenograms of the ankle be made with the foot in forced plantar flexion. If relaxation of the anterior structures of the ankle is demonstrated, then either tendons should be transferred to restore dorsiflexion or the ankle should be arthrodesed. Pyka, Coventry, and Moe noted 10 instances of anterior subluxation of the ankle in their study of 554 triple arthrodeses and presumed that subluxation might be caused by the technique of arthrodesis.

Foot stabilization is an orthopaedic procedure that requires exactness and precision; no other operation on the foot is so frequently performed that involves so many articular surfaces at one time. Thus an intimate knowledge of the normal structure and function of the foot is necessary. As Schwartz points out, roentgenographic analysis before surgery is important to determine individual variations in the foot; the operation may then be planned more intelligently. A paper tracing of the lateral roentgenogram may be made, and the tracing cut into three parts—the tibiotalar component, the calcaneal component, and the component comprising all of the bones of the foot distal to the midtarsal joints; these parts may then be reassembled with the foot in the desired position, and the size and shape of the wedges to be removed may be accurately determined.

The incision will vary somewhat with each particular deformity and with the experience and preference of the surgeon; those most frequently used are the anterolateral, the Kocher, and the Ollier or minor modifications of one of these (Chapter 2). Some surgeons also use an accessory short medial incision to expose the talonavicular joint; they believe that this reduces the operative time, lessens the amount of retraction of the skin edges incident to approaching this joint from the lateral side, and permits a more accurate fitting of the joint. However, in the Hoke and Dunn stabilizations, which use anterolateral incisions, the proximal navicular or cuneiform articular surfaces is easily excised, since the head and neck of the talus or the navicular or both are removed. In the Ryerson triple arthrodesis it may be difficult to excise all of the cartilage from the medial side of the talonavicular joint unless the exposure extends far enough on the anterolateral aspect of the talus or unless an accessory medial incision is used.

The operation must be performed with the accuracy and care of a cabinetmaker. Except when deformity is severe, the articular surfaces should be carefully denuded of cartilage and then accurately shaped so that alignment of the foot is proper and bony contact in the several joints is maximum and without dead spaces. The medial border of the foot should be straight, the heel and first and fifth metatarsal heads should be in the exact midposition; a mild valgus position of the heel will usually not harm the functional result, but a *varus position certainly will*. It should be remembered that the purpose of care after surgery is not to correct the position of the foot but only to maintain the position obtained at surgery.

The details of the operation will vary with the nature of the deformity. Uniformly satisfactory results will be obtained only when attention is given in each individual patient to the technical details applicable to each deformity. For example, stabilization for a paralytic equinocavovarus deformity will differ materially from stabilization for planovalgus. In talipes equinocavovarus there is bone hypertrophy to a varying extent of the anterolateral aspect of the calcaneus, the cuboid, and the head and neck of the talus. The head of the talus lies lateral in relation to the midline of the foot, the distal ends of the metatarsal shafts are directed medially and plantarward, and the shafts are rotated to some extent. In simple equinus deformity there is less fullness over the anterolateral aspect of the tarsus, but there is an overgrowth of the head and neck of the talus superiorly in the midline that blocks dorsiflexion of the foot even though the tendo calcaneus is lengthened. In sta-

bilizing a varus foot the head of the talus should be replaced slightly to the medial side of the midline of the foot, whereas in an equinocavus deformity the head of the talus is made smaller and is implanted deeply on the anterior end of the calcaneus in the midline.

The structural pathologic disorder in talipes planovalgus is the opposite of that just described for talipes equinovarus. On their medial and inferior aspects the head and neck of the talus and the navicular enlarge to varying degrees. When the deformity is marked, there is inferior subluxation or even dislocation of the head of the talus. Abduction of the forefoot and dropping of the longitudinal arch are associated with this plantar flexion of the talus. Thus the head of the talus must be raised from its deep bed on the medial side of the foot, and the anterior end of the calcaneus must be shifted medially beneath it. To permit this shift much of the head and neck of the talus must be excised, and a wedge must be removed from the medial side of the subtalar joint. However, the valgus deformity of the heel must not be overcorrected, for the forefoot has a tendency to supinate when the valgus heel is corrected. This supination should be corrected when the forefoot valgus is corrected and the longitudinal arch of the foot is reestablished. When necessary, the prominent tuberosity of the navicular is removed through a small medial incision. In fact, it is in this type of deformity that an accessory medial incision is most useful.

The muscle balance of the foot and ankle determines how much the foot should be displaced posteriorly. Posterior displacement of the foot transfers its fulcrum (the ankle) anteriorly to a position near its center and lengthens its posterior lever arm; this is of particular advantage when the triceps surae group is weak. When it is desirable to displace the foot as far posteriorly as possible, the procedure of Hoke or Dunn is used; the latter permits slightly more displacement than the former. When the dorsiflexors and plantar flexors of the ankle are about equally strong, Ryerson's triple arthrodesis may be used.

At the time of stabilization the foot must be placed in correct relationship to the ankle joint without regard to other deformities of the extremity such as knock-knee or tibial torsion. But these deformities must be corrected later; otherwise malalignment of the extremity may cause the foot deformity to recur despite stabilization.

When stabilizing the adult foot, no attempt should be made to materially change the weight-bearing alignment, since the added strain on the ligaments and other structures would often lead to an unsatisfactory result. Edema after operations on the foot is usually more severe in adults than in children and may persist for several months.

Marek and Schein called attention to the possibility of avascular necrosis of the body of the talus after triple arthrodesis and pantalar arthrodesis. This complication seems to be more likely in adolescents and adults than in young children and occurs most often after wide resection of the head and neck of the talus. Revascularization usually occurs in adolescents in 6 to 9 months; collapse of the body of the talus may be prevented by delaying weight bearing until then. When weight bearing is allowed too early, it compresses the body of the talus and damages the ankle joint; then secondary degenerative changes occur, and ankle fusion may ultimately be required for relief of pain.

Triple arthrodesis subjects the ankle joint to many minor medial, lateral, and rotary stresses and strains that would be dissipated by normal intertarsal joint motion. Ingram and Hundley found degenerative arthritic changes in the ankle joint in 40 of 90 patients (44.4%) with triple arthrodesis and posterior bone block of the ankle studied 5 to 27 years (average 18 years) after the operation. They believe these changes to be secondary to the arthrodesis rather than to the bone block. In 27 patients who had had tarsal arthrodesis 13 to 20 years previously, Drew observed limitation of ankle motion in most; in 10 patients the roentgenograms revealed degenerative arthritis, which was usually asymptomatic. He too thought it was the extra strain that tarsal arthrodesis places on both the proximal and distal joints that ultimately leads to degenerative arthritic changes.

According to Hoke a satisfactorily stabilized foot meets the following requirements: it looks natural in shoes, it does not turn laterally on its long axis when the patient is standing or walking, it does not require a brace to maintain a natural or nearly natural position, and when bare it appears natural or at least not grossly deformed. To these Thompson added the following: the weight is evenly distributed over the plantar surface during stance and gait, the axis of the ankle joint is well forward, and at a right angle to the long axis of the foot, the patient is able to control ankle joint motion, and there is no pain.

Crego and McCarroll studied a series of 1100 foot stabilizations for deformities secondary to poliomyelitis. Most were triple arthrodeses; deformity recurred after 212 (about 20%) of these operations. The most common cause of failure was muscle imbalance, although other deformities in the extremity and stabilization at too early an age were responsible for some. These authors suggest that unless completely paralyzed the tendons of the peroneus longus and brevis and of the tibialis anterior and posterior be transferred to the midline posteriorly and anteriorly; the only exception is the cavus deformity produced by paralysis of the intrinsic muscles of the foot while the extrinsic muscles remain normal. However, we believe that in conjunction with foot stabilization less radical tendon transfers will usually balance the foot well enough to prevent recurrence of deformity. But we agree with Peabody that correction of dynamic deformities cannot be maintained in a growing child by arthrodesis alone regardless of its extent.

In 1950 Patterson, Parrish, and Hathaway reported an evaluation of 305 stabilizing operations on the foot and ankle. Stabilization failed in 55 (18%); deformity or pseudarthrosis accounted for 51 of these. Over two thirds of the 39 failures caused by residual deformity were the result of incomplete correction at operation. Factors observed to be responsible in the 12 cases of recurrent deformity were (1) immobilization for an insufficient time to allow firm consolidation of bone, (2) failure to align the foot with the ankle mortise, (3) loss of position at the time of cast change, (4) pseudarthrosis, (5) muscle imbalance, and (6) operation before the bones of the foot were sufficiently mature. Pain resulted in most instances from pseudarthrosis, although in two patients painful callosities secondary to deformity were the cause.

One of the conclusions from this study by these authors was that the Hoke stabilization (see Fig. 66-5) can correct any foot deformity; it cannot be relied on alone to correct a footdrop, but a good result can be expected when sufficient muscle power is available for transfer to the dorsum of the foot. They also found that since the classical triple arthrodesis (see Fig. 66-1) does not allow backward displacement of the foot, because the head and neck of the talus are not resected, it is not as effective as the Hoke stabilization in correcting many deformities; nor is it as effective as the Lambrinudi procedure in correcting a fixed equinus deformity. The Lambrinudi procedure (see Fig. 66-23) in their experience surpasses all other stabilization procedures for correcting this deformity, but it cannot be expected to correct a footdrop unless lateral muscles are available for transfer. Pseudarthrosis of the talonavicular joint should be guarded against in this procedure by making the area of bony contact large and by continuing immobilization until there is roentgenographic evidence of solid fusion. Finally they found the results of two-joint arthrodesis much less satisfactory than those of the group as a whole. Both midtarsal wedge osteotomy and subtalar arthrodesis were responsible for failure in many instances because of the difficulty of obtaining complete correction without a three-joint arthrodesis.

Friedenbërg found pseudarthrosis in one or more joints in 15 (23%) of 65 three-joint stabilizations performed 1 to 8 years previously; it was most common in the talonavicular joint; the calcaneocuboid and talocalcaneal joints fused readily and regularly. Patterson, Parrish, and Hath-

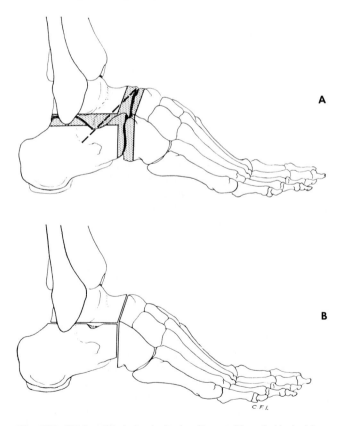

Fig. 66-1. Triple arthrodesis. **A,** *Broken line,* position of skin incision; *shaded area,* amount of bone resected. **B,** Position of bones after surgery.

away found pseudarthroses in 56 (18%) of their cases, and one fifth of these were rated failures because of severe pain. Most of these pseudarthroses (89%) were in the talonavicular joint. Wilson, Fay, Lanotte, and Williams found pseudarthroses in 31 (10.3%) of their 301 cases, and again most were in the talonavicular joint. Pseudarthrosis of this joint is best prevented by securing an accurate, snug contact between the talus and navicular and by immobilizing the joint accurately and efficiently in plaster long enough for bony union to occur.

Seltz and Carpenter in 1974 reviewed 66 triple arthrodeses carried out in 47 children whose average age at the time of surgery was 12.1 years and who were observed for at least 2 years after surgery. Pseudarthroses occurred in 9.1%, but the chief problem was residual deformity present to some extent in 57%; deformity was most common in spastic paralysis and painful flatfoot.

Hill, Wilson, Chevres, and Sweterditsch in 1970 studied the results of triple arthrodeses performed at ages younger than has been customary. They pointed out the advantage of early definitive surgery so that braces can be avoided during the childhood years. They studied 43 triple arthrodeses carried out in 37 children between the ages of 5 and 8 years who were observed for an average of 9.5 years. They sought to determine whether the operation when performed early would increase the incidence of pseudarthrosis, recurrent deformity, and excessive shortening of the foot. They deferred the operation until the ossification center of the navicular was large enough to provide a small area for union with the denuded talus. Pseudarthrosis occurred in 10 joints of the 43 feet, and in one instance it occurred at both the talonavicular and calcaneocuboid joints. Five feet required a revision later because the deformity was not fully corrected at the original operation. The average shortening of the foot was 2 cm, and the most marked was 5 cm after a wound infection and later a talectomy. In their opinion early stabilization properly carried out can avoid years of casting and bracing and can make the child more active.

TECHNIQUES

The technique we use for stabilizing the foot is a combination and modification of the technical principles developed by Davis, Ryerson, Hoke, and Campbell, and poularized by Kite, Irwin, and others.

TECHNIQUE. Make a straight incision (Fig. 66-1) centered over the sinus tarsi; extend it from the peroneus brevis tendon anteriorly toward the head of the talus and end it at the lateral border of the extensor tendons. Carry the incision directly down to the floor of the sinus tarsi. Cleanly elevate the periosteum of the calcaneus, the contents of the sinus tarsi, and the tendinous origin of the extensor digitorum brevis muscle from the calcaneus and the lateral aspect of the neck of the talus and retract them distally; when handled carefully, these tissues will provide a viable pedicle to obliterate the dead space remaining at the end of the operation. Incise the capsule of the calcaneocuboid joint; identify and remove the anterior articular process of the calcaneus parallel with the floor of the sinus tarsi. Save the bone for use later. Now cleanly remove the articular surfaces of the calcaneocuboid joint. Next incise the talonavicular joint and amputate the head of the talus at the

junction of the neck with the articular surface; make the plane of the osteotomy perpendicular to the long axis of the neck. Remove the proximal articular surface and subchondral bone plate of the navicular; shape and roughen the opposing bony surfaces for a snug fit with maximum contact. Next excise the articular surfaces of the sustentaculum tali and anterior facet of the talus.

Expose the subtalar joint by incising and reflecting the capsule along its anterior and lateral borders back to the dome of the posterior articular facet of the calcaneus. For better exposure of this joint, excise the anterior lip of the posterior facet of the talus level with the dome of the calcaneus. Now cleanly excise the articular surfaces of the subtalar joint. Remove wedges of bone as necessary to correct the deformity (Figs. 66-2 and 66-3) and roughen the bony surfaces for maximum contact. If the foot is to be displaced posteriorly, resect more of the neck of the talus.

In most adult feet, in children's feet when minimal resection of the head of the talus is required, and in feet with planovalgus deformity, approaching the talonavicular joint through an accessory medial incision is often wise; this incision allows thorough preparation of the talonavicular joint and easy removal of the tuberosity of the navicular when unduly prominent, both without excessive retraction of the anterolateral incision.

When the removed pieces of bone are not to be used as a posterior bone block, chip them up finely and pack them into the defects until maximum bony contact is obtained in all joints; these grafts are needed most at the talonavicular area, since this is the most likely site of pseudarthrosis. When desired, the tarsus may be held in the correct position by transfixing the joints with Kirschner wires that are removed later (Caldwell). Now rotate the soft tissue pedicle into the tarsal sinus and secure it with two interrupted figure-of-eight sutures. Subcutaneous sutures are usually unnecessary; close the skin with four or five interrupted vertical mattress sutures or more when necessary if a valgus deformity was present before operation.

A long leg plaster cast is now applied. An improperly applied cast may cause failure despite the most precise operation. It should be applied with the foot and leg suspended over the edge of the table; the foot is molded to the correct shape and is carefully aligned with the malleoli. First a padded cast is applied from the toes to the tibial tuberosity; when this has hardened, the tourniquet is removed, the leg is elevated, and the cast is extended to the proximal third of the thigh, with the knee at 20 degrees. A large window is marked over the anterior surface of the foot and leg to be cut out if circulation becomes impaired.

AFTERTREATMENT. The cast is suspended by slings to an overhead frame until all swelling has subsided. After 10 to 14 days the patient is prepared for general anesthesia and the cast is removed. If the alignment is satisfactory both clinically and roentgenographically, a snug boot cast is applied; otherwise the foot is manipulated with the patient under general anesthesia, for proper alignment must be obtained at this time; a boot cast is then applied. The patient is allowed up on crutches as tolerated; 6 weeks after operation the cast is removed, roentgenograms are made, and a walking boot cast is applied. This cast is worn until solid

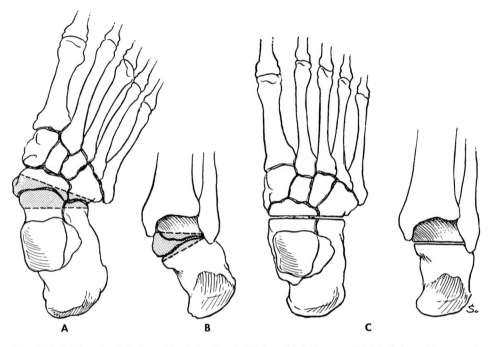

Fig. 66-2. Triple arthrodesis for valgus deformity. **A,** Wedge with its base medial *(shaded area)* is resected from midtarsal region to correct abduction deformity of forefoot. **B,** Wedge with its base also medial *(shaded area)* is resected from subtalar joint region to correct valgus deformity of hind foot. **C,** Position of bones after surgery.

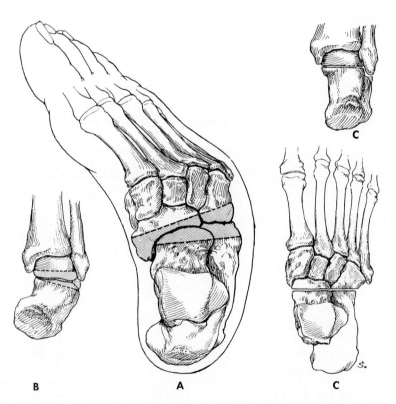

Fig. 66-3. Triple arthrodesis for varus deformity. **A,** Wedge with its base lateral *(shaded area)* is resected from midtarsal region to correct deformity of forefoot. **B,** Wedge with its base lateral *(shaded area)* is resected from subtalar joint region to correct varus deformity of hindfoot. **C,** Position of bones after surgery.

bony union is demonstrated both clinically and roentgenographically; this is usually 12 weeks after surgery.

• • •

Brittain discussed the Dunn stabilization exceptionally well and in considerable detail. What follows is the operative technique he used.

TECHNIQUE (DUNN-BRITTAIN). Make a straight incision beginning at a point 1.5 cm inferior to the lateral malleolus and ending at the base of the second metatarsal. Keep the skin and subcutaneous tissue flaps, particularly the superior one, as thick as possible to avoid necrosis. Dissect the extensor digitorum brevis from the underlying tarsus and retract it anteriorly and distally to expose the calcaneocuboid joint. Identify the peroneal tendons and divide them in a Z-plastic fashion. Now open the subtalar joint and divide the calcaneofibular and anterior talofibular ligaments. Retract the tendons of the extensor digitorum longus medially and expose the head of the talus. Now incise the talonavicular, naviculocuneiform, and calcaneocuboid joints. Gently elevate the soft tissues from the anteromedial aspect of the tarsus so that the foot can be broken open without excessive force. The great toe should "almost touch the shin." Carefully remove the navicular and excise the contents of the sinus tarsi. Now remove the cartilage from the tarsal bones in the following order if possible: the cuneiforms, the cuboid, the calcaneus, the head of the talus, and, finally, the inferior surface of the talus (Fig. 66-4, *A*). Brittain stresses the importance of removing all

of the cartilage from the posteromedial aspect of the posterior talar articular facet; the tendon of the flexor hallucis longus is usually exposed at this time. Brittain removed the cortex of the superior noncartilaginous surface of the calcaneus back to and including the sinus tarsi. More bone must be removed from the second cuneiform than from the bones on either side to form a bed for the head of the talus.

Now fit the foot together. If the operation has been done well, the head of the talus will articulate with the cuneiform bones (Fig. 66-4, *B*); otherwise the subtalar joint has been insufficiently mobilized, or the talonavicular capsule is hypertrophied. Greater correction can be obtained if the foot is more extensively mobilized by dividing the ligaments on the medial side of the tarsus or by removing more bone from the calcaneocuboid joint.

Unless the navicular is to be used for a posterior bone block, denude it of cartilage and cut it up finely; then pack the bone in and about the areas to be fused. Suture any remaining capsular tissue. Replace the extensor digitorum brevis over the capsule and suture the peroneal tendons. Apply a well-fitting long leg plaster cast; window it before the patient leaves the operating room.

AFTERTREATMENT. Aftertreatment is the same as for the routine foot stabilization (see above).

TECHNIQUE (HOKE). Make a skin incision from the lateral aspect of the head of the talus inferiorly and posteriorly to a point below the end of the fibula in the interval between the tendons of the peroneus tertius and longus (Fig. 66-5,

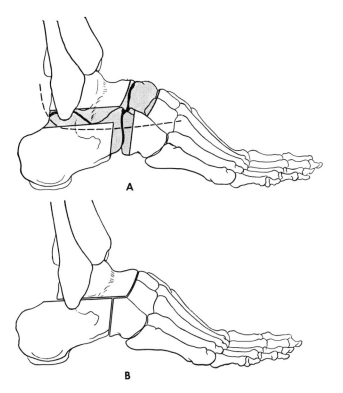

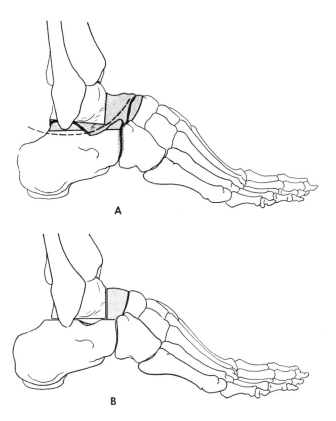

Fig. 66-4. Dunn arthrodesis. **A,** *Broken line,* position of skin incision; *shaded area,* amount of bone resected. **B,** Position of bones after surgery. Foot (except for talus) has been displaced posteriorly at subtalar joint so that head of talus is apposed to cuneiforms.

Fig. 66-5. Hoke arthrodesis. **A,** *Broken line,* position of skin incision; *shaded area;* amount of bone resected. **B,** Position of bones after surgery; head of talus has been reshaped and replaced.

A). Dissect the adipose tissue from the sinus tarsi and free the soft tissue from the superior surface of the neck of the talus. With a scalpel separate the head of the talus from the navicular by dividing the talonavicular ligament; begin laterally and sweep around the head medially. Next with an osteotome excise a part of the inferior surface of the body of the talus and the adjacent surface of the calcaneus. Sever the head and neck of the talus from the body, cut the soft tissue attachments of this fragment, and remove and preserve it in a sterile towel. Then with a small chisel denude the articular surface of the navicular and the facets on the superior surface of the calcaneus.

Now correct any lateral or rotary deformities of the foot and shift the calcaneus into satisfactory alignment; if desired, displace the foot posteriorly. Denude the head of the talus and replace it between the navicular and the body of the talus; the position of the head will depend on the type and degree of deformity. Then slightly dorsiflex the foot.

This description is based on Hoke's orginal paper. Kite, who was Hoke's associate for many years, included the calcaneocuboid joint in the arthrodesis and proceeded in the following order. First clean the sinus tarsi and excise the superolateral corner of the distal articular surface of the calcaneus to facilitate exposure. Then excise the calcaneocuboid joint and remove appropriate wedges of bone to correct any lateral deformity. Now remove the subtalar articular surfaces, including that of the sustentaculum tali. Using a knife denude the superior surface of the head and neck of the talus and divide the neck with an osteotome; sever the soft tissue attachments of the head and neck with a scalpel and scissors. Use a large curet to remove the head; then completely denude the posterior articular surface of the navicular. When there is a clubfoot deformity, divide the plantar calcaneonavicular (spring) ligament medially and inferiorly to permit better correction in this part of the foot. Kite also advocated fish scaling the denuded articular surfaces of the joints to be arthrodesed. After reshaping and reducing the size of the head-neck fragment of the talus, replace it in the defect in the desired position. Use the remaining bone fragments to fill any defect in the vicinity of the sinus tarsi.

AFTERTREATMENT. Aftertreatment is the same as for the routine foot stabilization (p. 2935).

Claw toes

Claw toe deformities, characterized by hyperextension of the metatarsophalangeal joints and flexion of the interphalangeal joints, are common features of a neuropathic clawfoot or talipes cavus. In poliomyelitis they may occur in either of two situations, and the responsible mechanism may be determined by careful analysis of the foot. In the first situation the deformities result when the long toe extensors are used to substitute for severely weakened ankle dorsiflexors; clawing is even more marked when the tendo calcaneus is contracted. Examination of the barefoot gait shows that during the swing phase the long toe extensors actively contract, producing the toe deformities; during the stance phase when weight is borne on the foot, these deformities are usually not apparent. The need for this substitution pattern may be eliminated and the deformities may be minimized by correcting the equinus deformity of the ankle and by transferring suitable tendons to restore

active dorsiflexion of the ankle. In the second situation the long toe flexors are used to substitute for a severely weakened triceps surae group in the propulsive or push-off phase of gait. Examination of the barefoot gait here shows clawing of the toes only when propulsion or push-off is attempted. The need for this substitution pattern may be eliminated by correcting any foot deformity and by suitable tendon transfers to restore active plantar flexion of the ankle; operation on the toes is then usually unnecessary.

All of the toes are usually affected, although the contracture of the great toe is the most severe. The flexed proximal interphalangeal joints are constantly irritated by the shoe, and painful metatarsal callosities develop. The deformity eventually becomes permanent.

When claw toe deformities are associated with a cavus deformity, the tarsal deformity should be corrected first by appropriate operations on bones and tendons, since clawing of the toes will then usually be corrected spontaneously.

In 1922 Stiles and Forrester-Brown described an operation to correct paralysis of the intrinsic muscles of the hand; the sublimis flexor tendons of the fingers are transferred into the extensor tendons. Forrester-Brown in 1938 described an analogous procedure to correct clawing of the great toe. According to Taylor, Girdlestone was the first to transfer the long flexor tendons of the toes into the dorsal expansions of the extensor tendons to correct claw toe deformities. This procedure enables the long flexor muscles of the toes to assume the function of the intrinsic muscles in producing active plantar flexion at the metatarsophalangeal joints and extension at the interphalangeal joints. Often the contracted extensor tendons must be tenotomized subcutaneously to permit correction of dorsal subluxation of the metacarpophalangeal joints; at times even capsulotomies of the joints are also necessary.

Taylor reports the results of this procedure as follows: of 38 patients with claw toe deformities associated with talipes cavus, 27 obtained a good result; 5 with some disability as a result of slight residual clawing of one or more of the toes obtained a fair result; 6 obtained only a poor result. Of 23 patients with claw toe deformities associated with a valgus deformity of the foot, 21 obtained a good result, 1 a fair result, and 1 a poor result. Of 7 patients without tarsal deformity, 2 obtained a good result, 4 a fair result, and 1 a poor result.

Pyper examined the results of the Girdlestone-Taylor operation on 45 feet (26 patients). The results were classed as good or excellent in 23, only fair in 8, and poor or bad in 14. Among the causes of residual disability were metatarsal pain and metatarsal callosities; when troublesome before surgery, these were not significantly improved after surgery. Stiffness of the interphalangeal joints was a frequent finding; in 60% of the feet, active and passive motion of the toes was limited, regardless of the position of the toes. This limitation did not necessarily impair the functional result. In almost 20% the extensor tendons regenerated and caused the deformity to recur; in these it appeared as though the operation had never been performed.

We have found that if the deformity at the metatarsophalangeal joint is not fixed, the long flexor tendon can be tenotomized through a short incision on the plantar aspect of the toe and the proximal end can be sutured to the plantar aspect of the proximal phalanx. This reinforces active flexion at the metatarsophalangeal joint, and when the muscle power is balanced at this joint, the distal joints assume a more normal posture.

CLAWING OF LATERAL TOES

Either of the two procedures described here has in our experience satisfactorily corrected clawing of the lateral four toes.

TECHNIQUE. Beginning distally at the level of the metatarsophalangeal joint, incise the skin dorsally between the second and third metatarsals for 4 to 5 cm. Retract the medial edge of the incision and by a long oblique or Z-plastic incision divide the long extensor tendon of the second toe. Expose and completely resect the dorsal capsule of the metatarsophalangeal joint. Then forcibly plantar flex the joint into an overcorrected position. Retract the lateral edge of the incision and correct the third toe in the same manner. Now make a second incision the same length between the fourth and fifth metatarsals, lengthen the extensor tendons to these toes, and resect the dorsal capsule of the fourth and fifth metatarsophalangeal joints. Do not suture the tendons, for they will reunite spontaneously.

TECHNIQUE. Through a plantar incision on each deformed toe expose the long flexor tendon as it courses beneath the proximal two phalanges to insert into the distal phalanx, and divide it at its insertion. Correct the clawing deformity of the interphalangeal joints by capsulotomy. Then securely attach the long flexor tendon to the plantar aspect of the proximal phalanx using a nonabsorbable suture. Immobilize the toes in the straight position for 2 weeks, and allow activities as tolerated thereafter.

CLAWING OF GREAT TOE

When clawing of the great toe is caused by insufficiency of the plantar flexors of the ankle and persists after appropriate foot stabilization and tendon transfers to restore active plantar flexion of the ankle, the dynamic clawing of the great toe can best be corrected by transfer of the flexor hallucis longus from the distal to the proximal phalanx and arthrodesis of the interphalangeal joint of the great toe using the technique described for the modified Jones procedure (see below). When clawing of the great toe is caused by insufficiency of the dorsiflexors or the ankle and contracture of the tendo calcaneus, a modified Jones operation is recommended.

The principles used in the Jones operation for clawfoot (attachment of the extensor hallucis longus tendon into the first metatarsal) and for hammertoe (resection and arthrodesis of the interphalangeal joint) may be combined to treat clawing of the great toe. The extensor hallucis longus tendon is divided proximal to the interphalangeal joint; its proximal segment is attached to the neck of the first metatarsal, and its distal segment is securely anchored to the soft tissues on the dorsum of the proximal phalanx. The interphalangeal joint may or may not be fused, depending on the age of the patient. Arthrodesis is preferable, but since the epiphysis in a child is largely cartilage, fusion is difficult to obtain before skeletal maturity.

The following modification of the Jones operation is satisfactory.

TECHNIQUE (JONES, MODIFIED). Expose the interphalangeal joint of the great toe through an L-shaped incision (Fig. 66-6). Retract the flap of skin and subcutaneous tissue medially and proximally and expose the tendon of the extensor hallucis longus. Cut the tendon transversely 1 cm prox-

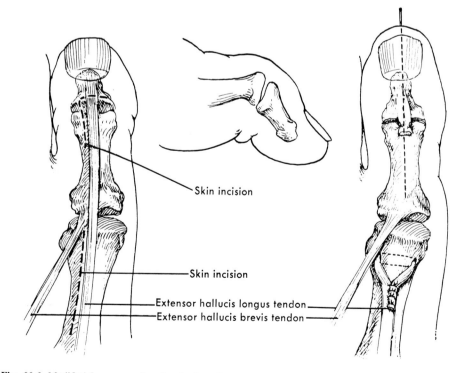

Skin incision

Skin incision

Extensor hallucis longus tendon

Extensor hallucis brevis tendon

Fig. 66-6. Modified Jones operation for clawing of great toe. Extensor hallucis longus tendon is attached to neck of first metatarsal; interphalangeal joint is arthrodesed and fixed by medullary wire and by suturing distal end of extensor hallucis longus tendon to soft tissues over proximal phalanx.

imal to the joint and expose the joint. Excise the cartilage and fit the joint surfaces together; immobilize the joint with a medullary Kirschner wire as recommended by O'Donoghue and Stauffer. Clip the wire off just beneath the skin (leave the rest in place until fusion of the joint is demonstrated roentgenographically). Now expose the neck of the first metatarsal through a 2.5 cm dorsomedial incision extending distally to the proximal extensor skin crease. Dissect free the extensor hallucis longus tendon but protect the short extensor tendon. Cleanly and carefully excise the sheath of the long extensor tendon throughout the length of the proximal incision. Beginning on the inferomedial aspect of the first metatarsal neck, drill a hole transverse to the long axis of the bone to emerge on the dorsolateral aspect of the neck. Now pass the tendon through the hole and suture it to itself with interrupted silk sutures.

This modification minimizes the chief objections to the Jones operation: the hypertrophic scar that frequently forms in the dorsal incision is eliminated by preserving a bridge of intact skin; pseudarthrosis is rare when medullary fixation and accessory cancellous bone are used; regeneration of the tendon, described by Fowler, is less likely when the tendon sheath is completely excised for 5 cm.

AFTERTREATMENT. A short leg cast is applied with the ankle in neutral position; walking on crutches is allowed in a few days. At 3 weeks the cast and skin sutures are removed and a walking short leg cast is applied. At 6 weeks the walking cast and Kirschner wire are removed and active exercises are started.

Cavus deformity and clawfoot

Clawfoot is a deformity caused by a poorly understood weakness or imbalance of one or several of the muscle groups, both intrinsic and extrinsic, which control the foot. The primary deformity is a drop or equinus of the forefoot, that is, a cavus foot. A secondary deformity is the typical clawing of the toes, with flexion of the interphalangeal joints and hyperextension of the metatarsophalangeal joints. Clawing of the toes disappears when a mild cavus deformity is corrected early but persists after correction of a more severe one of long duration. In severe cavus deformity large callosities or even ulcerations may develop beneath the metatarsal heads because of their plantar thrust, and clawing of the toes may cause dorsal dislocations of the metatarsophalangeal joints; in extreme cavus deformity all of the plantar structures may contract.

Although some clawfoot deformities are idiopathic, some result from poliomyelitis; they are therefore discussed in this chapter although the treatment usually depends on the type and severity of the deformity rather than on its cause. In idiopathic clawfoot several etiologic factors are thought to be active; usually no single factor can be held directly responsible. In most instances the cause is some lesion of the nervous system such as spina bifida and unrecognized poliomyelitis and less frequently Friedreich's ataxia, multiple sclerosis, and the progressive muscle atrophies.

Whether idiopathic or secondary to poliomyelitis or some other lesion of the nervous system, a cavus deformity is only a symptom of some primary lesion, not an entity in itself. When it is idiopathic, the triceps surae muscles are usually either normal or slightly contracted; when it is secondary to poliomyelitis, these muscles may be normal or may be contracted to varying degrees. However, a calcaneocavus deformity secondary to poliomyelitis is usually caused by weakness and overstretching of these muscles, and there is a drop of the hindfoot as well as the forefoot; a lateral roentgenogram made with the ankle held in maximal dorsiflexion by manual pressure beneath the metatarsal heads reveals the extent of both of these deformities. The treatment of paralytic calcaneocavus deformity is given on p. 2968.

The treatment of clawfoot usually depends on the type and severity of the deformity. When mild, the deformity is hard to distinguish from a normal foot with a high arch, for the cavus and slight clawing of the toes disappear with weight bearing. For this type of foot conservative measures such as a metatarsal bar on the shoe or an insole with a metatarsal pad for use by day and a splint with a metatarsal bar for use at night have been advised. But these measures will not prevent the deformity from increasing when the lesion is progressive; occasionally the progression ceases spontaneously.

Several operations have been recommended for mild cavus deformity or clawfoot, and each is based on a theory of muscle imbalance. According to Bentzon, the deformity is caused by an imbalance of the tibialis anterior and peroneus longus muscles; he recommends division of the peroneus longus tendon and imbrication of its proximal stump into the tendon of the peroneus brevis. This concept of imbalance is supported by Hallgrimsson, who notes that paralysis or weakness of the peroneus brevis muscle from overstretching or other causes is compensated for by hypertrophy of the peroneus longus; however, since the peroneus longus is inserted into the base of the first metatarsal and into the plantar aspect of the first cuneiform, this hypertrophy does not prevent varus of the hindfoot or pronation of the forefoot. Lambrinudi recommended arthrodesis of the interphalangeal joints of all toes (Fig. 66-7) on the basis that clawing of the toes is caused by paralysis or disturbance of function and balance of the intrinsic muscles of the foot, especially of the lumbrical and interosseus groups, and that the cavus deformity is secondary. The toes can no longer perform their normal functions of supporting the metatarsal heads and of propulsive action in walking. Thus, according to Lambrinudi, treatment should restore these functions, which are normally controlled by the combination action of the intrinsic muscles and the long toe flexors. After arthrodesis of the interphalangeal joints, the long flexor tendons are able to exert their whole effect on the metatarsophalangeal joints; thus the normal support of the metatarsal heads and propulsion by the toes are restored when the toes are pressed to the ground.

Garceau and Brahms also believe that pes cavus or clawfoot is caused by imbalance of the intrinsic muscles. In their opinion the chief offending muscles are the abductor hallucis, flexor hallucis brevis, flexor digitorum brevis, and quadratus plantae. They have described a technique for selective denervation of these muscles (p. 2968). In 22 of 28 patients who had this operation for cavus deformity after poliomyelitis, performance of the foot improved: bal-

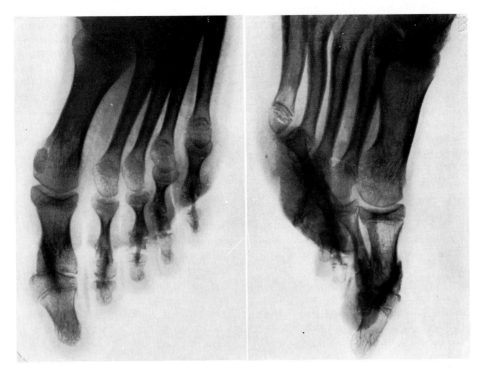

Fig. 66-7. Early cavus deformity and clawfoot may be treated by fusing interphalangeal joints with medullary autogenous grafts.

ance was better, gait was smoother, endurance on weight bearing was improved, and braces were worn with greater ease. In each patient the improvement could be attributed to correction of the deformity and to increased stability of the foot. Twelve patients had a large callosity under the base of the fifth metatarsal before surgery, and in only one did it persist after surgery. The best results are obtained when the operation is done in children before secondary skeletal deformities occur.

For the moderately severe deformity that progresses despite conservative measures and for the severe deformity in a patient too young for tarsal reconstruction, a Steindler plantar fasciotomy (see below) followed by wedging plaster casts may be indicated. Or the selective dernervation procedure of Garceau and Brahms, the osteotomy of the calcaneus as described by Dwyer (p. 2942) or the V-osteotomy of the tarsus described by Japas (p. 2946) may be used. If the dorsiflexors of the foot are weak, the Jones transfer of the extensor hallucis longus tendon (p. 2939) or the Hibbs transfer of the extensor digitorum longus tendons (p. 2943) or both are indicated.

Dwyer's operation for clawfoot or cavus deformity with varus deformity of the heel attacks the deformity of the hindfoot. It consists of dividing the contracted plantar fascia subcutaneously and removing a wedge of bone from the lateral aspect of the calcaneus to correct the varus heel; thus the foot is rendered plantigrade. Dwyer contends that after this operation weight bearing exerts a corrective influence that results in progressive decrease in the deformity. The operation is more effective before a structural deformity has developed and before the foot has stopped growing; however, he recommends the procedure routinely

for established cavus deformity. He reports 63 operations on 41 children from 3 to 16 years of age; according to him, the improvement has been striking: the gait is better, shoes are worn more normally, and the forefoot drop and clawing of the toes have decreased. For patients seen early with a high arch but with no varus of the heel he recommends plantar fasciotomy alone.

The severe deformities in skeletally mature feet are complicated by structural changes in the tarsal bones. When the hindfoot is not deformed, an anterior tarsal wedge resection is indicated. On the other hand, when there is a varus deformity of the heel, a plantar fasciotomy and stabilization of the foot by the procedure of Dunn (p. 2937), of Hoke (p. 2968), or of Siffert, Forster, and Nachamie (p. 2937) are indicated; 4 to 6 weeks later the tibialis posterior tendon is transferred to the dorsolateral aspect of the tarsus, and if indicated, deformities of the toes are corrected. Dwyer has treated older patients who have fixed deformities of the forefoot and varus of the heel by wedge osteotomy of the calcaneus and dorsal wedge resection of the tarsometatarsal region; thus not only is the deformity corrected, but also movement in the midtarsal joints is preserved.

STEINDLER OPERATION FOR CAVUS DEFORMITY

TECHNIQUE. Make a longitudinal incision along the medial side of the calcaneus and carry it distally to a point 4 cm anterior to the medial tubercle (Fig. 66-8). Separate the superficial and deep surfaces of the plantar fascia from the muscle and fat and free it throughout its breadth. Then incise the fascia transversely close to where it blends into the plantar surface of the calcaneus. With a blunt instrument strip from the periosteum of the calcaneus the muscles covered by the plantar fascia: from within outward, the abductor of the great toe, the short flexors of the toes, and the abductor of the fifth toe. Avoid removing cortical bone with the fascia and muscle attachments; otherwise new bone may form on the plantar surface of the calcaneus and cause pain on weight bearing. Continue the dissection distally to the calcaneocuboid joint and release the long plantar ligament, which extends from the calcaneus to the cuboid; this ligament is also contracted and produces a convexity of the lateral border of the foot. By dissecting close to the bone the plantar vessels are not injured. After all the structures have been released, force the foot into the corrected position. When this maneuver has not been easy, or when it has not wholly corrected the deformity, insert a Steinmann pin or Knowles pin longitudinally into the calcaneus from the tip of the heel. Close the skin with silk or wire as desired.

AFTERTREATMENT. When the deformity has been completely corrected at operation, a boot cast is applied. Seven to ten days later, the sutures are removed and a new boot cast is applied, with padding beneath metatarsal heads and over the dorsum of the foot to prevent pressure necrosis of the skin.

When the Steinmann pin or Knowles pin in the calcaneus has been used to help correct the deformity, the pin is incorporated in the cast; as the plaster hardens, the cast is molded to flatten the longitudinal arch. The cast is then gently wedged at intervals of 3 to 5 days until roentgenograms show the deformity to be corrected. This method is particularly useful in correcting a paralytic calcaneocavus deformity with elongation of the tendo calcaneus and ro-

tation of the calcaneus. In this instance the rotation of the calcaneus is the primary skeletal deformity, and unless the calcaneus is stabilized, the deformity is not only difficult to correct but is also likely to recur soon after surgery. Immobolization is continued for 3 weeks after complete correction has been obtained. The cast and pin are then removed, and a carefully molded walking boot cast is applied and is worn for 2 or 3 weeks. Metatarsal bars are then applied to the shoes, and plantar-stretching exercises are started.

OSTEOTOMY OF CALCANEUS FOR CAVUS DEFORMITY

TECHNIQUE (DWYER). First divide the plantar fascia subcutaneously to reduce the drop of the forefoot. Then expose the lateral aspect of the calcaneus through a curved incision paralleling the peroneus longus tendon but 1 cm posterior and inferior to it. Turn the entire flap anteriorly until the tendon of the peroneus longus muscle is exposed. Strip the periosteum from the superior, lateral, and inferior surfaces of the calcaneus. Now remove a wedge of bone from the calcaneus just inferior and posterior to the peroneus longus tendon and parallel with it (Fig. 66-9); make the base of the wedge 8 to 12 mm wide, and taper the wedge to but not through the medial cortex. Break the medial cortex and close the gap; bring the bony surfaces snugly together by pressing the forefoot into dorsiflexion against the pull of the tendo calcaneus. Failure to obtain closure of the gap is always caused by a small piece of bone left behind at the apex of the wedge. Now be certain that the varus deformity has been corrected and that the heel is in a neutral or even slightly valgus position; failure to correct the varus deformity completely will lead to an increase in

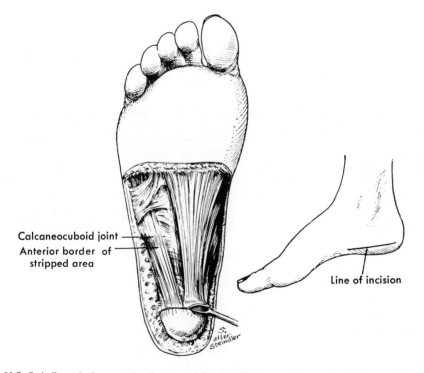

Calcaneocuboid joint
Anterior border of stripped area

Line of incision

Fig. 66-8. Steindler stripping operation for cavus deformity. *Right,* medial approach; *left,* subperiosteal stripping of long plantar ligament and origins of short plantar muscles. (Redrawn from Steindler, A.: J. Orthop. Surg. **2:**8, 1920.)

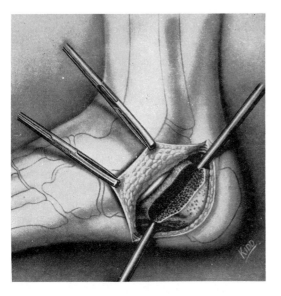

Fig. 66-9. Dwyer osteotomy of calcaneus for cavus deformity. Wedge of bone with its base lateral is resected just inferior and posterior to peroneus longus tendon and parallel to it. Medial cortex of calcaneus is not divided but is broken manually to close gap. (From Dwyer, F.C.: J. Bone Joint Surg. **41-B**:80, 1959.)

the deformity. Close the wound and immobilize the foot in a cast from the tibial tuberosity to the toes until the osteotomy is solid.

TENDON TRANSFERS FOR CLAW TOES AND CAVUS DEFORMITY

Tendon transfers are of particular advantage for cavus deformities with claw toes because they not only correct the deformities of the toes and the longitudinal arch but also may restore muscle balance. In most of these procedures the long extensor tendons of the toes are inserted into the heads of the metatarsals; thus these tendons dorsiflex the foot and ankle, and if the muscles are well balanced, the deformity does not recur.

Sherman in 1904 described such an operation and established the principles on which were based the more efficient operations of Watkins in 1912, Jones in 1916, Hibbs in 1919, and Heyman in 1932. Many minor variations of these techniques have been devised. The Jones operation for clawing of the great toe (p. 2939) and the Hibbs operation for clawing of the lateral toes (Fig. 66-10) are used most frequently.

TECHNIQUE (HIBBS). Separate the plantar structures from the calcaneus as described on p. 2941. By forcibly elevating the forefoot, correct the exaggerated arch and improve the position of the metatarsals. Now make a curved incision 7.5 to 10 cm long on the dorsum of the foot lateral to the midline and expose the common extensor tendons. Di-

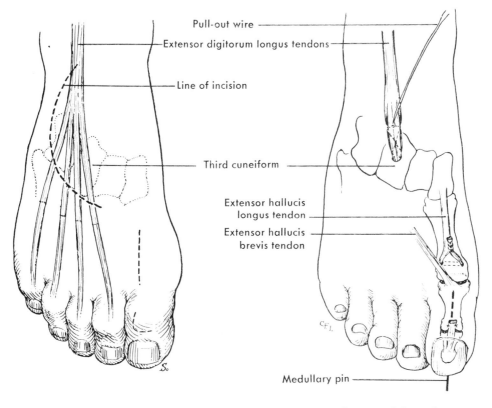

Fig. 66-10. Hibbs operation for cavus deformity and clawfoot. Tendons of extensor digitorum longus are divided, and their proximal ends are inserted as a group into third cuneiform by method of Cole. Extensor hallucis longus tendon is divided and fixed to neck of first metatarsal. Interphalangeal joint of great toe is arthrodesed and fixed with medullary pin.

vide the tendons as far distally as feasible, draw their proximal ends through a tunnel in the third cuneiform, and fix them with a nonabsorbable suture.

AFTERTREATMENT. With the foot in the corrected position, a plaster boot cast is applied and is worn for 6 weeks. Physical therapy is then started and is continued for an additional 6 weeks.

• • •

Sell, and Frank and Johnson recommend extensor shift operations in which the long toe extensor tendons are transferred to the necks or shafts of the metatarsals. In addition to increasing the power of dorsiflexion of the foot, any pronation or supination deformity of the forefoot can be corrected by anchoring the tendons to appropriate medial or lateral metatarsals (Fig. 66-11).

ANTERIOR TARSAL WEDGE OSTEOTOMY
FOR CAVUS DEFORMITY

Anterior tarsal wedge osteotomy is indicated for cavus deformity without varus of the calcaneus or gross muscle imbalance but in which the plantar structures may be contracted and the toes clawed. It corrects the cavus deformity

but preserves motion in the midtarsal and subtalar joints. It has the disadvantage of shortening the dorsum of the foot; therefore we prefer the V-osteotomy of Japas (p. 2946). Usually a Steindler plantar fasciotomy (p. 2941) is indicated as the first step in the operation. When the heel is in varus, the foot deformity must be corrected by triple arthrodesis (p. 2935), or the osteotomy may be combined with the Dwyer procedure (p. 2942).

TECHNIQUE (COLE). Make a dorsal longitudinal incision in the midline of the foot beginning just proximal to the midtarsal joints and extending distally to the level of the middle of the metatarsal shafts. Separate the extensor tendons, usually between those of the third and fourth toes. Incise the periosteum longitudinally and elevate it medially and laterally. Identify the tarsal bones with certainty. Now make an almost vertical transverse osteotomy from near the center of the navicular and cuboid to the inferior surface of the tarsus; then make a second osteotomy, beginning distal to the first and connecting with it at the inferior surface of the tarsus. The distance from the proximal to the distal osteotomy (the width of the wedge) is determined by the severity of the deformity to be corrected (Figs. 66-12 and 66-13). Then elevate the forefoot and

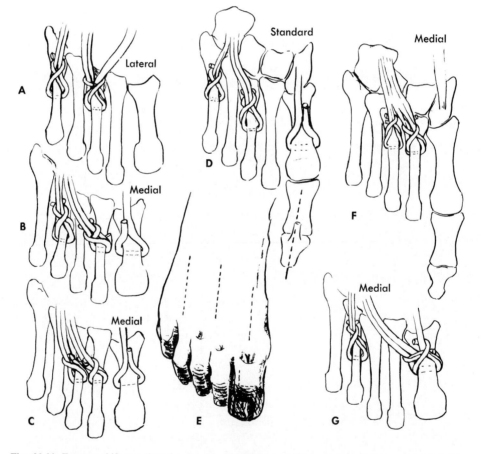

Fig. 66-11. Extensor shift operations for claw toe deformities in children. Any pronation or supination deformity is corrected by anchoring tendons to appropriate medial or lateral metatarsals. **A,** Lateral shift for supination deformity. **B,** and **C,** Medial shift for varying degrees of pronation deformity. **D,** Standard shift used in absence of pronation or supination deformity. **E,** *Broken lines,* skin incisions for standard shift. **F** and **G,** Additional medial shifts for pronation deformity. (From Frank, G.R., and Johnson, W.M.: South. Med. J. **59:**889, 1966.)

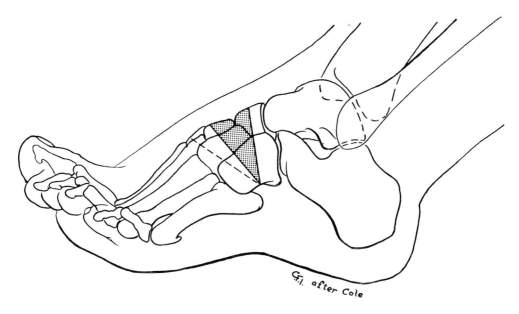

Fig. 66-12. Cole anterior tarsal wedge osteotomy for cavus deformity. *Shaded area,* wedge removed; *broken line,* distal limits of wedge. Midtarsal joints are preserved. (From Cole, W.H.: J. Bone Joint Surg. **22:**895, 1940.)

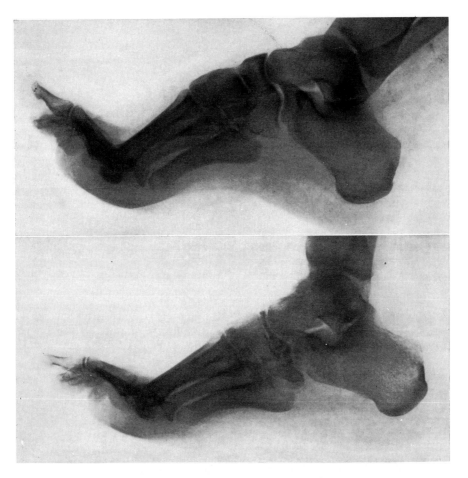

Fig. 66-13. Cavus deformity before and after anterior tarsal wedge osteotomy.

close the defect made by removal of the wedge. Close the periosteum with interrupted sutures. Apply a plaster cast from the toes to the knee.

Sometimes extensor tendons should be transferred; in these instances the tendons may be anchored into the osteotomy site at the midline of the foot. Usually, however, unless clawing of the toes is fixed, it disappears after correction of the cavus deformity.

V-OSTEOTOMY OF TARSUS FOR CAVUS DEFORMITY

The disadvantage of anterior tarsal wedge osteotomy is that the deformity is corrected by shortening the convex dorsal surface of the foot rather than by lengthening the concave plantar surface, and consequently the foot is shortened, widened, and thickened. Japas described a technique that should result in a more normal appearing foot. It consists of a V-osteotomy in which the apex of the V is proximal and at the highest point of the cavus, usually within the navicular. One limb of the V extends laterally through the cuboid to the lateral border of the foot and the other medially through the first cuneiform to the medial border. No bone is excised; instead the proximal border of the distal fragment of the osteotomy is depressed plantar-ward while the metatarsal heads are elevated, thus correcting the deformity and lengthening the plantar surface of the foot. The technique is recommended for children 6 years old or older in whom the deformity is only moderate. It too does not correct deformity of the hindfoot or midtarsal joint; any deformities in these areas should be corrected later by triple arthrodesis (p. 2935) or the Dwyer osteotomy (p. 2942).

TECHNIQUE (JAPAS). First perform a Steindler plantar fasciotomy through a medial incision on the heel (p. 2941). Then on the dorsum of the foot make a longitudinal incision 6 to 8 cm long (Fig. 66-14, *1*). Carry the dissection between the long extensor tendons of the second and third toes. Retract laterally the extensor digitorum brevis and expose extraperiosteally the dorsum of the foot from the talonavicular joint to the tarsometatarsal joints. Now using a power saw or chisel and osteotome, make the V-osteot-

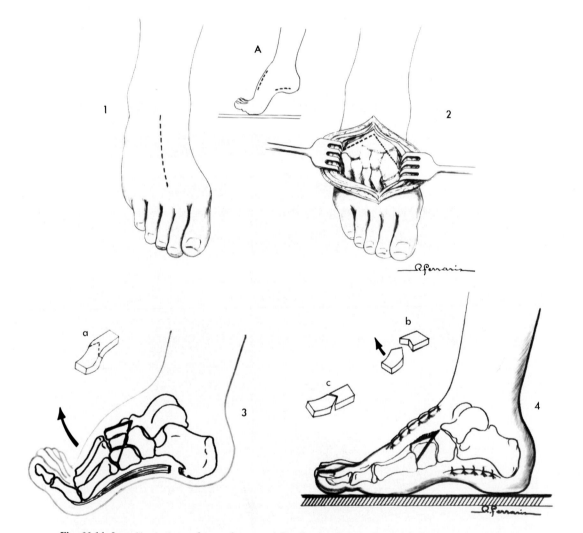

Fig. 66-14. Japas V-osteotomy of tarsus for cavus deformity. **1** and *A, Broken lines,* skin incisions. **2,** *Broken line,* location of osteotomy. **3** and *a,* Osteotomy has been completed and Steindler fasciotomy has been made. **4** and *b* and *c,* Proximal margin of distal fragment has been depressed and metatarsal heads have been elevated. (From Japas, L.M.: J. Bone Joint Surg. **50-A:**927, 1968.)

omy as follows (Fig. 66-14, *2*). Begin the medial limb of the osteotomy in the first cuneiform immediately proximal to the first metatarsocuneiform joint and the lateral limb in the cuboid immediately proximal to the joint between this bone and the fifth metatarsal; carry these limbs proximally to join in the midline of the foot at the apex of the cavus deformity, usually within the substance of the navicular. Take care not to enter the midtarsal joint. After the osteotomy has been completed, apply traction to the distal fragment and using a periosteal elevator depress its proximal margin plantarward while elevating the metatarsal heads (Fig. 66-14, *3* and *4*). If the first metatarsal is in marked equinus, carry the medial limb of the osteotomy through the base of this bone to correct the deformity. Correct any abduction or adduction deformity of the forefoot by simple manipulation. When proper alignment has been obtained, fix the osteotomy by one or two Steinmann pins inserted in a posterior direction. Remove the tourniquet, obtain hemostasis, and close the incisions. If lengthening of the tendo calcaneus is necessary, perform this procedure after the tarsal osteotomy. Apply a cast from the base of the toes to the tibial tuberosity.

AFTERTREATMENT. Immediately after surgery the limb is elevated. At 2 months the cast and Steinmann pins are removed and the foot is examined clinically and by roentgenograms. A walking boot cast is applied and is worn for 1 month. Then the cast is removed and physical therapy is started. Fig. 66-15 shows the results of a successful V-osteotomy.

DORSAL BUNION

In this deformity the shaft of the first metatarsal is dorsiflexed and the great toe is plantar flexed; it is usually the result of muscle imbalance, although occasionally there may be other causes. In its early stages the deformity is not fixed but is present only on weight bearing, especially walking; when the muscle imbalance is not corrected, however, it becomes fixed although it remains more pronounced on weight bearing.

Usually only the metatarsophalangeal joint of the great toe is flexed, and on weight bearing the first metatarsal head is displaced upward; thus the longitudinal axis of the metatarsal shaft may be horizontal or its distal end may even be directed slightly upward. The first cuneiform may

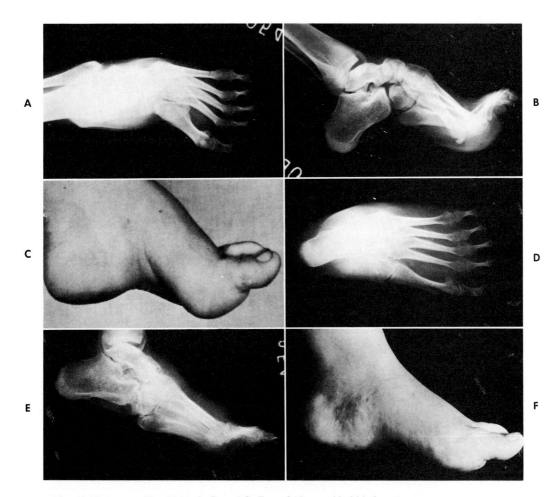

Fig. 66-15. Same as Fig. 66-14. **A, B,** and **C,** Foot of 15-year-old girl before V-osteotomy; note pes cavus. **D, E,** and **F,** Same foot 7 months after V-osteotomy; note that deformity has been corrected. (From Japas, L.M.: J. Bone Joint Surg. **50-A:**927, 1968.)

also be tilted upward. A small exostosis may form on the dorsum of the metatarsal head. When flexion of the great toe is severe enough, the metatarsophalangeal joint may even subluxate, and the dorsal part of the cartilage of the metatarsal head may eventually degenerate. The plantar part of the joint capsule and the flexor hallucis brevis muscle may both contract.

Two types of muscle imbalance may cause a dorsal bunion: the most common dorsiflexes the first metatarsal, and the plantar flexion of the great toe is secondary; the less common plantar flexes the great toe, and dorsiflexion of the first metatarsal is secondary.

The most common imbalance is between the tibialis anterior and peroneus longus muscles; normally the tibialis anterior raises the first cuneiform and the base of the first metatarsal, and the peroneus longus opposes this action. When the peroneus longus is weak, is paralyzed, or has been transferred elsewhere, the first metatarsal can be dorsiflexed by a strong tibialis anterior or by a muscle substituting for it. When the first metatarsal is dorsiflexed, the great toe becomes actively plantar flexed to establish a point of weight bearing for the medial side of the forefoot and to assist push-off in walking. Weakness of the dorsiflexor muscles of the great toe may also favor the development of this position of the toe. Lapidus and Hammond have observed that many dorsal bunions develop after ill-advised tendon transfers for residual poliomyelitis; the same has also been observed in this clinic. In such patients the opposing actions of the peroneus longus and tibialis anterior muscles on the first metatarsal had not been considered in the transfers. Before any transfer of the peroneus longus tendon, the effect of its loss on the first metatarsal must be carefully considered. When the tibialis anterior is paralyzed and tendon transfer is feasible, the peroneus longus tendon or the tendons of the peroneus longus and brevis should be transferred to the third cuneiform rather than to the insertion of the tibialis anterior; as an alternative Hammond suggests transferring the peroneus brevis tendon to the insertion of the tibialis anterior and leaving the peroneus longus tendon undisturbed. We believe that when the peroneus longus tendon is transferred, the proximal end of its distal segment should be securely fixed to bone at the level of division. When the triceps surae group is weak or paralyzed and the tibialis anterior and peroneus longus muscles are strong, the peroneus longus should not be transferred to the calcaneus unless the tibialis anterior is transferred to the midline of the foot. A dorsal bunion does not always follow ill-advised tendon transfers, for the muscle imbalance may not be severe enough to cause it. When the deformity is progressive, operation may simply consist of transferring the tibialis anterior (or the previously transferred peroneus longus) to the third cuneiform; correcting the deformity itself may then be unnecessary. But when the deformity is fixed, surgery must, of course, correct not only the muscle imbalance but also the deformity.

The second and less common muscle imbalance that can cause a dorsal bunion results from paralysis of all muscles controlling the foot except the triceps surae group, which may be of variable strength, and the long toe flexors,

which are strong. These strong toe flexors are used to help steady the foot in weight bearing and to sustain the push-off in walking. The flexor hallucis longus, of course, assumes a large share of this added function, and with active use of the great toe may be almost constantly plantar flexed; the first metatarsal head is then displaced upward to accommodate. A strong flexor hallucis brevis muscle may also help to produce the deformity. When this mechanism has caused a dorsal bunion, one of the operations described here may be used.

There are other less common causes for the deformity. It may develop in conjunction with a hallux rigidus in which dorsiflexion of the first metatarsophalangeal joint is painful. The articular surfaces become irregular, and the plantar part of the joint capsule gradually contracts; proliferation of bone on the dorsum of the first metatarsal head often becomes pronounced and blocks dorsiflexion of the joint. When walking, the patient may then unconsciously supinate the foot and plantar flex the great toe to protect the weight-bearing pad of the great toe. A dorsal bunion is also sometimes seen in a severe congenital flatfoot with a rocker-bottom deformity.

TECHNIQUE (LAPIDUS). Make a longitudinal incision over the dorsomedial aspect of the first metatarsohalangeal joint to expose the dorsal part of the capsule. Outline a dorsal tongue-shaped flap of capsular tissue with its base attached to the proximal phalanx; open the joint by reflecting this flap distally. With an osteotome remove any abnormal bone from the dorsum of the metatarsal head. Now make a second longitudinal incision along the dorsomedial border of the forefoot and expose the first metatarsocuneiform joint and if necessary also the first naviculocuneiform joint. If the tibialis anterior is overactive, detach its tendon and transfer it to the second or third cuneiform on the dorsum of the foot or into the navicular. Thus the action of the tibialis anterior in dorsiflexion of the first metatarsal shaft is eliminated. Now remove a wedge of bone from the first metatarsocuneiform joint and if necessary also from the first naviculocuneiform joint (Fig. 66-16, *A*); the base of the wedge or wedges should be inferior, and their size will depend on the severity of the deformity. Lapidus points out that a metatarsus primus varus deformity when present may be corrected at the same time by following the principles of his bunion operation (p. 883). Now detach the flexor hallucis longus tendon from its insertion and pull it proximally into the incision over the forefoot. Drill an oblique tunnel in the shaft of the first metatarsal from its proximal plantar aspect to its distal dorsal aspect. Bring the end of the flexor hallucis longus tendon dorsally through this tunnel into the wound over the toe; this converts the flexor hallucis longus into a plantar flexor of the first metatarsal and eliminates its action in plantar flexing the great toe. Completely correct the flexion contracture of the great toe by subcutaneous plantar tenotomy and capsulotomy of the first metatarsophalangeal joint just proximal to the sesamoids.

Overlap the dorsal capsular flap to place the great toe in a few degrees of dorsiflexion; if there is hallux valgus, suture the flap with more tension on its medial side. Then anchor the distal end of the transferred flexor hallucis lon-

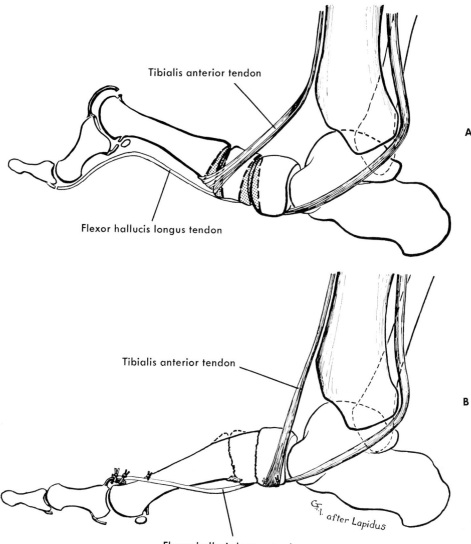

Tibialis anterior tendon

A

Flexor hallucis longus tendon

Tibialis anterior tendon

B

F.h.l. after Lapidus

Flexor hallucis longus tendon

Fig. 66-16. Lapidus operation to correct dorsal bunion. **A,** *Shaded areas,* bone to be resected and joints to be fused. **B,** Operation completed. Flexor hallucis longus has been converted to depressor of first metatarsal, and action of tibialis anterior as dorsiflexor of first metatarsal has been eliminated by transferring its insertion posteriorly. (Modified from Lapidus, P.W.: J. Bone Joint Surg. **22:**627, 1940.)

gus tendon into the capsular flap to passively reinforce the dorsal capsule. Also suture the tendon to the periosteum where it emerges from the metatarsal shaft (Fig. 66-16, *B*).

AFTERTREATMENT. A cast is applied from the toes to the knee, with the foot in the correct position. After 2 weeks it is replaced by an unpadded walking cast that permits flexion of the great toe; weight bearing is gradually resumed. Eight to ten weeks after surgery this cast is removed, an arch support is fitted in the shoe, and physical therapy is begun.

TALIPES EQUINUS

Talipes equinus is caused by a muscle imbalance at the ankle in which the plantar flexors are stronger than the dorsiflexors, or a completely flail foot may develop a fixed equinus deformity of the ankle with contracture of the tendo calcaneus and the posterior capsular structures caused by the forces of posture and gravity. If the onset of poliomyelitis is in early childhood and the muscle imbalance is great, the deformity is more severe than when the imbalance develops after skeletal maturity. When there is also a lateral muscle imbalance, an equinovarus or equinovalgus deformity will occur; management of these deformities is discussed in detail later in this chapter.

When talipes equinus cannot be corrected by conservative measures, the tendo calcaneus should be lengthened; when the deformity is of long standing and severe, a posterior capsulotomy of the ankle joint (p. 2952) may also be necessary. After the equinus deformity has been corrected, one of the following stabilizing operations should be done to prevent its recurrence: posterior bone block, Lambrinudi procedure, pantalar arthrodesis, or arthrodesis of the ankle joint. The aim of the first two operations is to make a footdrop brace unnecessary by eliminating plantar flexion at the ankle while retaining a desirable range of dorsiflexion.

Campbell devised a *posterior bone block* of the ankle in 1917 and reported it locally in 1919; in 1923 he published a report of 23 cases. In this procedure a bone block is constructed on the posterior aspect of the talus and the superior aspect of the calcaneus in such a manner that it will impinge on the posterior lip of the distal tibia and prevent plantar flexion of the ankle. In 1920 Toupet, working independently, used the same principle in an operation for equinus. The operation has been modified and popularized by Gill, Inclan, and others.

Ingram and Hundley in a long-term follow-up study (1951) of the posterior bone block in 90 patients treated at this clinic found the following complications.

1. *Recurrence of deformity.* The procedure failed in one third of those ankles in which the imbalance in the strength of the plantar flexor and dorsiflexor muscles of the ankle was severe. The results are best when the difference in strength of these muscle groups is two grades or less.

2. *Fibrous or bony ankylosis of the ankle joint.* This complication occurred in one fourth of the flail feet treated by this procedure. The construction of a massive bone block favors the development of ankylosis.

3. *Degenerative arthritis.* This was present to some extent in 40 (44.4%) of the 90 ankles studied. The changes were severe in two, with flattening of the body of the talus secondary to avascular necrosis. Mild arthritic changes were found in 19. Pain was not an important symptom, and in only one ankle with roentgenographic evidence of arthritis was endurance significantly limited. These degenerative changes in the ankle joint are probably secondary to the foot stabilization rather than to the posterior bone block.

4. *Flattening of the talus.* This occurred to some extent in 24 (26.7%) of the 90 ankles and was thought to be caused by avascular necrosis. Mild avascular necrosis cannot be distinguished roentgenographically from mild arthritic changes. Marek and Schein called attention to the fact that avascular necrosis of the body of the talus may also occur after triple arthrodesis or pantalar arthrodesis. Avascular necrosis has also occurred after the Lambrinudi procedure.

In the Lambrinudi procedure a wedge of bone is removed from the plantar and distal part of the talus so that the talus remains in complete equinus at the ankle joint while the rest of the foot is in the desired degree of plantar flexion.

MacKenzie studied 100 Lambrinudi procedures observed from 1 to 27 years; 37 were graded as good, 44 as fair, and 19 as failures. He found that many of the failures were caused by errors in technique. The significant complications that occurred in these patients were as follows.

1. *Recurrence of the deformity.* On follow-up examination 29 patients had more than 30 degrees of equinus deformity. In 7 it was caused by pseudarthrosis at the talonavicular joint and in the remaining 22 by stretching of the anterior ligaments of the ankle, which occurred as early as the first year in all age groups. About one third of the 29 patients had pain.

2. *Residual deformity of the foot.* Valgus deformity was severe enough to cause symptoms in 4 feet and varus in 26 feet. Some of the deformities were a result of technical errors at operation, but some slowly developed after surgery because the foot had not been balanced by tendon transfers.

3. *Tarsal arthritis.* Arthritis in the joints distal to the arthrodesis caused pain in five patients, but all had balanced power in the feet and led active lives. The shortest follow-up in this group was 11 years.

4. *Pseudarthrosis.* Fusion occurred in the subtalar joint in all patients, but in 13 the talonavicular joint and in 4 the calcaneocuboid joint failed to fuse. In those patients in whom the pseudarthrosis was painful, poor apposition of the bone surfaces was obvious on the roentgenograms made immediately after operation. The risk of pseudarthrosis is greater when the patient is over 20 years old at the time of operation.

5. *Arthritis of the ankle.* Roentgenograms showed arthritis of the ankle in 15 patients, but in only 12 was it painful. This complication was found in only 1 of 39 patients observed 5 years or less, but it was found in 11 of 51 patients observed more than 5 years.

6. *Flattening of the superior surface of the talus.* This complication occurred in 17 of 51 patients observed more than 5 years after the Lambrinudi procedure. It had been interpreted by Ingram and Hundley in their study of the posterior bone block as representing avascular necrosis of the talus.

When properly performed, either the posterior bone block of the ankle or the Lambrinudi procedure will produce good results in most correctly selected patients. However, the Lambrinudi procedure must be carefully planned with tracings before surgery, and this plan must be followed exactly or the results will often be unsatisfactory, whereas a posterior bone block will be successful more often than the Lambrinudi procedure when done by a surgeon who only occasionally performs foot stabilizations and blocking procedures. Either operation should be combined with suitable tendon transfers to restore active dorsiflexion of the ankle whenever possible; either alone will correct a deformity produced by gravity or by a minor muscle imbalance but cannot be expected to maintain correction against a severe muscle imbalance.

Flint and MacKenzie studied 60 feet with paralytic equinus deformity that had not been treated surgically and found anterior subluxation of the ankle in 43%. They recommend that before surgery lateral roentgenograms of the ankle be made with the foot in forced plantar flexion. If relaxation of the anterior structures of the ankle is demonstrated, then either tendons should be transferred to restore dorsiflexion or the ankle should be arthrodesed. Pyka, Coventry, and Moe noted 10 instances of anterior subluxation of the ankle in their study of 554 triple arthrodeses and presumed that this complication might in some way be related to the technique of arthrodesis.

Pantalar arthrodesis is the surgical fusion of the tibiotalar, talonavicular, and subtalar joints, and although the calcaneocuboid joint is not a joint of the talus, it is also fused. This operation is indicated as follows: (1) for patients who have calcaneus or equinus deformities combined with lateral instability of the foot, and whose leg muscles are not strong enough to control the foot and ankle when only the foot itself is stabilized, (2) for patients whose deformity has recurred after a posterior bone block or a Lambrinudi procedure, and (3) sometimes for patients with an unstable knee from paralysis of the quadriceps muscles.

Braces required for stability of the knee or foot may often be discarded after pantalar arthrodesis, and the gait becomes easier, smoother, and less fatiguing. However, the operation should not be done unless the knee will fully extend or even hyperextend a few degrees and unless there is some mechanism to protect it against recurvatum—usually functioning hamstrings, or occasionally functioning triceps surae in the absence of functioning hamstrings.

Steindler recommended a one-stage operation (p. 2956), but Leibolt and King recommended two stages, the first stabilizing the foot and the second fusing the ankle, because it is difficult to achieve and maintain the proper position of both the foot and the ankle at the same time, whereas after the foot has been stabilized in the proper weight-bearing position, the amount of equinus deformity at the ankle is relatively easy to handle.

The foot should be stabilized in a good weight-bearing position; the heel should be in the neutral position, although a little valgus is preferable to any varus. The ankle should be fused in equinus; the amount will vary with the sex of the patient and the condition for which the operation is done. Liebolt and King advise a position of 5 degrees for a man whose shoe heel is about 2 cm high and 15 degrees for a woman whose ordinary shoe heel is about 6 cm high. Thus when the foot has already been stabilized, as the first of two stages in a pantalar arthrodesis, the ankle should be fused in about 5 degrees more of equinus than when the ankle alone is fused for some condition such as traumatic arthritis (p. 1092). The correct amount of equinus may also be determined before surgery by a lateral roentgenogram made with the patient standing in shoes with heels of the desired height. However, when a pantalar arthrodesis has been done to stabilize the knee because of quadriceps weakness, the heel should not be quite high enough to compensate for the amount of equinus deformity in the ankle; thus the knee will be stabilized in full extension or even slight hyperextension on weight bearing. When there is talipes equinus or talipes calcaneus in addition to an unstable knee, whether pantalar arthrodesis will effectively stabilize the knee may be determined before surgery by applying a short leg walking cast with the foot in about 10 degrees of equinus deformity; if the cast stabilizes the knee, the knee will then be stable after surgery if the ankle is fused in the proper position.

Waugh, Wagner, and Stinchfield reviewed 116 pantalar arthrodeses in 97 patients observed for 2 to 22 years after surgery. In most instances the operation had been carried out for poliomyelitis. The results were the same regardless of whether the operation had been performed in one stage of two. Function was best when the ankle had been fused in 5 to 10 degrees of plantar flexion. The ideal patient for the operation was one with a flail foot and ankle and normal muscles about the hip and knee. But in patients with a flail limb, stability of the knee was increased by genu recurvatum when the foot had been placed in a little more plantar flexion than usual.

Arthrodesis of the ankle is rarely indicated for talipes equinus. Barr and Record, however, have found it a satisfactory method of stabilizing the ankle in adults whose muscle function is too weak to permit tendon transfers and tarsal arthrodesis aimed at restoring active dorsiflexion of the ankle.

In summary, other factors being equal, our preference among procedures to correct talipes equinus is in descending order as follows: (1) posterior bone block, (2) Lambrinudi procedure, (3) pantalar arthrodesis, and (4) arthrodesis of the ankle.

LENGTHENING OF TENDO CALCANEUS
BY INCOMPLETE TENOTOMY

White in 1943 described a method of lengthening the tendo calcaneus that he had used for many years. It is based on his observation that the tendon rotates about 90 degrees on its longitudinal axis between its origin and insertion; the rotation from the posterior view is from medial to lateral.

TECHNIQUE (WHITE). Expose the tendo calcaneus through a posteromedial longitudinal incision 10 cm long. Near its insertion divide the anterior two thirds of the tendon; while moderate force is applied to dorsiflex the foot, divide the medial two thirds of the tendon 5 to 8 cm proximal to the site of the first division. Dorsiflexion of the foot lengthens the tendon; suture of the tendon is unnecessary.

AFTERTREATMENT. Aftertreatment is the same as for Z-plastic tenotomy (p. 2952).

• • •

Cummins et al., who studied 100 calcaneal tendons, found varying degrees of rotation and classed them for convenience into three groups. In the first group (52%), those with the least rotation, the soleus composed one third of the posterior surface and the gastrocnemius two thirds. In the second group (35%) the soleus composed half of the posterior surface and the gastrocnemius half. In the third group (13%), those with extreme rotation, the soleus composed two thirds of the posterior surface and the gastrocnemius only one third. The rotation began about 12 to 15 cm proximal to the insertion of the tendon, that is, at about the level at which the soleus begins to contribute fibers to the tendon. From these observations Hauser devised the following lengthening operation.

TECHNIQUE (HAUSER). Expose the tendon through a posteromedial longitudinal incision. Incise the tendon transversely at a level 8 to 12 cm proximal to its insertion, depending on the amount of correction desired as follows. Insert a tenotome transversely into the tendon with the flat surfaces facing anteriorly and posteriorly and so that two thirds of the tendon is posterior to the blade; then turn the sharp edge of the blade posteriorly and cut through the tendon to its posterior surface. Then incise the tendon 1.2 cm proximal to its insertion as follows. Insert a curved tenotome anterior to the medial two thirds of the tendon and draw it posteriorly and medially to partially divide the tendon at this point. The tendon lengthens as the foot is dorsiflexed.

AFTERTREATMENT. Aftertreatment is the same as for Z-plastic tenotomy (see below).

Z-PLASTIC TENOTOMY OF TENDO CALCANEUS AND POSTERIOR CAPSULOTOMY

The procedures just described are often sufficient if the tendon has not been lengthened previously by surgery, but if it has, the resultant scarring requires a Z-plastic operation in either the anteroposterior or lateral plane. We usually prefer the lateral plane because the width of the tendon is thus preserved and the amount of residual exposed cut surface is less. When the deformity cannot be completely corrected by such a tenotomy, posterior capsulotomy of the ankle is indicated.

In an equinovarus deformity Z-plastic lengthening of the tendo calcaneus in the anteroposterior plane that leaves the lateral half attached to the calcaneus (see Fig. 61-27) is usually preferable because the tendon is often inserted medially and favors recurrence of the hindfoot varus deformity. Other structures, especially the tibialis posterior tendon, must usually also be lengthened to obtain satisfactory correction (see posteromedial release, p. 2641).

TECHNIQUE. Place the patient on the unaffected side or prone. Make a longitudinal incision 8 to 10 cm long medial to the tendo calcaneus, incise the tendon sheath, and grasp its edges with small hemostats for accurate closure later. With a knife divide the tendon longitudinally from side to side, beginning proximally and continuing distally for 8 to 10 cm. Proximally complete the division posteriorly and distally complete it anteriorly to leave a posterior flap of tendon attached to the calcaneus and an anterior flap attached to the gastrocnemius and soleus muscles. At this stage the foot can usually be fully dorsiflexed by manual force. While it is held in dorsiflexion, appose the raw surfaces of the tendon flaps and suture them together without tension. The only residual raw area of tendon is in the superior part of the wound, and it is covered when the sheath and subcutaneous fat are closed. Therefore the possibility that the tendon may adhere to the skin is reduced because its distal and more superficial part is smooth and uninterrupted posteriorly, whereas the raw area is proximal and relatively deep to the skin.

To lengthen the tendon in the anteroposterior plane make the division longitudinally in the midline of the tendon. Sever one half laterally at the proximal end and the other half medially at the distal end.

If the posterior part of the ankle capsule is contracted, dorsiflexing the foot completely may be impossible after division of the tendo calcaneus alone; in this instance continue the dissection in the midline posteriorly and retract medialward the flexor hallucis longus tendon, which passes obliquely across the capsule on the medial side. Protect the nerves, vessels, and tendons posterior to the medial malleolus. Then expose the capsule and incise it transversely to allow full dorsiflexion.

AFTERTREATMENT. A cast is applied from the midthigh to the toes with the knee in 30 degrees of flexion and the ankle in the desired degree of dorsiflexion. However, before the cast is applied, the skin over the tendo calcaneus just proximal to the heel must be carefully inspected with the foot in the desired position. If the skin is blanched or under undue tension, the edges of the wound may slough and expose the tendon, or the sloughing may even involve a part of the tendon itself and cause fibrosis, which will add to the danger that the deformity will recur. If the skin is taut, the deformity should be only partially corrected, and the foot should be held in this position in a cast until the acute reaction has subsided; thus sloughing is avoided. At 6 weeks the cast is removed, passive and active exercises are begun, and walking is allowed in a brace that permits dorsiflexion but prevents plantar flexion.

When an equinus deformity recurs after surgery, scarring may be marked and involve the skin and subcutaneous tissues as well as the deeper structures. This not only provides a poor field for surgery but also increases the possibility of repeated recurrence of the deformity. After correction of a recurrent equinus deformity, sloughs resulting from circulatory insufficiency are common. When the recurrent deformity is extreme, excising the superficial scar tissue and replacing it with a full-thickness skin graft may be advisable before correcting the equinus position.

POSTERIOR BONE BLOCK

This procedure is usually combined with a triple arthrodesis; thus the foot is stabilized against medial and lateral motions, but dorsiflexion in the ankle is preserved.

TECHNIQUE (CAMPBELL). Incise the skin along the medial border of the tendo calcaneus from its insertion on the calcaneus proximally in a straight line for 7.5 to 10 cm. If the tendo calcaneus is contracted, lengthen it by the Z-plastic method; otherwise retract it laterally. Now make a straight incision through the deep structures in the midline to the posterior surface of the ankle joint and retract the tendon of the flexor hallucis longus medially. Using a periosteal elevator, clear a pyramidal space and expose the posterior surfaces of the tibia, ankle joint, and subtalar joint and the superior surface of the calcaneus. Then dorsiflex the foot and bring the posterior surface of the talus into view. Resect this part of the talus and immediately below excavate a wedge from the superior aspect of the calcaneus so that the posterior surface of the remaining part of the talus makes a smooth coronal plane with one side of the cavity in the calcaneus (Fig. 66-17, *B*). Take great care to avoid denuding the posterior surface of the tibia; otherwise, the bone block may unit with it and fuse the ankle joint. The foot usually must be stabilized by a triple arthrodesis (p. 2935); the fragments of bone removed during this procedure may be used for the bone block. Denude them of cartilage and insert the largest, which is usually the head of the talus or the navicular, into the cavity prepared in the superior part of the calcaneus in close apposition to the ankle joint posteriorly. Then arrange small particles of bone in a pyramid above the wedge. Place the cartilage removed from the bone fragments in a mosaic fashion over the posterior, medial, and lateral aspects of the pyramid to help prevent adhesions to surrounding structures. However, using bone from the foot is by no means essential; the results are equally good when cancellous bone without cartilage is obtained elsewhere.

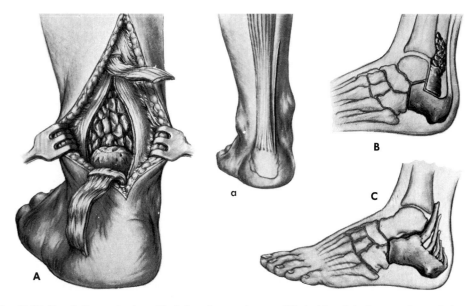

Fig. 66-17. Campbell posterior bone block for talipes equinus. **a,** Skin incision. Joint is exposed posteriorly be retracting tendo calcaneus or by dividing it by Z-plasty. **A,** Operation completed. Large block of bone is in place, and many small chips have been placed above it in shape of pyramid. **B,** Relation of grafts to subtalar and ankle joints and to posterior surface of tibia. **C,** Bone block operation has been carried out by reflecting bone superiorly and anteriorly from superior surface of calcaneus.

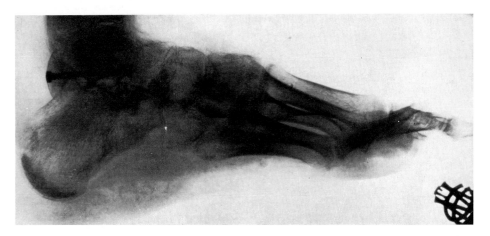

Fig. 66-18. Campbell posterior bone block. Block of bone obtained from excised head of talus has been placed beneath posterior lip of tibia and fixed with one screw.

Grafts of cancellous bone taken from the femur when correcting genu valgum and from the ilium when transferring its crest for flexion contractures of the hip have proved efficient. When only a single piece of bone is available, shape it to fit the defect and transfix it to the posterior surface of the talus with a single screw (Fig. 66-18). This modification assures union with the block in the proper position. Suture the soft tissue snugly to hold the transplants in place. Suture the tendo calcaneus if divided and close the fascia and skin.

When the foot has already been stabilized, another modification is to reflect several flaps of bone anteriorly and superiorly from the superior surface of the calcaneus (Fig. 66–17, *C*).

AFTERTREATMENT. The extremity is immobilized in a long leg cast with the ankle in neutral position or in slight dorsiflexion, the foot in proper alignment with the malleoli, and the knee in 20 degrees of flexion. When multiple bone chips are used, the foot must be held at exactly a right angle to the leg; otherwise either a calcaneus deformity will result or the bone block will not be effective. A window is cut in the cast on the anterior surface of the foot and leg to allow for swelling. The extremity is then elevated until all swelling has subsided.

At 10 to 14 days after the operation the patient is prepared for general anesthesia. The cast and sutures are removed, and roentgenograms in two planes are obtained. If the position of the foot is not satisfactory clinically and

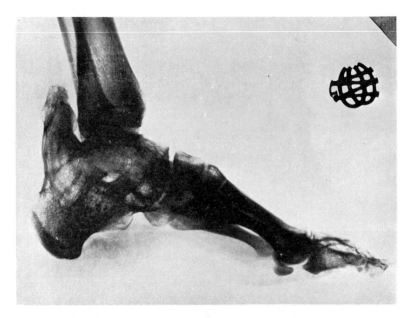

Fig. 66-19. Eighteen years after Campbell posterior bone block for talipes equinus.

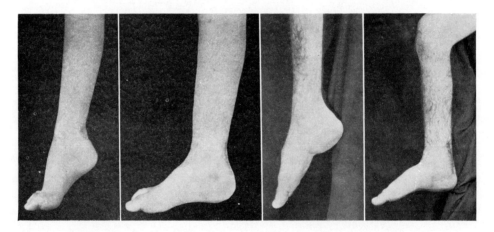

Fig. 66-20. Foot before and after Campbell posterior bone block in two patients.

roentgenographically, the patient is anesthetized and the foot is manipulated. A lightly padded boot cast is applied, and the patient is allowed up on crutches. Six weeks after operation a walking boot cast is applied to be worn until consolidation is complete; when either a triple arthrodesis or a posterior bone block or both have been done, this is usually a total of 3 months after operation. After the cast is removed, the bone block should be protected by a foot-drop brace that eliminates plantar flexion at the ankle yet allows dorsiflexion. The brace is usually worn for 6 months. Figs. 66-19 and 66-20 show the results of Campbell posterior bone block.

TECHNIQUE (GILL). Through a longitudinal skin incision divide the tendo calcaneus by a Z-shaped cut. After exposing the ankle and the superior aspect of the calcaneus, dorsiflex the foot as much as possible and bring into view the posterior part of the superior articular surface of the talus. Using a broad thin osteotome, lift up from posteriorly the

cartilage together with a thin layer of bone from the talus and appose it to the posterior lip of the tibia (Fig. 66-21). The apex of the wedge-shaped space thus formed lies beneath the cartilage anterior to the posterior lip of the tibia. Then remove a wedge of bone from the superior aspect of the calcaneus and drive it into the space, thus holding the foot in dorsiflexion. Suture the tendo calcaneus and the incision in the usual manner.

AFTERTREATMENT. The foot is immobilized in slight dorsiflexion with a plaster cast for 3 months.

• • •

Irwin modified the Gill procedure by inserting a bone peg into the talus to support the osteocartilaginous flap raised from the posterior surface of the talus. Inclan combined the principles of the Campbell and Gill techniques: an osteocartilaginous flap is elevated from the posterior aspect of the articular surface of the talus; this is held in

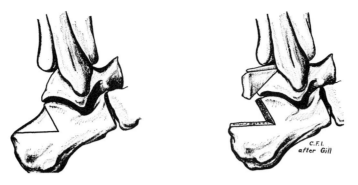

Fig. 66-21. Gill technique of posterior bone block for talipes equinus. (Redrawn from Gill, A.B.: J. Bone Joint Surg. **15**:166, 1933.)

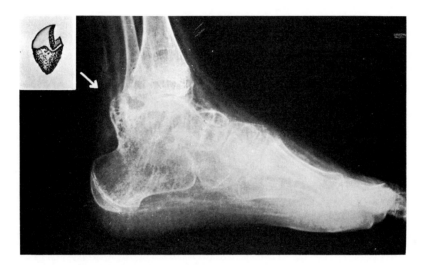

Fig. 66-22. Inclan technique of posterior bone block that combines principles of Campbell and Gill techniques. (Courtesy Dr. Alberto Inclan.)

position by the head of the talus, which has been excised during triple arthrodesis and fashioned into the shape of a cockscomb (Fig. 66-22). One raw surface comes in contact with the back of the body of the talus and another with the superior surface of the calcaneus. The posterior part of the block consists of the articular surface of the head of the talus and provides a smooth surface for the tendons.

LAMBRINUDI OPERATION

TECHNIQUE (LAMBRINUDI). With the foot and ankle in extreme plantar flexion make a lateral roentgenogram and trace the film. Cut the tracing into three pieces along the outlines of the subtalar and midtarsal joints; from these pieces the exact amount of bone to be removed from the talus can be determined with accuracy before operation. In the tracing the line representing the articulation of the talus with the tibia is of course left undisturbed, but that corresponding to its plantar and distal parts is to be so cut that when the navicular and the calcaneocuboid joint are later fitted to it the foot will be in slight equinus relation to the leg (Fig. 66-23). Five to ten degrees is best unless the extremity has shortened; more may then be desirable.

Expose the tarsus through a long lateral curved incision.

Section the peroneal tendons by a Z-shaped cut, open the talonavicular and calcaneocuboid joints, and divide the interosseous and fibular collateral ligaments of the ankle to permit complete medial dislocation of the tarsus at the subtalar joint. With a small power saw (more accurate than a chisel or osteotome) remove the predetermined wedge of bone from the plantar and distal parts of the neck and body of the talus. Remove the cartilage and bone from the superior surface of the calcaneus to form a plane parallel with the longitudinal axis of the foot. Next make a V-shaped trough transversely in the inferior part of the proximal navicular and denude the calcaneocuboid joint of enough bone to correct any lateral deformity. Firmly wedge the sharp distal margin of the remaining part of the talus into the prepared trough in the navicular and appose the calcaneus and talus. Take care to place the distal margin of the talus well medially in the trough; otherwise the position of the foot will not be satisfactory. (Obviously, no attempt should be made to compensate in the foot for any tibial torsion.) The talus is now locked in the ankle joint in complete equinus, and the foot cannot be further planter flexed. Suture the peroneal tendons and close the wound in the routine manner.

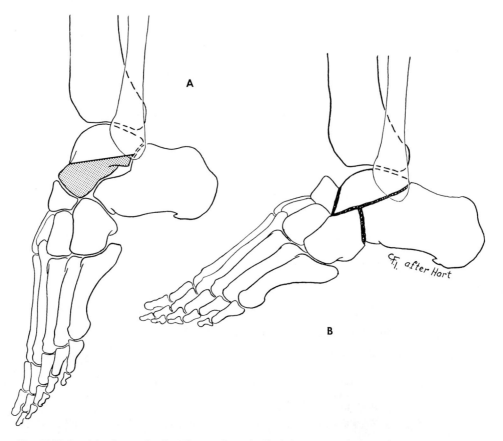

Fig. 66-23. Lambrinudi operation for talipes equinus. **A,** *Shaded area,* part of talus to be resected. **B,** Sharp distal margin of remaining part of talus has been wedged into prepared trough in navicular, and raw osseous surfaces of talus, calcaneus, and cuboid have been apposed. (From Hart, V.L.: J. Bone Joint Surg. **22:**937, 1940.)

AFTERTREATMENT. Aftertreatment is the same as for posterior bone block (p. 2953).

PANTALAR ARTHRODESIS

TECHNIQUE (STEINDLER). Make an anterolateral incision (Fig. 2-5) just anterior to the tip of the lateral malleolus; this incision is preferred here to Kocher's so as not to disturb the inferior ligaments of the talus any more than necessary and to protect the blood supply to the talus. Retract the toe extensors medially, divide the lateral ligaments of the ankle, and open the ankle joint by extreme supination and adduction of the foot, as in the Whitman talectomy. To expose the subtalar joint as well as the ankle joint, mobilize the talus by dividing all ligaments to the neighboring bones except the inferior ligament. Remove the articular cartilage of the tibia and fibula and of the body of the talus. Now pull the talus proximally and remove the cartilage from the subtalar joint, including the facet of the sustentaculum tali. Denude the talonavicular and calcaneocuboid joints. Correct any lateral deformity by removing bone from the subtalar and midtarsal joints.

TECHNIQUE (LIEBOLT)

Stage 1. This consists of stabilization of the foot by Hoke's method (p. 2937).

Stage 2—arthrodesis of the ankle. Approach the ankle joint through an anterior incision 12.5 cm long and divide the transverse crural and cruciate ligaments. Retract me-

dially the extensor hallucis longus and tibialis anterior tendons, the dorsalis pedis artery and vein, and the deep peroneal nerve; retract the extensor digitorum longus tendons laterally. Divide and ligate the anterior lateral malleolar artery and vein. Then remove the articular cartilage from the ankle joint along with enough bone to correct the deformity and to place the foot in the desired position. With a curved osteotome roughen the apposing surfaces for good bony contact between the talus and tibia. Next incise the periosteum over the distal tibial metaphysis but avoid stripping the periosteum over the epiphyseal cartilage. Remove some bone from the tibial metaphysis well proximal to the epiphyseal plate and wedge small chips of it into the ankle joint, especially between the talus and the malleoli, to fill the space created by removal of the cartilage; also place a few anteriorly over the ankle joint. If the distal tibial epiphyseal plate has not closed, every effort should be made to avoid damaging it.

AFTERTREATMENT. A cast is applied from the groin to the toes, immobilizing the knee in moderate flexion and the ankle in the desired equinus position; the forefoot should be in maximum dorsiflexion in relation to the hindfoot, for this is its weight-bearing position. Roentgenograms are made, and the amount of equinus is determined by the angle of intersection between a line drawn down the shaft of the tibia and another drawn from the inferior surface of the first metatarsal head to the lowest point of the calcaneus. If the position is not exactly as desired, the plaster should be wedged within a few days after surgery. At 6 weeks a short leg walking cast is applied. When fusion is sufficiently advanced, weight bearing is started. Immobilization is continued until roentgenograms reveal solid fusion.

ARTHRODESIS OF ANKLE

One technique for arthrodesis of the ankle for talipes equinus has just been described, and that for talipes equinovarus is described on p. 2961. Other techniques for arthrodesis of the ankle are described in Chapter 38.

TALIPES EQUINOVARUS

Talipes equinovarus caused by poliomyelitis is characterized by equinus deformity of the ankle, inversion of the heel, and at the midtarsal joints adduction and supination of the forefoot. When the deformity is of long duration, there is also a cavus deformity of the foot; clawing of the toes may develop secondary to substitution of motor patterns.

The pathogenesis of paralytic talipes equinovarus is as follows. The peroneal muscles are paralyzed or severely weakened, but the tibialis posterior is usually normal and thus stronger than the peroneals; the tibialis anterior may be weakened or it may be normal; the triceps surae is comparatively strong and becomes contracted by a combination of forces: motor imbalance, growth, gravity, and posture. The equinus position thus produced increases the mechanical advantage of the tibialis posterior; this in turn encourages the fixation of hindfoot inversion and forefoot adduction and supination. Cavus deformity and clawing of the toes develop when the toe extensors help a weak tibialis anterior to dorsiflex the ankle; after the triceps surae becomes contracted, clawing of the toes is even more pronounced. When there is external torsion of the tibia, a brace may also contribute to an equinovarus deformity unless this torsion is considered during construction of the brace. After the deformity is established, its rate of increase is determined by the forces of growth, muscle imbalance, and abnormal posture and weight bearing.

The treatment of paralytic talipes equinovarus depends on the age of the patient, the forces causing the deformity, the severity of the deformity, and its rate of increase.

When treating a skeletally immature foot, a brace may be indicated to help prevent the deformity; it is of the double bar type with a 90-degree ankle stop and an outside T-strap. When there is external tibial torsion, the shoe is attached to the brace in an externally rotated position; otherwise the deformity will be aggravated (if an equinus deformity has become fixed, the heel may have to be elevated). The plantar fascia and the posterior ankle structures are stretched regularly. If the deformity increases despite these measures, an attempt should be made to correct it with the wedging cast technique; this is usually successful when the deformity is not too severe. Rarely Steindler fascial stripping (p. 2941), tendo calcaneus lengthening (p. 2952), and posterior capsulotomy (p. 2952) may be necessary. After the deformity has been corrected, surgery is then indicated to prevent its recurrence. The tibialis posterior is usually strong, and *unless its influence is removed, the deformity will recur.* In most instances it should be

transferred anteriorly through the interosseous membrane to the anterolateral tarsal area, as recommended by Barr and Blount. Occasionally it may be transferred posteriorly to reinforce a weak triceps surae. When the tibialis posterior is weak, the tibialis anterior if strong enough may be split and a portion of it transferred to the insertion of the peroneus brevis as described by Hoffer et al. External tibial torsion of 30 degrees or more should be corrected by derotational osteotomies of the tibia and fibula (p. 2983).

When treating a skeletally mature foot for this deformity, the following plan is used: the foot is stabilized by a triple arthrodesis and the cavus is corrected at the same time by a Steindler plantar fasciotomy. If the operation does not completely correct the deformity, the cast is removed 10 days later, the foot is manipulated with the patient under general anesthesia, and a new long leg cast is then applied. If further correction is necessary, the cast may be wedged at 3- to 5-day intervals until the deformity is corrected both clinically and roentgenographically. Four to six weeks after the first operation the tendo calcaneus is lengthened, the extensor hallucis longus is transferred to the neck of the first metatarsal (modified Jones operation, p. 2939), and the tendon of the tibialis posterior is transferred to the anterolateral tarsal area through the interosseous membrane. When the tibialis posterior is weak, the tendon of the tibialis anterior is transferred to a point slightly lateral to the midline on the dorsum of the foot. External tibial torsion is corrected by derotational osteotomies of the tibia and fibula. A new long leg cast is then applied.

ANTERIOR TRANSFER OF TIBIALIS POSTERIOR TENDON

In paralytic talipes equinovarus anterior transfer of the tibialis posterior tendon serves two purposes: it removes a dynamic deforming force and aids in active dorsiflexion of the foot. Unfortunately active dorsiflexion is rarely restored satisfactorily by this transfer alone. When no other functional dorsiflexors are present or are available for transfer, anterior transfer of the tibialis posterior tendon should be combined with a triple arthrodesis and a posterior bone block of the ankle. The tendon is preferably transferred through the interosseous membrane, although it may be rerouted around the medial side of the tibia. According to Blount, Ludloff described in German the method of transfer through the interosseous membrane; in the United States Barr pointed out the merits of the procedure and advocated its use in properly selected patients. Watkins et al. have reported favorably on it; more recently Gunn and Molesworth, using a technique similar to that of Barr, reported satisfactory results in 49 of 50 transfers. However, Lipscomb and Sanchez reported satisfactory results in 9 of 10 feet in which the tendon was transferred around the medial side of the tibia according to the technique of Ober.

When the extensor digitorum longus is active, the transfer may be supplemented by the Hibbs operation for claw toes (p. 2943) to increase the power of dorsiflexion; however, triple arthrodesis and usually posterior bone block are still indicated if the foot is mature enough.

TECHNIQUE (BARR). Make a skin incision on the medial side of the ankle, beginning distally at the insertion of the tibialis posterior tendon and extending proximally over the tendon just posterior to the malleolus and from there proximally along the medial border of the tibia for 5 to 7.5 cm. Free the tendon from its insertion, preserving as much of its length as possible. Split its sheath and free it in a proximal direction until the distal 5 cm of the muscle has been mobilized. Carefully preserve the nerves and vessels supplying the muscle. Make a second skin incision anteriorly: begin it distally at the level of the ankle joint and extend it proximally for 7.5 cm just lateral to the tibialis anterior tendon. Carry the dissection deep between the tendons of the tibialis anterior and the extensor hallucis longus, carefully preserving the dorsalis pedis artery; expose the interosseous membrane just proximal to the malleoli. Now cut a generous window in the interosseous membrane but avoid stripping the periosteum from the tibia or fibula. Then pass the tibialis posterior tendon through the window between the bones with care that it is not kinked, twisted, or constricted and that the vessels and nerves to the muscle are not damaged. Pass the tendon beneath the cruciate ligament; the ligament may be divided if necessary to relieve pressure on the tendon. Expose the third cuneiform or the base of the third metatarsal through a transverse incision 2.5 cm long. Retract the extensor tendons, sharply incise the periosteum over the bone in a cruciate fashion, and fold back osteoperiosteal flaps. Now drill a hole through the bone in line with the tendon and large enough to receive it; anchor it in the bone with a pull-out wire according to the method of Cole (p. 12). Be sure that the button on the plantar surface of the foot is well padded. Now suture the osteoperiosteal flaps to the tendon with two figure-of-eight silk sutures. Close the incision and apply a plaster cast to hold the foot in calcaneovalgus position.

Instead of the long medial incision used by Barr, we make a short longitudinal one to free the tibialis posterior tendon at its insertion and withdraw it through another incision 5 cm long at the musculotendinous junction just posterior to the subcutaneous border of the tibia (Fig. 66-24). Further, we anchor the tendon by passing it through a hole drilled in the bone, looping it back, and suturing it to itself with nonabsorbable sutures. This fixation is more secure than that obtained by the method of Cole.

AFTERTREATMENT. The cast is removed at 3 weeks, the wounds are inspected, the sutures are removed, and a new boot walking cast is applied with the foot in the neutral position and the ankle in slight dorsiflexion. Six weeks after operation the cast is removed and a program of rehabilitative exercises is started that is continued under supervision until a full range of active resisted function is obtained. The transfer is protected for 6 months by a double bar foot drop brace with an outside T-strap.

TECHNIQUE (OBER). Through a medial longitudinal incision 7.5 cm long free the tibialis posterior tendon from its attachment to the navicular (Fig. 66-25). Now make a second longitudinal medial incision 10 cm long centered over the musculotendinous junction of the tibialis posterior. Withdraw the tendon from the proximal wound and free the muscle belly well up on the tibia. Strip the periosteum obliquely on the medial surface of the tibia so that when the tendon is moved into the anterior tibial compartment only the belly of the muscle will come in contact with denuded bone. The tendon *must not* be in contact with the tibia. Make a third incision over the base of the third metatarsal, draw the tibialis posterior tendon from the second into the third incision, and anchor its distal end in the base of the third metatarsal.

Hatt modified this procedure by anchoring the transferred tibialis posterior tendon in the second cuneiform. He used Cole's method (p. 12) to anchor it and reinforced the new insertion with several stay sutures.

AFTERTREATMENT. Aftertreatment is the same as for the Barr technique just mentioned.

TRANSFER OF TIBIALIS ANTERIOR TENDON FOR PARALYSIS
OF PERONEAL MUSCLES

This operation is perhaps the most successful of all tendon transfers about the foot.

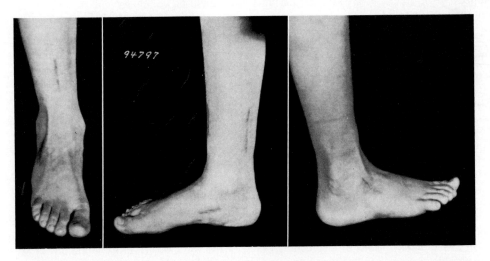

Fig. 66-24. Result of anterior transfer of tibialis posterior tendon through interosseous membrane. Foot is in mild valgus position, and result would have been better if transferred tendon had been anchored nearer midline of foot. Note small scar at normal insertion of tibialis posterior tendon and another over musculotendinous junction of tibialis posterior muscle just posterior to subcutaneous border of tibia.

TECHNIQUE. Make a longitudinal incision 5 cm long on the medial border of the foot at the joint between the first metatarsal and first cuneiform. Locate and divide the insertion of the tibialis anterior tendon on the undersurface of these bones (Fig. 66-26). Then incise the anterior surface of the distal third of the leg in the midline longitudi-

nally for 7.5 cm and expose in medial to lateral sequence the tendons of the tibialis anterior, extensor hallucis longus, and extensor digitorum longus. Open the sheath of the tibialis anterior tendon, elevate the tendon with a hemostat, and with steady traction withdraw it from the wound. Now make a third incision over the anterolateral

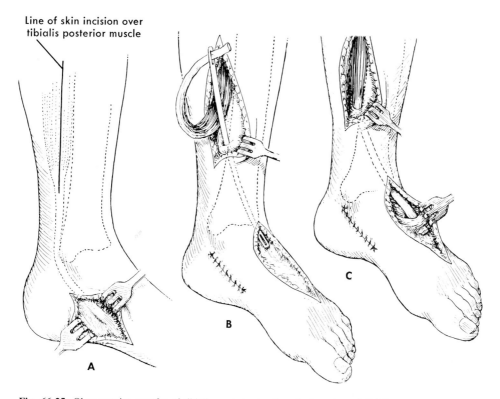

Fig. 66-25. Ober anterior transfer of tibialis posterior tendon. **A,** Insertion of tibialis posterior tendon has been exposed. Note line of skin incision over muscle. **B,** Tendon has been freed from its insertion and muscle has been dissected from tibia. **C,** Tendon and muscle have been passed through anterior tibial compartment to dorsum of foot, and tendon has been anchored in third metatarsal. (Redrawn from Ober, F.R.: N. Engl. J. Med. **209:**52, 1933.)

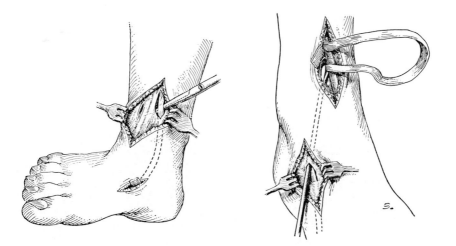

Fig. 66-26. Transfer of tibialis anterior tendon for paralysis of peroneal muscles. Tendon is freed at its insertion, is rerouted to lateral side of foot, and is attached to cuboid or to divided tendon of peroneus brevis muscle.

aspect of the foot and expose the midtarsal area. Carry the dissection toward the midline of the foot and incise the sheath of the extensor digitorum longus tendon. Pass a hemostat proximally within the sheath toward the second incision in the distal third of the leg; through this incision split the sheath over the end of the hemostat enough to admit the hemostat into the incision. Now grasp the free end of the tibialis anterior tendon with the hemostat and draw it through the sheath of the extensor digitorum longus into the wound on the anterolateral side of the foot. Determining exactly where the tendon should be anchored to the distal tarsus is important. When the tibialis posterior muscle is strong, the tendon should be anchored in line with the fourth ray; on the other hand, when this muscle is weak, the tendon should be anchored in line with the second or third ray. With a 4.3 mm drill and a curet next make a tunnel through the cuboid or second or third cuneiform, as indicated, from proximally and anteriorly in a distal, lateral, and plantar direction. Stitch a silk suture into the end of the tibialis anterior tendon; advance the suture proximally along the medial border of the tendon, across the tendon, and back distally along its opposite border. Draw the two ends of the suture through the tunnel in the bone from proximally to distally, using a wire loop. With the foot in dorsiflexion draw the tendon through the tunnel and when possible suture it on itself under physiologic tension. When the tendon is not long enough to fix in this manner draw it distally under moderate tension and fix it securely to bone by a platform type of staple. Or, if desired, omit drilling a hole in the cuboid: divide the tendon of the peroneus brevis behind the lateral malleolus, transpose its distal segment anteriorly, and suture it to the transferred tibialis anterior tendon. This method was described by White.

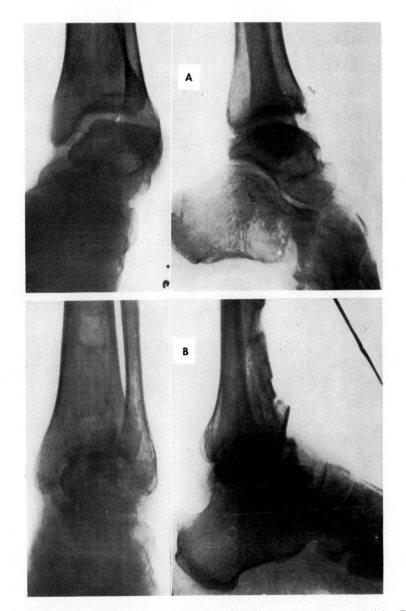

Fig. 66-27. A, Paralytic equinovarus deformity. Notice supination of body of talus in ankle joint. **B,** After anterior arthrodesis of ankle. (Courtesy Dr. J.A. Orris.)

AFTERTREATMENT. A boot cast is applied with the foot at a right angle to the leg. When the operation has consisted of the tendon transfer alone, the cast is bivalved after 3 weeks, and active and passive exercises are started, with care not to place the tendon under excessive strain. Six weeks after surgery an ankle brace that prevents plantar flexion is fitted. At night and between exercise periods the back half of the bivalved cast or a splint is worn to keep the foot at a right angle. Support is not discarded until active dorsiflexion of the foot to a right angle is possible; this usually requires at least 6 months.

When stabilizing procedures have supplemented the tendon transfer, muscle reeducation is delayed for 8 weeks; aftertreatment is as just described.

SPLIT TRANSFER OF TIBIALIS ANTERIOR TENDON

Hoffer et al. devised a new operation to correct varus deformity of the foot in cerebral palsy caused by overactivity of the tibialis anterior, called the split tibialis anterior tendon transfer. It has been carried out many times in children and adults with spastic cerebral palsy and in patients with other paralytic affections. The technique is described on p. 2869.

ARTHRODESIS OF ANKLE FOR EQUINOVARUS DEFORMITY

Barr and Record recommend ankle arthrodesis instead of triple arthrodesis and bone block or pantalar arthrodesis for severe paralytic equinovarus deformities in adults when muscles suitable for transfer are not available. They believe that the major deformity is supination of the body of the talus in the ankle joint (Fig. 66-27) and thus prefer not to disturb the tarsal joints.

TECHNIQUE (BARR AND RECORD). For a foot with a severe equinovarus and cavus deformity, subcutaneous plantar fasciotomy (p. 2941) and lengthening of the tendo calcaneus (p. 2952) are done first as a separate procedure.

Later the ankle is arthrodesed as follows. Expose the joint through an anteromedial skin incision that follows the tibialis anterior tendon. Incise the sheath and retract the tendon. By subperiosteal dissection strip the medial malleolus to release all ligamentous attachments. Next divide the tibialis posterior tendon. Free the talus and distal end of the tibia on their medial and anterior aspects of all soft tissue attachments. Make a second incision over the distal end of the fibula and remove the ligaments from the lateral malleolus and lateral aspect of the talus. Remove the articular cartilage from the ankle joint but sacrifice as little bone as possible. Now bring the foot to the neutral position and in normal external rotation in relation to the leg. Continue the arthrodesis by driving a bone graft through a tunnel in the lower metaphyseal region of the tibia and into a slot in the talus; preserve an anterior bridge of the metaphysis to hold the graft in place. Finally pack additional bone chips about the lateral recesses of the joint. If necessary, osteotomize the lateral malleolus and displace it medially for accurate apposition.

AFTERTREATMENT. A cast is applied from the groin to the toes with the knee at 20 degrees. The sutures are removed through a window in the cast on the tenth day. A short leg walking cast is applied at 6 weeks and partial weight bearing is permitted. Two weeks later full weight bearing is permitted, and at 10 weeks all immobilization is discontinued if fusion is complete.

TALIPES CAVOVARUS

Paralytic talipes cavovarus may be caused by an imbalance of the extrinsic muscles (see discussion of talipes equinovarus) or by persistent function of the short toe flexors and other intrinsic muscles when the foot is otherwise flail. Coonrad et al. observed that the plantar muscles play an important role in its development. They treat it by excising the short flexor muscles and a block of the plantar fascia and by resecting the motor branches of the lateral plantar nerve. These procedures may be done at the time of foot stabilization.

Garceau and Brahms, working independently, reached similar conclusions about the role of the intrinsic muscles. However, they resect the motor branches of both the medial and lateral plantar nerves; the sensory branches are spared to preserve sensation in the sole of the foot. This procedure was performed on 47 feet in 40 patients with encouraging results; it was found most useful for cavus deformity and talipes cavovarus after poliomyelitis; the results were also promising in the cavovarus deformity of recurrent congenital talipes equinovarus and in idiopathic clawfoot. The procedure was of no value in treating a cavovarus deformity secondary to arthrogryposis multiplex congenita. The best results were obtained in children before bone growth was advanced.

TECHNIQUE (GARCEAU AND BRAHMS). Use Henry's approach to the medial aspect of the foot, as follows. Begin the incision over the medial side of the first metatarsal neck and gently curve it anteriorly over the tuberosity of the navicular, and then plantarward and proximally toward the heel. Reflect a flap of skin and fascia plantarward and expose the abductor hallucis muscle and tendon. Elevate the anterior border of the muscle and free its belly proximally to its origin on the medial process of the calcaneal tuberosity. Incise the laciniate ligament and retract the tendons of the flexor hallucis longus and flexor digitorum longus. Now free the medial and lateral plantar nerves and locate their branches to the intrinsic muscles. Lift the branches with nerve hooks, identify them by electrical stimulation, and resect them. Spare the sensory branches. Now stimulate the main nerve trunks to be sure that all motor branches are divided. Close the incision in layers without a drain and apply a boot cast.

TALIPES EQUINOVALGUS

Talipes equinovalgus usually develops when the tibialis anterior and posterior muscles are weak, the peroneus longus and brevis are strong, and the triceps surae is strong and contracted. The triceps surae pulls the foot into equinus and the peroneals into valgus position; when the extensor digitorum longus and the peroneus tertius muscles are also strong, they help to pull the foot into valgus position on walking. Structural changes in the bones and ligaments follow the muscle imbalance; eventually the plantar calcaneonavicular ligament becomes stretched and attenuated, the weight-bearing thrust shifts to the medial border of the foot, the forefoot abducts and pronates, and the head and neck of the talus become depressed and prominent on the medial side of the foot. When a structural deformity begins to develop, prompt surgery is indicated to correct it and to prevent its recurrence by relieving the dynamic muscle imbalance.

Treatment of this deformity in a skeletally immature foot is difficult. A double bar brace with a 90-degree ankle stop and inside T-strap, a shoe with an arch support and a medial heel wedge, and repeated stretching exercises are necessary; despite these measures, wedging casts must occasionally be resorted to, and if correction is still not obtained, the tendo calcaneus may have to be lengthened. After correction, surgery is necessary to prevent recurrence. Subtalar arthrodesis by the method of Grice and Green and anterior transfer of the peroneus longus and brevis tendons will usually suffice until the bones are mature; if necessary a triple arthrodesis can then be done. Failure to transfer the tendons is the usual cause of recurrence.

Axer described an operation in which the talonavicular and subtalar joints are opened, the talus, the calcaneus, and the navicular are placed in their normal positions, and one or more of the deforming evertor muscles of the foot are transferred into the neck of the talus; when necessary, the tendo calcaneus is lengthened. In his experience this operation is best suited for correcting dynamic paralytic equinovalgus, valgus, and rocker-bottom deformities in children 3 to 6 years old. Of 24 cases reported in detail, the result was good or very good in 14, fair in 9, and poor in 3. Osmond-Clarke in 1956 described a similar operation for congenital vertical talus. We have had no experience with this procedure.

According to Fried and Hendel a dynamic valgus deformity is caused by paralysis of the tibialis anterior or the tibialis posterior or both.

Paralysis of the tibialis anterior alone usually causes only a moderate valgus deformity that is more pronounced during dorsiflexion of the ankle and may even disappear during plantar flexion. The long toe extensors dorsiflex the foot. First the extensor hallucis longus hyperextends the great toe at the metatarsophalangeal joint while the interphalangeal joint remains flexed; then the extensor digitorum longus pulls the foot into valgus deformity because of its anterolateral anchorage at the ankle and its insertion into the lateral toes. The pull of the extensor digitorum longus in everting the foot during dorsiflexion is comparable to that of the peroneals. According to Fried and Hendel this everting force should be corrected by a transfer of the peroneus longus to the first cuneiform (Biesalk and Mayer), by a similar transfer of the extensor digitorum longus, or by the Jones operation.

Paralysis of the tibialis posterior alone causes a planovalgus deformity. Normally this muscle inverts the foot during plantar flexion, and when it is paralyzed, a valgus deformity develops, which the long flexor muscles of the toes because of their lateral position are ineffective in preventing. Since most of the functions of the foot are performed during plantar flexion, loss of the tibialis posterior is a severe impairment. Moreover it is normally the principal support of the arch of the foot, for its tendon divides and inserts into the navicular and the metatarsals, and when this support is lost, the arch collapses, the valgus

deformity gradually increases, and the result is a planovalgus deformity. Fried and Hendel have devised a method of transferring the peroneus longus tendon to correct this imbalance: the tendon is severed at its insertion in the sole of the foot, is rerouted posterior to the ankle, and is inserted through the sheath of the paralyzed tibialis posterior tendon into the plantar aspect of the navicular. As alternatives they transfer the flexor digitorum longus or the flexor hallucis longus in the same manner or the extensor hallucis longus through the interosseous membrane and then through the tendon sheath to the navicular.

Fried and Moyseyev in 1970 reported 20 patients treated by tendon transfers to replace the paralyzed tibialis posterior. In 14 the peroneus longus and in 6 one of the long toe flexors or the extensor hallucis longus was transferred. In seven full correction was obtained and no further treatment was necessary. In the other 13 correction was good at first, but varus or valgus deformities developed later. Before surgery there was severe planovalgus deformity of the feet, and after surgery only one recurrent deformity was severe; the others were slight to moderate. In 12 feet with slight to moderate deformity further surgery could be postponed until the foot was mature enough for bony stabilization.

Paralysis of both the tibialis anterior and tibialis posterior results, according to Fried and Hendel, in extreme deformity. Convex pes planus is often the result, and the head of the talus is prominent on the plantar surface of the foot. The deformity is similar to congenital convex pes planus or rocker-bottom flatfoot. For such a deformity they recommend a transfer to replace the tibialis posterior and later if necessary another to replace the tibialis anterior.

Goldner has pointed out that clawing of the toes in equinovalgus (as in some other paralytic foot deformities) is the result of a substitution pattern in which the long toe extensors assist the weak tibialis anterior in dorsiflexing the ankle. Clawing of the lateral toes, unless fixed, will disappear after tarsal reconstruction, tendo calcaneus lengthening, and peroneal tendon transfer, but clawing of the great toe is corrected by the Jones operation (p. 2939).

Talipes equinovalgus in the skeletally mature foot requires triple arthrodesis and lengthening of the tendo calcaneus, followed in 4 to 6 weeks by anterior transfer of the peroneus longus and brevis tendons, the Jones operation, and arthrodesis of the interphalangeal joint of the great toe.

A valgus deformity without detectable calcaneus or equinus of the ankle occasionally occurs in people who have poliomyelitis after growth is complete. The triceps surae, tibialis anterior, and tibialis posterior are usually weak. Treatment consists of triple arthrodesis and the Jones operation followed in 6 weeks by posterior transfer of the peroneals to reinforce the triceps surae.

TARSAL RECONSTRUCTION FOR TALIPES EQUINOVALGUS

TECHNIQUE. The basic triple arthrodesis (p. 2935) is modified to meet the needs of the individual patient. Sufficient wedges of bone must be removed from the medial side of the talonavicular joint to correct abduction and pronation and of the subtalar joint to correct valgus deformity of the heel. A short medial longitudinal incision over the talonavicular joint makes exposure of this area easier and permits more precise correction. Bone chips should be packed in and about the calcaneocuboid joint to adduct and supinate the forefoot by elongating the lateral border of the foot; chips should also be packed into the lateral part of the subtalar joint. As in all foot stabilizations, the heel must be brought into a neutral position as to varus and valgus, and the heads of the first and fifth metatarsals must be made to lie on the same plane.

AFTERTREATMENT. Aftertreatment is the same as for the routine foot stabilization (p. 2935).

EXTRAARTICULAR ARTHRODESIS OF SUBTALAR JOINT
FOR TALIPES EQUINOVALGUS

This operation is indicated for equinovalgus deformity in children 4 to 12 years of age. However, the equinus must either be corrected before operation by wedging casts or at operation by lengthening the tendo calcaneus because equinus deformity of more than 15 degrees prevents the calcaneus from being brought far enough distally beneath the talus to allow correction of the valgus and abduction deformities. Four to six weeks after operation the peroneus longus and brevis tendons are transferred anteriorly to prevent recurrence.

The use of two trapezoidal bone grafts is the simplest and most effective method, especially in regard to fitting the grafts and adjusting the amount of correction. The grafts must be securely fixed under some compression at the end of the operation; if not, they will be displaced or absorbed or both—the most common complication from technical error. They must also provide exact correction—undercorrecting and overcorrecting are common errors. When the deformity is undercorrected, the heel is fused in valgus position, and the situation becomes analogous to the fixed valgus of congenital talocalcaneal coalition; as would be expected, such patients frequently develop peroneal muscle spasm and pain. However, it is better to fuse the heel in slight valgus position than to overcorrect the deformity, for even a slight varus deformity seems to increase with growth. An uncommon complication is absorption of the middle of the graft; this seems to occur when the grafts either are too long or are homogenous rather than autogenous.

Grice reviewed (1959) 52 feet in which this operation had been done at least 5 years previously. In 38 growth of the foot was completed by this time, and little if any change in its position could be expected later, but in the other 14, although all were over 11 years old on review, growth of the foot was incomplete, and final evaluation was impossible at the time. Of the 52 patients the result was satisfactory in 44 (17 were rated excellent and 27 good) and unsatisfactory in 8 (3 were rated fair and 5 poor). Six patients with an unsatisfactory result required a triple arthrodesis to improve either the function or the appearance of the foot; of these the deformity in three had been undercorrected and in three it had been overcorrected.

Studies of the results of subtalar extraarticular arthrodesis have been made and reported by Pollock and Carrell, Hunt and Brooks, Smith and Westin, Paluska and Blount, Lahdenranta and Pylkkänen, and Broms. Brindley and

Brindley reviewed 43 extraarticular subtalar arthrodeses. Although the results in simple pes planus were difficult to evaluate, in poliomyelitis the procedure accomplished its goals. Of 19 patients with adequate follow-up, only seven required subsequent surgery, usually triple arthrodesis, and in only two were the results considered unsatisfactory. In all, the results of the operation in more than 600 feet were analyzed and were found satisfactory in 60% to 70%. Unsatisfactory results were caused most frequently by varus deformity of the foot resulting either from improper positioning of the heel during surgery or from dynamic imbalance of muscle power in which the invertors of the foot were too strong and the evertors were too weak after peroneal tendon transfer. Sometimes, however, unsatisfactory results were caused by incomplete correction of equinus deformity, infection after surgery, or improper placement, pseudarthrosis, absorption, or fracture of grafts. Unrelated to the operation was valgus deformity of the ankle joint in which the talus was tilted in the ankle mortise observed by Smith and Westin and by Paluska and Blount; this deformity was treated by temporarily stapling the medial aspect of the distal tibial epiphyseal plate, and the preliminary results were satisfactory. Dorsal bunion (p. 2947) has occasionally developed after transfer of the peroneus longus tendon. Despite these complications, most of which will decrease in frequency as experience with the operation increases, extraarticular subtalar arthrodesis has proved to be of lasting benefit when properly performed.

In 1968 Brown and Seymour and Evans described a method of extraarticular subtalar arthrodesis suggested by Batchelor in which the sinus tarsi is not exposed. A graft taken from the fibula is inserted through the neck of the talus across the sinus tarsi into the calcaneus with the hindfoot in neutral position. In 1976 Hsu, O'Brien, Yau, and Hodgson reported the results of 64 feet treated by this type of arthrodesis for deformities in poliomyelitis. The results were unsatisfactory in 21 because of fusion in varus or valgus position or because of nonunion, fracture, or absorption of the graft. Gross also in 1976 reviewed his experience with the Bachelor arthrodesis in 34 feet observed for an average of 39 months. The rate of pseudarthrosis was 41%, and in only 18 (53%) were the results satisfactory. In his opinion the Grice procedure is more reliable. In 1972 Hsu et al. reported an earlier study of the Bachelor arthrodesis. In 28 instances in which the graft was removed from the distal third of the fibula, the bone failed to regenerate and valgus instability of the ankle resulted. In 16 ankles the distal fibular epiphysis migrated proximally. This is probably another reason why the procedure of Grice is better than that of Bachelor.

In 1976 Dennyson and Fulford reported the treatment of 48 feet with flexible pes planus using a modification of the Bachelor procedure in which, instead of a fibular graft, a long stainless steel screw was used to transfix the talus to the calcaneus in the corrected position; cancellous bone chips were packed in the sinus tarsi. In 45 feet solid union was obtained after an average of 7½ weeks in a short leg walking cast.

TECHNIQUE (GRICE AND GREEN). Make a short curved lateral incision directly over the subtalar joint. Expose the interosseous talocalcaneal ligament overlying the joint and cut it in the direction of its fibers. Dissect the fatty and ligamentous tissues from the sinus tarsi and reflect distally from the calcaneus the origin of the short toe extensors. The relationship of the calcaneus to the talus can now be determined, and the mechanism of the deformity can be demonstrated. After placing the foot in equinus position and inversion, the calcaneus can usually be rotated into its normal position beneath the talus, but if the deformity is severe and of long duration, it may be necessary to divide the posterior capsule of the subtalar joint or to remove a small amount of bone laterally from beneath the anterosuperior articular surface of the calcaneus before normal alignment can be restored. Insert an osteotome or a broad periosteal elevator into the sinus tarsi and block the subtalar joint to demonstrate the stability that the grafts will provide and to determine their size and optimum position. If the distal end of the calcaneus cannot be held beneath the talus despite correction of the valgus deformity, transfix the anterior talocalcaneal articulation with a screw inserted through a short anterior incision. To prepare beds for the grafts remove a thin layer of cortical bone from the inferior surface of the talus and superior surface of the calcaneus (Fig. 66-28). Now from the anteromedial surface of the proximal tibial metaphysis remove a block of bone (usually 3.5 to 4.5 cm long and 1.5 cm wide) large enough to provide two grafts. Cut the grafts like trapezoids to fit the prepared beds. Rongeur away the corners of the broad base of each graft so that each can be countersunk into cancellous bone, thus preventing their lateral displacement after operation. With their cancellous surfaces facing each other, place the grafts in the sinus tarsi with the foot held in a slightly overcorrected position; as the foot is ev-

erted, the grafts are locked in place. At this stage the foot is usually so stable that an equinus deformity, if present, can be corrected by lengthening the tendo calcaneus at the same operation.

Apply a long leg cast with the knee flexed, the ankle in maximum dorsiflexion, and the foot in the corrected position.

AFTERTREATMENT. Tendon transfer is usually indicated 6 to 8 weeks after the arthrodesis but should be deferred until any residual equinus has been corrected by wedging casts. Transfer of one of the peroneal tendons anteriorly to the base of the second metatarsal is usually sufficient to maintain correction of a mild or moderate deformity; Grice and Green have transferred the peroneus longus tendon around the medial border of the foot into the plantar aspect of the navicular medially to maintain correction of a severe deformity or even to help correct a recurrence of the deformity caused by relaxation of the ligments and valgus tilting of the talus in the ankle mortise. Plication or proximal advancement of the deltoid ligament is indicated when relaxation of ligaments is severe. Occasionally it is desirable to postpone tendon transfer until the foot has been mobilized and the muscles have regained their power. In a young child it may be advisable to defer tendon surgery until he is old enough to cooperate in reeducating the transferred muscle. Regardless of when the transfer is done, weight bearing is not allowed until the arthrodesis is solid (usually at 10 to 12 weeks).

PERONEAL TENDON TRANSFER FOR TALIPES EQUINOVALGUS

TECHNIQUE. Expose the tendons of the peroneus longus and brevis through an oblique incision paralleling the skin creases at a point midway between the distal tip of the lateral malleolus and the base of the fifth metatarsal. Divide the tendons as far distally as possible, securely suture the distal end of the peroneus longus to its tunnel to prevent the development of a dorsal bunion, and free the tendons proximally to the posterior border of the lateral malleolus. (When they are to be transferred at the time of foot stabilization, they can be divided through a short extension of the routine incision as shown in Fig. 66-1.) Make a second incision 5 cm long at the junction of the middle and distal thirds of the leg overlying the tendons. Gently withdraw the tendons from their sheaths with care not to disrupt the origin of the peroneus brevis muscle.

The new site of insertion of the peroneal tendons is determined by the severity of the deformity and the existing muscle power. When the extensor hallucis longus is functioning and is to be transferred to the neck of the first metatarsal, the peroneal tendons should be transferred to the third cuneiform; when no other functioning dorsiflexor is available, they should be transferred to the midline of the foot anteriorly.

Expose the new site of insertion of the tendons through a short longitudinal incision. Retract the tendons of the extensor digitorum longus and make a cruciate or H-shaped cut in the periosteum of the recipient bone. Raise and fold back osteoperiosteal flaps and drill a hole in the bone big enough to receive the tendons. Then bring the tendons out beneath the cruciate crural ligament into this incision and anchor them side by side and under equal ten-

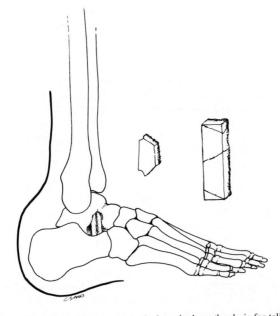

Fig. 66-28. Grice and Green extraarticular subtalar arthrodesis for talipes equinovalgus or planovalgus. Removing corners of base of grafts makes them easier to countersink into talus and calcaneus. Note their position in sinus tarsi. (Redrawn from Grice, D.S.: J. Bone Joint Surg. **34-A**:927, 1952.)

sion through a hole drilled in the bone, either by suturing them back on themselves or by securely fixing them to bone using a platform type of staple.

Irwin preferred to cut the peroneus brevis tendon at or immediately distal to its musculotendinous junction and to suture its proximal stump into the peroneus longus tendon; this tendon is then transferred anteriorly as just described.

When there is significant clawing of the great toe, the extensor hallucis longus tendon should be transferred to the neck of the first metatarsal, and the interphalangeal joint is fused after the method of Jones (p. 2939). Residual clawing of the lateral four toes is usually of little or no significance after transfer of the peroneal and extensor hallucis longus tendons.

TENDON TRANSFER FOR TIBIALIS POSTERIOR PARALYSIS

TECHNIQUE (FRIED AND HENDEL). In this operation the tendon of the peroneus longus, flexor digitorum longus, flexor hallucis longus, or extensor hallucis longus may be transferred to replace a paralyzed tibialis posterior.

When the *peroneus longus tendon* is to be transferred, make a longitudinal incision 5 to 8 cm long laterally over the shaft of the fibula. After incising the fascia of the peroneal muscles, inspect them: if their color does not confirm their preoperative grading, the transfer will fail. Now make a second incision along the lateral border of the foot over the cuboid and the peroneus longus tendon. Free the tendon, divide it as far distally in the sole of the foot as possible, suture its distal end in its tunnel, and withdraw the tendon through the first incision. By blunt dissection create a space between the triceps surae and the deep layer of leg muscles; from here make a wide tunnel posterior to the fibula and to the deep muscles and directed to a point proximal and posterior to the medial malleolus. Now make a small incision at this point and draw the peroneus longus tendon through the tunnel; it now emerges where the tibialis posterior tendon enters its sheath. Make a fourth incision 4 to 5 cm long over the middle of the medial side of the foot centered below the tuberosity of the navicular. Free and retract plantarward the anterior border of the abductor hallucis muscle and expose the tuberosity of the navicular and the insertion of the tibialis posterior tendon; proximal to the medial malleolus open the sheath of this tendon and into it introduce and advance a curved probe until it emerges with the tendon at the sole of the foot. Using the probe, pull the peroneus longus tendon through the same sheath, which is large enough to contain this second tendon. Now drill a narrow tunnel through the navicular, beginning on its plantar surface lateral to the tuberosity and emerging through its anterior surface. Pull the peroneus longus tendon through the tunnel in an anterior direction and anchor it with a Bunnell pull-out suture. Also suture it to the tibialis posterior tendon close to its insertion. Close the wounds and apply a boot cast with the foot in slight equinus and varus position.

When the *flexor digitorum longus tendon* is to be transferred, make the incision near the medial malleolus as just described but extend it for about 7 cm. Free the three deep muscles and observe their color; if it is satisfactory, make the incision on the medial side of the foot as just described. Free and retract the short plantar muscles and expose the flexor digitorum longus tendon as it emerges from behind the medial malleolus. Free the tendon as far distally as possible, divide it, and withdraw it through the first incision; now pass it through the sheath of the tibialis posterior tendon and anchor it in the navicular as just described.

When the *flexor hallucis longus tendon* is to be transferred, use the same procedure as described for the flexor digitorum longus.

When the *extensor hallucis longus tendon* is to be transferred, cut it near the metatarsophalangeal joint of the great toe. Suture its distal end to the long extensor tendon of the second toe. Withdraw the proximal end through an anterolateral longitudinal incision over the distal part of the leg. Open the interosseous membrane widely, as in the Peabody operation (p. 2974). Make the incision near the medial malleolus as previously described and with a broad probe draw the tendon through the interosseous space and through the sheath of the tibialis posterior tendon to the insertion of that tendon. Then continue with the operation as described for transfer of the peroneus longus tendon.

AFTERTREATMENT. At 10 days a rubber heel is applied to the cast, and walking is permitted. At 6 weeks the walking cast is removed, a splint is used at night, and muscle reeducation is started.

TALIPES CALCANEUS

Talipes calcaneus is a vicious, rapidly progressive paralytic deformity caused by paralysis of the triceps surae while the other extrinsic foot muscles, especially those that dorsiflex the ankle, remain functional.

The *pathogenesis* of the deformity is as follows. When the triceps surae is severely weakened or paralyzed, the calcaneus cannot be stabilized nor the body weight borne on the metatarsal heads; thus the spring or push-off in walking is immediately lost. Because the dorsiflexors of the ankle are unopposed, the tendo calcaneus becomes thin and elongated. When walking is attempted, the calcaneus then rotates, for its posterior end is pulled plantarward by the long and short toe flexors, the lumbricales, and the interossei; thus a cavus deformity develops. After this, gravity assists in the development of forefoot equinus deformity, while rotation of the calcaneus continues unopposed. Also, because of the position of their tendons, the peroneals and the tibials aggravate the deformity. The plantar fascia now becomes contracted, and with growth, structural changes occur in the bones and joints.

The *treatment* of talipes calcaneus is extremely difficult. Unfortunately no appliance will replace a paralyzed triceps surae nor prevent a calcaneus deformity from developing and increasing. However, a mild deformity in the skeletally immature foot should be treated conservatively until the rate at which the deformity is increasing can be determined. It is useful to apply an elevated and posteriorly extended heel that forces the foot into equinus position when it strikes the floor and an ankle brace with limited motion and an elastic posterior ankle strap. Exercises are also recommended that attempt to maintain normal alignment of the foot and ankle and to restore power in the triceps surae. When the deformity is progressing rapidly, especially in a young child, tendon transfers are indicated

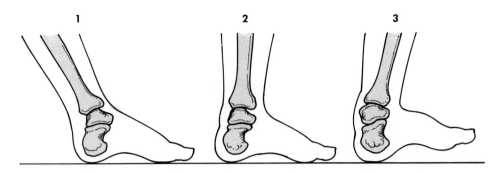

Fig. 66-29. Gait in presence of gastrosoleus paralysis and resulting calcaneus deformity: *1,* heel strike; *2,* stance; and *3,* toe rise at push-off, instead of heel lift. (Courtesy Dr. G.W. Westin.)

early; according to Irwin, this may be as early as 12 months after the onset of the disease. Again unfortunately muscles strong enough to restore normal push-off in walking are not available for transfer, and a limp usually persists after surgery. Only rarely is it possible to rise actively and without support on the ball of the affected foot after tendon transfers for complete paralysis of the triceps surae.

The purpose of surgery in the skeletally immature foot is to keep a deformity from increasing or to correct a severe one already present without damaging the bones. However, all concerned must understand that foot stabilization will be necessary after skeletal maturity. The plantar fascia should be stripped (p. 2941), and the tendons of the tibialis posterior and of the peroneus longus and brevis should be transferred to the calcaneus to restore active plantar flexion. When these muscles are too weak for useful transfer, posterior transfer of the tibialis anterior tendon (Peabody) is indicated. When the strength of the extensor hallucis longus and extensor digitorum longus is good or normal, both tibials and both peroneals can be transferred posteriorly; in this event, the extensor digitorum longus or extensor hallucis longus must be transferred proximally to prevent an equinus deformity. For talipes calcaneocavus Irwin recommended transferring the tibialis anterior tendon to the calcaneus (Peabody) to prevent excessive dorsiflexion at the ankle, although he recognized that this does not alter the cavus component of the deformity. For talipes calcaneovalgus he recommended early transfer of the peroneus longus and brevis tendons to the calcaneus as far posteriorly as possible and immediately lateral to its midline.

On analysis of gait in patients with paralysis of the gastrosoleus, Westin observed that normal push-off is lost at the end of stance phase, and instead of heel rise, the ankle rotates into dorsiflexion and ultimately into posterior subluxation and toe rise occurs (Fig. 66-29). He also noted a disproportionate inhibition of the rate of growth of the fibula in such ankles, so that the distal fibular epiphyseal plate frequently lies at the level of the distal tibial epiphyseal plate instead of in its normal position at the level of the joint line. Such ankles also frequently have thinning or wedging of the lateral portion of the distal tibial epiphysis and valgus deformity of the ankle.

For reasons previously mentioned, braces do not eliminate the calcaneal hitch in the gait, nor do they prevent progression of the deformity in the skeletally immature

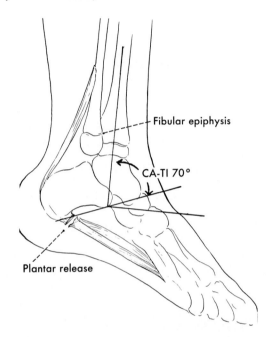

Fig. 66-30. Westin's calcaneal tenodesis to fibula. Calcaneotibial angle measures 70 degrees (see text). Plantar fascial release and calcaneal tenodesis have been completed. (Courtesy Dr. G.W. Westin.)

foot with gross plantar flexor insufficiency. If muscles of adequate power are available, tendons should be transferred early to improve function and to avoid progressive deformity. If adequate muscles are not available, Westin recommends tenodesis of the tendo calcaneus to the fibula.

Of 66 patients who underwent this procedure, deformity was caused in one by myelomeningocele at the L4 level and the rest by poliomyelitis. Six procedures were bilateral, and the average follow-up time was 5.7 years (range of 2 to 10.8 years). The calcaneal hitch was eliminated in all patients. Circumference and length of the fibula improved in 82% of the 66 feet studied, and length of the calcaneus improved in 83%.

The calcaneotibial angle (Fig. 66-30) is formed by the intersection of the axis of the tibia with a line drawn along the plantar aspect of the calcaneus. Normally this angle measures between 70 and 80 degrees; in equinus deformity it is greater than 80 degrees, and in calcaneus deformity it

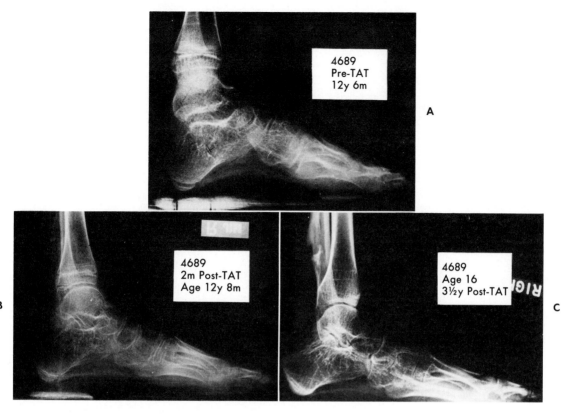

Fig. 66-31. Westin's calcaneal tenodesis to fibula. **A,** Preoperative. **B,** Immediately after operation. **C,** Three and one-half years after surgery. (Courtesy Dr. G.W. Westin.)

is less than 70 degrees. The average calcaneotibial angle before operation measured 55 degrees and at final follow-up was 76 degrees (Fig. 66-31). It was further noted that when the tenodesis was fixed at 70 degrees or more at the time of surgery, the patient tended to develop a progressive equinus deformity with growth. This complication occurred in 25 feet, and in 16 revision was required because of the equinus. Progressive equinus was also directly related to the patient's age at surgery: the younger the patient, the greater the calcaneotibial angle and the more likely the development of progressive equinus deformity with subsequent growth.

In three patients the tenodesis was inadequate: one had pulled away from the bone and two were loosely inserted. The former was corrected by reattachment and the latter two by subtalar or triple arthrodesis.

TECHNIQUE (WESTIN). Expose the tendo calcaneus through a 10 cm vertical incision immediately lateral to the palpable border of the tendon. Identify, protect, and retract the sural nerve, the lesser saphenous vein, and the peroneal tendons. Isolate the tendo calcaneus and divide it at a point that will permit it to be attached to the fibula so that the deformity is corrected snugly and the calcaneotibial angle is less than 70 degrees. Now expose the periosteum over the posterior aspect of the fibula and make in it a T-incision with a long vertical element. Elevate the periosteum, place the distal stump of the tendo calcaneus beneath it, and securely fix the tendon to the periosteum by inter-

rupted sutures. Close the wound as usual and apply a non-weight-bearing cast from toes to tibial tuberosity.

AFTERTREATMENT. After 6 weeks in a non-weight-bearing cast, the patient is fitted with a leg brace with elevated heel and dorsiflexion stop that is worn for 6 months or so. Any residual cavus deformity is corrected by plantar release, using a lateral incision 3 to 6 months after the tenodesis.

In the skeletally mature foot the initial surgery for talipes calcaneus consists of plantar fasciotomy (p. 2941) and Hoke stabilization (p. 2937) in which the calcaneus and cavus deformities are both corrected. Or the "beak" triple arthrodesis described by Siffert, Forster, and Nachamie for severe cavus deformity may be used (p. 2968). This operation was designed to preserve the circulation in the talar head, correct the calcaneus deformity, and by lengthening the plantar surface of the foot, make the shape of the foot more normal. Any foot stabilization for paralytic calcaneocavus should displace the foot as far posteriorly as possible to lengthen its posterior lever arm (the calcaneus) and thus to lessen the muscle power required to lift the heel. When the peroneals, for example, are transferred to the calcaneus, their function is improved so much by posterior displacement of the foot that not only is the anteroposterior balance of the foot better, but also the power exerted on the heel is considerable, even though the peroneals are weak when compared with the normal triceps surae. If the deformity cannot be satisfactorily corrected at operation the calcaneus is stabilized with a Knowles pin inserted through its long axis and incorporated in the cast; the deformity is then gradually corrected by wedging casts. Four to six weeks after stabilization the tendons of the peroneus longus and brevis and of the tibialis posterior are transferred to the calcaneus, and when the extensor digitorum longus is functional, it may be transferred to a cuneiform, and the tibialis anterior may also then be transferred to the calcaneus. Irwin recommended the following method for correcting talipes calcaneus in the skeletally mature foot: fusion of the interphalangeal joint of the great toe (first stage of the Jones operation), excision of a block of plantar fascia 2 to 3 cm square, and Hoke stabilization, and 4 weeks later transfer of the extensor hallucis longus into the first metatarsal neck (second stage of the Jones operation) and posterior transfer of the tendons just named.

Pantalar arthrodesis (p. 2956) is indicated for talipes calcaneocavus when instability is severe and muscles for effective tendon transfer are not available. This operation is technically more difficult than a triple arthrodesis. Considerable judgment and dexterity are required to resect the various bone wedges so accurately that the various components of the deformity are all corrected and all raw surfaces are exactly apposed. We prefer, as do Patterson, Parrish, and Hathaway, the two-stage method; they found a disproportionately high incidence of complications and poor results after one-stage pantalar arthrodesis. However, if the operation is done in one stage, Kirschner wires or staples are valuable in maintaining alignment and apposition.

We no longer use talectomy (astragalectomy) for talipes calcaneus, although the results have been good in many instances. Other less mutilating operations are available. However, the procedure is included in this section (see below) for completeness.

TRIPLE ARTHRODESIS FOR TALIPES CALCANEOCAVUS

TECHNIQUE. First strip the plantar fascia by the method of Steindler (p. 2941) to release the contracted soft tissues bridging the longitudinal arch. Then forcibly correct the cavus deformity as much as possible. Now expose the calcaneocuboid, talonavicular, and subtalar joints through the incision used for triple arthrodesis (p. 2935). With an osteotome remove from the talonavicular and calcaneocuboid joints a wedge-shaped or cuneiform section of bone with its base anterior and large enough to correct the cavus deformity that remains after the plantar fascial stripping. Then dorsiflex the forefoot and appose the raw surfaces to see if the cavus is corrected; if so, expose the subtalar joint and remove from it a wedge of bone with its base posterior to correct the deformity or rotation of the calcaneus (Fig. 66-32). Be sure that all bone surfaces fit together well and that the foot is in satisfactory position before closing the wound.

AFTERTREATMENT. A cast is applied with the foot in moderate equinus position and the knee in slight flexion. Firm pressure is exerted on the sole of the foot while the plaster is setting to stretch the plantar structures as much as possible.

Miller and Irwin and Goldner have advised postoperative manipulation of the foot after this stabilization. At 10

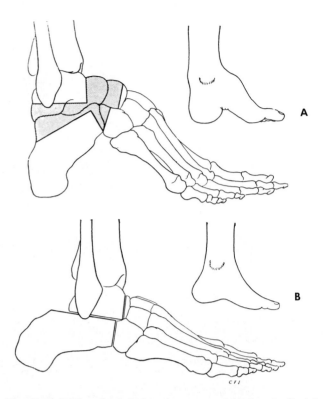

Fig. 66-32. Triple arthrodesis for calcaneocavus deformity. **A,** *Shaded area,* amount of bone resected. **B,** Position of bones after surgery; note that foot has been displaced posteriorly at subtalar joint.

to 14 days the cast and sutures should be removed, the foot should be inspected, and roentgenograms should be made. If the position is not satisfactory, the foot should be manipulated with the patient under general anesthesia. A new cast, snug but properly padded, is then applied and is molded to the contour of the foot.

TECHNIQUE (SIFFERT, FORSTER, NACHAMIE). Expose the calcaneocuboid, talonavicular, and subtalar joints through the incision used for ordinary triple arthrodesis (Fig. 66-1). Next denude of cartilage the calcaneocuboid and subtalar joints. Then excise the dorsal cortex of the navicular. Next plan the wedge of bone to be removed by osteotomy of the anterior aspect of the calcaneus, the posterior aspect of the navicular, and inferior aspect of the talar head and neck (Fig. 66-33, *A*); start the osteotomy inferiorly and carry it superiorly to the inferior surface of the talus. Then resect the inferior part of the talar head and neck to form a beak, leaving undisturbed the soft tissue structures on the superior aspect of the talus anterior to the ankle joint (Fig. 66-33, *B*). Displace the forefoot plantarward and lock the navicular beneath the remaining part of the talar head and neck (Fig. 66-33), *C*). When the bones fit together snugly, maintain the position manually by applying slight pressure beneath the forefoot while the cast is being applied; when the fit is not so snug, fix the navicular in proper relationship to the talus by a staple if desired; occasionally fixing the talus to the calcaneus may be wise.

AFTERTREATMENT. The aftertreatment is the same as described for triple arthrodesis for talipes calcaneocavus (see above).

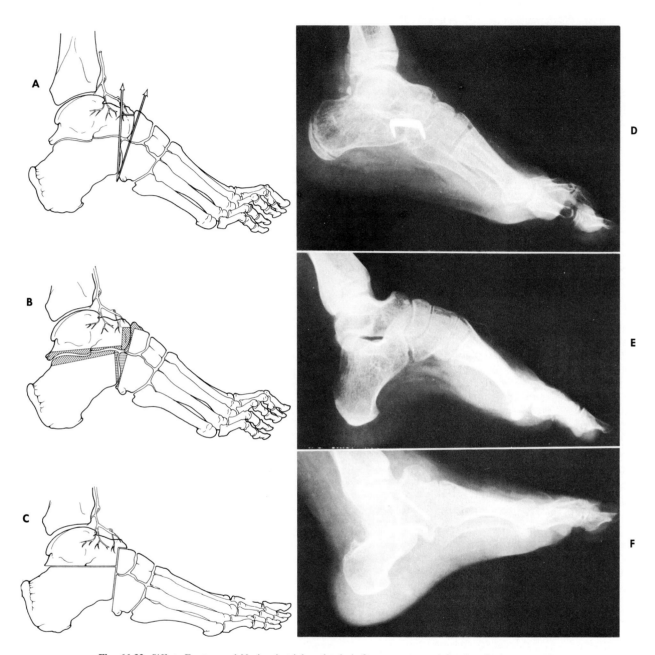

Fig. 66-33. Siffert, Forster, and Nachamie triple arthrodesis for severe cavus deformity. **A,** *Arrows,* wedge of bone to be removed by osteotomy. Note that superior part of talar head is retained to form ''beak.'' **B,** *Shaded areas,* bone to be resected from region of midtarsal and subtalar joints. Note that dorsal cortex of navicular is included. **C,** Final position of foot; forefoot has been displaced plantarward and navicular has been locked beneath remaining part of talar head. **D,** Lateral view of foot after arthrodesis for severe cavus deformity. Navicular lies beneath ''beak'' of talus. **E,** Lateral roentgenogram of foot made before surgery; note severe cavus deformity. **F,** Lateral roentgenogram of same foot after arthrodesis; cavus has been corrected 34 degrees (**A** to **C** courtesy Dr. Robert S. Siffert and Dr. Jacob F. Katz; **D** to **F** from Siffert, R.S., Forster, R.I., and Nachamie, B.: Clin Orthop. **45:**101, 1966.)

OSTEOTOMY AND LENGTHENING OF CALCANEUS FOR TALIPES
CALCANEOVALGUS (FLATFOOT)

In 1975 Evans described a technique used in 56 feet with talipes calcaneovalgus. This technique is based on his concept of the pathomechanics of relapsed clubfoot reported in 1961. In the normal foot the medial and lateral borders are about equal in length; however, in talipes equinovarus the lateral border is longer and in talipes calcaneovalgus the medial border is longer. He suggested that in treating either deformity the length of the borders be equalized. The technique described here consists of a transverse osteotomy of the calcaneus at a point 1.5 cm posterior and parallel to the calcaneocuboid joint and the insertion of a bone graft to open a wedge and thus to lengthen the lateral border of the foot.

The operation, first carried out in 1959, is used as an alternative to triple arthrodesis. The roentgenographic features indicating need for the operation are seen on the anteroposterior view of the foot made in the standing position: the talus points medially and the navicular is displaced laterally in relation to the head of the talus (the reverse of the deformity in clubfoot). The operation has been carried out in 56 feet, 21 in treating talipes calcaneovalgus in poliomyelitis. The ideal age for surgery is between 8 and 12 years; the operation can be done earlier but may have to be repeated. When deformity is severe, full correction may not be possible at the first operation but should be at a second operation 2 or 3 years later. The operation is contraindicated in spastic disorders because the deformity is often overcorrected and in spina bifida because the bone is too soft and the grafts tend to sink into it.

TECHNIQUE (EVANS). The operation is constant in principle, but details vary with the cause of the deformity (Fig. 66-34, *A*). Make an incision over the lateral surface of the calcaneus in line with and just proximal to the peroneal tendons, avoiding the sural nerve so that it will not be caught in the scar. Expose the anterior half of the calcaneus and identify the calcaneocuboid joint. With an osteotome divide the anterior end of the calcaneus through its narrow part distal to the peroneal tubercle. Make the line of division parallel to and 1.5 cm posterior to the calcaneocuboid joint (Fig. 66-34, *B*). Next by means of a spreader separate the cut surfaces of the calcaneus (Fig. 66-34, *D*) and insert a cortical tibial bone graft so that it keeps the bony surfaces separated (Fig. 66-34, *C* and *E*). Inspect the foot to be sure that the forefoot has been adducted, that the heel has been moved into varus position, and that extension of the ankle has become less free. Now insert additional grafts above and below the first one. Close the wound and immobilize the foot in a plaster cast in slight equinovarus position.

AFTERTREATMENT. The cast is worn for about 4 months to allow consolidation of bone, but weight bearing is allowed in the cast at 4 weeks. After the osteotomy is solid, no additional care is needed.

POSTERIOR TRANSFER OF PERONEUS LONGUS, PERONEUS BREVIS,
AND TIBIALIS POSTERIOR TENDONS

TECHNIQUE. Expose the peroneus longus and brevis tendons through an oblique incision 2.5 cm long midway between the tip of the lateral malleolus and the base of the fifth metatarsal. Divide the tendons as far distally as possible, and securely suture the distal end of the peroneus longus tendon to its tunnel. Then bring the tendons out through a second incision overlying the peroneal tendons at the junction of the middle and distal thirds of the leg. If desired, suture the peroneus brevis at its musculotendinous junction to the peroneus longus tendon and discard the distal end of the peroneus brevis tendon. Expose the tibialis posterior tendon through a short incision over its insertion; free its distal end and gently bring it out through a second incision 2.5 cm long at its musculotendinous junction. Then reroute all three tendons subcutaneously to and out of a separate incision lateral and anterior to the insertion of the tendo calcaneus. Drill a hole in the superior surface of the posterior part of the calcaneus just lateral to the midline and enlarge it enough to receive the tendons; anchor the tendons in the hole with a Cole suture (Fig. 1-8) while holding the foot in equinus and the heel in the corrected position. An axial pin in the calcaneus may also be required. With interrupted figure-of-eight sutures transfix the tendons to the tendo calcaneus near its insertion; close the wounds.

AFTERTREATMENT. The foot is immobilized in a long leg cast with the ankle in plantar flexion and the knee at 20 degrees. The pull-out sutures and cast are removed at 6 weeks, and physical therapy is started. Weight bearing is not allowed until active plantar flexion is possible and dorsiflexion to the neutral position is regained. The foot is protected for at least 6 more months by a reverse 90 degree ankle stop brace and an appropriate heel elevation.

TRANSFER OF TIBIALIS POSTERIOR, PERONEUS LONGUS, AND
FLEXOR HALLUCIS LONGUS TENDONS TO CALCANEUS

TECHNIQUE (GREEN AND GRICE). Place the patient prone for easier access to the heel. First, expose the tibialis posterior tendon through an oblique incision 3 or 4 cm long from just inferior to the medial malleolus to the plantar aspect of the talonavicular joint; open its sheath and divide it as close to bone as possible for maximum length. Then remove the peritenon from its distal 3 or 4 cm, scarify it, and insert a 1-0 or 2-0 braided silk suture into its distal end. When the flexor hallucis longus tendon is also to be transferred, expose it through this same incision where it lies posterior and lateral to the flexor digitorum longus tendon. At the proper level for the desired tendon length, place two braided silk sutures in the flexor hallucis longus tendon and divide it between them; suture the distal end of this tendon to the flexor digitorum longus tendon. Second, make a longitudinal medial incision usually about 10 cm long over the tibialis posterior muscle, extending distally from the junction of the middle and distal thirds of the leg. Open the medial compartment of the leg and identify the tibialis posterior and flexor hallucis longus muscle bellies. Using moist sponges deliver the tendons of these two muscles into this wound. Third, make an incision parallel to the bottom of the foot from about a fingerbreadth distal to the lateral malleolus to the base of the fifth metatarsal. Expose the peroneus longus and brevis tendons throughout the length of the incision and divide that of the peroneus longus between sutures as far distally as possible in the

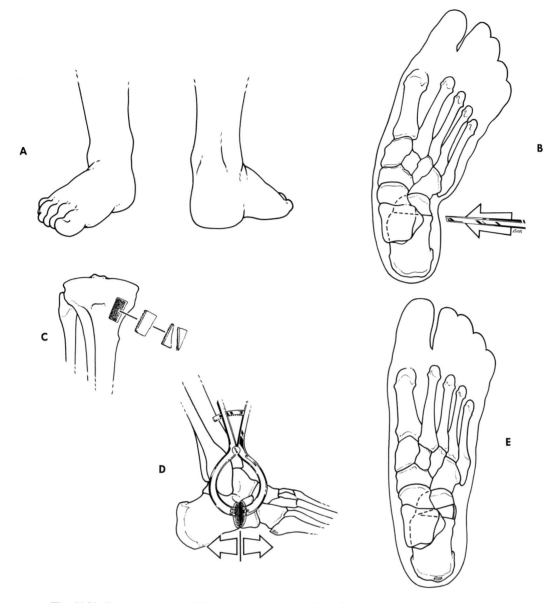

Fig. 66-34. Evans osteotomy and lengthening of calcaneus for talipes calcaneovalgus. **A,** The deformity. **B,** Plane of osteotomy. **C,** Rectangular graft from upper tibia, cut into measured wedges. **D,** Osteotomy spread and grafts inserted. **E,** Deformity corrected. (Redrawn from Evans, D.: J. Bone Joint Surg. **57-B:**270, 1975.)

sole of the foot and free its proximal end to behind the lateral malleolus. Then place a suture in the peroneus brevis tendon, detach it from its insertion on the fifth metatarsal, and suture it to the distal end of the peroneus longus tendon. Fourth, make a lateral longitudinal incision over the posterior aspect of the fibula at the same level as the medial incision and deliver the peroneus longus tendon into it. Fifth, make a posterior transverse incision 6 cm long over the calcaneus (Fig. 66-35, *A*) in the part of the heel that neither strikes the ground nor presses against the shoe. Deepen the incision, reflect the skin flaps subcutaneously, and expose the tendo calcaneus and calcaneus. Beginning laterally, partially divide the tendo calcaneus at its insertion and reflect it medially, exposing the calcaneal

epiphysis. With a %4-inch (3.57 mm) drill make a hole through the calcaneus, beginning in the center of its epiphysis and emerging through its plantar aspect near its lateral border. Enlarge the hole enough to receive the three tendons and ream its posterior end to make a shallow facet for their easier insertion.

Now through the medial wound on the leg (the second incision) incise widely the intermuscular septum between the medial and posterior compartments; insert a tendon passer through the wound and along the anterior side of the tendo calcaneus to the transverse incision over the calcaneus. Thread the sutures in the ends of the tibialis posterior and flexor hallucis longus tendons through the tendon passer and deliver the tendons at the heel. Now

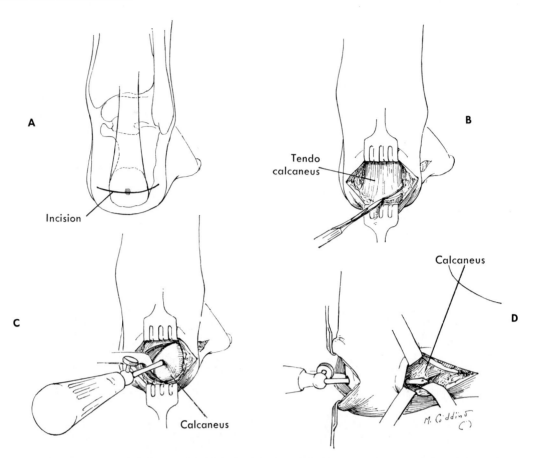

Fig. 66-35. Green and Grice tendon transfers to calcaneus. **A,** Transverse incision is made over calcaneus. **B,** Beginning laterally, tendo calcaneus is partially divided at its insertion. **C** and **D,** Hole is drilled through calcaneus, beginning in center of its epiphysis and emerging at its plantar aspect near its lateral border.

through the lateral wound on the leg (the fourth incision) open widely the intermuscular septum between the medial and posterior compartments in this area and pass the peroneus longus tendon to the heel. Pass all tendons through smooth tissues in a straight line from as far proximally as possible to avoid angulation. With a twisted wire probe (Fig. 66-35, *E*) bring the tendons through the hole in the calcaneus; suture them to the periosteum and ligamentous attachments where they emerge. When the dorsiflexors are weak, suture them under enough tension to hold the foot in 10 to 15 degrees of equinus and when they are strong in about 30 degrees of equinus position. Also suture the tendons to the epiphysis at the proximal end of the tunnel and to each other with 2-0 or 3-0 sutures. Replace the tendo calcaneus posterior to the transferred tendons and suture it in its original position. Close the wounds and apply a long leg cast with the foot in equinus.

AFTERTREATMENT. Usually at 3 weeks the cast is bivalved and exercises are started with the leg in the anterior half of the cast; the bivalved cast is reapplied between exercise periods. At first dorsiflexion exercises are not permitted, but later guided reciprocal motion is allowed. The exercises are gradually increased, and at 6 weeks the patient is allowed to stand but not to bear full weight on the foot. The periods of partial weight bearing on crutches are in-

creased depending on the effectiveness of the transfer, the cooperation of the patient, and his ability to control his motions. Usually at 6 to 8 weeks a single step is allowed, using crutches and an elevated heel; later more steps are allowed, using crutches and a plantar-flexion spring brace with an elastic strap posteriorly. Crutches are continued for a long time, sometimes for even a year or more.

POSTERIOR TRANSFER OF TIBIALIS ANTERIOR TENDON

Peabody described a method of posterior transfer of the tibialis anterior tendon that has been successful in many children at this clinic. Some have regained the ability to walk on tiptoe; in others the calcaneus limp has been materially lessened, and a progressive deformity of the foot has been prevented. In some the ankle could be actively or passively dorsiflexed only to the neutral position. This operation, of course, may be done long before the bones mature, and if stabilization is necessary later, there is little if any tarsal deformity to correct. The experience of Peabody, that a varus instability does not develop after this operation, has been verified in our series; varus instability would probably develop only when the peroneals are completely paralyzed and the tibialis posterior and the long toe flexors are normal. But when the tibialis posterior is weak and the peroneal muscles are normal, valgus instability

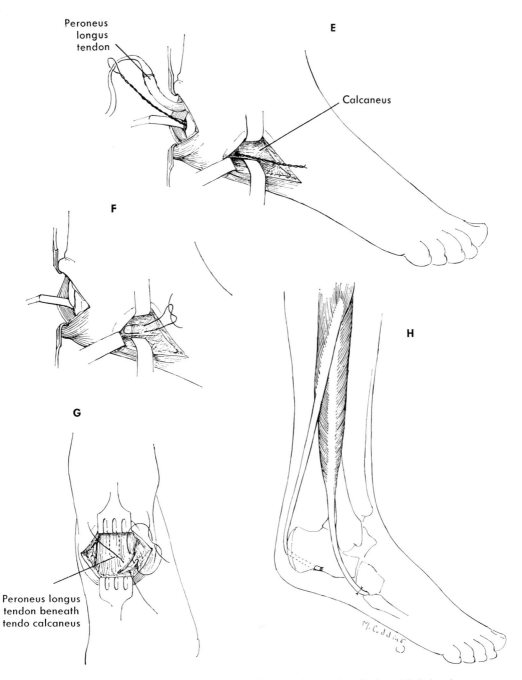

Fig. 66-35, cont'd. E, With a twisted wire probe, tendon or tendons are brought through hole in calcaneus, and **F,** are sutured to periosteum and ligamentous attachments. **G,** Tendo calcaneus is sutured in its original position. **H,** New course of peroneus longus muscle; peroneus brevis tendon has been sutured to distal stump of peroneus longus tendon. (Modified from Green, W.T., and Grice, D.S.: In American Academy of Orthopaedic Surgeons: Instructional course lectures, vol. 13, Ann Arbor, Mich. 1956, J.W. Edwards.)

will develop after the operation; this may be corrected by transferring the peroneus longus to the calcaneus. In such instances the distal stump of the peroneus longus should be sutured to the peroneus brevis tendon to prevent a dorsal bunion. Clawing of the toes from the action of the long toe extensors in dorsiflexing the foot has not occurred in this series, probably because function of the short toe flexors was preserved.

In 1971 Turner and Cooper studied their experience with posterior transfer of the tibialis anterior tendon through the interosseous membrane to restore strength of plantar flexion and to prevent calcaneus deformity and calcaneus gait. They concluded that the results of the operation should be satisfactory if the following conditions are met: (1) the tibialis anterior muscle rates 4+ or 5 (good or excellent), (2) the transfer is carried out before fixed talipes calcaneus develops, (3) the tibialis anterior tendon alone is transferred through the interosseous membrane, and (4) a window rather than a hole is made in the interosseous membrane through which to pass the tibialis anterior tendon.

TECHNIQUE (PEABODY). Make a small incision on the medial side of the foot over the insertion of the tibialis anterior tendon into the first cuneiform and cut the tendon as close to the bone as possible to preserve length. Through a long anterior longitudinal incision overlying the middle two thirds of the leg incise the sheath of the tibialis anterior parallel with the tibial crest. By gentle traction draw the tendon out from its distal sheath into the wound and protect it with a moist sponge. Mobilize the tendon and belly of the muscle in the anterior compartment proximal to the junction of the middle and proximal thirds of the leg; take care not to injure either the neurovascular bundle, which enters the muscle belly in its middle third, or the anterior tibial artery, which lies just lateral to the muscle against the interosseous membrane in the proximal half of the leg. (It will be noted that the posterior surface of the membrane is free although some fibers of the tibialis anterior muscle may take origin from its anterior surface.) Now make a long trapdoor in the interosseous membrane over the entire middle third of the leg as follows. Make a longitudinal incision in the membrane next to its tibial attachment and transverse incisions to the fibula proximally and distally. Then turn the flap laterally and tack it with a few fine plain catgut or silk sutures to the digital extensor aponeurosis so as to prevent its free edge from coming in contact with the transferred tendon (Blount recommends complete removal of the interosseous membrane). By blunt dissection create a tunnel from the trapdoor in the interosseous membrane along the paralyzed soleus muscle to the tendo calcaneus. Next make a posterolateral incision along the tendo calcaneus distally to the calcaneus and expose the tendon. Bring the tibialis anterior tendon through the interosseous space without angulation or torsion, taking care not to damage the vascular supply during this maneuver. While holding the foot in extreme plantar flexion, anchor the tendon into the calcaneus by the method of Cole (Fig. 1-8). Regardless of whether the transferred tendon is interwoven through or sutured to the tendo calcaneus, always anchor it in a tunnel in the bone with a pull-out wire suture.

AFTERTREATMENT. The extremity is immobilized in a long leg cast with the knee in slight flexion and the ankle in complete plantar flexion. At 3 weeks the cast is bivalved to permit muscle reeducation. Such reeducation after this operation is highly important, since the function and phase of the tibialis anterior muscle must be completely reversed. Six to eight weeks after surgery walking is started in an ankle brace that prevents dorsiflexion; the heel is elevated, or an adjustable calcaneus stop may be used that gradually decreases plantar flexion by a progressive reduction in heel height. When a neutral position is obtained, the brace should prevent further dorsiflexion for another 3 months.

KNEE

The disabilities caused by paralysis of the muscles acting across the knee joint are discussed under the following headings: (1) flexion contracture of the knee, (2) quadriceps paralysis, (3) genu recurvatum, and (4) flail knee.

Flexion contracture of knee

Flexion contracture of the knee may be caused by a contracture of the iliotibial band (p. 2984); in fact, contracture of this band may cause not only flexion contracture but also genu valgum and an external rotational deformity of the tibia on the femur. Yount, Forbes, and Irwin advised division of the band and of the lateral intermuscular septum proximal to the knee. When the deformity is of long duration, more extensive procedures are necessary (p. 2987).

Flexion contracture may also be caused by paralysis of the quadriceps muscle when the hamstrings are normal or only partially paralyzed. When the biceps femoris is stronger than the medial hamstrings, there may again be genu valgum and an external rotational deformity of the tibia on the femur; often the tibia subluxates posteriorly on the femur. A mild or moderate contracture may be treated by conservative means, but a severe fixed one may require posterior capsulotomy (Chapter 56) and lengthening of the hamstring tendons followed by use of wedging plaster casts. Harandi and Zahir point out that soft tissue release followed by wedging of the knee in extension, even though more troublesome and time-consuming for both the patient and the physician, is the best way to correct flexion contracture, especially in Asians to whom full flexion of the knee is important for cultural and social reasons. In contractures of 40 degrees or less, a long leg or spica cast is applied and 2 days later the cast is wedged; this is repeated every second or third day. The wedging must be monitored by frequent lateral roentgenograms of the knee to be sure that the tibia is not subluxating on the distal femur. Posterior capsulotomy of the knee is not recommended unless the contracture exceeds 40 degrees. When genu valgum remains after the contracture has been corrected, alignment may be restored later by supracondylar osteotomy of the femur.

We agree with Conner that subluxation of the tibia on the femur during the correction of a severe flexion contracture can usually be avoided by careful attention and by the use of a technique that attempts to pull the tibia anteriorly on the femoral condyles while the knee is being extended. He corrects the contracture by manipulating the knee with the patient under general anesthesia at intervals of 2 weeks and applies a long leg cast between manipulations. We have found the following method satisfactory. A Steinmann pin is inserted through the proximal tibia and is incorporated in a long leg cast. Then at weekly intervals the cast is wedged by leaving plaster hinges intact over the collateral ligaments while a wedge is opened posteriorly and a corresponding wedge is closed anteriorly. A conscious attempt is made to move the tibia anteriorly on the femoral condyles each time the cast is wedged.

Harandi and Zahir reported two patients who developed severe hypertension after flexion contracture of 90 to 100 degrees had been corrected. One had been treated by soft tissue release and wedging plaster casts and the second by a closing-wedge osteotomy of the distal femur. In both patients the blood pressure returned to normal after stretching of the tissues was discontinued and the deformity was allowed to recur.

Leong, Alade, and Fang observed that if a patient with marked weakness in the quadriceps develops a mild or moderate knee flexion deformity, a hand-knee gait is required. If the deformity is severe, the knee buckels on ambulation and walking is extremely difficult without mechanical aid. Based on their experience between 1970 and 1978 in treating 151 patients with knee flexion contractures following poliomyelitis, they have developed the following protocol: if the deformity is 15 degrees or less, it is corrected by exercises and wedging plaster casts; if between 15 and 50 degrees, the deformity is corrected by a one-stage closing-wedge recurvatum osteotomy of the distal femur; if greater than 50 degrees, a preliminary posterior release is done but without a posterior capsulotomy because it is frequently followed by posterior subluxation of the tibia. After the deformity has been corrected to less than 50 degrees, a supracondylar recurvatum osteotomy is done.

They studied 82 patients with 89 knee flexion deformities treated surgically and found 12 patients had residual flexion deformities of 5 to 20 degrees, and 6 of these had been incompletely corrected at surgery. Five were severe enough to warrant reoperation. Ten patients had residual recurvatum between 5 and 30 degrees; only one of these with 30-degree deformity was symptomatic, requiring continued use of a caliper. Residual range of motion was greater than 90 degrees in all but four cases. Six had significant pain on walking—two because of knee stiffness, two from posterior subluxation of the tibia, and one from recurvatum of 30 degrees. The following complications were reported: three superficial and three deep infections, the latter resulting in markedly decreased range of motion; two temporary peroneal nerve palsies; and two posterior tibial subluxations, attributed to posterior capsulotomy at the time of posterior soft tissue release of the knee.

TECHNIQUE OF SUPRACONDYLAR RECURVATUM OSTEOTOMY. Apply a pneumatic tourniquet high on the thigh. Expose the supracondylar portion of the femur through a lateral incision. Divide the fascia lata and the lateral intermuscular septum transversely if they are tight, and expose the femur subperiosteally. Avoid entering the surapatellar pouch. In the growing child carefully identify and then avoid the epiphyseal plate, performing the osteotomy 2.5 cm proximal to it. Using either a power saw or the multiple drill hole technique, remove a wedge of bone, base anterior, from the supracondylar portion of the femur, leaving the posterior cortex intact. Now close the wedge by manipulation. The intact posterior cortex aids stability, and the porosity of the bone permits impaction of the surfaces until the knee is extended fully or in a position of 5 degrees recurvatum. Close the wound over suction drains, and apply a long leg cast. Skeletal fixation is usually not necessary.

AFTERTREATMENT. The drains are removed after 2 or 3 days. Non-weight-bearing crutch walking is allowed after 5 to 7 days. At 2 weeks, the cast and sutures are removed and roentgenograms in two planes are obtained. If complete extension of the knee has not been obtained, the knee is manipulated into extension and a long leg cast is applied. Full weight bearing is allowed in the cast after 6 weeks, and the cast is removed when the osteotomy is solid, usually at 10 to 12 weeks. Early physical therapy is instituted and continued until 90 degrees of flexion has been obtained, usually for 3 weeks or so.

Quadriceps paralysis

Disability from paralysis of the quadriceps muscle is severe, for the knee may be exceedingly unstable, especially if there is the slightest fixed flexion contracture. When there is slight recurvatum, the knee may be stable if the triceps surae is active.

Tendons are transferred about the knee joint almost exclusively to reinforce a weak or paralyzed quadriceps muscle; transfers are not necessary for paralysis of the hamstring muscles because in walking gravity flexes the knee as the hip is flexed. Several muscles are available for transfer to the quadriceps tendon and patella: the biceps femoris, semitendinosus, sartorius, and tensor fasciae latae. When the power of certain other muscles is satisfactory, transfer of the biceps femoris has been the most successful. Transfer of one or more of the hamstring tendons is contraindicated unless one other flexor in the thigh and the triceps surae, which also acts as a knee flexor, are functioning. Transfer of the tensor fasciae latae and sartorius muscles, although theoretically more satisfactory, is usually insufficient because these muscles are not strong enough to replace the quadriceps. As will be mentioned later, Riska has transferred the iliotibial band to the patella and included in the transfer the tensor fasciae latae muscle and part of the gluteus maximus.

If a satisfactory result is to be expected after hamstring transfer, the power not only of the hamstrings but also of the hip flexors, the gluteus maximus, and the triceps surae must be fair or better; when the hip flexor muscles are less than fair, clearing the extremity from the floor may be difficult after surgery. Wray also came to these conclusions after reviewing 51 hamstring transfers in 47 patients for paralysis of the quadriceps muscle. No transfer was rated as excellent; 46.5% were rated as good, 14% as fair, and 39.5% as unsatisfactory. Dislocation of the patella occurred after five transfers and severe recurvatum after two. Schwartzmann and Crego in a review of 134 hamstring tendon transfers for quadriceps paralysis found that of 100 patients in whom the biceps femoris alone had been transferred, 29 developed lateral dislocation of the patella, 16 recurvatum of the knee, and 5 lateral instability of the knee; in 4 the transfer failed to function. However, of 30 patients in whom both the biceps femoris and semitendinosus tendons were transferred, none developed lateral dislocation of the patella; seven developed recurvatum, and one developed lateral instability of the knee; in one the transfer failed to function. Of four transfers of the semitendinosus alone, three were satisfactory; this procedure was done primarily to prevent recurrent flexion contracture of the knee from paralysis of the quadriceps and lateral hamstring muscles rather than to restore active extension of the knee.

Schwartzmann and Crego transfer the biceps and the semitendinosus together when muscle power is such that a brace will probably be unnecessary after surgery. But they point out that when the strength in one or more of the important muscle groups (hip flexors, gluteus maximus, hamstrings, and triceps surae) is below the optimal level, the result may be deficient in one particular respect. Even so, general functional improvement may be obtained. Ease in ascending or descending steps depends on the strength of the hip flexors and extensors. Strong hamstrings, of course, are necessary for active extension of the knee against gravity after the transfer; however, a weak medial hamstring may be transferred to serve as a checkrein on the patella to prevent its dislocating laterally. A normal triceps surae is desirable, for it aids in preventing genu recurvatum and remains as an active knee flexor after surgery; it may not, however, always prevent genu recurvatum, which can result from other factors—in only 6 of 23 patients in whom this deformity developed was the power in the triceps surae less than fair. Recurvatum after hamstring transfers can be kept to a minimum (1) if strength in the triceps surae is fair or better, (2) if the knee is not immobilized in hyperextension after surgery, (3) if talipes equinus when present is corrected before weight bearing is resumed, (4) if a brace that even slightly hyperextends the knee is avoided after operation, and (5) if physical therapy promotes active knee flexion.

Caldwell reported a method, devised by Durham, in which the insertion of the biceps femoris is detached, dissected proximally, and transferred through the medial intermuscular septum to the patella. Of 39 such transfers the result was good in 70%, fair in 15%, and poor in 15%. In no instance did the patella dislocate. Recurvatum occurred after surgery in two instances because the triceps surae and medial hamstrings were weak.

Kleinberg in 1957 reported in one patient the complete transplantation of the adductor longus muscle including its neurovascular pedicle to supplement the quadriceps. The transplanted muscle was attached proximally to the anterosuperior iliac spine and distally to the rectus femoris muscle. The immediate result was very satisfactory.

Riska in 1962 reported 63 transfers of the iliotibial band to the patella for quadriceps paralysis. He emphasized the importance of carefully mobilizing the band proximally and of including in the transfer not only the tensor fasciae latae muscle but part of the gluteus maximus muscle as well. He prefers osseous fixation of the distal end of the band to the patella. Of the 63 transfers, stability of the knee had definitely improved in 85% and power of extension of the knee had improved in 60%. Thus in 85% there had been at least some benefit from the operation.

Mestikawy and Zeier in 1971 reported anterior transfer of the iliotibial band into the patella along with either the semitendinosus or semimembranosus tendon. They separate the iliotibial band from the deep fascia of the thigh anteriorly and from the lateral intermuscular septum posteriorly, from the level of the tensor fasciae latae and gluteus maximus muscles proximally to the insertion of the band on the tibia distally where it is divided. Once the insertion of the band is divided, much of the flexion-abduction contracture of the hip disappears. The band is converted into a tube by rolling its edges from outside in and suturing them together. The tendon of the semitendinosus or of the gracilis is detached, and subcutaneous tunnels are constructed so that the new motors will follow straight courses. Two periosteochondral flaps are raised, and a longitudinal groove is then made on the anterior surface of the patella. The iliotibial band and the tendon are passed through the rectus femoris just proximal to the patella, are laid in the groove in the patella, and are sutured there.

This procedure not only corrects any flexion-abduction deformity of the hip but restores active extension of the knee as well.

Sutherland, Bost, and Schottstaedt reported an electromyographic study of 21 patients with paralysis of the lower extremities from poliomyelitis in whom 39 muscle transfers had been done for quadriceps insufficiency. Electromyograms and movies of gait were recorded simultaneously on the same film by special apparatus. In the 21 patients with poliomyelitis and in 6 normal persons as controls, the phasic activity of each muscle studied was plotted on polar coordinates. In the patients with poliomyelitis many phasic conversions were found in both nontransferred and transferred muscles. Conversion of hamstring activity from swing phase to stance phase and extension of the phasic activity of the gluteus maximus throughout most of the stance phase were observed in nontransferred muscles. Ten of fourteen hamstring transfers achieved stance-phase activity roughly comparable to that of the normal quadriceps; 2 of 11 sartorius transfers and 4 of 12 tensor fasciae latae transfers also achieved stance-phase activity. These results contrast with those of Close and Todd who found that conversion of the biceps femoris to stance-phase activity after transfer was infrequent.

Before tendon transfer about the knee any slight flexion contracture must be corrected; in fact, slight hyperextension is desirable. When the contracture is of 10 to 15 degrees only, supracondylar osteotomy may be made at the time of tendon transfer, or when the quadriceps is fairly strong and the flexion contracture only slight, supracondylar osteotomy alone will produce a relatively stable knee. Flexion contracture of the hip, genu valgum, and contracture of the tendo calcaneus are also common when the quadriceps is paralyzed. These also should be corrected before tendon transfer.

TRANSFER OF BICEPS FEMORIS AND SEMITENDINOSUS TENDONS

TECHNIQUE. Make an incision along the anteromedial aspect of the knee to conform to the medial border of the quadriceps tendon, the patella, and the patellar tendon. Retract the lateral edge of the incision and expose the patella and the quadriceps tendon. Then incise longitudinally the lateral side of the thigh and leg from a point 7.5 cm distal to the head of the fibula to the junction of the proximal and middle thirds of the thigh. Isolate and retract the common peroneal nerve, which is near the medial side of the biceps tendon. With an osteotome free from the head of the fibula the biceps tendon along with a thin piece of bone. Do not divide the fibular collateral ligament, which lies firmly adherent to the biceps tendon at its point of insertion. Free the tendon and its muscle belly proximally as far as the incision will permit; free the origin of the short head of the biceps proximally to where its nerve and blood supplies enter so that the new line of pull of the muscle may be as oblique as possible. Now create a subcutaneous tunnel from the first incision to the lateral thigh incision and make it wide enough for the transferred muscle belly to glide freely. To further increase the obliquity of pull of the transferred muscle divide the iliotibial band, the facia of the vastus lateralis, and the lateral intermuscular septum at a point distal to where the muscle will pass.

Beginning distally over the insertion of the medial hamstring tendons into the tibia, make a third incision longitudinally along the posteromedial aspect of the knee and extend it to the middle of the thigh. Locate the semitendinosus tendon: it is small and round, is inserted on the medial side of the tibia as far anteriorly as its crest, and lies posterior to the tendon of the sartorius and distal to that of the gracilis. Divide the insertion of the semitendinosus tendon and free the muscle to the middle third of the thigh. Now reroute this muscle and tendon subcutaneously to emerge in the first incision over the knee.

Make an I-shaped incision through the fascia, quadriceps tendon, and periosteum over the anterior surface of the patella and strip these tissues medially and laterally. Next with an $^{11}/_{64}$-inch (4.36 mm) drill make a hole transversely through the patella at the junction of its middle and proximal thirds; if necessary, enlarge the tunnel with a small curet. Then lace the biceps tendon in line with and anterior to the quadriceps tendon, the patella, and the patellar tendon. Suture the biceps tendon to the patella with the knee in extension or hyperextension. When only the biceps tendon is transferred, close the soft tissues over the anterior aspect of the patella and the transferred tendon. With interrupted sutures fix the biceps tendon to the medial side of the quadriceps tendon. When the semitendinosus is also transferred, place it over the biceps and suture the two together with interrupted sutures; place additional sutures proximally and distally through the semitendinosus, quadriceps, and patellar tendons.

Crego's technique differs from that just described. The

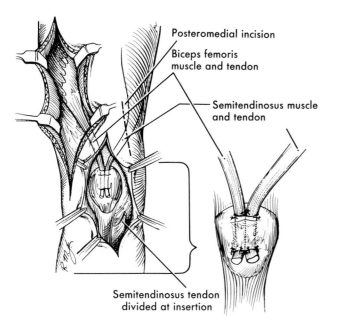

Fig. 66-36. Transfer of semitendinosus and biceps femoris tendons to patella for quadriceps paralysis. (Modified from Schwartzmann, J.R., and Crego, C.H., Jr.: J. Bone Joint Surg. **30-A:**541, 1948.)

insertion of the semitendinosus is detached from the tibia through an incision 2.5 cm long and is brought out through a posteromedial incision 7.5 cm long over its musculotendinous junction (Fig. 66-36). The enveloping fascia is incised to prevent acute angulation of the muscle, and the tendon is passed subcutaneously in a straight line to the patellar incision.

AFTERTREATMENT. With the knee in the neutral position a long leg cast is applied. To prevent swelling the extremity is elevated by raising the foot of the bed rather than by using pillows; otherwise flexion of the hip may put too much tension on the transferred tendons.

At 3 weeks physical therapy and active and passive exercises are started. Knee flexion is gradually developed, and the hamstring muscles are reeducated. At 8 weeks weight bearing is started, with the extremity supported by a controlled dial knee brace locked in extension. Knee motion is gradually allowed in the brace when the muscles of the transferred tendons are strong enough to extend the knee actively against considerable force. To prevent overstretching or strain of the muscles, a night splint is worn for at least 6 weeks and the brace for at least 12 weeks.

TRANSFER OF BICEPS FEMORIS TENDON

TECHNIQUE (CALDWELL AND DURHAM). Expose the biceps femoris muscle through a posterolateral longitudinal incision from a point 2.5 cm distal to the head of the fibula to the junction of the middle and proximal thirds of the thigh (Fig. 66-37, *A*). Free the insertion of the biceps tendon but protect the underlying common peroneal nerve. Free the tendon and muscle from their soft tissue attachments well proximally to the proximal third of the thigh. Detach from the femur the distal two thirds of the origin of the short head of the biceps; avoid damaging its nerve and blood supply, which enters it proximal third. Beginning at the most proximal point of detachment of the short head and extending distally 10 to 12 cm, strip the medial intermuscular septum from the linea aspera; preserve the perforating vessels. At several points divide the septum, which is tight and inelastic, to prevent constriction of the biceps muscle as it spirals posteriorly around the femur.

Now expose the patella and the quadriceps tendon through an anteromedial incision. Drill a tunnel in the patella as previously described, but make it longitudinal (Fig. 66-37, *C*). Then by blunt dissection create a tunnel extending proximally from the patella between the rectus femoris and the vastus medialis muscles and then in an obliquely posterior direction to the opening formed by stripping the medial intermuscular septum. The tunnel must be large enough to permit free passage of the biceps tendon and a part of its muscle belly. Now pass the tendon spirally around the femur posteriorly, medially, and distally and deep to the vastus medialis to the superior pole of the patella (Fig. 66-37, *B*). Using a heavy silk suture, pull the tendon through the tunnel in the patella and anchor it securely with multiple mattress sutures of silk. Split the quadriceps tendon, form an anterolateral flap, and bury the biceps tendon beneath it. This not only reinforces the attachment of the tendon but also aligns the pull of the trans-

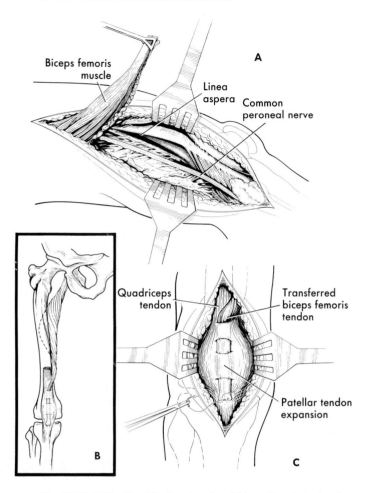

Fig. 66-37. Caldwell and Durham transfer of biceps femoris tendon for quadriceps paralysis. **A,** Insertion of biceps tendon has been freed, and tendon and muscle have been dissected proximally into proximal third of thigh. Common peroneal nerve has been protected. **B,** Biceps femoris tendon has been transferred. Note its direct line of pull. **C,** Method of inserting transferred biceps femoris tendon into quadriceps tendon and patella. (Redrawn from Caldwell, G.D.: J. Bone Joint Surg. **37-A:**347, 1955.)

ferred tendon more nearly with the normal movement of the patella. Apply a well-padded long leg cast with the knee in the neutral position.

AFTERTREATMENT. Aftertreatment is the same as for transfer of the biceps femoris and semitendinosus tendons (p. 2977).

TRANSFER OF SARTORIUS TENDON

TECHNIQUE. Begin an incision at the tibial tuberosity, curve it medially across the insertion of the sartorius muscle and thence proximally along the medial aspect of the thigh, and end it on the anterior surface of the thigh at the junction of its middle and proximal thirds. After subcutaneous dissection retract the distal sides of the skin incision laterally to expose the patellar tendon and medially to expose the sartorius muscle. Sever the insertion of the sartorius tendon, which is just anterior to the insertions of the semitendinosus and gracilis tendons, and free the tendon and muscle proximally to the middle of the thigh, leaving as much of the sheath intact as possible; several small ves-

sels must be divided during this procedure. Elevate and retract the saphenous nerve, which lies near the posterior border of the sartorius muscle. Now place a suture of braided silk in the distal end of the tendon and advance it along the medial border of the tendon for 5 cm and thence across and distally along its lateral border and back to the end of the tendon. The two ends of the suture should remain free. Then pass the tendon subcutaneously from the middle third of the thigh to the patella. Fix it to the quadriceps tendon, the patella, and the patellar tendon as described for transfer of the biceps femoris tendon (see above).

AFTERTREATMENT. Aftertreatment is the same as for transfer of the biceps femoris and semitendinosus tendons (p. 2977).

OTHER TRANSFERS FOR QUADRICEPS PARALYSIS

Muscles and combinations of muscles other than those mentioned above may be transferred for quadriceps paralysis. These transfers include those of the tensor fasciae latae and sartorius (Ober) and of the tensor fascia lata and biceps (Yount). The details of these operations are similar to those described for transfer of the biceps femoris and semitendinosus (p. 2976). The descriptions of these other transfers may be found in the original papers or in early editions of this book.

Genu recurvatum

In genu recurvatum the deformity is the opposite of that in a flexion contracture, for the knee is hyperextended. Mild genu recurvatum may cause some disability, but when the quadriceps is severely weakened or paralyzed, such a deformity is desirable because it stabilizes the knee in walking. However, severe genu recurvatum is materially disabling.

Genu recurvatum from poliomyelitis is of two types: the first is caused by structural bone changes following lack of power in the quadriceps and the second by relaxation of the soft tissues about the posterior aspect of the knee.

The cause of the first type is lack of enough power in the quadriceps to lock the knee in extension in walking. Usually the hamstrings remain normal and are not stretched; the triceps surae is normal, and the heel touches the floor when weight is borne on the extremity. By limiting dorsiflexion of the ankle and thus stabilizing the foot on the leg, the triceps surae stabilizes the knee and prevents it from buckling or giving way. But the pressures of weight bearing and gravity force eventual bone changes in the tibial condyles and in the proximal third of the tibial shaft. The condyles become elongated posteriorly, their anterior margins are depressed as compared with their posterior margins, and the angle of their articular surfaces to the long axis of the tibia, which is normally 90 degrees, becomes more acute. The proximal third of the tibial shaft usually bows posteriorly, and partial subluxation of the tibia may gradually occur.

The cause of the second type is weakness of the triceps surae and hamstring muscles. The knee becomes hyperextended from relaxation of the soft tissues: stretching of the hamstring and triceps surae muscles is followed by that of the posterior capsular ligaments. There is often a calcaneus or calcaneovalgus deformity of the foot on the same side, and the gait is characterized by a lack of spring in the step; with continued use of the extremity further stretching of the soft tissues occurs. This second type of recurvatum develops more rapidly than does the first.

Irwin, who described the two types of genu recurvatum, pointed out that operations to correct either type should aim to fulfill two requirements: first, the alignment of the extremity should be restored, and, second, the cause of the deformity should be corrected so that the deformity will not recur. The prognosis after correction of the first type is excellent; the skeletal deformity is corrected first, and then one or more of the hamstrings is transferred to the patella. The prognosis after the second type is questionable; because no muscles are available for transfer, the underlying cause cannot be corrected, and the deformity may recur. Although procedures that shorten the soft tissues may be successful for a time, these tissues may eventually become stretched again as after any tenodesis subject to the strain of supporting the body weight. Frequently a long leg brace is necessary to prevent the deformity from recurring; although arthrodesis of the knee would solve the mechanical problem, most patients prefer to use a brace permanently.

Perry, O'Brien, and Hodgson described an operation on the soft tissues, triple tenodesis of the knee, for correcting paralytic genu recurvatum. They point out that if the deformity is 30 degrees or less, prolonged bracing of the knee in flexion usually prevents an increase in deformity. However, when the deformity is severe, bracing is ineffective, the knee becomes unstable and weak, the gait is inefficient, and in adults pain is marked. They have carried out triple tenodesis in 16 extremities paralyzed by poliomyelitis and requiring surgery. In seven the deformity was less than 40 degrees and in nine it was greater. The patients were observed for an average of 51 months after surgery, and the average hyperextension at the knee was then between 5 and 6 degrees. Three had recurrence of recurvatum to 10 degrees and one to 15 degrees.

OSTEOTOMY OF TIBIA FOR GENU RECURVATUM

Irwin described an osteotomy of the proximal tibia to correct the first type of genu recurvatum, that is, that caused by structural bone changes. The operation is relatively simple and has been used in this clinic with uniform success. It is similar to the procedure described by Campbell.

Støren modified the Irwin osteotomy by immobilizing the fragments of the tibia with a Charnley clamp. After experience with three patients he thinks that with this modification the technique is easier, healing is faster and more certain, and because only a long leg cast is needed, morbidity is lessened.

TECHNIQUE (IRWIN). Through a short longitudinal incision remove a section of the shaft of the fibula about 2.5 cm long from just distal to the neck. Pack the defect with chips from the sectioned piece of bone. Close the periosteum and overlying soft tissues. Through an anteromedial incision expose and, without entering the joint, osteotomize the proximal fourth of the tibia as follows. With a thin osteotome or a power saw outline a tongue of bone, but

leave it attached to the anterior cortex of the distal fragment. Now at a right angle to the longitudinal axis of the knee joint and parallel to its lateral plane pass a Kirschner wire through the distal end of the proposed proximal fragment before the tibial shaft is divided. Then complete the osteotomy with a Gigli saw, an osteotome, or power saw. Lift the proximal end of the distal fragment from its periosteal bed and remove from it a wedge of bone of predetermined size, its base being the posterior cortex. Replace the tongue in its recess in the proximal fragment and push the fragments firmly together. Suture the periosteum, which is quite thick in this area, firmly over the tongue; this is enough fixation to keep the fragments in position until a cast can be applied.

AFTERTREATMENT. The patient is placed on a fracture table, and the extremity is suspended to an overhead arm with a chain or rope fastened through the Kirschner wire bow. The proximal fragment is hyperextended to its fullest extent by the weight of the extremity and by pressure applied to the anterior surface of the distal thigh. With the extremity in this position a long leg cast is applied. The position of the fragments and the general alignment of the extremity are checked by roentgenograms. When necessary, further changes in the position of the distal fragment are made by wedging the cast distal to the wire 10 to 14 days after surgery. The wire is removed at 6 weeks, and a new long leg cast is applied. At about 8 weeks the osteotomy is usually united, and the cast is removed. Full knee motion should be regained before any operation is done to correct the underlying cause of the recurvatum.

Fig. 66-38 shows correction of genu recurvatum by the Campbell technique.

SOFT TISSUE OPERATIONS FOR GENU RECURVATUM

Genu recurvatum of the second type, that is, caused by relaxation of the soft tissues posteriorly, may be corrected by a surgical procedure on the tendons, ligaments, and fascia. Heyman in 1924 was the first to describe such a procedure. In his original technique both collateral ligaments are reconstructed and attached on the femoral condyles as far posteriorly as possible. The operation is indicated only when the quadriceps is at least strong enough to lock the knee and when walking is possible without a brace. After seven of his original operations good stability was maintained in five knees; the recurrent deformity in these five was mild at most and did not require the use of a brace. The two failures were caused by severe osteoporosis of the femoral condyles that prevented secure fixation of the reconstructed ligaments.

Perry et al. listed the three following principles that must be considered if operations on the soft tissues for genu recurvatum are to be successful: (1) The fibrous tissue mass used for tenodesis must be sufficient to withstand the stretching forces generated by walking and thus all available tendons must be used. (2) Healing tissues must be protected until they are fully mature. The operation should not be undertaken unless the surgeon is assured that the patient will conscientiously use a brace that limits extension to 15 degrees of flexion for 1 year. (3) The alignment and stability of the ankle must meet the basic requirements of gait. Any equinus deformity must be

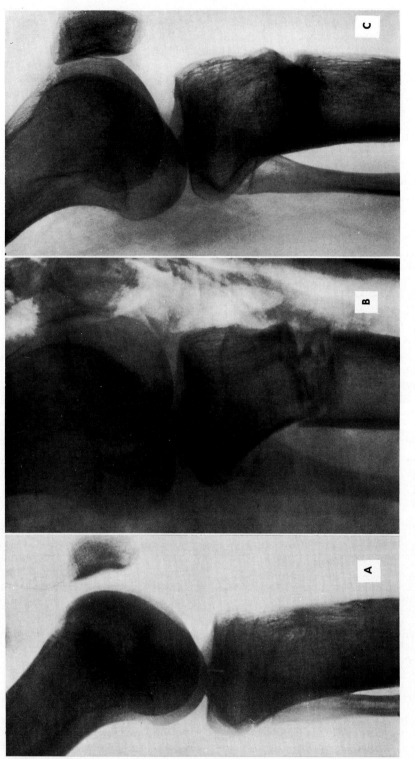

Fig. 66-38. A, Recurvatum secondary to anterior tilt of tibial plateau. **B,** After correction by Campbell technique. **C,** Five months after operation.

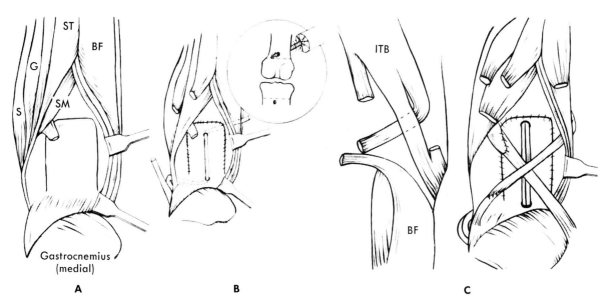

Fig. 66-39. Perry, O'Brien, and Hodgson operation for genu recurvatum. **A,** Origin of medial head of gastrocnemius has been released, leaving proximal strap. Broad flap of posterior capsule is released for future advancement. **B,** Semitendinosus and gracilis tendons are divided at musculotendinous junctions. Each is passed through tunnel in tibia, then across exterior of joint, and then through tunnel in femur. Flap of posterior capsule is advanced and sutured snugly with knee flexed 20 degrees. **C,** Cross straps are made with biceps femoris and iliotibial band (see text). *S,* Sartorius; *G,* gracilis; *ST,* semitendinosus; *SM,* semimembranosus; *BF,* biceps femoris; *ITB,* iliotibial band. (From Perry, J., O'Brien, J.P., and Hodgson, A.R.: J. Bone Joint Surg. **58-A:**978, 1976.)

corrected to at least neutral. If the strength of the soleus is less than good on the standing test, this defect must be corrected by tendon transfer, tenodesis, or arthrodesis of the ankle in the neutral position. Their operation for genu recurvatum is known as triple tenodesis.

TECHNIQUE (PERRY ET AL.). The operation consists of three parts: proximal advancement of the posterior capsule of the knee with the joint flexed 20 degrees, construction of a checkrein in the midline posteriorly using the tendons of the semitendinosus and gracilis, and creation of two diagonal straps posteriorly using the biceps tendon and the anterior half of the iliotibial band.

Place the patient prone, apply a tourniquet high on the thigh, and place a large sandbag beneath the ankle to flex the knee about 20 degrees. Make an S-shaped incision beginning laterally parallel to and 1 cm anterior to the biceps tendon, extend it distally 4 cm to the transverse flexion crease of the knee, then carry it medially across the popliteal fossa, and finally extend it distally for 4 or 5 cm overlying or just medial to the semitendinosus tendon. Identify the sural nerve and retract it laterally. Then identify the tibial nerve and the popliteal artery and vein and protect them with a soft rubber tape. Next identify and free the peroneal nerve and protect it in a similar manner. Retract the neurovascular bundle laterally and identify the posterior part of the joint capsule. Detach the medial head of the gastrocnemius muscle in a step cut fashion, preserving a long, strong proximal strap of the Z to be used in the tenodesis (Fig. 66-39, *A*). Next using a knife detach the joint capsule from its attachment to the femur just proximal to the condyles and the intercondylar notch. Detach the tendons of the gracilis and semitendinosus at their

musculotendinous junctions and suture their proximal ends to the sartorius. Be sure to divide these tendons as far proximally as possible because all available length will be needed. Next drill a hole in the tibia beginning at a point in the midline posteriorly inferior to the epiphyseal plate and emerging near the insertion of the pes anserinus; take care to avoid the epiphyseal plate. Next drill a hole in the femur beginning in the midline posteriorly proximal to the femoral epiphyseal plate and emerging on the lateral aspect of the distal femur (Fig. 66-39, *B*). Draw the tendons of the gracilis and semitendinosus through the hole in the tibia, pass them posterior to the detached part of the capsule, and pull them through the hole in the femur to emerge on the lateral aspect of the distal femur; suture the tendons to the periosteum here under moderate tension with heavy nonabsorbable sutures with the knee flexed 20 degrees. Now advance the free edge of the joint capsule proximally on the femur until all slack has disappeared and suture it to the periosteum in its new position using nonabsorbable sutures. Detach the biceps tendon from its muscle, rotate it on its fibular insertion, and pass it across the posterior aspect of the joint deep to the neurovascular structures and anchor it to the femoral origin of the medial head of the gastrocnemius under moderate tension (Fig. 66-39, *C*). Next detach the anterior half of the iliotibial band from its insertion on the tibia, pass it deep to the intact part of the band, the biceps tendon, and the neurovascular structures, and suture it to the semimembranosus insertion on the tibia under moderate tension. If one of the tendons being used is of an active muscle, then split that tendon and use only half of it in the tenodesis, leaving the other half attached at its insertion. Close the wound in layers and use suction drainage for 48 hours. Apply a well-padded cast from groin to toes with the knee flexed 30 degrees to avoid tension on the sutures.

AFTERTREATMENT. The cast is removed at 6 weeks, and a long leg brace that was fitted before surgery is applied. The brace is designed to limit extension of the knee to 15 degrees of flexion. Full weight bearing is allowed in the brace, and at night a plaster shell is used to hold the knee flexed 15 degrees. Twelve months after surgery the patient is readmitted to the hospital, and the flexion contracture of the knee is gradually corrected to neutral by serial plaster casts. Unprotected weight bearing is then permitted. According to Perry, O'Brien, and Hodgson, it is extremely important that the soft tissues are completely healed before being subjected to excessive stretching caused by unprotected weight bearing or by wedging plaster casts.

Flail knee

When the knee is unstable in all directions and muscle power sufficient to overcome this instability is not available for tendon transfer, either a long leg brace with a locking knee joint must be worn or the knee must be fused. Fusion of the knee in a good position not only permits a satisfactory gait but also improves it by eliminating the weight of the brace; on the other hand, fusion of the knee causes inconvenience while sitting. The policy at this clinic is to defer fusion until the patient is old enough to weigh its advantages and disadvantages and to make the decision himself. Some patients may be heavy laborers who would have trouble in maintaining a brace and for whom the advantages of being free of a brace would outweigh the advantages of being able to sit with the knee flexed in a brace; these individuals would select arthrodesis. Others who sit much of the time may prefer to use a brace permanently. When both legs are badly paralyzed, one knee may be fused and the other stabilized with a brace.

It is always wise to apply a cylinder cast on a trial basis, immobilizing the knee in the position in which it would be fused. Thus the patient can make an informed decision concerning the advantages and disadvantages of arthrodesis of the knee. The techniques of knee fusion are described in Chapter 38.

TIBIA AND FEMUR

Although angular and torsional deformities of the tibia and femur may be secondary to conditions other than poliomyelitis, they are included in this chapter because of their frequency after this disease. They may result from congenital or static abnormalities of the bones and joints or from disturbances in growth caused by infection or by disorders of metabolism. They may also be secondary to muscle imbalance, as in poliomyelitis or in the spastic type of cerebral palsy.

Valgus angulation of the tibia or femur, anterior or posterior tilting of the proximal tibial articular surface, and torsion of the tibia are the most common deformities of these bones after poliomyelitis.

Maintaining the normal alignment of the lower extremities, a major problem in managing the patient with poliomyelitis, requires constant attention beginning with the onset of the disease; correct positioning in bed, an intelligent

program of physical therapy and rehabilitation, and the use of braces, shoes, and other appliances as indicated are required. If a deformity develops despite these measures, it should be corrected surgically when proper support of the extremity in a brace becomes impossible.

In a study of osteotomies of the tibia and femur for deformities from poliomyelitis, Gailey, Musgrave, and Irwin found contracture of the iliotibial band in 54% of the patients they examined. The contractures produced external torsion of the tibia and valgus deformity of the distal femur or proximal tibia or both. In some patients a strong biceps in the presence of weak medial hamstrings seemed to aid in producing external tibial torsion. A limp from weakness of the hip abductors tended to produce a valgus deformity of the distal femur.

Angular deformity of tibia

Surgery to correct an angular deformity of the tibia should restore the longitudinal axis of the tibia to its normal plane perpendicular to the axis of the knee and the axis of the ankle to normal alignment with that of the knee. The osteotomy of the tibia should be made at the apex of the deformity, and of the fibula should be 4 to 5 cm distal to its head. An opening wedge osteotomy of the tibia that lengthens the extremity is preferable to a closing wedge osteotomy that further shortens an already shortened extremity. For the same reason asymmetric epiphyseal stapling to correct an angular deformity after poliomyelitis is not advisable.

Many techniques for osteotomy of the long bones have been described, and some of these have appeared in earlier editions of this book. Among these are the notching rotational osteotomy of the tibia, the Z-osteotomy of the tibia in which a wedge of bone based anteriorly is resected from the tibia to correct torsion, the matchstick osteotomy in which multiple vertical cuts are made in the tibia with an electric saw and the deformity is corrected by creating a greenstick fracture, and the orange peel osteotomy of Harandi in which the cortex of the tibia is excised, leaving the cancellous bone intact, and the deformity is corrected by creating a greenstick fracture of the cancellous bone. We have concluded that the simpler techniques of osteotomy are safer and more reliable. When possible the end of the distal fragment should be rounded so that a three-dimensional deformity can be corrected while maximum bone contact between the fragments is maintained.

The correction of anterior tilting of the proximal articular surface of the tibia (genu recurvatum) is discussed on p. 2978.

TECHNIQUE OF OPENING WEDGE TIBIAL OSTEOTOMY. Insert a Knowles pin into the medial surface of the tibia just distal to the proximal epiphyseal plate and parallel to the axis of the knee in both the anteroposterior and lateral planes. Then insert a second Knowles pin into the medial surface of the middle third of the tibia parallel to the axis of the ankle. The pins must engage both cortices but should project little beyond the lateral cortex.

Expose the shaft of the proximal tibia through an oblique incision just medial to the tibial crest and 4 cm distal to the proximal pin. Elevate the periosteum and drill multiple holes through the bone at the level of the proposed osteotomy. Now complete the osteotomy by cutting the bone with a narrow osteotome between the holes. Through a separate incision osteotomize the fibula at a point 4 to 5 cm distal to its head, with care to protect the peroneal nerve. Now align the Knowles pins so that the axes of both the knee and ankle are in proper relationship to each other in both the anteroposterior and lateral planes and close the wounds. Apply a long leg cast, with the knee in 30 degrees of flexion and incorporating the Knowles pins. When the patient is obese or when a severe deformity has been corrected, extend the cast to the crest of the ilium.

AFTERTREATMENT. The position of the fragments at the osteotomy is checked by roentgenograms at 10 days; if it is not satisfactory, the cast is wedged between the Knowles pins. In a child this osteotomy usually heals within 8 weeks.

Torsion of tibia

In torsion of the tibia the most common site for osteotomy is just distal to the tibial condyles, for in this area the fragments are less likely to be displaced and union is faster. When torsion is associated with varus or valgus an-

gulation, the osteotomy is made near or at the apex of the angulation. The fibula should also be osteotomized because the deformity is then less likely to recur.

TECHNIQUE. Insert the Knowles pins and make the osteotomy as just described for angular deformity. Make the osteotomy just distal to the flare of the proximal metaphysis unless there is also an angular deformity to correct; in this instance make the osteotomy at the apex of the angular deformity. Through a separate incision osteotomize the fibula 4 to 5 cm distal to its head. Align the Knowles pins as just described but rotate the distal fragment with its Knowles pin internally or externally to correct the torsion. Now close the wound.

AFTERTREATMENT. A plaster cast incorporating the pins is applied from the groin to the toes, with the knee in slight flexion. At 6 weeks the cast is removed; roentgenograms then usually reveal enough consolidation of the osteotomy to permit guarded weight bearing.

Angular deformity of femur

In an angular deformity of the femur a tibial osteotomy would improve the appearance of the extremity, but the

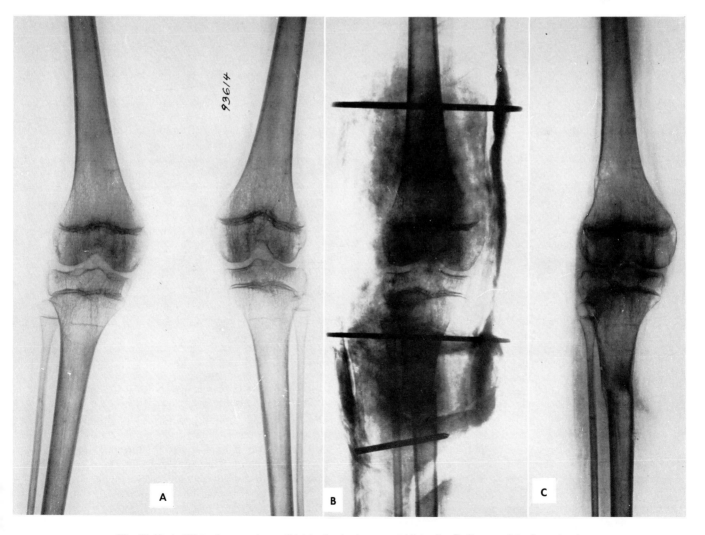

Fig. 66-40. A, Bilateral genu valgum; tibial torsion is also present bilaterally. **B,** Supracondylar femoral and proximal tibial osteotomies made at same operation to correct both angular and rotational deformities in one limb. **C,** Same limb as shown in **B,** after osteotomies have healed.

transverse axis of the knee would then be altered from its normal position perpendicular to the longitudinal axis of the tibia; thus the ligaments of the joint would then be stretched and secondary arthritic changes would eventually develop. Occasionally an angulation of the femur of 10 to 15 degrees may be corrected by a high tibial osteotomy, but more severe angulation must be corrected by a femoral osteotomy (Fig. 66-40).

We prefer an opening wedge supracondylar osteotomy with the base of the wedge lateral, because it adds length to the extremity; Irwin used a closing wedge supracondylar osteotomy with the base of the wedge medial.

TECHNIQUE. Insert a Knowles pin into the lateral supracondylar region of the femur at a right angle to the long axis of the bone. The pin should be long enough for its point to penetrate both cortices and for its head to remain 2.5 to 5 cm outside the skin. Then insert a second Knowles pin in a similar manner into the proximal part of the distal third of the femur. Expose the femur subperiosteally through a lateral longitudinal incision 5 cm long just proximal to the distal Knowles pin. Retract the vastus lateralis anteriorly and drill multiple holes in the femur parallel to the proximal Knowles pin. With an osteotome cut the bone between the holes, except in the medial cortex; complete the osteotomy manually. Now correct the deformity, and if desired pack the defect with cancellous bone chips. Close the wound and apply a single hip spica cast incorporating the pins.

AFTERTREATMENT. At 7 to 10 days two-plane roentgenograms of the osteotomy are made. If the alignment is not satisfactory, the cast is wedged between the pins. Immobilization is continued until the osteotomy is united (usually 8 weeks).

HIP

The disabilities caused by paralysis of the muscles about the hip are usually severe. They are discussed under the following headings: (1) contracture of the hip, (2) paralysis of the gluteus maximus and medius muscles, and (3) paralytic dislocation of the hip.

Contracture of hip

An abduction contracture is the most common deformity associated with paralysis of the muscles about the hip; it usually occurs in conjunction with flexion and external rotational contractures of varying degrees. Less often the contracture is one of adduction with flexion and internal rotation. When contractures of the hip are severe and bilateral, locomotion is possible only as a quadruped; the upright position is possible after the contractures are released.

INFLUENCE OF ILIOTIBIAL BAND ON FLEXION AND ABDUCTION CONTRACTURE OF HIP

The role of the iliotibial band (or tract) as a cause of deformities of the lower trunk and lower extremities after poliomyelitis involving these regions has received little attention in comparison with its importance. But Yount in 1926 observed that the iliotibial band is responsible for a triad of deformities: flexion and abduction contracture of the hip, flexion contracture of the knee, and genu valgum; Forbes (1928) and Fitchet (1933) may be cited, and Irwin (1949) has shown that even a mild contracture of the band

may be responsible for many deformities in the lower trunk and lower extremity.

Spasm of the hamstrings, the hip flexors, the tensor fasciae latae, and the hip abductors is common during the acute and convalescent stages of poliomyelitis. Straight leg raising is usually limited. The patient assumes the frog position, with the knees and hips flexed and the extremities completely rotated externally. When this position is maintained for even a few weeks, secondary soft tissue contractures occur; thus a permanent deformity develops, particularly when the gluteal muscles are weakened. The deformity puts the gluteus maximus at a disadvantage and prevents its return to normal strength. If the faulty position is not corrected, growth of the contracted soft tissues will fail to keep pace with bone growth, and the deformity will progressively increase. On the other hand, if positioning in bed is correct while muscle spasm is present, and if the joints are carried through a full range of motion at regular intervals after the muscle spasm disappears, contractures are prevented and soft tissues are kept sufficiently long and elastic to meet normal functional demands.

The large expanse of the fascia lata (the iliotibial band is a thickened part of this fascia) must be recognized before the deforming possibilities of the iliotibial band can be appreciated. Proximally the fascia lata arises from the coccyx, the sacrum, the crest of the ilium, the inguinal ligament, and the pubic arch and invests the muscles of the thigh and buttock. Either the superficial or the deep layer is attached to most of the gluteus maximus muscle and to all of the tensor fasciae latae muscle. All of the attachments of the fascia converge to form the iliotibial band on the lateral side of the thigh. This band is continuous throughout the length of the femur with the lateral intermuscular septum, which in turn is attached throughout to the linea aspera. The fact that the short head of the biceps takes origin in part from the lateral intermuscular septum and in part from the linea aspera further complicates the dynamic influence of the band. Distally the band is inserted into all of the prominences distal to the lateral side of the knee. Thus because of its long, strong distribution and its location in a plane anterior and lateral to the axis of the hip and posterior and lateral to the axis of the knee, the iliotibial band can produce deformities of these two joints through spasm of the biceps, gluteus maximus, and tensor fasciae latae muscles and through contracture of the band.

Contracture of the iliotibial band may contribute to the following deformities.

FLEXION, ABDUCTION, AND EXTERNAL ROTATIONAL CONTRACTURE OF HIP

A flexion and abduction deformity of the hip is readily attributable to contracture of the iliotibial band, since the band lies lateral and anterior to the hip joint. The position of external rotation is assumed for comfort; when this position is not corrected, however, the external rotators of the hip contract secondarily and contribute to the fixed deformity.

GENU VALGUM AND FLEXION CONTRACTURE OF KNEE

With growth, a contracted iliotibial band acts as a taut bowstring across the knee joint and gradually abducts and flexes the tibia. As the deformity increases, the mechanical advantage of the band also increases.

DISCREPANCY IN LEG LENGTH

Irwin believed that a contracted iliotibial band, which is attached to the femur by way of the lateral intermuscular septum, can to some extent slow the growth of both femoral epiphyses and of the proximal tibial epiphysis. Regardless of the cause, a contracted iliotibial band on one side is likely to be associated with considerable shortening of that extremity after years of growth.

EXTERNAL TIBIAL TORSION WITH OR WITHOUT SUBLUXATION OF KNEE JOINT

Because of its lateral attachment distally, the iliotibial band gradually rotates the tibia and fibula externally on the femur; this rotation may be increased if the short head of the biceps is strong. When the deformity becomes extreme, the lateral tibial condyle subluxates on the lateral femoral condyle, and the head of the fibula lies in the popliteal space.

SECONDARY TALIPES EQUINOVARUS

When there is external tibial torsion, the axes of the ankle and knee joints are no longer in the same plane. An improperly fitted brace that does not compensate for this torsion will force the foot into an equinovarus position; if the foot continues in this position, structural changes will eventually occur and require surgical correction.

EXTERNAL FEMORAL TORSION

When a flexion and abduction contracture is of long duration, the head and neck of the femur become anteverted as in congenital dislocation of the hip; that is, with the patella anterior the greater trochanter lies posteriorly.

PELVIC OBLIQUITY

When the band is contracted and the patient is supine with the hip in abduction and flexion, the pelvis may remain at a right angle to the long axis of the spine (Fig. 66-41, *A*). However, when the patient stands and the affected extremity is brought into the weight-bearing position, that is, parallel to the vertical axis of the trunk, the pelvis must assume an oblique position; the crest of the ilium is low on the contracted side and high on the opposite side. The lateral thrust forces the pelvis toward the unaffected side. Further, the trunk muscles on the affected side lengthen and those on the opposite side contract. If not corrected, the two contralateral contractures, that is, the band on the affected side and the trunk muscles on the unaffected side, hold the pelvis in this oblique position until skeletal changes fix the deformity (Fig. 66-41, *B*).

Bjerkreim reported seven instances of dysplasia and osteoarthritis of the adducted hip secondary to functional or fixed pelvic obliquity of long duration.

INCREASED LUMBAR LORDOSIS

Bilateral flexion contractures of the hip pull the proximal part of the pelvis anteriorly; for the trunk to assume an upright position, a compensatory increase in lumbar lordosis must develop.

PREVENTION AND TREATMENT OF FLEXION AND ABDUCTION CONTRACTURE OF HIP

A flexion and abduction contracture of the hip can be minimized or prevented in the early convalescent stage of poliomyelitis. The patient should be placed in bed with the hips in neutral rotation, slight abduction, and no flexion. All joints must be carried through a full range of passive motion several times daily; the hips must be stretched in extension, adduction, and internal rotation. To prevent rotation a bar similar to a Denis Browne splint is useful, especially when a knee roll is used to prevent a genu recurvatum deformity; the bar is clamped to the shoe soles to hold the feet in slight internal rotation. The contracture is carefully watched for in the acute and early convalescent stages; if found, it must be corrected before ambulation is allowed.

Irwin pointed out that secondary adaptive changes occur soon after the iliotibial band contracts and that the resulting deformity, regardless of its duration or of the patient's age, cannot be corrected by conservative measures; on the contrary, attempts at correction with traction will only increase the obliquity and hyperextension of the pelvis and cannot exert any helpful corrective force on the deformity.

Simple fasciotomies about the hip and knee may correct a minor contracture, but recurrence is common; they will not correct a severe contracture. Resecting a section of the iliotibial band and of the lateral intermuscular septum, first suggested by Yount, is a valuable part of the treatment, but the deformity frequently recurs when this procedure alone is used. Consequently, we follow the suggestion of Irwin and combine this procedure with one to release the hip. For a mild contracture the Yount procedure is combined with the Soutter fasciotomy; for a moderately severe one it is combined with soft tissue release as described in the Campbell operation (without resection of the crest of the ilium); and for a severe one it is combined with the complete Campbell transfer of the crest of the ilium.

Eberle reviewed 400 patients seen between June 1976 and April 1978 because of disabilities following poliomyelitis. Contractures about the hip were severe enough to require surgical release in 140, and of this group, 32 had unilateral abduction or flexion and abduction hip contracture and the opposite, "high side" hip was either subluxated or dislocated. In 11 patients the unstable hip was the site of either a flexion contracture or strong flexors in the presence of weak abductors. In 21 of the 32 patients the hip was flail, and in only 1 of the 400 was there an unstable hip without pelvic obliquity, the only patient in whom the dislocation was attributed to muscle imbalance alone.

Convinced of the overriding importance of pelvic obliquity in paralytic hip instability, Eberle found that surgical release of the contralateral abduction contracture alone was sufficient to correct the hip instability in the weight-bearing posture, and then the patient is usually able to walk without operation on the flail, previously unstable side.

His surgical technique consists of division of all tight fascial and tendinous structures about the anterolateral aspect of the hip until the deformity is completely corrected. This includes fascia lata, fascia over the gluteus medius and minimus, tensor fasciae latae, sartorius, rectus femoris, and occasionally the psoas tendon and anterolateral capsule. Muscle tissue is not divided; only its enveloping

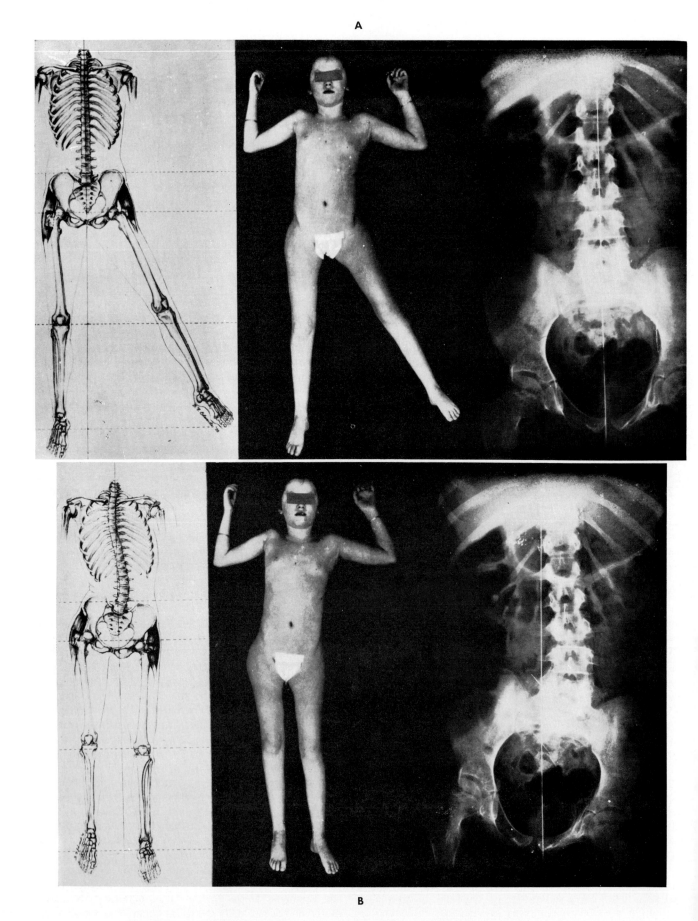

A

B

Fig. 66-41. A, In abduction contracture of hip, spine remains straight and pelvis level as long as hip is in abduction. **B,** When hip with abduction contracture is brought into weight-bearing position, pelvis must assume oblique position, causing scoliosis of lumbar spine. (Courtesy Dr. C.E. Irwin.)

fascial structures are. If the iliopsoas is strong and active, it is transferred after the fashion of Mustard and Sharrard, depending on the condition of the gluteus maximus.

Long leg casts with a short spreader bar are used after operation and nursing care is provided prone for 4 hours daily; the hip is passively stretched into extension and adduction.

If the dislocated hip is flail, it usually requires only closed reduction without surgery. If a flexion deformity is present, it is released. If the iliopsoas is normal or nearly so, it is transferred as above.

If scoliosis coexists in the patient with pelvic obliquity, the flexion and abduction contracture of the hip is corrected first and the pelvis is rendered level in the weight-bearing position. Then attention is directed to the scoliosis, if necessary, as described on p. 3224.

Yount in 1926 called attention to the tensor fasciae latae muscle as a cause of flexion and abduction contractures of the hip, flexion contracture of the knee, and abduction and external rotational contracture of the tibia on the femur. This combination of deformities often occurs in poliomyelitis. Unless it is severe and of long duration, Yount advocated dividing the iliotibial band proximal to the knee. Deformities of the hip of long duration require more extensive surgery (see below) in addition to this operation.

TECHNIQUE (YOUNT). Expose the fascia lata through a lateral longitudinal incision just proximal to the femoral condyle. Divide the iliotibial band and fascia lata posteriorly to the biceps tendon and anteriorly to the midline of the thigh at a level 2.5 cm proximal to the patella. Now at this level excise a segment of the iliotibial band and lateral intermuscular septum 5 to 8 cm long (Fitchet). Before closing the wound determine by palpation that all tight bands are divided.

AFTERTREATMENT. Aftertreatment is as described for posterior capsulotomy (Chapter 56). (See also the aftertreatment of Irwin, p. 2990)

For a *severe deformity* of the knee without a flexion deformity of the hip the following operation is used. Beginning 9 cm proximal to the knee over the biceps femoris tendon, make an incision proceeding anteriorly and distally over the iliotibial band to the lateral border of the patella and end it on the lateral surface of the leg just distal to the head of the fibula. Reflect the skin flap and expose the fascia lata and biceps tendon at their attachments distal to the knee. Lengthen the biceps tendon, and beginning at the tibial tuberosity, free all ligamentous structures, including the attachment of the iliotibial band, from the lateral condyle of the tibia proximally to the level of the joint by subperiosteal stripping. Free the lateral intermuscular septum and excise a segment of it 5 cm long. Detach a part of the fibular collateral ligament from the head of the fibula but avoid injuring the peroneal nerve. Then forcibly extend the knee and rotate it internally.

TRANSFER OF CREST OF ILIUM

Occasionally, forcible attempts to fully correct a flexion contracture of the hip without releasing all contracted structures have been fatal. Campbell devised a technique based on the Soutter operation that permits complete cor-

rection of the deformity; it is especially suitable for extreme flexion and abduction contracture after poliomyelitis.

TECHNIQUE (CAMPBELL). Incise the skin along the anterior one half or two thirds of the iliac crest to the anterosuperior spine and then distally for 5 to 10 cm on the anterior surface of the thigh. Divide the superficial and deep fasciae to the crest of the ilium. Strip the origins of the tensor fasciae latae and gluteus medius and minimus muscles subperiosteally from the wing of the ilium down to the acetabulum (Fig. 66-42, *A*). Then free the proximal part of the sartorius from the tensor fasciae latae. With an osteotome resect the anterosuperior iliac spine along with the origin of the sartorius muscle and allow both to retract distally and posteriorly. Next denude the anterior border of the ilium down to the anteroinferior spine. Free subperiosteally the attachments of the abdominal muscles from the iliac crest (or resect a narrow strip of bone with the attachments). Strip the iliacus muscle subperiosteally from the inner table. Free the straight tendon of the rectus femoris muscle from the anteroinferior iliac spine and the reflected tendon from the anterior margin of the acetabulum or simply divide the conjoined tendon of the muscle. Releasing these contracted structures will often allow the hip to be hyperextended without increasing the lumbar lordosis; this is a most important point because in this situation correction may be more apparent than real. If the hip cannot be hyperextended, other contracted structures must be divided. If necessary divide the capsule of the hip obliquely from proximally to distally and as a last resort free the iliopsoas muscle from the lesser trochanter by tenotomy. After the deformity has been completely corrected, resect the redundant part of the denuded ilium with an osteotome (Fig. 66-42, *B*). Now suture the abdominal muscles to the edge of the gluteal muscles and tensor fasciae latae over the remaining rim of the ilium with interrupted sutures. Suture the superficial fascia on the medial side of the incision to the deep fascia on the lateral side to bring the skin incision 2.5 cm posterior to the rim of the ilium.

To preserve the iliac epiphysis in a young child, modify the procedure as follows. Free the muscles subperiosteally from the lateral surface of the ilium. Detach the sartorius and rectus femoris as just described and if necessary release the capsule and iliopsoas muscle. Stripping the muscles from the medial surface of the ilium is unnecessary. Now with an osteotome remove a wedge of bone from the crest of the ilium distal to the epiphysis from anterior to posterior; its apex should be as far posterior as the end of the incision and its base anterior and 2.5 cm or more in width, as necessary to correct the deformity. Then displace the crest of the ilium distally to contact the main part of the ilium and fix it in place with sutures through the soft tissues.

AFTERTREATMENT. When the deformity has been mild, the hip is placed in hyperextension and about 10 degrees of abduction, and a spica cast is applied from the toes to the nipple line on the affected side and to above the knee on the opposite side. After 3 or 4 weeks the cast is removed, and the hip is mobilized (Fig. 66-43). Support may be unnec-

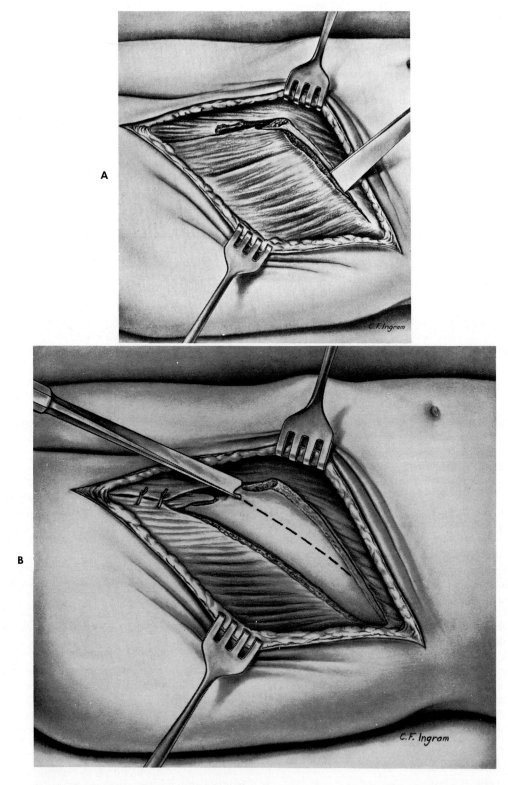

Fig. 66-42. Campbell transfer of crest of ilium for flexion contracture of hip. **A,** Origins of sartorius, tensor fasciae latae, and gluteus medius muscles are being detached from ilium. **B,** Redundant part of ilium is being resected.

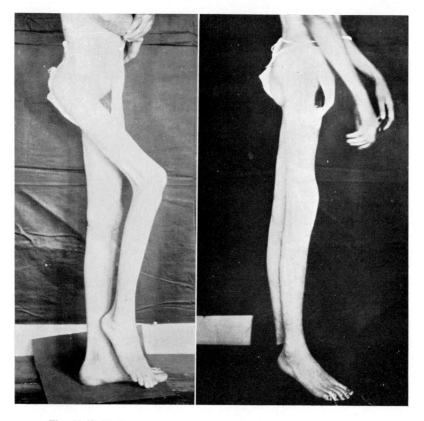

Fig. 66-43. Flexion contracture of hip released by transfer of crest of ilium.

essary during the day when the patient is on crutches; however, Buck's extension or an appropriate splint should be used at night. When the deformity has been moderate or severe, the aftertreatment of Irwin (p. 2990) is indicated.

SOFT TISSUE RELEASE OF HIP

TECHNIQUE (SOUTTER). Incise the skin as for an anterior iliofemoral approach (p. 59). Retract the subcutaneous tissue and divide the entire thickness of the fascia at a right angle to the skin incision from the anterosuperior iliac spine to the greater trochanter. Next retract the skin to expose the anterosuperior iliac spine. With an osteotome free the muscles and fascia subperiosteally from the spine medially, laterally, and inferiorly. Now hyperextend the hip and allow the tissues to retract distally. If the tension is still excessive, displace the periosteum and soft tissues from that part of the pelvis distal to the anterosuperior iliac spine with gauze or a blunt dissector.

AFTERTREATMENT. Aftertreatment is the same as for transfer of the crest of the ilium just described.

SOFT TISSUE RELEASE OF HIP AND THIGH

If the knee flexion deformity is 30 degrees or less, it can usually be corrected by wedging plaster casts, with care taken to prevent tibial subluxation. A flexion deformity of 30 degrees or less at the hip is usually not severe enough to require treatment.

TECHNIQUE (HUCKSTEP). Prepare and drape both lower ex-

tremities from the iliac crests to below the knees. Flex the unaffected hip fully throughout the procedure to flatten the lumbar spine against the table.

Make the first incision 2 cm proximal to the superior border of the patella over the midlateral aspect of the thigh. Insert the knife horizontally from laterally to medially until the tip of the blade touches the lateral femoral cortex. Now twist the blade 90 degrees so that its sharp edge points vertically anteriorly. Incise all soft tissues lateral to the femur and anterior to its midlateral point. If the flexion deformity of the knee is 30 degrees or more, make a short vertical incision over the biceps femoris tendon at the same level, identify, retract and protect the peroneal nerve, and then divide the biceps tendon and the lateral intermuscular septum down to the femur.

Then make a second incision at the midthigh, directly lateral and in the same manner as before. Again divide the tensor fascia lata and all tight structures from the midlateral aspect of the femur anteriorly. In severe contractures, instead of the midthigh incision, similar incisions can be made at the junctions of the middle and distal thirds of the thigh and of the middle and proximal thirds.

Make the final incision one finger breadth distal to the anterosuperior iliac spine, being careful to avoid the inguinal ligament and the femoral nerve, artery, and vein. Insert the blade 2 cm deep and then turn the cutting edge of the blade laterally through 90 degrees and divide all tight subcutaneous structures. If the flexion deformity is severe, divide all tight structures lateral to the femoral nerve down to the neck of the femur and posteriorly to the midlateral plane. Keep the hip in extension and adduction so that the tight structures are palpable, and, except those mentioned, leave no tight bands undivided.

AFTERTREATMENT. All blood clots should be repeatedly and completely expressed from the wounds by manual pressure during and on completion of the operation. Then simple dressings are applied using elasticized tape that does not encircle the extremity. Bilateral long leg casts are applied and then removed after 3 weeks. Braces and crutches are fitted and ambulation is permitted as tolerated.

• • •

After transfer of the crest of the ilium or the Soutter release for moderate or severe flexion and abduction contractures of the hip, the aftertreatment described by Irwin, as already mentioned, is indicated.

AFTERTREATMENT (IRWIN). A Kirschner wire is inserted into each femur just proximal to the condyles. Bilateral long leg casts are applied, incorporating the Kirschner wires and bows. The affected limb is flexed and abducted, and enough traction is applied to the normal limb to place the pelvis at a right angle to the longitudinal axis of the trunk (Fig. 66-44, *A*); a cast is then applied to the trunk and is attached to the cast on the normal limb to form a single spica (Fig. 66-44, *B*). The affected limb is now internally

rotated, extended, and adducted to the point of resistance, and the cast on this side is attached to the cast on the trunk (Fig. 66-44, *C*). Beginning at 2 weeks, the affected extremity is wedged every 3 to 5 days toward more adduction and extension to increase the correction. By this method, in contrast to well leg traction, the abduction and flexion contractures are corrected simultaneously beginning with the pelvis level and the lumbar spine flat; thus anterior tilting of the pelvis and exaggeration of lumbar lordosis are avoided.

Paralysis of gluteus maximus and medius muscles

One of the most severe disabilities from poliomyelitis is caused by paralysis of the gluteus maximus muscle or the gluteus medius or both; the result is an unstable hip and an unsightly and fatiguing limp. During weight bearing on the affected side when the gluteus medius alone is paralyzed, the trunk sways toward this side and the pelvis sags on the opposite side, and when the gluteus maximus alone is paralyzed, the body lurches backward. The strength of the gluteal muscles may be demonstrated by the Trendelenburg test: when a normal person bears weight on one extremity and flexes the other at the hip, the pelvis is held on a horizontal plane and the gluteal folds are on the same level; when the gluteal muscles are impaired and weight is borne on the affected side, the level of the pelvis on the normal side will drop lower than that on the affected side;

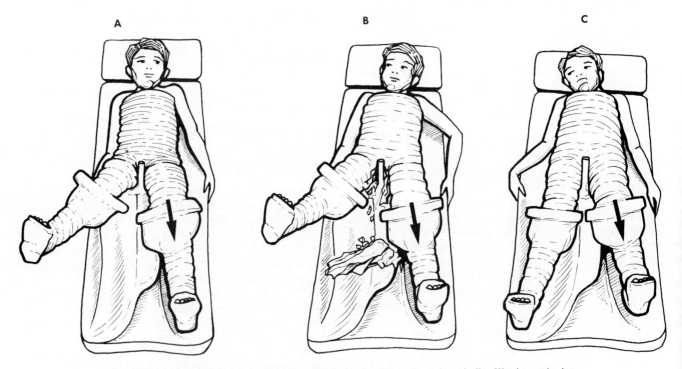

A **B** **C**

Fig. 66-44. A, Flexion-abduction contracture of right hip has been corrected surgically. Kirschner wire has been inserted into distal femur on left, and bilateral long leg casts have been applied; that on left incorporates Kirschner wire and bow. We insert Kirschner wire into each femur. Right limb has been flexed and abducted, and enough traction has been applied to left limb to place pelvis at right angle to longitudinal axis of trunk. **B,** With spine flat and pelvis level, cast is then applied to trunk and is attached to cast on left limb (normal one) to form single spica. Right hip is still abducted and flexed. **C,** Right limb (affected one) has been adducted and extended to point of resistance, and cast on this side has been attached to cast on trunk. After 2 weeks, affected limb will be wedged every 3 to 5 days toward more adduction and extension to increase correction.

when the gluteal paralysis is severe, the test cannot be made, for balance on the disabled extremity is impossible.

Because no apparatus will stabilize the pelvis when one or both of these muscles are paralyzed, function can be improved only by transferring muscular attachments to replace the gluteal muscles when feasible. Fritz Lange of Munich first used the erector spinae muscle under these circumstances; he lengthened the muscle with silk and inserted in into the greater trochanter. Kreuscher's technique is almost identical. Ober and Hey Groves improved and modified this operation by attaching the erector spinae muscle to the trochanter with a strip of fascia lata and by transferring the tensor fasciae latae muscle in a manner similar to that of Legg. Barr redefined the indications for this procedure and improved the technique of Ober and Hey Groves. This procedure was described in detail in previous editions of this book but is omitted here since it is both technically difficult to properly perform and its results are disappointing because it usually functions only by its tenodesing effect.

Lowman in 1947 described a method of attaching a part of the external oblique muscle to the greater trochanter with a strip of fascia lata. His results were encouraging: in 12 such transfers function improved from 25% to 80%; in all 12 fatigue while standing and walking was decreased, and in some the limp was markedly reduced. Thomas, Thompson, and Straub in 1950 also described a method of transferring the external oblique muscle for paralysis of the gluteus medius, but in this procedure all of the muscle belly is used. The muscle is freed from its normal insertion and is mobilized to its origin; the distal aponeurosis is then inserted into the most prominent part of the greater trochanter.

Mustard described another operation to restore stability and abduction of the hip; the iliopsoas tendon is transferred laterally to the greater trochanter. Our experience with this operation has been gratifying. When the power of the gluteus maximus muscle has been fair or better, we have seen the Trendelenburg test, which was positive before surgery, become negative after surgery. The gait and the stability and strength of the hip have consistently improved. However, function of the transfer may not become maximum until 12 to 18 months after surgery.

Sharrard modified Mustard's operation by transferring the iliopsoas posteriorly. This operation was designed for paralysis not only of the gluteus medius but of the gluteus maximus as well. Although it was conceived primarily for treating paralytic dislocation of the hip in meningomyelocele, it is also useful in poliomyelitis. In this operation the psoas tendon and the entire iliacus muscle are passed through a hole made in the posterior part of the ilium just lateral to the sacroiliac joint; the iliopsoas tendon is anchored to the greater trochanter and the origin of the iliacus muscle is sutured to the lateral surface of the ilium. Thus if the gluteus medius muscle is paralyzed and the gluteus maximus is not, the Mustard lateral transfer of the iliopsoas is indicated, but if both muscles are paralyzed, then the Sharrard posterior transfer of the iliopsoas is indicated.

Cabaud, Westin, and Connelly analyzed the results of tendon transfers about the hip to augment abductor power in 149 patients with flaccid paralysis. After the transfer operation 23 of 38 hips that had previously been subluxated or dislocated became stable in the reduced position. Every hip stable before operation remained so, and 37 patients previously brace dependent became brace free.

Of the 149 patients, 29 underwent erector spinae transfers before the procedure was abandoned because it was difficult to perform and its resulting function was primarily as a tenodesis. Psoas transfer was performed in 57 patients, while 98 underwent external oblique transfers. Either psoas or external oblique transfer to the greater trochanter improved hip stability as long as the contralateral hip abductor-extensor muscles were strong enough to provide a stable pelvic platform and support to permit the transferred muscle to function. Problems encountered after psoas transfer were weakness of hip flexion secondary to loss of primary flexor (all patients); avascular necrosis of femoral head (3); femoral nerve palsy (4); infection (7); femoral fracture (2); and abduction contracture (1). Problems following external abdominal oblique transfer were as follows: avascular necrosis of femoral head (1); infection (6); fractured femur (3); fascial hernia (1); transfer pulled out (1); and reefing of transfer required (30).

Gait analysis revealed that following external abdominal oblique transfer, single limb support was increased in each patient tested; additionally, it helped to better position the limb in terminal swing phase and in properly presenting the limb for stance phase.

Hammesfahr, Topple, Yoo, Whitesides, and Paullin, in a preliminary report of 37 external abdominal oblique transfers performed on poliomyelitis patients, found an 89% patient satisfaction rate; none of the patients who required a pelvic band brace before operation required one afterward. Most patients had an increase in abductor muscle power of two or three grades after operation, none had an abduction or a flexion contracture, and while the Trendelenburg test was not reversed, all exhibited considerable decrease in hip lurch on walking. Further, this procedure is relatively simple technically and is broadly applicable, since the muscle is innervated by the T4-12 nerve roots, which are not often affected in poliomyelitis and are unaffected in lumbar myelomeningocele patients. On the other hand, the Mustard and Sharrard procedures that transfer the psoas tendon to the greater trochanter have disadvantages. Mustard recommends that the procedure be restricted to patients who have good or normal power in the iliopsoas, the sartorius, the rectus femoris, and the gluteus maximus, a condition that frequently does not exist. In addition, the procedure is more difficult, it endangers the femoral nerve, and it especially weakens significantly active hip flexion.

Parker and Walker studied 44 children who underwent 72 posterior psoas transfer operations 1 to 8 years after operation, and they made these significant observations: 57% of the patients had an acceptable functional result in that they were able to sit down, stand up, and walk at least 25 meters unassisted; 49% of the hips were stable before operation, and 94% were stable at review.

Sharrard's original technique of psoas transfer was used with only a few modifications. A portion of the lesser trochanter was detached to retain length and make the insertion into bone easier; a large hole was made in the ilium to allow freedom of action of the transfer; the iliacus muscle was sacrificed, since its mobilization devitalized it; a wire stitch at the point of insertion subsequently marked the end of the tendon and, when avulsed, was readily apparent on roentgenograms; finally, any adduction contracture existing at the time of transfer was corrected by adductor tenotomy.

Complications included lower limb fractures in 22; sepsis in 9; marker stitch displacement in 9; ankylosis by heterotopic bone in 1; and avascular necrosis of the femoral head in 8, of which 4 had undergone open reduction.

A small redistribution of power occurred about the hips with flexion effectively reduced and abduction and extension marginally improved. Children with normal power at the L3-4 level (intact quadriceps) usually did well, while the results in those with more proximal involvement were less satisfactory.

These authors concluded (1) that the transfer should be done before adaptive joint changes become irreversible; (2) that in children more than 2 years of age it should be reserved for those with active power at L3-4 levels; and (3) that children who required trunk bracing because of instability rarely had a useful level of walking after operation.

These operations are only relatively successful. When the gluteal muscles are completely paralyzed, normal balance is never restored, and although the gluteal limp may be lessened, it remains; however, when the paralysis is only partial, the gait may be markedly improved.

TRANSFER OF EXTERNAL OBLIQUE MUSCLE FOR PARALYSIS OF GLUTEUS MEDIUS MUSCLE

Anatomically the external oblique muscle is a good substitute for paralyzed abductors of the hip. Because its nerve supply is from a different spinal segment than that of the gluteus medius and minimus muscles, it is less likely to be paralyzed when these muscles are. Its aponeurosis is long and broad, its surfaces are well adapted for gliding movement, and after transfer its mechanical action on the greater trochanter is direct. When it is strong enough for transfer, the other abdominal muscles are almost always strong enough to maintain the integrity of the abdominal wall. But the hip will be stable during weight bearing and active abduction will be restored by this procedure only when the transferred muscle is strong. When desired, a strong tensor fasciae latae in addition may be transferred posteriorly on the iliac crest (Legg), or the superior part of the gluteus maximus may be moved anteriorly to assist in active abduction. When the gluteus maximus and medius are both paralyzed, the Ober-Barr operation may be combined with transfer of the external oblique to restore both extension and abduction.

TECHNIQUE (THOMAS, THOMPSON, AND STRAUB). Make a skin incision beginning at the pubic tubercle and extending proximally over the crest of the ilium and ending at the costal margin in the posterior axillary line (Fig. 66-45, A). Make two incisions in the aponeurosis of the external oblique muscle 2 cm apart and parallel with each other and with the inguinal ligament; join the incisions at a point 1 cm proximal to the pubis. Then carry the superior incision proximally along the medial border of the muscle belly to the rib cage to free the muscle from the remainder of its aponeurosis; carry the inferior incision laterally to the anterosuperior iliac spine, pass a blunt dissector beneath the fibers of the external oblique, and incise them adjacent to their insertion into the ilium. Free the muscle from the underlying tissues by blunt dissection (Fig. 66-45, B). Now fold under and suture together the cut edges of the

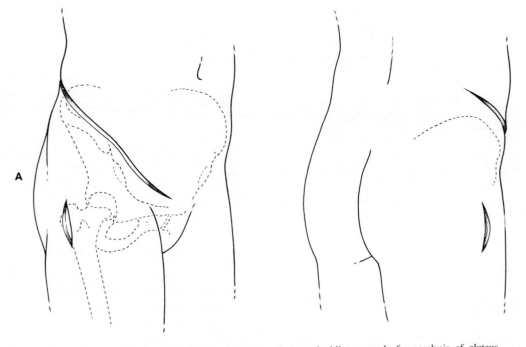

Fig. 66-45. Thomas, Thompson, and Straub transfer of external oblique muscle for paralysis of gluteus medius. **A,** Skin incisions as seen from anterolateral and posterolateral viewpoints.

muscle and its aponeurosis to form a cone-shaped structure. Beginning at the pubis, repair the remaining aponeurosis of the muscle as far laterally as possible (Fig. 66-45, *C*). Next suture the remaining free edge of the aponeurosis to the underlying internal oblique muscle. A small triangular defect remains in the outer layer of the anterolateral wall but seems to cause no trouble (Fig. 66-45, *D*).

Now make a 6 cm lateral incision over the most promi-

nent part of the greater trochanter. Through separate incisions in the fascia and periosteum, drill two holes 1 cm in diameter and at right angles to each other in the prominent part of the bone. Make a subcutaneous tunnel extending proximally to the original incision as far posteriorly as possible; it must be large where it crosses the ilium, for the transferred muscle will form a mass 5 to 6 cm in diameter at this level. Now pass the cone-shaped strip of the

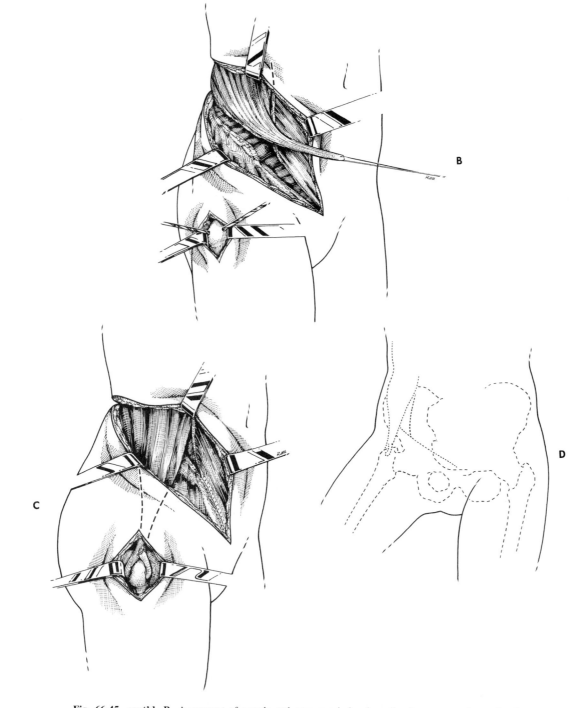

Fig. 66-45, cont'd. B, A segment of muscle and aponeurosis has been freed; greater trochanter has been exposed and holes have been drilled in it to receive transfer. **C,** and **D** Aponeurosis of external oblique muscle has been passed through subcutaneous tunnel and tunnel in trochanter and firmly sutured. (Redrawn from Thomas, L.I., Thompson, T.C., and Straub, L.R.: J. Bone Joint Surg. **32-A:**207, 1950.)

external oblique muscle distally through the tunnel; place the hip in wide abduction, pass the aponeurotic end of the strip (which serves as a tendon) through the holes in the trochanter, and suture it firmly to itself (Fig. 66-45, *D*). Close the wound and apply a spica cast, holding the hip in wide abduction and moderate extension.

AFTERTREATMENT. At 4 weeks the cast is removed, and underwater exercises and muscle reeducation are started; therapy is continued until maximum improvement has been obtained. Full weight bearing may usually be allowed after 8 weeks.

LATERAL TRANSFER OF ILIOPSOAS TENDON FOR PARALYSIS OF GLUTEUS MEDIUS MUSCLE

Mustard devised an operation for weakness of the hip abductors in which the tendon of the iliopsoas muscle is transferred to the greater trochanter. This muscle is strong enough to serve as an abductor, and the short-fibered iliacus is already a stabilizer.

The ideal patient for lateral iliopsoas transfer is one in whom the hip abductors are weak but the gluteus maximus, sartorius, iliopsoas, quadriceps, and abdominal muscles are good. However, in a follow-up of 50 such transfers for hip instability, Mustard included a number of patients who had not met these requirements, but who nevertheless obtained gratifying results. According to him, isolated paralysis of the hip abductors is uncommon; the gluteus maximus is usually also paralyzed to some extent. The results of the operation have been so satisfactory when both the abductors and the gluteus maximus are weak that he recommends the operation even for patients who have power only in the hip flexors. The limp resulting from hip instability is not only disfiguring, it gradually increases and may lead eventually to pain and even subluxation of the hip; this limp, he found, was always decreased when a normal iliopsoas muscle was transferred. Strength in the hip was definitely increased in all but one patient after the operation; in 28 the Trendelenburg test was converted to negative. Although the object of the operation is to stabilize the hip, the range of abduction was materially improved in most instances. The age of his patients varied from 3½ to 55 years, and age did not seem to affect the results.

TECHNIQUE (MUSTARD). Begin the skin incision lateral and posterior to the anterosuperior iliac spine, carry it anteriorly for about 7.5 cm (go a little more medially than in the Smith-Petersen incision), and curve it distally and posteriorly to cross the tensor fasciae latae at a point about two fifths of the way distally along the thigh. Find the plane between the tensor fasciae latae and the sartorius and resect the lateral femoral cutaneous nerve. Then incise the periosteum along the crest of the ilium and reflect subperiosteally the tensor fasciae latae and the remnants of the gluteal muscles; reflect also the attachment of the abdominal muscles until the iliacus is exposed. By subperiosteal dissection enter the pelvis on the lateral side of the iliacus muscle and make the anterosuperior spine stand out in relief; resect the spine, taking with it the origin of the sartorius muscle. Reflect this muscle distally and medially by dissecting boldly along its lateral border and carefully along its medial border until the nerve that enters its belly

is seen. Trace this nerve to the femoral nerve and carry the dissection distally until the branch of the femoral nerve to the rectus femoris is found; occasionally this branch originates more proximally than usual, and dissection between it and the femoral nerve is necessary to identify and ligate the circumflex vessels. Retract the femoral nerve and vessels medially, identify the apex of the lesser trochanter, and with the finger clear a space proximal and distal to it as well as beneath the iliacus. Beginning in a plane deep to the belly of the iliacus dissect distally until from the lateral aspect of the iliopsoas muscle the lesser trochanter can be felt; flex and externally rotate the hip to expose the trochanter. Now place a finger on the anteromedial aspect of the trochanter and use it to direct an osteotome to its deep superior edge; divide and deliver the trochanter into the wound. Shave off the remainder of the iliacus that is attached to the linea aspera; if the nerve to the rectus femoris seems to be in the way during this part of the operation, proceed distal to it. Now deliver the iliopsoas tendon and the iliacus muscle into the wound.

Now divide the tensor fasciae latae halfway between its origin and insertion and turn it posteriorly without injuring its nerve supply. Rotate the femur medially and expose the greater trochanter. Then cut a trough in the wing of the ilium including the base of the anterosuperior spine and large enough to accomodate the transferred muscle; cut it as far proximal and posterior as possible to allow a more direct line of pull for the muscle. Next observe the direction in which the iliopsoas will be placed, and either divide the remnants of the abductor muscles and lay the iliopsoas in this gutter or split the muscles so that the iliopsoas can be pulled through them with ease. Now transfer the iliopsoas laterally; with the thigh in full abduction and slight internal rotation and with powerful tension on the tendon, determine the site for its insertion into the femoral shaft. Cut a small window in the femur at this site and anchor the lesser trochanter in it. Suture the vastus lateralis to the edges of the iliopsoas tendon and the iliacus muscle and any remnants of the hip abductor muscles to the psoas. Then repair the tensor fasciae latae and anchor the anterosuperior spine to the crest of the ilium. Suture the tensor fasciae latae and the remainder of the abductor muscles to the abdominal muscles and close the incision. Apply a spica cast with the hip in internal rotation, slight flexion, and full abduction.

AFTERTREATMENT. Aftertreatment is the same as for transfer of the external oblique muscle (see above).

POSTERIOR TRANSFER OF ILIOPSOAS FOR PARALYSIS OF GLUTEUS MEDIUS AND MAXIMUS MUSCLES

Sharrard modified Mustard's operation by transferring the iliopsoas tendon and the entire iliacus muscle posteriorly. This operation is more extensive than Mustard's but is superior to it when the gluteus maximus and medius are both paralyzed. Sharrard emphasizes that open adductor tenotomy should always precede iliopsoas transfer.

TECHNIQUE (SHARRARD). Place the patient on an ordinary operating table slightly tilted to the side opposite the operation. Make an incision along the anterior two thirds of the iliac crest and extend it distally along the medial border of the sartorius muscle to the middle of the thigh. Dissect down to the deep fascia and define the iliac crest in the proximal half of the incision. Then define and incise the gluteal fascia along the middle and posterior thirds of the iliac crest. Divide the atrophic gluteus medius and minimus muscles and expose subperiosteally the outer surface of the ilium. Next expose the sartorius muscle in its proximal half (Fig. 66-46, *A*); do not release its origin unless there is a severe flexion contracture of the hip. Now identify the rectus femoris tendon but again, unless there is flexion contracture of the hip and extension contracture of the knee, do not divide it; if there is, then divide the tendon and allow it to retract. Next define the inferior border of the inguinal ligament, identify the femoral nerve as it emerges from the pelvis, and mobilize the nerve toward

the lateral side. Expose the inner surface of the false pelvis by detaching the abdominal muscles from the anterior two thirds of the iliac crest; in a young child do this by incising the iliac epiphysis anteriorly and gently prying it from the ilium posteriorly to its posterior end. Now flex and externally rotate the hip to bring the lesser trochanter anteriorly. During the next dissection preserve if possible the lateral femoral circumflex vessels. Identify the lesser trochanter and detach it from the femur along with that portion of the iliopsoas tendon that inserts on it. Then free the deeper parts of the tendon and mobilize the entire tendon proximally into the pelvis; a bursa deep to the psoas indicates the plane of separation. Identify and carefully preserve the branches of the femoral nerve that enter the iliacus muscle

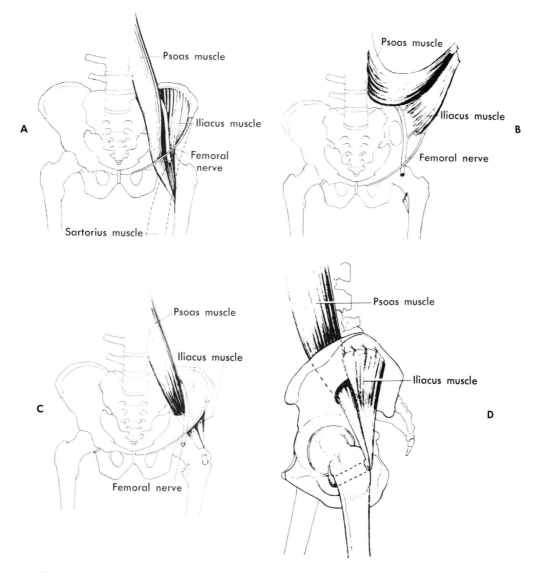

Fig. 66-46. Sharrard posterior transfer of iliopsoas for paralysis of gluteus medius and maximus muscles. **A,** Normal anatomy. **B,** Iliopsoas tendon and lesser trochanter have been detached, iliacus and psoas muscles have been elevated, origin of iliacus has been freed, and hole has been made in ilium. Note branches of femoral nerve entering iliacus. **C,** Iliopsoas tendon and entire iliacus muscle have been passed beneath femoral nerve and through hole in ilium. **D,** Iliopsoas tendon has been passed from posterior to anterior through hole in greater trochanter and anchored there. Origin of iliacus muscle has been sutured to outer surface of ilium. (Modified from Sharrard, W.J.W.: J. Bone Joint Surg. **46-B:**426, 1964.)

(Fig. 66-46, *B*); there are usually two, one being given off soon after the nerve enters the pelvis and the other about halfway along the course of the nerve in the pelvis. If necessary to mobilize it sufficiently, dissect the distal branch proximally away from the main nerve. With the hip still flexed to relax the femoral nerve, pass the iliopsoas tendon and attached part of the lesser trochanter beneath the nerve to its lateral side. Then by blunt and sharp dissection detach extraperiosteally the origin of the iliacus muscle from the inner aspect of the pelvis.

Now make a hole through the iliac wing just lateral to the sacroiliac joint (Fig. 66-46, *B*): make it oval with its long axis longitudinal, its width slightly more than one third of that of the iliac wing, and its length one and one-half times as long as its width. Then pass the iliopsoas tendon and the entire iliacus muscle through the hole (Fig. 66-46, *C*); pass the origin of the iliacus through the hole first and then its insertion, and the iliopsoas tendon will follow easily.

Pass a finger from the gluteal region distally and posteriorly into the bursa deep to the gluteus maximus tendon and identify by touch the posterolateral aspect of the greater trochanter; the transfer should be anchored here. By referring to this point expose the corresponding anterior aspect of the greater trochanter by dissecting through the fascia lata and the fatty and fibrous tissue over the trochanter. Now with awls and burrs and from anteriorly to posteriorly make a hole through the greater trochanter until it is big enough to receive the tendon. Using a clove hitch attach a strong silk suture to the fragment of the lesser trochanter and to the iliopsoas tendon. Then while the hip is held in abduction, extension, and neutral rotation, pass the end of the tendon through the buttock and from posteriorly to anteriorly through the tunnel in the greater trochanter (Fig. 66-46, *D*). With several strong sutures anchor the tendon securely and under good tension to the anterior surface of the trochanter. Now suture the origin of the iliacus muscle to the ilium just inferior to the iliac crest in the position corresponding to the origin of the gluteus medius.

Now suture the abdominal muscles and gluteal fascia to the iliac crest, and close the space between the inguinal ligament and the pubic bone by suturing the ligament to the iliopectineal line. Then suture the deep fascia and skin. With the hip in full abduction and extension and in neutral rotation, apply a spica cast that extends distally to the base of the toes on the affected side.

The following technical difficulties have been encountered in the operation: (1) exposing of the lesser trochanter by the approach between the femoral nerve and vessels; (2) separating the origin of the iliacus muscle from the most posterior and medial aspects of the inner surface of the ilium when the iliac wing is more vertical than usual; in these instances the approach must be extended farther posteriorly; and (3) passing the iliopsoas tendon from posteriorly to anteriorly through the greater trochanter; the tendon tends to jam at the entrance of the tunnel in the bone resulting in insufficient tension on the transfer. Sharrard has developed a cannula that makes this part of the operation easier.

AFTERTREATMENT. Immobilization is discontinued at 3½ weeks in children 2 to 4 years old, at 4 weeks in children 4 to 6 years old, and at 4½ weeks in children 6 to 10 years old. If the same operation is necessary on the opposite side, it may be performed the same day as the first operation if the condition of the patient permits, otherwise at 3 weeks.

Paralytic dislocation of hip*

If a child contracts poliomyelitis before the age of 2 years and the gluteal muscles become paralyzed but the flexors and adductors of the hip do not, then he is almost certain to develop paralytic dislocation of the hip before he is grown. That the combination of imbalance in muscle power, habitually faulty postures, and growth are important in producing deformity is illustrated nowhere better than in this situation. Since the factors predisposing to paralytic dislocation of the hip are similar in myelomeningocele and poliomyelitis, its management is similar. Dislocation of the hip associated with cerebral palsy is discussed in Chapter 65, p. 2905.

Jones notes that although paralytic dislocations of the hip are entirely different from congenital dislocations they have been given little consideration, probably because they are rare. In 1954 he reported a study of 22 paralytic dislocations in 14 patients. The distribution of these according to cause was as follows: poliomyelitis, 6 hips in 4 patients; spastic paraplegia, 12 hips in 7 patients; spastic hemiplegia, 2 hips in 2 patients; and meningomyelocele, both hips in 1 patient. In 1948 Miller and Irwin reported a series of only 20 paralytic dislocations of the hip among 5400 patients with poliomyelitis examined at the Georgia Warm Springs Foundation over a period of 15 years; their ages ranged from 8 to 30 years.

Only paralytic dislocations from poliomyelitis will be discussed here; those from cerebral palsy are discussed in Chapter 65 and from meningomyelocele later in this chapter.

Paralytic dislocations of the hip can usually be reduced easily, but the final results of treatment have been generally unsatisfactory. When seen early, the dislocation can be reduced by simply abducting the hip; later when a mild flexion and adduction contracture has developed, gentle, but prolonged traction in addition to abduction may be necessary; even later when the contracture and dislocation are more severe, adductor tenotomy (Chapter 65) and skeletal traction are necessary but are usually sufficient. When a dislocation is irreducible by closed methods, adductor tenotomy and skeletal traction are necessary before open reduction is attempted, and the traction must be continued until the femoral head is opposite the acetabulum and at least 30 degrees of abduction are possible. In the past, surgical treatment for paralytic dislocation was often followed by persistent deformity, recurrence of the dislocation, and pain and instability. But now a more rational program for treating this difficult problem is available because of Mustard's development of his iliopsoas transfer, Jones' description of his varus femoral osteotomy, Salter's and Pemberton's work on surgical deepening of the ace-

---

*See also Chapter 65.

tabulum (Chapter 62), and Sharrard's studies and his modification of Mustard's operation.

The primary cause of paralytic dislocation is imbalance of muscle power about the hip, and unless this imbalance is corrected the dislocation is likely to recur regardless of other treatment. Because the imbalance is characterized by weak abductors and extensors and by strong or relatively strong flexors and adductors, the aim of treatment must be the restoration of power of abduction and extension. The Mustard lateral transfer of the iliopsoas tendon (p. 2994) is indicated when the gluteus medius is paralyzed but the gluteus maximus is fair or better (which it usually is not). The Sharrard posterior transfer of the iliopsoas (p. 2994), which is a bigger operation, is indicated when the gluteus medius and maximus muscles are both paralyzed. These operations have the disadvantage of significantly weakening flexion of the hip. Therefore in consideration of transfer of the iliopsoas to restore abduction or extension, the presence of strong and active power in the tensor fasciae latae, the sartorius, and the rectus femoris is important.

Valgus deformity of the femoral neck is a secondary or adaptive skeletal change and in our experience is slowly and unrelentingly progressive. It is caused by the absence of or marked decrease in the upward traction exerted on the greater trochanter by the gluteal muscles and by the absence of or marked decrease in the downward thrust applied to the femoral head by the weight of the body during standing and walking. This downward thrust is further decreased by the absence of normal leverage present when strong gluteal muscles stabilize the pelvis over the femur. Any persistent valgus deformity of the femoral neck tends to cause subluxation or even recurrence of the dislocation by concentrating the forces of weight bearing in the lateral part of the acetabulum. Since 1949 we have recognized the need for varus osteotomies of the proximal femur and have made them many times (Fig. 66-47, A and B). When one is performed as an isolated operation, usually its benefits are only temporary because the valgus deformity tends to recur during growth; this has been confirmed by Jones and others. Thus the value of varus osteotomy as a definitive operation is limited to correcting valgus deformity of the femoral neck (and the usually associated anteversional deformity) before the iliopsoas is transferred to correct muscle imbalance. In children under 5 years old we fix the osteotomy at an angle of 105 degrees and in older children of 125 degrees. Samilson, Tsou, Aamoth, and Green found in treating dislocation of the hip in cerebral palsy that the osteotomy should be fixed at an angle of 90 to 100 degrees. When the angle exceeds 100 degrees, especially in a young child, subluxation or dislocation of the hip before skeletal maturity is likely. In infants we use a small, angled blade plate for internal fixation.

An increase in obliquity of the acetabular roof is also an adaptive skeletal change. It is caused by uneven pressure in the acetabulum and by persistent subluxation of the femoral head and may eventually lead to dislocation. This increased obliquity develops less frequently and also later than does valgus deformity of the femoral neck. Many operations have been designed to deepen the acetabulum, but in our experience the most satisfactory ones have been osteotomy of the innominate bone described by Salter (p.

2733) and pericapsular osteotomy of the ilium described by Pemberton (p. 2738). Such an operation is indicated when the acetabulum is insufficient to retain the femoral head after the normal angle between the femoral neck and shaft has been restored by varus osteotomy; it is carried out at the same time as iliopsoas transfer.

The pelvic support osteotomy (Schanz), as described by Milch, provides a painless stable hip and improves the gait (Fig. 66-47, C). However, it has the disadvantages of putting weight on movable extraarticular structures and of further shortening an already short extremity. It is indicated when a fixed pelvic obliquity is uncorrectable; in this instance it is on the high side of the pelvis that the hip is adducted and dislocated. As pointed out by Irwin, an abduction or a pelvic support osteotomy on this side shifts the weight-bearing axis of the limb medially and improves the ability of the limb to bear weight, especially if the opposite abducted limb either is shortened or its femoral neck is placed in more varus. We prefer pelvic support osteotomy to arthrodesis of the hip for a painful and unstable paralytic dislocation in a patient who is skeletally mature, especially when the opposite limb is also affected by poliomyelitis.

Arthrodesis of the hip may be indicated when a dislocation is irreducible by other methods, when other reconstructive procedures have failed, or when a dislocated hip in an adult has become painfully arthritic. Hallock reported a series of 20 patients in whom arthrodesis was done for a painful paralytic dislocation or for a severe limp caused by extensive paralysis about the hip; pain was relieved, stability was improved, and the hip limp was controlled far more satisfactorily than is possible by a shelf operation. The ligaments of the knee must be stable to withstand the additional strain that a stiff hip imposes on this joint. Although helpful, functional quadriceps power is not essential, but the knee must have no significant flexion contracture, especially when the quadriceps is weak. The foot and ankle must also be stable. Hip fusion is contraindicated when the abdominal muscles are severely paralyzed (Mayer). The joint should be fused in 35 degrees of flexion, neutral rotation, and neutral abduction-adduction unless the extremity is considerably shortened; in this instance 10 to 15 degrees of abduction are preferable. The hip should not be fused for a paralytic dislocation until the patient is old enough to consider the advantages and disadvantages of a stiff hip and to make his own decision.

Sharp, Guhl, Sorensen, and Voshell arthrodesed 16 hips in patients with poliomyelitis between the ages of 7½ and 16½ years and reported a number of complications after surgery: eight undisplaced supracondylar fractures of the femur, one fracture of the tibia, three pseudarthroses of the hip, three at least partial disruptions of the capital femoral epiphyseal plate, and three positional deformities of the hip severe enough to require femoral osteotomy. Thus arthrodesis of the hip is a major operation that may lead to complications, and the results of it, either good or bad, are permanent; it should not be considered lightly.

VARUS OSTEOTOMY

Varus osteotomy should not be done until the hip can be abducted enough for the femoral neck to make an angle

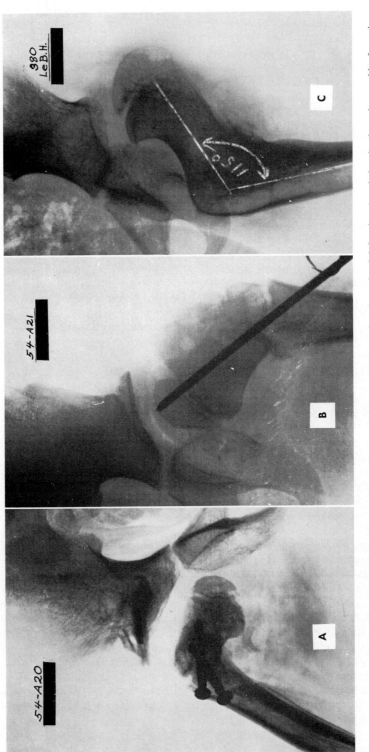
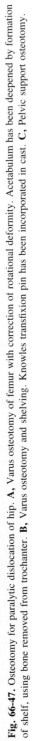

Fig. 66-47. Osteotomy for paralytic dislocation of hip. **A,** Varus osteotomy of femur with correction of rotational deformity. Acetabulum has been deepened by formation of shelf, using bone removed from trochanter. **B,** Varus osteotomy and shelving. Knowles transfixion pin has been incorporated in cast. **C,** Pelvic support osteotomy.

of 120 degrees or less with the midline of the body. Any contracted hip adductor muscles must first be released by tenotomy and stretching in an abduction plaster cast. In children under the age of 5 years we fix the osteotomy at an angle of 105 degrees and in older children of 125 degrees.

TECHNIQUE (BLUNDELL JONES). With the patient prone, expose the trochanteric region of the femur through a posterolateral approach. Remove a wedge of bone, its base medial, from as far distally in the femoral neck as possible; include in the base of the wedge the proximal half of the lesser trochanter and make the angle at the apex of the wedge equal to the desired angle of correction. Unless the bone is too small, fix the osteotomy with a blade plate or a plate shaped to fit the fragments and fix it to the bone with at least two screws through each fragment. Apply a double spica cast.

AFTERTREATMENT. The cast is removed when the osteotomy has united. When used, the blade plate is removed at 6 months before it becomes too deeply embedded in the growing bone.

PELVIC SUPPORT OSTEOTOMY

This is discussed in Chapter 62, p. 2749.

ARTHRODESIS OF HIP

This is discussed in Chapter 38, p. 1112.

OSTEOTOMY OF ILIUM (PEMBERTON)

This is discussed in Chapter 62, p. 2738.

OSTEOTOMY OF INNOMINATE BONE (SALTER)

This is discussed in Chapter 62, p. 2733.

TRUNK

To understand the deformities and disabilities that may occur after the muscles of the trunk and hips are affected by poliomyelitis requires a complex knowledge of the normal actions and interactions of these muscles. Otherwise the operations described here will have little meaning. Irwin describes as follows the actions of the hip abductors and of the lateral trunk muscles during weight bearing.

The different muscle groups, bone levers, and weight-bearing thrusts have a symmetric and triangular relationship as shown in Figs. 66-48 to 66-50. The line BC represents the abductor muscles of the hip; AB, the femoral head, neck, and trochanter, which provide a lever for the abductor muscles; AC, the weight-bearing thrust on the femoral head; DF and CF, the lateral trunk muscles; CE, the bone lever of the pelvis through which the trunk muscles act; FE, the weight-bearing thrust through the midline of the pelvis from above. When the body is balanced, the triangles above and below the pelvis are symmetric.

During normal walking the abductors of the hip on the weight-bearing side pull downward on the pelvis and the lateral trunk muscles on the opposite side pull upward; these two sets of muscles hold the pelvis at a right angle to the longitudinal axis of the trunk. The femoral head on the weight-bearing side serves as the fulcrum. The point of fixation of the trunk muscles (the ribs and spine) is less stable than that of the abductor muscles. Thus when DF

elevates the pelvis, CF must provide counterfixation; CF in turn depends on the abductors of the hip, BC, for counterfixation. Thus with each step the femur on the weight-bearing side is the central point of action for this coordinated system of fixation and counterfixation. Obviously then each part of the system depends on the others for proper pelvic balance during walking.

Pelvic obliquity

Irwin continues that when there is an abduction contracture of the hip, line BC is shortened; as the affected extremity is placed in the weight-bearing position, the femur, acting through the contracted abductor group, BC, depresses the pelvis on that side. During this motion the affected extremity and the pelvis act as a unit; the pelvis is displaced by the lateral thrust toward the opposite side, and thus the normal symmetry of the pelvis in relation to the weight-bearing thrust from above is altered. This thrust from above, FE, now closely approaches the affected hip, and the pelvis is tilted obliquely. The adducted position of the unaffected hip elongates the abductor muscles, DG, to about the same extent that the abductors on the affected side, BC, have been shortened so that even when the abductors, DG, are normal, their contractility and efficiency are diminished. Moreover, the demand on these weakened muscles is increased by the increase in the length of line DE.

The trunk muscles are also affected by this asymmetry. The lateral trunk muscles, CF, become elongated, and their efficiency is impaired. The elongation of the abductors, DG, alters their interrelation with the lateral trunk muscles, DF, in providing a fixed point for contracture of the lateral trunk muscles, CF. The lateral trunk muscles, CF, normally elevate the pelvis on that side, but their position now prevents efficient function. Shortening of the lever, EC, places the trunk muscles, CF, at a further disadvantage. All these alterations in function and structure disrupt the mechanics of walking. When the contracted lateral trunk muscles, DF, and contracted hip abductors, BC, hold the pelvis in this position for long enough, its obliquity becomes fixed through adaptive changes in the spine.

When pelvic obliquity is associated with paralysis of the legs severe enough to require two long leg braces, walking is even more difficult. When the quadriceps is strong on the side of the abduction contracture (the apparently long extremity), the brace may be unlocked to allow knee flexion, and walking is then possible although with a marked limp. When the brace on the affected side cannot be unlocked and the heel on the opposite side (the apparently short extremity) is not elevated, the affected extremity must be widely abducted in walking; otherwise weight is borne only on the affected extremity, and the opposite one becomes almost useless.

TREATMENT

According to Irwin most pelvic obliquities arise from contractures distal to the iliac crest and few from unilateral weakness of the abdominal and lateral trunk muscles. Therefore when contractures are absent distal to the iliac crest, a pelvic obliquity should not be considered a true one but one secondary to scoliosis.

The early origin of a true pelvic obliquity from contracture of the iliotibial band has already been discussed (p. 2985). Before starting treatment, the degree of fixation of the lumbar scoliosis should be determined by roentgenograms. When the deformity is mild and the lumbar scoliosis is not fixed, the pelvic obliquity is corrected by treating the flexion and abduction contracture of the hip (p. 2985). When the pelvic obliquity is moderately severe and the lumbar scoliosis is fixed, the scoliosis is corrected first by instrumentation as described in Chapter 71. After this treatment has been completed the contractures about the hip are released.

For adults with arthritic changes in the lumbar spine that make correction impossible, Irwin suggests that the weight borne on the adducted extremity (the apparently short one)

be shifted nearer the midline by valgus osteotomy; a severe unilateral weakness of the gluteus medius may also be treated in this way. This procedure may enable a patient to walk who could not do so before. When the pelvic obliquity is extreme and the femoral head of the abducted extremity (the apparently long one) is almost within the center of gravity, varus osteotomy of the femur is indicated. The osteotomy is usually done at the level of the lesser trochanter, and the fragments are immobilized by appropriate internal fixation.

Paralysis of muscles of abdomen, back, scapula, and neck

That severe disabilities may result from paralysis of the abdominal, back, scapular, and neck muscles has long been recognized; yet until 1932 the treatment consisted en-

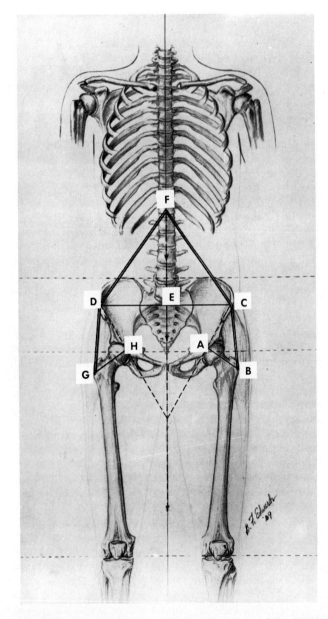

Fig. 66-48. Normal, balanced skeleton. (From Irwin, C.E.: JAMA **133**:231, 1947.)

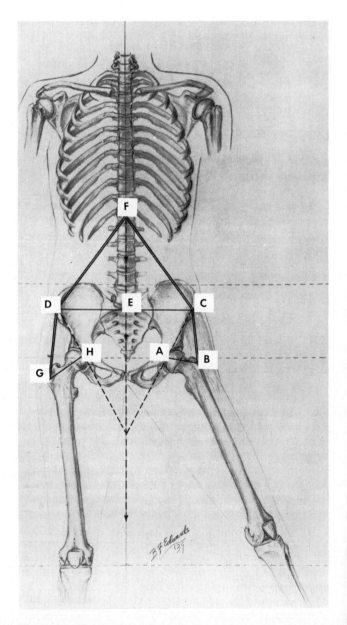

Fig. 66-49. Most true fixed pelvic obliquities are initiated by contractures below iliac crest (see text). (From Irwin, C.E.: JAMA **133**:231, 1947.)

tirely of muscle reeducation, physical therapy, support by apparatus, and spinal fusion for scoliosis. Lowman deserves great credit for taking the lead in this field by suggesting fascial transplants to compensate for the functional loss of these muscles; Dickson and Mayer have also made contributions.

The following are Lowman's conclusions about the influence of imbalance in the trunk and shoulder muscles.

1. Weakness or paralysis of the rectus abdominis produces an anterior tilt of the pelvis and an increase in lumbar lordosis that are exaggerated if the hip flexors are active.

2. Unilateral weakness of the quadratus lumborum produces a lateral deviation of the spine or a pelvic obliquity with secondary compensatory changes proximally. Unilat-

eral weakness of the latissimus dorsi may produce a similar effect.

3. When the serratus anterior and pectoralis major are active, the rhomboids weak, and the shoulder drooping, the weight of the shoulder girdle is thrown anterior to the angle of the ribs and together with the pull of the active muscles tends to flatten them.

4. Contractures of unopposed muscles that pull diagonally or laterally, such as the transversalis, serratus anterior, and abdominal obliques, together with an unbalanced pull of the pectoralis major, latissimus dorsi, and quadratus lumborum, contribute to rotary and lateral deformities of the spine and ribs.

Dickson pointed out that paralysis of various muscles about the shoulder may contribute to paralytic scoliosis in the cervical and upper thoracic spine, drooping and instability of the shoulder girdle, and deformity of the chest.

According to Mayer, a fascial transplant not only hypertrophies with use but grows in length as the patient grows; in patients observed from early childhood to late adolescence he noted a measurable lengthening of the transplants as the distance from the ribs to the iliac crests increased. But Gratz has shown that these transplants hypertrophy only along the line of tension and that the parts of the transplant not under tension may atrophy. Thus it seems that wide transplants are unnecessary.

MUSCLE TRANSFERS AND FASCIAL TRANSPLANTS FOR PARALYSIS OF SCAPULAR MUSCLES

Paralysis of the scapular muscles makes the scapula unstable and shoulder function inefficient; it may be indirectly responsible for high thoracic or cervicothoracic scoliosis. Numerous procedures to treat serratus anterior paralysis and trapezius and levator scapulae paralysis have been devised. Several are discussed later in this chapter (see next section).

SERRATUS ANTERIOR PARALYSIS

The following procedures were devised to treat this paralysis.

Dickson. A fascial transplant to anchor the inferior angle of the scapula to the inferior border of the pectoralis major.

Whitman. Multiple fascial transplants extending from the vertebral border of the scapula to the fourth, fifth, sixth, and seventh thoracic spinous processes.

Haas, after His. Transfer of the teres major tendon from the humerus to the fifth and sixth ribs (p. 3050).

Chaves. Transfer of the coracoid insertion of the pectoralis minor muscle to the vertebral border of the scapula (p. 3050).

Chaves-Rapp. Transfer of the coracoid insertion of the pectoralis minor to the inferior angle of the scapula (p. 3050).

Vastamäki. Transfer of pectoralis minor to distal third of scapula (p. 3050).

TRAPEZIUS AND LEVATOR SCAPULAE PARALYSIS

The following procedures are used to treat this paralysis.

Dickson. Fascial transplants extending from the spine of the scapula to the cervical muscles and to the first thoracic

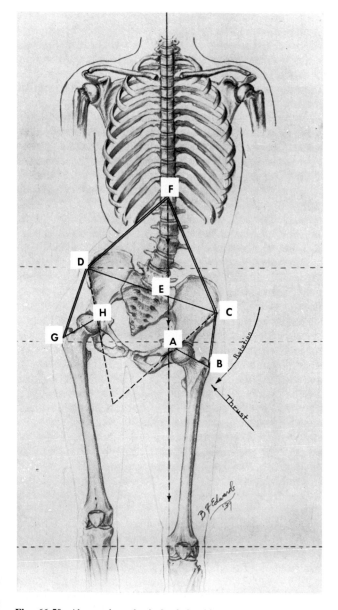

Fig. 66-50. Abnormal mechanical relationships are created when contracted hip is brought down into weight-bearing position (see text). (From Irwin, C.E.: JAMA **133**:231, 1947.)

spinous process. The inferior angle of the scapula is also anchored to the adjacent paraspinal muscles for stability.

Henry. Transplant of two fascial strips, one extending from the vertebral border of the scapula just proximal to its spine to the sixth cervical spinous process and the other from a point 6 cm distal to the first transplant to the third thoracic spinous process (p. 3048).

DeWar and Harris. A fascial transplant extending from the middle of the vertebral border of the scapula to the spinous process of the second and third thoracic vertebrae and transfer of the insertion of the levator scapulae muscle lateralward on the spine of the scapula to a point adjacent to the acromion (p. 3048).

Paralytic scoliosis

The treatment of paralytic scoliosis is discussed in Chapter 71.

Cervical spine fusion for paralysis of neck muscles

Perry and Nickel, and Perry, Nickel, and Garrett have called attention to the grave disability that results from instability of the head after severe paralysis of the cervical muscles. According to them, when paralysis of the flexors or extensors of the neck is significantly disabling and when the disability cannot be eliminated by tendon transfers or muscle transplants, the spine should be fused from the second cervical vertebra to the second thoracic. Then if strength of the capital extensors is poor or fair, capital fascial transplants are indicated, and they should be performed while the patient is still immobilized in a cast and halo after the fusion (Fig. 71-14, *A*), preferably 6 weeks before the halo is to be removed. On the other hand, if strength of the capital extensors is less than poor, then the spinal fusion should be extended superiorly to include the occiput. For a detailed discussion of the indications and techniques, we suggest that their excellent articles be read.

SHOULDER

The disability caused by paralysis of the muscles about the shoulder may be decreased to some extent by tendon and muscle transfers or by arthrodesis of the joint. The pattern and severity of the paralysis determine which method is most appropriate. But neither one is indicated unless the hand, forearm, and elbow have remained serviceable or have already been made so by reconstructive surgery.

Tendons and muscles are transferred to substitute for a paralyzed deltoid muscle or to reinforce a weak one. For these operations to be successful, power must be fair or better in the serratus anterior, the trapezius, and the short external rotators of the shoulder (for the trapezius tranfer, also in the pectoralis major, the rhomboids, and the levator scapulae). When the short external rotators are below functional level, the latissimus dorsi or teres major may be transferred to the lateral aspect of the humerus to reinforce them (Harmon). When the supraspinatus is below functional level, Saha transfers to the greater tuberosity the levator scapulae, sternocleidomastoid, scalenus anterior, scalenus medius, or scalenus capitis; he prefers the levator scapulae. When the subscapularis is below functional level, he transfers to the lesser tuberosity either the pecto-

ralis minor or the superior two digitations of the serratus anterior; or he transfers the latissimus dorsi or teres major posteriorly to a point exactly opposite the insertion of the subscapularis (here the action is backward although identical to that of the subscapularis after elevation above 90 degrees).

Arthrodesis of the shoulder may be indicated when the paralysis about the joint is extensive, provided that power in at least the serratus anterior and the trapezius is fair or better.

Tendon and muscle transfers for paralysis of deltoid

According to Haas, Hildebrandt in 1906 laid the foundation for tendon and muscle transfers about the shoulder for paralysis of the deltoid when he transferred the entire origin of the pectoralis major to the clavicle and acromion. Slomann in 1916 reported transferring the origin of the long head of the triceps to the acromion, and more recently Ober reported transferring the same origin and that of the short head of the biceps. Mayer transfers the insertion of the trapezius to or near the deltoid tuberosity of the humerus by means of a transplant of fascia lata. According to Steindler, most of the improvement in function after a trapezius transfer is caused by a tenodesis effect; he pointed out that the muscle is rarely functional after transfer. Ober and Harmon have both advised anterior transfer of the posterior part of the deltoid, when strong, to replace a paralyzed anterior part.

According to Haas, the Mayer transfer of the insertion of the trapezius is the most satisfactory operation for complete paralysis of the deltoid. Bateman modified the Mayer technique by resecting a part of the spine of the scapula and including it in the transfer; this permits fixation of the transfer with screws after the muscle is pulled like a hood over the head of the humerus (Fig. 66-51). Saha also modified and improved the technique. The superior and middle trapezius is completely mobilized laterally from its origin, and thus the transfer is made 5 cm longer without endangering its nerve or blood supply; this added length greatly increases leverage of the transfer on the humerus. The entire insertion of the trapezius is freed by resecting the lateral clavicle, the acromion, and the adjoining part of the scapular spine; these are then anchored to the humerus by screws (Fig. 66-52).

Saha in an excellent monograph on surgery of the paralyzed and flail shoulder developed a functional classification of the muscles about the joint and recommended careful assessment of their strength before surgery. Further, believing there is no indication for arthrodesis of paralyzed shoulders, he devised several rational transfers to improve their function.

A summary of Saha's classification of the muscles of the shoulder follows.

1. *Prime movers.* In this group are the deltoid and clavicular head of the pectoralis major that in lifting exert forces in three directions at the junction of the proximal and middle thirds of the humeral shaft axis.

2. *Steering group.* In this group are the subscapularis, the supraspinatus, and the infraspinatus. These muscles exert forces at the junction of the axes of the humeral head and neck and humeral shaft. As the arm is elevated the

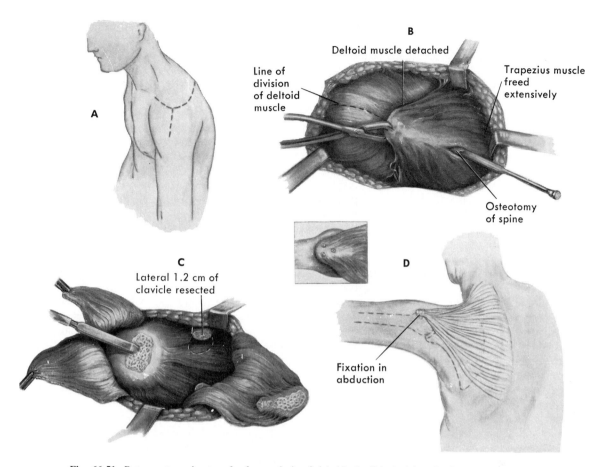

Fig. 66-51. Bateman trapezius transfer for paralysis of deltoid. **A.** Skin incision. **B,** Spine of scapula is osteotomized near its base in obliquely distal and lateral plane. *Broken line,* division of deltoid. **C,** Atrophic deltoid has been split, deep surface of acromion and spine and corresponding area on lateral aspect of humerus have been roughened, and lateral end of clavicle has been resected. **D,** Acromion has been anchored to humerus as far distally as possible with two or three screws. (Modified from Bateman, J.E.: The shoulder and environs, St. Louis, 1954, The C.V. Mosby Co.)

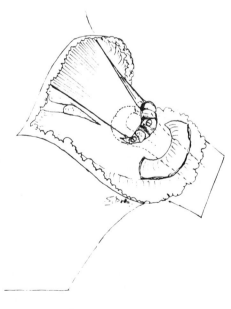

Fig. 66-52. Saha trapezius transfer for paralysis of deltoid. Entire insertion of trapezius along with attached lateral end of clavicle, acromioclavicular joint, and acromion and adjoining part of scapular spine have been anchored to lateral aspect of humerus distal to tuberosities by two screws. (From Saha, A.K.: Acta Orthop. Scand., suppl. 97, 1967.)

humeral head, by rolling and gliding movements, constantly changes its point of contact with the glenoid cavity. Although these muscles exert a little force in lifting the arm, their chief function is stabilizing the humeral head as it moves in the glenoid.

3. *Depressor group.* In this group are the pectoralis major (sternal head), latissimus dorsi, teres major, and teres minor. These muscles are intermediately located and exert their forces on the proximal fourth of the humeral shaft axis. During elevation they rotate the shaft, and in the last few degrees of this movement they depress the humeral head. They exert only minimal steering action on the head. Absence of their power would cause no apparent disability except that performance of the limb in lifting weights above the head would be decreased.

The classic methods of transferring a single muscle (or even several muscles to a common attachment) to restore abduction of the shoulder do not consider the functions of the steering muscles. Saha, confirming the observations of others, found that when the steering muscles are paralyzed and a single muscle has been transferred to restore functions only of the deltoid, the arm cannot be elevated more than 90 degrees and scapulohumeral motion is significantly disturbed. Thus for paralysis of the deltoid Saha transfers the entire insertion of the trapezius to the humerus to replace the anterior and middle parts of the muscle. But he carefully evaluates the subscapularis, the supraspinatus, and the infraspinatus, and when any two are found paralyzed, he restores their functions too because otherwise the effectiveness of the transferred trapezius as an elevator of the shoulder would be greatly reduced. As already mentioned, for paralysis of the subscapularis either the pectoralis minor or the superior two digitations of the serratus anterior can be transferred because either can be rerouted and anchored to the lesser tuberosity; or as an alternative procedure, the latissimus dorsi or the teres major can be transferred posteriorly to a point exactly opposite the lesser tuberosity. For paralysis of the supraspinatus the levator scapulae, sternocleidomastoid, scalenus anterior, scalenus medius, or scalenus capitis can be transferred to the greater tuberosity; of these the levator scapulae is the best because of the direction and length of its fibers. When suitable transfers are unavailable, the insertion of the trapezius can be anchored more anteriorly or posteriorly on the humerus to restore internal or external rotation.

Contractures of unopposed muscles about the shoulder are rarely severe enough to cause extreme disability; most can be corrected at the time of transfer or arthrodesis.

TRAPEZIUS TRANSFER FOR PARALYSIS OF DELTOID

The Mayer procedure was based on Lange's method in which numerous silk strands were threaded through the trapezius at its insertion, were passed distally, and were attached to the humerus at the insertion of the deltoid; instead of silk Mayer used a transplant of fascia lata. But Steindler, Haas, and others believed that the Mayer procedure resulted in a tenodesis. As time passed the range of motion of the shoulder gradually decreased because the transplanted fascia adhered to the acromion and the surrounding soft tissues. To minimize this problem Haas made a groove in the acromion process; Bateman osteo-

tomized the acromion and scapular spine, transferred them laterally, and anchored them directly to the humerus. Saha further modified the operation by mobilizing completely the superior and middle trapezius; this makes the transfer longer and allows it to be anchored more distally on the humerus, increasing its leverage on the bone.

TECHNIQUE (BATEMAN). With the patient prone, approach the shoulder through a T-shaped incision (Fig. 66-51, *A*): extend the transverse part around the shoulder over the spine of the scapula and the acromion and end it just above the coracoid process; extend the longitudinal limb distally over the lateral aspect of the shoulder and upper arm for 6 cm. Mobilize the flaps, split the atrophic deltoid muscle, and expose the joint. Free of soft tissue the undersurface of the acromion and spine of the scapula. Now osteotomize the spine of the scapula near its base in an obliquely distal and lateral plane; thus a broad cuff of the trapezius is freed, still attached to the spine and the acromion. Now resect the lateral 2 cm of the clavicle with care to avoid damaging the coracoclavicular ligament. Roughen the deep surface of the acromion and spine, abduct the arm to 90 degrees, and at the appropriate level on the lateral aspect of the humerus roughen a corresponding area. Now by firm traction bring the muscular cuff laterally over the humeral head and anchor the acromion to the humerus as far distally as possible with two or three screws. Immobilize the arm in a shoulder spica cast, with the shoulder abducted to 90 degrees.

AFTERTREATMENT. Immobilization is continued for 8 weeks, but at 4 to 6 weeks the arm and shoulder part of the spica is bivalved to allow some movement. When the transplanted acromion has united with the humerus, the arm is placed on an abduction humerus splint and is gradually lowered to the side, and the muscle is reeducated by exercises.

TECHNIQUE (SAHA). Make a saber-cut incision (Fig. 66-52) convex medially: begin it anteriorly a little superior to the inferior margin of the anterior axillary fold at about its middle, extend it superiorly, then posteriorly, and finally inferiorly, and end it slightly inferior to the base of the scapular spine and 2.5 cm lateral to the vertebral border of the scapula. Mobilize the skin flaps and expose the trapezius medially to 2.5 cm medial to the vertebral border of the scapula; expose the acromion, the capsule of the acromioclavicular joint, the lateral third of the clavicle, and the entire origin of the paralyzed deltoid muscle. Next detach and reflect laterally the origin of the deltoid, and locate the anterior border of the trapezius. Identify the coronoid ligament and divide the clavicle just lateral to it. Then palpate the scapular notch, identify the acromion and the adjoining part of the scapular spine, and with a Gigli saw and beveling posteriorly, resect the spine. Now elevate the insertion of the trapezius along with the attached lateral end of the clavicle, the acromioclavicular joint, and the acromion and adjoining part of the scapular spine. Then free the trapezius from the superior boder of the remaining part of the scapular spine medially to the base of the spine where the inferior fibers of the muscle glide over the triangular area of the scapula. Next free from the investing layer of deep cervical fascia the anterior border of the trapezius and raise the muscle from its bed for rerouting.

Denude the inferior surfaces of the bones attached to the freed trapezius insertion; then with forceps break these bones in several places but leave intact the periosteum on their superior surfaces. Denude also the area on the lateral aspect of the proximal humerus selected for attachment of the transfer. Then with the shoulder in neutral rotation and 45 degrees of abduction, anchor the transfer by two screws passed through fragments of bone and into the proximal humerus (Fig. 66-52). When suitable transfers are unavailable to replace any paralyzed external or internal rotators, anchor the muscle a little more anteriorly or posteriorly. Transfers for paralysis of the subscapularis, supraspinatus, or infraspinatus are discussed later; when indicated, they should be performed at the time of trapezius transfer.

AFTERTREATMENT. A spica cast is applied with the shoulder abducted 45 degrees, neutrally rotated, and flexed in the plane of the scapula. At 10 days the sutures are removed, and roentgenograms are made to be sure that the humeral head has not become dislocated inferiorly. At 6 to 8 weeks the cast is removed and active exercises are started.

TRANSFER OF DELTOID ORIGIN FOR PARTIAL PARALYSIS

In some patients the entire deltoid muscle is not paralyzed, and its unaffected part (usually the posterior) retains good power. Ober transferred the origin of this part into a more favorable position to improve the power of abduction. Harmon described the operation in detail and reported a good result in a patient with recurrent anterior dislocation of the shoulder. With proper indications for this operation, our results have been satisfactory.

TECHNIQUE (HARMON). Make a U-shaped incision 20 cm long, extending from the middle third of the clavicle laterally and posteriorly around the shoulder just distal to the acromion to the middle of the spine of the scapula. Raise flaps of skin and subcutaneous tissue proximally and distally. Detach subperiosteally from its origin the active posterior part of the deltoid and free it distally from the deep structures for about one half its length, with care to avoid injuring the axillary nerve and its branches. Expose subperiosteally the lateral third of the clavicle, transfer the muscle flap anteriorly, and anchor it against the clavicle with interrupted nonabsorbable sutures through the adjacent soft tissues (Fig. 66-53).

AFTERTREATMENT. A shoulder spica cast is applied, holding the arm abducted 75 degrees. At 3 weeks part of the cast is removed for massage and active exercise. At 6 weeks the entire cast is removed, and an abduction humerus splint is fitted to be worn for at least 4 months; supervised active exercises are continued during this time.

Harmon also reported a small series in which multiple tendons were transferred about the shoulder (Fig. 66-54). These operations consisted of combinations of the following procedures, selected according to the needs of each patient: (1) anterior transfer of a functional posterior part of the deltoid, as just described; (2) lateral transfer of the clavicular fibers of the pectoralis major; (3) transfer of the origin of the long head of the triceps and of the short head of the biceps to the tip of the acromion; and (4) transfer of the insertions of the latissimus dorsi and teres major to the lateral surface of the humerus to replace the external rota-

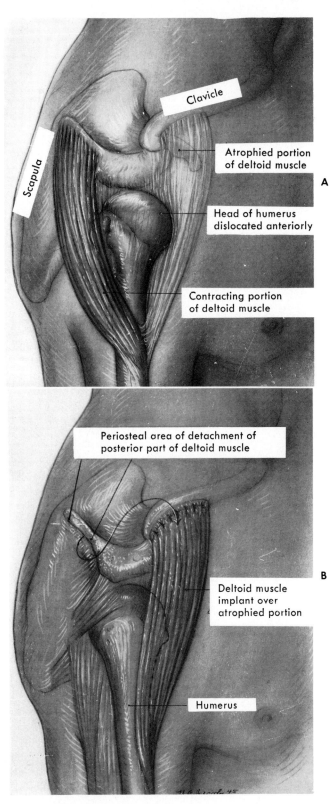

Fig. 66-53. Harmon transfer of origin of deltoid for partial paralysis. **A,** Posterior part of deltoid is functioning; middle and anterior parts are paralyzed. **B,** Transferred posterior part of deltoid is overlying atrophic anterior part. Transfer when it contracts prevents anterior dislocation of shoulder and exerts a more direct abduction force than in its previous posterior location. (From Harmon, P.H.: Surg. Gynecol. Obstet. **84:**117, 1947. By permission of Surgery, Gynecology & Obstetrics.)

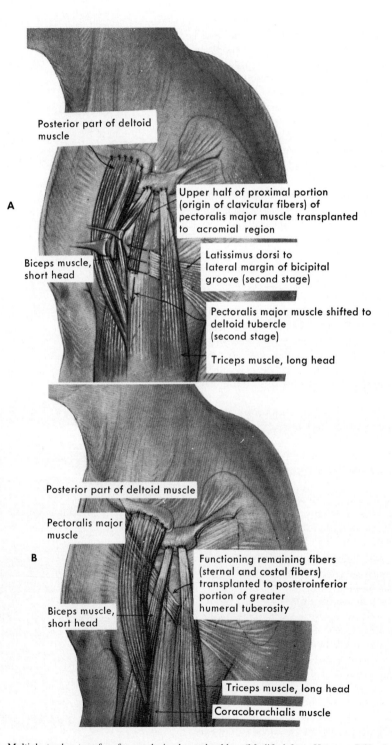

Fig. 66-54. Multiple tendon transfers for paralysis about shoulder. (Modified from Harmon, P.H.: J. Bone Joint Surg. **32-A:**583, 1950.)

tors. According to Harmon, the result in each patient was superior to that after arthrodesis of the shoulder.

Tendon and muscle transfers for paralysis of subscapularis, supraspinatus, or infraspinatus

Saha has emphasized the importance of transfers for paralysis of the subscapularis, supraspinatus, or infraspinatus. According to him, when as many as two of these three muscles are paralyzed, their functions must be restored by suitable transfers; this is just as necessary as the trapezius transfer for paralysis of the deltoid. Without the function of these muscles or their substitutes, the effectiveness of the transferred trapezius in elevating the shoulder would be markedly reduced. Muscles suitable for transfer are those whose distal ends can be carried to the tuberosities of the humerus and whose general directions of pull correspond to those of the muscles they are to replace. The transfers should be rerouted close to the end of the axis of the humeral head and neck, or the desired functions will not be restored. The nerve and blood supply to any transferred muscle must, of course, be protected. The various transfers described next, when indicated, are carried out at the same time as the Saha trapezius transfer for paralysis of the deltoid. Consequently, in each instance the sabercut incision will have been made, the lateral end of the clavicle and the acromion and adjoining part of the scapular spine will have been elevated, and the superior and middle trapezius will have been mobilized as already described for this transfer (p. 3004); further, the treatment after each is that described for the trapezius transfer (p. 3005).

TRANSFER OF SUPERIOR TWO DIGITATIONS OF SERRATUS ANTERIOR FOR PARALYSIS OF SUBSCAPULARIS

TECHNIQUE (SAHA). Expose the superior part of the vertebral border of the scapula and the insertion of the levator scapulae by reflecting the trapezius further superiorly and posteriorly. Define the superior and inferior borders of the levator scapulae and free subperiosteally the insertion of the muscle from the superior third of the vertebral border of the scapula; take care to avoid the nerve to the rhomboids and the vessels lying deeper and more medially. If necessary this muscle may be transferred for paralysis of the subscapularis or supraspinatus. Elevate the superior part of the vertebral border of the scapula and define the superior two digitations of the serratus anterior; hook these digitations with a blunt instrument or index finger inserted near the superior angle of the scapula between the serratus anterior and the subscapularis (Fig. 66-55, *A*). Free the insertion of the muscle from the vertebral border of the scapula from the superior angle of the bone distally to the level of the base of the spine. Now fold the freed insertion on itself, close its margins with three interrupted sutures, and place a strong mattress suture in the end of the transfer for rerouting the muscle (Fig. 66-55, *B*). Next elevate the arm 130 degrees and incise the floor of the axilla close to its posterior wall. Avoid the thoracodorsal nerve if the latissimus dorsi is not paralyzed; if necessary ligate the subscapularis vessels. Retract the neurovascular bundle superiorly and laterally and pull the end of the transfer anteriorly into the axilla. Then by blunt dissection poste-

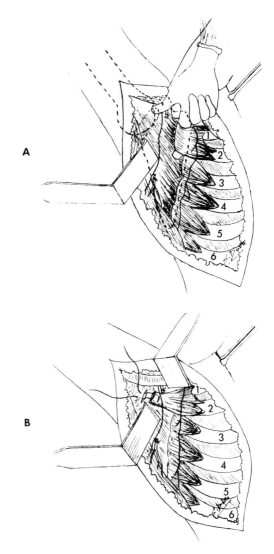

Fig. 66-55. Saha transfer of superior two digitations of serratus anterior for paralysis of subscapularis (see text). (From Saha, A.K.: Acta Orthop. Scand., suppl. 97, 1967.)

rior to the neurovascular bundle expose the lesser tuberosity. Finally reroute the muscle to this tuberosity and anchor it there by interrupted sutures.

TRANSFER OF LEVATOR SCAPULAE FOR PARALYSIS OF SUPRASPINATUS OR SUBSCAPULARIS

TECHNIQUE (SAHA). Carry out the operation as just described for transfer of the superior two digitations of the serratus anterior for paralysis of subscapularis until the superior and inferior borders of the levator scapulae have been defined and the insertion of the muscle has been freed from the vertebral border of the scapula. Then raise the superior skin flap a little more and expose the belly of the muscle to about its middle. Next fold the freed insertion of the muscle on itself and close its margins with interrupted sutures. Reroute the transfer and anchor it to either the greater or lesser tuberosity of the humerus (Fig. 66-56).

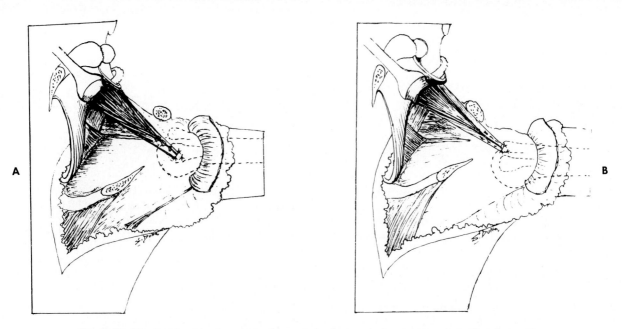

Fig. 66-56. Saha transfer of levator scapulae for paralysis of supraspinatus or subscapularis. Transfer may be anchored either to greater tuberosity, as in **A,** or to lesser tuberosity, as in **B** (see text). (From Saha, A.K.: Acta Orthop. Scand., suppl. 97, 1967.)

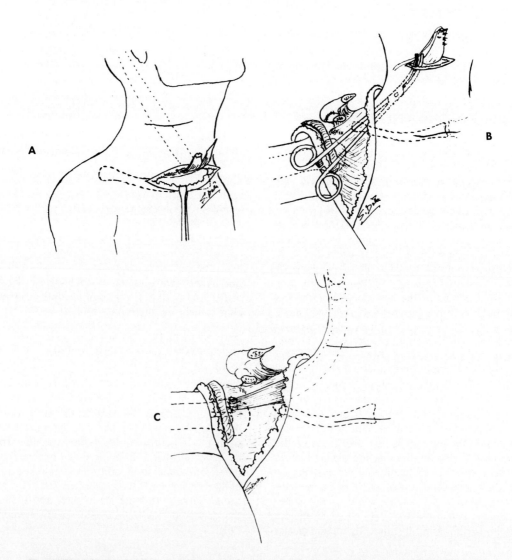

Fig. 66-57. Saha transfer of sternocleidomastoid for paralysis of supraspinatus (see text). (From Saha, A.K.: Acta Orthop. Scand., suppl. 97, 1967.)

TRANSFER OF PECTORALIS MINOR FOR PARALYSIS OF SUBSCAPULARIS

TECHNIQUE (SAHA). Expose the insertion of the pectoralis minor. Because the nerve supply of the muscle is more medial, it will not be injured. Free from the coracoid process the tendon of insertion and place in its end a strong mattress suture. Abduct and externally rotate the arm and bring into prominence the lesser tuberosity inferior to the retracted neurovascular bundle. Then reroute the muscle to the lesser tuberosity as described for transfer of the serratus anterior (p. 3007), and anchor it with heavy sutures.

TRANSFER OF STERNOCLEIDOMASTOID FOR PARALYSIS OF SUPRASPINATUS

Saha has transferred the sternocleidomastoid to the greater tuberosity to act as an elevator of the shoulder. The only disadvantage in the transfer is that while contracting it may cause webbing of the neck.

TECHNIQUE (SAHA). Beginning medially at the midline make an incision laterally over the clavicle to the junction of its medial fourth and lateral three fourths (Fig. 66-57, A). Free from the sternum and clavicle the two heads of origin of the sternocleidomastoid. Next retract the superior skin flap and free from the deep fascia the distal third of the muscle. Narrow the freed origin of the muscle by closing its margins with interrupted sutures, and place in its end a strong mattress suture. Now in the neck make another transverse incision at about the middle of the sternocleidomastoid. Through this incision and beginning superiorly, free the muscle inferiorly without injuring its vessels and nerves. Bring the freed part of the muscle out this last incision (Fig. 66-57, B), reroute it subcutaneously, and fix it to the greater tuberosity with heavy sutures (Fig. 66-57, C).

TRANSFER OF LATISSIMUS DORSI OR TERES MAJOR OR BOTH FOR PARALYSIS OF SUBSCAPULARIS OR INFRASPINATUS

TECHNIQUE (SAHA). Elevate the arm about 130 degrees. Then make an incision in the posterior axillary fold beginning in the upper arm about 6.5 cm inferior to the crease of the axilla and extending to the inferior angle of the scapula, crossing the crease in a zigzag manner. Expose and free the insertion of the latissimus dorsi and raise the muscle from its bed, taking care to preserve its nerve and blood supply. If the transfer is to be reinforced by the teres major, then free and raise both muscles. Next fold the freed insertion on itself and close its margins by interrupted sutures; place in its end a strong mattress suture. Next with a blunt instrument open the interval between the deltoid and long head of the triceps. Identify the tubercle at the inferior end of the greater tuberosity, carry the end of the transfer to this tubercle, and while holding the limb in neutral rotation, anchor the transfer there by interrupted sutures.

Arthrodesis

When paralysis about the shoulder is extensive, arthrodesis may be the procedure of choice, especially when there is a paralytic dislocation, the muscles of the forearm and hand are functional, and the serratus anterior and trapezius are strong. Motion of the scapula then compensates for lack of motion in the joint.

The Research Committee of the American Orthopaedic Association reported a survey of results after 101 shoulder fusions for poliomyelitis. These findings apply especially to fusions for paralysis but also apply to fusion for other conditions (Chapter 39). What follows is a summary.

1. The position of the humerus should be calculated in relation to the scapula rather than to the chest.

2. When function of the trapezius and serratus anterior is fair or good, the best position is one of 45 to 55 degrees of abduction, 15 to 25 degrees of flexion, and 15 to 25 degrees of internal rotation. Abduction of more than 45 degrees produces some winging of the scapula, although abduction up to 55 degrees is satisfactory for a boy under 12 years old.

3. Good power in the upper trapezius and upper two thirds of the serratus anterior muscles is necessary for satisfactory function. When the serratus anterior is paralyzed, the shoulder should be fused in no more than 30 degrees of abduction, for two reasons: (a) when function in the serratus anterior is absent, the upper trapezius can elevate the acromion while the shoulder girdle pivots on the sternoclavicular joint, but it can abduct the shoulder to only 45 degrees, and (b) if the shoulder is fused in more than 45 degrees of abduction when the serratus anterior is paralyzed, the weight of the arm may depress the lateral part of the scapula and overstretch and weaken the trapezius.

4. When the trapezius retains moderate power and all of the other muscles about the shoulder are paralyzed, some improvement in appearance and function may be restored by fusion.

5. Before the shoulder joint is positioned, any adduction contracture of the scapulohumeral joint must be corrected first; otherwise, proper positioning in abduction is impossible.

6. True abduction of the shoulder is measured by the angle between the vertebral border of the scapula and the humerus. Because of the tendency for this angle to change in the cast after surgery, internal fixation is advised. When roentgenograms show that fusion has begun, further changes in abduction will not occur.

7. Fusion of the shoulder in too much flexion causes winging of the scapula and stretching of the serratus anterior. When flexion is not more than 15 degrees, the weight of the arm will cause the scapula to lie flat against the thorax, even when the serratus anterior is paralyzed. But fusion without some flexion would result in poor function.

8. Too little internal rotation is worse than too much. When internal rotation is no more than 15 degrees, the hand may still be placed on top of the head, provided that abduction is 35 to 40 degrees. When the elbow and hand are weak, however, the shoulder may be fused in more internal rotation if the opposite arm is normal. Even so, internal rotation should not exceed 45 degrees.

9. Special problems, which include scoliosis, age, bilateral paralysis, and flail shoulder, must be given particular consideration.

a. *Scoliosis.* There is no definitive evidence that shoulder fusion adversely affects scoliosis, but on the other hand, scoliosis will limit the range of scapular motion and thus the range of shoulder motion after fusion. When there is a severe curve convex toward the shoulder to be fused, too much flexion must be avoided; otherwise the scapula will wing too much and will accentuate deformity.

b. *Age.* A greater range of motion is obtained after surgery if the shoulder is fused before the age of 12 years. There is little danger of epiphyseal damage. Makin in 1977 reported the results of arthrodesis of the shoulder in seven children 5 to 9 years old in whom the shoulder was flail but the hand and elbow were functional. The fusions became solid in all seven, and function of the shoulder was much improved. When the patients were examined as adults, little length of the humerus had been lost and the position of the fused shoulder had not changed. He recommends early arthrodesis of the flail shoulder and agrees that waiting for skeletal maturity is unnecessary.

c. *Bilateral paralysis.* When both shoulders must be fused, their positions should allow the patient to bring the hands together. When muscle power in the two shoulders differs, the weaker should be fused in more internal rotation. When power is about equal, the left shoulder in a right-handed patient should be fused in more internal rotation, and vice versa.

d. *Flail shoulder.* Fusing a flail shoulder offers the following advantages: greater ease in turning in bed and putting on a coat, better use of the hand, for example, to steady paper while writing, and a feeling of security or stability in the shoulder. Also a flail shoulder is usually carried higher than normal, and fusion restores its appearance and position. A weak or flail shoulder should be fused in only slight abduction. Fusion of the shoulder may improve the power of elbow flexion.

The techniques for shoulder arthrodesis are described in Chapter 39.

ELBOW

Most operations for paralysis of the muscles acting across the elbow are designed to restore active flexion or extension of the joint. Operations to correct deformity or those to stabilize the joint, such as posterior bone block or arthrodesis, are rarely necessary.

Muscle and tendon transfers to restore elbow flexion

There are several methods of restoring active elbow flexion. Here, as elsewhere, the actual and the relative power of the remaining muscles must be accurately determined before deciding on a given transfer. Also, because the function of the hand is more important than flexion of the elbow, these operations should not be done when the muscles controlling the fingers are paralyzed unless their function has been or can be restored by tendon transfers. The methods of restoring elbow flexion are as follows: (1) flexorplasty (Steindler), (2) anterior transfer of the triceps tendon (Bunnell and Carroll), (3) transfer of part of the pectoralis major muscle (Clark), (4) transfer of the sternocleidomastoid muscle (Bunnell), (5) transfer of the pectoralis minor muscle (Spira), (6) transfer of the pectoralis major tendon (Brooks and Seddon), and (7) transfer of the latissimus dorsi muscle (Hovnanian).

Ahmad reported restoration of active flexion of the el-

bow by detaching the flexor carpi ulnaris distally, carefully mobilizing it proximally to its neurovascular bundle, then turning it on itself and attaching it to the anterior surface of the humerus by two staples about 7.5 cm proximal to the elbow. The result was satisfactory in this patient.

STEINDLER FLEXORPLASTY

The Steindler flexorplasty consists of transferring the common origin of the pronator teres, the flexor carpi radialis, the palmaris longus, the flexor digitorum sublimis, and the flexor carpi ulnaris muscles from the medial epicondylar region of the humerus proximally about 5 cm. Its chief disadvantage is the frequent development of a pronation deformity of the forearm.

Flexorplasty is indicated when the biceps brachii and brachialis are paralyzed and the group of muscles arising from the medial epicondyle are fair or better in strength. The best results are obtained when the elbow flexors are only partially paralyzed and the finger and wrist flexors are normal. The strength in active flexion and the range of motion of the elbow after surgery do not compare favorably with the normal, but the usefulness of the arm is nonetheless increased. Kettelkamp and Larson studied the strength and range of motion after flexorplasty in 15 patients and found that in 9 patients 1 pound (0.5 kg) or more could be lifted to 110 degrees flexion. Strength was greatest when a flexion contracture of the elbow of 30 degrees or more was present. Thus if the object of the operation is to obtain maximum strength, the surgeon should aim at producing a contracture of 30 to 60 degrees; then the average result should be the ability to lift 2 pounds (1 kg) to 110 degrees of flexion. When only the flexor digitorum sublimis is active, the elbow can be flexed only if the fingers are strongly flexed; this, of course, interferes with the function of the hand, and another method should be used to restore elbow flexion. According to Mayer and Green, unsuccessful results from this procedure are usually caused by overestimating the strength of the muscles to be transferred. A practical way to test them is to hold the patient's arm at a right angle to the body, rotate it so as to eliminate the influence of gravity, and then determine whether the muscles to be transferred can flex the elbow in this position; if not, this type of transfer will fail, and another should be used. However, according to Segal, Seddon, and Brooks, when the pattern of paralysis is such that a free choice of procedures is possible, the Steindler flexorplasty is preferable. Carroll advises against transferring a muscle arising from the medial epicondyle to restore hand function until after any indicated flexorplasty has been done and the strength and function of the transferred muscles have been regained. In 1973 Lindholm and Einola studied the results of 61 Steindler flexorplasties, two thirds of which were followed for more than 6 years. Fifty elbows regained a range of flexion of at least 90 degrees, and the average flexion deformity was 25 degrees. A pronation deformity was found in almost one third of the patients and was considered secondary to imbalance of muscle power between the pronators and supinators present before the operation and not a result of it.

Dutton and Dawson recently studied 25 modified Steindler flexorplasties performed between 1952 and 1976. The

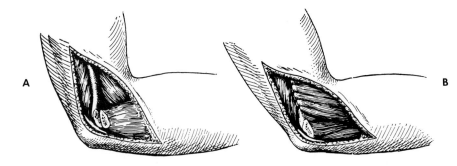

Fig. 66-58. Steindler flexorplasty for paralysis of flexor muscles of elbow joint. **A,** Common origin of flexor muscles is detached from medial epicondyle. **B,** Muscles are freed distally for 3.7 cm and with elbow in flexion are transferred 5 cm proximal to medial epicondyle between triceps and brachialis muscles.

resulting residual flexion deformity of the elbow averaged 36 degrees, with a residual arc of active flexion of 95 degrees starting from that point. The average loss of supination was 39 degrees with the mean active arc of supination being 51 degrees and pronation being 79 degrees. At final evaluation, a mean of 9.3 years after operation, 14 were judged as excellent; 6 as good; 4 as fair; and 1 as poor.

TECHNIQUE (STEINDLER). Make a curved longitudinal incision over the medial side of the elbow, beginning 7.5 cm proximal to the medial epicondyle and extending distally posterior to the medial condyle and thence anteriorly on the volar surface of the forearm along the course of the pronator teres muscle. Locate the ulnar nerve posterior to the medial epicondyle and retract it posteriorly. Detach en bloc the common origin of the pronator teres, flexor carpi radialis, palmaris longus, flexor digitorum sublimis, and flexor carpi ulnaris from the medial epicondyle close to the periosteum. Free these muscles distally for 4 cm; then with the elbow in flexion transfer them 5 cm proximal to the medial epicondyle to the intermuscular septum between the triceps and brachialis or to the periosteum of the humerus and fix them to the soft tissues with strong sutures (Fig. 66-58).

In an attempt to minimize the loss of supination following this procedure, Carroll and Gartland, Bunnell, and Mayer and Green have modified the Steindler flexorplasty by moving the origin of the medial muscle mass not only proximally, as above, but also laterally onto the anterior surface of the humerus.

AFTERTREATMENT. A cast is applied, with the elbow in acute flexion and the forearm in a position midway between pronation and supination. At 2 weeks the cast is replaced by a splint that holds the arm in this same position for at least 6 weeks; physical therapy and active exercises are then started and are gradually increased to strengthen the transferred muscles.

BUNNELL'S MODIFICATION OF STEINDLER FLEXORPLASTY

Bunnell modified the technique by transferring the common muscle origin laterally on the humerus by means of a fascial transplant. This largely eliminates the action of the transferred muscle group in pronating the forearm.

TECHNIQUE (BUNNELL). Do the operation as just described but prolong the common muscle origin with a free graft of

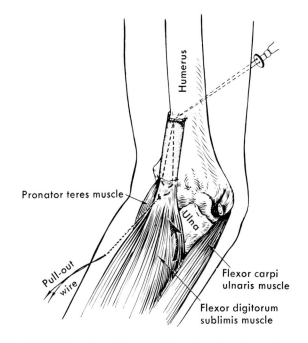

Fig. 66-59. Bunnell modification of Steindler flexorplasty. Common muscle origin is transferred laterally on humerus by means of fascial transplant. (Modified from Bunnell, S.: J. Bone Joint Surg. **33-A:**566, 1951.)

fascia lata. Then advance this origin 5 cm up the lateral side rather than the medial side of the humerus (Fig. 66-59). This results in a moderate although not complete correction of the tendency of the transfer to pronate the forearm. Should a pronation deformity persist after this procedure, it may be corrected by transferring the tendon of the flexor carpi ulnaris around the ulnar margin of the forearm into the distal radius (Steindler).

AFTERTREATMENT. Aftertreatment is the same as for the Steindler technique just described.

EYLER'S MODIFICATION OF STEINDLER FLEXORPLASTY

Eyler and Irwin also modified the Steindler procedure by using the "internervous" plane for easier mobilization and transfer of the common muscle origin.

TECHNIQUE (EYLER). Make an incision over the medial side of the elbow beginning 2.5 cm proximal to the medial epicondyle and gently curving distally on the medial side of the forearm for 7.5 cm. Reflect the anterior flap, divide the bicipital aponeurosis, and identify the median nerve. The brachial artery lies just lateral to the nerve and neither need be disturbed; the ulnar nerve lies medial to the incision and is not yet seen. In the distal end of the incision identify and open the intermuscular (internervous) plane between the flexor digitorum sublimis and the combined mass of the flexor carpi ulnaris and flexor digitorum profundus. By digital palpation and exploration carry the dissection proximally; this may be done without endangering the neurovascular structures. Just beneath the dissecting finger the ulnar nerve and artery become visible, lying on the profundus; the median nerve is safely beneath the sublimis and is easily seen without further dissection. By sharp and blunt dissection the muscle mass consisting of the flexor digitorum sublimis, palmaris longus, flexor carpi radialis, and superficial head of the pronator teres can now be quickly mobilized. Free their common origin from the medial epicondyle and insert it into the lateral side of the humerus by the method of Bunnell, using either a graft of fascia lata or a section of a long toe extensor tendon (the latter is more easily handled) to prolong the transfer. The transfer may be passed either superficial or deep to the cubital veins.

AFTERTREATMENT. Aftertreatment is the same as for the Steindler technique (p. 3011).

ANTERIOR TRANSFER OF TRICEPS

The triceps tendon will not reach the tuberosity of the radius, but it may be prolonged by a short graft of fascia or tendon.

TECHNIQUE (BUNNELL). Through a posterolateral incision expose the triceps tendon and divide it at its insertion. Dissect it from the posterior aspect of the distal fourth of the humerus and transfer it around the lateral aspect. Make an anterolateral curvilinear incision and retract the brachioradialis and pronator teres muscles to expose the tuberosity of the radius. Prolong the triceps tendon by a graft of fascia lata 4 cm long and wide enough to make a tube. Attach it to the roughened tuberosity of the radius with a steel pull-out suture passed to the dorsum of the forearm by way of a hole drilled through the tuberosity and the neck of the radius (Fig. 66-60). Flex the elbow, gently pull the suture taut to snug the tendon against the bone, and tie the suture over a padded button; immobilize the elbow in flexion.

Carroll described a similar method of triceps transfer. The tendon is passed superficial to the radial nerve and through a longitudinal slit in the biceps tendon and is sutured under tension with the elbow in flexion. Carroll and Hill in 1970 reported 15 transfers of the triceps muscle in seven patients with traumatic or paralytic loss of flexion of the elbow and in eight with arthrogryposis. Bilateral triceps transfers were not recommended because one functional triceps is required for toilet care and for assistance in rising from a chair. After surgery the average arc of active flexion was 116 degrees, and the average residual flexion contracture was 24 degrees. Excellent flexion against gravity was restored. The results were more predictable in paralytic or traumatic loss of flexion than in

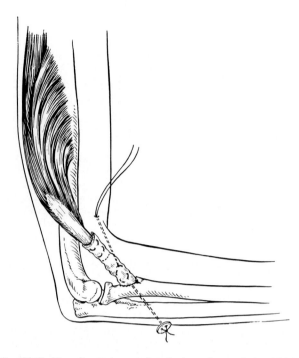

Fig. 66-60. Bunnell anterior transfer of triceps for paralysis of biceps. Triceps tendon is prolonged by short graft of fascia or tendon, is routed laterally, and is inserted into tuberosity of radius by pull-out suture. (From Bunnell, S.: J. Bone Joint Surg. **33-A:**566, 1951.)

patients with arthrogryposis, but in the latter the results were good enough to justify the operation.

AFTERTREATMENT. The pull-out wire is removed at 4 weeks; otherwise the aftertreatment is as described on p. 3011.

TRANSFER OF PART OF PECTORALIS MAJOR MUSCLE

In 1946 Clark described a method of restoring active elbow flexion by transferring the distal third of the pectoralis major. This part of the muscle has a nerve and blood supply separate from that of the proximal part and so may still be active when the latter is paralyzed.

Seddon reported the results of 16 of these operations in 15 patients; in most the paralysis was caused by a traction injury of the brachial plexus. In 11 patients the elbow flexors were not completely paralyzed but were too weak to act against gravity. In four patients the transfer was supplemented by the pectoralis minor muscle. Results in 15 of the 16 transfers were satisfactory enough to justify the operation: six were excellent, and in seven the elbow could be flexed against gravity and slight resistance.

Subsequently (1959) Segal, Seddon, and Brooks reported the results of 17 more of these transfers; in 5 the paralysis was from poliomyelitis and in 12 from brachial plexus injuries. The result was excellent or good in eight and only fair or a failure in nine. After this operation (as is true for the Brooks and Seddon procedure to be described later) flexion of the elbow frequently produces undesirable shoulder movements such as shrugging, adduction, or internal rotation of the arm so that the hand strikes

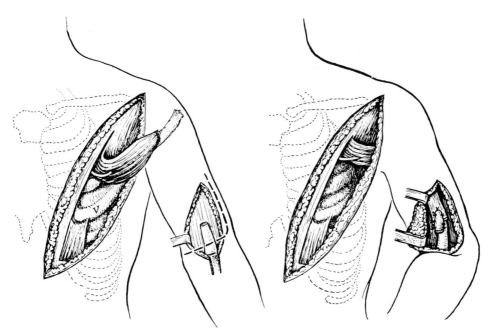

Fig. 66-61. Clark transfer of part of pectoralis major muscle for paralysis of biceps. Distal one third of pectoralis major is detached from its origin, including strip of sheath of rectus abdominis muscle. Nerve supply to transfer is preserved. Muscle is transferred subcutaneously into arm and sutured to biceps tendon. When biceps is completely paralyzed, its tendon may be divided as far proximally as possible, and transfer is sutured directly to it.

the chest wall; these movements occur when muscular control of the shoulder and scapula is poor, unless the shoulder has been fused. Thus when the muscles about the shoulder are appreciably paralyzed, the joint should be fused either before or after this type of transfer.

Samii reported a patient in whom he had detached the humeral insertion of the clavicular head of the pectoralis major, detached the tendon of the short head of the biceps from the coracoid process, and sutured the mobilized part of the pectoralis major to both heads of the biceps.

TECHNIQUE (CLARK). Place the patient supine, with the arm in moderate abduction and the elbow in complete extension. First make an incision distally from the axillary fold along the lateral border of the pectoralis major to the seventh rib; then make a second incision in the distal one fourth of the arm shaped like an L, with the transverse limb in the flexor crease of the elbow and the longitudinal limb extending proximally along the lateral margin of the biceps muscle (Fig. 66-61). Expose the pectoralis major and define its lateral border and distal costal attachment. Free the distal third (usually 6 cm wide) from the remainder of the muscle; also free the origin of this part of the muscle and elevate with it a part of the sheath of the rectus abdominis to lengthen the transfer and to serve as a tendon for insertion. While mobilizing the transfer proximally, protect a major terminal branch of the lateral anterior thoracic nerve that appears at the level of the third intercostal space; it courses distally along the deep surface of the transfer and innervates it; Seddon suggests that the nerve be located by electrical stimulation. Next through the arm

incision expose the distal biceps and its tendon. By blunt dissection create a large tunnel beneath the deep fascia between the two incisions. If the tunnel is too small, transferring the muscle will be difficult, and the blood supply to the transfer will be jeopardized. Now transfer the muscle to the arm, but take care that the neurovascular bundle, easily palpated beneath the muscle mass, is not taut. Close the thoracic incision; when oozing is considerable, drain the incision through a stab wound in the axilla. Now with the elbow flexed to 120 degrees and the forearm in supination, suture the transfer to the biceps tendon. When the pectoral transfer is short, suture its fascial prolongation to the underlying biceps muscle belly; this is a less desirable method of inserting the transfer. Close the arm incision, apply a posterior plaster splint holding the elbow flexed to 120 degrees, and immobilize the arm against the side of the chest with a light Velpeau dressing.

AFTERTREATMENT. Immobilization is continued for 3 weeks. Then a collar-and-cuff sling is fitted, and physical therapy and muscle reeducation are started. The sling is discarded at 6 weeks. Initially elbow flexion is accompanied by contraction of the entire pectoralis major muscle, but eventually independent flexion of the elbow is achieved (Seddon).

TRANSFER OF STERNOCLEIDOMASTOID MUSCLE

Bunnell devised another transfer to restore active elbow flexion when the biceps and brachialis muscles are paralyzed (Fig. 66-62).

TECHNIQUE (BUNNELL). Through the medial part of a transverse supraclavicular incision 6.5 cm long detach the sternoclavicular insertion of the sternocleidomastoid muscle. Gently mobilize the distal one half of the muscle by digital dissection. Expose the biceps tendon through an anterior L-shaped incision, its transverse limb in the flexor crease of the elbow and its longitudinal limb along the lateral aspect of the biceps muscle. Now through a longitudinal incision over the lateral aspect of the thigh obtain a fascial graft 4 cm wide and long enough to reach from the clavicle to the elbow (a graft of sufficient length and width cannot be obtained with a fascial stripper). Overlap one end of the fascial graft and the distal end of the sternocleidomastoid muscle and suture them together with multiple interrupted nonabsorbable sutures. Then pass the graft subcutaneously toward the elbow and close the supraclavicular incision. With the elbow in 115 degrees of flexion, attach the graft to the tuberosity of the radius with a pullout suture.

AFTERTREATMENT. The arm is immobilized in plaster with the elbow in 135 degrees of flexion. At 3 weeks the cast is removed, a posterior elbow splint with straps and buckles is applied, and muscle reeducation and physical therapy are started.

TRANSFER OF PECTORALIS MINOR MUSCLE

In a patient with complete paralysis of the pectoralis major, biceps brachii, and deltoid and marked weakness of the triceps, Spira detached the origin of the pectoralis minor, prolonged it with a tube of fascia lata, and attached it

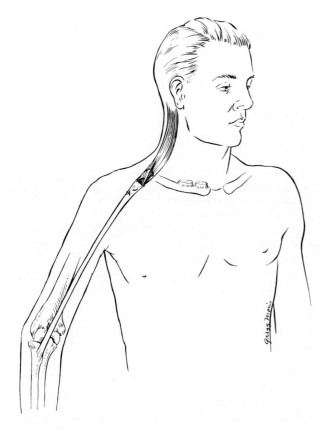

Fig. 66-62. Transfer of sternocleidomastoid muscle for paralysis of biceps and brachialis muscles. (From Bunnell, S.: J. Bone Joint Surg. **33-A:**566, 1951.)

to the tendon of the paralyzed biceps. Six months later flexion of the elbow was strong through a range of 135 degrees. In Spira's patient, although the pectoralis minor was rotated through almost 90 degrees, there seemed to be no undue tension on its nerves and vessels.

TECHNIQUE (SPIRA). Use the same incisions as for the Clark transfer of part of the pectoralis major muscle (p. 3013). Split the pectoralis major in line with its fibers and expose the pectoralis minor. Dissect the origin of the pectoralis minor from the third, fourth, and fifth ribs and elevate the muscle; the nerves can be seen entering the muscle on its lateral side. Through a lateral longitudinal incision over the thigh secure a fascial graft 30 cm long and 5 cm wide and with interrupted sutures attach it like a sleeve to the detached origin of the muscle. Now draw the elongated pectoralis minor subcutaneously from the incision over the chest to the one at the elbow and suture it under tension to the tendon of insertion of the biceps.

AFTERTREATMENT. Aftertreatment is the same as for transfer of the sternocleidomastoid muscle just described.

TRANSFER OF PECTORALIS MAJOR TENDON

Brooks and Seddon described an operation to restore elbow flexion in which the entire pectoralis major muscle is used as the motor, and its tendon is prolonged distally by means of the long head of the biceps brachii. This transfer is contraindicated unless the biceps is completely paralyzed; they recommend it when the Steindler flexorplasty is not applicable, when the distal part of the pectoralis major is too weak for the Clark transfer but the proximal part is strong, or when both parts of the muscle are so weak that the entire muscle is needed for transfer. To avoid undesirable movements of the shoulder during elbow flexion after this procedure (as after the Clark transfer), muscular control of the shoulder and scapula must be good or the shoulder must be fused.

TECHNIQUE (BROOKS AND SEDDON). Make an incision from the distal end of the deltopectoral groove distally to the junction of the proximal and middle thirds of the arm. Detach the tendon of insertion of the pectoralis major as close to bone as possible and by blunt dissection mobilize the muscle from the chest wall proximally toward the clavicle (Fig. 66-63, *A*). Then retract the deltoid laterally and superiorly and expose the tendon of the long head of the biceps as it runs proximally into the shoulder joint; sever this tendon at the proximal end of the bicipital groove and withdraw it into the wound. By blunt and sharp dissection free the belly of the long head of the biceps from that of the short head and ligate and divide all vessels entering it. Now make an L-shaped incision at the elbow, with its transverse limb in the flexor crease and its longitudinal limb extending proximally along the medial border of the biceps muscle. Now mobilize the long head of the biceps by dividing its remaining neurovascular bundles so that the tendon and muscle are completely freed distally to the tuberosity of the radius; withdraw the tendon and muscle through the distal incision (Fig. 66-63, *C*). (When the muscle belly is adherent to the overlying fascia, free it by sharp dissection.) Now replace the long head of the biceps in its original position and through the proximal incision pass its tendon and muscle belly through two slits in the

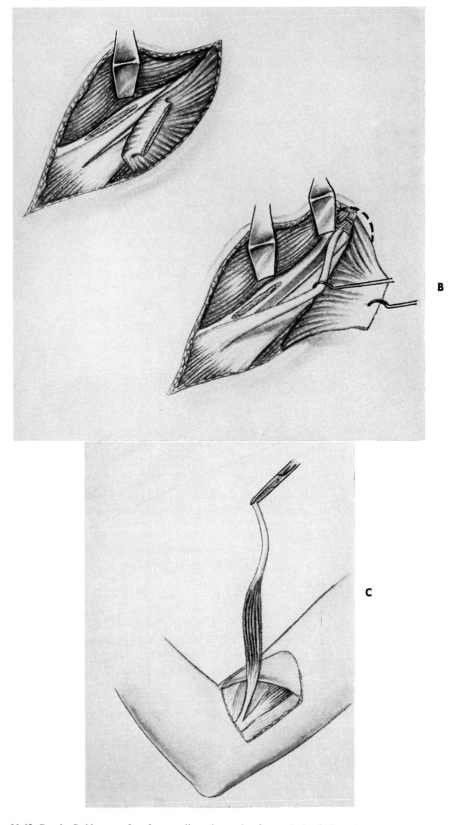

Fig. 66-63. Brooks-Seddon transfer of pectoralis major tendon for paralysis of elbow flexors. **A,** Insertion of pectoralis major is detached as close to bone as possible. **B,** Tendon of long head of biceps is exposed and divided at proximal end of bicipital groove. **C,** Tendon and muscle of long head of biceps are completely mobilized distally to tuberosity of radius by dividing all vessels and nerves that enter muscle proximal to elbow. *Continued.*

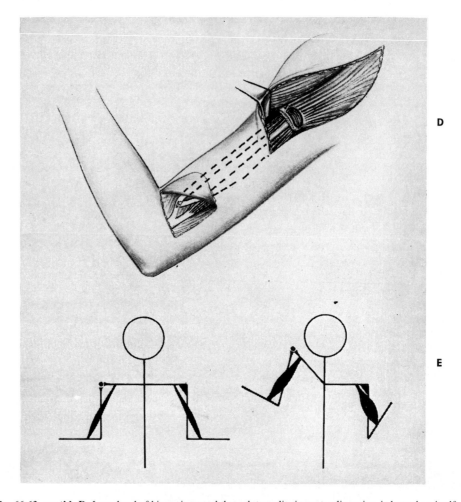

Fig. 66-63, cont'd. D, Long head of biceps is passed through two slits in pectoralis major, is looped on itself so that its proximal tendon is brought into distal incision, and is sutured through slit in its distal tendon. **E,** To avoid undesirable movements of shoulder during elbow flexion after this transfer, muscular control of shoulder and scapula must be good, or shoulder must be fused. Left shoulder shown is flail; right has been fused. When transfer on left contracts, some of its force is wasted because of lack of control of shoulder, but on right, transfer moves only elbow. (From Brooks, D.M., and Seddon, H.J.: J. Bone Joint Surg. **41-B:**36, 1959.)

tendon of the pectoralis major; loop the long head of the biceps on itself so that its proximal tendon is brought into the distal incision. Then, using silk, suture the end of the proximal tendon through a slit in the distal tendon (Fig. 66-63, *D*) and suture the tendon of the pectoralis major to the long head of the biceps at their junction. Close the incisions.

AFTERTREATMENT. Apply a posterior plaster splint with the elbow in flexion. At 3 weeks the splint is removed and muscle reeducation is started; care must be taken to extend the elbow gradually so that active flexion of more than 90 degrees is preserved. It may be 2 or 3 months before full extension is possible.

TRANSFER OF LATISSIMUS DORSI MUSCLE

Hovnanian described a method of restoring active elbow flexion by transferring the origin and belly of the latissimus dorsi to the arm and anchoring the origin near the radial tuberosity. This transfer is possible because the neurovascular bundle of the muscle is long and easily mobi-

lized (Fig. 66-64, *A*); a similar transfer in which the origin is anchored to the olecranon to restore active extension is also possible (p. 3018). In the latissimus dorsi transplantation described in 1955 by Schottstaedt, Larsen, and Bost, both the origin and insertion of the muscle are freed, the insertion is anchored to the coracoid process, and the origin is anchored to the biceps tendon. Zancolli and Mitre in 1973 reported eight patients with paralysis of the flexors of the elbow caused by brachial plexus palsy or poliomyelitis treated by transplantation of the latissimus dorsi muscle as described by Schottstaedt et al. Thirteen months to 6 years after surgery strength and flexion of the elbow were satisfactory. The amount of flexion regained in all eight patients was excellent, and according to Zancolli and Mitre, a comparable range of motion after flexorplasty is obtained only by transfers of the pectoralis major or triceps muscles.

TECHNIQUE (HOVNANIAN). Place the patient on his side with the affected extremity upward. Start the skin incision over the loin and extend it superiorly along the lateral border of

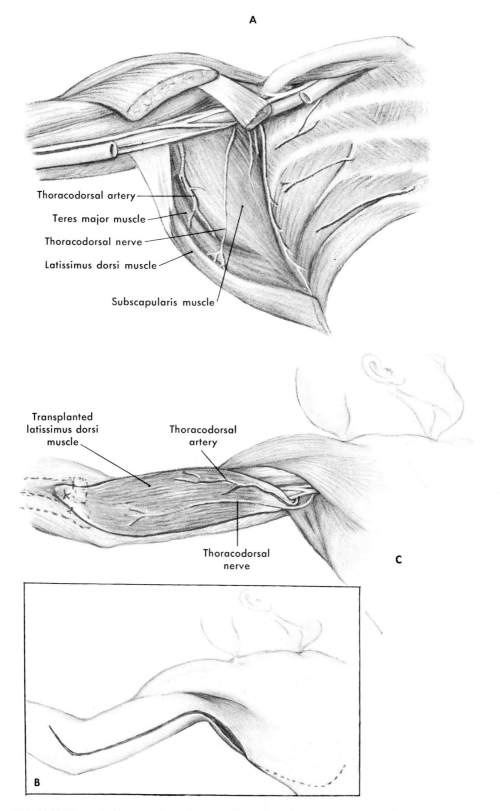

Fig. 66-64. Hovnanian transfer of latissimus dorsi muscle for paralysis of biceps and brachialis muscles. **A,** Normal anatomy of axilla; note that thoracodorsal nerve and artery are long and can be easily mobilized. **B,** Skin incision. **C,** Origin and belly of latissimus dorsi have been transferred to arm, and origin has been sutured to biceps tendon and to other structures distal to elbow joint. (From Hovnanian, A.P.: Ann. Surg. **143:**493, 1956.)

the latissimus dorsi to the posterior axillary fold, distally along the medial aspect of the arm, and finally laterally to end in the antecubital fossa (Fig. 66-64, *B*). Carefully expose the dorsal and lateral aspects of the latissimus dorsi, leaving its investing fascia intact. Then free the origin of the muscle by cutting across its musculofascial junction inferiorly and its muscle fibers superiorly (Fig. 66-66, *B*). Then gradually free the muscle from the underlying abdominal and flank muscles. Divide the four slips of the muscle that arise from the inferior four ribs and the few arising from the angle of the scapula. Carefully protect the neurovascular bundle that enters the superior third of the muscle. To prevent injury of the vessels to the latissimus dorsi, ligate their branches that anastomose with the lateral thoracic vessels. Identify and gently free the thoracodorsal nerve that supplies the muscle; its trunk is about 15 cm long and runs from the apex of the axilla along the deep surface of the muscle belly.

Next prepare a bed in the anteromedial aspect of the arm to receive the transfer. Carefully swing the transfer into this bed without twisting its vessels or nerve. To prevent kinking of the vessels, divide the intercostobrachial nerve and the lateral cutaneous branches of the third and fourth intercostal nerves; also free as necessary any fascial bands. Now suture the aponeurotic origin of the muscle to the biceps tendon and the periosteal tissues about the radial tuberosity, and the remaining origin to the sheaths of the forearm muscles and to the lacertus fibrosus (Fig. 66-64, *C*). Close the wound in layers and bandage the arm against the thorax with the elbow flexed and the forearm pronated.

AFTERTREATMENT. Exercises of the fingers are encouraged early. At 3 or 4 weeks the bandage is removed and passive and active exercises of the elbow are started.

Muscle transfers for paralysis of triceps

Weakness or paralysis of the triceps muscle is usually considered of little importance, since gravity will extend the elbow passively in most positions that the arm assumes. But a good triceps is essential to crutch walking or to shifting the body weight to the hands during such activities as moving from a bed to a wheelchair because it can lock the elbow in extension. To place the hand on top of the head when the patient is erect, the triceps must be strong enough to extend the elbow against gravity; thrusting and pushing motions with the forearm also require a functional triceps. In other respects, strong active extension of the elbow is relatively unimportant in comparison with strong active flexion.

For weakness of the triceps Ober and Barr devised a method of transferring the brachioradialis muscle from the lateral aspect of the elbow and forearm to a position posterior to the lateral humeral condyle; should the power of the brachioradialis be insufficient, added power is obtained by transferring the extensor carpi radialis longus muscle also.

Friedenberg reported the successful transfer of the biceps for triceps weakness, and d'Aubigne mentioned transferring the posterior part of the deltoid into the triceps to reinforce it. Many years ago Hohmann, Lange, and Harmon each proposed transfer of the insertion of the latissimus dorsi for triceps paralysis. In 1955 Schottstaedt, Larsen, and Bost described a transplantation of the latissimus

dorsi in which the origin of the muscle is anchored to the olecranon and the insertion is anchored to the acromion. In 1967 duToit and Levy described a similar operation. In 1956 Hovnanian described a transfer of the origin of the latissimus dorsi to the olecranon, leaving the insertion intact.

TRANSFER OF BRACHIORADIALIS MUSCLE FOR PARALYSIS OF TRICEPS

TECHNIQUE (OBER AND BARR). Begin the skin incision on the posterolateral aspect of the humerus 7.5 to 10 cm proximal to the lateral epicondyle, direct it distally just anterior to the epicondyle, and end it 10 cm distal to the head of the radius on the lateral side of the forearm; take care to avoid injuring the posterior cutaneous nerve of the forearm. Define the anterior margin of the brachioradialis muscle and free it distally and proximally until its nerve and blood supply are well isolated; carefully avoid the recurrent radial artery and the motor branches of the radial nerve. Roll the freed anterior margin of the muscle laterally and posteriorly and suture it to the fascia and periosteum along the subcutaneous border of the ulna and olecranon and to the triceps tendon (Fig. 66-65). Detaching the origin of the brachioradialis is unnecessary, for transferring its muscle belly to the posterior aspect of the elbow is enough to change its function from that of a flexor to that of an extensor.

AFTERTREATMENT. The arm is immobilized in a plaster splint, with the elbow in full extension and the forearm in full supination. At 10 days exercises are started and are continued as long as ability to extend the elbow increases.

TRANSFER OF LATISSIMUS DORSI MUSCLE FOR PARALYSIS OF TRICEPS

TECHNIQUE (HOVNANIAN). Place the patient on his side with the affected extremity upward. Begin the skin incision over the loin and extend it superiorly along the lateral margin of the latissimus dorsi to the posterior axillary fold, distally along the posteromedial aspect of the arm to the medial epicondyle, and then laterally to end over the posterior aspect of the ulnar shaft (Fig. 66-66, *A*). Free the origin of the muscle and elevate its belly as already described for transfer of the latissimus dorsi to restore flexion of the elbow (p. 3016); carefully preserve the nerve and blood supply to the muscle. Then prepare the posterior aspect of the arm and elbow for reception of the transfer. Suture the aponeurotic origin of the muscle to the triceps tendon, the periosteum of the olecranon, and the connective tissue septa on the extensor surface of the forearm (Fig. 66-66, *C*). Close the wound in layers and bandage the limb to the side of the body with the elbow in extension.

AFTERTREATMENT. Finger movements are encouraged early. At 3 or 4 weeks the bandage is removed, and active and passive exercises are started.

POSTERIOR DELTOID TRANSFER FOR TRICEPS PARALYSIS (MOBERG)

In 1975 Moberg described an operation to transfer the posterior third of the deltoid muscle to the triceps to restore active elbow extension in the quadriplegic patient. Patients with complete quadriplegia at the functioning

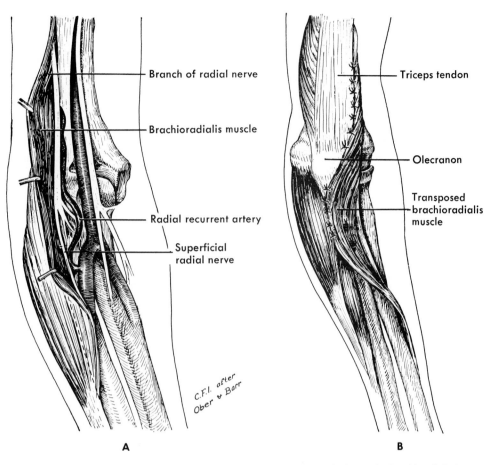

Branch of radial nerve

Brachioradialis muscle

Radial recurrent artery

Superficial radial nerve

Triceps tendon

Olecranon

Transposed brachioradialis muscle

C.F.I. after Ober & Barr

A

B

Fig. 66-65. Ober-Barr transfer of brachioradialis muscle for paralysis of triceps. **A,** Brachioradialis is retracted, showing its relation to radial nerve; nerve supply enters proximally. **B,** Position of muscle after transfer. (Redrawn from Ober, F.R., and Barr, J.S.: Surg Gynecol. Obstet **67**:105, 1938. By permission of Surgery, Gynecology & Obstetrics.)

level of C5 or C6 have active elbow flexion, shoulder flexion and abduction, and possibly wrist extension. Elbow extension is by gravity only, without triceps function (C7). Active extension is impossible. Ambulation is not a realistic goal in such patients. Rather, improved strength, mobility, and function were sought, as well as improved ability to reach overhead, to perform personal hygiene and grooming, to relieve ischial pressure from the wheelchair, to achieve driving ability and wheelchair use, and to eat and control eating utensils.

Satisfactory results in 19 such transfers performed on 18 patients were recently reported by Raczka, Braun, and Waters. The authors recommend that ample time (at least 10 months) after injury should elapse to allow recovery of the C7 nerve root. Further, the patient must be reliable and a proven rehabilitation candidate with good or normal deltoid power; cervical spine stability must be assured; range of motion in the shoulder and elbow should be full; and, especially, the patient must be willing to be immobilized a minimum of 15 weeks to assure complete healing of the tendon graft.

Castro-Sierra and Lopez-Pita have modified Moberg's procedure by the construction of tendinoperiosteal tongues proximally and distally instead of using the free tendon

grafts from the foot. The posterior belly of the deltoid muscle is freed, along with the most distal insertion of the muscle and including a strip of periosteum 1 cm wide and 3 cm in length, continuous with the muscle and its insertion. Next a 1.5 to 2 cm–wide tongue of the triceps tendon is developed by parallel incisions and including a continuous strip of periosteum similar to that above, if possible.

The length of the tendinoperiosteal tongues should be such that with the elbow extended and the arm adducted their deep surfaces should appose when the triceps tendon is folded over 180 degrees. The angle of tendinous reflection is reinforced by a narrow sheet of Dacron wrapped around the grafts and sutured to the tongues and to itself.

FOREARM

Operations on the forearm after poliomyelitis consist of tenotomy, fasciotomy, and osteotomy to correct deformities and tendon transfers to restore function.

Deformities of the forearm are seldom disabling enough in themselves to warrant surgery; the most common exception is a fixed pronation contracture from imbalance between the supinators and pronators. When the pronator teres is not strong enough to transfer to replace the paralyzed supinators, correcting the contracture alone is indi-

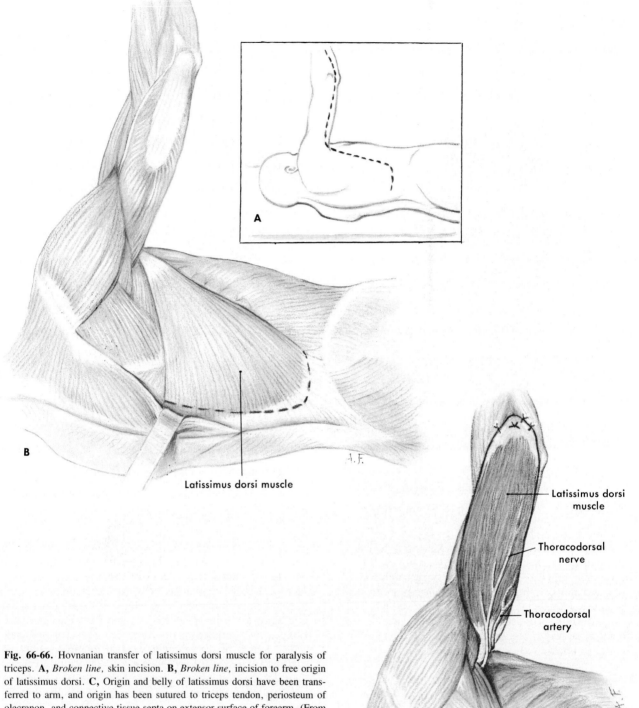

Fig. 66-66. Hovnanian transfer of latissimus dorsi muscle for paralysis of triceps. **A,** *Broken line,* skin incision. **B,** *Broken line,* incision to free origin of latissimus dorsi. **C,** Origin and belly of latissimus dorsi have been transferred to arm, and origin has been sutured to triceps tendon, periosteum of olecranon, and connective tissue septa on extensor surface of forearm. (From Hovnanian, A.P.: Ann. Surg. **143:**493, 1956.)

Latissimus dorsi muscle

Latissimus dorsi muscle

Thoracodorsal nerve

Thoracodorsal artery

cated, provided there is active flexion of the elbow. When the pronators of the forearm and the flexors of the wrist are active, however, function may be improved not only by correcting the pronation contracture but also by transferring the flexor carpi ulnaris after the method of Steindler or of Green and Banks (p. 369).

Blount called attention to the supination deformity of the forearm sometimes caused by poliomyelitis or obstetric palsy; it develops from muscle imblance in which usually the pronators and finger flexors are weak and the biceps and wrist extensors are strong. With the passage of time and with growth, soft tissue structures such as the interosseous membrane contract, the bones become deformed, and eventually the radioulnar joints may become dislocated. Inability to pronate the forearm from the position of supination is quite disabling. Schottstaedt, Larsen, and Bost mentioned rerouting the biceps tendon to change the biceps from a supinator to a pronator, and such an operation was described by Grilli. Zancolli has combined this operation with release of contracted soft structures, especially the interosseous membrane. To correct this deformity Bount uses manual osteoclasis of the middle third of the radius and ulna. This procedure is specifically indicated when muscle power is insufficient for tendon transfers but never after age 12 years. The deformity should be overcorrected, for it will recur to some extent after the cast is removed and with further growth; in several of Blount's patients correcting the deformity a second time was necessary because the initial correction was lost.

Owings, Wickstrom, Perry, and Nickel in 1971 reported 26 operations in which the biceps tendon was rerouted to correct supination deformity and to establish a pronating force to counteract the supinator muscles. The operation was carried out in three steps as follows: (1) When supination deformity was fixed, the interosseous membrane was stripped from the ulna. (2) When the biceps muscle was the only active supinator, it was transferred to the ulna. If both the biceps and the supinator muscles were active, as was usually true, the Zancolli rerouting of the biceps tendon as described here was performed. (3) When bowing of the forearm was so severe that pronation was impossible, or if the bones were locked in pronation, either the distal end of the ulna was resected or the ulna was osteotomized. They found that up to 4 cm of the distal ulna could be resected without impairing stability of the forearm. When bowing was severe and resection of more than 4 cm of the ulna would be required to correct deformity, the ulna was osteotomized and fixed by a medullary nail. The results were good in 9 patients, satisfactory in 11, and poor in 2; 4 patients were unavailable for evaluation.

Rerouting of biceps tendon for supination deformities of forearm

TECHNIQUE (ZANCOLLI). If full passive pronation is already possible before surgery, omit the first part of the operation. Otherwise make a longitudinal incision on the dorsum of the forearm over the radial shaft (Fig. 66-67, *A*, *1*). By

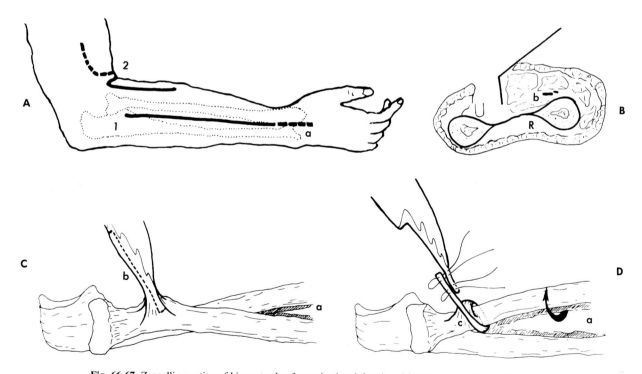

Fig. 66-67. Zancolli rerouting of biceps tendon for supination deformity of forearm. **A,** *1,* Dorsal skin incision is extended distally to *a* when distal radioulnar joint requires capsulotomy. *2,* Anterior incision to expose biceps tendon and radial head. **B,** Exposure of interosseous membrane by retracting dorsal muscles radially (see text). **C,** *Broken line* at *b,* Z-plasty incision to be made in biceps tendon. Interosseous membrane has been divided at *a.* **D,** At *c* biceps tendon has been divided by Z-plasty, distal segment has been rerouted around radial neck medially, and ends of tendon are being sutured together. Traction on tendon will now pronate forearm as indicated by arrow. (From Zancolli, E.A.: J. Bone Joint Surg. **49-A:**1275, 1967.)

blunt dissection expose the interosseous membrane and retract the dorsal muscles radialward to protect the posterior interosseous nerve (Fig. 66-67, *B*). Then divide the interosseous membrane throughout its length close to the ulna. If the dorsal ligaments of the distal radioulnar joint are contracted, extend the incision distally and perform a capsulotomy of this joint. If necessary, release the supinator muscle after identifying and protecting the posterior interosseous nerve in the proximal part of the incision. At this point in the operation full passive pronation of the forearm should be possible. Now make a second incision: begin it on the medial aspect of the arm proximal to the elbow and extend it distally to the flexion crease of the joint, then laterally across the joint in the crease, and then distally over the anterior aspect of the radial head (Fig. 66-67, *A,* 2). Identify and retract the median nerve and brachial artery. Divide the lacertus fibrosus and expose the insertion of the biceps tendon on the radial tuberosity. Now divide the biceps tendon by a long Z-plasty (Fig. 66-67, *C*). Then reroute the distal segment of the tendon around the radial neck medially, then posteriorly, and then laterally so that traction on it will pronate the forearm (Fig. 66-67, *D*). Then place the ends of the biceps tendon side-by-side and suture them together under tension that will maintain full pronation and yet allow extension of the elbow. If the radial head is subluxated or is dislocated, reduce it if possible and hold it in place by capsulorrhaphy of the radiohumeral joint; if the radial head cannot be reduced, then excise it and transfer the proximal segment of the biceps tendon to the brachialis tendon. Close the incisions and apply a cast with the elbow flexed 90 degrees and the forearm moderately pronated.

AFTERTREATMENT. At about 3 weeks the cast and sutures are removed and passive and active exercises are begun.

Osteoclasis for supination deformities of forearm

TECHNIQUE (BLOUNT). Abduct and externally rotate the affected arm to bring the wrist near the shoulder. Place the forearm in as near midpronation as possible, with the dorsum of the hand toward the table (in this position there are no important structures between the bones) and a padded sharp wedge beneath the middle of the forearm. Stand on a low stool, grasp the forearm on each side of the wedge, and with a quick straight arm thrust, fracture the bones. Then reverse the force to complete the fractures; bend the midforearm backward and forward several times to be sure the fractures are complete. Then pronate the forearm between 45 and 90 degrees and apply a cast from the axilla to the metacarpophalangeal joints with the elbow at 90 degrees; continue the immobilization for 6 to 8 weeks. When the deformity cannot be fully corrected without excessive displacement of the bones at the time of osteoclasis, the forearm may be manipulated again after 10 to 14 days.

WRIST AND HAND

The treatment of disabilities of the wrist and hand caused by paralysis is discussed in Chapter 12.

Spina Bifida

Recent advances in medicine, surgery, and the allied sciences have greatly reduced both mortality and morbidity in patients born with severe defects of the central nervous system. The challenge of the orthopaedic surgeon is to assist these patients in attaining the best possible function within the limitations imposed on them by their physical handicap.

In spina bifida abnormalities are found that have in common a separation of midline elements occurring in a genetically susceptible embryo. These abnormalities may be found within the neuroectoderm, ectoderm, mesoderm, and endoderm, resulting in a variety of clinical manifestations. Genetic studies reveal no more than a ''polygenetically inherited predisposition'' and the precise cause of spina bifida remains unknown. Since experimental teratology can reproduce the affection, it is likely caused by some environmental factor. The structural abnormalities are established by the twenty-eighth day of embryonic development, and secondary intrauterine forces may produce further deformity. Therefore a wide range of abnormalities may be found in the skin, muscle, bone, and nervous system.

The following classification of spina bifida was suggested by Bucy* in 1939 and has been in general use since:

A. Spina bifida anterior
B. Spina bifida posterior
   1. Spina bifida occulta
   2. Spina bifida cystica
      a. Meningocele
      b. Meningomyelocele
      c. Myelocele
C. Cranium bifidum

We limit the discussion here to spina bifida posterior, both occulta and cystica. Spina bifida occulta is characterized by incomplete closure of the laminae of one or more vertebrae in the absence of a posterior cystic mass. Spina bifida cystica is characterized by incomplete closure of posterior elements of vertebrae and the presence of a cystic mass that protrudes posteriorly over the bony defect. Only one type of spina bifida cystica, myelomeningocele (meningomyelocele), is discussed here. A myelomeningocele is a saclike structure containing cerebrospinal fluid and neural tissue, and because neural tissue is included, a neurologic defect results that varies in extent and severity with the location and severity of the lesion.

SPINA BIFIDA OCCULTA

James and Lassman described a syndrome in spina bifida occulta that they call *spinal dysraphism*. Lichtenstein used the same term to describe congenital defects in the lumbosacral area in which midline structures posteriorly fail to develop properly. He pointed out that in spina bifida occulta the tissues involved may be cutaneous, muscular, osseous, vascular or neural separately or together. Thus

---

*From Bucy, P.C.: Spina bifida and associated malformations. In Brennemann, J., editor: Practice of pediatrics, Hagerstown, Md., 1939, W.F. Prior Co., Inc.

there may be defects in neural tissue without any in the other tissues, and conversely, defects in the other tissues without any in neural tissue. However, defects in all these tissues tend to occur together.

In the syndrome of spinal dysraphism, asymmetric and progressive neurologic abnormalities develop in the lower extremities, usually in a growing child. The syndrome may begin at any age but is seen most often between the ages of 4 and 6 years. The most common finding is asymmetry of the calves with a cavovarus deformity of one foot with or without shortening of the leg. There may be sensory alterations, and sometimes trophic ulcers develop. Examination early reveals an abnormality in the gait in which the forepart of the shoe is twisted and later an overpull of the invertor muscles of the foot that results in cavovarus deformity. A patch of hair, a nevus, a sacral dimple, or a sacral lipoma was found in only 13 of the 24 patients of James and Lassman. Incontinence of bladder or bowel is fairly common and occasionally paraplegia develops. Roentgenograms reveal a spina bifida that is more extensive than a simple longitudinal defect in the first sacral vertebra. Myelography computed tomography, and magnetic resonance imaging are recommended to aid in diagnosis.

The treatment of spinal dysraphism consists of laminectomy and exploration of the extradural and intradural areas and of the spinal cord, cauda equina, and filum terminale. This treatment was carried out by James and Lassman in 24 patients, and in 22 a variety of congenital lesions was found. Sixteen patients were better after surgery and none were worse.

In 1953 Garceau described patients with *tethered cord syndrome (filum terminale syndrome* or *cord-traction syndrome)* associated with spina bifida occulta who had progressive neurologic deficits involving the lower extremities or bladder or both and who improved following section of a thick, tight, filum terminale discovered at laminectomy. In 1956 Jones and Love reported six patients, and later James and Lassman described the entity further. Characteristically these patients have many abnormalities, including deformities of the feet, abnormalities of gait, weakness or sensory loss in the lower extremities, difficulty in micturition, and usually back or leg pain. Hoffman, Hendrick, and Humphreys in 1976 presented an excellent survey of 31 children with spina bifida occulta who had back pain, scoliosis, a progressive neurologic deficit involving the lower extremities, or a neurogenic bladder. All were found to have a tethered spinal cord. Release of the tight filum terminale relieved pain in all patients and frequently corrected a progressive scoliosis, arrested or improved neurogenic foot deformities, and improved the neurogenic bladder. Fourteen of the 31 patients had cutaneous manifestations of spina bifida in the lumbosacral area such as a patch of hair, an angioma with a dimple, or a fat pad. Typically symptoms occurred during spurts of growth: in 12 patients under age 5 years, in 7 between ages 6 and 10 years, in 4 at age 11 or 12 years, and in 8 between ages 13 and 16 years. In all patients myelography was carried out, and often when the patient was prone, the myelogram was normal. However, when the patient was turned supine, a thickened filum and a low position of the conus could be better demonstrated. In those patients in whom the myelograms were normal, the symptoms were so characteristic that laminectomy was carried out, and the pathologic condition was found. At surgery the thickened filum was identified and divided between silver clips. Upward movement of the proximal filum or cord always occurred, and this ranged from 1 to 2.5 cm. After surgery pain disappeared in all patients. Parents often commented on how much more mobile the children were and that they could jump, hop, run, and touch their toes, which they could not do before surgery.

In summary, the tethered spinal cord syndrome must be borne in mind in any child with spina bifida occulta in the lumbosacral region who has back or leg pain, scoliosis, neurogenic foot abnormality, or sphincter disturbance. This is especially true in children with cutaneous manifestations, such as those just mentioned. The diagnosis therefore requires a strong clinical suspicion and careful myelographic studies.

Diastematomyelia is a congenital anomaly in which the spinal cord or filum terminale or both are split from dorsal to ventral into two parts, usually separated by an osseous or fibrocartilaginous septum. The two halves of the split spinal elements are unequal in their neuronal contents and therefore do not constitute a diplomyelia. The two parts are usually joined caudally but may remain split. The signs and symptoms of this affection usually begin in the developmental years and include abnormality of gait, unilateral or bilateral weakness or atrophy of the legs, discrepancy in leg lengths, abnormal reflexes in the lower extremities, deformities of the feet, cutaneous abnormalities on the back such as a patch of hair or a dimple, and possibly abnormalities of micturition. Evidence of a progressive neurologic deficit should be sought, and therefore the diagnosis may not be made early without careful, regular, and repeated examinations. The roentgenographic abnormalities include (1) prominent spinous processes at the level of the septum, (2) abnormalities of the laminae, (3) widened interpedicular distances, and (4) vertebral body abnormalities. Any bony septum may be difficult to see on an ordinary roentgenogram. The diagnosis of diastematomyelia is made by myelography. Typically the column of dye splits for a variable distance, producing a diamond-shaped defect, and the septum, if osseous, can be seen in the center of this defect.

It is important that diastematomyelia be diagnosed and treated early; because the spinal cord is transfixed by the osseous or fibrocartilaginous septum, it cannot ascend normally during growth, and consequently traction is exerted on it. The gradual increase in traction on the cord is thought to be the cause of the progressive nature of the neurologic abnormalities often reported in diastematomyelia. Treatment consists of laminectomy and excision of the septum, mobilization of the dural sac, and release of any tight filum terminale.

MYELOMENINGOCELE

A myelomeningocele, as already stated, is a saclike structure containing cerebrospinal fluid and neural tissue; because the neural tissue is included, a neurologic deficit results that varies in extent and severity with the location and severity of the lesion.

Epidemiology

The natural incidence of myelomeningocele varies considerably around the world but the average is 2 per 1000 live births. There are seasonal variations, racial differences, and environmental and genetic factors. The chance of a neural tube defect occurring in siblings born after a child with myelomeningocele is about 5%; after two children so malformed the chances are between 10% and 15%. The stillbirth rate for all infants with myelomeningocele is about 25%.

Prevention

Studying a normal constituent of fetal serum and amniotic fluid known as alpha fetoprotein, Brock and Sutcliffe observed its presence in excessive amounts when the fetus had an open neural tube defect. This excess is most marked between the sixteenth and eighteenth weeks of pregnancy and is determined by sampling the amnoiotic fluid. Since it is impractical to carry out amniocentesis in all pregnancies, this test is useful chiefly in preventing the birth of infants with myelomeningocele in high-risk families. This has therefore resulted in the study of alpha fetoprotein present in maternal serum, and in a few research centers the development of a simple blood test to be performed between the fourteenth and eighteenth weeks of pregnancy is likely. The upper limit of normal of this substance in the amniotic fluid is 40 μg/ml; higher values require a decision regarding termination of pregnancy. Ultrasonographic studies assist in determining the condition of the intrauterine fetus.

General considerations

The medical management of a child with spina bifida is most complex not only because of the wide variation in the extent and the degree of the causative neurologic lesion, but also because of the impairment of multiple organ systems imposed as a result of the neurologic defect. Appropriate treatment in a timely manner can best be rendered when a spina bifida team establishes the diagnosis, goals of treatment, and priorities in management and provides long-term supervisory and supportive care whose ultimate goal is to assist the individual to achieve his optimal role as a productive member of society. One of the earliest and best known of such teams is the Royal Melbourne Children's Hospital Spina Bifida Clinic, whose chief orthopaedic surgeon is Mr. Malcolm B. Menelaus. Menelaus' monograph on the orthopaedic management of spina bifida cystica is recognized as an authoritative source on the subject; the reader is referred to this book for a more complete exposition of the subject. It is based on experience with more than 900 affected patients extending over nearly 4 decades.

Mortality in the Melbourne series is approximately 40%. Of these, 40% die by the age of 1 month, 84% by the age of 1 year, and 90% by the age of 2 years. Thus if the child is 2 years of age, death in childhood is unlikely, and the orthopaedic surgeon should develop a plan of treatment for childhood and into adult life.

The defect is usually closed within the first 24 hours of life. This is accomplished by approximating in layers the dural sac, fascia, and skin. Although early closure does not improve the neurologic problem, it does prevent the slow progression of paralysis that follows nonoperative treatment. Many authors, including the Melbourne group, aware of the poor prognosis in grossly and severely handicapped patients with spina bifida, regard the presence of the following as contraindications for early sac closure: infected sac at presentation; cervical and thoracic lesions, especially if kyphosis is present; hydrocephalus at birth; meningitis; and multiple congenital anomalies or other life-threatening diseases. In such circumstances the situation, including the prognosis, is explained to the family; it is usually agreed that symptomatic and simple nursing care only be rendered. Should the baby thrive, matters are reevaluated and a more active treatment program is instituted. These decisions are usually made by the family on the advice of the clinic coordinator and the neurosurgeon; the orthopaedic surgeon is not involved until the neurologic problem is stabilized and the baby is thriving.

Hydrocephalus occurs in three fourths of all patients and is more common in those whose lesions are more cephalad. Of those with this complication, it is present at birth in one fourth and by 1 month of age in three fourths. It rarely develops after 6 months of age. Any ventricular shunt insertion performed to stabilize the process is usually done in the first 2 months of life.

Urinary diversion for incontinence is usually necessary and is most frequently done between the ages of 3 and 5 years, since less than 10% of patients have sufficiently low lesions to permit urinary and fecal continence. If diversion is done before renal function is impaired, then impaired renal function is less certain and more delayed. Still, renal deterioration before adulthood occurs in three fourths of those without and in one third of those with surgical diversion; it is the quality of renal function that largely determines survival and longevity after the second year of life.

The spina bifida team, then, as a minimum, includes the clinic coordinator, who is a pediatric generalist; a neurosurgeon; a urologist; an orthopaedic surgeon; physical and occupational therapists; a psychologist; a medical social worker; an orthotist; and such other specialists as may be deemed necessary from time to time. To conserve time and effort, to increase the benefits as much as possible, and to minimize expense, inconvenience, travel, and hospitalization for the patient, all treatment programs should be planned and coordinated before they are presented to the patient and the family.

The ultimate prognosis for patients with spina bifida depends on many factors, the most important being the level of neurological involvement. The more cephalad the neurologic lesion, the less likely is functional ambulation and the more likely is the patient to have hydrocephalus, mental retardation, perceptual visual problems, and difficulty in performing fine motor skills. Also important in ambulation are motivation, the absence of obesity, and the general health and well-being of the child.

Neurologic lesion and deformity

In 1964 Sharrard first correlated the level of the neurologic lesion with the presence or absence of deformity of the hip in 183 children, thus establishing the rationale on

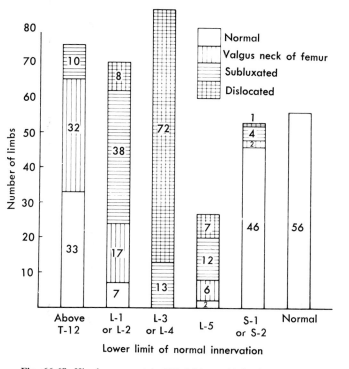

Fig. 66-68. Hip derangement in 183 children with lumbar myelomeningocele. Correlation of level of lesion, power of muscles controlling hip, and presence or absence of deformity of hip. Six groups described in text appear in order from left to right. (From Sharrard, W.J.W.: J. Bone Joint Surg. **46-B:**426, 1964.)

which treatment is presently based. The children were grouped as follows, depending on the level of the lesion (Fig. 66-68). In group 1 there was paralysis below the twelfth thoracic nerve root and thus complete paralysis of the lower extremities. Of the 75 hips included, 32 developed only valgus deformity of the femoral neck, 10 subluxated, but none dislocated. In group 2 there was paralysis below the first or second lumbar nerve root. The flexors of the hip were strong or moderately so, and the adductors were weak or at best moderately strong. All other muscles about the hip were paralyzed. Of the 70 hips included, most developed progressive flexion-adduction deformity and valgus deformity of the femoral neck, 38 became moderately or severely subluxated, and 8 became dislocated. In group 3 there was paralysis below the third or fourth lumbar nerve roots. The flexors and adductors of the hip were normal, and the abductors and extensors were completely paralyzed; the quadriceps was normal, and in a few hips the tensor fasciae latae was active. Of the 85 hips included, most developed valgus deformity of the femoral neck, 72 became dislocated by the end of the first year, and the remaining 13 became moderately or severely subluxated and, when left untreated, always became dislocated. In group 4 there was paralysis below the fifth lumbar nerve root. The flexors and adductors of the hip were normal, the abductors were weak to moderately strong, and the extensors were paralyzed; the quadriceps was normal. Of the 27 hips included, 6 developed only valgus deformity of the femoral neck and all developed a slowly progressive flexion-adduction deformity that caused sub-

luxation in 12 and, by the end of the first year, dislocation in 7. When left untreated, the subluxated hips became dislocated later, although sometimes as late as the fifth or sixth year. In group 5 there was paralysis below the first sacral nerve root. The only weakness of the hip was in extension. Included were 53 hips, and all remained normal or at most developed a mild subluxation. In group 6 were 56 patients in whom one limb was normal. No abnormality developed later in any of these limbs.

In recent years it has become clear that the neurologic lesion is usually not so clear and precise. Upper motor neuron lesions frequently coexist with lower motor neuron lesions in the lower limbs and may be present in the upper limbs. Frequently no precise level of demarcation exists between normal function and absent function; muscles innervated proximal to the major lesion may be weak, and there may be "skips," with areas of diminished function existing distal to the major lesion. Asymmetric cord involvement is frequently associated with asymmetric limb involvement. Finally, the neurologic lesion is not always stationary; in patients with progressive neurologic lesions such as hydromyelia, tethering of neural structures or diastematomyelia, progressive loss of neurologic function can occur, especially during the growth period. Thus it is important that the neurologic examination be thorough and complete. It must also be carefully recorded and repeated at least annually during the growth period to verify its residual, nonprogressive nature.

As in other musculoskeletal disabilities and diseases, deformity is usually the result of imbalanced muscle power, plus habitually faulty body posture, plus growth. As in arthrogryposis or multiple congenital contractures, when the paralysis is intrauterine at onset, it can be associated with lack of intrauterine mobility added to faulty intrauterine position. The resulting deformity is more fixed because of rigidity, thickening, and lack of elasticity of the soft tissue structures. Deformities developing after birth are more responsive to prevention and treatment and are less likely to recur once appropriate treatment has been rendered. To prevent deformity the attending orthopaedic surgeon must be alert to which particular neurologic lesion is likely to produce which specific faulty habitual body posture and which resulting deformity (Fig. 66-69). Based on the works of Sharrad and of Menelaus the following body postures are determined by the principal lesion.

The infant with cord function down to, but not below, the twelfth thoracic root (Fig. 66-70, *A*) has no muscle activity and no deformity in the lower limb, and the hip does not dislocate. The child assumes the frog-leg position in bed with flexion and abduction of the hips, flexion of the knees, external rotation of the legs, and equinovarus at the ankles. Unless the posture is corrected by positioning, splinting, support, and passive exercises, it becomes fixed.

If the first lumbar root is intact (Fig. 66-70, *B*), the infant assumes the position just described and has weak power in the iliopsoas, sartorius, and tensor fascia femoris.

When the second lumbar root is intact (Fig. 66-70, *C*), the resting position is as above and the iliopsoas, sartorius, rectus femoris, and adductors of the hip are stronger but not normal. There is a trace of power in the quadriceps but none in the hamstrings.

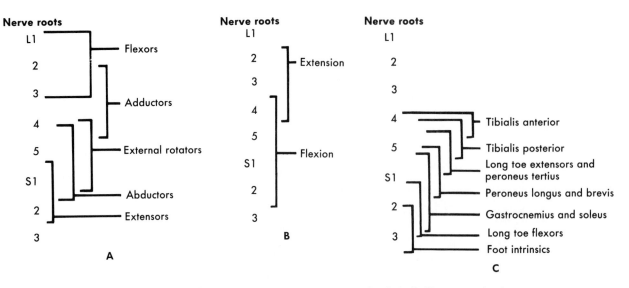

Fig. 66-69. **A,** Nerve roots that innervate motors of hip (an approximation). **B,** Nerve roots that innervate motors of knee (an approximation). **C,** Nerve roots that innervate motors of foot (an approximation). (From Menelaus, M.B.: The orthopaedic management of spina bifida cystica, ed. 2, New York, 1980, Churchill-Livingstone.)

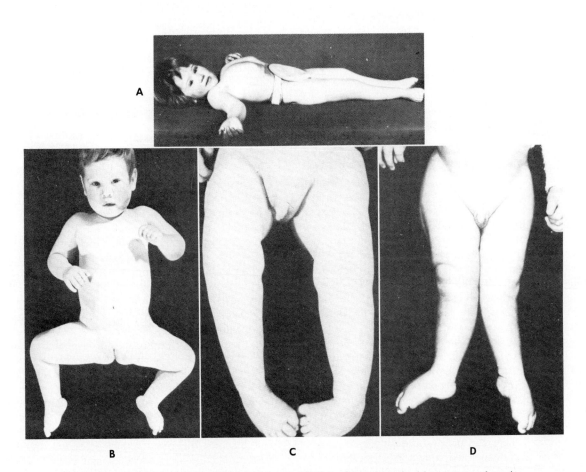

Fig. 66-70. **A,** Paralysis below twelfth thoracic nerve. Position of legs determined by posture and gravity. **B,** Paralysis below first lumbar roots. Flexion and abduction of hips become fixed with growth, posture, and time. **C,** Paralysis below second lumbar root on right (fourth on left). Right hip is abducted and flexed. **D,** Paralysis below third lumbar root. Hips are flexed and abducted, knees are extended, and feet are flail.

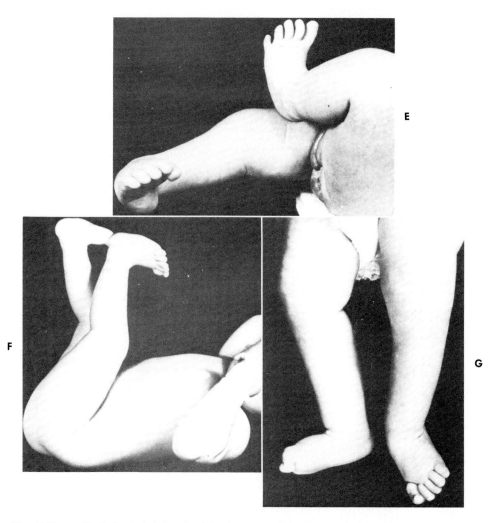

Fig. 66-70, cont'd. E, Paralysis below fourth lumbar root on right. There is flexion, abduction, and external rotation of hip, extension of knee, and equinovarus of foot. **F,** Paralysis below fifth lumbar roots. Hips are flexed, there is some flexion of knees, and feet are in calcaneus position. **G,** Paralysis below first sacral segment on right results in flattening of foot and clawing of toes. Left foot demonstrates peroneal spasticity, a manifestation of an upper motor neuron lesion. (From Menelaus, M.B.: The orthopaedic management of spina bifida cystica, ed. 2, New York, 1980, Churchill-Livingstone.)

If the third lumbar root is intact (Fig. 66-70, *D*), the hip flexors are normal and hip adductors and quadriceps are near normal. Hip subluxation leading to dislocation is frequent.

If the fourth lumbar nerve root is intact (Fig. 66-70, *E*), hip flexion and adduction and quadriceps function are normal. Hip subluxation and dislocation are likely unless appropriately treated. A trace of power is present in the hamstrings, less in the tibialis anterior and posterior muscles. If other conditions are favorable, these patients become community ambulators with below-knee orthoses at the most.

When the fifth lumbar nerve root is intact (Fig. 66-70, *F*), some power is present in the gluteus medius and minimus and more normal power in the hamstrings, tibialis anterior and posterior muscles, and toe extensors. The child lies with the hip and knee flexed and the foot in calcaneovarus position. The peroneals are weak. Ambulation is achieved.

If the first sacral root is intact (Fig. 66-70, *G*), some power is present in the gluteus maximus, gastrocsoleus, and toe flexors, and more power is present in the peroneals. Prognosis for ambulation is excellent.

If the second sacral nerve root is functioning, the chief limb weakness is in the intrinsics of the foot manifested as clawing of the toes. Ambulation is not impaired.

Orthopaedic management

Menelaus points out that the aim of orthopaedic management of the spine and lower limbs (Fig. 66-71) is the establishment and maintenance of a stable posture, and in these patients a stable posture requires some hyperextension of the hips and knees. If this situation exists, then the patient can stand for prolonged periods with relative stability and with one or even both hands free for independent use. Flexion deformity of the hips, on the other hand, is a position of instability, since it imposes flexion at the

Management

Birth	Assessment commences with view to determining realistic aims
↓	Posturing to correct deformity
Head control	Developmental stimulation
Head control	Encourage sitting balance
↓	
Sitting	Encourage hand skills and coordination
Sitting	Encourage upper limb strength and coordination hand function
↓	
Prone mobility	Provide sitting aids
Prone mobility	Continued assessment
↓	Increased social stimulation
Upright stance	Provide standing orthosis
Upright stance	Physiotherapy and bracing appropriate to the neurosegmental level
	Soft tissue releases for hip deformity
	Open tenotomy of psoas and adductors
	Reduction of hip dislocation (in combination with appropriate soft tissue procedure)
	Iliopsoas transfer
	Pemberton osteotomy
Upright mobility	Tendon excision of deforming foot tendons
2½ years	Kyphosis surgery
	Grice procedure
	Correction of fixed flexion at knees
	Quadriceps release
6 years	Chiari procedure
6 years	Correction of the early developing scoliosis (Surgery for recurrent hip and foot deformity)
↓	
10 years	
10 years	Scoliosis and lordosis surgery
	Osteotomy for fixed hip and knee deformity
16 years	Foot stabilization

Fig. 66-71. Orthopaedic management related to age, maturation, and development (From Menelaus, M.B.: The orthopaedic management of spina bifida cystica, ed. 2, New York, 1980, Churchill-Livingstone.)

knees, a tendency to collapse and fall forward, and thus a requirement that one or both upper limbs be constantly used while standing to ensure stability. Since 60% of spina bifida patients have some neurologic abnormalities in the arms with resulting functional impairment, the achievement of a stable standing posture becomes doubly important for them.

In recent years the integrity of the quadriceps muscles has been used by Menelaus and by others as an indicator for the appropriateness of complex reconstructive surgery. If the quadriceps is intact and at full strength, the paralysis is at or below the fourth lumbar nerve root and ambulation should ultimately be possible with below-knee orthoses as a maximum. Thus definitive surgical procedures on the feet and hips should be carried out when indicated. On the other hand, patients with little or no power in the quadriceps do not, as a rule, become functional ambulators. They usually revert to wheelchair locomotion in adoles-

cence, especially if obesity has supervened, as it usually has.

Thus children with strong quadriceps who have weak gluteals or deformity and muscle imbalance of the feet or knees can benefit most from complex surgical procedures. If adequate bilateral quadriceps power is not present, complex and complicated surgical procedures are not indicated; rather, simple soft tissue releases, tenotomies, or tendon excisions will correct deformities and muscle imbalance. At the same time sure and definitive steps should be taken to permanently prevent recurrence of deformity.

Menelaus enumerates additional principles of orthopaedic management: multiple procedures should be done while the patient is under a single anesthetic; plaster immobilization, especially in recumbency, should be minimized because it fosters skeletal demineralization and secondary fractures; the orthopaedic treatment program must be integrated with the total treatment program; the absence of sensation, the increased likelihood of pathologic fracture, and the increased danger of infection secondary to urinary problems must be constantly borne in mind; institutionalization must be kept at a minimum; and finally the sacrifices demanded of the family in terms of time, effort, expense, and separation must be minimized, lest these individual demands become collectively overwhelming.

As previously mentioned, in the first few months of life neurosurgical matters are of first priority, when treatment is indicated. The orthopaedic surgeon should see and examine the patient initially and repeat these examinations as often as is necessary to determine as precisely as possible the extent and degree of the neurologic and musculoskeletal abnormalities. He should institute and supervise a program of positioning and passive exercises aimed at the prevention or correction of deformity. Once the handicap has been defined, a program of orthopaedic treatment must be planned and proposed for integration into the total treatment program, with due regard for the importance of fostering the development of maximum independence in standing and walking, with orthoses as needed, by 2 years of age if possible.

FOOT

EQUINOVARUS DEFORMITY

When foot deformity is present, it is usually talipes equinovarus. Frequently the deformity is severe, rigid, and prone to recurrence, as in arthrogrypotic deformity. It should be treated soon after birth by carefully and adequately padded plaster casts along with subcutaneous or closed tendo calcaneus tenotomy, which can normally be done without anesthesia in these anesthetic feet. The cast should be changed every few days while the patient is in hospital and every 2 or 3 weeks after discharge. Nonoperative treatment rarely produces complete or permanent correction, and posterior or posteromedial release is usually required. The timing of surgical correction must be coordinated with the full treatment program and, when possible, multiple procedures should be done while the patient is under a single anesthetic. As in the treatment of arthrogrypotic deformity, complete correction of the deformity must be obtained at the time of surgery, and the foot must be plantigrade and in slight calcaneus at its termination. If the deformity is not fully corrected by surgery, it will probably not be improved by "corrective casts" in the postoperative period.

Menelaus no longer performs tibialis anterior or posterior tendon transfers in myelomeningocele patients because of poor results. He now excises a portion of these tendons along with the long toe flexor tendons as part of a posteromedial release, even if no active power is known to exist in these muscles. Additionally, as part of the posteromedial release, tendo calcaneus tenotomy, division of deep fascia, capsulectomy of the posteromedial aspects of the ankle, subtalar, and talonavicular joints, and division of posterior fibers of the medial and lateral aspects of the ankle and tibiofibular ligaments should be done, if necessary, for full correction.

If, after the above complete posteromedial release procedure, the deformity is not fully correctable, the cuboid is either decancellated or excised to correct varus, and the talus is either decancellated (Verebelyi-Ogston) or excised for persistent equinus and varus. The aim of treatment is the complete correction of the deformity and the elimination of possible future dynamic deforming factors; this goal must have been accomplished when the surgical procedure is completed.

If the deformity recurs during the growth period, then repetition of the extensive posteromedial release is preferred by Menelaus to talectomy. He now reserves talectomy for grossly and rigidly deformed feet that present late in treatment in children who are still too young for a triple arthrodeses. On the other hand, Trumble, Banta, Raycraft, and Curtis reviewed the results in 17 talectomized feet observed for an average of 7 years and found the hindfoot correction to be good in 15 and poor in 2, while the forefoot correction was good in 8, fair in 1, and poor in 8. The following factors were important to the success of the operation: meticulous and complete excision of the talus, to avoid recurrence of deformity from retained fragments; full and complete correction of deformity at operation, including forefoot varus and supination; posterior displacement of the foot on the tibia; and postoperative plaster immobilization for 6 months followed by protective orthoses until skeletal maturity. We have used talectomy successfully when deformity has recurred after the second posteromedial soft tissue release in children who are still skeletally immature.

Talectomy (astragalectomy). Whitman's talectomy, a stabilizing rather than an arthrodesing operation, has been condemned by many surgeons. Davis noted that to remove the talus weakens the foot, further deforms an already deformed foot, and further shortens an already shortened extremity. Another disadvantage is that painful pseudarthrosis may develop between the tibia and the foot that would require a difficult arthrodesis. Also, although talectomy may be done at an earlier age than a Hoke or Dunn arthrodesis, it is a definitive procedure than cannot be revised as easily or as satisfactorily as can an arthrodesis. The only treatment for unsuccessful talectomy is fusion of the calcaneus to the tibia.

The advantage of talectomy is the stability it provides, especially when combined with tendon transfer. The tendons of available functioning muscles may be transferred

to the tendo calcaneus and calcaneus early and will usually prevent a marked deformity. Thompson studied the procedure from the records of the Hospital for Special Surgery, where it was devised by Whitman, and has listed the causes of complete and partial failure after its use. These were as follows: (1) the tibialis anterior muscle was too strong, (2) an equinus or varus deformity existed before surgery, (3) the gastrocsoleus muscle group was too strong, (4) the patient was too young or too old (under 5 or over 15 years), or (5) errors were made in the operative procedure. Thompson stressed the importance of limiting talectomy to patients between the ages of 5 and 15 years with calcaneus or calcaneovalgus deformities or with flail feet without a tendency toward equinus or varus deformity. Incidentally, Evans has recommended it for calcaneus deformities after an unsuccessful lengthening of the tendo calcaneus in spastic paraplegia or hemiplegia.

Successful talectomy corrects or partially corrects the deformity and reestablishes satisfactory function. By displacing the foot posteriorly it brings the distal end of the tibia over the center of the weight-bearing area, eliminates lateral instability, and produces good contact between the foot and the ground. It also limits motion between the foot and the leg, especially in dorsiflexion; the range of passive motion between dorsiflexion and plantar flexion is usually 10 to 15 degrees and is made smooth by the thick pads of fibrous tissue in the spaces between the tibia and the foot. Usually only 2 to 3 degrees of lateral motion are possible. A permanent ankle brace should never be necessary after talectomy if the hip and thigh muscles are functional.

Holmdahl examined 153 feet after talectomy for various indications. Anatomically the results were good in 18.3%, fairly good in 47%, and poor in 34.7%; functionally the results were good in 32%, fairly good in 56.9%, and poor in 11.7%. Of the group with a varus deformity before talectomy, those with an associated equinus component obtained a clearly better result than those with a calcaneus component; why the results in these instances were different from those observed by other investigators was not explained; the difference did not seem related to the presence of ankylosis (Figs. 66-73 and 66-72, *A* and *B*), which was common in this series (bony ankylosis occurred in 34% and clinical ankylosis in an additional 38.5%). Complete posterior displacement of the foot is very important, according to Holmdahl: if it is not obtained at operation, the result is likely to be poor.

At this clinic talectomy has been used fairly frequently in the treatment of severe talipes equinovarus deformity in arthrogryposis and myelomeningocele. In the paralytic foot, however, it has been almost completely replaced by tendon transfer of available functioning leg muscles. This is supplemented when necessary by careful bracing to prevent a marked deformity of the foot and later by Hoke or Dunn foot stabilization (Fig. 66-72, *C* and *D*); when indicated, the ankle is also fused (p. 1091). This more conservative plan avoids shortening a leg that is frequently already shortened by residual paralysis.

TECHNIQUE (WHITMAN AND THOMPSON). Expose the talus through a long Kocher incision (Fig. 2-7, *A*) and divide the tendons of the peroneus longus and brevis. Incise the calcaneofibular ligament of the ankle and turn the foot me-

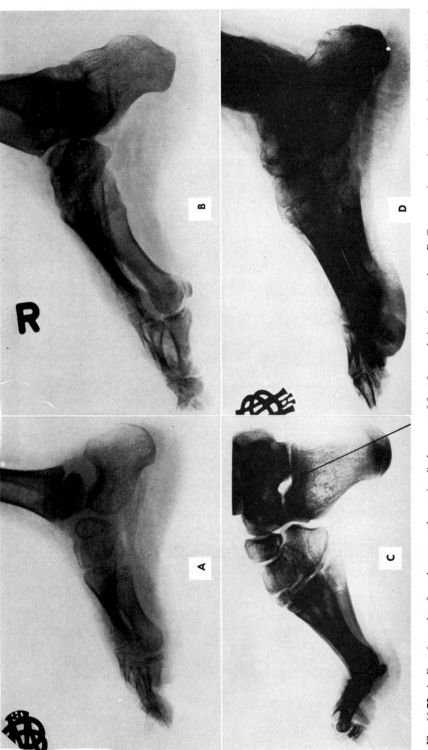

Fig. 66-72. A, Foot 6 months after talectomy and posterior displacement of foot for paralytic calcaneovalgus. **B,** Ten years later calcaneus has fused with tibia, and forefoot is in moderate valgus, causing pain on medial side of foot with weight bearing. Steindler stripping and tarsal reconstruction are indicated; temporarily fixing calcaneus with pin through its long axis will help to maintain its position. **C,** Foot with calcaneocavus deformity in patient 11 years of age. Line indicates correct position of pin in calcaneus. **D,** Same foot as shown in **C** after Hoke arthrodesis and tendon transfer; results are better than after talectomy.

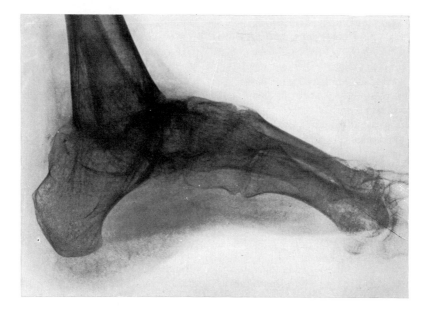

Fig. 66-73. Talectomy followed by osseous ankylosis of tibia to calcaneus. Disability was no greater than that after ankle fusion.

dially to permit easy delivery of the talus. Excise the talus, preferably in one piece; allow no fragments to remain. Strip the ligaments from both malleoli and from the distal 1.3 cm of the tibial metaphysis so that the foot may be easily displaced posteriorly. Remove the articular cartilage from both malleoli, reshape their deep surfaces to fit the calcaneus, and denude small areas of the medial and lateral surfaces of the extreme anterior part of the calcaneus. After the foot is displaced posteriorly, the medial malleolus should lie against the navicular and the lateral malleolus against the calcaneocuboid joint. To place the foot in this position rotate it externally on the leg; often 30 or 40 degrees of rotation are necessary, since the foot must be aligned with the ankle mortise rather than with the patella. Thus the new transverse axis will extend between the malleoli at a right angle to the long axis of the foot. When the tibialis anterior is strong, either release it by excising a long segment of its tendon or transfer it to some other position. Now suture the peroneal tendons. Evans and Steindler mentioned transferring these tendons to the tendo calcaneus when their muscles are active; Thompson, however, found that when any power remains in the triceps surae or in the tibialis anterior or posterior muscles, a varus or an equinus deformity will almost surely occur.

AFTERTREATMENT. A long leg cast is applied, with the knee in flexion and with the foot displaced well posteriorly and in marked equinus and valgus position. Any attempt to correct external rotation of the foot will produce a varus deformity. At 2 or 3 weeks the cast is changed, the position of the foot is observed, and if necessary minor changes in position are made. A snug short leg cast is applied, with the foot still in equinus, slight valgus, and external rotation. A few weeks later a rubber heel is applied to the cast, and weight bearing is allowed. Twelve weeks after the operation the cast is removed, and a shoe is fitted. The heel of the shoe is raised 2.5 to 4 cm and a

lateral wedge is applied if there has been or is the slightest tendency toward varus deformity. When necessary, a short double bar brace with a calcaneus ankle stop and an outside T-strap to hold the foot in valgus position is used temporarily. The patient is forbidden to walk barefoot for at least a year after surgery. If the patient cannot compensate for the external rotation of the foot by internal rotation of the entire extremity, a tibial derotation osteotomy may be done later.

• • •

The Verebelyi-Ogston procedure, described by Freeman in 1974, is mentioned here for completeness, since we have had no experience with it. It is recommended for severe or recurrent equinovarus in the infant under 2 or 3 years of age. Through an incision over the neck of the talus, as much as possible of its cancellous contents is curetted away, and the lateral wall of the hollow cartilaginous shell is incised to facilitate its collapse. Through a short incision over the cuboid, its cancellous contents are curetted away, and the foot is manipulated into calcaneus and valgus, in so doing, crushing the talus and cuboid bones.

The Dwyer osteotomy of the calcaneus (p. 2942) has proved successful in our hands in moderate deformity for patients between 5 and 10 years of age. If significant cavus is also present, it should be accompanied by a plantar release (p. 2941). Severe forefoot equinus frequently requires frontal plane osteotomy of the affected metatarsals at their bases, or an osteotomy through the midtarsal area with excision of a dorsal wedge and depression of the distal fragment.

Triple arthrodesis (p. 2935) remains the best and most definitive corrective procedure in the feet of myelomeningocele patients in our experience. When possible, the operation should be deferred until about 11 years of age, although Menelaus prefers age 14. If done earlier, the foot, which is usually already shortened in this condition, is likely to be further shortened. After the appropriate joints have been exposed by capsulectomy, wedges of bone are excised as required to completely correct the deformity, and the deforming tendons are tenotomized. The foot is immobilized in a position of slight calcaneovalgus until solid bony union has occurred.

Calcaneovalgus deformity. If the tibialis anterior is functioning at a "good" or normal level of power, it can be detached, transferred posteriorly through the interosseus membrane, and attached to the calcaneus through a vertical hole drilled immediately anterior and lateral to the tendo calcaneus insertion. This insertion should be reinforced by suturing it to the adjacent tendo calcaneus at its insertion. If the tibialis anterior tendon is only fair or poor in power, its transfer should be supplemented by tenodesing the tendo calcaneus to the tibia (Banta, Sutherland, and Wyatt) or to the fibula (Westin) if there is valgus at the ankle.

Grice subtalar fusion (p. 2963) can be performed between 4 and 10 years of age, after all deforming muscle imbalance has been corrected by tenotomy or tendon transfer. Because of the likelihood of fracture, tibial bone is no longer used as a source for the graft. Rather, a graft is removed from the fibula or the ilium, or banked bone is used to block the subtalar joint.

Menelaus has described a form of triple arthrodesis that he prefers for valgus deformity (Fig. 66-74) in which a precisely measured rectangle of bone is removed from the anterolateral aspect of the midtarsal joint at the junction of the calcaneus, the cuboid, the navicular, and the talus. A rectangle of cortical bone of similar size is then removed from the upper tibia and countersunk into the surgical defect thus prepared. The subtalar joint is also "harried" and cancellous bone is packed into it. The advantages claimed for the procedure are (1) no loss of length of the foot, (2) increased stability of the foot, and (3) a high rate of healing. We have no experience with this procedure, being satisfied with our results following triple arthrodesis.

The vertical talus or convex pes valgus deformity associated with myelomeningocele requires more extensive anterolateral and posterior releases through anterolateral and posteromedial surgical approaches. The operation includes lengthening of the peroneals, toe extensors, and tibialis anterior, as well as the tendo calcaneus and posterior capsule; open reduction of the joints between the calcaneus, talus, navicular, and cuboid; and internal fixation under direct

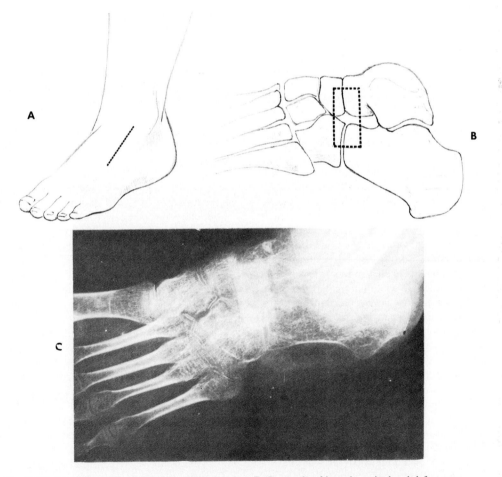

Fig. 66-74. Menelaus triple arthrodesis. **A,** Skin incision. **B,** Rectangle of bone is excised and defect accurately filled with bone graft after "harrying" subtalar joint. **C,** Oblique roentgenogram of foot on cast removal 3 months after operation. (From Menelaus, M.B.: The orthopaedic management of spina bifida cystica, ed. 2, New York, 1980, Churchill-Livingstone.)

vision using small pins placed as follows: one is drilled in a retrograde direction through the first metatarsal, medial cuneiform, and navicular and into the talus; and the second is drilled forward through the calcaneus and into the cuboid while the joint is held in a reduced position. A Grice fusion may be done at the same time. The placement of the two pins in precisely this manner is necessary to control both inversion and eversion of the subtalar joint, and abduction-adduction and pronation-supination of the midtarsal joint. Once the foot is thus stabilized, the position of the ankle can be controlled by plaster immobilization. The pins are left in place for 8 weeks, and plaster immobilization is continued at least 12 weeks, followed by orthoses as indicated. The position of the bones must always be verified by two-plane roentgenograms before the wounds are closed, and if their position is not satisfactory, the pins must be removed and the bones openly repositioned and fixed in satisfactory position as finally demonstrated by intraoperative roentgenograms.

KNEE

The most common knee deformities seen in myelomeningocele are flexion or extension, usually attributable to muscle imbalance. Valgus, varus, and rotational deformities occur most often as a result of faulty intrauterine position, fracture, or epiphyseal separation, whether recognized or not. Except in the mildest deformities, conservative measures usually do not fully correct the problem, and surgery is indicated if the deformity is severe or disabling. As mentioned before, when possible, multiple procedures should be done at the same time to minimize surgical settings. When necessary, knee surgery is usually done between 2 and 5 years of age.

Because of its influence on posture while standing or walking, full extension of the knee is highly desirable, but unless the knees can flex through at least 20 degrees arising is difficult, especially from a low seat, and the legs protrude when the child is seated. When severe and unresponsive to conservative measures, an extension contracture can be corrected by division of the vastus intermedius, V-Y lengthening of the rectus after it has been separated from the vastus medialis and lateralis, and reattachment to the rectus in its lengthened position. If necessary, the joint capsule can be divided by vertical parapatellar incisions continuous with those that detached the vastus medialis and lateralis from the rectus femoris.

Flexion is the most common deformity found at the knee in myelomeningocele patients, and it is associated with muscle imbalance with or without an element of spasticity in the flexor muscles. When flexion is 20 degrees or less at birth, correction by nonsurgical treatment can be expected, such as passive stretching, gentle manipulation, and splinting in the corrected position. More severe deformities frequently respond to frequent gentle manipulations and plaster cast changes. If the deformity is greater than 20 degrees and unresponsive to nonoperative methods, we favor lengthening the biceps and semimembranosus tendons and proximal transfer of the tendons of the gracilis and semitendinosus to the posterior surface of the intermuscular septum proximal and posterior to the adductor longus insertion. If the knee cannot

easily be placed at 10 degrees of recurvatum at surgery, posterior capsulotomy is indicated. Again, full correction permitted by neurovascular structures must be obtained at surgery. Recurvatum osteotomy of the femur is a useful procedure at or following skeletal maturity. If recurvatum osteotomy is done during the growth period, the deformity promptly recurs, as a rule.

HIP

According to Menelaus the aims of treatment of hip deformity and disability are to treat dislocation and deformity vigorously only in those children who will thrive and benefit significantly from such treatment, to perform only a single operation on each hip, and to minimize postoperative immobilization. This means that major surgery is appropriate only for those children who have strong power in their quadriceps muscles bilaterally because, under favorable conditions, they can expect to become community ambulators with or without below-knee orthoses. Children who do not have strong bilateral quadriceps power, on the other hand, rarely remain community ambulators; thus their requirements are permanent correction of the hip flexion and adduction deformity, and a level pelvis and straight spine. Dislocations and subluxations of the hip are not in themselves severely disabling to these patients; rather it is the fixed progressive flexion deformity that renders them incapable of ambulation, and this is caused by strong hip flexors and adductors and weak abductors and extensors. In these patients the power of the iliopsoas should be removed permanently or the tendon should be transferred, and the adductors must be either radically lengthened or transferred posteriorly.

Sharrard's posterolateral transfer of the iliopsoas (p. 2994) for instability of the hip in myelomeningocele was widely accepted at first, but in recent years enthusiasm for the procedure has waned somewhat. Although this transfer is distinctly valuable in removing a strong deforming element of the hip deformity, the loss of active hip flexion combined with the lack of active hip abduction or extension has caused some to question its value. Drummond, Moreau, and Cruess reviewed 17 posterior iliopsoas transfers and found that by itself the procedure did not necessarily achieve hip stability, improve walking ability, or improve power of the hip in extension. On the other hand, Benton, Salvati, and Root reported 31 hips in 17 patients who had undergone adductor transfer to the ischium along with Sharrard's iliopsoas transfer, with satisfactory results in correcting flexion-adduction deformity, increasing the range of abduction, and adding stability to the hips. Regarding motor power in abduction and extension, 20 were improved and the others retained about the same power.

Bunch and Hakala examined 32 hips in 17 children with an L4-level deficit 4 to 14 years after Sharrard's transfer. Of the transfers, 29 were active, 21 had abduction, and 15 had active extension against gravity. The results were more consistent in the 10 patients who had varus osteotomy combined with the transfer.

Parker and Walker reviewed 72 posterior iliopsoas transfers performed in 44 children 1 to 8 years after operation. Of the 44 children 20 had good, 5 fair, and 19 poor results. Twelve hips had definitely increased abduction and extension power, and all had reduced flexion power. They recommend the procedure be done before 2 years of age. After that time it should only be done in children with activity in the L3 or L4 segment of the lumbar cord.

In 1972 Carroll and Sharrard reviewed 53 children with myelomeningocele 5 to 10 years after hip surgery. In 58 hips of 33 children a posterior iliopsoas transfer had been performed. At review 34 hips were stable, 23 were unstable, and 1 was fused. These authors believed it important not only to restore muscle balance but also to correct, at the same time, associated adaptive changes such as maldirected acetabulum, valgus femoral neck, or lax capsule.

Dias and Hill, on the other hand, found iliopsoas transfer not necessary to achieve stable reduction and to prevent dislocation in hip subluxations in meningomyelocele. They were able to achieve stability by varus trochanteric osteotomy (p. 2729). They recommended varus positioning at 100 to 110 degrees in patients under 4 year of age, or else remodeling will occur with growth. If the acetabulum is dysplastic and its index is above 30 degrees, Chiari's acetabular reconstruction (p. 2748) is indicated.

Wissinger, Turner, and Donaldson compared the results of nonsurgical treatment of a group of 200 children with the results of Sharrard's transfer in 54 neurogenically dislocated hips in 33 children. They found that when properly performed the muscle transfer was capable of balancing forces about the hip and maintaining reduction. Further, while the balanced hip did not always improve patient function, the untreated, unbalanced hip always decreased function. All fixed deformity about the hip must be eliminated before or at the time of the transfer.

Yngve and Lindseth reviewed the results of muscle transfers on 35 hips and measured such results using radiographic indices. The operations were intended to augment the abductor power, to weaken the adductor power, or both. They found best results when posterior adductor transfer was accompanied by abductor augmentation by either iliopsoas or external abdominal oblique transfer. Because iliopsoas transfer produces weakness of active hip flexion and the external oblique transfer does not, they preferred the latter. The intact iliopsoas did not cause troublesome flexion deformity in this study. They recommend external olique transfer, especially in patients with unilateral hip subluxation before dislocation occurs, and, if pelvic obliquity is present, its cause must be identified and corrected before or at the time the transfer is done.

Menelaus recommends that, as a rule, deformity and dislocation of the hip be corrected between 18 and 24 months of age, and he usually uses one or more of the following procedures:

1. Radical hip release to correct the flexion, abduction, and external rotation as seen in children whose distal neurologic function ends with the first lumbar nerve root. He uses a vertical 8 cm incision centered over the tip of the greater trochanter; divides the short external rotators and posterior capsule while the hip is internally rotated; divides the fascia replacing the gluteus muscles, the tensor fasciae latae, and the sartorius muscles, and the rectus femoris and psoas tendons; and reefs the anterior capsule. The procedure is done bilaterally with the patient under the same anesthetic, and nursing care is provided with the child on a frame with the hips adducted and extended for 6 weeks.

2. Division of the adductors and the iliopsoas with excision of part of the psoas to prevent its reattachment. This operation is intended to prevent progressive flexion deformity and dislocation of the hip in children with high lumbar lesions, or in others with poor prognosis for ambulation, and is done before flexion deformity becomes severe or fixed. An adductor approach is used. The adductors are divided using electrocautery until at least 60 degrees of hip abduction is obtained. Through the same incision the lesser trochanter is identified and 1 cm of the psoas tendon is excised. The hip is immobilized in an abduction type of walking cast for 6 weeks.

3. Anterior hip release to correct flexion deformity and to prevent its recurrence. This is done on children with high lumbar lesions who have developed fixed flexion deformity. The iliac apophysis is split longitudinally, and the two halves are allowed to retract, one medially and the other laterally. The contracted anterior structures, including the capsule, are divided as necessary and 1 cm of psoas tendon is excised. The protuberant triangle of anterior iliac wing is excised, and the wound is closed over suction drainage. The operation is reminiscent of the Campbell transfer of the crest of the ilium (p. 2987).

4. Division of the adductors and psoas transfer. This is now recommended only for children who are otherwise thriving and who have function down to and including the fourth or fifth lumbar level as manifested by strong quadriceps, hip flexors, and adductor muscles. Menelaus has modified the procedure by using two incisions. The first, vertical over the adductors, allows release of the adductors as described above and identification and then division of the lesser trochanter, which is freed and mobilized upward to the brim of the pelvis. The second incision parallels the iliac crest and is 1 cm distal to it. The iliac crest is detached and retracted medially, and the psoas sheath is opened; the psoas tendon and lesser trochanter are then passed proximally into the upper operative area, and the psoas tendon is transferred according to Sharrard's technique.

5. Acetabuloplasty. This is usually reserved for children with neurologic function, including lumbar four or five roots and acetabular dysplasia. If the acetabulum is long and shallow, it can be deepened by Pemterton's osteotomy (p. 2738), using a segment of the ilium or rib as a graft. Usually, however, the acetabulum is actually deficient rather than elongated, and Chiari's osteotomy is required for its correction.

Canale, Hammond, Cotler, and Snedden reported satisfactory results in 19 of 21 hips that underwent Chiari's pelvic displacement osteotomy for chronic hip dislocation at an average age of 8¾ years. Gains were measured in ease of bracing, reduced pelvic obliquity, and gait pattern. They recommended the procedure in either unilateral or bilateral subluxation in children 4 years or older with deficient acetabulum (see Fig. 62-41). Postoperative immobilization in a spica cast is continued for 3 weeks if internal fixation was used and for 6 weeks if no internal fixation was used.

Several authors have pointed out that bilateral hip dislocation by itself has little or no influence on ambulation in myelomeningocele patients despite its undesirable appearance on roentgenograms. Thus we have previously recommended that such a condition be ignored in the child older than 5 years of age or in the child with a neurologic level of function at L3 or above. Unilateral dislocation of the hip should be treated more energetically, since lower limb shortening, pelvic obliquity, and scoliosis may result and thus interfere significantly with standing or sitting ability. A dislocated hip in the presence of fixed pelvic obliquity occurs on the ''high side'' of the pelvis and cannot be successfully treated without correction of the pelvic obliquity, whether its cause is an abduction deformity of the opposite hip on the ''low side'' or a fixed lumbosacral scoliotic curve of suprapelvic causation.

The first principles of treatment for paralytic dislocation of the hip are correction of fixed deformity, establishment of balanced motor power, and the prevention of recurrence of the deformity. We have discussed procedures to correct hip deformity, and we still prefer Sharrard's transfer (mentioned above). To correct the adaptive skeletal changes we prefer Chiari's pelvic osteotomy (p. 2748). Valgus of the femoral neck and femoral anteversion do not usually require correction if preceded by pelvic osteotomy. If subluxation or dislocation recurs after Chiari's osteotomy, a varus derotational osteotomy of the femur (p. 2729) can be done, using secure internal fixation.

Arthrogryposis Multiplex Congenita— Multiple Congenital Contractures

Arthrogryposis multiplex congenita (AMC), or multiple congenital contractures (MCC), is a nonprogressive syndrome characterized by (1) deformed and rigid joints, (2) atrophy or absence of muscles or muscle groups, (3) cylindric, fusiform, or cone-shaped involved extremities with diminished skin creases and subcutaneous tissue, (4) contracture and densification of joint capsular and periarticular tissues, (5) dislocation of joints, especially of the hip and knee, and (6) intact sensation and mentality. It was originally described by Otto in 1841, and for many years the condition was considered to be a discrete clinical entity or diagnosis. In recent years greater awareness and further studies have revealed that more than 150 specific entities can be associated with what has been called AMC in the past. Thus, as suggested by Swinyard and Bleck multiple congenital contractures (MCC) is a more appropriate name for the condition and the one we will subsequently use in this book.

ETIOLOGY

Several factors contribute to the cause of MCC. The deformities appear to be the result of intrauterine immobilization of joints at various stages of their development because of neurogenic, myogenic, skeletal, or environmental factors. The myopathic aspect, accounting for 10% or less of cases, appears to be transmitted as an autosomal recessive characteristic. Most cases are neurogenic in origin and

result from a congenital or acquired defect in the organization or the number of anterior horn cells, roots, peripheral nerves, or motor end plates, producing muscular weakness and resultant joint immobility at critical stages of intrauterine development. Some of the mechanical factors that can limit intrauterine movement are structural abnormalities of the uterus, oligohydramnios, amniotic bands, and simultaneous multiple pregnancies.

Wynne-Davies, Williams, and O'Connor studied 132 patients from the United Kingdom, Australia, and the United States and concluded that MCC is a nongenetic disease of early pregnancy associated with a variety of unfavorable intrauterine factors, possibly including a viral environmental agent. The maternal age was found to be higher and the gestational period tended to be abnormal in that 14% of gestations were less than 38 weeks and 25% were 42 weeks or more. There was an excess of breech presentations (36.9%) and a high incidence of oligohydramnios (25.7%). Bleeding during the first trimester was noted in 18.5% (normal 7%), and an unusually high incidence of other adverse factors or complications was reported as occurring during the pregnancies. The mothers almost always noted diminished fetal movements compared with previous normal pregnancies.

CLINICAL MANIFESTATIONS

Brown, Robson, and Sharrard carefully studied a group of 16 patients with MCC to learn whether neurosegmental levels of involvement could be found corresponding to typical and consistent patterns of manifestations. They identified two patterns of upper extremity involvement and six patterns of lower extremity involvement, each corresponding to a specific level of central nervous system involvement (Table 66-1). The segmental innervation charts are shown in Fig. 66-75, and the patterns of deformity are shown in Figs. 66-76 and 66-77. Although evidence currently available indicates that in most instances the deformities present at birth were paralytic in nature and thus required surgical procedures to balance muscle activity, it must be remembered that the associated contracture and thickening of capsular and periarticular tissues render the deformities extremely difficult to correct and quite prone to recur, especially in the presence of unbalanced muscle power, habitually faulty posture, and growth.

Usually the deformities are symmetric and are more severe distally. The most common topographic involvement is quadriplegic (all four extremities), followed by bimelic involvement of the lower extremities. Bimelic involvement confined to the upper extremities is quite rare, and the trunk is frequently spared, although scoliosis is found in about 20% of patients. Webbing of the skin and soft tissues at the concave aspect of the deformity is sometimes seen, especially at the knee. When present, webbing adds another difficult dimension to treatment because the contained nerves and vessels are structurally shortened and refractory to lengthening by stretching.

DIAGNOSIS

As indicated previously, at least 150 specific clinical entities are characterized by MCC; thus an accurate diagnosis is necessary for proper understanding of the causative

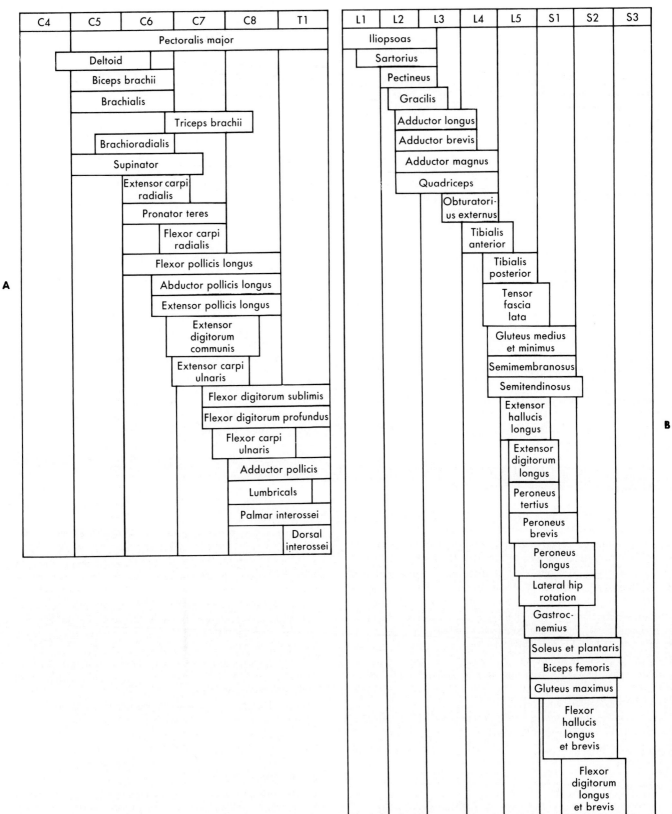

Fig. 66-75. A, Segmental innervation of upper limb muscles. **B,** Segmental innervation of lower limb muscles. (**A** modified from Carpenter, M.B.: Human neuroanatomy, ed. 7, Baltimore, 1976, Williams & Wilkins; and Hoppenfeld, S.: Orthopaedic neurology: a diagnostic guide to neurological levels, Philadelphia, 1977, J.B. Lippincott, Co. **B** modified from Sharrad, W.J.W.: Br. J. Surg. **44:**471, 1957.)

pathologic process and its natural history. Only then can the treating physician develop and implement a therapeutic program reasonably expected to decrease as much as possible the physical handicap and increase as much as possible the patient's function and independence. As in other neuromuscular disabilities, an accurate diagnosis requires a careful medical history, physical examination, and appropriate laboratory procedures.

The medical history should include details of the family history, the mother's reproductive history, and a careful and detailed search for unfavorable intrauterine factors during the specific pregnancy in question, in line with the observations by Wynne-Davies et al. previously mentioned.

In addition to a detailed tabulation and description of the various deformities observed, a careful neurologic exami-

Table 66-1. Deformities found in 11 patients with arthrogryposis multiplex congenita

Pattern of deformity	Level	Number of limbs affected
Upper limb		
Type I: adduction and/or medial rotation of shoulder, extension of elbow, pronation of forearm, flexion and ulnar deviation of wrist. (In addition, 2 had weak intrinsic muscles of the hand, indicating T1 involvement.)	C5, C6	13
Type II: adduction and/or medial rotation of shoulder, flexion deformity of elbow, flexion and ulnar deviation of wrist. (In addition, 2 had weak intrinsic muscles indicating T1 involvement.)	Partial C5, C6, partial C7	3
Lower limb		
Type III: flexion and adduction of hip (with dislocation in five limbs), extension of knee, equinovarus of foot. (In addition, 2 had weak intrinsic muscles indicating S3 involvement.)	L4, L5, S1	11
Type IV: flexion of knee, equinovarus of foot.	L3, L4, partial L5	1
Type V: flexion and abduction of hip, flexion of knee, equinovarus of foot.	L3, L4, patchy S1-2	2
Type VI: flexion of hip, extension of knee with valgus, equinus of foot.	L4, L5	2
Type VII: equinus of foot.	L4	2
Type VIII: equinovarus of foot, weak intrinsic muscles of foot.	L4, patchy L5, S3	1

From Brown, L.M., Robson, M.J.. and Sharrard, W.J.W.: J. Bone Joint Surg. **62-B**:4, 1980.

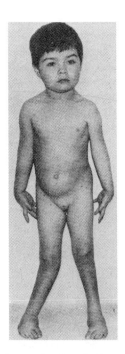

Fig. 66-76. Patient with neurogenic arthrogryposis at 4 years of age. (From Brown, L.M., Robson, M.J., and Sharrard, W.J.W.: J. Bone Joint Surg. **62-B**:291, 1980.)

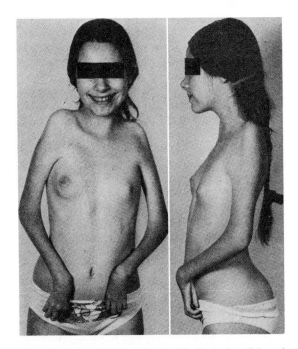

Fig. 66-77. Type II deformity. There is adduction and medial rotation of shoulders, flexion deformity of elbows, flexion and ulnar deviation of wrists, and weak intrinsic muscles of hands. (From Brown, L.M., Robson, M.J., and Sharrard, W.J.W.: J. Bone Joint Surg. **62-B**:291, 1980.)

nation is necessary, especially evaluating sensation, deep tendon reflexes, presence or absence of postural reflexes, and presence and degree of muscle power in the affected extremities. Although it is impossible to quantitate accurately the power in the affected extremities of the infant, with careful observation and repeated testing it is usually possible to state whether active muscular contraction is or is not present in the various motor groups.

The most important laboratory procedure is muscle biopsy, for it permits accurate differentiation between neurogenic and myogenic processes. Thompson and Bilenker prefer to perform the muscle biopsy at 3 or 4 months of age, if the infant's health permits, unless corrective surgery is anticipated shortly thereafter, in which case biopsy is performed at the time of the scheduled surgery. The muscle undergoing biopsy should be involved in the process but still functional. The quadriceps or deltoid is favored, although any skeletal muscle can be used, and biopsies are also taken of muscles encountered in the operative field for confirmation of the diagnosis.

In performing the biopsy on the preferred quadriceps muscle, the Thompson and Bilenker technique calls for a bloodless field controlled with a tourniquet and exposure of the middle third of the vastus medialis muscle where the small motor nerve branches from the femoral nerve cross its muscle fibers. The site chosen for biopsy is where these nerve fibers enter the muscle; muscle clamps are used to maintain length of the fibers. The specimen is taken along the long axis of the fibers with the nerve centrally located and the motor end plate included. The specimen is studied by the neuropathologist by light microscopy as well as histochemical and ultrastructural analysis.

Roentgenographic examination is indicated to assess the integrity of the skeletal system, especially the presence or absence of scoliosis, spinal rachischisis, dislocated hips or knees, or other skeletal malformations.

Electrophysiologic studies, including electromyographic and nerve conduction studies, are sometimes helpful in distinguishing between neurogenic or myogenic lesions, but they seldom permit a precise diagnosis.

Chromosome analysis is usually chiefly indicated in infants with extensive central nervous system involvement or with multisystem defects.

TREATMENT

As early as possible the diagnosis should be accurately established, the extent and degree of the various contractures recorded, and a careful search made to determine the presence and extent of any associated disabilities.

Palmer, McEwan, Bowen, and Palmer have devised a program of passive stretching exercises for each contracted joint to be carried out by the parents daily at four 30-minute sessions followed by serial splinting with individually fashioned thermoplastic splints that are frequently readjusted. The exercise program is regularly reviewed in detail by both the physical therapist and the orthopaedic surgeon. Significant gains in extremity function are claimed, and thus the need for corrective surgical procedures in young affected children has been diminished under this protocol. Most orthopaedic surgeons, however, have found that any improvement occurring after a physical therapy program is transient at best, and the deformity usually recurs all too promptly.

Orthopaedic treatment

Drummond, Sellers, and Cruess, as well as Williams, have enumerated some principles of orthopaedic management for patients with MCC, including the following:

1. Muscle balance should be established, if functioning muscles (motors) are available for transfer.
2. Recurrence of deformity is the rule because the dense, inelastic soft tissues about the joints do not properly elongate with growth.
3. Tenotomies should be accompanied by capsulotomy and capsulectomy on the concave side of the joint, followed by prolonged plaster and then orthotic support to prevent, or at least delay, recurrence of deformity.
4. Maximum safely obtainable correction should be achieved at the time of surgery. The use of "wedging" or "corrective" casts after surgery is usually of little additional benefit.
5. Osteotomies to correct deformity or transfer the range of motion to a more useful arc are beneficial, but only at or near skeletal maturity, or the deformity will promptly recur with growth.

FOOT AND ANKLE

The foot deformity in MCC is rigid and usually is either in the equinovarus– or planovalgus–vertical talus position. The realistic goal of treatment cannot be a normal foot. Rather, the surgeon and the patient must be satisfied with the conversion of a rigid deformed foot into a rigid plantigrade foot.

Factors essential for ambulation in severe MCC were studied in 36 affected patients by Hoffer, Swank, Eastman, Clark, and Tietge at Rancho los Amigo Rehabilitation Center. Functional ambulation in these patients required (1) hip extension range and power or ability to use crutches as a substitute for that power, (2) knee extension range and power or knee-ankle-foot orthosis as a substitute for that power, and (3) plantigrade feet. Progressive spinal deformity was the most common cause of decreased ambulatory ability once ambulation was achieved. Thus these authors contend that rational goals for ambulation should include evaluation of these factors; patients not capable of achieving these criteria should have their treatment emphasis placed on sitting (straight spine, hip flexion, and knee flexion) plus activities of daily living.

If the planovalgus foot is plantigrade, it is usually satisfactory without treatment. If not, surgical correction is indicated, usually between 3 and 6 months of age. Multiple extensive capsulectomies are required, along with generous lengthening of contracted tendons, the corrected position being maintained by internal fixation using Kirschner wires for 6 or 8 weeks. Plaster immobilization in the corrected position is continued for at least 3 months, followed by use of orthoses for prolonged periods until the tendency of the deformity to recur is past. Surgical treatment by open reduction is difficult at best, and the results leave much to be desired.

The most common foot deformity is equinovarus. The

foot is rigid, most difficult to correct, and relentless in its tendency to recur.

Initially, it should be treated by carefully padded, snugly applied plaster casts, changed at intervals of 4 to 7 days, depending on the infant's general health and rate of growth. An attempt should be made to correct first the forefoot adduction and heel varus, while maintaining slight pressure against the equinus contracture. As the forefoot and heel deformities gradually correct, attention is directed to the equinus. While complete correction by plaster casts is rare, the skin and subcutaneous tissue contractures are improved and corrective surgery is made easier by a period of 3 or 4 months of passive stretching by this technique.

When necessary, corrective surgery should be performed between the ages of 6 and 12 months, depending on the infant's physical condition and treatment priorities. Simple tendon lengthenings, adequate in other neuromotor deformities, are inadequate in MCC and are destined to early and complete failure.

Posteromedial release should include resection of a 1 cm segment of both the gastrosoleus and the tibialis posterior tendons, generous lengthening of all other tendons posterior to the medial malleolus, posterior capsulectomy of the ankle and subtalar joints, and capsulectomy of the talocalcaneal, talonavicular, and calcaneocuboid joints. The maximum correction permitted by the neurovascular structures should be obtained at surgery and maintained by Kirschner wires.

Correction of forefoot adduction and heel inversion can be maintained by Kirschner wires inserted in the axis of the first and of the fifth metatarsals, transfixing the talonavicular and calcaneocuboid joints. Dorsiflexion can be maintained by a similar wire inserted vertically through the sole of the foot, the calcaneus, and the talus and into the tibia. Satisfactory position of the foot and wires must be demonstrated by intraoperative roentgenograms before wound closure and long leg cast application. The wires are left in place at least 6 and usually 8 weeks. Plaster cast immobilization is continued for a total of 3 to 4 months as a minimum, followed by orthoses during periods of sleep.

If the deformity recurs in a young child or is severe and cannot be corrected by posterior and medial soft tissue re-

leases, talectomy is indicated (p. 3029); the tendency to recurrence is unrelenting. Drummond and Cruess obtained permanent and lasting hindfoot correction in 5 of 11 primary talectomies, and 1 other foot was improved by revision talectomy. A common cause of recurrence is retention and subsequent growth of a fragment of the talus; thus adequate surgical exposure and meticulous removal of the entire talus are necessary, along with capsulectomy, soft tissue correction, and internal fixation as previously described. Guidera and Drennan reported 14 talectomies in 7 patients; all eventually obtained good results. Green, Fixsen, and Lloyd-Roberts obtained satisfactory results in 24 (71%) of 34 feet treated by talectomy for equinovarus deformity. Relapse of deformity was attributable to either a retained fragment of talus or an inadequate tendo calcaneus release. Another common problem is allowing the calcaneus to displace forward under the tibia, resulting in a less prominent heel, fixed in equinus.

Likewise Hsu, Jeffray, and Leong have reported satisfactory results in 9 of 15 feet treated by talectomy, 7 of which developed spontaneous tibiocalcaneal fusion.

Gross has recently described the technique of cancellectomy of the talus and cuboid, which rendered them hollow cartilaginous shells, followed by manipulation of the foot into the desired position of correction by crushing the treated bones. He credits the original description of the procedure to Verebelyi in 1879; Ogston in 1902 and Kopits in 1974 reported its use in feet deformed by myelomeningocele. The procedure is performed by creating a window in the dorsal cortex of the cuboid and in the lateral cortex of the neck and body of the talus. All cancellous bone is carefully curetted away and the deformity is corrected by manual manipulation. We have had no experience with this procedure (Fig. 66-78).

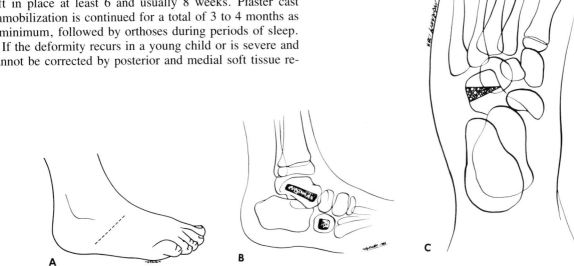

Fig. 66-78. Cancellectomy of talus and cuboid. **A,** Dorsolateral oblique skin incision over sinus tarsi for exposure of talus and cuboid. **B,** Windows in cartilaginous shells of talus and cuboid to expose cancellous bone. **C,** If necessary, closing wedge excision may be performed on cartilaginous shell and ossific nucleus of cuboid to facilitate collapse and correction. (**A** from Gross, R.H.: Clin. Orthop. **194:**99, 1985. **B** and **C** from Spires, T.D., Gross, R.H., Low, W., and Berringer, W.: J. Pediatr. Orthop. **4:**706, 1984.)

Spontaneous fusion of the calcaneus to the tibia is a frequent occurrence following talectomy, and recurrent deformity in this instance can be corrected by osteotomy of the fusion mass.

The most dependable method of correction of equinovarus in the MCC foot is triple arthrodesis. Again, capsulectomy and soft tissue correction are required, and since elongation of the short or contracted side of the deformity is usually only partially successful, wedge resection through the midtarsal or subtalar joint is frequently necessary to correct the adaptive skeletal deformities that have occurred. Likewise, excision of the navicular is sometimes required. Again, intraoperative roentgenograms should demonstrate the correction; if necessary it should be maintained by internal fixation left in place for 6 weeks. External fixation by plaster casts in the corrected position should be maintained until solid bony union occurs, usually after 3 months. As a rule, triple arthrodesis should be deferred until skeletal maturity for two reasons: (1) to prevent foot shortening from surgically inhibited growth and (2) to prevent recurrence of deformity in the growing foot. In some feet that display relentless recurrence of deformity despite surgery, we have resorted to triple arthrodesis in younger children, even as young as 6 years of age, with a satisfactory plantigrade, although shortened, foot.

KNEE

In MCC, knee deformity is most frequently in flexion, although extension deformity is not unusual. The *flexed* knee is caused by contracture of the hamstrings and posterior knee capsule, and when popliteal webbing is present, some neurovascular shortening and posterior displacement are also present. It is treated by serial splinting or casting in progressive degrees of extension changed at weekly intervals, being careful to avoid posterior subluxation of the tibia on the femur. If complete correction has not been obtained by 4 to 6 months of age, surgical correction is indicated.

The popliteal structures should be exposed through longitudinal posteromedial and posterolateral incisions, and then the popliteal vessels and tibial and peroneal nerves are exposed and retracted. The medial and lateral hamstring tendons are tenotomized, and the posterior capsule of the knee is divided and partially excised. When complete correction cannot be obtained, Williams advises that exploration of the anterior knee joint frequently reveals a fibrofatty plug filling the joint and limiting knee extension. This should be excised. Occasionally inspection of the femoral condyles reveals them to be flattened, apparently from lack of normal movement, and thus soft tissue surgery is not beneficial. In these instances a femoral osteotomy can be done at skeletal maturity to transfer the range of motion to a more useful arc, but procedures aimed at increasing the range of motion in such knees have been disappointing in our experience. Femoral shortening and extension osteotomy are required when knee webbing is present, after maximum permissible correction has been obtained by soft tissue release and posterior capsulotomy.

The *extended* and *hyperextended* knee is associated with contracture of the quadriceps mechanism, with or without fixation of the patella to the anterior aspect of the distal femur. It should be treated by the application of a splint or a plaster cast to the extensor aspect of the thigh and leg and then serially and progressively flexed by bending the splint or changing the plaster cast at intervals of 3 or 4 days. Since the femur in such knees is frequently externally rotated, sometimes as much as 90 degrees, it is imortant to determine the proper direction to move the leg to obtain knee flexion. This can usually be done by palpating the posterior surface of the femoral condyles and then flexing the knee so that the tibia courses over the condyles as it flexes. After full flexion has been obtained, it should be maintained for 2 or 3 weeks; afterward, correction should be maintained by orthoses during sleeping hours until the possibility of deformity is past.

If the deformity does not respond to conservative treatment by 4 to 6 months of age, surgical correction is indicated.

The quadriceps is exposed through a straight anterior incision, and the vastus medialis and lateralis are dissected from the rectus tendon, which is usually severely contracted. The rectus is transversely divided at or sightly above its musculotendinous junction. The patella is freed and mobilized, dividing the anterior capsule laterally and medially by parapatellar incisions if necessary. The knee is flexed to 90 degrees and the quadriceps is reconstructed in its lengthened position by interrupted sutures. The knee is immobilized in the corrected position for 3 weeks, and then active exercises are allowed while using an orthosis that holds the knee at 90 degrees during sleeping hours for 6 to 9 months.

HIP

The hip is involved in approximately 80% of patients with MCC. The method and results of treatment vary, depending on the presence of deformity, stiffness, subluxation, or dislocation of the hip. These four factors may exist singly or in any combination, and each profoundly affects treatment and ultimately the ambulatory status of the patient.

St. Clair and Zimbler found deformity of the hip to be largely of two distinct patterns characterized as types 3 and 5 (as described by Brown, Robson, and Sharrard). The most common presentation was Brown type 5, the "frog" position of flexion, abduction, and external rotation of the hips. Of their 17 patients, 9 exhibited this deformity, and 4 of them had subluxation or dislocation of the hips. The second most common pattern, Brown type 3, was manifested as hyperflexion of the hips with hyperextension of the knees. Of 17 patients, 4 had this deformity, and all also had either subluxation or dislocation of the hips.

Generally speaking, deformity of the hip should be treated by passive stretching exercises carried out by the family four times daily beginning in infancy. The family must be supervised frequently by the physical therapist and regularly by the orthopaedist. If the deformities do not respond to this treatment, more intensive conservative methods should be used, such as intermittent skin traction or the application of a spica cast with frequent gradual changes in position. If conservative measures fail, as they do in about one fourth of the patients, surgical correction should be deferred until after the feet, and then the knees, have been corrected either with or without surgery. According to Huurman and Jacobson, a hip flexion deformity of 35 degrees or less is acceptable in MCC patients, since it can be compensated for by lumbar lordosis.

Severe stiffness of the hip in the presence of disabling deformity is usually not correctable by conservative measures and requires either anterior or anterolateral surgical hip release for correction. The realistic goal of treatment must be the conversion of a stiff hip in a deformed position to a stiff hip in a functional position. Postoperative plaster spica immobilization is necessary for 6 weeks or so, followed by passive stretching and orthotic support as indicated.

A unilateral dislocation of the hip, whether mobile or stiff, should be openly reduced and placed in functional position; otherwise there will be limb shortening, pelvic tilt leading to obliquity, and possibly spinal involvement and interference with daily activities while sitting.

Based on extensive experience with individuals who have MCC, Williams states that if the hips are bilaterally stiff and dislocated but not greatly deformed they should not be reduced, for under the best of circumstances, such operation will convert them from stiff and dislocated to stiff and reduced, and while the roentgenographic appearance may be improved, the functional result will not be significantly changed. Numerous authors agree with Williams on this point. St. Clair and Zimbler on the other hand disagree and, convinced that bilateral dislocations are not consistent with a good gait, they recommend that a one-stage open reduction, varus derotational and shortening osteotomy of the femur, with pelvic osteotomy if needed, be performed during the first year of life. We tend to agree with the latter opinion.

The mobile subluxated hip should be treated by correction of the primary skeletal abnormality, be it in the femur or in the pelvis. The stiff subluxated hip does not require treatment, since it does not usually progress to dislocation. The MCC patient applies significantly less stress to his hips than normally, and thus minor biomechanical defects are better tolerated than by normal people.

UPPER LIMB

Although the extent and degree of involvement vary widely, typically the shoulder girdle is underdeveloped, the arms are small with limited abduction and external rotation, the elbows are stiff either in flexion or in full extension, the wrist is in flexion and ulnar deviation, and the thumb is small and rigidly clutched into the palm, with variable stiffness and flexion of the fingers. Webbing may be present at the axilla and the flexor surface of the elbow.

According to Williams, the primary goal of treatment is the achievement of a range of function that permits independence in the performance of toileting, feeding, crutch walking, and the essential activities of daily living. Treatment of the upper limb should be deferred until ambulation has been achieved, and before undertaking any surgical program the patient and the surgeon must be aware of the functions that will be lost, as well as the functions to be achieved, as a result of surgery. As affected children grow and mature, they develop compensatory or trick patterns of motor activity to enable them to perform daily activities; it is a good idea to have the patient studied carefully by an occupational therapist who will tabulate his functional abilities and functional needs and make them well understood before a surgical program is developed.

While awaiting the development and implementation of a surgical treatment program, an individualized nonoperative treatment program should be developed using passive stretching and range-of-motion exercises carried out four times daily by the parents, adjustable splints and orthoses, wedging plaster casts when indicated, and "educational toys" aimed at improving psychomotor, eye-hand, and manual skills.

Finally, the upper extremity must be considered as a total unit, not as isolated components, whose principal goal is to permit its terminal member, the hand, to function optimally in the performance of the tasks of daily living.

Shoulder. Weakness and stiffness about the shoulder do not add significantly to the patient's disability and thus usually require no treatment. The internal rotation deformity is occasionally bilateral and severe enough that the dorsum of the hand presents to the perineum, and the patient cannot attend to his toilet needs. It is readily corrected by a derotational osteotomy of the humerus with internal fixation using a plate and screws. The decision to operate is sometimes more difficult than its performance, since factors to be considered are the strength of the shoulder adductors, abductors, and rotators; the desired degree of correction; and its influence on the function of the elbow, wrist, and hand, as well as on the previously developed patterns of motor activity used in daily living.

Elbow. The articular surfaces at the elbow are normal at birth, but the surfaces gradually adapt to the stresses applied to them, so that with growth and the absence of motion, they become flattened, with the result that the joint may function as a simple hinge with a limited range of motion.

Deformity of the elbow is usually either stiffness in flexion or stiffness in extension.

The stiff flexed elbow generally exhibits a limited range of useful motion centered about the right-angle position. The biceps muscle is intact and strong, the triceps is weak or absent, and elbow extension through the limited range is achieved by gravity. Surgery is not indicated in these patients, since the disability caused by the elbow deformity is not severe.

The elbow that is stiff in extension constitutes a greater problem. The biceps is usually absent, while the triceps is strong. The forearm is usually pronated, and the wrist is in flexion and ulnar deviation with variable involvement of the hand. Since the deformity is usually bilateral, the major functional handicap is the inability of the patient to bring the hand to the mouth or face, and surgery is usually indicated to remedy this problem. If, however, the child will require leg orthoses and crutches for ambulation, surgery should be deferred until ambulation without arm support is possible. A relatively high degree of patient cooperation and effort is required for postoperative muscle reeducation; for this reason surgery should be deferred until the child is about 5 years of age.

According to Williams the surgical options available for the rigid extended elbow are tricepsplasty, triceps transfer, Steindler flexorplasty, and pectoralis major transfer.

Lengthening the triceps mechanism and posterior capsulotomy of the elbow are the most reliable and most durable of available surgical procedures. These are relatively simple and, if performed in the early years of life, restore a full range of passive flexion. A mild nondisabling flexion deformity frequently occurs with growth. Although active flexion is not rendered possible, these patients learn to achieve flexion by shoulder movements or by fixing the forearm and leaning the body toward it.

According to Williams, triceps transfer has not been as successful long term as it originally appeared short term because of the gradual development of a flexion deformity and the gradual diminution in the arc of flexion. In some instances the loss of function rendered the patient incapable of reaching the perineum, a problem solved by extension supracondylar humeral osteotomy and the transfer of the arc of motion to a more useful range of extension.

Williams now recommends a tricepsplasty on one side (the toilet arm) and a triceps transfer on the opposite side (the feeding arm). With this combination not only can the basic activities be performed, but the hands can be brought into apposition for bimanual activity.

The Steindler flexorplasty is rarely indicated in MCC because the wrist flexors are usually both inactive and contracted.

Pectoralis major transfer is more often indicated to confer active elbow flexion because it is usually strong. Since the biceps tendon is rudimentary or absent, a long tongue of fascia must be used to prolong the transplant so it can be securely fixed to the radius. As a separate procedure, the elbow must be mobilized by tricepsplasty before the muscle transfer for active flexion is undertaken.

Wrist and hand. As mentioned previously, the wrist is usually in pronation, flexion, and ulnar deviation. The wrist extensor musculature is usually without function, and the flexors are contracted, weak, or absent. Rarely is adequate controllable muscle power available for transfer. Function of the fingers and hand is likewise variable but limited and not readily susceptible to improvement by surgery.

Wrist stabilization at the optimal functional position is probably the most valuable single surgical contribution to the function of the upper extremity in MCC, but great care must be used to determine the best position for function. The preoperative trial use of splints and casts will usually reveal that slight ulnar deviation and flexion between 5 and 20 degrees constitute the optimum position. After skeletal maturity, wrist fusion can be achieved by traditional methods or by wedge resection of the (usually) fused carpal mass. In the younger child Williams recommends scarifying the carpal bones and radius and insertion of a medullary nail through the third metacarpal, the carpals, and the radius. Since fusion of the immature carpals is difficult to achieve in this situation, the nail should be left in situ permanently.

Obstetric Paralysis

Obstetric paralysis is caused by injury of the brachial plexus during birth. Fortunately, with improved obstetric care its frequency has decreased; according to Adler and Patterson it occurred on the obstetric service of the New York Hospital 1.56 times per 1000 live births in 1938 and only 0.38 times per 1000 in 1962. In obstetric paralysis the birth usually has been difficult and traumatic, and of the patients reported by Adler and Patterson it had been considered "normal" in only 10%; the birth weight of the affected infants had averaged 9 pounds 8 ounces as compared to the average birth weight in the United States of 7 pounds 8 ounces.

The findings in this condition, as will be discussed later, depend on which roots of the brachial plexus have been injured and on the extent of the injury. Wickstrom, in a careful study of 87 patients, found involvement of the fifth and sixth cervical nerve roots in 54, of the eighth cervical and first thoracic nerve roots in 11, and of all of the components of the brachial plexus in 22. In 46 patients the injury was minimal, in 26 moderate (3 had sensory deficiency as well as motor paralysis), and in 15 severe. Of the severe injuries, Horner's syndrome was present in 4, involvement of the dorsal scapular or anterior thoracic nerve in 7, and a sensory deficit in 12. Thus the presence of any of these three features, especially the first or second, indicates a severe injury and consequently a poor prognosis. A minimal injury responds well to conservative treatment and, although recovery may require as long as 18 months, usually residual disability or deformity is slight. But when the injury is more severe, characteristic deformities usually develop promptly. The shoulder becomes flexed, internally rotated, and slightly abducted; active abduction of the joint decreases; and external rotation disappears. The shoulder becomes posteriorly subluxated and eventually dislocated, or the humeral head loses its spheric shape and becomes flattened against the glenoid cavity.

Adler and Patterson found deformity of the elbow in 38 of their 88 patients. In 24 there was a flexion contracture and in 11 of these it was greater than 45 degrees. The radial head was dislocated posteriorly in 14, and in these the ulna was usually bowed. In the most severe deformities the elbow progressively dislocated posteriorly and medially; they were unable to explain these dislocations or to treat them successfully.

Obstetric paralysis is classified according to the location of injury in the brachial plexus. The three chief types are the following.

1. *Upper plexus or arm type (named for Erb and for Duchenne).* The muscles most frequently paralyzed are the supraspinatus and infraspinatus, apparently because the suprascapular nerve is fixed at the suprascapular notch (Erb's point). In patients more severely involved other muscles innervated by the fifth and sixth cervical nerve roots may also be affected, namely, the deltoid, biceps, brachialis, supinator, and subscapularis. This type of injury was present in 54 of the 87 patients studied by Wickstrom.

2. *Whole plexus or arm type.* There is complete sensory and motor paralysis of the entire extremity because of severe injury in all the roots of the brachial plexus. This type

of injury was present in 22 of the 87 patients studied by Wickstrom.

3. *Lower plexus or arm type (named for Klumpke).* The muscles of the forearm and hand together with parts served by the cervical sympathetic chain are paralyzed because of injury of the eighth cervical and first thoracic nerve roots. This type of injury was present in 11 of the 87 patients studied by Wickstrom.

TREATMENT

The aim of treatment in the initial stages of this paralysis should be to prevent contractures of muscles and joints while awaiting any neurologic recovery. The parents are shown gentle passive exercises to maintain a full range of passive motion of all the joints of the upper extremity. It is especially important to maintain full extension of the fingers, hand, and wrist, full pronation and supination of the forearm, full extension of the elbow, and full abduction, extension, and external rotation of the shoulder. Therefore it is important that the parents demonstrate to the surgeon that they understand the exercise program and will carry it out effectively for at least 2 or 3 minutes each time the diaper is changed.

During the initial examination the extent and severity of the involvement must be estimated as accurately as possible and any other associated handicap should be discovered. During the first 6 to 9 months the patient should be seen by the orthopaedic surgeon at intervals of about 1 month for evaluation of the neurologic status and of the range of motion of the joints, and thereafter less frequently. Spontaneous recovery usually continues until about the age of 18 months.

In our experience exploring the brachial plexus (p. 2809) rarely alters the course of the paralysis. Often maximum function will not return until 18 months after birth. Others, however, believe that when only slight muscle power has developed after 3 months, exploring the plexus is justified, especially in the whole-plexus type of paralysis. Then if neurolysis alone is found to be advisable, there is some hope for improvement, but if nerve suture or graft is indicated, there is little or no hope for improvement.

Shoulder

If patients with obstetric paralysis are first seen only after they are 2 or 3 years old, physical therapy and other conservative measures are indicated. Motion of the shoulder in both abduction and external rotation is demonstrably limited, and in some patients the joint has become subluxated posteriorly. The acromion is usually elongated anteriorly and inferiorly, and the scapula is rotated and elevated. Any surgery necessary to correct deformity and restore function of the shoulder should be deferred until the age of 4 unless the deformity is progressing rapidly despite conservative treatment.

Babbitt and Cassidy reported a rare complication in obstetric paralysis. They described two patients with anteroinferior dislocation of the shoulder that had developed within the first few months of life. Such a dislocation was described in 1953 by Liebolt and Furey, and we have seen patients with this complication. Clinically the shoulders

were fixed in abduction and the scapulas were winged. Conservative treatment and attempts at closed reduction of the dislocations failed. In each, open reduction of the shoulder revealed much thickening of the anteroinferior part of the joint capsule. After this part of the capsule had been divided, reduction of the dislocation was easy and stable. In the patient of Liebolt and Furey the tendon of the long head of the biceps was tight and required division before reduction was possible. The dislocation occurred in our patient, an infant who had been immobilized almost constantly on an airplane splint for several months. When conservative treatment failed and open reduction was carried out, the humeral head was found in the infraglenoid position. After the capsule had been divided, reduction of the dislocation was relatively easy.

CORRECTING INTERNAL ROTATION AND ADDUCTION CONTRACTURE BY OPERATION ON SOFT TISSUES

In 1913 Fairbank described an operation to correct internal rotation deformity of the shoulder in obstetric paralysis. Using the deltopectoral approach, he divided the superior part of the pectoralis major tendon, the entire subscapularis tendon, and the adjacent part of the shoulder joint capsule; when necessary, he also divided the coracohumeral ligament, the supraspinatus tendon, and the coracoid process. In 1916 Sever published his modification of this operation "following suggestions made by Fairbank." (Toft credits Slomann with describing the operation independently at the same time.) The Sever operation differs from that of Fairbank in that (1) the entire pectoralis major tendon is divided, (2) the capsule of the shoulder joint is not divided, (3) the coracobrachialis and the short head of the biceps are released when contracted, and (4) the coracoid and acromion are divided if either is found to interfere with the motion of the shoulder (Fig. 66-79). The operation as now performed is virtually that described by Sever. His modification of Fairbank's operation is best suited for patients in whom the shoulder joint is not subluxated and the humeral head is not deformed and in whom function can be demonstrated in the external rotators and abductors of the shoulder. When motion has been extremely limited, the results of this operation look good (Fig. 66-80), but when motion has been only mildly limited, the results are likely to disappoint the child's parents because the improvement is not so striking. The operation does not improve the strength of the shoulder.

When contractures of the latissimus dorsi and teres major muscles also interfere with abduction of the shoulder, Steindler added to the Sever operation by dividing the insertions of these muscles through an incision along the posterior axillary fold.

Carrying Steindler's addition a step farther, L'Episcopo transferred these insertions to a more lateral position on the humeral shaft, thus converting the muscles into external rotators of the shoulder. As a preliminary step, L'Episcopo performed the Sever operation, but when the capsule of the shoulder joint was contracted, he divided it as originally recommended by Fairbank. More recently Zachary has modified the transfer of the latissimus dorsi and teres major tendons by approaching the humerus posteriorly through the interval between the long and lateral heads of the triceps, rather than approaching it medial to the entire triceps muscle; thus during operation retraction of the triceps need not be so vigorous.

Wickstrom reported 28 operations on the soft tissues to correct deformity; 5 Sever operations were carried out and the result was satisfactory in 2 and poor in 3; of 16 L'Episcopo operations, the result was good in 10, satisfactory in 5, and poor in 1; and of 7 modified Fairbank operations, the result was good in 5, satisfactory in 1, and poor in 1.

Although we have not carefully studied the results of our treatment of shoulders with the upper plexus type of obstetric paralysis, we have the distinct impression that the traditional operations described here leave much to be desired. In our experience, even after the most carefully planned surgical treatment, motion, both active and passive, remains limited (especially in abduction and external rotation), the muscles controlling these motions are significantly weak, and scapulohumeral rhythm is impaired.

Since the publication of Saha's excellent monograph, *Surgery of the Paralyzed and Flail Shoulder,* we have concluded that usually the chief cause of shoulder disability in the upper arm type of obstetric paralysis is loss of ability

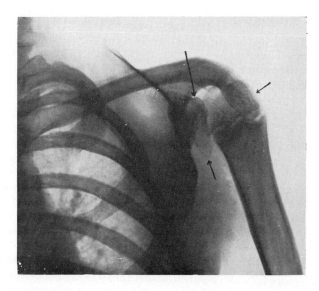

Fig. 66-79. Osseous deformity in severe obstetric paralysis of whole plexus or arm type. Note that scapula is underdeveloped, coracoid is markedly enlarged, acromion is elongated anteriorly and inferiorly, and head of humerus and glenoid cavity of scapula are hypoplastic. Head is subluxated posteriorly.

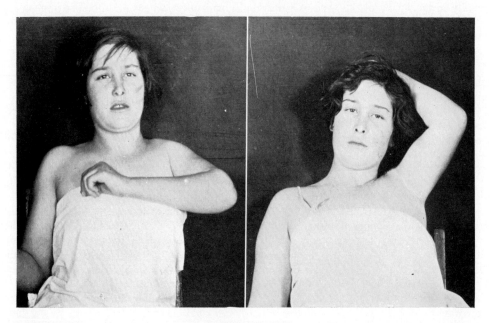

Fig. 66-80. Range of abduction and external rotation possible before and after Sever modification of Fairbank operation.

to stabilize the humeral head against the glenoid cavity caused by paralysis of the supraspinatus and infraspinatus muscles. According to Saha, the function of these two muscles acting with the subscapularis (these are the three "steering muscles") is to stabilize, steer, and fix the humeral head against the glenoid cavity while the deltoid and clavicular head of the pectoralis major (these are the "prime movers") supply power and the normal range of active motion of the shoulder joint. It follows then that paralysis of the supraspinatus and infraspinatus muscles will produce an imbalance in strength in this group of stabilizing muscles, and that the unopposed subscapularis will become contracted. This contracture leads to a progressive adduction and internal rotation deformity, and the loss of support posteriorly causes posterior subluxation and ultimately posterior dislocation of the humeral head.

Being convinced that Saha's concept of the pathogenesis of shoulder deformities is correct, we have developed a different operation for this paralysis. Because our experience with the operation has been limited by the infrequency of obstetric paralysis and because our results have been somewhat disappointing, the procedure has not yet been fully developed nor has it been published. At present the following technique is used. With the child in the semilateral position the shoulder is approached through a modified saber cut incision (Fig. 2-64) beginning just distal to the coracoid process and extending superiorly and posteriorly so that the deltoid is detached completely from the clavicle, the acromion, and the spine of the scapula to its posterior end. Likewise the trapezius is detached completely beginning anteriorly and continuing posteriorly. Then under direct vision the shoulder is put through a range of motion and the contracted and deforming structures are identified and closely studied. The muscles are also examined with a neuroelectric stimulator to determine their viability. The pectoralis major, which is almost always contracted, is detached from the humerus in a step-cut fashion so that later it can be reattached more proximally on the humerus and thus be effectively lengthened. The subscapularis tendon is incised obliquely beginning superficially and medially and ending deeply and laterally so that when sutured it will also have been lengthened. If the supraspinatus and infraspinatus muscles are contracted, they can be lengthened by either moving the insertion of the external rotator cuff more proximally on the humeral head or by elevating the bodies of the muscles from the supraspinatus and infraspinatus fossae and allowing them to retract laterally as the shoulder is adducted. Next the coracoid process is identified along with the origins of the coracobrachials and short head of the biceps. That part of the process at which these muscles originate is resected and is allowed to retract distally. Care is taken not to damage the musculocutaneous nerve, which is near the coracoid process at this stage in the operation.

Several combinations of transfers have been used in attempts to substitute for the lost power of the supraspinatus and infraspinatus muscles. The insertion of the levator scapulae on the superomedial corner of the scapula can be identified, detached, and rerouted, and sutured to the supraspinatus tendon. A slip of the latissimus dorsi or of the teres minor can be detached, rerouted, and sutured to the tendon of the infraspinatus at its insertion on the humerus. The deltoid and trapezius muscles are then reattached, and the extremity is immobilized on a splint that holds the shoulder in abduction for 3 or 4 weeks. Then physical therapy is started. We are not satisfied with the results of this operation, but they are at least better than after the other operations we have used. Motor function remains impaired but the deformity is corrected well.

TECHNIQUE (FAIRBANK, SEVER). Make an incision on the anterior aspect of the shoulder distally from the tip of the acromion to a point distal to the tendinous insertion of the pectoralis major muscle (Fig. 66-81); divide this tendon parallel to the humerus. Then retract the anterior margin of the deltoid laterally and the pectoralis major medially and expose the coracobrachialis muscle. With the shoulder externally rotated and abducted, trace the coracobrachialis superiorly to the coracoid process. If the coracoid is elongated, resect 0.5 to 1 cm of its tip together with the insertions of the coracobrachialis, the short head of the biceps, and the pectoralis minor muscles; this resection increases the range of motion of the shoulder in external rotation and abduction. Now locate the inferior edge of the subscapularis tendon at its insertion on the lesser tuberosity of the humerus, elevate it with a grooved director, and divide it completely without incising the capsule. External rotation and abduction of the shoulder should then be almost normal.

A curved prolongation of the acromion may interfere with abduction and with reduction of any mild posterior subluxation of the joint; in this event either resect this obstructing part or divide the acromion and elevate this part.

AFTERTREATMENT. An abduction humerus splint that holds the shoulder in abduction and mild external rotation is applied and is worn constantly for 2 weeks and intermittently for another 4 weeks. Active exercises are started early and are continued until maximum improvement has occurred.

TECHNIQUE (L'EPISCOPO, ZACHARY). This procedure consists of two steps.

Step 1. Perform the Sever operation but also (1) completely divide the capsule of the shoulder joint anteriorly if necessary and (2) free the tendons of insertion of the latissimus dorsi and teres major muscles.

Step 2. Make a curved longitudinal incision over the posterior aspect of the proximal third of the arm, retract the posterior margin of the deltoid muscle anteriorly, and expose the proximal part of the triceps muscle. Define and develop the interval between the long and lateral heads of the triceps and identify and carefully retract the radial nerve. Now transfer the previously freed latissimus dorsi and teres major tendons through a slit in the proximal part of the lateral head of the triceps (Fig. 66-82) and with the shoulder in full external rotation fix these tendons to the posterolateral aspect of the humerus beneath a thin osteoperiosteal flap. L'Episcopo found it unnecessary to anchor the tendons beneath a heavy flap or a trapdoor lifted from the bone.

AFTERTREATMENT. With the shoulder in full external rotation, slight abduction, and slight flexion, a shoulder spica cast is applied and is worn for 3 weeks.

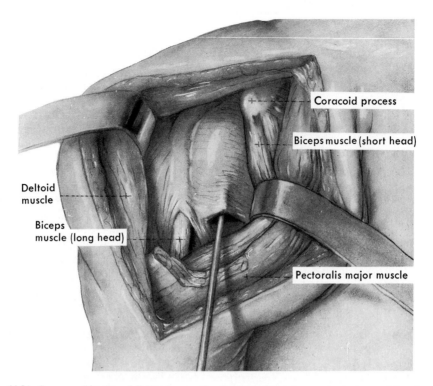

Fig. 66-81. Sever modification of Fairbank operation for internal rotation contracture caused by obstetric paralysis (see text). (Modified from Horsley, J.S., and Bigger, I.S.: Operative surgery, ed. 6, St. Louis, 1953, The C.V. Mosby Co.)

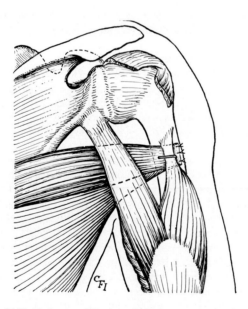

Fig. 66-82. Zachary modification of L'Episcopo operation (see text).

CORRECTING INTERNAL ROTATION DEFORMITY OF ARM BY OSTEOTOMY OF HUMERUS

Rogers and others made an osteotomy of the proximal shaft of the humerus to correct an internal rotation deformity of the arm when the humeral head itself is neither retroverted nor subluxated. This operation improves the appearance of the limb but usually fails to restore function

as well as the Sever operation does. Wickstrom has treated by osteotomy of the humerus nine shoulders in which the humeral head was flattened and fixed in internal rotation, and the result was satisfactory in all.

TECHNIQUE (ROGERS). Approach the humerus anteriorly between the deltoid and pectoralis major muscles. With the arm abducted, make an osteotomy 5 cm distal to the joint. Under direct vision externally rotate the distal fragment of the humerus 90 degrees; be sure the fragments are then apposed. Close the wound.

AFTERTREATMENT. With the shoulder abducted 90 degrees, the elbow flexed 90 degrees, and the forearm supinated, a shoulder spica cast is applied and is worn for 8 weeks.

CORRECTING POSTERIOR DISLOCATION OF HUMERAL HEAD BY SEVER OPERATION AND GRAFTING POSTERIORLY

Inserting a graft in the posterior part of the glenoid to prevent recurrence of posterior displacement (luxation) of the humeral head was devised by J.R. Moore; it is contraindicated until the age of 8 years. First the Sever modification of the Fairbank operation is performed to correct the internal rotation deformity of the arm; then 6 weeks later the graft is inserted. The day before grafting, two casts are applied—one to the body and the other to the arm. Enough space is left between them for surgical access to the posterior axillary fold. We recommend that the scapular neck be osteotomized incompletely and that the articular surface of the glenoid fossa be bent anteriorly and inferiorly by producing a greenstick fracture. A triangular wedge of bone usually obtained from the spine of the scapula is then inserted into the defect and fixed in position by heavy catgut sutures. Age is not a contraindication for this operation, and we have performed it in children as young as 2 years of age. Likewise the operation is not indicated as a separate procedure but can be combined with any other operation indicated.

TECHNIQUE (J.R. MOORE). Place the patient prone and abduct the shoulder 90 degrees. Make an incision along the posterior axillary fold. Identify the long head of the triceps and trace it superiorly to where it passes between the teres major and teres minor muscles. Retract the posterior border of the deltoid superolaterally. Separate the teres minor and infraspinatus muscles throughout their length and expose the scapula subperiosteally. Then by sharp dissection separate these muscles from the capsule of the shoulder joint. Displace the humeral head anteriorly and posteriorly and note how far posteriorly it has been subluxated; then hold the head displaced anteriorly. Drive a chisel 1 cm wide into the articular surface of the glenoid at a point 3 mm anterior to its posterior border and make a cleft 1 cm deep. Then cut a graft 1 cm wide and 2.5 cm long from the axillary border of the scapula. With its slight concave surface toward the humeral head, drive one-half the length of this graft into the cleft.

AFTERTREATMENT. With the shoulder abducted 90 degrees, extended 15 degrees, and externally rotated 45 degrees, join the casts on the arm and body to form a shoulder spica. At 8 weeks the cast is bivalved, and physical therapy and exercises, especially of the deltoid and external rotators, are begun. Two weeks later an abduction humeral splint is applied and is worn from 3 to 6 months while the exercises are continued. During this period the arm is brought to the side daily to prevent a permanent abduction contracture.

IMPROVING MUSCLE BALANCE BY TRANSFERRING POSTERIORLY PART OF DELTOID

B.H. Moore observed that in most patients with the upper plexus type of paralysis, the anterior part of the deltoid retains much power, whereas the posterior part is often weak; consequently strength for flexing the shoulder is greater than for abducting or extending it. He therefore transferred the origin of some of the anterior part posteriorly to replace the paralyzed or weakened part. But before this operation is performed, internal rotation contracture of the shoulder, unless slight, must be corrected by the Sever modification of the Fairbank operation. Transferring a part of the deltoid posteriorly will not correct any posterior displacement of the humeral head, and any instability that this displacement causes will impair the function of the transferred muscle. Since the transferred muscle acts chiefly as an external rotator and not as an abductor, Moore, to improve abduction, sometimes also transferred a part of the trapezius into the greater tuberosity of the humerus.

We have found partial paralysis of the deltoid muscle to be rare in obstetric paralysis but have occasionally mobilized the origin of the muscle and moved it where needed to establish better mechanical leverage, usually in combination with some other operation.

TECHNIQUE (B.H. MOORE). Place the patient on his side with the affected shoulder upward. Begin an incision over the clavicle medial to the acromioclavicular joint and extend it around the acromion to the middle of the spine of the scapula; if necessary, continue the anterior end of the incision inferiorly for 2.5 to 5 cm. Dissect the skin flap from the muscle distally for 5 cm. Now expose the lateral 4 cm of the spine of the scapula subperiosteally and prepare on it a bed to receive the transferred muscle. Then free the acromial origin and some of the clavicular origin of the deltoid by removing a thin osteoperiosteal layer from the underlying bone. Then free this flap of deltoid distally as far as possible without endangering the axillary nerve.

Should there be a mild internal rotation contracture of the shoulder, the subscapularis tendon may be divided at this time because it is now exposed in the floor of the wound. Abduct and externally rotate the shoulder and transfer the flap of deltoid posteriorly to the prepared bed on the spine of the scapula; anchor the flap to the periosteum with interrupted sutures and to the bone with similar sutures passed through holes drilled in it.

AFTERTREATMENT. A shoulder spica cast is applied to hold the shoulder appropriately flexed, abducted, and externally rotated, the elbow flexed 90 degrees, and the forearm pronated. At about 2 weeks the part of the cast that encases the shoulder and limb is bivalved, and the sutures are removed. At 6 weeks the superior shell of the bivalved part is discarded; then the shoulder is passively exercised by abducting and externally rotating it, and the elbow is exercised by flexing and extending it. At 8 weeks the part of the cast that encases the body is bivalved and the exercises are increased, but the cast is replaced between periods of exercise; 2 weeks later the whole cast is discarded. Then an abduction humeral splint is worn between exercise periods until full adduction of the shoulder is attained.

Elbow

In obstetric paralysis limitation of motion and even deformity of the elbow are usually disregarded. However, of 107 patients with the upper plexus type of obstetric paralysis, Aitken found osseous deformity of the elbow in 33 (30.8%). In 6 of these 33 patients he found anterior dislocation of the radial head, thought to have been present at birth. In the remaining 27 patients he found posterior dislocation of the radial head of varying severity and usually deformity of other structures of the elbow and forearm. Posterior dislocation he found chiefly in patients with severe paralysis, and this deformity could be observed in infants only as a clubbing of the proximal radial metaphysis associated with progressive bowing of the ulna. By the fifth to the eighth year, he pointed out, the radial head can become completely dislocated posteriorly, and that part of the capitulum that articulates with the radial head becomes flattened. It is only at some time between the eighth and fourteenth years that the proximal radial epiphysis becomes visible on roentgenograms. It is then seen to be flattened and smaller than normal.

According to Aitken, these deformities are caused chiefly by the effect of muscle imbalance; prolonged immobilization in an extremely abnormal position, however, may also be a factor. When these deformities are known to be developing, he recommends that the splint be changed so that the shoulder is moderately abducted and externally rotated, the elbow is extended past 90 degrees, and the forearm is neither pronated nor supinated; the splint must be removed regularly and often, and the limb must be exercised both actively and passively through full ranges of motion.

Excision of the radial head alone, at any stage of growth, does little in this situation to improve the range of motion of the elbow and supination of the forearm. Aitken therefore recommends that in addition an osteotomy be made through the proximal third of the ulna to establish a more normal relationship between the shaft of the ulna and that of the radius. Excision of the radial head should, of course, be deferred when feasible until growth is complete.

Of 88 patients with obstetric paralysis, Adler and Patterson found deformity in the elbow in 38. In 6 there was flexion contracture, in 14 posterior dislocation of the radial head, and in a few an unexplained progressive posteromedial dislocation of the elbow joint.

Forearm, wrist, and hand

Of 150 patients with obstetric paralysis, Zaoussis found the forearm fixed in pronation in 14% and in supination in 10%. He noted that for fixed supination deformity Lange in 1951 made an osteotomy of the radial neck 2 cm distal to the radial head, rotated the distal fragment into full pronation, and permitted the bone to heal. Zaoussis carried out a similar operation in six patients, and the result was good in five and poor in one. Through a Boyd approach (p. 100) he made the osteotomy just distal to the radial tuberosity, and when the supinator muscle was found contracted, as it usually was, he released its origin. Despite synostoses that developed between the proximal radius and ulna in two patients, function and appearance were both improved. Zancolli has described an operation for supination deformity that reroutes the biceps muscle and converts it from a supinator of the forearm to a pronator (p. 3021). Blount has described an osteoclasis of the forearm for supination deformities (p. 3022).

Any useful operations on the wrist and hand are considered in the discussion of the paralytic hand in Chapter 12.

Paralysis Caused by Peripheral Nerve Lesions

The principles for managing paralysis caused by lesions of peripheral nerves are similar to those for managing paralysis caused by other lower motor neuron lesions, such as poliomyelitis, spina bifida, and myelomeningocele, previously described in this chapter. A few such lesions occur frequently enough that their incidence gives them importance, and they will be discussed separately.

TENDON TRANSFER FOR PARALYSIS OF SPINAL ACCESSORY NERVE

Although the spinal accessory nerve is often sectioned for anastomosis with the facial nerve to restore function to the latter and is occasionally injured during operations in the posterior triangle of the neck, its paralysis rarely

causes a severe disability. Should a disabling drop shoulder and limitation of elevation of the arm develop, surgery is indicated. Henry, Dewar and Harris, Eden, and Lange have described operations for this disability.

Henry used two longitudinal incisions, one located over the lower cervical and upper dorsal spinous processes and the other over the vertebral border of the scapula. Two holes, each 0.7 cm in diameter, are made in the scapula near its vertebral border, one 2 cm from this border at a point just proximal to the spine of the scapula and the second 2 cm from this border at a point 6 cm distal to the spine of the scapula. A strip of fascia lata 2 cm wide is looped through the proximal hole and is routed subcutaneously through and around the spinous process of the sixth cervical vertebra and thence back to the scapula where it is tied and sutured to itself under proper tension. A second fascial strip is inserted similarly through the distal hole in the scapula and around the spinous process of the third dorsal vertebra. An abduction humerus splint is worn constantly for 4 weeks and intermittently for 4 more weeks.

In the technique of Dewar and Harris the scapular insertion of the levator scapulae is transferred laterally. A single L-shaped incision is used. A strip of fascia lata 5 cm wide is passed through a hole in the scapula near its vertebral border and through the spinous processes of the second and third dorsal vertebrae (Fig. 66-83). This anchor-

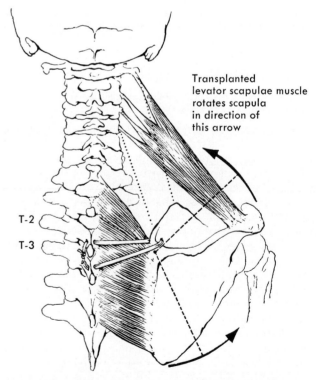

Transplanted levator scapulae muscle rotates scapula in direction of this arrow

T-2

T-3

Lower fibers of serratus anterior muscle rotate scapula in direction of this arrow

Fig. 66-83. Dewar and Harris operation to restore function of shoulder in paralysis of spinal accessory nerve (see text). (Modified from Dewar, F.P., and Harris, R.I.: Ann Surg. **123:**1111, 1950.)

age substitutes for the stabilizing and tethering action of the middle part of the trapezius. The scapular insertion of the levator scapulae muscle is transferred laterally on the spine of the scapula to a point near the acromion, and the muscle thus serves as a substitute for the superior part of the trapezius. After surgery the shoulder is held in moderate abduction for 8 weeks. After rehabilitation the scapula, anchored to the midline of the back by the fascial loop, exhibits movement that approaches normal in strength, range, and direction when it is acted on by the serratus anterior and by the laterally transferred levator scapulae. According to Dewar, the procedure has been used in 11 patients and has been satisfactory in all.

Eden and later Lange developed an operation in which both the levator scapulae and rhomboid muscles are transferred. Langenskiöld and Ryoppy reported success in three patients treated by this method. A curved incision extending from the acromion to the inferomedial angle of the scapula is made. The levator scapulae is detached along with a piece of bone from its scapular attachment, is mobilized proximally by blunt dissection, and is fixed laterally to the scapula near the acromioclavicular joint with nonabsorbable sutures. The infraspinatus muscle is then elevated subperiosteally from the scapula, and the rhomboid muscles are detached from the medial border of the scapula along with a piece of bone. The rhomboid muscle mass is pulled laterally and is attached under moderate tension to the scapula with nonabsorbable sutures passed through holes drilled in the bone. Then the infraspinatus muscle is reattached over the rhomboid muscle mass. The shoulder is immobilized in a spica cast in 35 to 45 degrees of abduction for 4 weeks. Then active exercises are started. Normal daily activities are resumed in 8 to 10 weeks.

ORTHOPAEDIC RECONSTRUCTION FOR PARALYSIS CAUSED BY INJURY OF BRACHIAL PLEXUS

Some injuries to the brachial plexus do not recover spontaneously or respond to surgical treatment. Usually traction injuries are unsuitable for repair because of the extensive intraneural damage commonly present. Further extensive root avulsions rarely if ever improve after surgery. Bonney studied 29 patients with supraclavicular traction injuries; no function returned in the wrist or finger extensors or in the intrinsic muscles of the hand. Tracy and Brannon studied 16 patients, most of whom were seen late after traction injuries in which one or more roots were avulsed. They recommended reconstructive operations in partial plexus injuries and considered total plexus avulsion as unsalvageable and an indication for amputation. In discussing reconstructions they emphasized stability of the shoulder, flexibility of the elbow, opposition of the thumb, and grasp of the hand. Yeoman and Seddon studied the problem of the flail arm after brachial plexus injuries in 36 patients. When all roots were damaged distal to the ganglia, they explored the plexus early; if lesions in continuity were found, recovery was considered possible. If the trunks were ruptured, then repair was considered impossible. Additional unfavorable findings included avulsion of nerve roots, severe damage from high-velocity missiles, severe spasmodic pain, and Horner's syndrome. They compared the results after reconstruction of the upper ex-

tremity by tenodesis of the fingers, posterior bone block of the elbow, and arthrodesis of the shoulder in 8 patients, amputation through the arm and arthrodesis of the shoulder in 17 patients, and no operative treatment at all in 12 patients. They concluded that results were better after treatment by combined amputation and arthrodesis than after other reconstructions or after no operative treatment. They also concluded that delay between injury and amputation had an adverse effect on the result. A long period of disuse causes osteoporosis of the humerus and shoulder joint and the development of a one-handed habit pattern, both of which interfere with proper use of the prosthesis.

Obviously an orderly classification of the disabilities caused by paralysis from injury of the brachial plexus and the operations suitable to correct them is impossible because of the variable location and extent of the paralysis, the variable distribution of anesthesia, and the common presence of complicating contractures of joints and fibrosis of muscles. Details of reconstruction must vary with the individual patient and his occupation.

If reasonable sensation is preserved, function superior to that provided by a prosthesis can often be restored. Because the aim of reconstruction is to restore function of the hand, it is best to begin with procedures on the hand. Amputation should not be considered until after an earnest effort to improve the extremity, even though the patient may request amputation. A carefully planned combination of operations on the hand, wrist, elbow, and shoulder, such as arthrodeses, tenodeses, tendon transfers, and bone blocks, is often helpful. For detailed discussions of the indications and techniques for these operations, the text of Bunnell and the articles of Hendry, Thompson, Luckey and McPherson, Brooks, Riordan, and others listed in the references at the end of this chapter, Chapter 12, and the section on poliomyelitis earlier in this chapter should be consulted.

RECONSTRUCTION FOR PARALYSIS OF LONG THORACIC NERVE

The serratus anterior muscle alone is occasionally paralyzed by injury to the long thoracic nerve. Such injuries may result from either sharp or blunt trauma or from traction when the head is forced acutely away from the shoulder or when the shoulder is depressed as when carrying heavy weights. Other causes include exposure to cold, viral infections, and placing patients in the Trendelenburg position with shoulder braces that compress the supraclavicular areas. When the serratus anterior is paralyzed, the patient cannot fully flex the arm above the level of the shoulder anteriorly, and active abduction may also be restricted. When the patient attempts to exert forward pushing movements with the hands, "winging" of the scapula occurs and its vertebral border and inferior angle become unduly prominent.

When the nerve has been stretched rather than severed, it is usually enough to immobilize the shoulder girdle in extension with the arm against the chest. Care should be taken to avoid contractures of the shoulder, elbow, and wrist while awaiting recovery. According to Sunderland, the nerve may recover after 3 to 12 months. If paralysis persists or if the nerve has been severed, the prognosis for

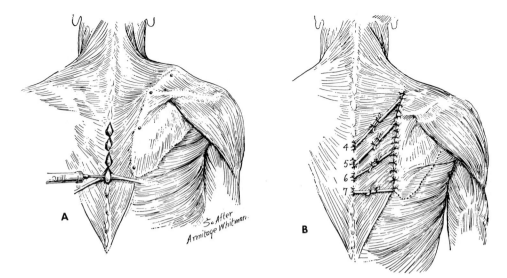

Fig. 66-84. Whitman operation for paralysis of serratus anterior. **A,** Exposure of displaced scapula and of spinous processes. Holes are drilled through vertebral border of scapula and spinous processes of fourth, fifth, sixth, and seventh dorsal vertebrae. **B,** Operation completed. Strips of fascia lata have been passed through corresponding holes in scapula and spinous processes; with scapula drawn inferiorly and medially, strips are tied under tension. (Redrawn from Whitman, A.: JAMA **99:**1332, 1932.)

recovery is poor, and one of the following operations may be indicated (see also the discussion of muscle transfers and fascial transplants for paralysis of the scapular muscles in poliomyelitis presented earlier in this chapter (p. 3001). There are no significant reports of results following suture of the long thoracic nerve.

TECHNIQUE (WHITMAN). Expose the superior and vertebral borders of the scapula through an incision extending from the acromion along the superior border and thence down the vertebral border. Drill four holes through the scapula, one at each of the following points: the superior border at the medial angle, the junction of the spine and the vertebral border, the middle of the vertebral border, and the inferior angle. Also drill holes in the spinous processes of the fourth, fifth, sixth, and seventh dorsal vertebrae. Pass strips of fascia lata through these corresponding holes (Fig. 66-84) and suture them under tension while the scapula is retracted inferiorly and medially.

AFTERTREATMENT. A shoulder spica cast is applied with the arm in 45 degrees of abduction. At 4 weeks the cast is removed, and motion is started.

TECHNIQUE (HAAS, AFTER HIS). Expose the tendon of the teres major muscle through a curved incision along the posterior border of the axilla; define and release its humeral insertion. Through the same incision prepare a bed on the chest wall in the region of the digitations of the serratus anterior muscle on the fifth and sixth ribs. Split the tendon and pass each half subperiosteally through a rib or anchor it to a rib beneath a trapdoor raised from the bone.

• • •

Chaves described a technique for paralysis of the serratus anterior muscle that uses the pectoralis minor. The tendon of this muscle is detached from its insertion on the coracoid and is prolonged with a fascial strip. This strip is inserted into the scapula through two holes chiseled in the bone near its vertebral border at the junction of its middle and distal thirds and is sutured to itself and to the fascia covering the subscapularis. The arm is immobilized in 90 degrees of abduction for 6 weeks. Rapp reported a successful result after this operation; however, he inserted the fascial strip at the inferior angle of the scapula (Fig. 66-85). Horwitz also reported a success with the operation as modified by Rapp.

Marmor and Bechtol described a technique for paralysis of this muscle in which a part of the pectoralis major is prolonged with a fascial strip and is inserted into the inferior angle of the scapula through a hole made in the bone.

Zeier reported success in two patients whom he treated by combining transfer of the pectoralis minor with a fascia lata extension and transfer of the humeral attachment of the teres major to the sixth and seventh ribs (Figs. 66-86 and 66-87).

Vastamäki has recently called attention again to transfer of the pectoralis minor to correct serratus anterior paralysis. It was previously described by Chaves (1951), Rapp (1954), and Trunchly (1981). Vastamäki uses a folded plantaris tendon graft to prolong the transfer. If conservative treatment has been unsuccessful after about 2 years and if disability is severe enough, the operation is indicated.

TECHNIQUE (VASTAMÄKI). Position the patient on the operating table with the unaffected side down. Expose the coracoid process by a short incision. Identify, isolate, and detach from the scapula the pectoralis minor tendon insertion, bringing with it a small piece of bone. Then free the upper part of the muscle belly, being careful to preserve its neurovascular bundle. Expose the lateral portion of the distal third of the scapula. Now gently create a tunnel under the pectoralis major muscle to the exposed part of the

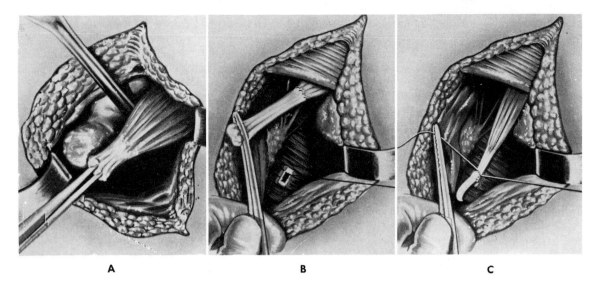

A   **B**   **C**

Fig. 66-85. Chaves and Rapp transfer of pectoralis minor for serratus anterior paralysis. **A,** Pectoralis minor tendon is freed from its coracoid insertion; periosteal elevator is freeing muscle from chest wall but preserving innervation. **B,** Kocher clamp holds fascial prolongation of pectoralis minor tendon to be passed through window in inferior angle of scapula, indicated by silk suture. **C,** Prolongation of pectoralis minor tendon has been passed through window in scapula and is being sutured to itself. (From Rapp, I.H.: J. Bone Joint Surg. **36-A:**852, 1954.)

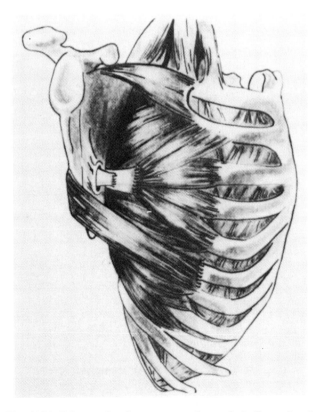

Fig. 66-86. Zeier transfers for serratus anterior paralysis. Pectoralis minor with fascia lata extension is transferred to window in interomedial border of scapula, and humeral attachment of teres major is transferred to sixth and seventh ribs. (From Zeier, F.G.: Clin. Orthop. **91:**128, 1973.)

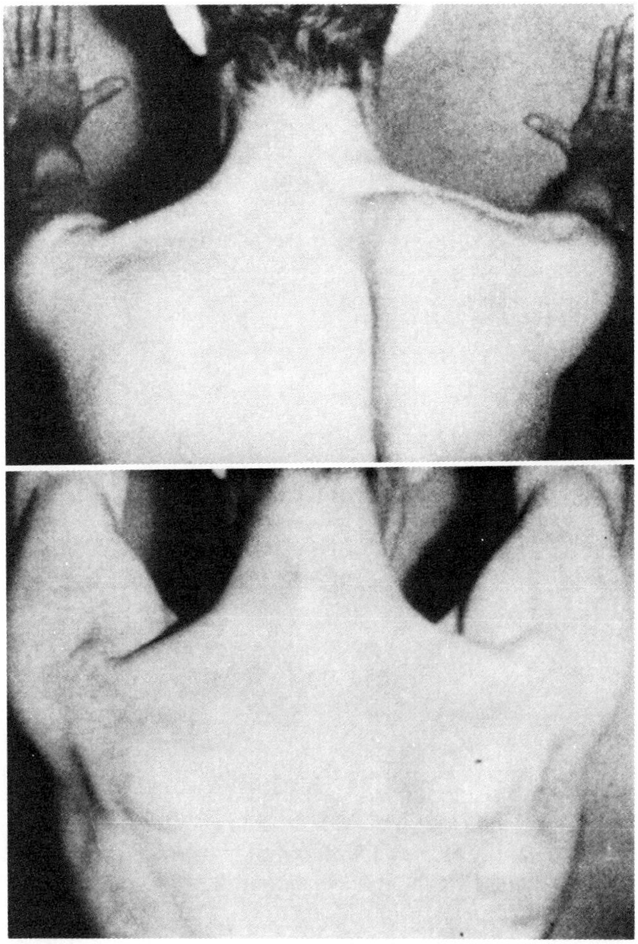

Fig. 66-87. Same technique as Fig. 66-86. **A,** Before surgery; showing winging of right scapula, **B,** After surgery; winging has disappeared. (From Zeier, F.G.: Clin Orthop. **91:**128, 1973.)

scapula. The pectoralis minor must not be overstretched. Usually there is a gap of 2 to 4 cm, and this is filled by a free graft of plantaris tendon folded over six to eight times and securely bridging the defect between scapula and transferred tendon end. Passive movement of the shoulder and scapula should be unrestricted, and the scapular winging should be corrected at surgery.

AFTERTREATMENT. A Velpeau type of bandage is worn for 4 weeks, and gentle active and passive exercises are then instituted.

TENDON AND MUSCLE TRANSFERS FOR PARALYSIS OF DELTOID

These tendon and muscle transfers are discussed in the section on poliomyelitis earlier in this chapter (p. 3002).

RECONSTRUCTION FOR PARALYSIS IN LOWER EXTREMITY

Orthopaedic operations to rehabilitate the lower extremity after irreparable peripheral nerve injury should be directed primarily toward correcting deformity to restore stability and endurance and secondarily toward restoring motion and replacing muscle function. The principles of treatment and the operative techniques described earlier for poliomyelitis (p. 2926) are generally applicable here. Unfortunately muscles strong enough to justify their transfer to reinforce the muscles controlling the hip, the knee, and the ankle are often unavailable. But a patient who can lock the joints of the limb in a satisfactory weight-bearing position can walk surprisingly well despite extensive paralysis. In quadriceps paralysis anterior transfer of one or more hamstrings is often helpful, but any slight flexion contracture of the knee seriously impairs the function of the transferred muscle.

For reconstruction to be satisfactory the limb, especially the foot, must be painless. Painful scars, adhesions, and tender neuromas must be excised, and a durable skin must be provided on which to bear weight. The foot must act as a stable pedestal during stance and as a strong lever during walking. For complete paralysis below the knee or fixed functional deformity of the foot, the foot should be stabilized as described earlier (p. 2930).

For partial paralysis below-knee tendon transfer with or without foot stabilization may be helpful. In adults with irreparable peroneal nerve injury a light footdrop brace is helpful, but to rid the patient of a brace stabilization of the foot is necessary. Anterior transfer of a normal tibialis posterior tendon to the dorsolateral aspect of the tarsus by the method of Ober or of Barr removes the deforming influence of this muscle and furnishes some dorsiflexion that in turn improves the appearance of the gait. When no suitable tendons are available for transfer, arthrodesis of the ankle is a satisfactory procedure. If a posterior bone block is used, the deformity may recur in one third of the patients. Tenodesis of the tendons anterior to the ankle joint or the Lambrinudi stabilization is usually unsatisfactory here. Cavus deformity with clawfoot usually develops after irreparable injury to the tibial nerve in the calf, although in adults it usually does not become severe. It may be relieved by arthrodesis or resection and capsulotomy of the interphalangeal joints. When it is severe, the long toe ex-

tensor tendons may be transferred to the midline of the tarsus or to the metatarsal necks, and a plantar fasciotomy may be performed.

REFERENCES
General references

Barr, J.S.: The management of poliomyelitis: the late stage. In Poliomyelitis, First International Poliomyelitis Congress, Philadelphia, 1949, J.B. Lippincott Co.

Bick, E.M.: Source book of orthopaedics, ed. 2, Baltimore, 1948, The Williams & Wilkins Co.

Broderick, T.F., Jr., Reidy, J.A., and Barr, J.S.: Tendon transplantations in the lower extremity: a review of end results in poliomyelitis: Part II. Tendon transplantations at the knee. J. Bone Joint Surg. **34-A:**909, 1952.

Brooks, D.M.: Symposium on reconstructive surgery of paralyzed upper limb: tendon transplantation in the forearm and arthrodesis of the wrist, Proc. R. Soc. Med. **42:**838, 1949.

Codivilla, A.: SVR trapianti tendinei nella practica orthopaedica, Arch. Orthop. **16:**225, 1899.

Close, J.R., and Todd, F.N.: The phasic activity of the muscles of the lower extremity and the effect of tendon transfer, J. Bone Joint Surg. **41-A:**189, 1959.

Elmslie, R.C.: In Turner, G.G., editor: Modern operative surgery, ed. 2, London, 1934, Cassell & Co., Ltd.

Green, W.T., and Grice, D.S.: The management of chronic poliomyelitis. In American Academy of Orthopaedic Surgeons: Instructional course lectures, vol. 9, Ann Arbor, Mich., 1952, J.W. Edwards.

Helferich, H.: Über Muskeltransplantation beim menschen, Verhandl. Deutsch. GlsEllsch. Chir., 1882.

Henderson, M.S.: Reconstructive surgery in paralytic deformities of the lower leg, J. Bone Joint Surg. **11:**810, 1929.

Herndon, C.H.: Tendon transplantation at the knee and foot. In American Academy of Orthopaedic Surgeons: Instructional course lectures, vol. 18, St. Louis, 1961, The C.V. Mosby Co.

Huckstep, R.L.: Poliomyelitis: a guide for developing countries, including appliances and rehabilitation for the disabled, Edinburgh, 1975, Churchill-Livingstone.

Irwin, C.E., and Eyler, D.L.: Surgical rehabilitation of the hand and forearm disabled by poliomyelitis, J. Bone Joint Surg. **33-A:**679, 1951.

Kuhlmann, R.F., and Bell, J.F.: A clinical evaluation of tendon transplantations for poliomyelitis affecting the lower extremities, J. Bone Joint Surg. **34-A:**915, 1952.

Lange, F.: Über periostale sehnenverpflanzung bei Lähmungen, münch. med. Wchnschr. **47:**486, 1900.

Lambrinudi, C.L., and Stamm, T.T.: A report of work in the orthopaedic department of Guy's Hospital, Guy's Hosp. Rep. **89:**184, 1939.

Mayer, L.: Tendon transplantations on the lower extremity. In American Academy of Orthopaedic Surgeons: Instructional course lectures, vol. 6, Ann Arbor, Mich., 1949, J.W. Edwards.

Milliken,: A new operation for deformities, N.Y. Med. Rec., Oct. 26, 1895.

Nicoladoni, K.: Nachtragzum Pes calcaneus und zur Transplantation der peronealsehnen, Arch. Klin. Chir. **27:**660, 1881.

Ober, F.R.: Tendon transplantation in the lower extremity, N. Engl. J. Med. **209:**52, 1933.

Parrish, B.F.: A new operation for paralytic talipes valgus, N.Y. Med. J. **56:**402, 1892.

Peabody, C.W.: Tendon transposition: an end-result study, J. Bone Joint Surg. **20:**193, 1938.

Salvia: Sultrapiantamentode; muscoli, Gaz. degli. Ospedal; 1885.

Scaglietti, O.: Ricupero funzionale di un arto poliomielitico, Boll. Mem. Soc. Emiliano-Romagnola Chir. **1:**4, 1935.

Seddon, H.J.: Reconstructive surgery of the upper extremity. In Poliomyelitis, Second International Poliomyelitis Congress, Philadelphia, 1952, J.B. Lippincott Co.

Steindler, A.: Orthopedic operations: indications, technique, and end results, Springfield, Ill., 1940, Charles C. Thomas, Publisher.

Velpeau, A.A.: Nouveaux Éléments de médicine opératoire, ed. 2, Paris, 1839.

von Baeyer: Described by Peabody, C.W.: Personal communication.

Vulpius, O.: Zur Kasuistik der Schnen transplantation, Münch. med. Wchnsche. **16:**1897.

Foot and ankle

Albert, E.: Einige Fálle leünstliche Ankylosenbildung an paralytischen Gliedmassen, Wien. Med. Press. 23, 1882.

Andersen, J.G.: Foot drop in leprosy and its surgical correction, Acta Orthop. Scand. **33**:151, 1962-1963.

Axer, A.: Into-talus transposition of tendons for correction of paralytic valgus foot after poliomyelitis in children, J. Bone Joint Surg. **42-A**:1119, 1960.

Barr, J.S.: Transference of posterior tibial tendon for paralytic talipes equinovarus. (Personal communication, July and October 1954).

Barr, J.S., and Record, E.E.: Arthrodesis of the ankle for correction of foot deformity, Surg. Clin. North Am. **27**:1281, 1947.

Barr, J.S., and Record, E.E.: Arthrodesis of the ankle joint, N. Engl. J. Med. **248**:53, 1953.

Bentzon, P.G.K.: Pes cavus and the M. peroneus longus, Acta Orthop. Scand. **4**:50, 1933.

Bényi, P.: A modified Lambrinudi operation for drop foot, J. Bone Joint Surg. **42-B**:333, 1960.

Biesalk, K., and Mayer, L.: Die physiologische Sehenverpflanzung, vol. 14, Berlin, 1916, Julius Springer.

Blount, W.P.: Forward transference of posterior tibial tendon for paralytic talipes equinovarus. (Personal communication, July 1954.)

Brewster, A.H.: Countersinking the astragalus in paralytic feet, N. Engl. J. Med. **209**:71, 1933.

Brindley, H., Sr., and Brindley, H., Jr.: Extra-articular subtalar arthrodesis, Orthop. Trans. **6**:188, 1982.

Brittain, H.A.: Architectural principles in arthrodesis, ed. 2, Edinburgh, 1952, E. & S. Livingstone, Ltd.

Broms, J.D.: Subtalar extra-articular arthrodesis: follow-up study, Clin. Orthop. **42**:139, 1965.

Brown, A.: A simple method of fusion of the subtalar joint in children, J. Bone Joint Surg. **50-B**:369, 1968.

Caldwell, G.A.: Arthrodeses of the feet. In American Academy of Orthopaedic Surgeons: Instructional course lectures, vol. 6, Ann Arbor, Mich., 1949, J.W. Edwards.

Campbell, W.C.: An operation for the correction of ''drop-foot,'' J. Bone Joint Surg. **5**:815, 1923.

Campbell, W.C.: End results of operation for correction of drop-foot, JAMA **85**:1927, 1925.

Carayon, A., Bourrel, P., Bourges, M., and Touze, M.: Dual transfer of the posterior tibial and flexor digitorum longus tendons for drop foot: report of thirty-one cases, J. Bone Joint Surg. **49-A**:144, 1967.

Carmack, J.C., and Hallock, H.: Tibiotarsal arthrodesis after astragalectomy: a report of eight cases, J. Bone Joint Surg. **29**:476, 1947.

Cholmeley, J.A.: Elmslie's operation for the calcaneus foot, J. Bone Joint Surg. **35-B**:46, 1953.

Cole, W.H.: The treatment of claw-foot, J. Bone Joint Surg. **22**:895, 1940.

Coonrad, R.W., and Irwin, C.E.: The short toe flexors as an important deforming factor in the paralytic equinovarus foot, Duke Correspondence Club Letter, Sept. 11, 1950.

Coonrad, R.W., Irwin, C.E., Gucker, T., III, and Wray, J.B.: The importance of plantar muscles in paralytic varus feet: the results of treatment by neurectomy and myotenotomy, J. Bone Joint Surg. **38-A**:563, 1956.

Cummins, E.J., et al.: The structure of the calcaneal tendon (of Achilles) in relation to orthopedic surgery, with additional observations on plantaris muscle, Surg. Gynecol. Obstet. **83**:107, 1946.

Crego, C.H., Jr., and McCarroll, H.R.: Recurrent deformities in stabilized paralytic feet: a report of 1100 consecutive stabilizations in poliomyelitis, J. Bone Joint Surg. **20**:609, 1938.

Davis, G.G.: Wedge-shaped resection of the foot for the relief of old cases of varus, N.Y. J. Med. **56**:379, 1892.

Davis, G.G.: The treatment of hollow foot (pes cavus), Am. J. Orthop. Surg. **11**:231, 1913.

Dennyson, W.G., and Fulford, G.E.: Subtalar arthrodesis by cancellous grafts and metallic internal fixation, J. Bone Joint Surg. **58-B**:507, 1976.

Dickson, F.D., and Diveley, R.L.: Operation for correction of mild clawfoot, the result of infantile paralysis, JAMA **87**:1275, 1926.

Drew, A.J.: The late results of arthrodesis of the foot, J. Bone Joint Surg. **33-B**:496, 1951.

Dunn, N.: Suggestions based on ten years' experience of arthrodesis of the tarsus in the treatment of deformities of the foot. In Robert Jones birthday volume, London, 1928, Oxford University Press.

Dwyer, F.C.: Osteotomy of the calcaneum for pes cavus, J. Bone Joint Surg. **41-B**:80, 1959.

Evans, D.: Relapsed club foot, J. Bone Joint Surg. **43-B**:722, 1961.

Evans, D.: Calcaneo-valgus deformity, J. Bone Joint Surg. **57-B**:270, 1975.

Evans, E.L.: Astragalectomy. In Robert Jones' birthday volume, London, 1928, Oxford University Press.

Fitzgerald, F.P., and Seddon, H.J.: Lambrinudi's operation for dropfoot, Br. J. Surg. **25**:283, 1937.

Flint, M.H., and MacKenzie, I.G.: Anterior laxity of the ankle: a cause of recurrent paralytic drop foot deformity, J. Bone Joint Surg. **44-B**:377, 1962.

Forrester-Brown, M.F.: Tendon transplantation for clawing of the great toe, J. Bone Joint Surg. **20**:57, 1938.

Frank, G.R., and Johnson, W.M.: The extensor shift procedure in the correction of clawtoe deformities in children, South. Med. J. **59**:889, 1966.

Fried, A., and Hendel, C.: Paralytic valgus deformity of the ankle: replacement of the paralyzed tibialis posterior by the peronaeus longus, J. Bone Joint Surg. **39-A**:921, 1957.

Fried, A., and Moyseyev, S.: Paralytic valgus deformity of the foot: treatment by replacement of paralyzed tibialis posterior muscle: a long-term follow-up study, J. Bone Joint Surg. **52-A**:1674, 1970.

Friedenbérg, Z.B.: Arthrodesis of the tarsal bones: a study of failure of fusions, Arch. Surg. **57**:162, 1948.

Garceau, G.J., and Brahms, M.A.: Selective plantar denervation (a preliminary report on a new and direct approach in the treatment of cavus deformity), Q. Bull. Ind. Univ. Med. Center **17**:3, 1955.

Garceau, G.J., and Brahms, M.A.: A preliminary study of selective plantar-muscle denervation for pes cavus, J. Bone Joint Surg. **38-A**:553, 1956.

Gill, A.B.: An operation to make a posterior bone block at the ankle to limit foot-drop, J. Bone Joint Surg. **15**:166, 1933.

Goldner, J.L.: Paralytic equinovarus deformities of the foot, South. Med. J. **42**:83, 1949.

Goldner, J.L., and Irwin, C.E.: Paralytic deformities of the foot. In American Academy of Orthopaedic Surgeons: Instructional course lectures, vol. 5, Ann Arbor, Mich., 1948, J.W. Edwards.

Goldner, J.L., and Irwin, C.E.: Clawing of the great toe in paralytic equinovalgus: mechanism and treatment, Duke Correspondence Club Letter, July 7, 1949.

Goldthwait, J.E.: An operation for the stiffening of the ankle joint in infantile paralysis, Am. J. Orthop. Surg. **5**:721, 1907-1908.

Green, W.T., and Grice, D.S.: The surgical correction of the paralytic foot. In American Academy of Orthopaedic Surgeons: Instructional course lectures, vol. 10, Ann Arbor, Mich.,1953, J.W. Edwards.

Green, W.T., and Grice, D.S.: The management of calcaneus deformity. In American Academy of Orthopaedic Surgeons: Instructional course lectures, vol. 13, Ann Arbor, Mich., 1956, J.W. Edwards.

Grice, D.S.: An extra-articular arthrodesis of the subastragalar joint for correction of paralytic flat feet in children, J. Bone Joint Surg. **34-A**:927, 1952.

Grice, D.S.: Further experience with extra-articular arthrodesis of the subtalar joint, J. Bone Joint Surg. **36-A**:246, 1955.

Grice, D.S.: The role of subtalar fusion in the treatment of valgus deformities of the feet. In American Academy of Orthopaedic Surgeons: Instructional course lectures, vol. 16, St. Louis, 1959, The C.V. Mosby Co.

Gross, R.H.: A clinical study of the Batchelor subtalar arthrodesis, J. Bone Joint Surg. **58-A**:343, 1976.

Gunn, D.R., and Molesworth, B.D.: The use of tibialis posterior as a dorsiflexor, J. Bone Joint Surg. **39-B**:674, 1957.

Hallgrimsson, S.: Studies on reconstructive and stabilizing operations on the skeleton of the foot, with special reference to subastragalar arthrodesis in treatment of foot deformities following infantile paralysis, Acta Chir. Scand. (suppl. 78) **88**:1, 1943.

Hammond, G.: Elevation of the first metatarsal bone with hallux equinus, Surgery **13**:240, 1943.

Hart, V.L.: Arthrodesis of the foot in infantile paralysis, Surg. Gynecol. Obstet. **64**:794, 1937.

Hart, V.L.: Lambrinudi operation for drop-foot, J. Bone Joint Surg. **22**:937, 1940.

Hatt, R.N.: Quoted by Thompson, T.C.: Personal communication.

Heyman, C.H.: The operative treatment of clawfoot, J. Bone Joint Surg. **14**:335, 1932.

Hibbs, R.A.: An operation for "claw-foot," JAMA **73**:1583, 1919.

Hill, N.A., Wilson, H.J., Chevres, F., and Sweterlitsch, P.R.: Triple arthrodesis in the young child, Clin. Orthop. **70**:187, 1970.

Hoffer, M.M., et al.: The split anterior tibial tendon transfer in the treatment of spastic varus hindfoot of childhood, Orthop. Clin. North Am. **5**:31, 1974.

Hoke, M.: An operation for stabilizing paralytic feet, J. Orthop. Surg. **3**:494, 1921.

Holmdahl, H.C.: Astragalectomy as a stabilising operation for foot paralysis following poliomyelitis: results of a follow-up investigation of 153 cases, Acta Orthop. Scand. **25**:207, 1956.

Hsu, L.C.S., O'Brien, J.P., Yau, A.C.M.C., and Hodgson, A.R.: Valgus deformity of the ankle in children with fibular pseudarthrosis: results of treatment by bone-grafting of the fibula, J. Bone Joint Surg. **56-A**:503, 1974.

Hsu, L.C.S., O'Brien, J.P., Yau, A.C.M.C., and Hodgson, A.R.: Batchelor's extra-articular subtalar arthrodesis, J. Bone Joint Surg. **58-A**:243, 1976.

Hsu, L.C.S., Yau, A.C.M.C., O'Brien, J.P., and Hodgson, A.R.: Valgus deformity of the ankle resulting from fibular resection for a graft in subtalar fusion in children. J. Bone Joint Surg. **54-A**:585, 1972.

Hunt, J.C., and Brooks, A.L.: Subtalar extraarticular arthrodesis for correction of paralytic valgus deformity of the foot: evaluation of forty-four procedures with particular reference to associated tendon transference, J. Bone Joint Surg. **47-A**:1310, 1965.

Hunt, W.S., Jr., and Thompson, H.A.: Pantalar arthrodesis: a one-stage operation, J. Bone Joint Surg. **36-A**:349, 1954.

Inclan, A.: Artrorisis posterior y anterior del tibilo, La Habana, Cuba, 1939.

Inclan, A.: End results in physiological blocking of flail joints, J. Bone Joint Surg. **31-A**:748, 1949.

Ingersoll, R.E.: Transplantation of peroneus longus to anterior tibial insertion in poliomyelitis, Surg. Gynecol. Obstet. **86**:717, 1948.

Ingram, A.J., and Hundley, J.M.: Posterior bone block of the ankle for paralytic equinus: an end-result study, J. Bone Joint Surg. **33-A**:679, 1951.

Irwin, C.E.: The calcaneus foot, South. Med. J. **44**:191, 1951.

Irwin, C.E.: Equinovalgus deformity in the immature foot: extra-articular subtalar arthrodesis, Piedmont Orthopaedic Society Letter, 1954.

Irwin, C.E.: The calcaneus foot: a revision. In American Academy of Orthopaedic Surgeons: Instructional course lectures, vol. 15, Ann Arbor, Mich., 1958, J.W. Edwards.

Japas, L.M.: Surgical treatment of pes cavus by tarsal V-osteotomy; preliminary report, J. Bone Joint Surg. **50-A**:927, 1968.

Jones, R.: The soldier's foot and the treatment of common deformities of the foot: Part II. Claw-foot, Br. Med. J. **1**:749, 1916.

King, B.B.: Ankle fusion for correction of paralytic drop foot and calcaneus deformities, Arch. Surg. **40**:90, 1940.

Kite, J.H.: Treatment of congenital club feet, J. Bone Joint Surg. **21**:595, 1939.

Kleinberg, S., Horwitz, T., and Sobel, R.: Pes cavus, Bull. Hosp. Joint Dis. **10**:252, 1949.

Lahdenranta, U., and Pylkkänen, P.: Subtalar extra-articular fusion in the treatment of valgus and varus deformities in children: a review of 162 operations in 136 patients, Acta Orthop. Scand. **43**:438, 1972.

Lambrinudi, C.: New operation on drop-foot, Br. J. Surg. **15**:193, 1927.

Lapidus, P.W.: "Dorsal bunion": its mechanics and operative correction, J. Bone Joint Surg. **22**:627, 1940.

Liebolt, F.L.: Pantalar arthrodesis in poliomyelitis, Surgery **6**:31, 1939.

Lipscomb, P.R., and Sanchez, J.J.: Anterior transplantation of the posterior tibial tendon for persistent palsy of the common peroneal nerve, J. Bone Joint Surg. **43-A**:60, 1961.

MacAusland, W.R., and MacAusland, A.R.: Astragalectomy (the Whitman operation) in paralytic deformities of the foot, Ann. Surg. **80**:861, 1924.

MacKenzie, I.G.: Lambrinudi's arthrodesis, J. Bone Joint Surg. **41-B**:738, 1959.

Mann, R.A.: Tendon transfers and electromyography, Clin. Orthop. **85**:64, 1972.

Marek, F.M., and Schein, A.J.: Aseptic necrosis of the astragalus following arthrodesing procedures of the tarsus, J. Bone Joint Surg. **27**:587, 1945.

McFarland, B.: Paralytic instability of the foot (editorial), J. Bone Joint Surg. **33-B**:493, 1951.

Miller, O.L.: Surgical management of pes calcaneus, J. Bone Joint Surg. **18**:169, 1936.

Mortens, J., Gregersen, P., and Zachariae, L.: Tendon transplantation in the foot after poliomyelitis in children, Acta Orthop. Scand. **27**:153, 1957-1958.

Mortens, J., and Pilcher, M.F.: Tendon transplantation in the prevention of foot deformities after poliomyelitis in children, J. Bone Joint Surg. **38-B**:633, 1956.

Niery, K.: Zur Behandlung der Fussdefoemitäten bei ausagedehnten Lähnungen, Arch. Orthop. Unfall. Chir. **3**:60, 1905.

O'Donoghue, D.H., and Stauffer, R.: An improved operative method for obtaining bony fusion of the great toe, Surg. Gynecol. Obstet. **76**:498, 1943.

Osmond-Clarke, H.: Elmslie's operation for the calcaneus foot. (Personal communication, October 1954.)

Osmond-Clarke, H.: Congenital vertical talus, J. Bone Joint Surg. **38-B**:334, 1956.

Paluska, D.J., and Blount, W.P.: Ankle valgus after the Grice subtalar stabilization: the late evaluation of a personal series with a modified technic, Clin. Orthop. **59**:137, 1968.

Patterson, R.L., Jr., Parrish, F.F., and Hathaway, E.N.: Stabilizing operations on the foot: a study of the indications, techniques used, and end results, J. Bone Joint Surg. **32-A**:1, 1950.

Peabody, C.W.: Tendon transposition in the paralytic foot. In American Academy of Orthopaedic Surgeons: Instructional course lectures, vol. 6, Ann Arbor, Mich., 1949, J.W. Edwards.

Pollock, J.H., and Carrell, B.: Subtalar extra-articular arthrodesis in the treatment of paralytic valgus deformities: a review of 112 procedures in 100 patients, J. Bone Joint Surg. **46-A**:533, 1964.

Pyka, R.A., Coventry, M.B., and Moe, J.H.: Anterior subluxation of the talus following triple arthrodesis, J. Bone Joint Surg. **46-A**:16, 1964.

Pyper, J.B.: The flexor-extensor transplant operation for claw toes, J. Bone Joint Surg. **40-B**:528, 1958.

Reidy, J.A., Broderick, T.F., Jr., and Barr, J.S.: Tendon transplantations in the lower extremity: a review of end results in poliomyelitis: Part I. Tendon transplantations about the foot and ankle, J. Bone Joint Surg. **34-A**:900, 1952.

Ryerson, E.W.: Arthrodesing operations on the feet, J. Bone Joint Surg. **5**:453, 1923.

Saunders, J.T.: Etiology and treatment of claw-foot: report of results in 102 feet treated by anterior tarsal resection, Arch. Surg. **30**:179, 1935.

Scheer, G.E., and Crego, C.H., Jr.: A two-stage stabilization procedure for correction of calcaneocavus, J. Bone Joint Surg. **38-A**:1247, 1965.

Schwartz, R.P.: Arthrodesis of subtalus and midtarsal joints of the foot: historical review, preoperative determinations, and operative procedure, Surgery **20**:619, 1946.

Sell, L.S.: Pes cavus, Spectator Correspondence Club Letter, Dec. 11, 1961 (mimeographed).

Seltz, D.G., and Carpenter, E.B.: Triple arthrodesis in children: a ten-year review, South. Med. J. **67**:1420, 1974.

Seymour, N., and Evans, D.K.: A modification of the Grice subtalar arthrodesis, J. Bone Joint Surg. **50-B**:372, 1968.

Sharrard, W.J., and Grosfield, I.: The management of deformity and paralysis of the foot in myelomeningocele, J. Bone Joint Surg. **50-B**:456, 1968.

Sherman, H.M.: The operative treatment of pes cavus, Am. J. Orthop. Surg. **2**:374, 1904-1905.

Siffert, R.S., Forster, R.I., and Nachamie, B.: "Beak" triple arthrodesis for correction of severe cavus deformity, Clin. Orthop. **45**:101, 1966.

Smith, J.B., and Westin, G.W.: Subtalar extra-articular arthrodesis, J. Bone Joint Surg. **50-A**:1027, 1968.

Steindler, A.: Stripping of the os calcis, J. Orthop. Surg. **2**:8, 1920.

Steindler, A.: The treatment of the flail ankle: panastragaloid arthrodesis, J. Bone Joint Surg. **5**:284, 1923.

Stiles, H.J., and Forrester-Brown, M.F.: Treatment of injuries of the spinal peripheral nerves, London, 1922, H. Frowde and Hodder & Stoughton.

Taylor, R.G.: The treatment of claw toes by multiple transfers of flexor into extensor tendons, J. Bone Joint Surg. **33-B**:539, 1951.

Thompson, T.C.: Astragalectomy and the treatment of calcaneovalgus, J. Bone Joint Surg. **21**:627, 1939.

Toupet, R.: Technique d'enchevillement du tarse, Réalisant C'arthrodêse de torsion et la Limitation des movements d'extension dupied. J. Chir. (Paris) **16**:268, 1920.

Turner, J.W., and Cooper, R.R.: Posterior transposition of tibialis anterior through the interosseous membrane, Clin. Orthop. **79:**71, 1971.

Turner, J.W., and Cooper, R.R.: Anterior transfer of the tibialis posterior through the interosseus membrane, Clin. Orthop. **83:**241, 1972.

Von Baeyer, H.: Translokation der Sehnen, Zbl. Chir. **58:**140, 1931.

Von Baeyer, H.: Translokation von Sehen, Z. Orthop. Chir. **56:**552, 1932.

Von Lesser, L.: Ueberoperative Behandlung des Pes varus paralyticus, Zbl. Chir. **6:**497, 1879.

Watkins, M.B., Jones, J.B., Ryder, C.T., Jr., and Brown, T.H., Jr.: Transplantation of the posterior tibial tendon, J. Bone Joint Surg. **36-A:**1181, 1954.

Waugh, T.R., Wagner, J., and Stinchfield, F.E.: An evaluation of pantalar arthrodesis: a follow-up study of one hundred and sixteen operations, J. Bone Joint Surg. **47-A:**1315, 1965.

Westin, W.: Tendo Achilles tenodesis to the fibula, update. (Personal communication, 1985.)

White, J.W.: Disorganization of the foot. In American Academy of Orthopaedic Surgeons: Instructional course lectures, vol. 1, Ann Arbor, Mich., 1944, J.W. Edwards.

Whitman, R.: The operative treatment of paralytic talipes of the calcaneus type, Am. J. Med. Sci. **122:**593, 1901.

Wilson, F.C., Jr., Fay, G.F., Lamotte, P., and Williams, J.C.: Triple arthrodesis: a study of the factors affecting fusion after three hundred and one procedures, J. Bone Joint Surg. **47-A:**340, 1965.

Zachariae, L.: The Grice operation for paralytic flat feet in children, Acta Orthop. Scand. **33:**80, 1963.

Knee

Caldwell, G.D.: Transplantation of the biceps femoris to the patella by the medial route in poliomyelitic quadriceps paralysis, J. Bone Joint Surg. **37-A:**347, 1955.

Conner, A.N.: The treatment of flexion contractures of the knee in poliomyelitis, J. Bone Joint Surg. **52-B:**138, 1970.

Crego, C.H., Jr., and Fischer, F.J.: Transplantation of the biceps femoris for the relief of quadriceps femoris paralysis in residual poliomyelitis, J. Bone Joint Surg. **13:**515, 1931.

Forbes, A.M.: The tensor fasciae femoris as a cause of deformity, J. Bone Joint Surg. **10:**579, 1928.

Harandi, B.A., and Zahir, A.: Severe hypertension following correction of flexion contracture of the knee: a report of two cases, J. Bone Joint Surg. **56-A:**1733, 1974.

Heyman, C.H.: A method for the correction of paralytic genu recurvatum: report of a bilateral case, J. Bone Joint Surg. **6:**689, 1924.

Heyman, C.H.: Operative treatment of paralytic genu recurvanum, J. Bone Joint Surg. **29:**644, 1947.

Heyman, C.H.: Operative treatment of paralytic genu recurvatum, J. Bone Joint Surg. **44-A:**1246, 1962.

Irwin, C.E.: Genu recurvatum following poliomyelitis: controlled method of operative correction, JAMA **120:**277, 1942.

Kleinberg, S.: The transplantation of the adductor longus in its entirety to supplement the quadriceps femoris, Bull. Hosp. Joint Dis. **18:**117, 1957.

Leong, J.C., Alade, C.O., and Fang, D.: Supracondylar femoral osteotomy for knee flexion contracture resulting from poliomyelitis, J. Bone Joint Surg. **64-B:**198, 1982.

Mestikawy, M., and Zeier, F.G.: Tendon transfers for poliomyelitis of the lower limb in Guinean children, Clin. Orthop. **75:**188, 1971.

Ober, F.R.: Tendon transplantation in the lower extremity, N. Engl. J. Med. **209:**52, 1933.

Perry, J., O'Brien, J.P., and Hodgson, A.R.: Triple tenodesis of the knee: a soft-tissue operation for the correction of paralytic genu recurvatum, J. Bone Joint Surg. **58-A:**978, 1976.

Riska, E.B.: Transposition of the tractus iliotibialis to the patella as a treatment of quadriceps paralysis and certain deformities of the lower extremity after poliomyelitis, Acta Orthop. Scand. **32:**140, 1962.

Schwartzmann, J.R., and Crego, C.H., Jr.: Hamstring-tendon transplantation for the relief of quadriceps femoris paralysis in residual poliomyelitis: a follow-up study of 134 cases, J. Bone Joint Surg. **30-A:**541, 1948.

Støren, G.: Genu recurvatum: treatment by wedge osteotomy of tibia with use of compression, Acta Chir. Scand. **114:**40, 1957.

Sutherland, D.H., Bost, F.C., and Schottstaedt, E.R.: Electromyographic study of transplanted muscles about the knee in poliomyelitic patients, J. Bone Joint Surg. **42-A:**919, 1960.

Wray, J.B.: Hamstrings transfer in the management of paralysis of the quadriceps due to poliomyelitis, March 1, 1955 (mimeographed).

Yount, C.C.: An operation to improve function in quadriceps paralysis, J. Bone Joint Surg. **20:**314, 1938.

Zarzecki, C.A., and Irwin, C.E.: Paralytic genu recurvatum and its treatment, Duke Correspondence Club Letter, Nov. 14, 1949.

Tibia and femur

Gailey, H.A., Jr., Musgrave, R.E., and Irwin, C.E.: Correction of deformities about the knee resulting from poliomyelitis, Duke Correspondence Club Letter, April 1, 1953.

Harandi, B.A.: Personal communication, 1977.

Lucas, L.S., and Cottrell, G.W.: Notched rotation osteotomy: a method employed in the correction of torsion of the tibia and other conditions, West. J. Surg. **57:**5, 1949.

O'Donoghue, D.H.: Controlled rotation osteotomy of the tibia, South. Med. J. **33:**1145, 1940.

Hip

Barr, J.S.: Poliomyelitic hip deformity and the erector spinae transplant, JAMA **144:**813, 1950.

Bjerkreim, I.: Secondary dysplasia and osteoarthrosis of the hip joint in functional and in fixed obliquity of the pelvis, Acta Orthop. Scand. **45:**873, 1974.

Cabaud, H.E., Westin, G.W., and Connelly, S.: Tendon transfers in the paralytic hip, J. Bone Joint Surg. **61-A:**1035, 1979.

Campbell, W.C.: Transference of the crest of the ilium for flexion contracture of the hip, South. Med. J. **166:**235, 1912.

Eberle, C.F.: Pelvic obliquity and the unstable hip after poliomyelitis, J. Bone Joint Surg. **64-B:**300, 1982.

Fitchet, S.M.: ''Flexion deformity'' of the hip and the lateral intermuscular septum, N. Engl. J. Med. **209:**74, 1933.

Forbes, A.M.: The tensor fasciae femoris as a cause of deformity, J. Bone Joint Surg. **10:**579, 1928.

Groves, E.W.H.: Some contributions to the reconstructive surgery of the hip. Br. J. Surg. **14:**486, 1926-1927.

Hallock, H.: Surgical stabilization of dislocated paralytic hips: end-result study, Surg. Gynecol. Obstet. **75:**742, 1942.

Hallock, H.: Arthrodesis of the hip for instability and pain in poliomyelitis, J. Bone Joint Surg. **32-A:**904, 1950.

Hammesfahr, R., Topple, S., Yoo, K., Whitesides, T., and Paullin, A.M.: Abductor paralysis and the role of the external abdominal oblique transfer, Orthopedics **6:**315, 1983.

Hogshead, H.P., and Ponseti, I.V.: Fascia lata transfer to the erector spinae for the treatment of flexion-abduction contractures of the hip in patients with poliomyelitis and meningomyelocele: evaluation of results, J. Bone Joint Surg. **46-A:**1389, 1964.

Irwin, C.E.: The iliotibial band, its role in producing deformity in poliomyelitis, J. Bone Joint Surg. **31-A:**141, 1949.

Johnson, E.W., Jr.: Contractures of the iliotibial band, Surg. Gynecol. Obstet. **96:**599, 1953.

Jones, G.B.: Paralytic dislocation of the hip, J. Bone Joint Surg. **36-B:**375, 1954.

Jones, G.B.: Paralytic dislocation of the hip, J. Bone Joint Surg. **44-B:**573, 1962.

Kreuscher, P.H.: The substitution of the erector spinae for paralyzed gluteal muscles, Surg. Gynecol. Obstet. **40:**593, 1925.

Lange, F.: Die Technik dés orthopädischen Eingriffs, P.J. Eriacher, Vienna, 1928, Julius Springer.

Lange, F.: Epidemic infantile paralysis, Munich, 1930, J.F. Lehmanns Verlag.

Lange, F.: American and German orthopedic surgery, J. Bone Joint Surg. **13:**479, 1931.

Lange, M.: Die Bedeutung and Behandlung der Hüftbeugekontraktur nach Poliomyelitis, Z. Orthop. Chir. **47:**86, 1925.

Legg, A.T.: Transplantation of tensor fasciae femoris in cases of weakened gluteus medius, JAMA **80:**242, 1923.

Legg, A.T.: Tensor fasciae femoris transplantation in cases of weakened gluteus medius, N. Engl. J. Med. **209:**61, 1933.

Lowman, C.L.: Lateral transplant for controlling a gluteus medius limp, Physiother. Rev. **27:**355, 1947.

Milch, H.: Osteotomy of the long bones, Springfield, Ill., 1947, Charles C Thomas, Publishers.

Miller, G.R., and Irwin, C.E.: Paralytic dislocations of the hip, Duke Correspondence Club Letter, Sept. 6, 1948.

Mustard, W.T.: Iliopsoas transfer for weakness of the hip abductors: preliminary report, J. Bone Joint Surg. **34-A**:647, 1952.

Mustard, W.T.: A follow-up study of iliopsoas transfer for hip instability, J. Bone Joint Surg. **41-B**:289, 1959.

Ober, F.R.: An operation for relief of paralysis of the gluteus maximus muscle, JAMA **88**:1063, 1927.

Parker, B., and Walker, G.: Posterior psoas transfer and hip instability in lumbar myelomeningocele, J. Bone Joint Surg. **57-B**:53, 1975.

Parsons, D.W., and Seddon, H.J.: The results of operations for disorders of the hip caused by poliomyelitis, J. Bone Joint Surg. **50-B**:266, 1968.

Samilson, R.L., Tsou, P., Aamoth, G., and Green, W.M.: Dislocation and subluxation of the hip in cerebral palsy: pathogenesis, natural history and management, J. Bone Joint Surg. **54-A**:863, 1972.

Sharp, N., Guhl, J.F., Sorensen, R.I., and Voshell, A.F.: Hip fusion in poliomyelitis in children: a preliminary report, J. Bone Joint Surg. **46-A**:121, 1964.

Sharrard, W.J.: Posterior iliopsoas transplantation in the treatment of paralytic dislocation of the hip, J. Bone Joint Surg. **46-B**:426, 1964.

Smith, E.T., Pevey, J.K., and Shindler, T.O.: The erector spinae transplant—a misnomer, Clin. Orthop. **30**:144, 1963.

Soutter, R.: A new operation for hip contractures in poliomyelitis, Boston Med. Surg. J. **170**:380, 1914.

Speed, J.S.: End results in transference of the crest of the ilium for flexion contracture of the hip, J. Bone Joint Surg. **10**:202, 1928.

Thomas, L.I., Thompson, T.C., and Straub, L.R.: Transplantation of the external oblique muscle for abductor paralysis, J. Bone Joint Surg. **32-A**:207, 1950.

Tohen, A., Carmona, J., Rosas, J., and Conzueo, S.: Supracondylar osteotomy of the femur for retroversion of the femoral head in the paralytic hip, Clin. Orthop. **59**:177, 1968.

Wagner, L.C., and Rizzo, P.C.: Stabilization of the hip by transplantation of the anterior thigh muscles, J. Bone Joint Surg. **18**:180, 1936.

Weissman, S.L.: Capsular arthroplasty in paralytic dislocation of the hip: a preliminary report, J. Bone Joint Surg. **41-A**:429, 1959.

Weissman, S.L., Torok, G., and Khermosh, O.: Intertrochanteric osteotomy in fixed paralytic obliquity of the pelvis: a preliminary report, J. Bone Joint Surg. **43-A**:1135, 1961.

Yount, C.C.: The role of the tensor fasciae femoris in certain deformities of the lower extremity, J. Bone Joint Surg. **8**:171, 1926.

Trunk

Axer, A.: Transposition of gluteus maximus, tensor fasciae latae and iliotibial band for paralysis of lateral abdominal muscles in children after poliomyelitis: a preliminary report, J. Bone Joint Surg. **40-B**:644, 1958.

Chaves, J.P.: Pectoralis minor transplant for paralysis of the serratus anterior, J. Bone Joint Surg. **33-B**:228, 1951.

Clark, J.M.P., and Axer, A.: A muscle-tendon transposition for paralysis of the lateral abdominal muscles in poliomyelitis, J. Bone Joint Surg. **38-B**:475, 1956.

Dickson, F.D.: Fascial transplants in paralytic and other conditions, J. Bone Joint Surg. **19**:405, 1937.

Eaton, G.O.: Results of abdominal stabilizations, South. Med. J. **34**:443, 1941.

Gratz, C.M.: Tensile strength and elasticity tests on human fascia lata, J. Bone Joint Surg. **13**:334, 1931.

Irwin, C.E.: Subtrochanteric osteotomy in poliomyelitis, JAMA **133**:231, 1947.

Lowman, C.L.: Abdominal fascial transplants, Los Angeles, 1954, privately printed.

Mayer, L.: The significance of the iliocostal fascial graft in the treatment of paralytic deformities of the trunk, J. Bone Joint Surg. **26**:257, 1944.

Perry, J., and Nickel, V.L.: Total cervical-spine fusion for neck paralysis, J. Bone Joint Surg. **41-A**:37, 1959.

Perry, J., Nickel, V.L., and Garrett, A.L.: Capital fascial transplants adjunct to spine fusion in flaccid neck paralysis, Clin. Orthop. **24**:128, 1962.

Rapp, I.H.: Serratus anterior paralysis treated by transplantation of the pectoralis minor, J. Bone Joint Surg. **36-A**:852, 1954.

Weissman, S.L., Torok, G., and Khermosh, O.: Intertrochanteric osteotomy in fixed paralytic obliquity of the pelvis: a preliminary report, J. Bone Joint Surg. **43-A**:1135, 1961.

Williamson, G.A., Moe, J.H., and Basom, W.C.: Results of the Lowman operation for paralysis of the abdominal muscles, Minn. Med. **25**:117, 1942.

Shoulder

Barr, J.S., Freiberg, J.A., Colonna, P.C., and Pemberton, P.A.: A survey of end results on stabilization of the paralytic shoulder, report of the research committee of the American Orthopaedic Association, J. Bone Joint Surg. **24**:699, 1942.

Bateman, J.E.: The shoulder and environs, St. Louis, 1954, The C.V. Mosby Co.

Dewar, F.P., and Harris, R.I.: Restoration of function of the shoulder following paralysis of the trapezius by fascial sling fixation and transplantation of the levator scapulae, Ann. Surg. **132**:1111, 1950.

Haas, S.L.: The treatment of permanent paralysis of the deltoid muscle, JAMA **104**:99, 1935.

Haas, S.L.: Serratus anterior paralysis, Orthopaedic Correspondence Club Letter, March 15, 1949.

Harmon, P.H.: Anterior transplantation of the posterior deltoid for shoulder palsy and dislocation in poliomyelitis, Surg. Gynecol. Obstet. **84**:117, 1947.

Harmon, P.H.: Surgical reconstruction of the paralytic shoulder by multiple muscle transplantations, J. Bone Joint Surg. **32-A**:583, 1950.

Henry, A.K.: An operation for slinging a dropped shoulder, Br. J. Surg. **15**:95, 1927.

Hohmann, G.: Ersatz des gelähmten Biceps brachii durch den pectoralis major, München. Med. Wschr. **65**:1240, 1918.

Makin, M.: Early arthrodesis for a flail shoulder in young children, J. Bone Joint Surg. **59-A**:317, 1977.

Mayer, L.: The physiological method of tendon transplantation, Surg. Gynecol. Obstet. **22**:182, 1916.

Ober, F.R.: An operation to relieve paralysis of the deltoid muscle, JAMA **99**:2182, 1932.

Ober, F.R.: Transplantation to improve the function of the shoulder joint and extensor function of the elbow joint. In American Academy of Orthopaedic Surgeons: Instructional course lectures, vol. 2, Ann Arbor, Mich., 1944, J.W. Edwards.

Saha, A.K.: Surgery of the paralyzed and flail shoulder, Acta Orthop. Scand., suppl. 97, 1967.

Schottsdaet, E.R., Larsen, L.J., and Bost, F.C.: Complete muscle transplantation, J. Bone Joint Surg. **37-A**:897, 1955.

Schottsdaet E.R., Larsen L.J., and Bost, F.C.: The surgical reconstruction of the upper extremity paralyzed by poliomyelitis, J. Bone Joint Surg. **40-A**:633, 1958.

Slomann: Ueber die Bahandlung der Deltoidenslähmheit, Z. Orthop. Chir. **35**:1916. Cited by Haas, S.L.: The treatment of permanent paralysis of the deltoid muscle, JAMA **104**:99, 1935.

Steindler, A.: The reconstruction of upper extremity in spinal and cerebral paralysis. In American Academy of Orthopaedic Surgeons: Instructional course lectures, vol. 6, Ann Arbor, Mich., 1949, J.W. Edwards.

Steindler, A.: Reconstruction of the poliomyelitic upper extremity, Bull. Hosp. Joint Dis. **15**:21, 1954.

Vastamäki, M.: Pectoralis minor transfer in serratus anterior paralysis, Acta Orthop. Scand. **55**:293, 1984.

Whitman, A.: Congenital elevation of scapula and paralysis of serratus magnus muscle, JAMA **99**:1332, 1932.

Elbow and forearm

Ahmad, I.: Restoration of elbow flexion by a new operative technique, Clin. Orthop. **106**:186, 1975.

d'Aubigne, R.M.: Treatment of residual paralysis after injuries of the main nerves (superior extremity), Proc. R. Soc. Med. **42**:831, 1949.

Blount, W.P.: Osteoclasis for supination deformities in children, J. Bone Joint Surg. **22**:300, 1940.

Brooks, D.M., and Seddon, H.J.: Pectoral transplantation for paralysis of the flexors of the elbow: a new technique, J. Bone Joint Surg. **41-B**:36, 1959.

Bunnell, S.: Restoring flexion to the paralytic elbow, J. Bone Joint Surg. **33-A**:566, 1951.

Burns, R.E.: Orthopaedic Correspondence Club Letter, 1946.

Carroll, R.E.: Restoration of flexor power to the flail elbow by transplantation of the triceps tendon, Surg. Gynecol. Obstet. **95**:685, 1952.

Carroll, R.E., and Gartland, J.J.: Flexorplasty of the elbow: an evaluation of a method, J. Bone Joint Surg. **35-A**:706, 1953.

Carroll, R.E., and Hill, N.A.: Triceps transfer to restore elbow flexion: a study of fifteen patients with paralytic lesions and arthrogryposis, J. Bone Joint Surg. **52-A**:239, 1970.

Castro-Sierra, A., and Lopez-Pita, A.: A new surgical technique to correct triceps paralysis, Hand **15:**42, 1983.

Clark, J.M.P.: Reconstruction of biceps brachii by pectoral muscle transplantation, Br. J. Surg. **34:**180, 1946.

duToit, G.T., and Levy, S.J.: Transposition of latissimus dorsi for paralysis of triceps brachii: report of a case, J. Bone Joint Surg. **49-B:**135, 1967.

Dutton, R.O., and Dawson, E.B.: Elbow flexorplasty: an analysis of long-term results, J. Bone Joint Surg. **63-A:**1064, 1981.

Eyler, D.L.: Modified Steindler flexorplasty. (Personal communication, September 1954.)

Eyler, D.L., and Irwin, C.E.: Modification of Steindler flexorplasty, Duke Correspondence Club Letter, October 19, 1950.

Friedenberg, Z.B.: Transposition of the biceps brachii for triceps weakness, J. Bone Joint Surg. **36-A:**656, 1954.

Green, W.T., and Banks, H.H.: flexor carpi wuloris transplant in cerebral palsy, J. Bone Joint Surg. **44-A:**1343, 1962.

Grilli, F.P.: Il trapianto del bicipite brachiale in funzione pronatoria, Arch. Putti **12:**359, 1959.

Harmon, P.H.: Muscle transplantation for triceps palsy: the technique of utilizing the latissimus dorsi, J. Bone Joint Surg. **31-A:**409, 1949.

Hohmann, G.: Ersatz des gelähmten Biceps brachii durch den Pectoralis major, Munch. Med. Wochenschr. **65:**1240, 1918.

Hovnanian, A.P.: Latissimus dorsi transplantation for loss of flexion or extension at the elbow: a preliminary report on technic, Ann. Surg. **143:**493, 1956.

Kettelkamp, D.B., and Larson, C.B.: Evaluation of the Steindler flexorplasty, J. Bone Joint Surg. **45-A:**513, 1963.

Lange, F.: Die Technik des orthopädischen Eingriffs, P.J. Eriacher, Vienna, 1928, Julius Springer.

Lange, F.: Epidemic infantile paralysis, Munich, 1930, J.F. Lehmanns Verlag.

Lange, F.: American and German orthopedic surgery, J. Bone Joint Surg. **13:**479, 1931.

Lindholm, T.S., and Einola, S.: Flexorplasty of paralytic elbows: analysis of late functional results, Acta Orthop. Scand. **44:**1, 1973.

Mayer, L., and Green, W.: Experiences with the Steindler flexorplasty at the elbow, J. Bone Joint Surg. **36-A:**775, 1954.

Moberg, E.: Surgical treatment for absent single hand grip and elbow extension in quadriplegia, J. Bone Joint Surg. **57-A:**196, 1975.

Nyholm, K.: Elbow flexorplasty in tendon transposition: an analysis of the functional result in 26 patients, Acta Orthop. Scand. **33:**30, 1963.

Ober, F.R., and Barr, J.S.: Brachioradialis muscle transposition for triceps weakness, Surg. Gynecol. Obstet. **67:**105, 1938.

Owings, R., Wickstrom, J., Perry, J., and Nickel, V.L.: Biceps brachii rerouting in treatment of paralytic supination contracture of the forearm, J. Bone Joint Surg. **53-A:**137, 1971.

Raczka, R., Braun, R., and Waters, R.L.: Posterior deltoid-to-triceps transfer in quadriplegia, Clin. Orthop. **187:**163, 1984.

Samii, K.: Transplantation of the clavicular head of the pectoralis major for paralysis of the elbow flexors, Am. Dig. Foreign Orthop. Lit., 2nd qtr., p. 61, 1970.

Schottstaedt, E.R., Larsen, L.J., and Bost, F.C.: Complete muscle transposition, J. Bone Joint Surg. **37-A:**897, 1955.

Schottstaedt, E.R., Larsen, L.J., and Bost, F.C.: The surgical reconstruction of the upper extremity paralyzed by poliomyelitis, J. Bone Joint Surg. **40-A:**633, 1958.

Seddon, H.J.: Transplantation of pectoralis major for paralysis of the flexors of the elbow, Proc. R. Soc. Med. **42:**837, 1949.

Segal, A., Seddon, H.J., and Brooks, D.M: Treatment of paralysis of the flexors of the elbow, J. Bone Joint Surg. **41-B:**44, 1959.

Spira, E.: Replacement of biceps brachii by pectoralis minor transplant: report of a case, J. Bone Joint Surg. **39-B:**126, 1957.

Steindler, A.: Muscle and tendon transplantation at the elbow. In American Academy of Orthopaedic Surgeons: Instructional course lectures, vol. 2, Ann Arbor, Mich., 1944, J.W. Edwards.

Zancolli, E.A.: Paralytic supination contracture of the forearm, J. Bone Joint Surg. **49-A:**1275, 1967.

Zancolli, E., and Mitre, H.: Latissimus dorsi transfer to restore elbow flexion: an appraisal of eight cases, J. Bone Joint Surg. **55-A:**1265, 1973.

Spina bifida occulta

Bucy, P.C.: Spina bifida and associated malformations. In Brennemann, J., editor: Practice of pediatrics, Hagerstown, Md., 1939, W.F. Prior Co., Inc.

Dawson, C.W., and Dreisbach, J.H.: Diastematomyelia and acquired club foot deformity: reports of two cases indicate that early surgical procedures offer children the possibilities of normal gait and stance, JAMA **175:**569, 1961.

Garceau, G.J.: Filum terminale syndrome (cord traction syndrome), J. Bone Joint Surg. **35-A:**711, 1953.

Hilal, S.K., Marton, D., and Pollack, E.: Diastematomyelia in children: radiographic study of 34 cases, Radiology **112:**609, 1974.

Hoffman, H.J., Hendrick, E.B., and Humphreys, R.P.: The tethered spinal cord: its protean manifestations, diagnosis and surgical corrections, Child's Brain **2:**145, 1976.

Holman, C.B., Svien, H.J., Bickel, W.H., and Keith, H.M.: Diastematomyelia, Pediatrics **15:**191, 1955.

James, C.C., and Lassman, L.P.: Spinal dysraphism: the diagnosis and treatment of progressive lesions in spina bifida occulta, J. Bone Joint Surg. **44-B:**828, 1962.

Jones, P.H., and Love, J.G.: Tight filum terminale, Arch. Surg. **73:**556, 1956.

Lichtenstein, B.W.: Spinal dysraphism: spina bifida and myelodysplasia, Arch. Neurol. Psychiat. **44:**792, 1940.

Love, J.G., Daly, D.D., and Harris, L.E.: Tight filum terminale: report of condition in three siblings, JAMA **176:**31, 1961.

Neuhauser, E.B., Wittenborg, M.H., and Dehlinger, K.: Diastematomyelia, Radiology **54:**659, 1950.

Ogston, A.: A new principle of curing club-foot in severe cases in children a few years old, Br. Med. J. **1:**1524, 1902.

Perret, G.: Diagnosis and treatment of diastematomyelia, Surg. Gynecol. Obstet. **105:**69, 1957.

Perret, G.: Symptoms and diagnosis of diastematomyelia, Neurology **10:**51, 1960.

Verebelyi, L.: Angeborner Klupfuss, dirch: subperios tales evidement des talus gehult, Pester Med. Chir. Presse **14:**224, 1877.

Myelomeningocele

Allan, J.H.: The challenge of spina bifida cystica. In Adams, J.P., editor: Current practice in orthopaedic surgery, vol. 1, St. Louis, 1963, The C.V. Mosby Co.

American Academy of Orthopaedic Surgeons: Symposium on myelomeningocele, St Louis, 1972, The C.V. Mosby Co.

Aprin, H., and Kilfoyle, R.M.: Extension contracture of the knees in patients with meningomyelocele, Clin. Orthop. **144:**260, 1979.

Asher, M., and Olson, J.: Factors affecting the ambulatory status of patients with spina bifida cystica, J. Bone Joint Surg. **65-A:**350, 1983.

Banta, J.V., Sutherland, D.H., and Wyatt, M.: Anterior tibial transfer to the os calcis with Achilles tenodesis for calcaneal deformity in myelomeningocele, J. Pediatr. Orthop. **1:**125, 1981.

Benton, L.J., Salvati, E.A., and Root, L.: Reconstructive surgery in the myelomeningocele hip, Clin. Orthop. **110:**261, 1975.

Brock, D.J.H., and Sutcliffe, R.G.: Alpha-fetoprotein in the antenatal diagnosis of anencephaly and spina bifida, Lancet **2:**197, 1972.

Brocklehurst, G., editor: Spina bifida for the clinician, Philadelphia, 1976, J.B. Lippincott Co.

Bunch, W.H., and Hakala, M.W.: Iliopsoas transfers in children with myelomeningocele, J. Bone Joint Surg. **66-A:**224, 1984.

Bunch, W.H., et al.: Modern management of myelomeningocele, St. Louis, 1972, Warren H. Green, Inc.

Burney, D.W., Jr., and Hamsa, W.R.: Spina bifida with myelomeningocele, Clin. Orthop. **30:**167, 1963.

Canale, S.T., Hammond, N.L., III, Cotler, J.M., and Snedden, H.E.: Pelvic displacement osteotomy for chronic hip dislocation in myelodysplasia, J. Bone Joint Surg. **57-A:**177, 1975.

Carroll, N.C., and Sharrard, W.J.W.: Long-term follow-up of posterior iliopsoas transplantation for paralytic dislocation of the hip, J. Bone Joint Surg. **54-A:**551, 1972.

Carter, C.O., Laurence, K.M., and David, P.A.: The genetics of the major central nervous system malformations. Based on the South Wales Sociogenetic Investigation, Dev. Med. Child Neurol. (suppl. 13) **9:**30, 1967.

Cruess, R.L., and Turner, N.S.: Paralysis of hip abductor muscles in spina bifida: results of treatment by the Mustard procedure, J. Bone Joint Surg. **52-A:**1364, 1970.

Curtis, B.H.: The hip in the myelomeningocele child, Clin. Orthop. **90:**11, 1973.

Curtis, B.H., and Fisher, R.L.: Congenital hyperextension with anterior subluxation of the knee: surgical treatment and long-term observations, J. Bone Joint Surg. **51-A:**255, 1969.

Dias, L.: Surgical management of knee contractures in myelomeningocele, J. Pediatr. Orthop. **2:**127, 1982.

Dias, L.S., and Hill, J.S.: Evaluation of treatment of hip for subluxation in myelomeningocele by intertrochanteric varus derotation femoral osteotomy, Orthop. Clin. North Am. **11:**31, 1980.

Donaldson, W.F.: Hip problems in the child with myelomeningocele. In American Academy of Orthopedic Surgeons: Symposium on myelomeningocele, St. Louis, 1972, The C.V. Mosby Co.

Drennan, J.C., and Sharrard, W.J.W.: The pathological anatomy of convex pes valgus, J. Bone Joint Surg. **53-B:**455, 1971.

Drummond, D.F., Moreau, M., and Cruess, R.L.: The results and complications of surgery for the paralytic hip and spine in myelomeningocele, J. Bone Joint Surg. **62-B:**49, 1980.

Duckworth, T., and Smith, T.W.D.: The treatment of paralytic convex pes valgus, J. Bone Joint Surg. **56-B:**305, 1974.

Dupré, P., and Walker, G.: Knee problems associated with spina bifida, Dev. Med. Child Neurol. (suppl. 27) **14:**152, 1972.

Dwyer, A.F., Newton, N.C., and Sherwood, A.A.: An anterior approach to scoliosis: a preliminary report, Clin. Orthop. **62:**192, 1969.

Feiwell, E.: Surgery of the hip in myelomeningocele as related to adult goals, Clin. Orthop. **148:**87, 1980.

Feiwell, E.: Selection of appropriate treatment for patients with myelomeningocele, Orthop. Clin. North Am. **12:**101, 1981.

Freehafer, A.A., Vessely, J.C., and Mack, R.P.: Iliopsoas muscle transfer in the treatment of myelomeningocele patients with paralytic hip deformities, J. Bone Joint Surg. **54-A:**1715, 1972.

Freeman, J.M.: Practical management of meningomyelacele, Baltimore, 1974, University Park Press.

Hay, M.C., and Walker, G.: Plantar pressures in healthy children and in children with myelomeningocele, J. Bone Joint Surg. **55-B:**828, 1973.

Hayes, J.T., and Gross, P.H.: Orthopaedic implications of myelodysplasia, JAMA **184:**762, 1963.

Hayes, J.T., Gross, P.H., and Dow, S.: Surgery for paralytic defects secondary to myelomeningocele and myelodysplasia, J. Bone Joint Surg. **46-A:**1577, 1964.

Hogshead, H.P., and Ponseti, I.V.: Fascia lata transfer to the erector spinae for the treatment of flexion-abduction contractures of the hip in patients with poliomyelitis and meningomyelocele: evaluation of results, J. Bone Joint Surg. **46-A:**1389, 1964.

Hoppenfeld, S.: Congenital kyphosis in myelomeningocele, J. Bone Joint Surg. **49-B:**276, 1967.

Jackson, R.D., Padgett, T.S., and Donovan, M.M.: Posterior iliopsoas transfer in myelodysplasia, J. Bone Joint Surg. **61-A:**40, 1979.

Kilfoyle, R.M., Foley, J.J., and Norton, P.L.: Spine and pelvic deformity in childhood and adolescent paraplegia: a study of 104 cases, J. Bone Joint Surg. **47-A:**659, 1965.

Laurence, K.M.: The genetics of spina bifida occulta, Dev. Med. Child Neurol. **9:**645, 1967.

Laurence, K.M.: The recurrence risk in spina bifida cystica and anencephaly, Dev. Med. Child Neurol. (suppl. 20) **11:**23, 1969.

Laurence, K.M., and Carter, C.O.: Some environmental factors in the incidence of central nervous system malformations in South Wales, Dev. Med. Child Neurol. (suppl. 15) **10:**83, 1968.

Levitt, R.L., Canale, S.T., and Gartland, J.J.: Surgical correction of foot deformity in the older patient with myelomeningocele, Orthop. Clin. North Am. **5:**19, 1974.

London, J.T., and Nichols, O.: Paralytic dislocation of the hip in myelodysplasia: the role of the adductor transfer, J. Bone Joint Surg. **57-A:**501, 1975.

Lorber, J.: Some paediatric aspects of myelomeningocele, Acta Orthop. Scand. **46:**350, 1975.

Lorber, J., Stewart, C.R., and Ward, A.M.: Alpha-fetoprotein in antenatal diagnosis of anencephaly and spina bifida, Lancet **1:**1187, 1973.

Menelaus, M.: The orthopaedic management of spina bifida cystica, ed. 2, Edinburgh, 1980, Churchill-Livingstone.

Menelaus, M.B.: Talectomy for equinovarus deformity in arthrogryposis and spina bifida, J. Bone Joint Surg. **53-B:**468, 1971.

Menelaus, M.B.: Progress in the management of the paralytic hip in myelomeningocele, Orthop. Clin. North Am. **11:**17, 1980.

Parker, B., and Walker, G.: Posterior psoas transfer and hip instability in lumbar myelomeningocele, J. Bone Joint Surg. **57-B:**53, 1975.

Parsch, K., and Manner, G.: Prevention and treatment of knee problems in children with spina bifida, Dev. Med. Child Neurol. (suppl. 37) **18:**114, 1976.

Parsons, D.W., and Seddon, H.J.: The results of operations for disorders of the hip caused by poliomyelitis, J. Bone Joint Surg. **50-B:**266, 1968.

Rueda, J., and Carroll, N.C.: Hip instability in patients with myelomeningocele, J. Bone Joint Surg. **54-B:**422, 1972.

Sharrard, W.J.W.: Posterior iliopsoas transplantation in the treatment of paralytic dislocation of the hip, J. Bone Joint Surg. **46-B:**426, 1964.

Sharrard, W.J.W.: Paralytic deformity in the lower limb, J. Bone Joint Surg. **49-B:**731, 1967.

Sharrard, W.J.W.: Spinal osteotomy for congenital kyphosis in myelomeningocele, J. Bone Joint Surg. **50-B:**466, 1968.

Sharrard, W.J.W.: The orthopaedic surgery of spina bifida, Clin. Orthop. **92:**195, 1973.

Sharrard, W.J.W.: The orthopaedic management of spina bifida, Acta Orthop. Scand. **46:**356, 1975.

Sharrard, W.J.W., and Drennan, J.C.: Osteotomy-excision of the spine for lumbar kyphosis in older children with myelomeningocele, J. Bone Joint Surg. **54-B:**50, 1972.

Sharrard, W.J.W., and Grosfield, I.: The management of deformity and paralysis of the foot in myelomeningocele, J. Bone Joint Surg. **50-B:**456, 1968.

Sharrard, W.J.W., Zachary, R.B., and Lorber, J.: The long-term evaluation of a trial of immediate and delayed closure of spina bifida cystica, Clin. Orthop. **50:**197, 1967.

Sharrard, W.J.W., Zachary, R.B., and Lorber, J.: Survival and paralysis in open myelomeningocele with special reference to the time of repair of the spinal lesion, Dev. Med. Child Neurol. (suppl. 13) **9:**35, 1967.

Sharrard, W.J.W., Zachary, R.B., Lorber, J., and Bruce, A.M.: A controlled trial of immediate and delayed closure of spina bifida cystica, Arch. Dis. Child **38:**18, 1963.

Smithells, R.W., D'Arcy, E.E., and McAllister, E.F.: The outcome of pregnancies before and after the birth of infants with nervous system malformations, Dev. Med. Child Neurol. (suppl. 15) **10:**6, 1968.

Smyth, B.T., Piggot, J., Forsythe, W.I., and Merrett, J.D.: A controlled trial of immediate and delayed closure of myelomeningocele, J. Bone Joint Surg. **56-B:**297, 1974.

Stillwell, A., and Menelaus, M.: Walking ability after transplantation of the iliopsoas, J. Bone Joint Surg. **66-B:**656, 1984.

Trumble, T., Banta, J.V., Raycroft, J.F., and Curtis, B.H.: Talectomy for equinovarus deformity in myelodysplasia, J. Bone Joint Surg. **67-A:**21, 1985.

Walker, G.: The early management of varus feet in myelomeningocele, J. Bone Joint Surg. **53-B:**462, 1971.

Wissinger, L.A., Turner, T., and Donaldson, W.F.: Posterior iliopsoas transfer: a treatment for some myelodysplastic hips, Orthopedics **3:**865, 1980.

Yngve, D.A., and Lindseth, R.E.: Effectiveness of muscle transfers in myelomeningocele hips measured by radiographic indices, J. Pediatr. Orthop. **2:**121, 1982.

Arthrogryposis multiplex congenita

Banker, B.Q.: Neuropathologic aspects of arthrogryposis multiplex congenita, Clin. Orthop. **194:**30, 1985.

Bayne, L.G.: Hand assessment and management in arthrogryposis multiplex congenita, Clin. Orthop. **194:**68, 1985.

Brown, L.M., Robson, M.J., and Sharrard, W.J.W.: The pathophysiology of arthrogryposis multiplex congenita neurologica, J. Bone Joint Surg. **62-B:**291, 1980.

Carlson, W.O., Speck, G.J., Vicari, V., and Wenger, D.R.: Arthrogryposis multiplex congenita: a long-term follow-up study, Clin. Orthop. **194:**115, 1985.

Drummond, D.S., and Cruess, R.L.: The management of the foot and ankle in arthrogryposis multiplex congenita, J. Bone Joint Surg. **60-B:**96, 1978.

Drummond, D.S., Siller, T.N., and Cruess, R.L.: The management of arthrogryposis multiplex congenita. In American Academy of Orthopaedic Surgeons: Instructional course lectures, vol. 23, St. Louis, 1974, The C.V. Mosby Co.

Green, A.D.L., Fixsen, J.A., and Lloyd-Roberts, G.C.: Talectomy for arthrogryposis multiplex congenita, J. Bone Joint Surg. **66-B:**697, 1984.

Gross, R.H.: The role of the Verebelyi-Ogston procedure in the management of the arthrogrypotic foot, Clin. Orthop. **194:**99, 1985.

Guidera, K.J., and Drennan, J.C.: Foot and ankle deformities in arthrogryposis multiplex congenita, Clin. Orthop. **194:**93, 1985.

Hahn, G.: Arthrogryposis: pediatric review and habilitative aspects, Clin. Orthop. **194:**104, 1985.

Hall, J.G.: Genetic aspects of arthrogryposis multiplex congenita, Clin. Orthop. **194:**44, 1985.

Hoffer, M.M., Swank, S., Eastman, F., Clark, D., and Teitge, R.: Ambulation in severe arthrogryposis, J. Pediatr. Orthop. **3:**293, 1983.

Hsu, L.C.S., Jaffray, D., and Leong, J.C.Y.: Talectomy for clubfoot in arthrogryposis, J. Bone Joint Surg. **66-B:**694, 1984.

Huurman, W.W., and Jacobsen, S.T.: The hip in arthrogryposis multiplex congenita, Clin. Orthop. **194:**81, 1985.

Kopits, S.: Orthopaedic management. In Freeman, J., editor: Practical management of meningomyelocele, Baltimore, 1974, University Park Press.

Ogston, A.: A new principle of curing club-foot in severe cases in children a few years old, Br. Med. J. **1:**1524, 1902.

Otto, A.G.: Monstrorum SEC centorum deseriptio anatomica in vratislaviae museum, Anatomico-Pathologicum Vratislaviae, 1841.

Palmer, P.M., MacEwan, G.D., Bowen, J.R., and Mathews, P.A.: Passive motion for infants with arthrogryposis, Clin. Orthop. **194:**54, 1985.

St. Clair, H.S., and Zimbler, S.: A plan of management and treatment results in the arthrogrypotic hip, Clin. Orthop. **194:**74, 1985.

Swinyard, C.A., and Bleck, E.E.: The etiology of arthrogryposis (multiple congenital contracture), Clin. Orthop. **194:**15, 1985.

Thomas, B., Schopler, S., Wood, W., and Oppenheim, W.L.: The knee in arthrogryposis, Clin. Orthop. **194:**87, 1985.

Thompson, G.H., and Bilenker, R.M.: Comprehensive management of arthrogryposis multiplex congenita, Clin. Orthop. **194:**6, 1985.

Williams, P.F.: The management of arthrogryposis, Orthop. Clin. North Am. **6:**967, 1978.

Williams, P.F.: Management of upper limb problems in arthrogryposis, Clin. Orthop. **194:**60, 1985.

Williams, P.F.: Personal communication, 1985.

Wynne-Davies, R.W., Williams, P.F., and O'Connor, J.B.F.: The 1960's epidemic of arthrogryposis multiplex congenita, J. Bone Joint Surg. **63-B:**76, 1981.

Obstetric paralysis

Adler, J.B., and Patterson, R.L., Jr.: Erb's palsy: long-term results of treatment in eighty-eight cases, J. Bone Joint Surg. **49-A:**1052, 1967.

Aitken, J.: Deformity of the elbow joint as a sequel to Erb's obstetrical paralysis, J. Bone Joint Surg. **34-B:**352, 1952.

Babbitt, D.P., and Cassidy, R.H.: Obstetrical paralysis and dislocation of the shoulder in infancy, J. Bone Joint Surg. **50-A:**1447, 1968.

Chung, S.M.K., and Nissenbaum, M.M.: Obstetrical paralysis, Orthop. Clin. North Am. **6:**393, 1975.

Déjerine-Klumpke, A.: Des polynévrites en général et des paralysies et atrophies saturnines en particulier. Etude clinique et anatomo-pathologique, Paris, 1889, Ancienne Librairie Germer Baillière et Cie.

Duchenne, G.B.: De l'électrisation localisée, et de son application à la pathologie et à la thérapeutique, 1855.

Duchenne, G.B.: Physiologie des mouvements démontrée à l'aide de l'expérimentation électrique et de l'observations clinique et applicable à l'étude des paralysies et des déformations, 1867.

Duchenne, G.B.: Physiology of motion demonstrated by means of electrical stimulation and clinical observation and applied to the study of paralysis and deformities (translated and edited by Emanuel B. Kaplan), Philadelphia, 1949, J.B. Lippincott Co.

L'Episcopo, J.B.: Restoration of muscle balance in the treatment of obstetrical paralysis, N.Y. J. Med. **39:**357, 1939.

Fairbank, H.A.T.: Birth palsy: subluxation of the shoulder-joint in infants and young children, Lancet **1:**1217, 1913.

Kendrick, J.I.: Changes in the upper humeral epiphysis following operations for obstetrical paralysis, J. Bone Joint Surg. **19:**473, 1937.

Kleinberg, S.: Reattachment of the capsule and external rotators of the shoulder for obstetric paralysis, JAMA **98:**294, 1932.

Klumpke, A.: Contribution à l'étude des paralysies radiculaires du plexus branchial. Paralysies radiculaires totales, paralysies radiculaires inférieures. De la participation des filets sympathiques oculopupillaires dans ces paralysies. Étude clinique et expérimentale, Rev. Méd., 1885, pp. 591, 736 (Mémoire couronné par l'Académie de Médecine, prix Godard, 1886).

Liebolt, F.L., and Furey, J.G.: Obstetrical paralysis with dislocation of the shoulder: a case report, J. Bone Joint Surg. **35-A:**227, 1953.

Lombard, P.: La paralysie dite obstetricale du membre superieur (The so-called obstetrical paralysis of the upper extremity), Rev. Orthop. **33:**235, 1947.

Moore, B.H.: A new operative procedure for brachial birth palsy—Erb's paralysis, Surg. Gynecol. Obstet. **61:**832, 1935.

Moore, B.H.: Brachial birth palsy, Am. J. Surg. **43:**338, 1939.

Moore, J.R.: Bone block to prevent posterior dislocation of the shoulder, personal communication.

Rogers, M.H.: An operation for the correction of the deformity due to "obstetrical paralysis," Boston Med. Surg. J. **174:**163, 1916.

Saha, A.K.: Surgery of the paralyzed and flail shoulder, Acta Orthop. Scand. (suppl.) **97:**5, 1967.

Scaglietti, O.: Lesioni obstetriche della spalla, Chir. Organi Mov. **22:**183, 1936.

Sever, J.W.: Obstetric paralysis, Am. J. Dis. Child. **12:**541, 1916.

Sever, J.W.: The results of a new operation for obstetrical paralysis, Am. J. Orthop. Surg. **16:**248, 1918.

Sever, J.W.: Obstetric paralysis, JAMA **85:**1862, 1925.

Sever, J.W.: Obstetric paralysis, Surg. Gynecol. Obstet. **44:**547, 1927.

Slomann, H.C.: Kobenhavns Med. Selskabs Forhandl., 1916-1917, p. 95. Quoted by Toft, G.: On obstetrical paralysis of the upper extremities, Acta Orthop. Scand. **13:**218, 1942.

Steindler, A.: Orthopedic operations, Springfield, Ill., 1940, Charles C Thomas, Publisher.

Steindler, A.: Post-graduate lectures on orthopedic diagnosis and indications, vol. II, Springfield, Ill., 1951, Charles C Thomas, Publisher.

Taylor, A.S.: Results from surgical treatment of brachial birth palsy, JAMA **48:**96, 1907.

Taylor, A.S.: Brachial birth palsy and injuries of similar type in adults, Surg. Gynecol. Obstet. **30:**494, 1920.

Thomas, T.T.: Laceration of the axillary portion of the capsule of the shoulder-joint as a factor in the etiology of traumatic combined paralysis of the upper extremity, Ann. Surg. **53:**77, 1911.

Thomas, T.T.: Obstetrical or brachial birth palsy, Am. J. Obstet. **73:**577, 1916.

Thomas, T.T.: Traumatic brachial paralysis with flail shoulder joint, Ann. Surg. **66:**532, 1917.

Thomas, T.T.: Brachial birth palsy: a pseudoparalysis of shoulder-joint origin, Am. J. Med. Sci. **159:**207, 1920.

Toft, G.: On obstetrical paralysis of the upper extremities, Acta Orthop. Scand. **13:**218, 1942.

Wickstrom, J.: Birth injuries of the brachial plexus: treatment of defects in the shoulder, Clin. Orthop. **23:**187, 1962.

Wickstrom, J., Haslam, E.D., and Hutchinson, R.H.: The surgical management of residual deformities of the shoulder following birth injuries of the brachial plexus, J. Bone Joint Surg. **37-A:**27, 1955.

Zachary, R.B.: Transplantation of teres major and latissimus dorsi for loss of external rotation at shoulder, Lancet, **2:**757, 1947.

Zancolli, E.A.: Paralytic supination contracture of the forearm, J. Bone Joint Surg. **49-A:**1275, 1967.

Zaoussis, A.L.: Osteotomy of the proximal end of the radius for paralytic supination deformity in children, J. Bone Joint Surg. **45-B:**523, 1963.

Paralysis caused by peripheral nerve injuries
Spinal accessory nerve

Dewar, F.P.: Personal communication, October 1954.

Dewar, F.P., and Harris, R.I.: Restoration of function of the shoulder following paralysis of the trapezius by fascial sling fixation and transplantation of the levator scapulae, Ann. Surg. **132:**1111, 1950.

Eden, R.: Zur Behandlung der Trapeziuslähmung mittels Muskelplastik, Deutsch. Z. Chir. **183:**387, 1924. (Cited in Lange, M.: Orthopadisch-Chirurgische Operationslehre, München, 1951, J.F. Bergmann.)

Henry, A.K.: An operation for slinging a dropped shoulder, Br. J. Surg. **15:**95, 1927-1928.

Lange, M.: Orthopädisch-Chirurgische Operations-lehre, München, 1951, J.F. Bergmann.

Langenskiöld, A., and Ryöppy, S.: Treatment of paralysis of the trapezius muscle by the Eden-Lange operation, Acta Orthop. Scand. **44:**383, 1973.

Brachial plexus

Barnes, R.: Traction injuries of the brachial plexus in adults, J. Bone Joint Surg. **31-B:**10, 1949.

Bonney, G.: The value of axon responses in determining the site of lesion in traction injuries of the brachial plexus, Brain **77:**588, 1954.

Brooks, D.M.: Tendon transplantation in the forearm and arthrodesis of the wrist, Proc. R. Soc. Med. **42:**838, 1949.

Brooks, D.M.: Open wounds of the brachial plexus. In Seddon, H.J., editor: Peripheral nerve injuries, London, 1954, Her Majesty's Stationery Office.

Bunnell, S.: Tendon transfers in the hand and forearm. In American Academy of Orthopaedic Surgeons: Instructional course lectures, vol. 6, Ann Arbor, Mich., 1949, J.W. Edwards.

Bunnell, S.: Surgery of the hand, ed. 3, Philadelphia, 1956, J.B. Lippincott Co.

Hendry, A.M.: The flail limb, Proc. R. Soc. Med. **42:**835, 1949.

Hendry, A.M.: The treatment of residual paralysis after brachial plexus injuries, J. Bone Joint Surg. **31-B:**42, 1949.

Luckey, C.A., and McPherson, S.R.: Tendinous reconstruction of the hand following irreparable injury to the peripheral nerves and brachial plexus, J. Bone Joint Surg. **29:**560, 1947.

Riordan, D.C.: Tendon transplantation in median nerve and ulner nerve paralysis, J. Bone Joint Surg. **35-A:**312, 1953.

Thompson, T.C.: Orthopedic measures for use in irreparable nerve injury, Int. Surg. **9:**116, 1946.

Tracy, J.F., and Brannon, E.W.: Management of brachial-plexus injuries (traction type), J. Bone Joint Surg. **40-A:**1031, 1958.

Yeoman, P.M., and Seddon, H.J.: Brachial plexus injuries: treatment of the flail arm, J. Bone Joint Surg. **43-B:**493, 1961.

Long thoracic nerve

Chaves, J.P.: Pectoralis minor transplant for paralysis of the serratus anterior, J. Bone Joint Surg. **33-B:**228, 1951.

Haas, J.: Muskelplastik bei Serratuslähmung, Z. Orthop. **55:**617, 1931.

Haas, S.L.: Serratus anterior paralysis, Orthopaedic Correspondence Club Letter, March 15, 1949.

Marmor, L., and Bechtol, C.O.: Paralysis of the serratus anterior due to electric shock relieved by transplantation of the pectoralis major muscle: a case report, J. Bone Joint Surg. **45-A:**156, 1963.

Rapp, I.H.: Serratus anterior paralysis treated by transplantation of the pectoralis minor, J. Bone Joint Surg. **36-A:**852, 1954.

Trunchly, G.: Reconstruction of the "winging scapula" deformity: an improvement of an old procedure, SICOT-81 Rio, XV World Congress, Abstracts, pp. 175-176.

Whitman, A.: Congenital elevation of scapula and paralysis of serratus magnus muscle, JAMA **99:**1332, 1932.

Zeier, F.G.: The treatment of winged-scapula, Clin. Orthop. **91:**128, 1973.

CHAPTER 67

Inheritable progressive neuromuscular diseases

Fred P. Sage

Inheritable progressive neuromuscular diseases are characterized by progressive muscular weakness, with some progressing more rapidly than others. They may be caused by muscle disease or by neuron disease with the muscle secondarily involved.

Only those diseases that may require orthopaedic treatment are discussed in this chapter.

Muscle weakness caused by muscle disease must be differentiated from that caused by diseases of nerves. The prognoses are different and in most cases predictable, and the treatment goals in each are distinct, although some procedures are applicable to both muscle and nerve diseases.

Distinguishing between the two kinds of diseases is usually accomplished by a good history, including a genetic inquiry; physical examination; electrodiagnostic studies, including an electromyogram and an electrocardiogram;

blood chemistry analyses, including serum enzyme assays; and a muscle biopsy with appropriate histochemical studies. The orthopaedic surgeon in most instances needs consultation with a pediatric neurologist and a pathologist skilled in muscle tissue evaluation.

The treatment of these diseases involves a team of physicians and paramedical personnel, which may include a pediatric neurologist, an orthopaedic surgeon, a psychiatrist or psychologist, a physician skilled in physical medicine and rehabilitation, a physical therapist, an occupational therapist, a speech and hearing therapist, an orthotist, rehabilitation engineers, nurses, and a social worker. Late in the course of some of these diseases a physician specializing in respiratory diseases and a cardiologist will definitely be needed; ophthalmologists and specialists in gastroenterology may also be needed.

DIFFERENTIATION OF MUSCLE DISEASE FROM NERVE DISEASE

In addition to the history, physical examination, and routine laboratory studies, special tests such as the electromyogram, muscle tissue biopsy, and serum enzyme studies help differentiate between the two diseases.

Electromyographic studies

In an electromyogram of normal muscle, resting muscles are usually relatively electrosilent; on voluntary contraction of a normal muscle the electromyogram shows a characteristic frequency, duration, and amplitude action potential (Fig. 67-1). In a myopathy the electromyogram shows increased frequency, decreased amplitude, and decreased duration of the motor action potentials. In a neuropathy is shows decreased frequency and increased amplitude and duration of the action potentials. In a neuropathy nerve conduction velocities are usually slowed; in a myopathy the nerve conduction velocities are usually normal. Myotonic dystrophy is characterized by an increase in frequency, duration, and amplitude of the action potentials on needle electrode insertion, which gradually decrease over time (Fig. 67-2). These action potentials when amplified create the "dive-bomber" sound that is almost universal in this disease.

Muscle tissue biopsy

Skillful interpretation of the muscle tissue biopsy not only will differentiate myopathy from neuropathy but also will differentiate the various types of congenital dystrophy from one another. In addition to the usual hematoxylin and

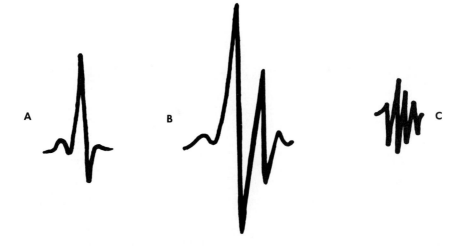

Fig. 67-1. Motor units seen in electromyography. **A,** Normal triphasic motor unit potential. **B,** Large polyphasic motor units as seen in neurogenic disorders such as spinal muscular atrophy, in which they are also reduced in number. **C,** Small polyphasic motor units as seen in muscular dystrophy. These are usually of normal number. (Courtesy Dr. Tulio E. Bertorini.)

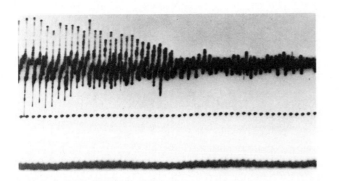

Fig. 67-2. Motor unit potential as seen in myotonic dystrophy. Action potentials increase in frequency, duration, and amplitude on needle insertion. This gradually decreases over time. (From Lenman, J.A.R., and Ritchie, A.E.: Clinical electromyography, Philadelphia, 1970, J.B. Lippincott, Co.)

eosin stain, special stains and techniques, such as the Gomori modified trichrome stain and the alizarin red S stain, are helpful. Electron microscopy is also beneficial.

Histopathologic study of muscle affected by myopathy shows an increased fibrosis in and between muscle spindles, with necrosis of the fibers (Fig. 67-3, *B*). Later, deposition of fat within the fibers occurs, accompanied by hyaline and granular degeneration of the fibers. The number of nuclei is increased with migration of some nuclei to the center of the fibers. Some small groups of inflammatory cells may also be seen, and in polymyositis inflammatory cells are markedly increased. Special histochemical stains that can demonstrate muscle fiber type show a preponderance of type I fibers. In normal skeletal muscle the ratio of type I to type II fibers is 1:2 (Fig. 67-3, *A*). In some dystrophies other than Duchenne's there is fiber splitting. Calcium accumulation in muscle fibers has also been demonstrated.

The microscopic picture in neuropathy is quite different

(Fig. 67-3, *C*). There is little or no increase in fibrous tissue, and small, angular, atrophic fibers are present between groups of normal-sized muscle fibers. Special stains that demonstrate fiber type show that 80% of the fibers are type II.

An adequate biopsy must be done. Muscles that are totally involved should not be used; biopsies of muscles suspected of early involvement are indicated. As an example the muscle bellies of the gastrocnemius in a patient with Duchenne's muscular dystrophy are usually involved early and are a poor site to obtain material for a biopsy, whereas the quadriceps (especially the vastus lateralis at midthigh) and rectus abdominis usually show early involvement without total replacement of the muscle spindles by fibrous tissue or fat. Biopsies of these muscles are usually the most reliable.

One must be careful when securing a biopsy specimen that the muscle is maintained at its normal length between clamps (Fig. 67-4) or sutures (Fig. 67-5) and that the biopsy specimen has not been violated by a needle electrode while performing an electromyogram or infiltrated with a local anesthetic before the biopsy.

Regional block anesthesia is preferred; a general anesthetic carries with it the possibility of complications.

TECHNIQUE. Block the area regionally with 1% lidocaine, and make a 1.5 cm incision through the skin and subcutaneous tissues. Carefully split the enveloping fascia to clearly expose the muscle bundles from which the biopsy specimen is to be taken. Using a special double clamp (Fig. 67-4) or silk sutures approximately 2 cm apart (Fig. 67-5), grasp the muscle and section around the outside of the arms of the clamp or sutures. Prevent bleeding within the muscle, and take only small biopsy specimens. Take more than one specimen, since different stains need different preservative techniques; for example, some histochemical changes are best demonstrated on fresh frozen sections that have had special staining. The pathologist should

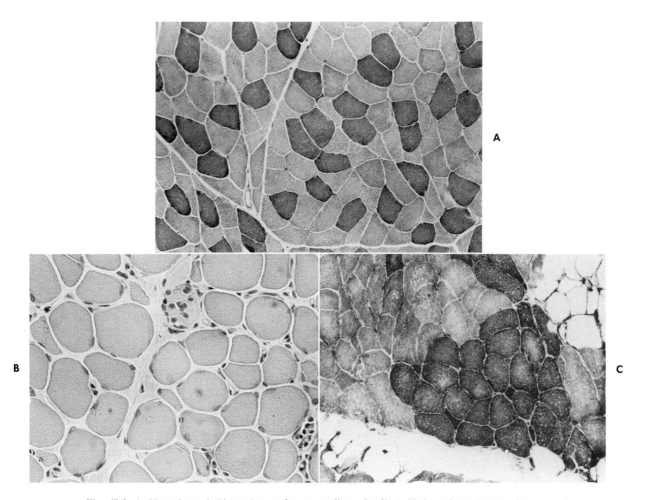

Fig. 67-3. A, Normal muscle biopsy (except for one small angular fiber). Notice polygonal shape of myofibrils, normal distribution of type I and type II fibers, and normal endomysiel connective tissue. (NADH-TR stain, 125×) **B,** Muscular dystrophy. Fibers are more rounded, some fibers have internalized nuclei, and others are atrophic. One muscle fiber is necrotic and is undergoing phagocytosis. Connective tissue between fibers is increased. (H & E stain, 295×) **C,** Chronic neurogenic atrophy (juvenile spinal muscular atrophy). Notice grouping of fibers of same type and some atrophic angular fibers. Fat is increased between muscle fascicles. (NADH-TR stain, 125×.) (Courtesy Dr. Tulio E. Bertorini.)

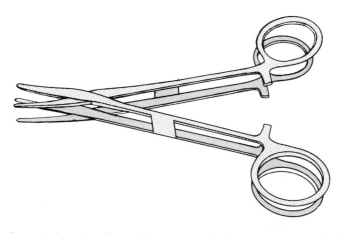

Fig. 67-4. Two hemostats bound together used in preserving length when securing muscle biopsy. (From Cruess, R.L., and Rennie, W.R.J.: Adult orthopaedics, New York, 1984, Churchill Livingstone.)

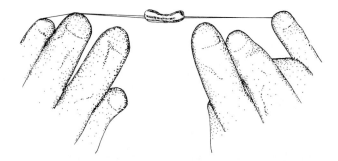

Fig. 67-5. Muscle length maintained by muscle biopsy done on outer side of previously placed sutures. (From Curtis, B.: In American Academy of Orthopaedic Surgeons: instructional course lectures, vol. 19, St. Louis, 1970, The C.V. Mosby Co.)

know in advance that a muscle biopsy is to be done so that special fixative techniques, such as freezing with liquid nitrogen, are readily available when the specimen is received.

Serum enzyme assays

Serum enzyme assays are extremely helpful, especially the level of serum creatine phosphokinase in the blood. Serum glutamic-oxaloacetic transaminase and serum glutamic-pyruvic transaminase levels are less specific, for although elevated, they are also elevated in other conditions, such as myocardial infarction, myocardial myopathy, or liver disease, as is lactic dehydrogenase.

The creatine phosphokinase elevation is extremely important in the diagnosis in the early stages of Duchenne's dystrophy. It is usually not elevated in liver disease. It is elevated in myocardial infarction but not to the level seen in the patient with early muscular dystrophy. In the affected newborn and the child in the first year of life, the creatine phosphokinase level may be 200 to 300 times the normal level. The level may fall in the later stages of the disease, when the greater muscle mass has already deteriorated and there is less breakdown of muscle mass than in the early stage. This test is extremely beneficial in detecting the carrier state of Duchenne's and Becker's dystrophies because it is usually elevated in the carrier female. Recently, a muscle provocation test has been advocated to detect the female carrier state. In the carrier female the creatine phosphokinase levels rise higher after strenuous exercise than in noncarrier females.

Blood and urine chemistry studies are beneficial in making a diagnosis. Skeletal muscles produce creatinine in their metabolism of creatine. In dystrophic muscles, serum creatine is not used as much as usual, and creatinine is not produced in as great a quantity. This leads to excess creatine in the blood and thus in the urine. Urine creatine is excessive in dystrophic patients in the active stage of muscle breakdown. Any process that causes muscle breakdown, however, can cause an excess urine creatine, such as excessive exercise, diabetes mellitus, starvation where carbohydrate intake is reduced, and also the neuropathies. In myotonic dystrophy, because of the reduced ability of the liver to produce creatine phosphate, there is decreased blood creatine.

The most diagnostic features in all these conditions are the classic clinical picture and the genetic history.

MUSCULAR DYSTROPHY

Muscular dystrophy is a broad, inclusive term that needs to be defined. Siegel says it is "the general designation for a group of chronic diseases whose most prominent characteristic is progressive degeneration of skeletal musculature leading to weakness, atrophy, contracture, deformity, and progressive disability." Muscular dystrophy is most often inherited, although in approximately 30% of patients with Duchenne's dystrophy, the disease occurs as a result of spontaneous gene mutation; in other words, it occurs without any carrier state.

There is no known cause for the disorder and no known cure. It is agreed, however, that something happens to the normal cell membrane in Duchenne's muscular dystrophy, making it more permeable to the extracellular fluids and to the loss of some intracellular elements as well. Calcium is often deposited in the fibers. Bertorini et al. found the calcium content elevated in the muscles of two aborted male fetuses that were at risk for muscular dystrophy. In a premature infant who later developed Duchenne's muscular dystrophy, calcium levels in the muscle were found to be elevated two to three times above normal. Bertorini and associates believed that excessive calcium deposition in the muscles of newborns precedes the onset of clinical weakness in Duchenne's muscular dystrophy. Abnormalities in the permeability of the cell membrane of erythrocytes of patients with Duchenne's muscular dystrophy, and of the carrier states of females who also have an elevated creatine phosphokinase level have also been found.

Although we cannot cure these disabling conditions, we can treat them and often keep them from deteriorating so swiftly; we can enhance the patients' functional abilities, make them more comfortable, and probably even prolong the lives of a significant number of patients. Supportive treatment enhances their outlook on life from one of abandonment and death to one of a better and maybe longer life. The longer we keep dystrophic patients alive, the greater the chance that we will devise a cure during their lifetimes.

Some believe that, although life may be prolonged by an intensive rehabilitation program of bracing, physical therapy, and surgery, the lifestyle of patients with muscular dystrophy and those of their families become so regimented and arduous as to make it hardly worth the effort. Bleck advocates a motto, "Not a life of treatment—but a life."

Supportive and palliative treatment, including limited surgery with limited morbidity, has certainly made life a little easier for the child and the caretaker in these disabling disorders.

Sex-linked muscular dystrophies

There are two types of sex-linked muscular dystrophy, Duchenne's muscular dystrophy and Becker's muscular dystrophy. These are alike in that the pattern of muscle weakness progresses in a similar geographic distribution (Fig. 67-6), but Becker's muscular dystrophy begins later in life, progresses more slowly, and is not nearly as fre-

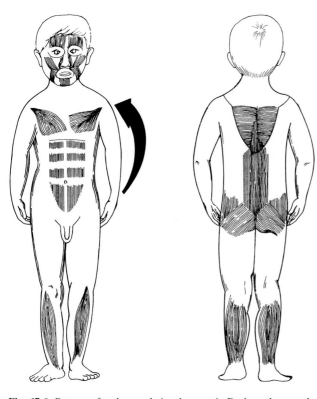

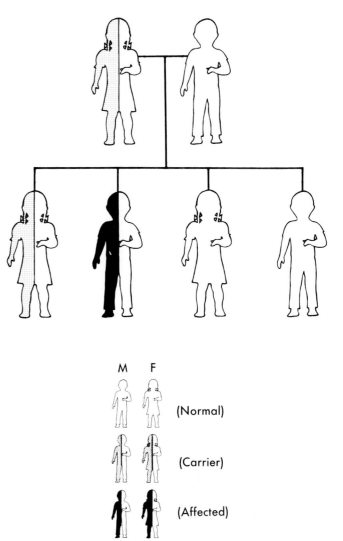

Fig. 67-6. Patterns of early muscle involvement in Duchenne's muscular dystrophy. (From Siegel, I.M.: Clinical management of muscle disease, London, 1977, William Heineman Medical Books, Ltd.)

Fig. 67-7. Pattern of inheritance in sex-linked dystrophy. Mother is carrier. There is 50% chance that male offspring will have disease. There is 50% chance that each female offspring will be carrier.

quent as Duchenne's muscular dystrophy. The outcome of these two diseases is the same, however: a slow, progressive weakness, usually to wheelchair confinement, and a premature death. Myocardial involvement is common in Duchenne's muscular dystrophy and is usually the cause of death; myocardial involvement is uncommon in Becker's muscular dystrophy.

DUCHENNE'S MUSCULAR DYSTROPHY

Duchenne's muscular dystrophy is a sex-linked dystrophy for which the mother is the carrier (Fig. 67-7). It usually occurs in the male offspring and almost never occurs in the female offspring, although a few such patients have been reported. Being a sex-linked disease means that there is a 50% chance of each male child of the mother having the disease and a 50% chance that each female child will be a carrier of the disease. In about two thirds of the patients the disease is inherited, and in about one third it results from a spontaneous gene mutation. It is estimated that more than 10,000 males with Duchenne's muscular dystrophy are alive in the United States at any given time. The risk of having a male child with Duchenne's muscular dystrophy is about 270 per 1 million live male births.

Although the child with Duchenne's muscular dystrophy appears to be normal at birth, he is already affected, as evidenced by a very high creatine phosphokinase enzyme level during the first year of life. This apparently normal appearance is probably because the muscles have not become weakened enough for the disease to be clinically

manifest. For weakness to be detected clinically in axial and limb musculature, approximately 30% to 50% of muscle mass must have been lost. Usually a child will have a history of early walking problems, and over 50% of children with Duchenne's muscular dystrophy do not walk until they are older than 17 months. The parent by this time has usually noticed some little abnormality, however, and a significant number of the children have been seen by a physician for flatfoot, toe walking, or clumsiness. It has been recommended that a creatine phosphokinase level be obtained in any male child who fails to walk by 18 months. If an elevated creatine phosphokinase level confirms the presence of Duchenne's muscular dystrophy by 18 months, then genetic counseling can be given to the family and a number of at-risk births probably can be prevented.

Amniotic fluid studies and fetal blood samples done early enough to give the parents a choice of termination of

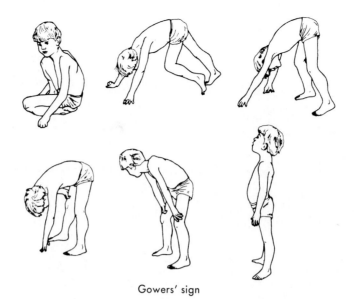

Gowers' sign

Fig. 67-8. Gower's sign. Child must use his hands to arise from sitting. (From Siegel, I.M.: Clinical management of muscle disease, London, 1977, William Heineman Medical Books, Ltd.)

the pregnancy have not proved to be reliable in forecasting affected offspring. However ultrasound studies of a fetus in a carrier mother may be made to determine the sex of the child, and then, since a male offspring would run a 50% risk of having Duchenne's muscular dystrophy, the family has the choice of terminating the pregnancy.

At age 3 to 5 years, the child usually is clumsy, has difficulty climbing stairs and arising from a sitting position (Gower's sign) (Fig. 67-8), seats himself too rapidly when attempting to sit, and has other complaints indicative of proximal lower extremity weakness.

The pattern of progressive weakness is fairly constant, from proximal to distal in the axial and limb muscles. The first weakness is usually in the neck flexors and then the shoulder and hip extensors. This results in a posture pattern of forward flexion of the neck, stabilized by gravity and the neck extensors, retraction of the shoulders, and a lumbar lordosis (Fig. 67-9). Hip flexion occurs, throwing the center of gravity in the front of the knee joint, and the child assumes an equinus gait to centralize weight bearing from hip to knee to ankle. The hip abductors and the quadriceps become weak, and for the child to walk he must waddle, swinging his trunk from side to side to elevate the leg and swing it forward. The calves hypertrophy, but this is a false hypertrophy, or pseudohypertrophy, since the muscles are replaced by fibrous tissue and fat infiltration. Tendo calcaneus contractures develop, as does tighteness of the iliotibial bands and hip flexors, from the flexed, abducted hip and equinus ankle posture. As the gait becomes more unstable and balance less certain, the child falls increasingly often and ultimately will choose to sit at about 8 to 10 years of age. Broken bones are not uncommon. Once the child assumes a sitting posture, there is little likelihood of his walking again. The child and the family are fearful of his falling, and the child has probably already sustained fractures. At complete rest, strength is lost at the rate of 3% per day; a short period of inactivity,

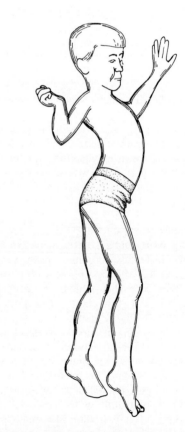

Fig. 67-9. Typical posture of child with Duchenne's muscular dystrophy. Head is flexed, shoulders are retracted, spine is lordotic, hips and knees are flexed (and abducted), and feet are in equinus.

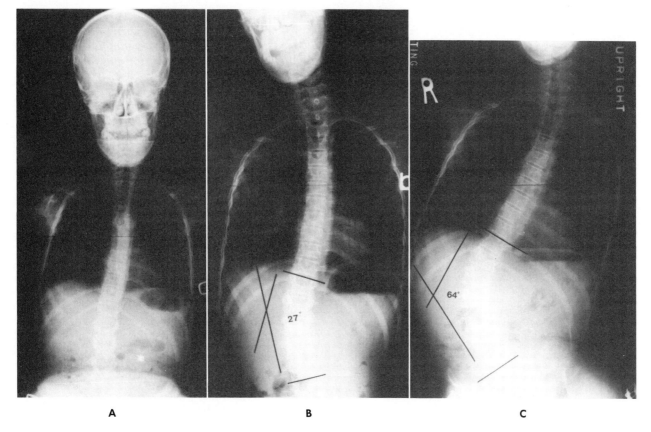

A   B   C

Fig. 67-10. Progressive scoliosis in wheelchair patients. **A,** Spine in patient with muscular dystrophy on first assuming wheelchair existence. **B,** Spine shown seated after 18 months in wheechair. **C,** Spine 2 years later after refusing spine-stabilizing operation.

even 2 to 3 weeks, may topple the balance between retaining enough strength to stay upright and having to sit. Once the child assumes a sitting posture, his axial muscles further deteriorate from inactivity and he usually becomes obese. He develops further flexion contractures of the hips and knees and equinus contractures of the ankles, which make wheelchair transfers difficult. He develops scoliosis, which is usually progressive (Fig. 67-10).

Approximately three fourths of the wheelchair patients with Duchenne's muscular dystrophy develop a severe collapsing scoliosis, usually convex toward the side of the dominant hand, since this is the side to which they lean to control their mobility device (most commonly an electric wheelchair). Kurz et al. have shown that for each 10-degree increase in the thoracic scoliosis, the vital capacity is decreased by 4%. Progressive muscular weakness also decreases the vital capacity in Duchenne's muscular dystrophy by about 4% per year. Thus an early attempt to prevent scoliosis is important and the best way to prevent it is by keeping the patient upright and walking. Theoretically, while walking, the lumbar lordosis locks the lumbar facets into the extended position and retricts lateral bending of the spine.

Orthotics have been of little help in preventing progressive scoliosis. Special wheelchair inserts to keep the lumbar spine in a lordotic position have likewise been of little benefit, because the child will usually lean forward with his elbows on the arm supports, thus flexing his lumbar spine in spite of the inserts.

Keeping the patient ambulatory as long as possible has become the treatment of choice. It seems to prolong the overall life of the child with Duchenne's muscular dystrophy from a few months to 5 years, a significant period when the total life span is usually less than 20 years.

Pneumonitis is responsible for 90% of the deaths in Duchenne's muscular dystrophy. In addition to a decreased maximum vital capacity, the child with this disease has a decreased maximum ventilatory volume, with impaired swallowing and a weak cough. About 80% of the children with Duchenne's muscular dystrophy develop cardiomyopathy, and a mild congestive heart failure may be enough to trigger a fatal pneumonitis. Congestive heart failure in itself may be fatal.

TREATMENT. The life of a child with Duchenne's muscular dystrophy has been divided into three stages: ambulation, transition, and wheelchair confinement.

The stage of ambulation lasts from birth through the time the child is a household and community walker. The transitional stage occurs when community ambulation becomes a problem and the patient requires some assistance to get about the community. The third stage begins when the patient is permanently confined to a wheelchair and needs assistance to stand and transfer.

Treatment by the orthopaedic surgeon is aimed at prolonging walking and standing by preventing contractures and deformity or by releasing contractures so that the extremity is adaptable to orthoses once weakness has become severe. In general, surgical releases require orthotic bracing in the postoperative period. Since wasting is so prone to occur with inactivity, any surgery should cause limited morbidity so that the child can stand the day of surgery and walk the following day.

In general, correct timing of the surgical procedures depends on the patient's ability to walk without falling. Surgery should be performed just before the child would refuse to walk. This is usually determined by the number of falls a child sustains each day. When weakness and contractures become such that the patient is so unstable that he falls three or four times a day, he is soon going to sit down and not try to walk.

During the walking stage attempts are made to prevent contractures by the use of judicious physical therapy aimed at preventing hip flexion-adduction contractures, knee flexion contractures, and ankle equinus or equinovarus. Night splints in the form of polypropylene ankle-foot orthoses will retard slightly the progression of equinus (Fig. 67-11). If some quadriceps strength remains and equinus is minimal, corrective casting may overcome the equinus contracture. Ultimately, however, at age 7 to 8 years, an equinus contracture will occur that requires a tendo calcaneus lengthening or an anterior transfer of a tibialis posterior tendon, which usually has retained almost normal strength. After tendo calcaneus lengthening, a floor-reaction ankle-foot orthosis is needed, because the quadriceps is weak and a slight equinus position of the foot is needed in walking to lock the knee in extension (Fig. 67-12). Once the patient reaches the transitional stage, hip, knee, and ankle surgery may be needed to keep him ambulatory with the aid of orthoses. Tenotomy of the hip flexors and abductors, iliotibial band tenotomies above the knee, and tenotomy of the tendo calcaneus and tibialis posterior tendon

may all be needed. In a gross equinovarus deformity, the skin medially is extremely tight. Triple arthrodesis or talectomy will not allow early weight bearing, so alternative procedures must be used. These include percutaneous tenotomy of the tendo calcaneus and the tibialis posterior tendon, and enucleation of the distal talus and distal calcaneus or cuboid. The distal ends of the talus and calcaneus or cuboid are merely curetted of all cancellous bone through a small incision, and then osteoclasis places the foot in the corrected position. This preserves the articular cartilage, and weight bearing can usually be begun the next day. Swelling may be severe following this operation, however.

Again it is important to remember that there should never be a period of longer than 24 hours when the patient is not standing or walking. Postoperative long leg casts with the knees in extension and the ankles in neutral position (right angle) are preferred to placing the child in previously fabricated knee-ankle-foot orthoses at the time of surgery. Casts cannot be removed by parents as easily as braces, and parents are prone to release or remove braces when postoperative pain is a problem. In long leg casts with the heels well padded or pounded soft to prevent heel pressure the patient can stand the day of surgery. The day after, walking should be supervised by a physical therapist, since these children (immediately postoperatively) need support as well as parallel bars or a walker to assist them. Usually, the upper extremities have become so weak that crutch walking or the use of canes is not feasible. To walk, the child needs to shift his torso from side to side as he walks with a stiff-legged gait. He should remain hospitalized until he is walking independently. If he is al-

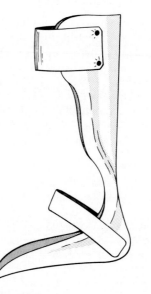

Fig. 67-11. Heat-molded, petroplastic ankle-foot orthoses.

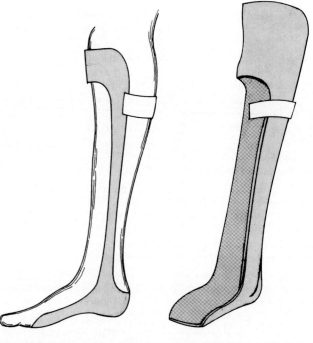

Fig. 67-12. Floor-reaction, ankle-foot orthosis (Saltiel brace). (Redrawn after Saltiel, J.: Orthot. Prosthet. **23**:71, 1969.)

lowed to return home before he is walking unassisted, it is extremely unlikely that he will ever walk independently again.

When the casts are removed at 3 to 6 weeks, knee-ankle-foot orthoses should have already been fabricated for walking and as nighttime splints. The orthoses should be fabricated of lightweight plastic with little metal (Fig. 67-13). The upper thigh bands in the knee-ankle-foot orthoses should be rigid enough to sit on because these children use them to bear trunk weight when standing and shifting weight from one side to the other. Weight bearing should be encouraged for as long as possible. Standing or walking for 2 to 4 hours each day is desirable. As already mentioned, if these children continue to stand and walk, scoliosis is retarded in its appearance and progression.

Once the wheelchair stage is reached, the lower extremities require primarily tenotomies of the tendo calcaneus and tibialis posterior tendons to correct the position of the feet so that shoes and ankle-foot orthoses can position the feet to transfer to and from the wheelchair. Occasionally, the deformity will be so severe that a tarsal enucleation is required.

The greatest concern once the wheelchair period has

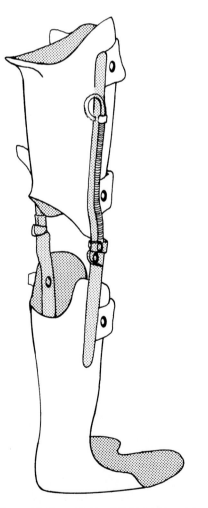

Fig. 67-13. Knee-ankle-foot orthosis of lightweight metal and plastic. (Redrawn from Drennan, J.C., and Bondurant, M.: Atlas of orthopaedics, St. Louis, 1985, The C.V. Mosby Co.)

been reached is to prevent and treat scoliosis. The aim is to keep the pelvis level and the back as straight as possible. This is best accomplished with a seat that is firm and a backrest that keeps the spine extended. Various types of thoracic lumbar spine orthoses have been devised, but their value is questionable. They are usually poorly tolerated by patients with Duchenne's muscular dystrophy because they often restrict respiratory efforts, they may be uncomfortable because of body heat retention, and pressure areas may develop over the bony prominences. If used, they should be molded to the pelvis and trunk when the spine is extended to its fullest, and they should be made of a lightweight petroplastic material. Lateral side supports in wheelchairs are of little benefit. Their positioning is uncertain, and they may interfere with functional posturing. Hsu et al. have shown that the thoracic lumbar spine orthosis may be capable of slowing the progression of curves of less than 25 degrees but has no slowing effect whatsoever on larger curves. For patients whose curves are large or are progressing, internal fixation and fusion appear to offer the best alternative if pulmonary function is adequate enough to withstand the surgery. Internal fixation and fusion with Harrington rods require postoperative external support in the form of a cast or a jacket, which is poorly tolerated by these patients. Recently, the Luque rod–segmental wire fixation and fusion have become the method of choice for spinal stabilization in these patients, since it does not require external support postoperatively or prolonged recumbency. Sussman reviewed internal fixation of the dystrophic spine in 11 patients. In his opinion spine surgery on patients with Duchenne's muscular dystrophy should be done at an early age (by the time the curve reaches 30 degrees), because pulmonary function is better in this group and correction of the curves and pelvic balance are better obtained than they are later. According to Sussman, by using contoured Luque rods with segmental wiring, the thoracic kyphosis and lumbar lordosis can be controlled, thereby preventing a decrease in the vital capacity that occurs when the thoracic kyphosis disappears. Maintaining the thoracic kyphosis also allows the patient to maintain his neck in flexion by gravity, stabilized by the still active neck extensors.

BECKER'S MUSCULAR DYSTROPHY

Muscle weakness in Becker's muscular dystrophy follows a pattern similar to that in Duchenne's muscular dystrophy, although it is later in onset and more slowly progressive; heart involvement is less common, although conduction defects in the myocardium have been described in some patients. The mode of inheritance is the same as in Duchenne's muscular dystrophy, and about 10% to 20% of the sex-linked dystrophies are Becker's muscular dystrophy. Serum creatine phosphokinase levels are highest in the years before clinically apparent muscle weakness and may be 10 to 20 times higher than normal. Onset of the disease is usually after 7 years of life, and patients may live to their mid 40s or later. Becker's muscular dystrophy has been termed "benign muscular dystrophy" because of its slow progression. As already stated, the weakness progresses in a pattern similar to that in Duchenne's muscular dystrophy, and during the last few years of a patient's life he may be wheelchair bound. Weakness develops first in the hip flexors and the tibialis anterior muscles. Pseudo-hypertrophy of the calves develops later, and equinus ankle contractures are common. Progressive scoliosis is not as common in Becker's muscular dystrophy as it is in Duchenne's muscular dystrophy because the patients remain ambulatory during the years of growth of the spine.

TREATMENT. The treatment for this muscular dystrophy generally follows that described for Duchenne's muscular dystrophy (p. 3067).

ANESTHESIA IN DYSTROPHIC PATIENTS

The use of general anesthesia in dystrophic patients is a serious step. With decreased vital capacity, decreased expiratory ability, decreased maximum ventilatory volume, decreased cough, and poor swallowing, aspiration pneumonia is common postoperatively. Cardiomyopathy with conduction defects and congestive heart failure to the point of cardiorespiratory arrest are encountered. Hyperpyrexia and malignant hyperthermia are more common in this group than in the uninvolved population.

When general anesthesia is to be used, preoperative respiratory function studies are mandatory. A reduced vital capacity of less than 30% of the predicted volume may well produce difficulty in weaning a patient from the endotracheal tube or assisted ventilation in the recovery room or intensive care unit. Some patients may never be weaned from either and die a respiratory death. Tracheostomy may be needed intraoperatively or postoperatively, and weaning the patient from the tracheostomy tube postoperatively may be impossible.

The patient must be closely observed for malignant hyperthermia. Mortality is reported as 50% or more in this condition, although the use of dantrolene sodium for hyperthermia has decreased the mortality. Doses of dantrolene sodium of 1 mg/kg of body weight should be given intravenously when hyperpyrexia occurs and should be repeated at intervals as long as it persists. Depolarizing drugs, such as succinylcholine, should not be used because rhabdomyolysis may occur, leading to myoglobinuria and renal failure. Depolarizing drugs may cause release into the blood of potassium in excessive amounts, with production of conduction defects in the heart. General anesthesia is necessary in spine surgery, but these complications may occur, and the family should be so informed. Appropriate procedures should be undertaken to combat these complications if they do occur.

Malignant hyperthermia may occur from local anesthetics, but it is much less likely than with general anesthetics. Local anesthetics are safer, and in surgery of limited scope they should be used as much as possible. The amount of local anesthetic that can be tolerated is limited and the dosage should stay on the low side of the maximum allowable dosage. Dilute solutions of local anesthetic, such as 0.25% to 0.5% lidocaine, can increase the amount of the surgery permitted. Bilateral hip flexor abductor tenotomies, iliotibial band tenotomies in the lower thighs, and tenotomies of the tibialis posterior tendons and the tendo calcaneus have all been done simultaneously with the patient under local anesthesia. In doing tendo calcaneus and tibialis posterior tenotomies with local anesthesia, the only discomfort occurs when the ankles are dorsiflexed. This discomfort can be moderated by an intravenous tranquilizing agent or a synthetic narcotic substitute.

SURGICAL TECHNIQUES
PERCUTANEOUS TENDO CALCANEUS TENOTOMY

TECHNIQUE. Do not use a tourniquet. Prepare and drape the foot and ankle up to the upper calf. Infiltrate the skin and tendo calcaneus with a local anesthetic agent about 1 cm above the insertion of the tendon onto the calcaneus. Insert a small No. 11 knife blade or a tenotome with the blade held vertically through the skin and subcutaneous tissue into the tendo calcaneus. Then turn the blade medially and laterally and sweep it back and forth until the foot can be dorsiflexed at the ankle. Apply pressure over the incision for 5 minutes to stop all bleeding. Then apply a sterile dressing and a long leg cast with the ankle in 10-degrees of dorsiflexion and the knee in maximum extension. Cut out the heel of the cast, pound it soft, and replace it to avoid heel pressure during the postoperative period.

AFTERTREATMENT. The patient stands the evening of surgery and walks the next day. At 3 weeks, the cast is removed and a previously fabricated ankle-foot orthosis is applied.

PERCUTANEOUS TENDO CALCENEUS LENGTHENING

Percutaneous lengthening of the tendo calcaneus is useful in the ambulatory child with equinus contractures in whom some quadriceps function is still retained. Usually a floor-reaction orthosis is needed to assist in locking the knee in extension postoperatively (see Fig. 67-12). The procedure can be done with the patient under local anesthesia supplemented with an intravenous tranquilizer or narcotics.

TECHNIQUE (HSU AND HSU) (see Fig. 65-8). Surgically prepare and drape the limb so that the knee can be extended. Dorsiflex the ankle maximally to put the tendo calcaneus on stretch. Insert a small, slender knife blade or tenotome medially just above the insertion of the tendo calcaneus onto the calcaneus. Turn the blade laterally, and sever the tendon through one half of its width. Then move proximally 5 to 6.2 cm above the first incision, and, again medially, sever one half of the tendon.

With the ankle still dorsiflexed, now move midway between the two incisions but on the lateral side of the tendon. Pass the blade from the lateral side medially through one half the width of the tendon. Thus three cuts are made in the tendon, and the lateral half of this tendon is cut at an equal distance from the medial two cuts. Forcefully dorsiflex the ankle, and an audible and palpable release of the tendon will take place. In making the three small percutaneous punctures, hold the knife blade with its cutting edge vertical. This keeps the small incisions vertical and prevents gaping of the skin as it is stretched when the ankle is dorsiflexed. Take care not to buttonhole the skin as the cuts are made in the tendon.

Apply pressure to the area for 5 minutes to minimize any postoperative hematoma and apply a sterile dressing. Do not insert any sutures. Apply a long leg cast with the knee in full extension.

An alternative to this technique is to make all skin penetrations directly over the midline of the tendon. Then sweep the blade or tenotome laterally or medially to make the cuts in the tendon.

AFTERTREATMENT. Aftertreatment is the same as that described for percutaneous tendo calcaneus tenotomy (p. 3070).

SUBCUTANEOUS TIBIALIS POSTERIOR TENOTOMY

Subcutaneous tibialis posterior tenotomy is used when the tibialis posterior is the deforming force, pulling the foot into equinus and varus. It may be, and usually is, combined with tenotomy of the tendo calcaneus; it may be combined also with release beneath the toes of the flexor hallucis longus and flexor digitorum communis tendons if on dorsiflexion of the foot, the toe flexor tendons are tight. Any talipes cavus can be treated with a limited percutaneous plantar release. Talipes cavus may be present in Becker's muscular dystrophy, and if only this requires correction, (no equinus contracture) a short leg cast may be used after surgery.

TECHNIQUE. Prepare and drape the foot, ankle, and lower leg. Do not use a tourniquet. Infiltrate the skin and subcutaneous tissue with a local anesthetic agent just above and posterior to the medial malleolus for a distance of about 2 cm. Make a 0.6 to 1.0 cm incision vertically along the posterior border of the tibia just above the medial malleolus. Now dorsiflex and abduct the foot and palpate the movement of or tension in the tibialis posterior tendon. As this is done make a small hole in the tendon sheath and identify the movement of the tendon. With a right-angled gallbladder clamp or a small hemostat, slip behind the tendon and bring it forward into but not out of the wound. Sever the tendon under direct vision, and let its ends retract beneath the skin. Apply pressure over the incision for 5 minutes and apply a sterile dressing and a cast.

If a percutaneous plantar fasciotomy is indicated, make a stab wound over the center of the distal end of the calcaneal fat pad, where the plantar fascia attaches to the calcaneus. Through this small, midline incision, sweep the knife or tenotome laterally and medially close to the bone until the insertion of the plantar fascia has been severed. This procedure can be carried out using regional anesthetic block of the tibial nerve above the ankle, with a small amount of supplemental local anesthetic applied over the lateral third of the plantar fascia and overlying subcutaneous tissue.

AFTERTREATMENT. A short leg cast is applied with the foot in the corrected position.

ANTERIOR TRANSFER OF TIBIALIS POSTERIOR TENDON

Hsu and others have recommended an anterior transfer of the tibialis posterior tendon early in the equinovarus deforming stages of the disease. This procedure is useful mainly in the patient with Becker's muscular dystrophy. In the Duchenne's muscular dystrophy patient, often a tenotomy will suffice without the need for transfer of the tibialis posterior tendon anteriorly. Postoperatively an ankle-foot orthosis will be needed. If additional dorsiflexion power of the ankle is desirable, however, then the tendon may be transferred anteriorly through the interosseous membrane or released from behind the medial malleolus and slipped anteriorly subcutaneously and anchored in the midfoot. After this latter procedure the tendon still has its fulcrum around the medial border of the tibia and will exert some varus pull on the foot as it dorsiflexes the ankle. Either procedure requires a general anesthetic.

TECHNIQUE (BARR). See p. 2957.
TECHNIQUE (OBER). See p. 2958.

MEDULLOSTOMY OF TARSAL BONES FOR SEVERE EQUINOVARUS DEFORMITY

In severe equinovarus of long duration, the skin medially may be tight enough to prevent any significant correction unless the lateral border and dorsal aspect of the foot are shortened. This may be accomplished by removing the cancellous bone from the head and neck of the talus, the distal calcaneus, and the cuboid through a small incision along the lateral border of the head and neck of the talus (Fig. 67-14). After the bones have been curetted of cancellous bone, the foot can then be forcibly dorsiflexed and abducted at the midfoot. This causes the enucleated bones to collapse, allowing correction. This procedure will allow the patient to stand the day of surgery and to begin walking the day after; however, the surgery may be followed by severe swelling. It is wise to bivalve the cast before leaving the operating room. The tibialis posterior tendon and the tendo calcaneus should be left intact until after the osteoclasis has taken place, since they act as tethers through which the force to collapse the foot laterally and dorsally can act.

This procedure is useful in severe deformities of long duration in which the use of shoes and orthoses is needed in transfer. It may be indicated in patients with congenital dystrophy who develop severe equinovarus contractures from failure to use foot supports on their wheelchairs. Without foot supports, the feet naturally fall into an equinovarus position, and the deformity may be severe enough to prevent the wearing of shoes.

RELEASE OF HIPS

Opinions differ as to whether the hips should be released when the knees are released in the patient with Duchenne's muscular dystrophy or Becker's muscular dystrophy. Siegel believes that in most instances both the hips and the knees require release. Some degree of hip flexion contracture is compatible with walking (probably 15 to 20 degrees) and can be compensated for by an exaggerated lumbar lordosis. Certainly, hip flexion contractures, along with knee flexion contractures and weak quadriceps mechanisms, are incompatible with walking without falling. Siegel has devised a formula to determine when to release the hips and knees when an equinovarus foot deformity must be corrected (Fig. 67-15). He tests the ability to extend the hip against gravity while prone, noting the hip extensor lag in degrees. He then tests the functional extension in the knee with the patient supine. This gives the extensor lag in the knee in degrees. When these two measurements are added together and exceed 90 degrees, he believes that walking will cease and surgical releases are indicated.

Spencer has long been an advocate of early knee and ankle releases, before cessation of walking, in patients

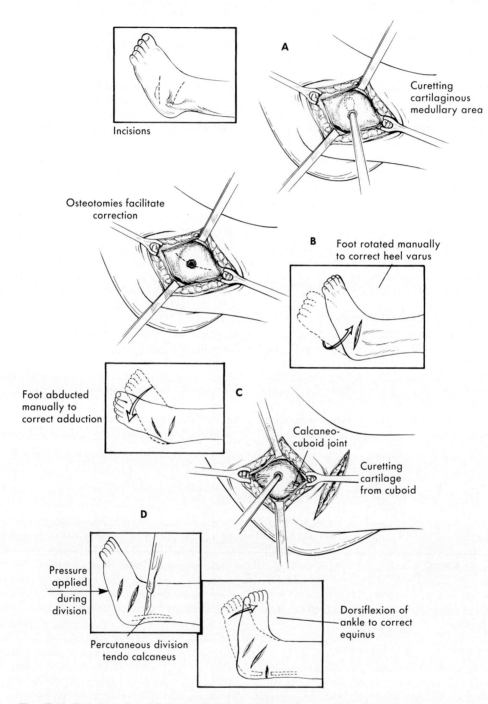

Fig. 67-14. Technique of medullostomy of tarsal bones for equinovarus deformity. (From Freeman, J.M.: Practical management of meningomyelocele, Baltimore, 1974, University Park Press.)

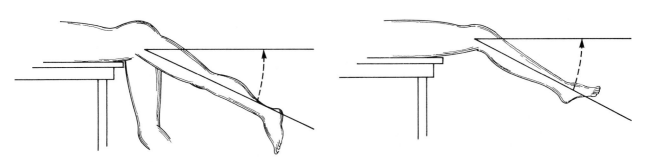

Fig. 67-15. Testing for hip and knee extensor lag. (From Siegel, I.M.: The clinical management of muscle disease. London, 1977, William Heinemann Medical Books, Ltd.)

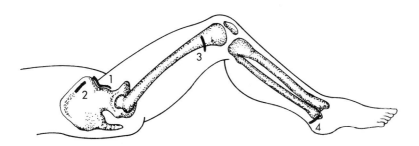

Fig. 67-16. Tenotomy sites for release of hip flexors, *1*, tenor fasciae latae and fascia lata, *2* and *3*, and tendo calcaneus, *4*. (From Siegel, I.M.: Clin. Pediatr. **19**:386, 1980.)

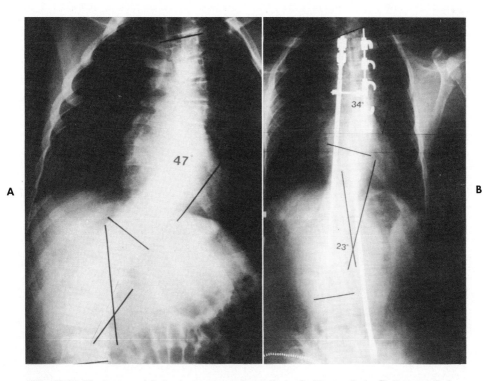

Fig. 67-17. Harrington rod fusion in neuromuscular scoliosis. **A,** Preoperatively. **B,** Postoperatively.

with Duchenne's muscular dystrophy, prolonging ambulation in some up to 5 years. He does not release the hips, believing that this is unnecessary for walking with long leg braces.

Vignos and associates have developed a series of functional and biochemical tests in an attempt to forecast the success of resuming ambulation of Duchenne's muscular dystrophy patients in braces after surgery. They found that they could predict with a reasonable degree of certainty whether such ambulation would be successful by measuring the remaining muscle strength in percentages of normal, the vital capacity, and the creatinine coefficient (the daily excretion of creatinine in the urine measured in milligrams divided by the body weight expressed in kilograms) and by attempting to assess the motivation of the patient and parents for bracing and walking.

With release of the hips, knees, and ankles by subcutaneous tenotomy, Siegel, Miller, and Ray have prolonged ambulation from 10 months to 22 months in 21 patients.

TECHNIQUE (SIEGEL). The procedure may be done with the patient under local or general anesthesia, using proper precautions to provide adequate ventilation and to prevent potassium overload and gastric dilation, which should compromise postoperative respiratory movements; cardiac monitoring is mandatory.

After a 24-hour presurgical skin preparation and with the patient supine on a fracture table, prepare and drape from the abdomen distally (Fig. 67-16). Have on hand an adequate supply of appropriate tenotomes so that each is used only once for each release. If desired carry out the same releases on each side as follows. Mark the femoral vessels and nerves at the hip and the common peroneal nerve at the knee, and avoid these areas during the release procedures. Release the hip flexors subcutaneously, flexing the contralateral hip. Insert the tenotome at the anterosuperior iliac spine and sweep it distally and posteriorly. This releases the sartorius and the straight head of the rectus femoris. Through the same stab wound sweep the tenotome laterally along the outer iliac crest to release the insertion of the tensor fasciae latae. Keep the tenotome close to the bone. This leaves only the iliopsoas and anterior hip capsule unreleased and usually allows 50% correction of any hip flexion deformity present.

Next release the iliotibial band just above the knee, avoiding the common peroneal nerve. Make a stab wound with another tenotome in the distal third of the thigh just above the supracondylar area of the femur. Incise the iliotibial band anteriorly and posteriorly just under the subcutaneous fat. Next sever the intermuscular septum down to the bone. The palpable ends of the severed iliotibial band separate approximately 2 cm. Apply pressure over the area to avoid a hematoma, but do not suture the wound. In the presence of an equinus contracture, do a percutaneous tendo calcaneus tenotomy at the same time.

AFTERTREATMENT. A toe-to-groin cast is applied with the ankles in neutral position and the knees in 5 degrees of flexion. The plantar surface of the cast is flattened against a board or another firm object to permit better ambulation. The cast is "fishmouthed" at the back of the heel, and the heel portion of the cast is pounded soft and then reapplied loosely. The patient stands at his bedside on the day of surgery and the next day begins walking in the physical therapy department; passive hip-stretching exercises also are begun. Extensive physical therapy instruction will allow the patient to gain walking ability in the cast and should be accomplished before discharge from the hospital. Family cooperation in the postoperative period is essential for success. At 3 weeks, the cast is removed and a

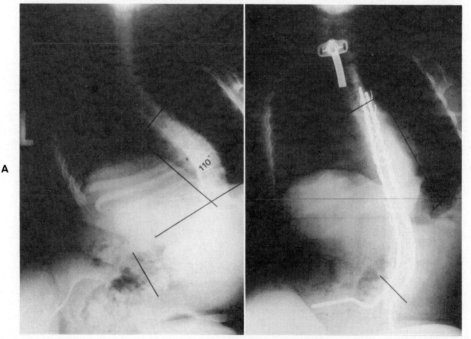

Fig. 67-18. Luque rod and segmental wire fixation in neuromuscular scoliosis. Curve measured 110 degrees preoperatively, **A**, and 71 degrees postoperatively, **B**.

lightweight knee-ankle-foot orthosis that has been fabricated preoperatively is applied.

• • •

Spencer et al. have performed, with the patient under general anesthesia, open surgical procedures on the knees and ankles, including releases and anterior transfers of the tibialis posterior tendons, in 44 patients, doing either one or all of the procedures bilaterally with two operating teams. They have had no anesthetic complications and few surgical complications. They have performed open fasciotomies just above the knees, tendo calcaneus tenotomies, and anterior transfers of the tibialis posterior tendon. They followed a strict postoperative physical therapy routine, so that the child was standing at least 3 hours each day in the week following surgery. Physical therapy was continued at home for an additional 2 weeks while the patient was in the long leg casts with the knees in maximum extension and the ankles dorsiflexed 10 degrees. When braces were fitted at 3 weeks, the patient was readmitted to the hospital for instruction in independent walking by a physical therapist.

SCOLIOSIS

Standing and walking patients usually do not develop scoliosis, so every attempt is made to see that standing and walking are continued as long as possible. Hsu studied the natural history of scoliosis in 6 nonambulatory patients with Duchenne's muscular dystrophy whose families refused efforts in any form to correct the spinal curve. He observed these six patients for an average of 5 years. The curve, usually a long C-shaped curve, involved the thoracic and lumbar vertebrae. In all six patients the curves progressed to exceed 40 degrees, and the function of the

patients in self-care and upright activities became more limited. In curves exceeding 80 degrees the curve became fixed and sitting at length was uncomfortable. Vital capacity was limited in all these patients. Other studies have shown that vital capacity decreases about 4% for each increase of 10 degrees in the scoliotic curve. It is likely that a curve greater than 30 degrees will increase in increments of 10 degrees each year.

Generally, it is wise to fit a wheelchair patient early with a thoracic lumbar spine orthosis that affords as much stability as possible without abdominal compression and to fit the wheelchair with appropriate inserts to prevent scoliosis, as well as to monitor regularly the patient's sitting spine roentgenograms. Evidence shows that, in curves of less than 30 degrees, a thoracic lumbar spine orthosis will help retard their progression; however, when the scoliosis reaches 30 degrees one should anticipate the need for a fusion and prepare the family for it. When the curve reaches 40 degrees and the vital capacity is greater than 30% of the expected volume, spine stabilization using any appropriate type of internal fixation is indicated (Fig. 67-17). This should improve wheelchair posture, make wheelchair use more comfortable, decrease the loss in vital capacity, and actually improve functional use of the wheelchair for the remaining life span.

That pulmonary function studies be evaluated preoperatively in scoliotic patients is especially important. If the vital capacity is less than 30% of the predicted value, the surgery probably should not be done. In these instances more difficulty will be encountered in getting the patient off the endotracheal tube or assisted respiration and in removing secretions from the tracheobronchial tree; thus postoperative pneumonitis is more likely to develop.

There is a strong possibility that the vital capacity for a

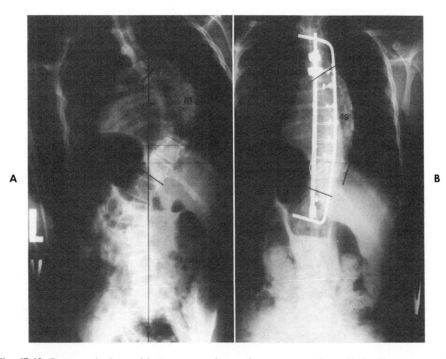

Fig. 67-19. Drummond wires and buttons over rods to reduce neuromuscular scoliosis. Curve measured 81 degrees preoperatively, **A**, and 49 degrees postoperatively, **B**.

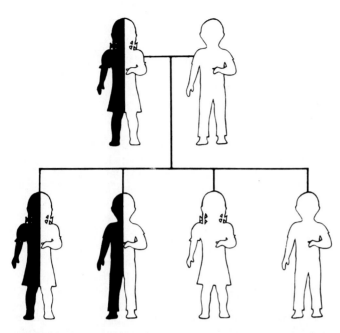

Fig. 67-20. Pattern of inheritance in musculofascial dystrophy, autosomal dominant inheritance. Either parent may have or transmit the disease. There is 50% chance of any offspring having disease and 50% chance that any offspring will be a carrier. (See Fig. 67-7, bottom, for key.)

limited period of time postoperatively and sometimes permanently will be less than before the operation. Straightening the spine may alter temporarily the strength in the remaining intercostal muscles and until they readjust to the change in their tension they do not function as well. Obliteration of the thoracic kyphosis by the fixation can reduce permanently the vital capacity, and it is wise to contour the rods to retain some dorsal kyphosis. Loss of the dorsal kyphosis may also make wheelchair transfers more difficult and impair function while sitting in a wheelchair. In addition, it may interfere with the delicate balance in neck and head control, since the neck must be thrust forward suspended by the active neck extensors to remain stable.

The method of fusion of the spine depends on the training and experience of the surgeon but should be one that requires minimum external immobilization.

Excellent results have been reported in patients whose spines were fused by Harrington rods and, more recently, by the Luque rods and segmental wiring techniques (Fig. 67-18). Success with the segmental wiring with Harrington rods has been reported, and some spine surgeons are using the Drummond wire and button modification of the segmental wiring technique (Fig. 67-19). At present the preference seems to be for the Luque technique. Considering possible complications, the technique requiring the least time in bed and the least external immobilization is the procedure of choice.

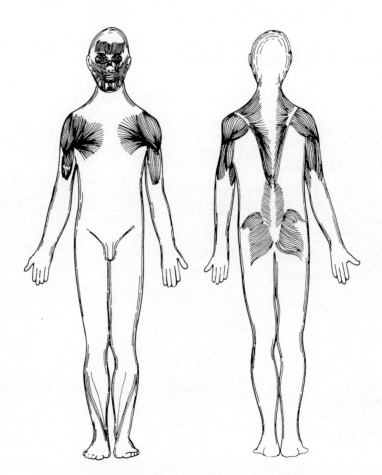

Fig. 67-21. Pattern of weakness in fascioscapulohumeral dystrophy.

TECHNIQUE FOR HARRINGTON INSTRUMENTATION AND FUSION. See Chapter 71.

TECHNIQUE FOR LUQUE RODS AND SEGMENTAL WIRING. See Chapter 71.

TECHNIQUE FOR DRUMMOND WIRES AND BUTTON. See Chapter 71.

Facioscapulohumeral dystrophy

Facioscapulohumeral dystrophy (Landouzy-Déjerine disease) is an autosomal dominant, inherited muscular dystrophy (Fig. 67-20). Since either parent may have the disease and transmit it, there is a 50% chance of any child having the disease, regardless of the sex, and there is a 50% chance that any offspring will be a carrier. Sporadic cases do appear occasionally but not as often as in Duchenne's muscular dystrophy.

The onset may be in very early childhood; in such patients the disease runs a rapid, progressive course and usually by 8 to 9 years of age the child becomes wheelchair bound. More often, the age of onset is from 15 to 35 years, and the disease is more slowly progressive. Periods of rapid progression may occur, however. The weakness is usually not as severe as in other forms of childhood muscular dystrophy, and the patient may lead a relatively normal life. The greatest functional disability is the inability to abduct and flex the arm at the glenohumeral joint (Fig. 67-21). This occurs not from weakness of the deltoid (which is usually relatively spared) but from an inability to stabilize the scapula on the thorax. This weakness may be asymmetric and thus may result in a scoliosis that requires spinal stabilization.

The clinical manifestation is usually one of facial weakness with an inability to whistle, purse the lips, wrinkle the brow, or blow out the cheeks. Children with facioscapulohumeral dystrophy may sleep with their eyes partially open, being unable to fully close them. Shoulder girdle weakness is also present, with atrophy of the trapezius, rhomboids, serratus anterior, serratus posterior, and latissimus dorsi (Fig. 67-21). The deltoid and forearm muscles are preserved, but the biceps and triceps become atrophic.

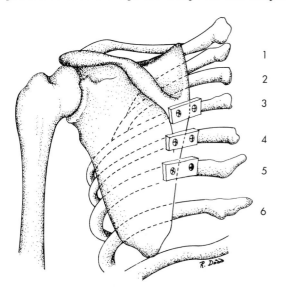

Fig. 67-22. Scapular stabilization with tibial struts. (Redrawn from Copeland, S.A., and Howard, R.C.: J. Bone Joint Surg. **60-B:**549, 1978.)

This results in the peculiar appearance of a "Popeye forearm." As the disease progresses, the lower extremities become weak, with weakness in the tibialis anterior and peroneal muscles and sometimes in the quadriceps. This requires either ankle-foot orthoses or knee-ankle-foot orthoses as determined by the weakness.

TREATMENT

Usually only the instability of the scapula requires orthopaedic treatment. As the deltoid attempts to abduct the shoulder, the scapula moves on the thorax, riding superiorly and anteriorly. Thus the motion occurs in the thoracoscapular area, rather than in the glenohumeral joint. In this disorder, scoliosis can progress and become severe enough to warrant spinal stabilization by any one of the techniques previously discussed. The lower extremities rarely require surgery, and the footdrop can usually be handled by a spring-loaded dorsiflexion assisted ankle-foot orthosis.

SCAPULOTHORACIC FUSION

Stabilization of the scapula on the thorax may be accomplished by fusing the scapula to the ribs or by fastening some tethering sling between the vertebral border of the scapula and the dorsal spine. The scapula should be stabilized in the neutral position, with the vertebral border parallel with the spine. This procedure usually results in an excellent cosmetic and functional result. Brachial plexus weakness may result if too great an effort is made to pull the scapula distalward.

TECHNIQUE (COPELAND AND HOWARD) (Fig. 67-22). With the patient under general anesthesia, prepare and drape one leg from groin to toes. Under tourniquet control, remove a 9 × 1 cm cortical graft from the anteromedial surface of the proximal tibia and curet cancellous bone from the proximal metaphysis. Close the wound in a routine fashion. Apply a long leg cast after the second stage of the procedure.

Turn the patient prone, and allow the arm to hang from the side of the table. Prepare and drape the upper back, shoulder, and upper arm to allow movement of the arm and access to the thoracic spine. Make an incision along the vertebral border of the scapula. Divide the underlying muscles, and denude for 2 cm the underside of the vertebral border of the scapula along most of its length.

Now denude by subperiosteal dissection the soft tissues of three ribs (usually the fourth, fifth, and sixth); this includes the periosteum, the intercostal muscles, and the parietal pleura. Expose enough of the ribs so that one half of the length of the cortical grafts (the original graft is divided into three segments 3 cm long) will lie against the denuded ribs. Drill a hole at each end of each graft, and fix the grafts with screws to the three ribs and to the underside of the medial aspect of the scapula. Protect the parietal pleura from penetration by a drill bit or screw. Fill any gap between the scapula and the chest wall with the cancellous bone removed from the tibia. Close the wound with drainage, and carefully turn the patient supine. Apply a shoulder spica cast with the arm in 30 degrees of forward flexion, 80 degrees of abduction, and the hand in front of the mouth.

AFTERTREATMENT. The patient is kept in a seated position. The arm section of the cast is removed at 3 months to allow abduction, and once abduction can be controlled, the entire cast is removed. A triangular pillow is placed between the inner arm and the thorax, and its size is gradually decreased to allow gradual adduction of the arm to the side. As soon as the cast is removed physical therapy is begun to help gain glenohumeral movement and deltoid strength.

The operation may be modified, according to Drennan, by screwing the scapula directly to the ribs and filling the area between the vertebral border of the scapula and the ribs with cancellous bone. This eliminates the need to remove the tibial cortical graft.

An alternative to fusion of the scapula to the chest wall is stabilization of the vertebral border of the scapula to the dorsal spine by a fascia lata sling. However, these slings have been known to stretch and cause recurrence of the shoulder instability. For this reason, and to decrease the extent of the procedure, we prefer to use a Dacron femoral artery prosthesis to tether the scapula to the spine. The prosthesis is well tolerated and does not stretch. It can, however, saw itself out of the dorsal spine or the scapula.

TECHNIQUE (WHITMAN). See Chapter 66, p. 3050.

Limb-girdle dystrophy

Limb-girdle dystrophy has an autosomal recessive inheritance pattern (Fig. 67-23), that is, for the disease to occur both parents must carry the trait. There is a 25% chance that any offspring of such a couple will have the disease (regardless of the sex of the child), and there is a 50% chance of any offspring carrying the defective gene. Occasionally, sporadic cases occur.

The disease may occur in the first to the fourth decade of life. The later the onset, the more rapid the progression.

The weakness may be in the muscles about either the shoulders or the pelvis (Fig. 67-24). Because the disease is usually slowly progressive and large muscle masses are not degenerating during any single period of time, the creatine phosphokinase level is not markedly elevated, although it is usually elevated to some extent. Electromyographic studies of involved muscles show the myopathic pattern, but nerve conduction studies are normal.

Involved members of a single family generally show the same degree of involvement. Contractures are uncommon. The diagnosis is made primarily on the clinical picture of muscle weakness and the inheritance pattern, which should include both parents' pedigrees.

The pattern of weakness of the lower extremities may be widespread throughout the pelvic girdle musculature. The gluteus maximus, the iliopsoas, and the quadriceps may be involved, causing marked hip instability and a waddling, knee-swinging gait. Pseudohypertrophy of the calves occurs in one out of five patients.

In the upper extremity weakness develops about the scapula, where the trapezius, the serratus anterior, the rhomboids, the latissimus dorsi, and the pectoralis major become involved. Some weakness may develop in the prime movers of the fingers and wrists as well. Since these patients are ambulatory into adulthood, scoliosis is seldom significant, although they may develop a degenerative arthritis of the spine as well as an exaggerated, painful lumbar lordosis. Death usually occurs by late in the third decade of life.

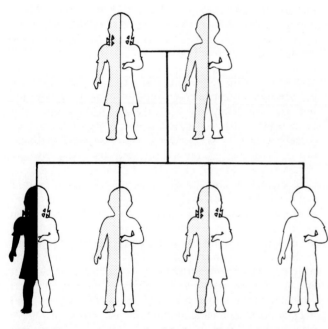

Fig. 67-23. Autosomal recessive inheritance. Both parents must carry trait. There is 25% chance that any offspring of such a couple will have disease and 50% chance that any offspring will carry trait. (See Fig. 67-7, bottom, for key.)

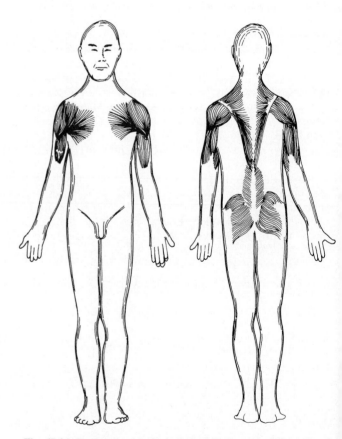

Fig. 67-24. Pattern of weakness in limb-girdle dystrophy. (From Siegel, I.M.: Clinical management of muscle disease, London, 1977, William Heinnemann Medical Books, Ltd.)

Little surgery is needed. The glenohumeral joint is stable, but the scapula may wing and occasionally require stabilization to the ribs or to the vertebrae, as in facioscapulohumeral dystrophy. Back pain may require a contoured back support, but surgical stabilization is seldom necessary. Muscle transfers about the wrist are rarely needed. In a slowly progressive pattern the brachioradialis muscle is usually spared, and this muscle may be used as a transfer to augment wrist or finger strength.

Congenital dystrophies

There are a number of types of congenital dystrophy. The differentiation is based primarily on special muscle stains that differentiate fiber types and show special characteristics of fiber abnormalities.

Some of the congenital muscular dystrophies are nemaline dystrophy, central core myopathy, myotubular myopathy, congenital fiber disproportion, and multicore and minicore disease. Electron microscopy may be needed to differentiate some of the types. Some show an inheritance pattern, whereas others may not, but usually the family history is positive. Some of the congenital muscular dystrophies are slowly progressive, and others are not. As a group they are infrequent. Because of weakness and contractures present at birth, the child may be born with dislocated hips and clubfeet or other deformities.

The patient is usually a hypotonic infant whose mother noted decreased fetal movements in utero. These infants often have marked respiratory weakness and, because of weakness of pharyngeal muscles, may have difficulty with feeding and swallowing. Their appearance is dysmorphic, with kyphoscoliosis, chest deformities, a long face, and a high palate. As the child becomes older, the muscle tissue is replaced by fibrous tissue and contractures may become severe.

The creatine phosphokinase level is usually moderately to well elevated at birth, since the disease process has begun in utero.

TREATMENT

Treatment is aimed at keeping the patient ambulatory and preventing contractures by exercises and orthotic splinting. As the disease progresses, hip and knee flexion contractures may develop. Equinus and varus deformities of the feet that prevent ambulation occur, as described in Duchenne's muscular dystrophy. These may require releases to allow the child to stand or walk. In some instances if hip flexion contractures can be eliminated, the LSU reciprocating brace may be used for walking. This is a cable-activated hip joint orthosis that includes the trunk and legs. The hips are activated reciprocally by extending the hip joint and shifting the weight to the contralateral side. This brace is ineffectual, however, in the presence of hip flexion contractures.

Congenital dislocations of the hip and clubfeet that are present at birth are difficult to treat and tend to recur, not unlike those in arthrogryposis. Treatment of these disorders is conventional, with a high rate of recurrence expected. Bracing may be required longer after correction, and follow-up must be more attentive than in the otherwise normal child.

Myotonic dystrophy

Myotonic dystrophy is characterized by an inability of the muscles to relax after contraction. It is progressive and usually is present at birth, although it may develop in later childhood. It is most often transmitted by an autosomal dominant pattern (Fig. 67-20), with the mother most frequently the carrier. The presentation may be autosomal recessive, however (Fig. 67-23).

Clinically, the muscles are unable to relax once they are stimulated. Tapping the thenar eminence with a reflex hammer will elicit a sustained contraction of the thenar muscles. This sustained contraction may also be demonstrated on the pronator-extensor muscle masses of the upper forearm or on the tongue where a sustained dimpling appears.

In addition to the inability of the muscles to relax, weakness that usually causes the most functional impairment is also present. Other defects are also present, including hyperostosis of the skull, frontal and temporal baldness, gonadal atrophy, dysphasia, dysarthria, electrocardiographic abnormalities, and mental abnormalities including retardation and depression. A low basal metabolic rate, impaired glucose tolerance, and impaired gastrointestinal mobility are also frequent.

The creatine phosphokinase level may be highly elevated early. Muscle biopsy shows a fatty degeneration and fibrous replacement.

These infants usually have a characteristic face at birth, with a tent-shaped mouth, facial diplegia, and a dull affect. Other members of the family may have similar faces. Approximately 50% of the infants have a talipes equinovarus, and some have hip dysplasia and scoliosis. The equinovarus may be accompanied by a peculiar deformity of the hallux that may ultimately require surgery. It is not unusual to see a child who has signs of a central nervous system insult as well. This is probably because more of these children with severe respiratory problems are being saved in neonatal intensive care units, and they have also suffered central nervous system injuries in the early neonatal period.

A characteristic myotonic electomyogram has been described and is especially striking (see Fig. 67-2). At the time of needle electrode insertion there is an increased frequency of a series of spiked action potentials at a high frequency, which then gradually diminishes until it is silent. If amplified on audio, this makes a characteristic "dive-bomber sound."

TREATMENT

The hip dysplasia can be treated as any dysplasia in the newborn, but because of capsular laxity it may not respond as readily as in an otherwise uncomplicated hip dysplasia.

An early equinovarus deformity has been found to be readily correctable by serial casting, but it is prone to recur and at times to change to a planovalgus deformity. Postoperative corrective bracing is indicated and must be used longer in this condition than in the otherwise uncomplicated clubfoot. With frequent recurrence in spite of posteromedial releases, a triple arthrodesis is often needed at skeletal maturity.

The peculiar hallux deformity of the big toe usually does not respond to soft tissue surgery, and an interphalangeal or a metatarsophalangeal joint fusion of the McKeever type may be necessary to align the toe.

Any surgical decision must take into account that serious cardiac abnormalities are frequent. Respiratory function studies are mandatory. The results of cardiac and respiratory studies may lead to the decision that surgery is too dangerous. A high incidence (33%) of surgical and anesthetic complications has been reported in those patients who undergo general surgical or obstetric and gynecologic procedures.

HERITABLE PROGRESSIVE NEUROPATHIC DISEASES

There is a mosaic of progressive neurologic conditions, usually inherited, that seem to be somewhat related. Almost a linear progression exists in the clinical appearance and pathologic findings. Some seem to be primarily diseases of the peripheral nerves; others are seen as a peripheral neuropathy with some involvement of the spinal cord; and others occur with spinal cord and brain involvement. Their eponyms are numerous.

Some order has been made in the delineation of the Charcot-Marie-Tooth variants in a classification by Dyck and Lambert. Greenfield has, in addition, classified the types of spinocerebellar atrophies. An unbroken link from one disease to the other is indicated.

Dyck and Lambert classification of Charcot-Marie-Tooth variants

HYPERTROPHIC NEUROPATHY

Hypertrophic neuropathy (classic Charcot-Marie-Tooth disease) is an autosomal dominant disease in which the peripheral nerves are enlarged and onion-bulb formations develop from segmental demyelinization and remyelinization as seen on electron microscopy of the peripheral nerves. Conduction velocities in the nerves are low.

Clinically, hypertrophic neuropathy occurs in the first or second decade of life, usually with foot abnormalities in the form of a high arch and clawed toes. The legs below the knees become progressively weak, and fine motor activity in the hands may be lost at the same time. Cavus or cavovarus deformity develops in the feet. With atrophy of the short toe flexors and intrinsic muscles of the foot, the arch rises. This cavus is at first flexible but then becomes fixed. Then the ankle dorsiflexors become weak and the toes claw. The first metatarsal pronates in relation to the hindfoot. As the toe extensors, along with the tibialis anterior and peroneal muscles, become weak, a footdrop may develop. Proprioceptive, light touch, and vibratory sensibilities in the feet are decreased. The deep tendon reflexes are absent in the lower extremities and decreased in the upper. As the disease progresses, not only do the intrinsic muscles of the hands atrophy, but the muscles on the back of the forearm, innervated by the radial nerve, also atrophy. Enlargement of the peripheral nerves may be palpable. The weakness is slow and progressive and the electromyographic pattern is one of a neuropathy while the creatine phosphokinase value is usually only slightly elevated. In the spinal cord the dorsal column degenerates with loss of cells in the dorsal nerve ganglia. Ventral horn cells in the lower spine may be smaller than normal.

ROUSSY-LÉVY SYNDROME

Roussy-Lévy syndrome (hereditary areflexic dystaxia) is also an autosomal dominant disease and carries with it the same clinical characteristics of a classic Charcot-Marie-Tooth disease; however, a static tremor occurs in the hands. The disease seems to become arrested at puberty.

DÉJERINE-SOTTAS SYNDROME

Déjerine-Sottas syndrome (familial interstitial hypertrophic neuritis) is an autosomal recessive disease, but it may show an autosomal dominant inheritance with poor expressivity. It usually begins in infancy but may appear in adolescence. The classic pes cavus deformity develops, but there is marked sensory loss in all four extremities. The patient may have a clubfoot or a kyphoscoliosis as well.

REFSUM'S SYNDROME

Refsum's syndrome is an autosomal recessive disorder beginning in childhood or at puberty and in it the spinal fluid protein is increased. The prognosis is poor. It is accompanied by retinitis pigmentosa and is characterized by a hypertrophic neuropathy with ataxia and areflexia. The course is unpredictable, with repeated reactivations and remissions. There is distal sensory and motor loss in the hands and feet.

NEURONAL TYPE OF CLASSIC CHARCOT-MARIE-TOOTH DISEASE

The neuronal type of classic Charcot-Marie-Tooth disease is an autosomal dominant disease whose onset is usually late in life, at middle age or later. The small muscles of the hands are not as weak but the muscles of the ankles and the plantar muscles of the feet are much weaker and more atrophic. Conduction velocities in the peripheral nerves are usually not diffusely slow.

CHARCOT-MARIE-TOOTH DISEASE WITH PROGRESSIVE SPINAL MUSCULAR ATROPHY

In addition to the classic pattern, patients with Charcot-Marie-Tooth disease with progressive spinal muscular atrophy have marked weakness in the muscles of the lower thigh and leg, and the distal forearm and hand show marked atrophy as well. Sensory deficits are absent. Although the reflexes may be diminished in the lower extremities, they are normal in the upper extremities.

• • •

All of these conditions are seen by the orthopaedist in most instances for gait problems, with loss of balance, cavus and varus feet, and occasionally equinus ankles.

DEGENERATIVE SPINOCEREBELLAR DISEASES
Greenfield's classification of spinocerebellar ataxias

    I. Spinal forms
        A. Friedreich's ataxia
            1. Pure forms
            2. Associated with peroneal muscular atrophy: Roussy-Lévy syndrome (hereditary areflexic dystaxia) or familial clawfoot, with absent tendon jerks, of Symonds and Shaw

3. Posterior column ataxia of Biemond
   B. Hereditary spastic ataxia
   C. Hereditary spastic paraplegia
   II. Spinocerebellar forms
   A. Menzel type of hereditary ataxia (olivopontocerebellar degeneration)
   B. Subacute spinocerebellar degeneration
   III. Cerebellar forms
   A. Holmes type of hereditary ataxia (cerebelloolivary or late cortical cerebellar atrophy of Marie Foix and Alajouanine; subacute familial type of akelaitis)
   B. Diffuse atrophy of Purkinje's cells (toxic and carcinogenic)

The spinal forms of hereditary ataxia are of interest primarily because they tend to cause foot deformities such as cavus, equinovarus, and claw toes and progressive scoliosis.

The main pathologic condition occurs in the long ascending and descending tracts of the spinal cord (the dorsal columns, the spinocerebellar tracts and the pyramidal tracts). The dorsal roots lose their larger fibers, more markedly in the lower spine. The spinocerebellar tracts are usually atrophied throughout their course, whereas the pyramidal tracts appear almost normal at the base of the medulla but show a progressive pallor as they descend through the spinal cord. Atrophy in the cerebellum, the medulla, and other parts of the brain and spinal cord has been reported.

In a few families, Friedreich's ataxia is associated with progressive deafness and optic atrophy. The heart is involved in most patients with Friedreich's ataxia, with an interstitial myocarditis with necrosis. A myopathy in the form of a granular degeneration of some muscle fibers and hypertrophy of others may occur.

In most patients the disease begins before the age of 20 years and may appear after an acute infection in childhood. The primary symptoms are an ataxic gait and pes cavus, which may be followed by clumsiness in the use of the hands, dysarthria, and nystagmus. The knee jerks and ankle jerks may be lost quite early, and with kyphoscoliosis often much deformity of the chest develops as the disease progresses.

The course of the disease is usually progressive, and most patients become unable to walk a few years after onset. Death is usually caused by cardiac failure during the third decade. Sudden cardiac death is not unusual. Extensive plantar responses occur, making wheelchair transfers difficult.

Spastic paraplegia is a condition that lies far down on the spectrum of these related diseases. Autosomal dominant disease is more common, but autosomal recessive inheritance through consanguineous marriages has been reported, as has a sex-linked inheritance pattern.

Spastic paraplegia is characterized by slowly progressive weakness and spastic paralysis in the lower extremities. Usually, disease that is autosomal recessive in inheritance is more rapidly progressive than that in autosomal dominant inheritance. The onset is usually in the first decade in the recessive type and in the second decade in the autosomal dominant type. The spinal cord shows corticospinal tract degeneration. From the level of the pyramids in the

medulla, there is progressive posterior column degeneration without loss of posterior root fibers. This condition is most often called a cerebral palsy, but it is not cerebral in origin and is progressive in nature.

TREATMENT

The orthopaedist is concerned primarily with the correction of pes cavus, pes cavovarus, and the associated claw toes that can develop. The cavus at first is flexible in the immature foot. This appears to be a result of atrophy of the intrinsic muscles of the foot, as well as of the flexor digitorum brevis in the sole of the foot. The loss of this muscle mass makes the arch appear to be higher, and early in the disease the pes cavus can be corrected easily by pressure exerted on the plantar surface of the metatarsal heads. Some think that the peroneus longus exerts an unopposed pull on the first metatarsal shaft, since the tibialis anterior muscle weakens earlier, and this force pulls the forefoot into equinus position in relation to the hindfoot.

Conservative treatment consisting of serial casting and an orthosis might suffice early in pes cavus; however, the deformity will continue to progress, and an extensive plantar release eventually may be needed to correct it. Once bony changes have developed, with the apex of the cavus at the midfoot, a procedure on the bone, such as dorsal wedge osteotomy (p. 2499) or a truncated osteotomy of the forefoot as advocated by Jahss (p. 3085), will be required.

The Jones procedure (see Fig. 67-27, *D*) (that is, a transfer of the extensor hallucis longus to the neck of the first metatarsal and fusion of the interphalangeal joint of the great toe) will aid in dorsiflexion of the first metatarsal and decrease clawing of this toe. The Hibbs procedure will likewise decrease the clawing of the lateral four toes and help elevate the metatarsal heads if each of the extensor tendon slips is inserted into the neck of the metatarsals. If the toe extensor tendons are inserted into the second or third cuneiform, it will elevate the midfoot and consequently the forefoot but will have no dynamic effect on changing the angle between the longitudinal axis of the first metatarsal and the longitudinal axis of the talus as seen on the lateral roentgenogram.

In the cavovarus foot one must determine whether the varus of the heel is fixed or if the varus is merely secondary to the forefoot deformity of pronation of the shaft of the first metatarsal; that is, the shaft of the first metatarsal is plantar flexed in relation to the hindfoot. This determination is best done by the Coleman block test (Fig. 67-25). The foot, except for the first ray, rests with weight bearing on a block of wood 1 cm thick. The first metatarsal is allowed to hang free from the medial side of the block. If, as weight is borne on the foot, the calcaneus realigns into a neutral or slightly valgus position in relation to the tibia, the heel varus is not fixed. If the calcaneus does not realign with the block test, the heel varus is fixed.

When heel varus is not fixed, surgery in the form of a plantar release (Fig. 67-26), an osteotomy of the first metatarsal, or an osteotomy of the medial cuneiform after the manner of Fowler and Brooks may be done.

If the varus is fixed, then some procedure on the bones of the hindfoot must be done, such as a valgus closing wedge calcaneal osteotomy as advocated by Dwyer (p.

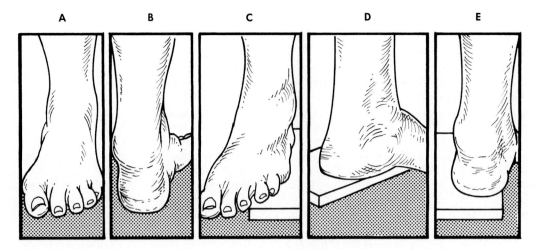

Fig. 67-25. Coleman block test to differentiate fixed from nonfixed heel varus. **A** and **B,** Supinated forefoot and varus heel. **C** and **D,** Foot, except for first metatarsal, rests on 1 cm block of wood. **E,** If heel realigns to neutral or slight valgus, varus is not fixed. (Redrawn after Coleman, S.S.: Complex foot deformities in children, Philadelphia, 1983, Lea & Febiger.)

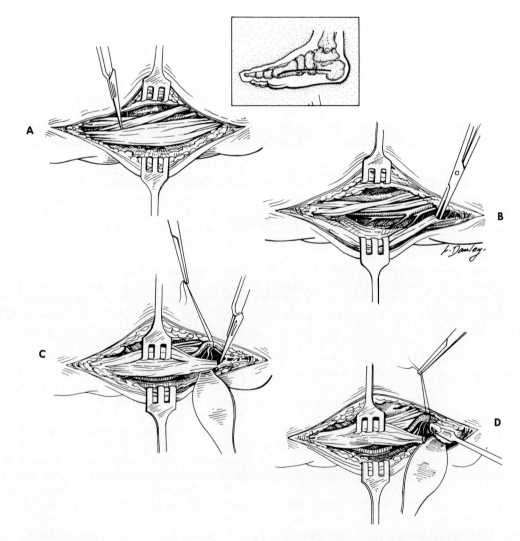

Fig. 67-26. Plantar release of cavovarus foot. **A,** Skin incision. **B,** Exposure of abductor hallucis over its entire length. **C,** Release of abductor hallucis from calcaneus. Identification and protection of plantar nerves and vessels. **D,** Release of long and short plantar ligaments, keeping neurovascular structures protected. (Redrawn after Coleman, S.S.: Complex foot deformities in children, Philadephia, 1983, Lea & Febiger.)

2942) or a subtalar arthrodesis (p. 2019). Transfer of the tibialis posterior tendon anteriorly to the midfoot may prevent recurrence of the heel varus and aid in dorsiflexion of the foot.

A cavovarus deformity and metatarsus adductus may be treated best by a medial plantar release, Dwyer's lateral calcaneal osteotomy, and multiple osteotomies of the metatarsal bases to correct the adducted forefoot (Berman's or Gartland's procedure) (see Fig. 67-20).

All these procedures may result in inadequate correction or recurrence of the deformity if the foot is immature or if muscle dynamics remain unbalanced.

A triple arthrodesis (p. 2935) may be required as a salvage procedure or as a primary procedure when the deformities have become fixed (Fig. 67-27).

Levitt and associates reviewed 15 children who had either Charcot-Marie-Tooth disease or Friedreich's ataxia. All had undergone soft tissue or bony procedures on the feet exclusive of a triple arthrodesis and none of these procedures had stood up over time; the deformities recurred in some form after all procedures. Only a triple arthrodesis was found to be satisfactory. They recommend that the other soft tissue and bony procedures be done as a first stage, followed by a triple arthrodesis done at a later time.

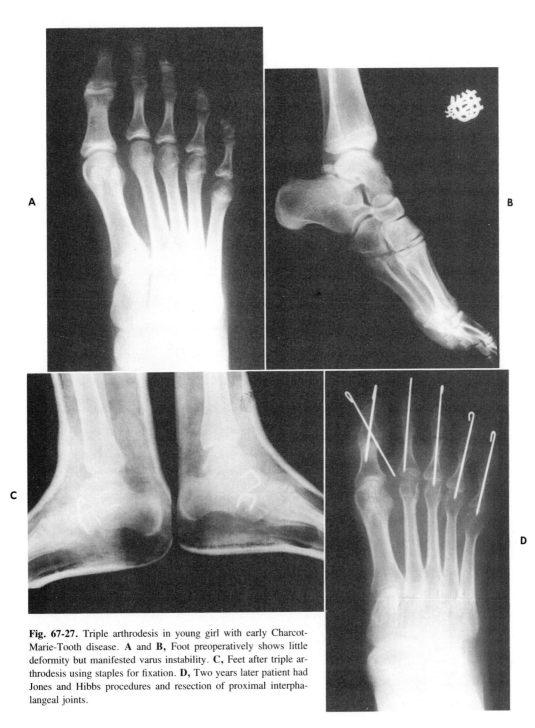

Fig. 67-27. Triple arthrodesis in young girl with early Charcot-Marie-Tooth disease. **A** and **B**, Foot preoperatively shows little deformity but manifested varus instability. **C**, Feet after triple arthrodesis using staples for fixation. **D**, Two years later patient had Jones and Hibbs procedures and resection of proximal interphalangeal joints.

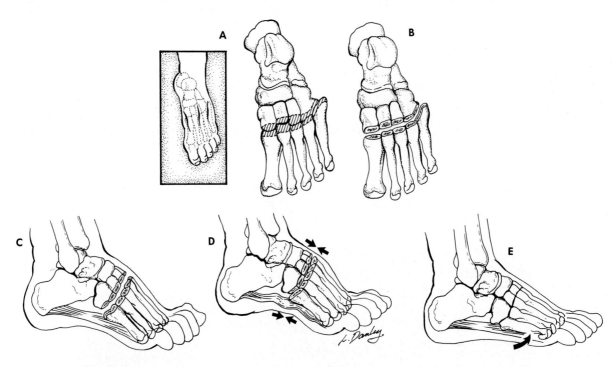

Fig. 67-28. Truncated dorsal wedge osteotomy of Jahss. (Redrawn from Jahss, M.: J. Bone Joint Surg. **62-A:**718, 1980.)

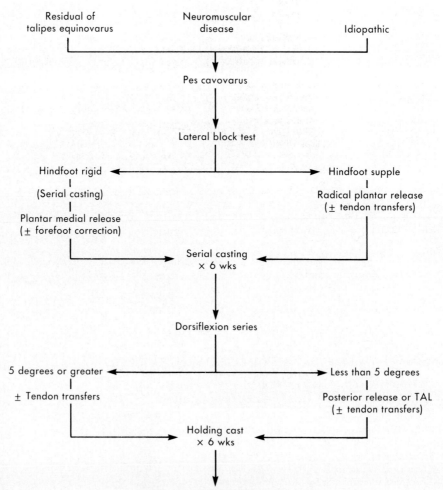

Fig. 67-29. Flow chart for diagnosis and treatment of pes cavovarus. (Redrawn from Paulos, L.E., Coleman, S.S., and Samuelson, K.M.: J. Bone Joint Surg. **62-A:**942, 1980.)

Rochelle, Bowen, and Ray have presented a rational approach to the correction of forefoot deformities in the progressive cavovarus neuromuscular foot. They recommend, in the flexible cavus foot a Steindler stripping of the plantar fascia (p. 2941) and postoperative serial cast correction. In fixed midfoot cavus with a heel varus that is flexible, they combine a plantar fascial release with either a truncated dorsal wedge osteotomy as advocated by Jahss or a dorsal wedge osteotomy of the tarsal bones (p. 2944) made at the apex of the deformity (Fig. 67-28). In severe fixed cavovarus feet, triple arthrodesis and plantar release, at times supplemented by a second stage anterior transfer of the tibialis posterior tendon through the interosseous membrane, is recommended. For the foot with heel equinus in addition to the cavovarus deformity, Lambrinudi's type of triple arthrodesis (p. 2955) is recommended. Claw toes, if flexible, are treated by transfer of the long toe flexors into the extensor expansions. The fixed great toe that is rigid in hyperextension should be treated by a Jones procedure (p. 2939) and a dorsal capsulotomy of the metatarsophalangeal joint.

Paulos, Coleman, and Samuelson have produced a flowchart to be used in the treatment of the cavovarus foot deformity (Fig. 67-29). The use of such a chart is an excellent idea.

Fowler devised a procedure to lengthen the medial border of the foot and correct the plantar flexion of the first metatarsal in the cavus foot. An opening wedge osteotomy of the medial cuneiform is done after a medial plantar release. The opening wedge in the osteotomy is trapezoidal, with the wider bases plantarward and medialward.

Sometimes in Friedreich's ataxia the plantar reflex is so great that when standing is attempted, the feet and toes immediately plantar flex and the tibialis posterior tendon pulls the forefoot into equinovarus. Such a response can be elicited simply by trying to put on socks and shoes. This effort makes dressing a monumental task. In such instances, in the face of myocardial involvement or other life-threatening conditions that would make a general anesthetic unduly hazardous, tenotomies of the heel cords, the tibialis posterior tendons at the ankles, and the toe flexors at the plantar side of the metatarsophalangeal joints can be done with the patient under local anesthesia and will make putting on shoes and wheelchair transfers easier.

Although scoliosis often develops to a significant degree (80%) in patients with Friedreich's ataxia (see Fig. 67-17), it rarely develops in patients with any of the variations of Charcot-Marie-Tooth disease. When it does develop the scoliosis is hard to control with any type of orthosis. The Milwaukee brace is poorly tolerated by such patients. The rate of progression of the scoliosis may be slowed by a thoracic lumbar spine orthosis of some type, but the progression does not stop; even after the patient becomes skeletally mature progression continues. Spinal stabilization and posterior fusion are being done with increasing frequency on patients with Friedreich's ataxia, using either the Harrington instrumentation, Luque rod, or Drummond wire technique. The latter two techniques require less postoperative immobilization, but any of the three can improve sitting balance and tolerance and aid in wheelchair transfers.

The techniques for these spine stabilization procedures are discussed in Chapter 71.

REFERENCES
Myopathic disease—general

Berman, A.T., et al.: Muscle biopsy: proper surgical technique, Clin. Orthop. **198**:240, 1985.

Bowker, J.H., and Halpin, P.J.: Factors determining success in reambulation of the child with progressive muscular dystrophy, Orthop. Clin. North Am. **9**:431, 1978.

Brink, J.D., and Hoffer, M.M.: Rehabilitation of brain injured children, Orthop. Clin. North Am. **9**:451, 1978.

Drennan, J.C.: Neuromuscular disorders. In Lovell, W.W., and Winter, R.B. (editors): Pediatric orthopaedics, ed. 2, vol. 2, Philadelphia, 1986, J.B. Lippincott Co.

Drennan, J.C.: Orthopaedic management of neuromuscular disorders, Philadelphia, 1984, J.B. Lippincott Co.

Gardner-Medwin, D.: Clinical features and classification of muscular dystrophies, Br. Med. Bull. **36**:109, 1980.

Hsu, J.D., Groolman, T.B., Hoffer, M.N., et al.: The orthopaedic management of spinal muscular atrophy, J. Bone Joint Surg. **55-B**:663, 1973.

Kottke, F.J.: The effects of limitation of activity upon the human body, JAMA **196**:10,117, 1966.

Lehman, J.B.: Biomechanics of ankle-foot orthoses: prescription and design, Arch. Phys. Med. Rehabil. **60**:200, 1979.

O'Neill, D.L., and Harris, S.R.: Developing goals and objectives for handicapped children, Phys. Ther. **62**:295, 1982.

Shapiro, F., and Bresnan, M.J.: Current concepts review: orthopaedic management of childhood neuromuscular disease. Part II: Diseases of muscle, J. Bone Joint Surg. **64-A**:1102, 1982.

Siegel, I.M.: Diagnosis, management, and orthopaedic treatment of muscular dystrophy. In American Academy of Orthopaedic Surgeons: Instructional course lectures, vol. 30, St. Louis, 1981, The C.V. Mosby Co.

Siegel, I.M.: The clinical management of muscle disease: a practical manual of diagnosis and treatment, London, 1977, William Heinemann Medical Books, Ltd.

Spencer, G.E., Jr.: Orthopaedic care of progressive muscular dystrophy, J. Bone Joint Surg. **49-A**:1201, 1967.

Spencer, G.E., Jr., and Vignos, P.J., Jr.: Bracing for ambulation in childhood progressive muscular dystrophy, J. Bone Joint Surg. **44-A**:234, 1962.

Swinyard, C.A.: Progressive muscular dystrophy and atrophy and related conditions: diagnosis and management, Pediatr. Clin. North Am. **7**:703, 1960.

Zellweger, H., Durnin, R., and Simpson, J.: The diagnostic significance of serum enzymes and electrocardiogram in various muscular dystrophies, Acta Neurol. Scand. **48**:87, 1972.

Duchenne's muscular dystrophy

Bertorini, T.E., et al.: Calcium and magnesium content in fetuses at risk and prenecrotic Duchenne muscular dystrophy, Neurology **34**:1436, 1984.

Bleck, E.E.: Mobility of patients with Duchenne muscular dystrophy (letter), Develop. Med. Child Neurol. **21**:823, 1979.

Brown, J.C.: Muscular dystrophy, Practitioner **226**:1031, 1982.

Brownell, A.K.W., et al.: Malignant hyperthermia in Duchenne muscular dystrophy, Anesthesiology **58**:180, 1983.

Cooper, R.R.: Skeletal muscle and muscle disorders. In Cruess, R.L., and Rennie, W.R.J.: Adult orthopaedics, vol. I, New York, 1984, Churchill Livingstone.

Cornelio, F., and Dones, I.: Muscle fiber degeneration and necrosis in muscular dystrophy and other muscle diseases: cytochemical and immunocytochemical data, Ann. Neurol. **16**:694, 1984.

Crisp, D.E., Ziter, F.A., and Bray, P.F.: Diagnostic delay in Duchenne's muscular dystrophy, JAMA **247**:478, 1982.

Curtis, B.H.: Orthopaedic management of muscular dystrophy and related disorders. In American Academy of Orthopaedic Surgeons: Instructional course lectures, vol. 19, St. Louis, 1970, The C.V. Mosby Co.

Douglas, R., Larson, P.F., D'Ambrosia, R., and McCall, R.E.: The LSU reciprocation-gait orthosis, Orthopedics **6**:834, 1983.

Drennan, J.C., and Bondurant, M.: Paralytic disorders. In American Academy of Orthopaedic Surgeons: Atlas of orthotics, ed. 2, St. Louis, 1985, The C.V. Mosby Co.

Dubowitz, V.: The female carrier of Duchenne muscular dystrophy, Br. Med. J. **284**:1423, 1982.

Falcão-Conceicão, D.N., Goncalves-Pimentel, M.M., Baptista, M., and Ubatuba, S.: Detection of carriers of X-linked gene for Duchenne muscular dystrophy by levels of creatine kinase and pyruvate kinase, J. Neurol. Sci. **62**:171, 1983.

Fletcher, R., Blennow, G., Olsson, A.-K., Ranklev, E., and Tornebrandt, K.: Malignant hyperthermia in a myopathic child: prolonged postoperative course requiring dantrolene, Acta Anaesth. Scand. **26**:435, 1982.

Florence, J.M., Brooke, M.H., and Carroll, J.E.: Evaluation of the child with muscular weakness, Orthop. Clin. North Am. **9**:409, 1978.

Firth, M.A.: Diagnosis of Duchenne muscular dystrophy: experiences of parents of sufferers, Br. Med. J. **286**:700, 1983.

Firth, M., Garder-Medwin, D., Hosking, G., and Wilkinson, E.: Interviews with parents of boys suffering from Duchenne muscular dystrophy, Develop. Med. Child Neurol. **25**:466, 1983.

Fowler, W.M., Jr., and Taylor, M.: Rehabilitation management of muscular dystrophy and related disorders: Part I. The role of exercise, Arch. Phys. Med. Rehabil. **63**:319, 1982.

Fowler, W.M., Jr.: Rehabilitation management of muscular dystrophy and related disorders: Part II. Comprehensive care, Arch. Phys. Med. Rehabil. **63**:322, 1982.

Gardner-Medwin, D.: Controversies about Duchenne muscular dystrophy: Part II. Bracing for ambulation, Develop. Med. Child Neurol. **21**:659, 1979.

Gardner-Medwin, D., and Johnston, H.M.: Severe muscular dystrophy in girls, J. Neurol. Sci. **64**:79, 1984.

Gibson, D.A., Koreska, J., Robertson, D., Kahn, A., III, and Albisser, A.M.: The management of spinal deformity in Duchenne's muscular dystrophy, Orthop. Clin. North Am. **9**:437, 1978.

Golbus, M.S., Stephens, J.D., Mahoney, M.J., et al.: Failure of fetal creatine phosphokinase as a diagnostic indicator of Duchenne muscular dystrophy, N. Engl. J. Med. **300**:860, 1979.

Harper, D.C.: Adjustment of adolescents with Duchenne muscular dystrophy (abstract), Orthop. Trans. **8**:120, 1984. Presented at the Annual Meeting of the American Academy for Cerebral Palsy and Developmental Medicine, Chicago, Illinois, October 3-5, 1983.

Headings, V.E., Anyaibe, S.I.O., Akindele, J., and Onaga, M.: An erythrocyte membrane antigen associated with X-linked muscular dystrophy, Arch. Neurol. **40**:300, 1983.

Hsu, J.D.: The natural history of spine curvature progression in the non-ambulatory Duchenne muscular dystrophy patient, Spine **8**:771, 1983.

Hsu, J.D.: Management of foot deformity in Duchenne's pseudohypertrophic muscular dystrophy, Orthop. Clin. North Am. **7**:979, 1976.

Hsu, J.D., et al.: Control of spine curvature in the Duchenne muscular dystrophy (DMD) patient. In Proceedings of the Scoliosis Research Society, Denver, Scoliosis Research Society, 1982.

Hsu, J.D., and Lewis, J.E.: Challenges in the care of the retarded child with Duchenne muscular dystrophy, Orthop. Clin. North Am. **12**:73, 1981.

Hsu, J.D., and Hsu, C.L.: Motor unit disease. In Jahss, M.H. (editor): Disorders of the foot, Philadelphia, 1982, W.B. Saunders Co.

Johnson, E.W., and Yarness, S.K.: Hand dominance and scoliosis in Duchenne muscular dystrophy, Arch. Phys. Med. Rehabil. **57**:462, 1976.

Jones, G.E., and Witkowski, J.A.: Membrane abnormalities in Duchenne muscular dystrophy, J. Neurol. Sci. **58**:159, 1983.

Kelfer, H.M., Singer, W.D., and Reynolds, R.N.: Malignant hyperthermia in a child with Duchenne muscular dystrophy, Pediatrics **71**:118, 1983.

Kurz, L.T., Murbarak, S.J., Schultz, P., Park, S.M., and Leach, J.: Correlation of scoliosis and pulmonary function in Duchenne muscular dystrophy, J. Pediatr. Orthop. **3**:347, 1983.

Lane, R.J.M., Robinow, M., and Roses, A.D.: The genetic status of mothers of isolated cases of Duchenne muscular dystrophy, J. Med. Genet. **20**:1, 1983.

Leterrier, F., et al.: A spin label study of the erythrocyte membrane in mothers and sisters of patients suffering from Duchenne muscular dystrophy, Clin. Chim. Acta **143**:99, 1984.

Linter, S.P.K., Thomas, P.R., Withington, P.S., and Hall, M.G.: Suxamethonium associated hypertonicity and cardiac arrest in unsuspected pseudohypertrophic muscular dystrophy, Br. J. Anaesth. **54**:1331, 1982.

Lutter, L.D., Carlson, M., Winter, R.B., and Zarling, V.R.: Spine curvatures in progressive muscular dystrophy. Presented at the Annual Meeting of the Pediatric Orthopaedic Society, Vancouver, B.C., Canada, May 21-23, 1984.

Marchildon, M.B.: Malignant hyperthermia: current concepts, Arch. Surg. **117**:349, 1982.

Melkonian, G.J., Cristofaro, R.L., Perry, J., and Hsu, J.D.: Dynamic gait electromyography study in Duchenne muscular dystrophy (DMD) patients, Foot Ankle **1**:78, 1980.

Miller, G.M., Hsu, J.D., Hoffer, M.M., and Rentfro, R.; Posterior tibial tendon transfer: a review of the literature and analysis of 74 procedures, J. Pediatr. Orthop. **2**:363, 1982.

Milne, B., and Rosales, J.K.: Anaesthetic considerations in patients with muscular dystrophy undergoing spinal fusion and Harrington rod insertion, Can. Anaesth. Soc. J. **29**:250, 1982.

Monckton, G., Zatz, M., Mion, C.S., and Marusyk, H.: Results of blind testing a method to detect carriers of the Duchenne muscular dystrophy gene, Am. J. Hum. Genet. **36**:926, 1984.

Moseley, C.F., Koreska, J., and Miller, F.: Treatment of spinal deformity in Duchenne muscular dystrophy. Presented at the Annual Meeting of the American Academy of Orthopaedic Surgeons, January 26, 1985, Las Vegas, Nev.

Moser, H.: Duchenne muscular dystrophy: pathogenetic aspects and genetic prevention, Hum. Genet. **66**:17, 1984.

Mubarak, S.J., Kurz, L., Schultz, P., and Park, S.M.: Correlating scoliosis and pulmonary function in Duchenne muscular dystrophy. Presented at the American Academy for Cerebral Palsy and Developmental Medicine Annual Meeting, 1983.

Nicholson, G.A., and Sugars, J.: An elevation of lymphocyte capping in Duchenne muscular dystrophy, J. Neurol. Sci. **53**:511, 1982.

Nomura, H., and Hizawa, K.: Histopathological study of the conduction system of the heart in Duchenne progressive muscular dystrophy, Acta Pathol. Jpn. **32**:1027, 1982.

Nordal, H.J., Andersson, T.R., and Dietrichson, P.: Lymphocyte capping: a diagnostic method in progressive muscular dystrophy? Acta Neurol. Scand. **65**:442, 1982.

Nørregaard-Hansen, K., and Hein-Sørensen, O.: Significance of serum myoglobin in neuromuscular disease and in carrier detection of Duchenne muscular dystrophy, Acta Neurol. Scand. **66**:259, 1982.

Nowak, T.V., Ionasescu, V., and Anuras, S.: Gastrointestinal manifestations of the muscular dystrophies, Gastroenterology **82**:800, 1982.

Oka, S., et al.: Malignant hyperpyrexia and Duchenne muscular dystrophy: a case report, Can. Anaesth. Soc. J. **29**:627, 1982.

Olson, B.J., and Fenichel, G.M.: Progressive muscle disease in a young woman with family history of Duchenne's muscular dystrophy, Arch. Neurol. **39**:378, 1982.

Perloff, J.K., Henze, E., and Schelbert, H.R.: Alterations in regional myocardial metabolism, perfusion, and wall motion in Duchenne muscular dystrophy studied by radionuclide imaging, Circulation **69**:33, 1984.

Rabbani, N., Moses, L., Anandavalli, T.E., and Anandraj, M.P.J.S.: Calcium-activated neutral protease from muscle and platelets of Duchenne muscular dystrophy cases, Clin. Chim. Acta **143**:163, 1984.

Renshaw, T.S.: Treatment of Duchenne's muscular dystrophy (letter), JAMA **248**:922, 1982.

Renshaw, T.S.: Treatment of Duchenne's muscular dystrophy, JAMA **248**:922, 1982.

Robin, G.C.: Scoliosis in Duchenne muscular dystrophy, Isr. J. Med. Sci. **13**:203, 1977.

Rochelle, J., Bowen, J.R., and Ray, S.: Pediatric foot deformities in progressive neuromuscular disease, Contemp. Orthop. **8**:41, 1984.

Saltiel, J.: A one-piece laminated knee locking short leg brace, Orthot. Prosthet. **23**:68, 1969.

Seeger, B.R., Caudrey, D.J., and Little, J.D.: Progression of equinus deformity in Duchenne muscular dystrophy, Arch. Phys. Med. Rehabil. **66:**286, 1985.

Seeger, B.R., Sutherland, A. D'A., and Clark, M.S.: Orthotic management of scoliosis in Duchenne muscular dystrophy, Arch. Phys. Med. Rehabil. **65:**83, 1984.

Shelborne, S.A.: Duchenne's muscular dystrophy (letter), JAMA **247:**496, 1982.

Siegel, I.M.: Maintenance of ambulation in Duchenne muscular dystrophy: the role of the orthopedic surgeon, Clin. Pediatr. **19:**383, 1980.

Siegel, I.M.: Equinocavovarus in muscular dystrophy: treatment by percutaneous tarsal medullostomy and soft tissue release, Isr. J. Med. Sci. **13:**198, 1977.

Siegel, I.M.: Prolongation of ambulation through early percutaneous tenotomy and bracing with plastic orthoses, Isr. J. Med. Sci. **13:**192, 1977.

Siegel, I.M., Miller, J.E., and Ray, R.D.: Subcutaneous lower limb tenotomy in the treatment of pseudohypertrophic muscular dystrophy: description of technique and presentation of twenty-one cases, J. Bone Joint Surg. **50-A:**1437, 1968.

Sussman, M.D.: Advantage of early spinal stabilization and fusion in patients with Duchenne muscular dystrophy, J. Pediatr. Orthop. **4:**531, 1984.

Swank, S.M., Brown, J.C., and Perry, R.E.: Spinal fusion in Duchenne's muscular dystrophy, Spine **7:**484, 1982.

Vignos, P.J., Wagner, M.B., Kaplan, J.S., and Spencer, G.E., Jr.: Predicting the success of reambulation in patients with Duchenne muscular dystrophy, J. Bone Joint Surg. **65-A:**719, 1983.

Weimann, R.L., Gibson, D.A., Moseley, C.F., and Jones, D.C.: Surgical stabilization of the spine in Duchenne muscular dystrophy, Spine **8:**776, 1983.

Wheeler, S.D.: Pathology of muscle and motor units, Phys. Ther. **62:**1809, 1982.

Yoshida, M., Ando, K., and Satoyoshi, E.: Abnormalities of erythrocytes in Duchenne muscular dystrophy, Ann. Neurol. **13:**649, 1983.

Becker's muscular dystrophy

Becker, P.E., Kiener, F.: Eine neue x-chromosomale Muskeldystrophie, Arch. Psychiatr. Nervenkr. **193:**427, 1955.

Curtis, B.H.: Orthopaedic management of muscular dystrophy and related disorders. In American Academy of Orthopaedic Surgeons: Instructional course lectures, vol. 19, St. Louis, 1970, The C.V. Mosby Co.

Emery, A.E.H., and Skinner, R.: Clinical studies in benign (Becker type) X-linked muscular dystrophy, Clin. Genet. **10:**189, 1976.

Florence, J.M., Brooke, M.H., and Carroll, J.E.: Evaluation of the child with muscular weakness, Orthop. Clin. North Am. **9:**409, 1978.

Fowler, W.M., Jr.: Rehabilitation management of muscular dystrophy and related disorders: II. Comprehensive care, Arch. Phys. Med. Rehabil. **63:**322, 1982.

Grimm, T.: Genetic counseling in Becker type X-linked muscular dystrophy: I. Theoretical considerations, Am. J. Med. Genet. **18:**713, 1984.

Grimm, T.: Genetic counseling in Becker type X-linked muscular dystrophy: II. Practical considerations, Am. J. Med. Genet. **18:**719, 1984.

Herrmann, F.H., and Spiegler, A.W.J.: Carrier detection in X-linked Becker muscular dystrophy by muscle provocation test (MPT), J. Neurol. Sci. **62:**141, 1983.

Khan, R.H., and MacNicol, M.F.: Bilateral patellar subluxation secondary to Becker muscular dystrophy: a case report, J. Bone Joint Surg. **64-A:**777, 1982.

Kloster, R.: Benign X-linked muscular dystrophy (Becker type): a kindred with very slow rate of progression, Acta Neurol. Scand. **68:**344, 1983.

Zellweger, H., and Hanson, J.W.: Slowly progressive X-linked recessive muscular dystrophy (Type IIIb), Arch. Intern. Med. **120:**525, 1967.

Facioscapulohumeral dystrophy

Copeland, S.A., and Howard, R.C.: Thoracoscapular fusion for facioscapulohumeral dystrophy, J. Bone Joint surg. **60-B:**547, 1978.

Fowler, W.M., Jr.: Rehabilitation management of muscular dystrophy and related disorders: II. Comprehensive care, Arch. Phys. Med. Rehabil. **63:**322, 1982.

McGarry, J., Garg, B., and Silbert, S.: Death in childhood due to facioscapulo-humeral dystrophy, Acta Neurol. Scand. **68:**61, 1983.

Padberg, G., et al.: Linkage studies in autosomal dominant facioscapulohumeral muscular dystrophy, J. Neurol. Sci. **65:**261, 1984.

Limb-girdle dystrophy

Fowler, W.M., Jr.: Rehabilitation management of muscular dystrophy and related disorders: II. Comprehensive care, Arch. Phys. Med. Rehabil. **63:**322, 1982.

Fowler, W.M., Jr., and Nayak, N.N.: Slowly progressive proximal weakness: limb-girdle syndromes, Arch. Phys. Med. Rehabil. **64:**527, 1983.

Congenital dystrophy

Fowler, W.M., Jr.: Rehabilitation management of muscular dystrophy and related disorders: II. Comprehensive care, Arch. Phys. Med. Rehabil. **63:**322, 1982.

Jones, R., Khan, R., Hughes, S., and Dubowitz, V.: Congenital muscular dystrophy: the importance of early diagnosis and orthopaedic management in the long-term prognosis, J. Bone Joint Surg. **61-B:**13, 1979.

McMenamin, J.B., Becker, L.E., and Murphy, E.G.: Fukuyama-type congenital muscular dystrophy, J. Pediatr. **100:**580, 1982.

McMenamin, J.B., Becker, L.E., and Murphy, E.G.: Congenital muscular dystrophy: a clinicopathologic report of 24 cases, J. Pediatr. **100:**692, 1982.

Takada, K., Nakamura, H., and Tanaka, J.: Cortical dysplasia in congenital muscular dystrophy with central nervous system involvement (Fukuyama type), J. Neuropathol. Exper. Neurol. **43:**395, 1984.

Myotonic dystrophy

Bégin, R., Bureau, M.A., Lupien, L., Bernier, J.-P., and Lemieux, B.: Pathogenesis of resiratory insufficiency in myotonic dystrophy: the mechanical factors, Am. Rev. Respir. Dis. **125:**312, 1982.

Brumback, R.A., and Wilson, H.: Cognitive and personality function in myotonic muscular dystrophy (letter), J. Neurol. Neurosurg. Psych. **47:**888, 1984.

Gottdiener, J.S., et al.: Left ventricular relaxation, mitral valve prolapse, and intracardiac conduction in myotonia atrophica: assessment by digitized echocardiography and noninvasive His bundle recording, Am. Heart J. **104:**77, 1982.

Hawley, R.J., Gottdiener, J.S., Gay, J.A., and Engel, W.K.: Families with myotonic dystrophy with and without cardiac involvement, Arch. Intern. Med. **143:**2134, 1983.

O'Brien, T.A., and Harper, P.S.: Course, prognosis and complications of childhood-onset myotonic dystrophy, Develop. Med. Child. Neurol. **26:**62, 1984.

Ray, S., Bowen, J.R., and Marks, H.G.: Foot deformity in myotonic dystrophy, Foot Ankle **5:**125, 1984.

Steinbeck, K.S., and Carter, J.N.: Thyroid abnormalities in patients with myotonic dystrophy, Clin. Endocrinol. **17:**449, 1982.

Neuropathic disease—general

Coleman, S.S., and Chestnut, W.J.: A simple test for hind foot flexibility in the cavovarus foot, Clin. Orthop. 123:60, 1977.

Drennan, J.C.: Neuromuscular disorders. In Lovell, W.W., and Winter, R.B. (editors): Pediatric orthopaedics, ed. 2, vol. 2, Philadelphia, 1986, J.B. Lippincott Co.

Dyck, P.J., and Lambert, E.H.: Lower motor and primary sensory neuron diseases with peroneal muscular atrophy: I. Neurologic, genetic, and electrophysiologic findings in hereditary polyneuropathies, Arch. Neurol. **18:**603, 1968.

Dyck, P.J., and Lambert, E.H.: Lower motor and primary sensory neuron diseases with peroneal muscular atrophy: II. Neurologic, genetic, and electrophysiologic findings in various neuronal degenerations, Arch. Neurol. **18:**619, 1968.

Swinyard, C.A.: Progressive muscular dystrophy and atrophy and related conditions: diagnosis and management, Pediatr. Clin. North Am. **7:**703, 1960.

Charcot-Marie-Tooth disease

Bost, F.C., Schottstaedt, E.R., and Larsen, L.J.: Plantar dissection: an operation to release the soft tissues in recurrent or recalcitrant talipes equinovarus, J. Bone Joint Surg. **42-A:**151, 1960.

Charcot, J.M., and Marie, P.: Sur une forme particuliére d'atrophie musculaire souvent familiale débutant par les pied et les jambes et atteignant plus tard les mains. Rev. Med. 1886, pp. 96-138.

Coleman, S.S., Complex foot deformities in children, Philadelphia, 1983, Lea & Febiger.

Dwyer, F.C.: The treatment of relapsed club foot by the insertion of a wedge into the calcaneum, J. Bone Joint Surg. **45-B:**67, 1963.

Dyck, P.J., and Lambert, E.H.: Lower motor and primary and sensory neuron diseases with peroneal muscular atrophy (I), Arch. Neurol. **18:**603, 1968.

Dyck, P.J., and Lambert, E.H.: Lower motor and primary sensory neuron diseases with peroneal muscular atrophy (II), Arch. Neurol. **18:**619, 1968.

Evans, D.: Relapsed club foot, J. Bone Joint Surg. **43-B:**722, 1961.

Gartland, J.J.: Posterior tibial transplant in the surgical treatment of recurrent club foot, J. Bone Joint Surg. **46-A:**1217, 1964.

Greenfield, J.G.: Diseases of the lower motor and sensory neurones (of uncertain pathogenesis). In Blackwood, W., McMenemey, W.H., Meyer, A., Normal, R.M., and Russell, D.S.: Greenfield's neuropathy, Baltimore, 1967, Williams and Wilkins Co.

Hsu, J.D.: Surgical correction of valgus feet in the young, ambulatory neuromuscular patients. Presented at the Annual Meeting of the American Orthopaedic Foot and Ankle Society, Inc., Jan. 23, 1985, Las Vegas, Nev.

Hughes, J.T., and Brownell, B.: Pathology of peroneal muscular atrophy (Charcot-Marie-Tooth disease), J. Neurol. Neurosurg. Psych. **35:**648, 1972.

Ibrahim, K.: Cavus feet deformity in children-a comprehensive approach. Presented at the Annual Meeting of the American Academy of Orthopaedic Surgeons, Jan. 24, 1985, Las Vegas, Nev.

Ibrahim, K.: Comprehensive approach for cavus foot deformity in children. Presented at the American Academy for Cerebral Palsy and Developmental Medicine Annual Meeting, 1984.

Jacobs, J.E., and Carr, C.L.: Progressive muscular atrophy of the peroneal type (Charcot-Marie-Tooth disease): orthopaedic management and an end-result study, J. Bone Joint Surg. **32-A:**27, 1950.

Jahss, M.H.: Tarsometatarsal truncated-wedge arthrodesis for pes cavus and equinovarus deformity of the fore part of the foot, J. Bone Joint Surg. **62-A:**713, 1980.

Karlholm, S., and Nilsonne, U.: Operative treatment of the foot deformity in Charcot-Marie-Tooth disease, Acta Orthop. Scand. **39:**101, 1968.

Lambrinudi, C.: New operation on drop-foot, Brit. J. Surg. **15:**193, 1927.

Levitt, R.L., Canale, S.T., Cooke, A.J., Jr., and Gartland, J.J.: The role of foot surgery in progressive neuromuscular disorders in children, J. Bone Joint Surg. **55-A:**1396, 1973.

Ma, S.M., Moreland, J.R., and Westin, G.W.: Long term results in Grice subtalar arthrodesis. Presented at the Annual Meeting of the American Academy of Orthopaedic Surgeons, January 24, 1985, Las Vegas, Nev.

Ober, F.R.: Tendon transplantation in the lower extremity, N. Engl. J. Med. **209:**52, 1933.

Paulos, L., Coleman, S.S., and Samuelson, K.M.: Pes cavovarus: review of a surgical approach using selective soft-tissue procedures, J. Bone Joint Surg. **62-A:**942, 1980.

Rochelle, J., Bowen, J.R., and Ray, S.: Pediatric foot deformities in progressive neuromuscular disease, Contemp. Orthop. **8:**41, 1984.

Ryerson, E.W.: Arthrodesing operations on the feet, J. Bone Joint Surg. **5:**453, 1923.

Sabir, M., and Lyttle, D.: Pathogenesis of Charcot-Marie-Tooth disease: gait analysis and electrophysiologic, genetic, histopathologic, and enzyme studies in a kinship, Clin. Orthop. **184:**223, 1984.

Siffert, R.S., and del Torto, U.: "Beak" triple arthrodesis for severe cavus deformity, Clin. Orthop. **181:**64, 1983.

Siffert, R.S., Forster, R.I., and Nachamie, B.: "Beak" triple arthrodesis for severe cavus deformity, Clin. Orthop. **45:**101, 1966.

Wilcox, P.G., and Weiner, D.S.: Midtarsal dome osteotomy in the treatment of rigid pes cavus. Presented at the Annual Meeting of the American Academy of Orthopaedic Surgeons, Jan. 27, 1985, Las Vegas, Nev.

Friedreich's ataxia

Holmes, G.L., and Shaywitz, B.A.: Strumpell's pure familial spastic paraplegia: case study and review of the literature, J. Neurol. Neurosurg. Psych. **40:**1003, 1977.

Ibrahim, K.: Cavus feet deformity in children—a comprehensive approach. Presented at the Annual Meeting of the American Academy of Orthpaedic Surgeons, Jan. 24, 1985, Las Vegas, Nev.

Labelle, H., Tohme, S., Frassier, F., Duhaime, M., and Poitras, B.P.: Natural history of scoliosis in Friedreich's ataxia. Presented at the Annual Meeting of the American Academy of Orthopaedic Surgeons, Jan. 26, 1985, Las Vegas, Nev.

Lemieux, B., Giguére, R., and Shapcott, D.: Studies on the role of taurine in Friedreich's ataxia, Can. J. Neurol. Sci. **11:**610, 1984.

Levitt, R.L., Canale, S.T., Cooke, A.J., Jr., and Gartland, J.J.: The role of foot surgery in progressive neuromuscular disorders in children, J. Bone Joint Surg. **55-A:**1396, 1973.

Ma, S.M., Moreland, J.R., and Westin, G.W.: Long term results of Grice subtalar arthrodesis. Presented at the Annual Meeting of the American Academy of Orthopaedic Surgeons, Jan. 24, 1985, Las Vegas, Nev.

Makin, M.: The surgical management of Friedreich's ataxia, J. Bone Joint Surg. **35-A:**425, 1953.

Paulos, L., Coleman, S.S., and Samuelson, K.M.: Pes cavovarus: review of a surgical approach using selective soft-tissue procedures, J. Bone Joint Surg. **62-A:**942, 1980.

Rochelle, J., Bowen, J.R., and Ray, S.: Pediatric foot deformities in progressive neuromuscular disease, Contemp. Orthop. **8:**41, 1984.

Rothschild, H., Shoji, H., and McCormick, D.: Heel deformity in hereditary spastic paraplegia, Clin. Orthop. **160:**48, 1981.

Rotschild, H., Happel, L., Rampp, D., and Hackett, E.: Autosomal recessive spastic paraplegia: evidence for demyelination, Clin. Genet. **15:**356, 1979.

Shapcott, D., Giguére, R., and Lemieux, B.: Zinc and taurine in Friedreich's ataxia, Can. J. Neurol. Sci. **11:**623, 1984.

Tyrer, J.H., and Sutherland, J.M.: The primary spino-cerebellar atrophies and their associated defects, with a study of the foot deformity, Brain **84:**289, 1961.

PART XVII

The Spine

CHAPTER 68

Spinal anatomy and surgical approaches

Allen S. Edmonson

CIRCULATION OF SPINAL CORD

The arterial supply to the spinal cord has been determined from gross anatomic dissection, latex arterial injections, and intercostal arteriography. Dommisse has contributed most significantly to our knowledge of the blood supply, stating that the principles that govern the blood supply of the cord are constant, whereas the patterns vary with the individual. He emphasized the following factors:

1. *Dependence on three vessels:* these are the anterior median longitudinal arterial trunk and a pair of posterolateral trunks near the posterior nerve rootlets.

2. *Relative demands of gray matter and white matter:* the longitudinal arterial trunks are largest in the cervical and lumbar regions near the ganglionic enlargements and are much smaller in the thoracic region. This is because the metabolic demands of the gray matter are greater than those of the white matter, which contains fewer capillary networks.

3. *Medullary feeder (radicular) arteries of the cord:* these reinforce the longitudinal arterial channels. There are from 2 to 17 anteriorly and 6 to 25 posteriorly. The vertebral arteries supply 80% of the radicular arteries in the neck; those in the thoracic and lumbar areas arise from the aorta. The lateral sacral arteries, as well as the fifth lumbar, the iliolumbar, and the middle sacral arteries, are important in the sacral region.

4. *Supplementary source of blood supply to the spinal cord:* the vertebral and posteroinferior cerebellar arteries are an important source of arterial supply. Sacral medullary feeders arise from the lateral sacral arteries and accompany the distal roots of the cauda equina. The flow in these vessels seems reversible and the volume adjustable in response to the metabolic demands.

5. *Segmental arteries of the spine:* at every vertebral level a pair of segmental arteries supplies the extraspinal and intraspinal structures. The thoracic and lumbar segmental arteries arise from the aorta; the cervical segmental arteries arise from the vertebral arteries as well as the costocervical and thyrocervical trunks. In 60% of people an additional source arises from the ascending pharyngeal branch of the external carotid artery. The lateral sacral arteries and to a lesser extent the fifth lumbar, iliolumbar, and middle sacral arteries supply segmental vessels in the sacral region.

6. *"Distribution point"* of the segmental arteries: the segmental arteries divide into numerous branches at the intervertebral foramen, which has been termed the distribution point (Fig. 68-1). A second anastomotic network lies within the spinal canal in the loose connective tissue of the extradural space. This occurs at all levels, with the greatest concentration in the cervical and lumbar regions. Undoubtedly the presence of the rich anastomotic channels offers alternative pathways for arterial flow, preserving spinal cord circulation after the ligation of segmental arteries.

7. *Artery of Adamkiewicz:* the artery of Adamkiewicz is the largest of the feeders of the lumbar cord; it is located on the left side, usually at the level of T9 to T11 (in 80% of people). It is clear that the anterior longitudinal arterial channel of the cord rather than any single medullary feeder is crucial. Equally clear is that the preservation of this large feeder does not ensure continued satisfactory circulation for the spinal cord. In principle it would seem of practical value to protect and preserve each contributing artery as far as is surgically possible.

8. *Variability of patterns of supply of the spinal cord:* the variability of is striking feature, yet there is absolute conformity with a principle of a rich supply for the cervical and lumbar cord enlargements. The supply for the thoracic cord from approximately T4 to T9 is much poorer.

9. *Direction of flow in the blood vessels of the spinal cord:* the three longitudinal arterial channels of the spinal cord can be compared to the circle of Willis at the base of the brain, but it is more extensive and more complicated, although it functions with identical principles. These channels permit reversal of flow and alterations in the volume of blood flow in response to metabolic demands. This internal arterial circle of the cord is surrounded by at least two outer arterial circles, the first of which is situated in the extradural space and the second in the extravertebral

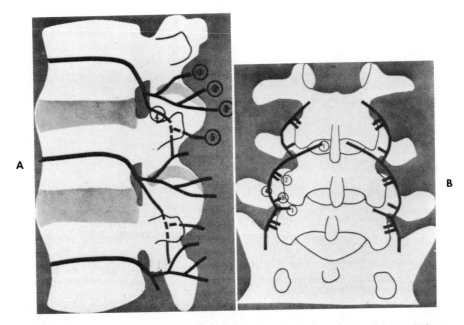

Fig. 68-1. Disposition of major muscular branches of lumbar arteries. **A,** Lateral view. *1,* Interarticular artery. *2* and *3,* Superior articular arteries. *4,* Communicating branch. *5,* Inferior articular artery. **B,** Posterior view showing relation of arteries to surgical exposure. *1,* Interarticular artery is immediately lateral to pars interarticularis. *2,* Two superior articular arteries lie just lateral to tip of superior articular facet. *4,* Large communicating artery lies just lateral to superior articular facet on dorsum of transverse process. *5,* Inferior articular artery lies in angle formed by transverse process and superior articular fact. (From Macnab, I., and Dall, D.: J. Bone Joint Surg. **53-B:**628, 1971.)

tissue planes. It is by virtue of the latter that the spinal cord enjoys reserve sources of supply through a degree of anastomosis lacking in the inner circle. The "outlet points," however, are limited to the perforating sulcal arteries and the pial arteries of the cord.

In summary, the blood supply to the spinal cord is rich, but the spinal canal is narrowest and the blood supply is poorest from T4 to T9. This should be considered the critical vascular zone of the spinal cord, a zone in which interference with the circulation is most likely to result in paraplegia.

It has been assumed that spinal cord dysfunction as a result of avascularity is caused by interference with the radicular arteries at T4 to T10. However, studies of these arteries have shown that attempts at direct occlusion push them into the soft cord tissue rather than compressing them: therefore their lumens are retained. Also the abundance of anastomotic arteries suggests an adequate circulation, and the size of the bony canal in which the coordinate blood supply lies is considered an additional factor in compromising cord function; the thoracic vertebral canal is relatively small compared to the cervical and lumbar. Kardjiev et al. found that arteriographic injection of the right fifth intercostal artery produced spinal pain followed in several hours by neurologic changes. A catheter at this level must be withdrawn immediately. Pasternak et al. emphasized maintenance of a systolic blood pressure above 120 mm Hg to avoid spinal cord ischemia at the time of cross-clamping the thoracic aorta.

The dominance of the anterior spinal artery system has

been challenged by the fact that much anterior spinal surgery has been performed in recent years with no increase in the incidence of paralysis. This would seem to indicate that a rich anastomotic supply does exist and that it protects the spinal cord. Dwyer has extended his fixation from as high as T3 to L3 without evidence of cord damage. The evidence suggests that the posterior spinal arteries may be as important as the anterior system but are as yet poorly understood.

During anterior spinal surgery, we empirically follow these principles: (1) ligate segmental spinal arteries only as necessary to gain exposure; (2) ligate segmental spinal arteries near the aorta rather than near the vertebral foramina; (3) ligate segmental spinal arteries on one side only when possible, leaving the circulation intact on the opposite side; and (4) limit dissection in the vertebral foramina to a single level when possible so that collateral circulation is disturbed as little as possible.

SURGICAL APPROACHES
Anterior approaches

With the posterior approach for correction of spinal deformities well established, in recent years more attention has been placed on the anterior approach to the spinal column. Many pioneers in the field of anterior spinal surgery recognized that anterior spinal cord decompression was necessary in spinal tuberculosis and that laminectomy not only failed to relieve anterior pressure but also removed important posterior stability and produced worsening of kyphosis. Advances in major surgical procedures, includ-

Table 68-1. Indications for anterior approach*

I. Absolute
   A. Scoliosis with deficient posterior spinal elements
      1. Congenital—myelomeningocele
      2. Acquired—after extensive laminectomy
   B. Severe rigid congenital scoliosis
      1. Unilateral unsegmented bar
      2. Hemivertebrae
   C. Severe kyphosis
      1. Congenital
         Anterior hemi- or microvertebrae
         Anterior unsegmented bar
      2. Acquired
         Posttraumatic
         Inflammatory (tuberculosis)
         Postirradiation
   D. Hyperlordosis
      After lumboperitoneal shunts with tethered spinal cord
II. Relative
   A. Cervical spondylosis
   B. Some paralytic curves with lordosis (cerebral palsy)
   C. Thoracolumbar scoliosis
   D. Spondylolisthesis (without neurologic deficit)
   E. Thoracic idiopathic scoliosis

*From Hall, J.E.: Orthop. Clin. North Am. **3:**81, 1972.

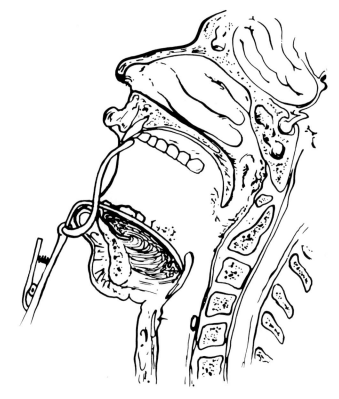

Fig. 68-2. Anterior approach from occiput to C2. With splitting and retraction of palate, C1, C2, and upper part of C3 are available for surgical manipulation. (From Perry, J.: In Pierce, D.S., and Nickel, V.H., editors: The total care of spinal cord injuries, Boston, 1977, Little, Brown & Co.)

ing anesthesia and intensive care, have made it possible to perform spinal surgery with acceptable safety.

Common use of the anterior approach for spinal surgery did not evolve until the 1950s. Leaders in the anterior approach to the cervical and lumbar areas have been Cloward, Southwick and Robinson, Bailey and Badgley, Harmon, and Wiltberger. The transthoracic approach to the thoracic spine has developed more slowly. Nachlas and Borden, and Smith, von Lackum, and Wylie were among the first to report their experiences; however, the major proponents of this technique were Hodgson et al. of Hong Kong. Their reports of success with this method received worldwide acceptance.

Hall's indications for an anterior approach to the spine are outlined in Table 68-1.

In anterior approaches to the spine it is advantageous to have the help of a thoracic or general surgeon during both the intraoperative and the postoperative period. The orthopaedic surgeon still must have a working knowledge of the overlying viscera, fluid balance, physiology, and other elements of intensive care. Anterior spinal surgery is usually performed by experienced spinal surgeons in medical centers. As a rule, this type of surgery is not appropriate for the surgeon who only occasionally does spinal techniques.

Correction of severe spinal deformities by the anterior approach involves several major risks. The potential dangers include excessive angulation or compression of the cord by rapid correction of the deformity at the time of resection, intolerable distraction of the cord with an opening wedge procedure, and interference with the circulation of the spinal cord. There is therefore a high risk of significant morbidity, and this approach must be used with care and only in appropriate circumstances.

An excellent review of all anterior approaches to the spine has been presented by Perry. Much of the following discussion is based on her work.

ANTERIOR APPROACH FROM OCCIPUT TO C2

This approach to the more proximal cervical vertebrae is used by otolaryngologists in draining retropharyngeal abscesses. Its primary disadvantage in "clean" cases is a higher infection rate.

TECHNIQUE (PERRY). Administer endotracheal anesthesia through a tracheostomy with a cuffed endotracheal tube. Place the patient in the Trendelenburg position and insert a mouth gag to provide the best retraction (Fig. 68-2). Approach the junction of C1 and C2 through the mouth using a midline splitting incision of the posterior pharyngeal wall. Postretraction paresis of the soft palate is less apt to occur if the soft palate is split along its median raphe (Fig. 68-3). Make the posterior pharyngeal wall incision approximately 5 cm in length and center it 1 fingerbreadth below the anterior tubercle of the atlas. This midline is not particularly vascular. Continue the midline dissection down to bone and reflect the tissue laterally to the outer margins of the lateral masses representing the facet articulations of the atlas and axis. Immediately beyond these margins are the vertebral arteries; take care not to harm them. Keep this limitation in mind when creating a bed for a bone graft within the lateral masses. Central grafting is restricted by the small amount of cancellous bone present in the ring of the atlas. To expose the atlantooccipital joint, extend the

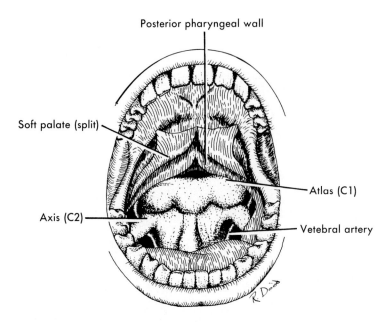

Posterior pharyngeal wall

Soft palate (split)

Atlas (C1)

Axis (C2)

Vetebral artery

Fig. 68-3. Anterior approach from occiput to C2. Soft palate and posterior pharyngeal wall are split (see text). (From Perry, J.: In Pierce, D.S., and Nickel, V.H., editors: The total care of spinal cord injuries, Boston, 1977, Little, Brown & Co.)

soft palate incision more proximally. Southwick and Robinson reach the junction of C2 and C3 through the mouth with vigorous tongue retraction, which allows exposure of the top of the third cervical vertebra and the anterior structures to the base of the skull.

ANTERIOR APPROACH FROM C3 TO T2

Whether the approach should be from the right or the left side is a question with advocates on both sides. Bailey and Badgley recommend the right side approach and protection of the recurrent laryngeal nerve, whereas Southwick and Robinson prefer the left side to avoid exposing this nerve.

TECHNIQUE (PERRY, ROBINSON). Support the head with 5 pounds (2.2 kg) of head halter or skull traction. The direction of the skin incision depends on the number of vertebra to be exposed. Whenever possible, make a transverse incision, which is most acceptable cosmetically but more limited in extent of exposure. Expose the platysma muscle, sharply incise it in the direction of the wound, and separate it bluntly from the underlying structures. Dissect along the anterior border of the sternocleidomastoid and retract it laterally to expose a middle layer of the cervical fascia. Divide the fascia longitudinally to expose the omohyoid muscle in the midportion of the neck; mobilize and retract this muscle inferiorly or superiorly, or transect it in its midtendinous segment. Identify the carotid sheath and gently retract it laterally with the sternocleidomastoid (Fig. 68-4). This exposes the anterior surface of the cervical spine with the esophagus lying just posterior to the trachea or, more superiorly in the neck, the larynx. Next incise the prevertebral fascia longitudinally in the midline and retract it medially and laterally to avoid interference with the cervical sympathetic chain, the vertebral artery, and the vascular

longus colli muscles. Elevate the longus colli muscles from the vertebral bodies and intervertebral discs. Considerable bleeding may occur as the nutrient vessels are torn in passing from muscles to bone. Pack the area with Surgicel or use a cautery as the preferred method of hemostasis. Maintain the exposure with self-retaining or hand-held retractors, avoiding prolonged carotid retraction (Fig. 68-5).

In the anterior approach to the most proximal segments of the cervical spine, important structures must be identified and preserved. These include the superior laryngeal nerve and artery, the hypoglossal artery, and the external carotid artery with its branches (Fig. 68-6).

• • •

To expose both the upper and lower cervical areas through a single approach, Whitesides and Kelly have used the classic approach of Henry to the vertebral artery, in which the sternocleidomastoid is everted and retracted posteriorly, and then have carried the dissection posterior to the carotid sheath (Fig. 68-7, *A*).

TECHNIQUE (WHITESIDES AND KELLY). Make a longitudinal incision along the anterior margin of the sternocleidomastoid and at the superior end of the muscle carry the incision posteriorly across the base of the temporal bone. Divide the muscle at its mastoid origin. Partially divide the insertion of the splenius capitis at its insertion into the same area. Then evert the sternocleidomastoid and identify the spinal accessory nerve as it approaches and passes into the muscle; divide and ligate the vascular structures that accompany the nerve. Now develop the approach posterior to the carotid sheath, which is retracted anteriorly, and anterior to the sternocleidomastoid muscle, which is retracted posteriorly (Fig. 68-7, *A*). At this point in the operation

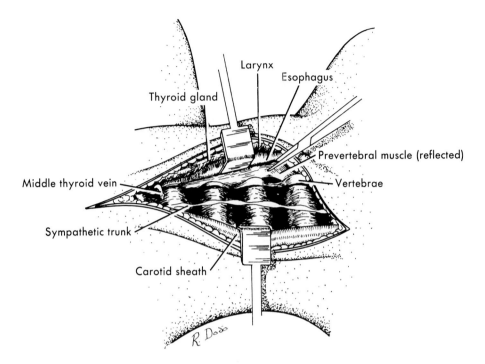

Fig. 68-4. Anterior approach from C2 to T2 (see text). (From Perry, J.: In Pierce, D.S., and Nickel, V.H., editors: The total care of spinal cord injuries, Boston, 1977, Little, Brown & Co.)

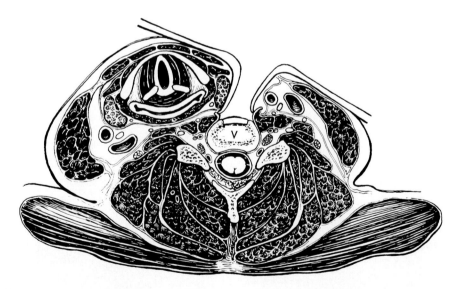

Fig. 68-5. Anterior approach to cervical spine. Thyroid gland, trachea, and esophagus have been retracted laterally from midline, and carotid sheath and its contents laterally in opposite direction.

the transverse processes of all the cervical vertebrae are exposed. By further dissection along the anterior aspect of the transverse processes and by dividing Sharpey's fibers, expose the anterior aspect of the cervical vertebrae. In this manner the spine can be exposed from the anterior ring of the first cervical vertebra to the anterior surface of the first thoracic vertebra.

ANTERIOR APPROACH TO CERVICOTHORACIC AREA

The cervicothoracic area is without ready anterior access. The rapid transition from cervical lordosis to thoracic kyphosis results in an abrupt change in the depth of the wound. Also this is a confluent area of vital structures that are not readily retracted. The three approaches to this area include (1) high transthoracic, (2) low anterior cervical, and (3) sternal splitting.

TECHNIQUE. A kyphotic deformity of the thoracic spine tends to force the cervical spine into the chest, in which instance a high transthoracic approach is a logical choice. Make a periscapular incision and remove the second or third rib; removing the latter is necessary to provide sufficient working space in a child or if a kyphotic deformity is present. This exposes the interval between C6 and T4 (Fig. 68-8). Excision of the first or second rib is adequate in adults or in the absence of an exaggerated kyphosis.

The low anterior cervical approach provides access to

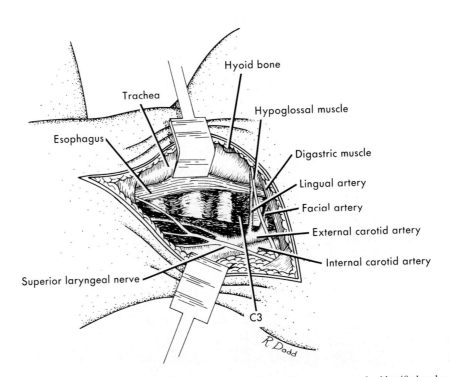

Fig. 68-6. Anterolateral approach to upper cervical spine. Important structures must be identified and protected (see text). (From Perry, J.: In Pierce, D.S., and Nickel, V.H., editors: The total care of spinal cord injuries, Boston, 1977, Little, Brown & Co.)

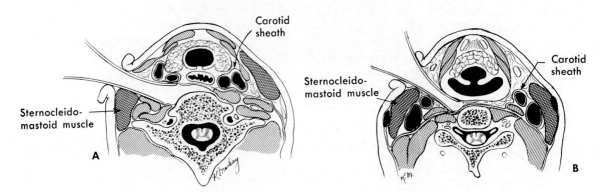

Fig. 68-7. Anterior approach to cervical spine. **A,** Whitesides and Kelly approach anterior to sternocleidomastoid muscle and posterior to carotid sheath (see text). **B,** Usual approach anterior to sternocleidomastoid muscle and medial to carotid sheath; same approach as shown in Fig. 68-5. (From Whitesides, T.E., Jr., and Kelly, R.P.: South. Med. J. **59:**879, 1966.)

T1 and T2 to permit embedding a graft in these bodies, as well as to the cervical vertebrae above. Enter on the left side by a transverse incision placed 1 fingerbreadth above the clavicle. Extend it well across the midline, taking particular care when dissecting about the carotid sheath in the area of entry of the thoracic duct. The latter approaches the jugular vein from its lateral side, but variations are not uncommon. Further steps in exposure follow those of the conventional anterior cervical approach.

For equal exposure of the thoracic and cervical spine from C4 to T4, the sternal splitting approach presented by Fang et al. is recommended; it is commonly used in cardiac surgery (Fig. 68-9). Make a Y-shaped incision with the vertical segment passing along the midsternal area from the suprasternal notch to just below the xiphoid process. Now extend the proximal end diagonally to the right and left along the base of the neck for a short distance. To avoid entering the abdominal cavity, take care to keep the dissection beneath the periosteum while exposing the distal end of the sternum. At the proximal end of the sternal notch take care to avoid the inferior thyroid vein. By blunt dissection reflect the parietal pleura from the posterior surfaces of the sternum and costal cartilages, and develop a space. Pass one finger or an instrument above and below the suprasternal space, insert a Gigli saw, and split the sternum. Now spread the split sternum and gain access to the center of the chest. In children the upper portion of the exposure will be posterior to the thymus and bounded by the innominate and carotid arteries and their venous coun-

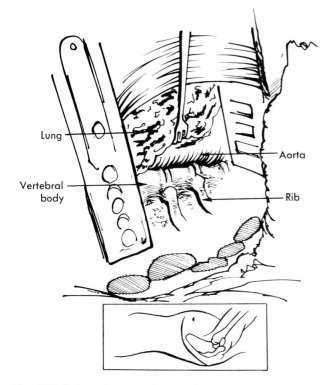

Fig. 68-8. Periscapular approach to anterior cervicothoracic spine area (see text). *Inset,* Skin incision. (From Perry, J.: In Pierce, D.S., and Nickel, V.H., editors: The total care of spinal cord injuries, Boston, 1977, Little, Brown & Co.)

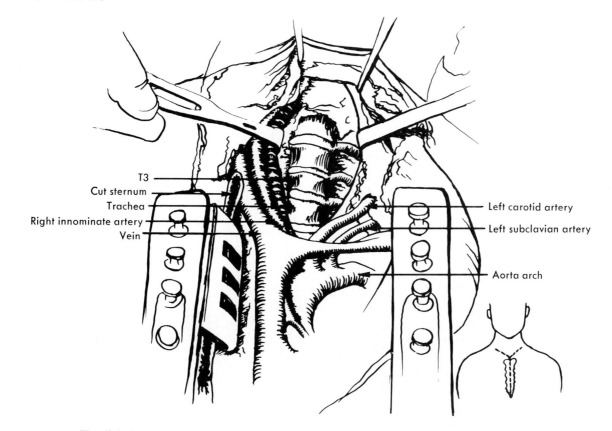

Fig. 68-9. Sternal splitting anterior approach to cervicothoracic spine area (see text). (From Perry, J.: In Pierce, D.S., and Nickel, V.H., editors: The total care of spinal cord injuries, Boston, 1977, Little, Brown & Co.)

terparts. Now develop the left side of this area bluntly. In patients with kyphotic deformity the innominate vein may now be divided as it crosses the field; it may be very tense and subject to rupture. This division is recommended by Fang et al. The disadvantage of ligation is that it leaves a slight postoperative enlargement of the left upper extremity that is not apparent unless carefully assessed. This approach provides limited access, and its success depends on accuracy in preoperative interpretation of the deformity and a high degree of surgical precision.

ANTERIOR APPROACH TO THORACIC SPINE

Most surgeons prefer to enter the chest on the left because the aorta is more tolerant of handling than the thin-walled vena cava. Although the vessels feeding the spinal cord are generally found to enter from the left, descriptions in the literature of many anterior procedures have shown no relationship between the site of entry and the subsequent spinal cord function.

The level of exposure should be two ribs above the vertebral level sought. For example, if a lesion is in T7, the fifth rib on the left is removed (Fig. 68-10).

TECHNIQUE. Although thoracic surgeons prefer entering through an intercostal space, rib resection provides a larger working aperture and the rib provides any necessary graft. If possible, use a retropleural approach, which in our experience has resulted in less morbidity; this is easier in children than in adults. To avoid penetrating the lung in a transpleural approach, nick the pleura with a knife, insert a finger, and continue the splitting with a partially opened scissors. Pack off the lung in 20-minute intervals between periods of full inflation. The latter consists of adequate

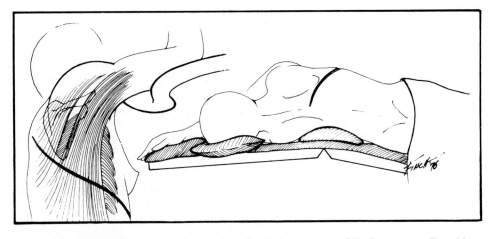

Fig. 68-10. Anterior approach to thoracic spine through right thoracotomy at fifth rib (see text). (From Moe, J.H., et al.: Scoliosis and other deformities, Philadelphia, 1978, W.B. Saunders Co.)

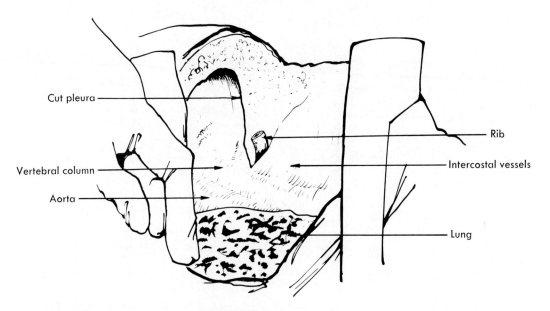

Fig. 68-11. Transthoracic anterior approach to spine. Lung is deflated. (From Perry, J.: In Pierce, D.S., and Nickel, V.H., editors: The total care of spinal cord injuries, Boston, 1977, Little, Brown & Co.)

aeration to remove all cyanotic spots and make the lung fully pink again (Fig. 68-11).

Use blunt and sharp dissection to mobilize the areolar tissue between the great vessels and vertebral bodies and reflect it as a protective layer to form a pocket in which to place retractors. This reduces the pressure on the aorta and also protects the thoracic duct. Continue dissection to the vertebral bodies and identify intercostal vessels as they adhere to the waist of each vertebra (Fig. 68-12). Clamp and ligate each one in situ and section them near the midline. Do not ligate them near the distribution point of Dommisse at the foramen.

Reflect the periosteum of the adjacent vertebrae, the anterior longitudinal ligament, and the outer layer of anulus as a single layer. Alternatively only the anulus and disc may be removed to minimize bleeding when the entire front of the body need not be exposed. This is applicable when bone chips or blocks are placed at individual levels rather than using a long slotted rib or fibular graft. Take particular care in exposing the posterior margin of the vertebra and the adjacent pedicle (Fig. 68-13). Excise the disc and cartilaginous plates and expose the vertebral end plates. An entire cross section of the vertebral body is thus developed, and the anterior margin of the neural canal is identified with the posterior longitudinal ligament lying in the slight concavity on the back of the vertebral body. Expose sufficient segmental vessels and disc spaces to accomplish the intended procedure. Colletta and Mayer have reported a chylothorax that followed a single-level T10 to T11 anterior interbody fusion.

ANTERIOR APPROACH TO THORACOLUMBAR SPINE

TECHNIQUE. Place the patient in the right lateral decubitus position and place supports beneath the buttock and shoulder (Fig. 68-14, *A*). Make the incision curvilinear with ability to extend either the cephalad or caudal end. To best gain access to the interval of T12 to L1, resect the tenth rib, which allows exposure between T10 and L2. The only difficulty is in identifying the diaphragm as a separate structure; it tends to closely approximate the wall of the thoracic cage, allowing the edge of the lung to penetrate into the space beneath the knife as the pleura is divided. Now take care in entering the abdominal cavity. Since the transversalis fascia and the peritoneum do not diverge, dissect with caution and identify the two cavities on either side of the diaphragm. To achieve confluence of the two cavities, reflect the diaphragm from the lower ribs and the crus from the side of the spine (Fig. 68-14, *B*). Alternatively, incise the diaphragm 2.5 cm away from its insertion and tag it with sutures for later accurate closure (Fig. 68-15). Incise the prevertebral fascia in the direction of the spine. Take care to identify the segmental arteries and veins over the waist of each vertebral body. Isolate these, ligate them in the midline, and expose the bone as previously described.

Expose L1 to L3 through the eleventh or twelfth rib. Because ribs vary in their obliquity, such as in kyphosis, which brings the ribs to a lower level, the exact rib may vary from one patient to another. The approach is similar to that in the lumbar area except that the kidney rather than the ureter is the most posterior structure reflected and the

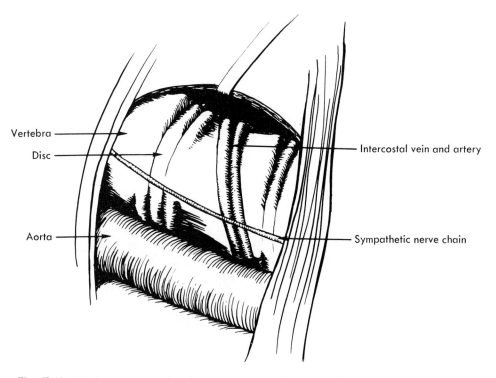

Fig. 68-12. Anterior approach to thoracic spine (see text). (From Perry, J.: In Pierce, D.S., and Nickel, V.H., editors: The total care of spinal cord injuries, Boston, 1977, Little, Brown & Co.)

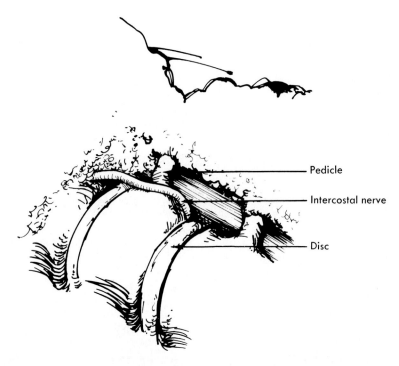

Pedicle

Intercostal nerve

Disc

Fig. 68-13. Anterior approach to thoracic spine (see text). (From Perry, J.: In Pierce, D.S., and Nickel, V.H., editors: The total care of spinal cord injuries, Boston, 1977, Little, Brown & Co.)

crus of the diaphragm extends as a longitudinal fibrous tongue that is reflected with the anterior longitudinal ligament and periosteum. Remember that the proximal dissection will enter the pleural cavity and will require careful closure at the end of the procedure. Reflection of the aorta is a bit more difficult at this level, since the crura are really extensions of the aortic foramen in the diaphragm, tying the aorta more closely to the vertebrae in this area.

ANTERIOR APPROACH TO LUMBAR AND LUMBOSACRAL SPINE

TECHNIQUE. Place the patient in the right lateral decubitus position and approach from the left. To reach the lumbar spine between the sacrum and L3, make a midflank incision from the midline anteriorly to midline posteriorly or any portion thereof (Fig. 68-16). This usually is on a line midway between the umbilicus and the symphysis pubis passing laterally and posteriorly in the interval between the ribs and the iliac crest. Divide the abdominal oblique muscles in line with the incision and cauterize the bleeders as they are identified. Proceed laterally, identifying the latissimus dorsi as it adds another layer while the deeper transverse abdominis muscle becomes quite inconspicuous posteriorly. Now identify the transversalis fascia and the peritoneum, which are so closely approximated anteriorly that separation is difficult. Their sheaths diverge posteriorly as the transversalis fascia lines the trunk wall and the peritoneum turns anteriorly to encase the viscera. The dissection, in this plane posteriorly, gains access to the spine without entering the abdominal cavity. Any entry into the peritoneum should be repaired immediately as it may not be identifiable later. Reflect all the fat-containing areolar

tissue back to the transversalis and lumbar fascia, reflecting the ureter along with the peritoneum. Since fat may contain hidden vital structures, careful dissection is mandatory. Again, as in the thoracic cavity, the prevertebral fascia (now called the lumbar fascia) with its underlying fat covers three columns. Nearer the midline find the major vessels (the aorta on the left and the vena cava on the right); next, partly covered by the great vessels, is the vertebral column; and most lateral is the outline of the psoas with the roots of the femoral nerve on its posterior surface. Divide the lumbar fascia with care to avoid the underlying segmental arteries and veins, and ligate these vessels in situ to control hemorrhage. Excise the disc and expose the vertebral body as previously described.

If spinal alignment is normal, a transperitoneal exposure or a lateral retroperitoneal approach can be used. In kyphosis the wound depth is exaggerated and thus a lateral approach is preferable. Long-standing lordosis makes the anterior approach more appropriate, since the spine is close to the anterior abdominal wall and displaces the great vessels laterally. The transperitoneal approach is convenient for operations on the lumbosacral disc or for wedge resection of a lordotic spine, but it is seldom indicated in management of spinal injuries except at the L5 body. The lumbosacral segment of the spine lies distal to the bifurcation of the aorta into the right and left common iliac arteries accompanied by their veins (Fig. 68-17). The major disadvantage of the transperitoneal approach at the lumbosacral level is that upward extension and exposure cannot be accomplished without generous mobilization of the vessels so that one can alternately work above and be-

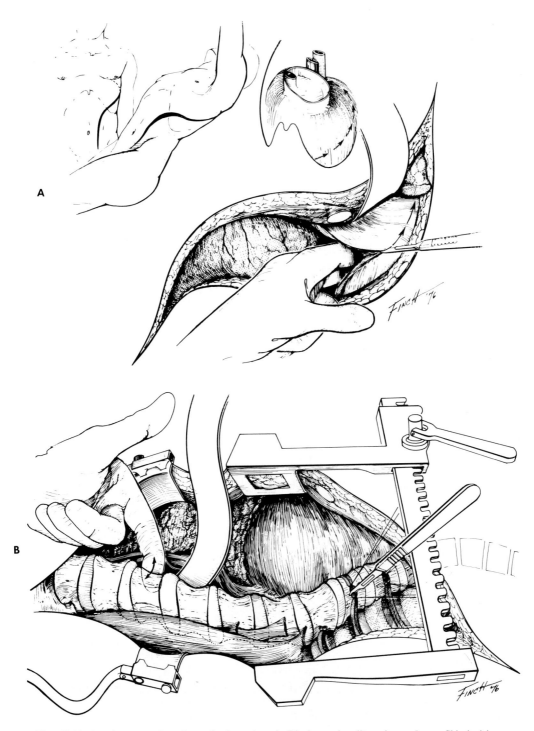

Fig. 68-14. Anterior approach to thoracolumbar spine. **A,** Diaphragm is split as shown. *Insets,* Skin incision and incision in diaphragm. **B,** Deeper dissection of thoracolumbar approach (see text). (From Moe, J.H., et al.: Scoliosis and other deformities, Philadelphia, 1978, W.B. Saunders Co.)

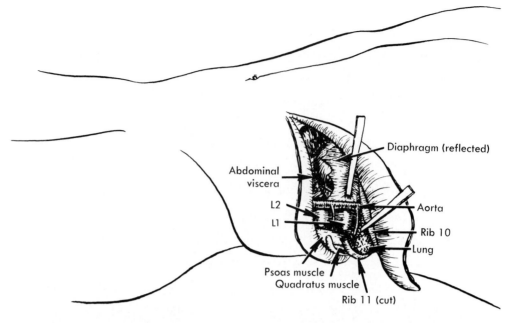

Fig. 68-15. Anterior approach to thoracolumbar spine. Eleventh rib has been resected and diaphragm has been incised and reflected. (From Perry, J.: In Pierce, D.S., and Nickel, V.H., editors: The total care of spinal cord injuries, Boston, 1977, Little, Brown & Co.)

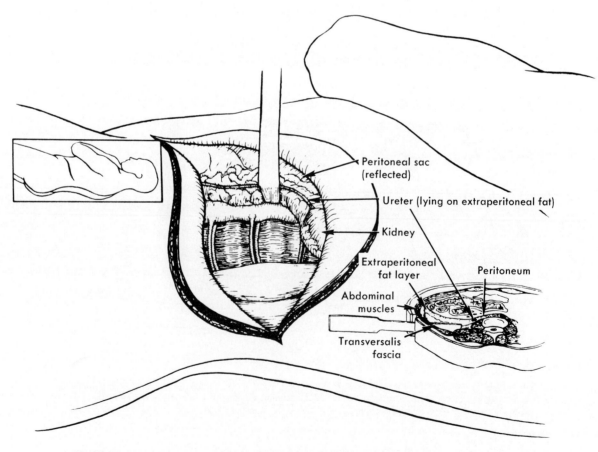

Fig. 68-16. Anterior approach to lumbar spine (see text). (From Perry, J.: In Pierce, D.S., and Nickel, V.H., editors: The total care of spinal cord injuries, Boston, 1977, Little, Brown & Co.)

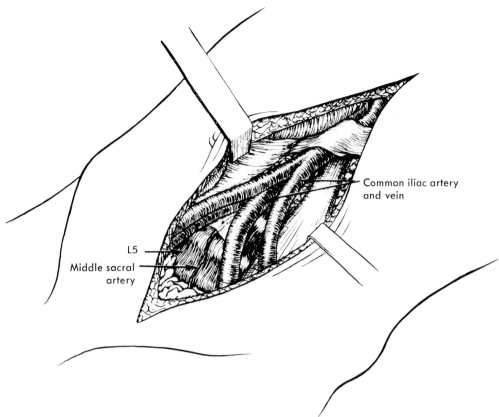

Fig. 68-17. Anterior approach to lumbosacral spine (see text). (From Perry, J.: In Pierce, D.S., and Nickel, V.H., editors: The total care of spinal cord injuries, Boston, 1977, Little, Brown & Co.)

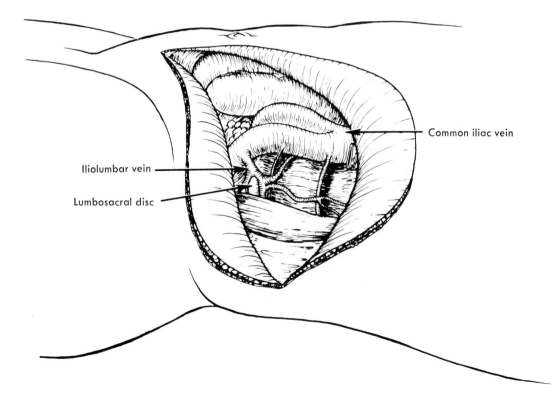

Fig. 68-18. Oblique lateral approach to lumbosacral spine (see text). (From Perry, J.: In Pierce, D.S., and Nickel, V.H., editors: The total care of spinal cord injuries, Boston, 1977, Little, Brown & Co.)

low them. The second vascular obstacle is the middle sacral artery, which originates from the bifurcation and traverses distally over the midline of the spine; it can cause considerable hemorrhage if attention is not paid to it. The oblique lateral approach is preferred for spinal injuries because it makes visible a greater area (Fig. 68-18). In the lateral approach to the lumbosacral joint the iliolumbar artery must be anticipated; it extends as a branch from the common iliac artery crossing the lumbosacral area diagonally to reach the iliac area. This artery must be identified and handled to prevent considerable hemorrhage. Further development of the exposure then proceeds as in the approach to the lumbar spine.

ANTERIOR APPROACH TO CERVICAL, CERVICODORSAL, DORSAL, AND LUMBAR SPINE (HODGSON ET AL.)

This approach is discussed on p. 3333.

APPROACH TO DORSAL SPINE BY COSTOTRANSVERSECTOMY

This approach is discussed on p. 3330.

APPROACH TO DORSAL SPINE FOR ANTEROLATERAL DECOMPRESSION

This approach is discussed on p. 3341.

Posterior approaches

POSTERIOR APPROACH TO CERVICAL SPINE

TECHNIQUE. Place the patient prone with the head supported well, taking care to avoid eye pressure. Make a longitudinal midline incision. Use self-retaining retractors to keep the tissues under constant tension and incise the nuchal ligament (Fig. 68-19). Continue slowly along this wandering avascular ligament and avoid the highly vascular muscle. At the area of C2 and C3 proceed carefully downward to the atlantoaxial membrane, removing muscle attachments with a twisting rather than pulling motion of the elevator. Proceed cautiously in the lateral direction

avoiding the nerve roots and the vertebral artery (Fig. 68-20). The lateral margins of the facets are the safe lateral extent of dissection (Fig. 68-21). Identify the large C2 spinous process distally with bifid processes below. In this region continue a midline dissection as above; then carry it laterally over the bifid process. Remove the bifid process with a rongeur if necessary avoiding large bites into the vascular muscle (Fig. 68-22).

POSTERIOR APPROACH TO THORACIC SPINE

For the posterior approach to the thoracic spine see the discussion in Chapter 71.

POSTERIOR APPROACH TO LUMBAR SPINE

Hibbs and others have recommended this approach, and Wagoner has described the technique in detail.

TECHNIQUE (WAGONER). Make a longitudinal incision over the spinous processes of the appropriate vertebrae and incise the superficial fascia, the lumbodorsal fascia, and the supraspinous ligament longitudinally, precisely over the tips of the processes. With a scalpel, divide longitudinally the ligament between the two spinous processes in the most distal part of the wound. Insert a small, blunt periosteal elevator through this opening so that its end rests on the junction of the spinous process with the lamina of the more proximal vertebra. Move the handle of the elevator

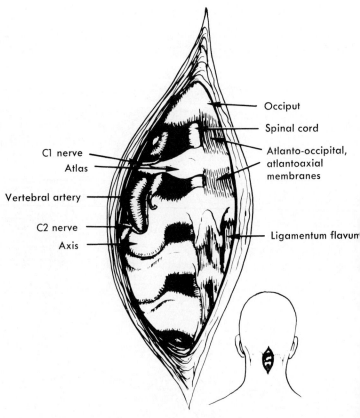

Fig. 68-20. Posterior approach to cervical spine. Dissection is carried laterally (see text). (From Perry, J.: In Pierce, D.S., and Nickel, V.H., editors: The total care of spinal cord injuries, Boston, 1977, Little, Brown & Co.)

Labels on figure: Occiput, Spinal cord, Atlanto-occipital, atlantoaxial membranes, Ligamentum flavum, C1 nerve, Atlas, Vertebral artery, C2 nerve, Axis

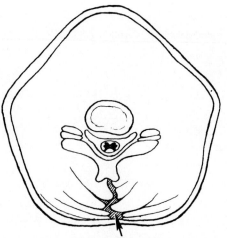

Nuchal ligament

Fig. 68-19. Posterior approach to cervical spine. Nuchal ligament is irregular. To maintain dry field, surgeon must stay within ligament. (From Perry, J.: In Pierce, D.S., and Nickel, V.H., editors: The total care of spinal cord injuries, Boston, 1977, Little, Brown & Co.)

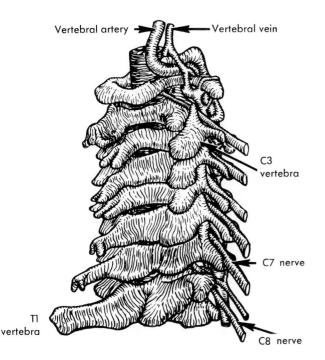

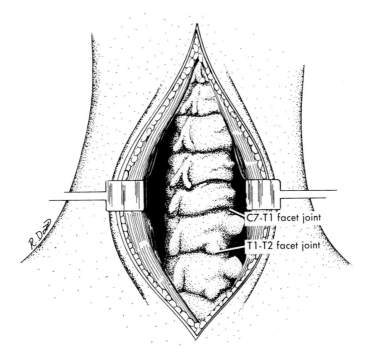

proximally and laterally to place under tension the muscles attached to this spinous process. Then with a scalpel moving from distally to proximally strip the muscles subperiosteally from the lateral surface of the process. Then place the end of the elevator in the wound so that its end rests on the junction of the spinous process with the lamina of the next most proximal vertebra and repeat the procedure as described. Repeat the procedure until the desired number of vertebrae has been exposed (Fig. 68-23). For operations requiring exposure of both sides of the spine, use the same technique on each side.

This approach exposes the spinous processes and medial part of the laminae. Increase the exposure, if desired, by further subperiosteal reflection along the laminae; expose the posterior surface of the laminae and the articular facets. Pack each segment with a tape sponge immediately after exposure to lessen bleeding. Divide the supraspinous ligament precisely over the tip of the spinous processes and denude subperiosteally the sides of the processes because this route leads through a relatively avascular field; otherwise the arterial supply to the muscles will be encountered (Fig. 68-23, *1*). Blood loss may be further decreased by using an electrocautery and a suction apparatus. Replace blood as it is lost. Expose the spinous processes from distally to proximally as just described because the muscles may then be stripped from the spinous processes in the acute angle between their insertions and the bone. If exposure in the opposite direction is attempted, the knife blade or periosteal elevator will tend to follow the direction of the fibers into the muscle and divide the vessels, thus increasing hemorrhage.

Fig. 68-21. Posterior approach to cervical spine. Posterolateral view of cervical spine to show relationship of vertebral artery and cervical nerve roots. (From Perry, J.: In Pierce, D.S., and Nickel, V.H., editors: The total care of spinal cord injuries, Boston, 1977, Little, Brown & Co.)

Fig. 68-22. Posterior approach at cervicothoracic junction. Note abrupt change in alignment between cervical and thoracic facet columns that occurs at T1. (From Perry, J.: In Pierce, D.S., and Nickel, V.H., editors: The total care of spinal cord injuries, Boston, 1977, Little, Brown & Co.)

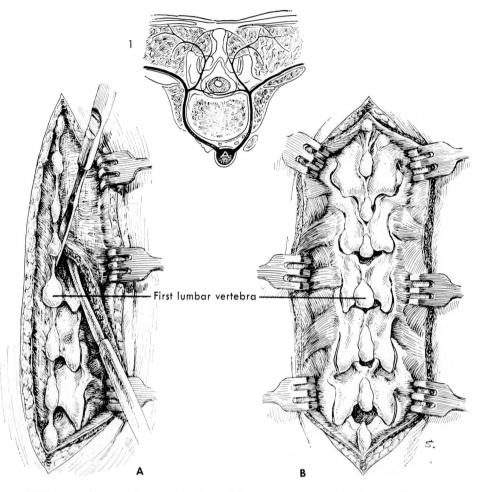

First lumbar vertebra

A   **B**

Fig. 68-23. Approach to posterior aspect of spine. **A,** Muscle insertions are freed subperiosteally from lateral side of spinous processes and interspinous ligaments; dissection proceeds proximally, the periosteal elevator being held against bases of spinous processes. **B,** Spinous processes, laminae, and articular facets exposed. **1,** Courses of arteries supplying posterior spinal muscles, showing proximity of internal muscular branches to spinous processes. (Modified from Wagoner, G.: J. Bone Joint Surg. **19:**469, 1937.)

REFERENCES
Circulation of spinal cord

Di Chiro, G.: Angiography of obstructive vascular disease of the spinal cord, Radiology **100:**607, 1971.

Dommisse, G.F.: The blood supply of the spinal cord: a critical vascular zone in spinal surgery, J. Bone Joint Surg. **56-B:**225, 1974.

Kardjieve, V., Symeonov, A., and Chankov, I.: Etiology, pathogenesis, and prevention of spinal cord lesions in selective angiography of the bronchial and intercostal arteries, Radiology **112:**81, 1974.

Keim, H.A., and Hilal, S.K.: Spinal angiography in scoliosis patients, J. Bone Joint Surg. **53-A:**904, 1971.

Macnab, I., and Dall, D.: The blood supply of the lumbar spine and its application to the technique of intertransverse lumbar fusion, J. Bone Joint Surg. **53-B:**628, 1971.

Pasternak, B.M., Boyd, D.P., and Ellis, F.H., Jr.: Spinal cord injury after procedures on the aorta, Surg. Gynecol. Obstet. **135:**29, 1972.

Surgical approaches

Bailey, R.W., and Badgley, C.E.: Stabilization of the cervical spine by anterior fusion, J. Bone Joint Surg. **42-A:**565, 1960.

Bonney, G., and Williams, J.P.R.: Trans-oral approach to the upper cervical spine: a report of 16 cases, J. Bone Joint Surg. **67-B:**691, 1985.

Burrington, J.D., et al.: Anterior approach to the thoracolumbar spine: technical considerations, Arch. Surg. **111:**456, 1976.

Cauchoix, J., and Binet, J.P.: Anterior surgical approaches to the spine, Ann. R. Coll. Surg. **21:**237, 1957.

Cloward, R.B.: The anterior approach for ruptured cervical discs, J. Neurosurg. **15:**602, 1958.

Codivilla, A.: Sulla scoliosi congenita, Arch. di Ortop. **18:**65, 1901.

Colletta, A.J., and Mayer, P.J.: Chylothorax: an unusual complication of anterior thoracic interbody spinal fusion, Spine **7:**46, 1982.

Compere, E.L.: Excision of hemivertebrae for correction of congenital scoliosis: report of two cases, J. Bone Joint Surg. **14:**555, 1932.

Fang, H.S.Y., Ong, G.B., and Hodgson, A.R.: Anterior spinal fusion: the operative approaches, Clin. Orthop. **35:**16, 1964.

Fraser, R.D.: A wide muscle-splitting approach to the lumbosacral spine, J. Bone Joint Surg. **64-B:**44, 1982.

Hall, J.E.: The anterior approach to spinal deformities, Orthop. Clin. North Am. **3:**81, 1972.

Hall, J.E., Denis, F., and Murray, J.: Exposure of the upper cervical spine for spinal decompression by a mandible and tongue-splitting approach: case report, J. Bone Joint Surg. **59-A:**121, 1977.

Harmon, P.C.: Results from the treatment of sciatica due to lumbar disc protrusion, Am. J. Surg. **80:**829, 1950.

Hodgson, A.R., et al.: Anterior spinal fusion: the operative approach and pathological findings in 412 patients with Pott's disease of the spine, Br. J. Surg. **48:**172, 1960.

Johnson, R.M., and McGuire, E.J.: Urogenital complications of anterior approaches to the lumbar spine, Clin. Orthop. **154:**114, 1981.

Michele, A.A., and Krueger, F.J.: Surgical approach to the vertebral body, J. Bone Joint Surg. **31-A:**873, 1949.

Mirbaha, M.M.: Anterior approach to the thoraco-lumbar junction of the spine by a retroperitoneal-extrapleural technic, Clin. Orthop. **91:**41, 1973.

Nachlas, I.W., and Borden, J.N.: The cure of experimental scoliosis by directed growth control, J. Bone Joint Surg. **33-A:**24, 1951.

Perry, J.: Surgical approaches to the spine. In Pierce, D.S., and Nickel, V.H., editors: The total care of spinal cord injuries, Boston, 1977, Little, Brown & Co.

Riley, L.H., Jr.: Surgical approaches to the anterior structures of the cervical spine, Clin. Orthop. **91:**16, 1973.

Riseborough, E.J.: The anterior approach to the spine for the correction of deformities of the axial skeleton, Clin. Orthop. **93:**207, 1973.

Robinson, R.A., and Riley, L.H., Jr.: Techniques of exposure and fusion of the cervical spine, Clin. Orthop. **109:**78, 1975.

Royle, N.D.: The operative removal of an accessory vertebra, Med. J. Australia **1:**467, 1928.

Smith, A.D., von Lackum, W.H., and Wylie, R.: An operation for stapling vertebral bodies in congenital scoliosis, J. Bone Joint Surg. **36-A:**342, 1954.

Southwick, W.O., and Robinson, R.A.: Surgical approaches to the vertebral bodies in the cervical and lumbar regions, J. Bone Joint Surg. **39-A:**631, 1957.

von Lackum, H.L., and Smith, A.F.: Removal of vertebral bodies in the treatment of scoliosis, Surg. Gynecol. Obstet. **57:**250, 1933.

Wagoner, G.: A technique for lessening hemorrhage in operations on the spine, J. Bone Joint Surg. **19:**469, 1937.

Whitesides, T.E., Jr., and Kelly, R.P.: Lateral approach to the upper cervical spine for anterior fusion, South. Med. J. **59:**879, 1966.

Wiltberger, B.R.: Resection of vertebral bodies and bone grafting for chronic osteomyelitis of the spine, J. Bone Joint Surg. **34-A:**215, 1952.

Wiltberger, B.R.: The dowel intervertebral-body fusion as used in lumbar disc surgery, J. Bone Joint Surg. **39-A:**284, 1957.

Wiltse, L.L.: The paraspinal sacrospinalis-splitting approach to the lumbar spine, Clin. Orthop. **91:**48, 1973.

CHAPTER 69

Fractures, dislocations, and fracture-dislocations of spine

Barney L. Freeman III

CERVICAL SPINE FRACTURES

Fractures and dislocations of the cervical spine are serious injuries and, unfortunately, usually occur in young people. The neurologic effects of a severe cervical injury can be devastating. In the Edwin Smith papers from ancient Egypt, traumatic quadriplegia was considered untreatable. Fortunately our ability to treat cervical spine fractures and dislocations has improved greatly during the past 20 to 30 years, partly as a result of improved emergency medical techniques. More patients with severe neck injuries are arriving at the emergency room without the disastrous consequences of a significant neurologic injury.

Consequently it is imperative that any fracture be detected early so that proper treatment can be instituted without delay. Bohlman in a study of 300 cervical spine fractures found that one third had not been discovered on initial evaluation.

Evaluation of cervical spine injury
HISTORY

A detailed history of the mechanism of injury will frequently help in planning the appropriate treatment for the specific type of fracture. Any history of transient paralysis should be taken seriously. Any patient with a head or neck injury should be suspected of having a cervical spine fracture. Care especially should be taken in patients with a decreased level of consciousness for any reason and in those with multiple injuries. Certainly comatose patients and those intoxicated from alcohol should be suspects for neck injury until proven otherwise.

PHYSICAL EXAMINATION

Any evidence of head injury, such as lacerations or abrasions of the face or scalp, should draw attention to the cervical spine. Is there any voluntary motion of the upper or lower extremities? Is there any sign of nuchal rigidity? Frequently cervical spine injuries occur in combination with other major life-threatening injuries, and these latter injuries should be evaluated as in any multiply traumatized patient. The spine, of course, should be protected during this system review.

NEUROLOGIC EVALUATION

Stauffer emphasizes the importance of accuracy in evaluating the patient with spinal cord injury. The presence of an incomplete or complete lesion must be determined by careful assessment of the sacral segments (Fig. 69-1). A complete lesion is characterized by absence of perianal sensation and loss of voluntary control of the sacral-innervated muscles, the toe flexors, or the rectal sphincter. If this condition persists for 24 hours, 99% of patients will have no functional recovery. Conversely, any evidence of sparing of the sacral segments, such as retained perianal skin sensation, toe flexion, or sphincter control, indicates an incomplete lesion with the possibility for significant recovery. The period of complete lumbar and sacral areflexia (spinal shock) is quite transient and usually persists less than 24 hours. Return of the bulbocavernosus reflex or anal wink, normal cord-mediated reflexes, signifies its termination (Figs. 69-2 and 69-3). The lesion cannot be con-

3109

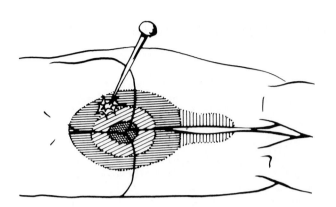

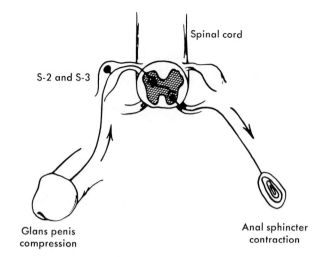

Fig. 69-1. Examination of perianal skin for sensation in cervical cord injury. Discrimination between sharpness and dullness may be only indication of incomplete injury. (From Stauffer, E.S.: Clin. Orthop. **112**:9, 1975.)

Fig. 69-2. Bulbocavernosus reflex (see text). (From Stauffer, E.S.: Clin. Orthop. **112**:9, 1975.)

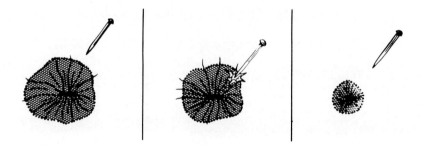

Fig. 69-3. Anal wink. Contracture of external sphincter caused by pinprick (see text). (From Stauffer, E.S.: Clin. Orthop. **112**:9, 1975.)

sidered complete until one or both of these reflexes return. Further examination of patients with complete lesions will then accurately define the level of injury. Ninety percent of the lesions in surviving complete quadriplegics are at the C5, C6, or C7 level. Even in complete quadriplegics the prognosis for return of the nerve roots at the level of the fracture is good.

ROENTGENOGRAPHIC EXAMINATION

Weir, in a study of 360 normal adults, established criteria for roentgenographic evaluation of the cervical spine. This included the prevertebral soft tissue shadow, which should not exceed 5 mm in depth at the level of the antero-inferior border of the third cervical vertebra. Depths in excess of this strongly suggest injury with swelling and require thorough roentgenographic evaluation of the entire cervical spine. He has shown that loss of the cervical lordotic curve is not in itself indirect evidence of cervical spine injury with resultant muscle spasm but may be only a normal variant.

The initial roentgenographic views of the injured neck should include standard anteroposterior, lateral, and oblique projections with the patient immobilized and un-moved during the examination. If these standard views do not reveal the pathologic condition, specialized views, including the pillar views or laminagrams or both, should be obtained. The pillar views are taken with the central roentgen beam centered over the midcervical area with a 35-degree cephalocaudal tilt. The head is rotated 45 degrees to the right to view the left pillars and 45 degrees to the left to view the right pillars. Rotation of the head moves the chin out of the way of the roentgen beam. This movement of the head should be within the limits of the patient's comfort. These views can be taken without head rotation, but superimposition of the cranial vault compromises the examination. Lateral flexion and extension roentgenograms can be made to check for instability secondary to comminuted unilateral fracture of the pillar of the subluxing segment or a severe injury to the ligaments and supporting structures of the apophyseal joints.

Weir has found a wide variation in the height of the pillars from individual to individual and also within the same spine. This variation can lead to false diagnosis of occult fractures. Because of the normal posteroinferior inclination of the apophyseal joints at 35 degrees, a horizontal pillar in the anteroposterior view is strong evidence of a pillar fracture. A comminuted pillar fracture can occur with subluxation up to 50% of the width of the vertebral

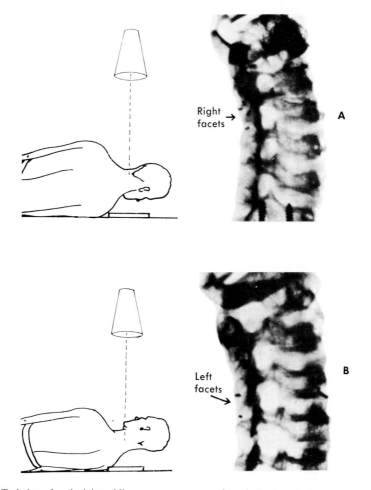

Fig. 69-4. Technique for obtaining oblique roentgenograms of cervical spine. **A,** Patient is placed in right oblique semiprone position, and roentgenogram so produced shows *right* facets and intervertebral foramina. **B,** Patient is placed in right oblique semisupine position, and roentgenogram so produced reveals left facets and intervertebral foramina. (From Beatson, T.R.: J. Bone Joint Surg. **45-B:**21, 1963.)

body, but usually the subluxation is in the 2 to 4 mm range.

In unilateral facet dislocations a lateral view shows an anterior offset of less than 50% of one vertebral body on another. Bilateral facet dislocations result in displacement of 50% or more.

Sometimes a fracture-dislocation in the lower cervical spine is overlooked because the roentgenograms do not include this area. In stocky people with short necks, satisfactory lateral roentgenograms are difficult to make; laminagrams may be necessary, but usually the lower cervical area will be included if the patient's arms are pulled distally and the cassette is placed lateral to the shoulder. Care should certainly be taken during this maneuver if one strongly suspects a significant cervical spine injury. A swimmer's view can also be obtained. Braakman and Vinken reported 36 patients with unilateral or bilateral dislocation of the articular facets, mostly in the lower cervical area; 25 had already sought medical assistance and had been examined roentgenographically, but the correct diagnosis had not been made. According to them, the following points are helpful in interpreting anteroposterior roent-

genograms: (1) in bilateral dislocations the spinous processes are farther apart than normal, and (2) in unilateral dislocations, the spinous process deviates toward the side of the dislocation. Beatson emphasized the importance of oblique views and described the technique for making them (Fig. 69-4).

White et al. have described the "stretch test," which is a safe way to assess possible instability in an injured cervical spine. This test should be performed under the supervision of a physician. After an initial lateral cervical spine roentgenogram has been made and examined, traction is applied either through a head halter or skull tongs. A film is placed at the standard distance from a patient's neck to obtain a lateral roentgenogram. Fifteen pounds of weight are added to the traction, and another lateral roentgenogram is made. The weight is increased in 10-pound increments, every 5 or more minutes, with lateral roentgenograms made at each step, until either one third of the body weight or 65 pounds is reached. After each additional weight is applied, any change in neurologic status or any abnormal separation of the anterior and posterior elements of the vertebrae should be noted. The test is considered positive if either of these occurs; it is used only in cervical spine injuries where the stability of a fracture is in question. It is unnecessary in obviously unstable injuries.

Computed axial tomography of the cervical spine can supply additional information concerning fractures and other injuries. It can be especially useful in demonstrating any bone fragment protruding into the spinal canal with subsequent compression of the spinal cord. It is also helpful in evaluating lateral mass fractures and fractures of the articular facets. This special examination should be done, however, only after thorough routine roentgenographic evaluation of the cervical spine has been carried out.

Cattell and Filtzer have described several normal anatomic variations that can lead to misinterpretation of instability on roentgenograms of the cervical spine in children under the age of 8 years. In flexion the atlas often shifts 3 to 4 mm anterior to the odontoid process and in extension it can override the process so that more than two thirds of the anterior arch is above its superior margin. Ligamentous laxity at C2-3 and C3-4, plus the horizontal configuration of the facets, can permit pseudosubluxation at these levels. The base of the odontoid synchondrosis is present in one half of children aged 4 to 5 years. Sixteen percent of normal children in the study of Cattell and Filtzer had significant angulation at only one level, and with a history of trauma it would have been consistent with a posterior ligamentous injury. Therefore the roentgenographic findings in a child under age 8 should correlate with the physical findings and with the history of the injury.

Spinal cord syndromes

Spinal cord syndromes resulting from incomplete traumatic lesions have been described by Schneider and Kahn and Bosch, Stauffer, and Nickel. The following generalizations can be made from their investigations: (1) the greater the sparing of motor and sensory functions distal to the injury, the greater the expected recovery; (2) the more rapid the recovery, the greater the amount of recovery; and (3) when new recovery ceases and a plateau is reached, no further recovery can be expected. Ninety percent of incomplete lesions will produce one of three clinical syndromes: (1) the central cord syndrome, (2) the Brown-Séquard syndrome, or (3) the anterior cervical cord syndrome.

The *central cord syndrome* is the most common. It consists of gray matter destruction and central spinothalamic and pyramidal tract destruction (Fig. 69-5). Prognosis is variable, but more than 50% of patients will have return of bowel and bladder control, will become ambulatory, and will have improved hand function (Table 69-1). This syndrome is usually the result of a hyperextension injury in a person with preexisting osteoarthritis of the spine. The spinal cord is pinched between the vertebral body anteriorly and the infolding of the ligamentum flavum posteriorly. The patient will have an incomplete lesion with greater involvement of the upper extremities than of the lower.

The *Brown-Séquard syndrome* is characterized by total paralysis on the ipsilateral side and hypesthesia on the contralateral side of the injury to the cord. Prognosis is better than in other incomplete lesions. The patient can recover control of bowel or bladder, most become ambulatory, and almost all have marked recovery of hand function, although hand strength is less than normal (Table 69-2).

The *anterior cervical cord syndrome* is characterized by complete motor loss and loss of pain and temperature discrimination below the level of the injury, but deep touch,

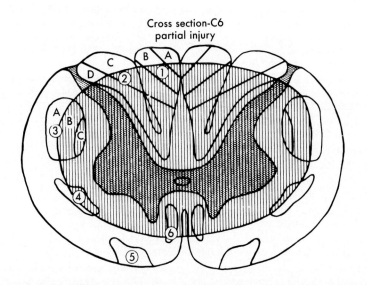

Fig. 69-5. Cross section of C6 level of spinal cord indicating an incomplete cord injury of the central cord syndrome type. *A*, Sacral; *B*, lumbar; *C*, thoracic; *D*, cervical; *1*, fasciculus gracilis; *2*, fasciculus cuneatus; *3*, tractus corticospinalis lateralis; *4*, tractus spinothalamicus lateralis; *5*, tractus spinothalamicus anterior; *6*, tractus corticospinalis anterior. Note specifically the sparing of sacral portions of the corticospinal tract (motor) and spinothalamic tract (pain and temperature). The long tracts of the white matter may show progressive recovery. The damage to the gray matter, however, resulting in upper extremity paralysis, is usually profound and permanent. (From Stauffer, E.S.: Clin. Orthop. **112:**9, 1975.)

position sense, and vibratory sensation remain intact throughout. Prognosis for significant neurologic recovery in this injury is poor (Table 69-3). Anterior cord syndrome is usually caused by a hyperflexion or teardrop fracture, a hyperextension injury, posterior displacement of fragments in a comminuted vertebral body fracture, or an extrusion of intervetebral disc material. The injury to the cord may be secondary to direct trauma from bone fragments or extruded material or may possibly be secondary to some compromise in the anterior spinal artery system.

In Stauffer's experience, if complete paralysis and the absolute loss of pain and temperature discrimination (including the sacral segments) remain for 48 hours after the return of the bulbocavernosus reflex, some roots in the immediate area of the injury may recover, but there is never significant motor or sensory recovery below that level. Thus the spinal cord injury is complete.

Soft tissue injuries of cervical spine

Most patients with injuries of the cervical spine have only soft tissue damage and initially should receive nonoperative treatment; surgical treatment should be considered after 12 months if there is an established discogenic pain pattern. Macnab has found that 45% of persons with extension injuries of the cervical spine still had symptoms on later evaluation, but most were of a nuisance nature and did not cause a significant disability. In patients with continued disability after injury, a discogram should be performed. If the symptoms are reproduced by the discogram at one level, then anterior disc excision and replacement by bone grafting may be indicated.

In soft tissue injuries with neurologic deficit, the type of neurologic pattern determines the surgical approach. Early computed tomography or a myelogram is indicated to demonstrate any defect that correlates with the clinical findings. In the anterior cord syndrome, anterior decompression of the spinal cord is indicated if an anterior defect is noted on the myelogram or scan. In the central cord syndrome with cervical spondylosis, skeletal traction usually results in partial recovery. In a young patient with a flexion injury, a soft disc protrusion must be considered if symptoms persist; however, a laminectomy is not indicated, but a myelogram should be made to show the level of the lesion. A decision can then be made, based on the myelogram, as to whether decompression is indicated.

Fractures, dislocations, or both without neurologic deficit

In cervical fractures without neurologic deficit, the surgeon must decide whether the lesion is stable or unstable. White, Southwick, and Panjabi have defined clinical instability as loss of the ability of the spine under physiologic loads to maintain relationships between vertebrae in such a way that there is neither damage nor subsequent irritation to the spinal cord or nerve roots and, in addition, no painful deformity. Deciding whether a specific spine fracture is stable or unstable is sometimes difficult. White et al. have presented an excellent guide for making this decision (Table 69-4). Although only a guide, it is helpful when considering a specific fracture pattern.

In general, stable fractures are treated nonoperatively; unstable injuries should be considered for possible surgical stabilization. All unstable fractures without neurologic deficit are treated initially by skeletal traction, and many can be reduced by this treatment alone. If reduction is unsuccessful, then open reduction, internal fixation, and fusion, if possible, should be considered. Opinions differ as to

Table 69-1. Function attained following central cord lesion*

	Admission (%)	Present at discharge (%)	Follow-up (%)
Ambulation	33.3	77	59
Hand function	26	42	56
Bladder function	17	—	53
Bowel function	9.5	—	53

From Bosch, A., Stauffer, E.S., and Nickel, V.L.: JAMA **216:**473, 1971.
*Chronic sequelae of central cord damage: (1) increased spasticity and pyramidal tract involvement, (2) incidence of 23.8%, (3) prognosis poor with progressive neurologic loss.

Table 69-2. Function attained following hemisection cord lesion

	Admission (%)	Present at discharge (%)	Follow-up (%)
Ambulation	60	100	80
Hand function	60	80	100
Bowel function	80	80	100
Bladder function	100	100	100

From Bosch, A., Stauffer, E.S., and Nickel, V.L.: JAMA **216:**473, 1971.

Table 69-3. Function attained following anterior cord lesion

	Admission (%)	Present at discharge (%)	Follow-up (%)
Ambulation	0	0	0
Hand function	16	16	16
Bladder function	0	0	0
Bowel function	0	0	0

From Bosch, A., Stauffer, E.S., and Nickel, V.L.: JAMA **216:**473, 1971.

Table 69-4. Checklist for the diagnosis of clinical instability in the lower cervical spine*

Element	Point value
Anterior elements destroyed or unable to function	2
Posterior elements destroyed or unable to function	2
Relative sagittal plane translation >3.5 mm	2
Relative sagittal plane rotation >11 degrees	2
Positive stretch test	2
Medullary (cord) damage	2
Root damage	1
Abnormal disc narrowing	1
Dangerous loading anticipated	1

From White, A.A., Southwick, W.O., and Panjabi, M.M.: Spine **1:**15, 1976.
*Total of 5 or more = unstable.

whether surgery is necessary in unstable fractures. Munro has taken issue with those who use open reduction too often. He bases his opinion on the higher mortality and the number of undesirable side effects after surgery and on the fact that simple skeletal traction is usually effective. In our experience, however, ligamentous healing in unstable fractures cannot be relied on routinely after treatment by skeletal traction, and internal fixation and fusion have been satisfactory. Further, as surgical and anesthesiologic techniques have improved, the mortality and morbidity after surgery have decreased substantially.

Fractures, dislocations, or both with neurologic deficit

Accurate initial examination of patients with a neurologic deficit is essential to determine whether the deficit is complete or incomplete. Complete quadriplegics do poorly with immediate operative treatment, and their condition should be allowed to stabilize medically before surgery is considered. In most patients with incomplete quadriplegia, the fracture-dislocation should be reduced promptly by traction; early aggressive anterior decompression and stabilization or posterior stabilization may be indicated based on myelographic findings.

In quadriplegics, survival itself may be the major issue, requiring prompt measures for respiratory and abdominal difficulties. The problem is to decide whether an operation is indicated and, if so, when; this decision and further treatment may require both an orthopaedic surgeon and a neurosurgeon and occasionally other specialists. The amount of neurologic improvement that may eventually occur has usually been determined at the time of injury; the compressive pathologic condition is almost always anterior. The spine should be stabilized externally by skeletal traction as quickly as feasible. If decompression is indicated, it should be performed either anteriorly or posteri-

orly, depending on which side of the cord the defect is located.

Skeletal traction for fractures, dislocations, or fracture-dislocations of cervical spine

Crutchfield has described the use of skeletal traction in both recent and old fracture-dislocations of the cervical spine. For this purpose he devised special tongs that are applied to the vertex of the skull. They are efficient, make nursing care easier, and cause few complications. With Crutchfield tongs, skeletal traction may be used not only for patients with fresh fracture-dislocations, with or without cord injury, but also for patients with old fractures or fracture-dislocations of the cervical spine for which insufficient or no treatment was given at the time of injury.

Gardner-Wells tongs are now being used with equally good results and have largely replaced Crutchfield tongs. Their ease of application and their self-contained tension device are definite advantages. They are also less likely than Crutchfield tongs to dislodge. For patients in whom long-term immobilization in the halo cast is required, the halo itself can be used for initial traction.

TECHNIQUE (CRUTCHFIELD). After preparing the patient's head, paint two lines on the scalp, one in the midline of the skull and the other across it in line with the mastoid processes. These lines aid in the proper placement of the tongs. With the traction bar resting on the midline (Fig. 69-6), place the tongs on the transverse line and mark the points of contact for the placement of stab wounds. Inject the two areas with lidocaine (Xylocaine) and make a stab wound down to the skull in each just large enough to admit a drill. Use a special drill point with a flange at the distal end that allows the drill to penetrate only the outer table of the skull; in children the depth is 3 mm and in adults 4 mm. Now fit the points of the tongs into the holes in the

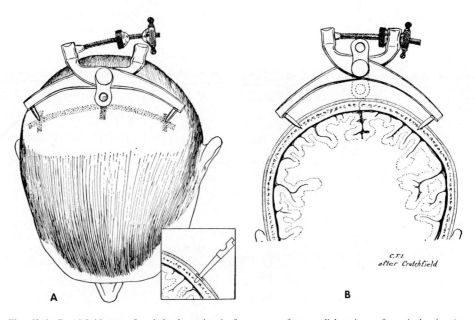

A

B

C.F.I.
after Crutchfield

Fig. 69-6. Crutchfield tongs for skeletal traction in fractures or fracture-dislocations of cervical spine (see text). *Inset,* Special drill constructed with flange that allows it to penetrate outer table only. (Redrawn from Crutchfield, W.G.: Am. J. Surg. **38:**592, 1937.)

Table 69-5. Traction recommended for levels of injury

Level	Minimum weight in pounds (kg)	Maximum weight in pounds (kg)
First cervical vertebra	5 (2.3)	10 (4.5)
Second cervical vertebra	6 (2.7)	10-12 (4.5-5.4)
Third cervical vertebra	8 (3.6)	10-15 (4.5-6.8)
Fourth cervical vertebra	10 (4.5)	15-20 (6.8-9.0)
Fifth cervical vertebra	12 (5.4)	20-25 (9.0-11.3)
Sixth cervical vertebra	15 (6.8)	20-30 (9.0-13.5)
Seventh cervical vertebra	18 (8.1)	25-35 (11.3-15.8)

skull and hold them in position until the tongs have been locked. Dress the stab wounds with a collodion dressing.

Check the tongs daily to see that they are firmly in place; tighten them if necessary. To-and-fro movements will result in local irritation, enlargement of the holes, and eventual disengagement of the tongs. On the other hand, routine tightening of the tongs, whether needed or not, may result in perforation of the inner table of the skull. Crutchfield recommends the amount of traction for each cervical level as given in Table 69-5.

TECHNIQUE (GARDNER-WELLS). The following instructions are found on the metal tag that is an integral part of the Gardner-Wells tong system. Be certain that the points of the tongs are needle sharp and wipe them with an antiseptic. Spray the hair and scalp with an aerosol antiseptic, and rub in the antiseptic at the temple ridges. Inject a local anesthetic, spray the area again, and apply the tongs. Tighten the system until the indicator protrudes 1 mm (Fig. 69-7). Tilt the tongs back and forth to set the points. After 24 hours do not tighten the tongs further.

TECHNIQUE (PERRY AND NICKEL). The halo orthosis was first used on the body jacket by Perry and Nickel in 1959. It is now an important device in the treatment of many cervical spine injuries.

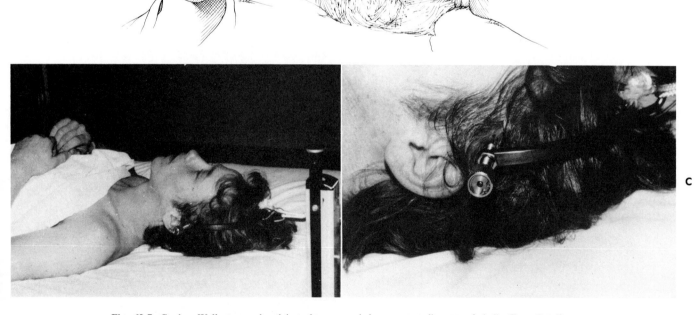

Fig. 69-7. Gardner-Wells tongs placed just above ears, below greatest diameter of skull. (From Stauffer, E.S.: Management of cervical spine injuries. In Evarts, C.M., editor: Surgery of the musculoskeletal system, New York, 1983, Churchill Livingstone.)

The halo ring comes in six sizes. The circumference of the skull is measured just above the ears, and the manufacturer's chart is consulted for proper ring size. The halo and pins should be kept sterilized when stored. The application of the halo requires two people. With the patient supine, the head is supported just over the end of the stretcher by an assistant or by one of the application devices, which is attached to the stretcher and which will also hold the halo itself. The skin and scalp where the pins are to be placed are prepared by washing the hair with a surgical preparation such a povidone-iodine (Betadine). Usually cutting the hair is unnecessary. The halo of appropriate size is then supported about the patient's head by another assistant or by the application device. The halo must be held below the area of greatest diameter of the skull. It should be just above the eyebrows and about 1 cm above the tips of the ears (Fig. 69-8).

Inject a local anesthetic into the four areas selected for pin insertion. Then place the two anterior pins in bare skin and not within the hairline. The bone is extremely thin just anterior to the ears, and anchorage here is not good. Further, the supraorbital nerve should be avoided; it can be located by palpating its foramen. The most medial halo channels are usually chosen for the pin sites anteriorly. Posteriorly, the central channels are usually the best sites. Introduce the pins and tighten two diagonally opposed pins simultaneously. Continue this until all four pins just engage the skin and bone. It is important that, as the pins are being tightened, the patient keeps his eyes closed to make certain that the skin on the forehead is not anchored in such a way as to prevent the eyelids from closing after application of the halo. Continue tightening diagonal pairs of pins with a torque screwdriver. Using only the fingertips and not the palm on the short screwdriver will give final tension of about 5½ inch pounds. Alternate tightening of the pins to prevent migration of the halo to an asymmetric position. After all pins are tightened to 5½ inch pounds, unscrew each about one quarter of a turn. This allows the rotary stretch of the skin to return to a relaxed position, preventing skin necrosis. Finally secure the pins to the halo with appropriate lock nuts or set screws.

AFTERTREATMENT. The halo pins should be cleansed at the pin-skin interface with hydrogen peroxide daily, inspected, and kept dry. They should not be tightened daily as has been the habit with the Crutchfield tongs, since the pins rarely enter the skull more than 2 mm but rather act as a wedge forcing the halo from the skull. The indications for changing the pins are serous drainage, inflammation, or a clicking sensation. The pins should otherwise be undisturbed. If a pin must be replaced, this is achieved by inserting a new sterilized pin into an adjacent hole before removal of the offending pin. Three pins alone will not hold a halo.

In our experience the cervical spine is not held as stable in the halo vest as in a halo body jacket. The halo vest is useful, however, in quadriplegic patients with loss of sensibility.

• • •

Following the application of skeletal traction, rapid reduction of a dislocation or fracture-dislocation is not advisable, because the force sufficient to accomplish this may increase the soft tissue injury and endanger the spinal cord. Rather, minimal corrective pull is applied, giving immediate protection to the cord and beginning the reduction. Reduction may be complete within an hour but need not be checked roentgenographically until the next day. If strong traction is advisable, portable roentgenograms are made at 15-minute intervals, or at least once an hour, until the surgeon is certain that the force is not too strong. No further weight is added after the vertebrae have been distracted enough for them to slip back into position. Following reduction, the weight is decreased to 5 to 7 pounds (2.3 to 3.2 kg) to maintain the corrected position.

The preceding discussion has been concerned mainly with reduction of fractures or fracture-dislocations in the cervical spine. However, one must not forget that the primary object of reduction is to restore the anteroposterior diameter of the spinal canal, thus decompressing the spinal cord. Complete reduction is most desirable but not always possible. According to Rogers, satisfactory reductions are those with less than 3 mm of decrease in the anteroposte-

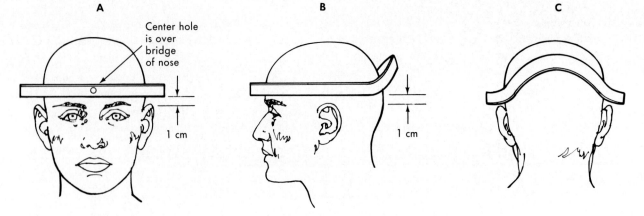

Fig. 69-8. When one is applying halo ring, pin sites should be 1 cm above lateral one third of eyebrows and same distance above tops of ears in occipital area (mastoid area). (From Young, R., and Thomassen, E.H.: Orthop. Review **3**:62, 1974.)

rior diameter of the canal. After satisfactory reduction has been obtained, maintaining it for 8 to 12 months may be a problem. Roentgenograms after 3 months may show a remarkably good reduction, but if the patient does not return again for regular checkups for an additional 4 to 6 months, the original deformity may recur. Although we agree with Munro that many injuries of the cervical spine can be treated conservatively, many are unstable and difficult to hold in an acceptable position. No one can be sure which lesions will remain stable and heal satisfactorily and which will not. Some fracture-dislocations of the cervical spine spontaneously develop a bridge of bone anteriorly, resulting in an interbody fusion; others show little evidence of union and are a source of worry for months. To aid in deciding which injury should be treated conservatively we offer these suggestions. When the injury is chiefly ligamentous and any fracture is only minor, the dislocation is likely to recur and early Rogers fusion is indicated. On the other hand, when the injury is chiefly osseous and osseous

union can be expected, as for example, in fractures of the pedicles of C2, union will stabilize the spine and fusion is unnecessary.

Specific fractures

FRACTURE OF C1

Jefferson first described burst fractures of C1 in 1920. Patients with this fracture usually have neck pain or stiffness without a neurologic deficit. Roentgenographically, the fracture is detected in the open-mouth odontoid view, which reveals displacement of the lateral masses of the atlas laterally beyond the articular surfaces of the axis. Computed axial tomography of C1 is often helpful in further delineating the exact displacement of the fragments (Fig. 69-9). Spence, Decker, and Sell have determined that if the lateral masses overhang the articular surfaces of the axis more than 7 mm, then the transverse ligament is likely to be torn (Fig. 69-10); this fracture is therefore considered unstable and should be treated in a halo cast or skeletal traction for 3 months. If the overhang is less than 7 mm, then the fracture is stable and should be treated in a rigid support, such as a cervicothoracic brace, for 3 months.

ROTARY SUBLUXATION OF C1 ON C2

Fielding and Hawkins have described atlantoaxial rotary subluxation. Patients with this injury are seen clinically with torticollis and restricted neck motion, and frequently the diagnosis has been delayed. The diagnosis is suggested by asymmetry of the lateral masses as seen on the open-mouth odontoid view and is confirmed by cineradiography or computed axial tomography. In the cineradiography, in the lateral views, the posterior arches of the atlas and axis move as a unit during attempted neck motion. Four types of rotary subluxation of C1 on C2 are described (Fig. 69-11). Usually the deformity is easily correctible, but sometimes it becomes fixed and requires treatment in skull traction. Then if reduction takes place, the patient is kept in traction or a halo cast for 3 months. Recurrence of deformity is possible, however, even with this treatment. Rotary subluxations of longer than 3 months are best treated

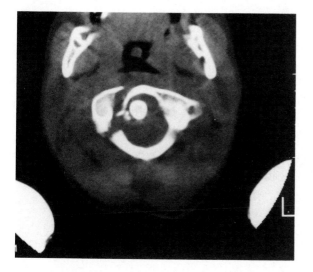

Fig. 69-9. Computed tomographic scan of ring of C1 demonstrating Jefferson's fracture of C1.

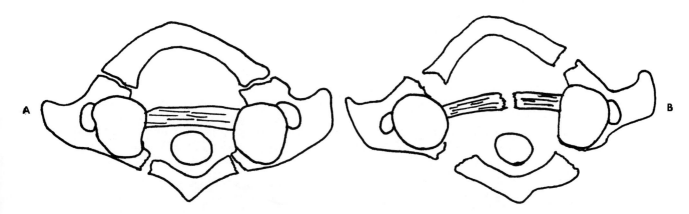

Fig. 69-10. A, Drawing indicating axial view of stable Jefferson's fracture (transverse ligament intact). **B,** Drawing indicating axial view of unstable Jefferson's fracture (transverse ligament ruptured). (From Schlicke, L.H., and Callahan, R.: Clin. Orthop. **154:**18, 1981.)

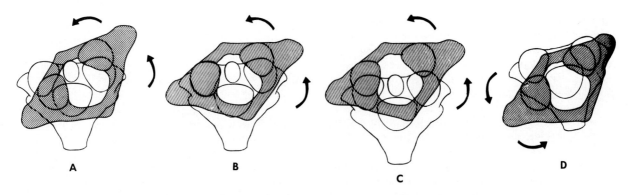

Fig. 69-11. Four types of rotary fixation. **A,** Type I: rotary fixation with no anterior displacement and odontoid process acting as pivot. **B,** Type II: rotary fixation with anterior displacement of 3 to 5 mm, with one lateral articular process acting as pivot. **C,** Type III: rotary fixation with anterior displacement of more than 5 mm. **D,** Type IV: rotary fixation with posterior displacement. (From Fielding, J.W., and Hawkins, R.J.: J. Bone Joint Surg. **59-A:**37, 1977.)

by C1, C2 fusion (p. 3119). The fusion should be preceded by 2 to 3 weeks of skeletal traction. After fusion, traction is continued for 6 weeks or a halo cast is used.

ANTERIOR DISLOCATION OF C1 ON C2 WITH RUPTURED TRANSVERSE LIGAMENT

Fielding, Cochran, Lawsing, and Hohl have shown that widening of 3 to 5 mm of the space between the anterior arch of C1 and the odontoid process implies injury to the transverse ligament. Widening greater than 5 mm implies injury to both the transverse ligament and the alar ligaments. A patient with traumatic anterior subluxation of C1 on C2 should be immobilized with the head in extension. Early elective posterior C1, C2 fusion is indicated since healing of the ligaments cannot be relied on to provide adequate stability and any instability at this level is potentially fatal.

ODONTOID PROCESS FRACTURES

Anderson and D'Alonzo have classified odontoid process fractures into three types (Fig. 69-12). Type I fractures are uncommon, and even if nonunion occurs, no instability results. Type II fractures are the most common and, in the study of Anderson and D'Alonzo, had a 36% nonunion rate for both displaced and nondisplaced fractures. Type III fractures have a large cancellous base and healed without surgery in 90% of the patients. Our treatment program follows these guidelines. We most commonly use surgical wiring and fusion for type II fractures. When surgery is not used, rigid immobilization such as with the halo cast is preferred to prolonged hospitalization in tong traction. Type III fractures are also treated with a halo cast for more rapid rehabilitation.

The reported success in achieving fusion between the atlas and the axis varies widely in the literature. Schatzker, Rorabeck, and Waddell have reported successful union in 13 of 15 patients treated by primary wiring and fusion. Fried, however, achieved primary union in only 2 of 10 of his patients, and the others required additional surgery or prolonged immobilization. Our results are similar to those of McGraw and Rusch, who reported success in 14 of 15 fractures compared to 16 of 18 in our series.

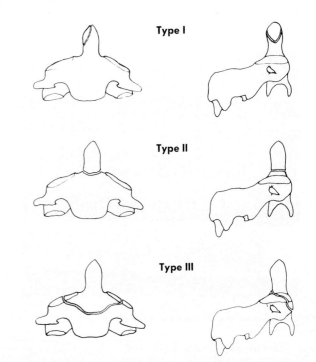

Fig. 69-12. Three types of odontoid process fractures as seen in anteroposterior and lateral planes. Type I is oblique fracture through upper part of odontoid process. Type II is fracture at junction of odontoid process and body of second cervical vertebra. Type III is fracture through upper body of vertebra. (From Anderson, L.D., and D'Alonzo, R.T.: J. Bone Joint Surg. **56-A:**1663, 1974.)

Fractures of the odontoid process can occur in children and are usually a separation through the synchondrosis at the junction of the odontoid process with the body of C2. These fractures usually heal well when treated by rigid external fixation such as in a halo cast.

FRACTURE THROUGH PEDICLES OF C2

These fractures, termed "hangman's fractures," commonly result from a distraction-extension force applied to the head and neck and are usually not associated with a neurologic deficit. Undisplaced fractures of the pedicles of

C2 without injury to the disc can be treated in a rigid support, such as a Somi brace. Displaced fractures of the pedicles of C2 are usually accompanied by injury to the disc and are potentially unstable; these should be treated in a halo cast for 12 weeks.

UNILATERAL FACET DISLOCATIONS

Unilateral facet dislocations are usually the result of a flexion-rotation injury of the cervical spine. The most common site of dislocation is between C5 and C6 and may cause nerve root damage. In general, unilateral facet dislocations associated with neurologic damage or facet fracture are clinically unstable. On the other hand, some unilateral facet fractures may be considered stable, especially when they are difficult to reduce by skeletal traction, which implies an intact anulus fibrosus and ligamentum falvum. In our experience, however, a stable unilateral facet dislocation will require open reduction; this then renders the dislocation unstable, and it should be accompanied by a Rogers wiring and posterior fusion. In unstable unilateral facet dislocations, reduction, Rogers wiring, and posterior fusion are also indicated. Before reduction, roentgenograms must be made and carefully studied for the type and location of any fracture that may be present. A dislocation uncomplicated by a fracture of any consequence should be treated immediately with gradual reduction by skeletal traction.

BILATERAL FACET DISLOCATIONS

Bilateral facet dislocations are also usually the result of a flexion-rotation injury of the neck. They are more frequently associated with neurologic injury than unilateral dislocations. All are considered unstable and require closed or open reduction followed by Rogers wiring and posterior fusion (Fig. 69-13).

WEDGE COMPRESSION FRACTURES OF CERVICAL VERTEBRAE

Compression fractures are caused by flexion forces applied to the cervical spine. In minimally displaced wedge fractures, significant posterior ligamentous disruption does not take place and the injuries are stable. These should heal satisfactorily when treated by 12 weeks of immobilization in a rigid orthosis or halo cast. One should be certain, however, that the posterior ligamentous structures are intact by applying the principles of White, Southwick, and Panjabi, or the ''stretch test'' (p. 3111).

COMMINUTED BURST FRACTURES

A comminuted burst fracture is usually caused by axial loading plus a flexion moment and often results from diving injuries. It is markedly unstable and is frequently complicated by disastrous neurologic sequelae as a result of damage to both the anterior and posterior columns of the cervical spine. The vertebral body is comminuted, and bony fragments are retropulsed into the spinal canal, injuring the cord. This fracture should be reduced as soon as possible by skeletal traction. After the patient's condition has stabilized, a decision should be made as to whether the spinal cord should be decompressed surgically. Stauffer has emphasized the potential problems encountered in anterior vertebral body excision and fibular or iliac crest strut

grafting in the face of associated posterior ligamentous injury. If decompression is indicated and the posterior interspinous ligaments can be demonstrated to be intact, then anterior vertebral body excision and grafting with an iliac bone strut are indicated. If, however, posterior ligamentous instability is present, a Rogers wiring and fusion should be performed to stabilize the posterior structures; then an anterior decompression can be carried out. The neck should be immobilized after surgery in a halo vest or cast, or skeletal traction can be used instead.

OTHER FRACTURES OF CERVICAL SPINE

Fractured laminae, lateral masses, or pedicles, if isolated injuries, are usually associated with intact ligamentous structures. Immobilization in a rigid cervical orthosis or halo cast is the only treatment necessary.

Surgical techniques

ATLANTOAXIAL FUSION

There are many variations of two basic techniques of atlantoaxial fusion. Fielding and Hawkins and others have reported successful results using a Gallie type of fusion, but Griswold, Albright, Schiffman, Johnson, and Southwick found in their series a higher nonunion rate with this method and now recommend the method described by Brooks and Jenkins. The major advantage of the latter type of fusion is its greater resistance to rotational movement and lateral bending. Its major disadvantage is that the two wires are passed beneath the C2 lamina rather than through the C2 spinous process as in the simpler midline Gallie type of fusion. For a fractured odontoid process with anterior displacement of the process requiring extension for reduction, we prefer the Gallie fusion. For a fractured odontoid process with posterior displacement we prefer to avoid any extension at the C1, C2 level and use the Brooks and Jenkins fusion.

TECHNIQUE (GALLIE). Carefully intubate the patient in the supine position while the patient is still in bed and then carefully place him prone on the operating table using a headrest. In turning the patient take care to maintain the head-thoracic relationship. Then make cervical spine roentgenograms while the patient is on the operating table to be certain of the status of the fracture.

Prepare and drape the operative field in the usual fashion. Inject a 1:500,000 epinephrine solution intradermally to help with hemostasis. Then make a midline incision from the occiput to the fourth or fifth cervical vertebra. Using a cutting current and sharp dissection, expose the spinous processes and laminae. By subperiosteal dissection, expose the posterior arch of the atlas and the laminae of C2 and gently remove all soft tissue from the bony surfaces. The upper surface of the arch of C1 should be exposed no further laterally than 1.5 cm from the midline in adults and 1 cm in children to avoid the vertebral arteries. Decortication of C1 and C2 is generally not needed. Now pass a no. 18 or no. 20 wire loop from below upward under the arch of the atlas either directly or with the aid of a Mersiline suture; the suture can be passed using an aneurysm needle if necessary. Pass the free ends of the wire through the loop, thus grasping the arch of C1 in the loop (Fig. 69-14). Take a corticocancellous graft from the iliac

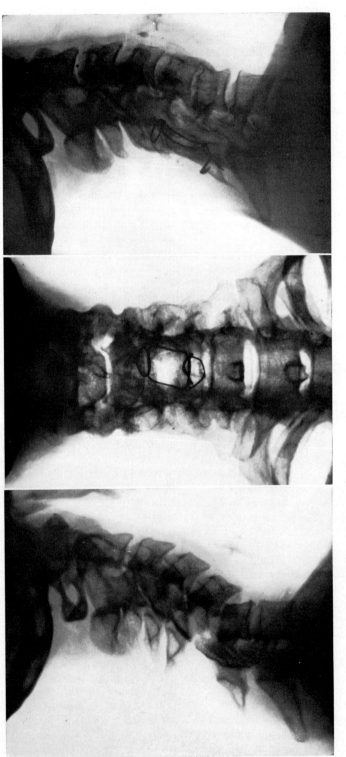

Fig. 69-13. Dislocation of fifth on sixth cervical vertebra. Neurologic symptoms were temporary. Two and one-half years after open reduction and Rogers wiring and fusion there is a solid bony bridge from fourth through sixth spinous processes. Bodies of fifth and sixth cervical vertebrae subsequently fused.

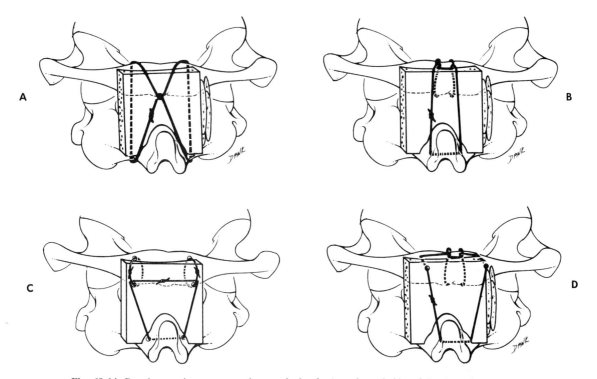

Fig. 69-14. Drawings to demonstrate various methods of using wire to hold graft in place. **A,** Wire passes under lamina of atlas and axis and is tied over graft. **B,** Wire passes through holes drilled in lamina of atlas and through spine of axis; holes are drilled thorugh graft. **C,** Wire passes under lamina of atlas and through spine of axis and is tied over graft. This is method we use most frequently. **D,** Wire passes under lamina of atlas and through spine of axis; holes are drilled through graft. (From Fielding, J.W., Hawkins, R.J., and Ratzan, S.A.: J. Bone Joint Surg. **58-A:**400, 1976.)

crest and place it against the lamina of C2 and the arch of C1 beneath the wire. Then pass one end of the wire through the spinous process of C2 and twist the wire on itself to secure the graft in place. Irrigate the wound and close it in layers over suction drainage tubes.

AFTERTREATMENT. The patient is mobilized as soon as possible. Skeletal traction is maintained immediately after surgery until it is certain that no significant swelling has occurred. The patient is then placed in a cervicothoracic type of orthosis, or if fixation is unstable a halo cast is applied. Immobilization is continued for 12 weeks.

TECHNIQUE (BROOKS AND JENKINS). Intubate and turn the patient on the operating table as in the Gallie fusion just described. Prepare and drape the patient in the same manner. Expose the C1, C2 level through a midline incision, as in the Gallie fusion (Fig. 69-15, *A*). Using an aneurysm needle, pass a no. 2 Mersiline suture on each side of the midline in a cephalad-to-caudad direction, first under the arch of the atlas and then under the lamina of the axis (Fig. 69-15, *B*). These serve as guides to introduce two doubled no. 20 stainless steel wires into place. Obtain two full-thickness rectangular bone grafts approximately 1.25 × 3.5 cm (Fig. 69-15, *C*) from the iliac crest. Bevel the grafts to fit in the interval between the arch of the atlas and each lamina of the axis. While holding the grafts in position on each side of the midline and maintaining the width of the interlaminal space, tighten the doubled wires over them and twist and tie the wires to secure the grafts

(Fig. 69-15, *D* and *E*). Irrigate and close the wound in layers over suction drains.

AFTERTREATMENT. The aftertreatment is the same as described for the Gallie fusion (see above).

OCCIPITOCERVICAL FUSION

The technique described here for occipitocervical fusion includes features and procedures used by Cone and Turner, Rogers, and Willard and Nicholson.

TECHNIQUE OF OPEN REDUCTION AND FUSION. Approach the base of the occiput and the spinous processes of the second, third, fourth, and fifth cervical vertebrae and expose the entire field subperiosteally. If reduction has not been obtained, apply traction and manipulation to the first cervical vertebra and reduce the dislocation if possible. If a laminectomy is needed for relief of pressure on the cord, extend the grafts from the occiput to the third or fourth cervical vertebra (Fig. 69-16). With a Hudson burr make openings in the occipital bone on each side of the midline about 2.5 cm superior to the posterior arch of the foramen magnum. Through these openings, separate the dura from the skull and protect it while drilling additional holes for wire loops. Pass short lengths of wire through the holes in the occiput and through the foramen magnum. Next pass wires beneath the posterior arch of C1 on either side if the arch is intact. Then drill holes through the base of the spinous processes of the second and third cervical vertebrae and pass short lengths of wire through these holes. Obtain

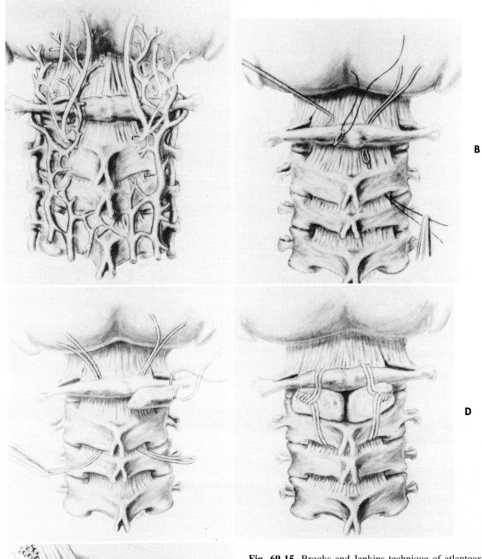

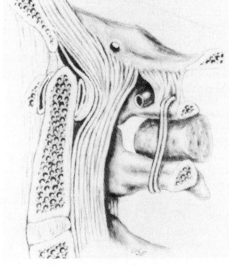

Fig. 69-15. Brooks and Jenkins technique of atlantoaxial fusion. **A,** Position of vertebral arteries and occipital nerves. With midline approach they are fairly well protected by neck muscles. **B,** Insertion of wires under atlas and axis. **C,** Wires are in place, and one graft is being inserted. **D,** and **E,** Grafts are secured by wires. (From Brooks, A.L., and Jenkins, E.B.: J. Bone Joint Surg. **60-A:**279, 1978.)

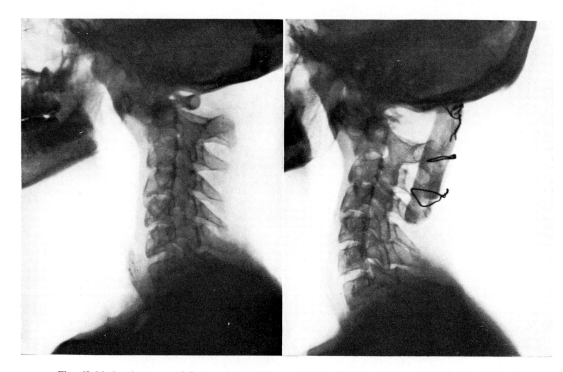

Fig. 69-16. Laminectomy of first cervical vertebra and fusion from occiput to second, third, and fourth vertebrae for old dislocation of first cervical vertebra (see text).

corticocancellous iliac grafts, drill holes in each and pass one end of each wire through each hole. Lay the grafts against the occiput and the lamina of C2 and C3 and tighten the wire loops, holding each graft in place. Alternatively, as described by Robinson and Southwick, pass individual wires beneath the lamina on each side of the spinous processes of C2 and C3. Then pass the ends of these wires through the corticocancellous graft on each side to hold them in place (Fig. 69-17).

AFTERTREATMENT. The patient is kept in skeletal traction until his condition has stabilized. Then if mobilization is desired, a halo cast is applied and is worn for 12 weeks.

OPEN REDUCTION AND FUSION OF CERVICAL SPINE
BELOW ATLAS

TECHNIQUE OF OPEN REDUCTION AND FUSION FOR CERVICAL DIS-LOCATION. Closed methods usually fail to reduce a dislocation. Traction may disengage the articular facets until reduction is almost possible; the addition of more weight, however, still does not allow reduction to occur. Open reduction is then the only recourse.

Administer general anesthesia with the patient in the supine position, and carefully perform intubation, preferably through the nasal route. If available, oral fiberoptic intubation is an excellent technique. Then turn the patient prone on the operating table, maintaining skeletal traction, and prepare and drape in a routine manner. It is suggested that the towels and drapes be sutured in place so that roentgenographic detail will not be obscured by towel clips. Assuming that the lesion is a dislocation of the fifth or sixth cervical vertebra, expose the area through a longitudinal midline incision (Fig. 69-18, A). Usually the proper level can easily be determined, since the sixth cervical vertebra has the last bifid spinous process. The anatomy here, however, is not constant, nor is the spinous process of the seventh cervical vertebra always the most prominent. The first dorsal vertebra may be more prominent. The only accurate method of determining the vertebral level consists of inserting a needle or pin into an exposed spinous process and checking its position with a lateral roentgenogram. After the dislocated articular facets are exposed, carefully hook a curved periosteal elevator under the superior articular facet; while traction is constantly exerted on the head, lever the facets into normal position. If reduction cannot be accomplished by this maneuver, remove a portion of the superior articular facet. Because the interspinous ligament and the ligamentum flavum are almost always torn, these dislocations are usually unstable and especially so if a facet has been removed. Therefore we routinely combine reduction of the dislocation with Rogers fusion (Fig. 69-13). Reduce the weight to 5 pounds (2.3 kg), wire the affected two or more vertebrae as described for the Rogers fusion (p. 3126), and add bone grafts that extend across the laminae of the involved vertebrae. Grafts from the ilium are most suitable.

AFTERTREATMENT. Cervical spine traction with the neck slightly hyperextended is continued for several days. Then a cervical spine brace with a chin-occiput piece is fitted, and the patient is allowed to walk. The brace should be worn during sleep, or after the patient is horizontal, it may be removed and a light halter traction applied. The brace is reapplied before the patient sits up. It is worn until the fusion is solid, usually at 3 to 4 months.

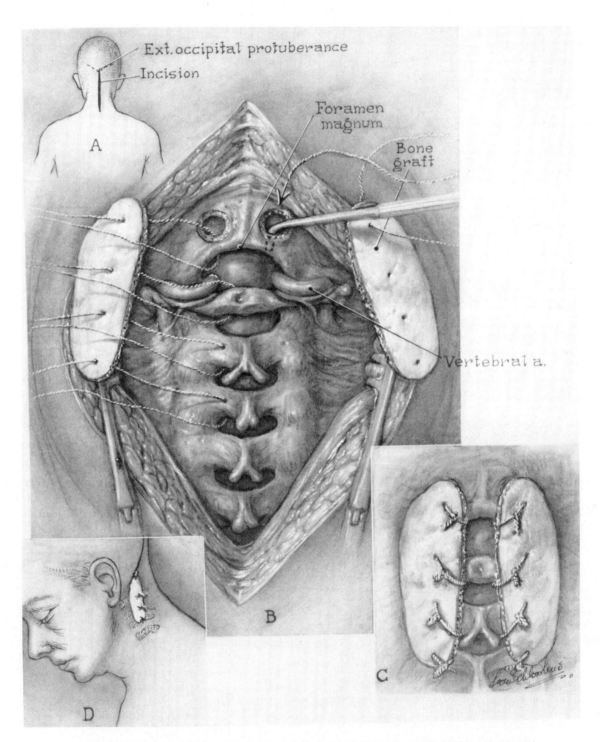

Fig. 69-17. Method of occipitocervical fusion, particularly useful if posterior arch of C1 has to be partly removed to relieve dural and cord compression. (From Robinson, R.A., and Southwick, W.O.: In American Academy of Orthopaedic Surgeons: Instructional course lectures, vol. 17, St. Louis, 1960, The C.V. Mosby Co.)

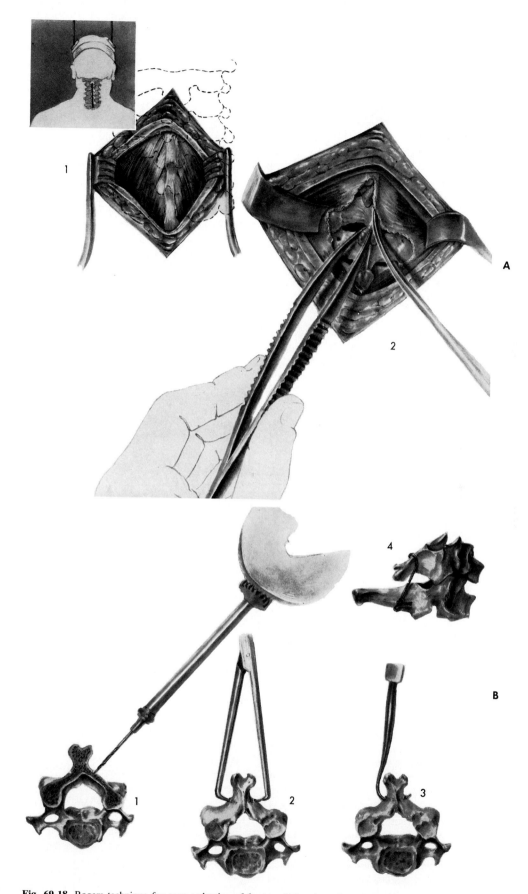

Fig. 69-18. Rogers technique for open reduction of fracture-dislocation of cervical spine. **A,** *1*, Incision; *2*, subperiosteal approach to posterior aspect of vertebrae. **B,** *1*, Hole is drilled in bone on each side of base of spinous process; *2* and *3*, hole through base is completed with vulsellum forceps and small hook; *4*, vertebrae are fixed with wire loop as described in text.

Continued.

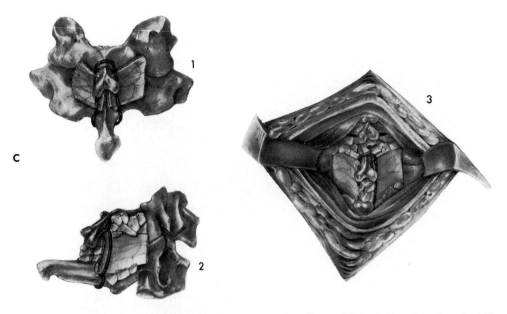

Fig. 69-18, cont'd. C, Iliac grafts are applied (see text). (From Rogers, W.A.: J. Bone Joint Surg. **24**:245, 1942.)

TECHNIQUE OF OPEN REDUCTION AND FUSION FOR FRACTURE-DIS-LOCATION (ROGERS). Make an incision in the midline from the prominent spinous process of the seventh cervical vertebra to the easily palpable spinous process of the second (Fig. 69-18, *A*). When the first, second, or third vertebra is involved, extend the incision toward the occiput. Identify the spinous processes in preparation for subperiosteal exposure of the posterior aspect of one vertebra above and one below the involved vertebra. Insert a needle or pin into this spinous process and check its location by a lateral roentgenogram. Expose by sharp subperiosteal dissection the spinous processes, laminae, and posterior articulations; if the neural arch has been fractured, be careful during the exposure to prevent cord damage. Steady the spinous process of the unstable vertebra with forceps during this dissection. Then accomplish the reduction by gentle traction with forceps. If the articular facets are dislocated, manipulate them into position using the procedure just described for dislocation.

Fix the fracture internally as follows. Usually two and sometimes three vertebrae are included in the internal fixation and fusion. If it is a dislocated vertebra only, fix the involved vertebra to the one below. Sometimes, however, the spinous processes (especially of the third, fourth, and fifth vertebrae) are small and fixation is insecure. In these instances, fix three or four vertebrae. When a fusion is being done for a fracture-dislocation, extend the fusion area from the first intact vertebra above to the first intact vertebra below the level of injury. Make a hole in the base of the spinous process of each vertebra to be included in the fusion. Use a towel clip to start the hole and complete it with a Lewin clamp. This is safer than using a drill that can slip and damage the cord. By sharp dissection, removal all soft tissue from the spinous process and lamina of each vertebra to be fused; a small ronguer or pituitary

forceps is helpful. Loop a wire through these holes as illustrated in Fig. 69-18, *B*. Place the wire around the superior border of the superior process and insert the ends in opposite directions through the hole in this process. Then pass the ends of the wires distally and parallel along the spinous processes to the last process to be fused, and then through the hole in this spinous process in opposite directions, and loop them around the distal border of this process. Now lay transversely two iliac grafts bridging each interspace and tighten the wire. Force the edges of the graft beneath the wire to ensure maintenance of position (Fig. 69-18, *C*). Pack multiple chips of cancellous bone wherever possible to reinforce the larger grafts. When the spine is unstable, subperiosteal exposure is dangerous, and decortication of the laminae is even more so. The latter is unnecessary, since the cancellous grafts will fuse satisfactorily to the laminae and spinous processes without this additional step.

AFTERTREATMENT. Aftertreatment is the same as described for open reduction of dislocations (p. 3123).

ANTERIOR CERVICAL VERTEBRECTOMY

TECHNIQUE OF ANTERIOR CERVICAL VERTEBRECTOMY (BOHL-MAN). If anterior decompression in a comminuted vertebral body fracture, such as a burst fracture, is necessary, this can be performed by surgically removing the vertebral body through an anterior approach. The patient is given a general anesthetic and carefully intubated, with the cervical spine protected by skeletal traction during this procedure.

Use an anterior approach to the cervical spine (p. 3094). Identify the fractured vertebral body either clinically or by a lateral roentgenogram. Remove the disc material above and below the body by incision of the anterior longitudinal ligament and curettage of the disc material. Then using the

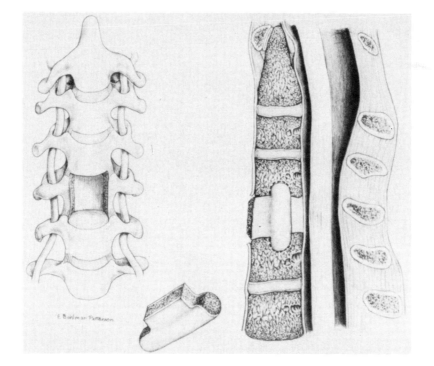

Fig. 69-19. Anterior cervical vertebrectomy. *Left,* Drawing of anterior part of cervical spine shows extent of vertebral body resection in which vertebral body was removed back to posterior longitudinal ligament, sparing lateral cortices to protect vertebral arteries. Posterior longitudinal ligament is not violated, and no instruments enter spinal canal. *Right,* Full-thickness iliac-crest graft is inserted to replace resected vertebra, with cortical surface of crest placed posteriorly. This procedure corrects kyphotic deformity and relieves spinal cord compression. (From Bohlman, H.H.: J. Bone Joint Surg. **61-A:**1119, 1979.)

ronguer or curet, remove the anterior aspect of the fractured vertebra. Remove the remaining disc material above and below back to the posterior longitudinal ligament. Make every effort to leave this ligament intact, since it serves as some protection for the spinal cord, which is just posterior. At this point, using a ronguer, curet, or dental burr, remove the bone back to the posterior cortex of the vertebral body. Then gently remove the posterior cortex from the posterior longitudinal ligament with curets. If necessary, traction under direct vision is suggested to reduce the deformity of the cervical spine. Remove the central portion of the end plates of the vertebra above and the vertebra below to produce two holes to accept the ends of an iliac or fibular graft. Take a full-thickness corticocancellous iliac graft and shape it as a short T to fit into the holes in the vertebrae (Fig. 69-19). Tamp the graft into place with the three-sided cortical portion of the iliac crest facing posteriorly. Then trim off any excess bone from the graft smooth with the anterior cervical spine. Drain and close the area in the routine fashion. If desired, a fibular graft can be used. The advantage of such a graft is that it is structurally stronger; the disadvantage is that it requires a longer time for incorporation into the vertebrae than does an iliac graft.

AFTERTREATMENT. The patient is kept in traction during the immediate postoperative period and then is allowed to walk in a rigid cervicothoracic orthosis; if stability is questionable, a halo cast or vest can be used instead. The sur-

geon must be sure that the posterior interspinous ligaments are intact or that the posterior structures have been surgically stabilized; otherwise, anterior vertebrectomy will further decrease stability of the spine.

FUSION AFTER LAMINECTOMY

TECHNIQUE FOR FLEXION INJURIES (ROBINSON AND SOUTHWICK). Expose the involved area through a longitudinal incision (p. 3094). Reduce a unilateral dislocation, bilateral dislocation, or fracture-dislocation as described previously in this chapter. While maintaining the reduction by traction on the spinous process of the proximal vertebra in a dorsal and inferior direction, open slightly a facet at the level of the dislocation with a narrow osteotome inserted into the joint space. Then turn the osteotome slightly on its side, allowing the entrance of a neurosurgical sucker tip just lateral to the ligamentum flavum. Do the same procedure with the opposite facet and with those at the level above (and sometimes below). Now drill a hole through each of the inferior facets into the joint space at these levels (Fig. 69-20, *A*) and pass a no. 20 stainless steel wire through each. Grasp the end of each wire with a hemostat and draw it out through the distal part of the facet joint. Now pull the wires distally like reins to the level of the seventh cervical or first dorsal vertebra and firmly anchor them there to maintain reduction (Fig. 69-20, *C* and *D*). Place bone grafts posteriorly and laterally across the facets (or later do an anterior fusion).

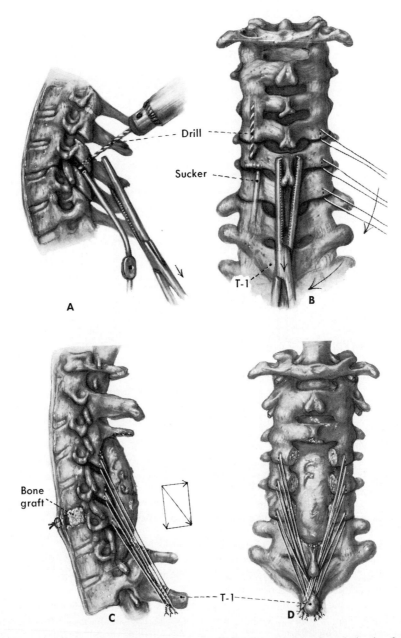

Fig. 69-20. Robinson and Southwick technique for laminectomy and fusion of cervical spine for flexion injuries (see text). (From Robinson, R.A., and Southwick, W.O.: South. Med. J. **53**:565, 1960.)

TECHNIQUE FOR EXTENSION OR VERTICAL INJURIES (ROBINSON AND SOUTHWICK). Do the procedure as just described and insert wires through the inferior facets. However, do not use the wires as reins, since tightening them around the seventh cervical or first dorsal vertebra in this instance would exaggerate the cervical deformity. Perform a laminectomy and use the wires to anchor the graft on either side of the laminectomy site, with the graft being on the facets. Tighten the inferior loops over the iliac or tibial grafts to hold the vertebrae anteriorly, superior to the level of the fracture-dislocation (Fig. 69-21, A), thus flattening to some extent the cervical lordosis, and then tighten the other wire loops.

AFTERTREATMENT. Skeletal traction is reduced to about 5 pounds (2.3 kg) and is continued during the period of bed rest. Usually if the cord has not been damaged, the patient should remain in bed for 4 to 6 weeks. When the patient is allowed up, a neck brace is fitted and is worn until the fusion is complete, usually 4 to 6 months after operation. If early mobilization is desirable, a halo cast or vest can be used.

TECHNIQUE (CALLAHAN). Callahan and associates have reviewed the experience of Robinson and Southwick with their posterolateral facet fusion following laminectomy. Fusion is indicated after laminectomy in the high-risk group, including children and adults less than 25 years old.

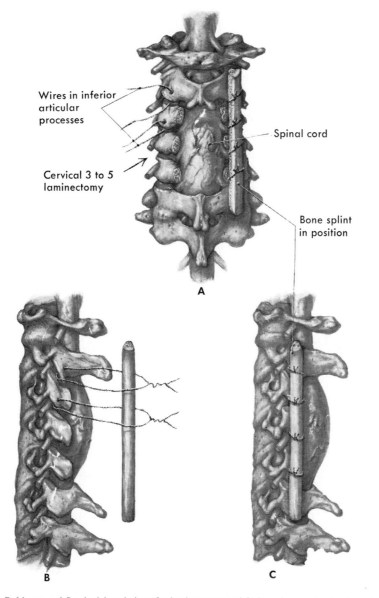

Wires in inferior
articular
processes

Spinal cord

Cervical 3 to 5
laminectomy

Bone splint
in position

A

B   C

Fig. 69-21. Robinson and Southwick technique for laminectomy and fusion of cervical spine for extension or vertical injuries. (From Robinson, R.A., and Southwick, W.O.: South. Med. J. **53:**565, 1960.)

Even for one-level laminectomy, fusion should be considered. Callahan et al. have modified the surgical techniques based on their findings:

1. Although more time consuming, careful wiring of the graft at each level (Fig. 69-22, *A*) results in a higher incidence and greater speed of union with fewer structural complications.
2. It is necessary to extend the fusion one segment below the lower end of the laminectomy to the first intact spinous process, whereas at the upper end of the laminectomy, the fusion should extend only to the last exposed articular facet.
3. No structural deformities occur below the caudal end of the fusion.
4. A corticocancellous graft from the outer table of the

posterior iliac crest with two concave surfaces is preferred. However, a rib having the same biconcave configuration can be used (Fig. 69-22, *B*).

DORSAL AND LUMBAR SPINE FRACTURES

The treatment of unstable fracures and fracture-dislocations of the dorsal and lumbar spine has been controversial for years. Many authors, such as Guttmann and Bedbrook, have advised nonoperative treatment. In the recent literature, authors such as Kaufer and Hayes, Kelly and Whitesides, Flesch et al., Jacobs et al., Soref et al., Dickson and associates, and Bradford have emphasized the many advantages of surgical reduction and stabilization of these injuries.

Paul of Aegina, 625 to 690 AD, first introduced laminec-

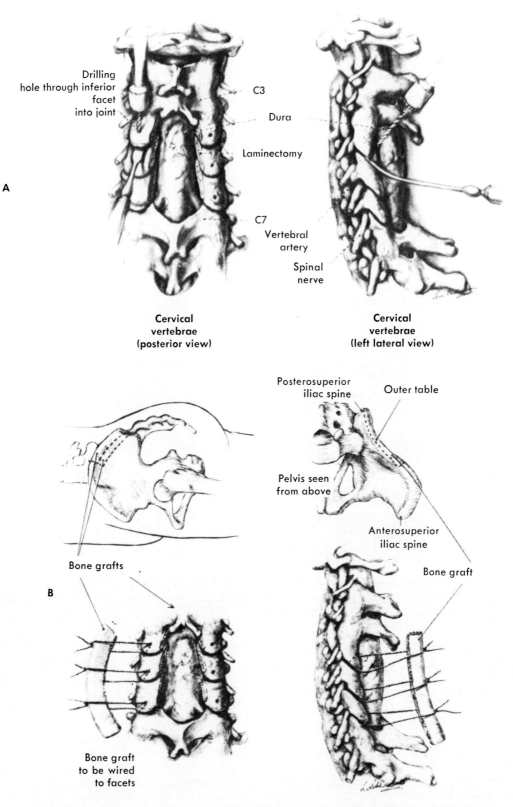

Drilling
hole through inferior
facet
into joint

C3

Dura

Laminectomy

C7

Vertebral
artery

Spinal
nerve

A

Cervical
vertebrae
(posterior view)

Cervical
vertebrae
(left lateral view)

Posterosuperior
iliac spine

Outer table

Pelvis seen
from above

Anterosuperior
iliac spine

Bone graft

Bone grafts

B

Bone graft
to be wired
to facets

Fig. 69-22. Technique of Callahan et al. similar to that shown in Fig. 69-21. **A,** Holes are drilled through inferior facets into joints. **B,** Curved grafts are obtained from posterior iliac crest for grafts, and wires are inserted through holes in inferior facets. **C,** Grafts are wired in place. (From Callahan, R.A., et al.: J. Bone Joint Surg. **59-A:**991, 1977.)

tomy for spinal cord injury, unaware of the controversy this would cause. The seventeenth century saw an increase in its use that has continued to the present. Munro, in the late 1930s, advised that laminectomy be delayed and reserved for selected patients. Guttmann condemned the routine use of early laminectomy and certain forms of internal fixation and advocated a conservative program of postural reduction by extension of the spine. Holdsworth agreed about the dangers of routine laminectomy but preferred early open reduction and internal fixation for certain injuries of the dorsolumbar and lumbar spine. Morgan, Wharton, and Austin have pointed out that laminectomy offers little benefit in these injuries and is not without morbidity and mortality. We also believe that laminectomy alone is contraindicated in fracture-dislocations since it fails to relieve the anterior compression and increases spinal instability.

Types of fractures

An unstable fracture is one in which the bony fragments or the dislocation of the spinal column is capable through movement of producing neural damage during healing. A stable fracture is one in which such movement is unlikely. We basically use the two-column concept in determining the stability of individual fractures of the dorsal and lumbar spine. The anterior column is the weight-bearing column of the spine and includes the anterior longitudinal ligament, the intervertebral discs, the vertebral bodies, and the posterior longitudinal ligament. The posterior column consists of the neural arches, the interspinous ligaments, and the facet joint capsules and is a tension-resisting mechanism. Acute instability is possible if both columns are disrupted.

We agree with Holdsworth's basic classification of fractures and fracture-dislocations of the dorsal and lumbar spine. An anterior wedge fracture occurs as a result of *pure flexion*. The posterior ligamentous structures are not ruptured because there is no rotation involved in the injury (Fig. 69-23, *A*). These fractures are generally stable, and surgery is usually not needed. It should be noted, however, that if the wedge compression defect anteriorly is 50% or more of the posterior height of the vertebral body, posterior facet malalignment can occur with the possibility of late pain and deformity requiring surgical stabilization. Patients with this degree of compression can initially be considered surgical candidates.

Flexion and rotation produce an unstable fracture-dislocation with rupture of the posterior ligament complex. This is the type of fracture Holdsworth has termed the "slice fracture." A fracture of the upper border of the lower vertebra and dislocation of the articular processes of the upper vertebra characterize this injury (Fig. 69-23, *C*). It frequently produces neurologic damage, and operative stabilization is required (Fig. 69-24, *C* and *D*).

A *flexion-distraction* force produces a distraction injury of the spinal column. This is usually caused by sudden

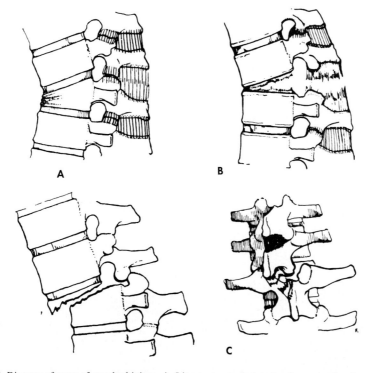

Fig. 69-23. Diagram of types of vertebral injury. **A,** Ligaments remain intact and compression fracture results. **B,** Ligaments rupture and dislocation results. **C,** Ligaments rupture, one superior facet dislocates over corresponding inferior one, and shearing fracture of superior surface of distal vertebra occurs. This injury is produced by torsional forces superimposed on flexion forces. It is the most common type of injury that causes paraplegia. (From Holdsworth, F.W.: In Platt, H., editor: Modern trends in orthopaedics, second series, London, 1956, Butterworth & Co., Ltd.)

deceleration in a person wearing a seat belt, which transfers the fulcrum of flexion anteriorly and applies a distraction force to the spine. Smith and Kaufer have described two basic types of this fracture (Figs. 69-25 and 69-26). If the injury occurs entirely through bone (a Chance fracture), it can generally be treated in a body cast. Rapid healing of the cancellous bone can be expected, and the

spine will be stable. The damage, however, can traverse the posterior ligamentous structures rather than bone, and if significant ligamentous injury results, the best treatment is by stabilization with a Harrington compression system.

A burst fracture is caused by *axial loading* of the spine, and bone or disc material is retropulsed into the spinal canal. Holdsworth originally considered all burst fractures

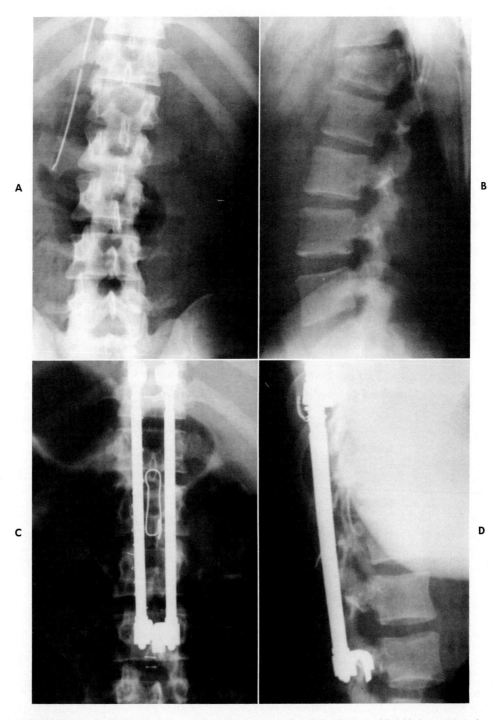

Fig. 69-24. A and **B,** Anteroposterior and lateral roentgenograms of slice fracture of L1. Notice rotation of spinous processes on anteroposterior view as well as fracture of facet. **C** and **D,** Postreduction roentgenograms after Harrington distraction rod fixation. Excellent reduction as well as stabilization is obtained. Note interspinous wire at level of posterior ligament disruption to prevent slight overdistraction of posterior elements.

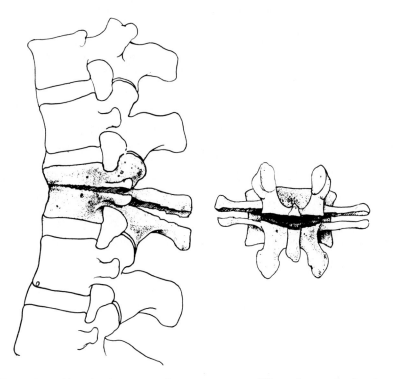

Fig. 69-25. Drawings of lateral and anteroposterior roentgenograms of Chance fracture showing characteristic features. (From Smith, W.S., and Kaufer, H.: J. Bone Joint Surg. **51-A:**239, 1969.)

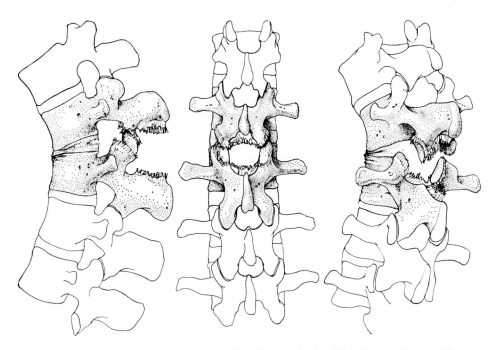

Fig. 69-26. Extensive ligament tearing is outstanding feature of this variety of seat-belt injury. Surgical exploration demonstrates gross instability caused by rupture of lumbodorsal fascia, interspinous ligaments, ligamentum flavum, capsules, joint between articular processes, and posterior longitudinal ligament. (From Smith, W.S., and Kaufer, H.: J. Bone Joint Surg. **51-A:**239, 1969.)

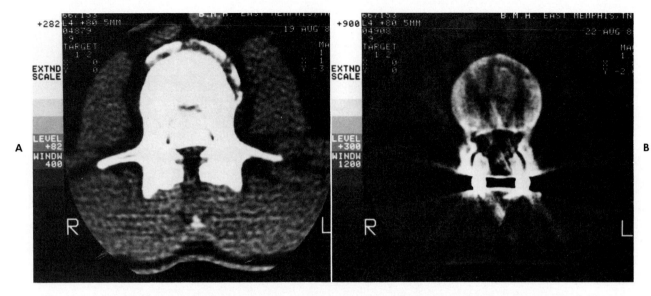

Fig. 69-27. A, Preoperative computed tomographic scan of patient with acute burst fracture of L1. Note typical retropulsed table of bone in spinal canal. **B,** Postoperative scan showing reduction of bony table with Harrington distraction rods posteriorly. Limited laminectomy was performed at time of surgery to confirm decompression of canal. Posterolateral approach to spine was not necessary in this case.

to be stable, but in our experience, many lead to chronic instability and are often associated with neurologic injuries. These latter have been termed "unstable burst fractures" by McAfee, Yuan, and Lasada. Computed axial tomography is helpful in evaluation here and will frequently show fragments retropulsed into the spinal canal that could not be seen on standard roentgenograms or tomograms. Significant spinal canal intrusion by a bony plug is consistent with an unstable burst fracture (Fig. 69-27). Evidence of posterior column disruption, in addition to the anterior column damage, may also indicate instability. Further, if loss of vertebral body height is greater than 50%, the possibility of an unstable fracture should be considered. Unstable burst fractures are best treated by reduction, internal fixation, and fusion.

An *extension* force causes rupture of the intervertebral disc and anterior longitudinal ligament. A dislocation occurs that almost always reduces spontaneously and is stable in flexion. Often a small fragment is avulsed from the anterior border of the dislocated vertebra. This type of injury is rare in the lumbar spine.

Shearing forces result in anterior displacement of the whole vertebra and frequently produce an unstable fracture of the articular processes or pedicles. The anterior longitudinal ligament is usually torn. Frequently, significant compression of the bony column anteriorly is absent. This unstable injury is probably best treated by reduction and stabilization with a compression type of system or posterior wiring and fusion (Fig. 69-28).

When paralysis from cord injury is immediate and complete and has lasted for more than 24 hours, appreciable recovery is rare and there is little controversy over treatment. When paralysis is incomplete, however, opinions vary considerably as to the best treatment. If the wisest orthopaedic surgeons and neurosurgeons studied the treat-

ment used for patients who have partially or completely recovered from cord injuries, opinions would vary even more as to which particular form of treatment contributed most to the recovery.

Because of the variations in diameter of the spinal canal, the damage to the cord or its related structures caused by fractures and fracture-dislocations is determined to some extent by the level of the injury. The spinal canal in the thoracic area is small, but because of the support supplied by the ribs in this region, fractures in the thoracic spine, except at the eleventh and twelfth vertebrae, are usually not displaced enough to impinge on the cord. We have seen several cases of severe displacement of thoracic vertebrae without paraplegia. Laminography or computed axial tomography of this area often shows that the fracture has occurred through the pedicles and the posterior elements have remained aligned, effecting autodecompression. These fractures have stabilized, and the patients remained pain free after nonoperative cast immobilization, except in one patient who underwent posterior fusion with an excellent result. Generally speaking, thoracic fractures are stabilized by the ribs and seldom need stabilization unless a laminectomy has been performed.

Fractures or fracture-dislocations of the lumbar spine may show marked displacement, lateral as well as anteroposterior, and still produce little neurologic deficit. Not only is the canal in this region large, but also the cord ends at the first lumbar vertebra and the cauda equina is less vulnerable than the cord above.

Neurologic deficit and roentgenographic evaluation

The extent of the neurologic deficit, its improvement or lack of improvement, and the roentgenograms all provide important data for treatment and prognosis. However, errors are possible in interpreting the roentgenograms. The

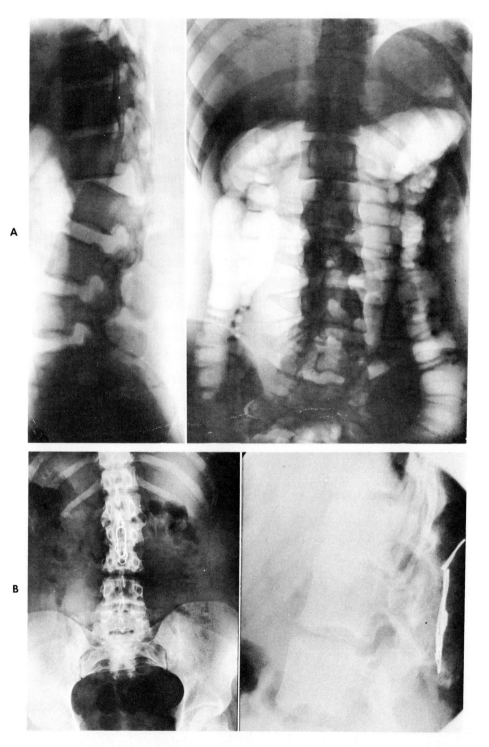

Fig. 69-28. A, Dislocation of lumbar spine with intact but locked articular facets and no neurologic deficit. Patient was in automobile accident, wearing a lap seat belt. **B,** Eighteen months after open reduction, wiring of spinous processes as described by Rogers. Iliac bone grafting, and application of plaster jacket. Fusion is solid, and symptoms are absent. This compression arthrodesis is useful in Chance fracture also.

roentgenograms may show only moderate displacement of the vertebrae when the cord is completely severed or severely injured, or the cord may remain intact even when the angulation and displacement of the vertebrae are severe. Since the injuring forces and the degree of initial displacement are unknown quantities, it is important to assess spinous process alignment in both the anteroposterior and lateral planes. Excessive separation and malalignment of these on the emergency room roentgenograms indicate rupture of the posterior ligament complex and therefore instability.

Holdsworth has emphasized that neurologic recovery is a function of the injury to the cord, to the roots, or to both. Since the roots are peripheral nerves, some may indeed recover, whereas the cord injury usually does not. The ultimate degree of recovery seems to depend almost entirely on the extent of neurologic damage at the time of injury and little on the method of subsequent treatment.

Internal fixation of spinal fractures

The methods of internal fixation of spinal fractures have included wire loops, spinal plates, Weiss springs, methylmethacrylate reinforcement with steel mesh, Harrington instrumentation, and anterior stabilization. In our experience the Harrington instrumentation system is best for most unstable fractures and fracture-dislocations. The goal of internal fixation in these injuries is to stabilize the spine, relieve pain, facilitate union, prevent late deformity and further neurologic deterioration with movement of the spine, and allow earlier upright activity. In deciding whether to use a distraction or a compression system, the surgeon must keep in mind the biomechanical principles of both the injury and the fixation systems. If the injury is basically ligamentous, such as a pure dislocation, the anterior bony column is intact and can resist compressive forces. Under these circumstances the injury is suitable for posterior compression fixation, which will replace the absent posterior ligamentous structures. On the other hand, if the vertebral body is disrupted and is unable to withstand compressive loads, a distraction system is needed. In using the distraction system, several basic biomechanical principles must be kept in mind. For successful use of the Harrington distraction system, the anterior longitudinal ligament must be intact. The system also requires a three-point fixation principle for reduction of the fracture, and therefore proper contouring of the Harrington rods to accommodate the normal lumbar lordosis may be needed.

We have found that early stabilization (within 10 days of the injury) allows anatomic restoration of alignment in most patients. Less than anatomic alignment is obtained in patients whose surgery is delayed beyond this time for various reasons. We agree with Guttmann and Bedbrook that the neural tissue damage occurs at the time of injury and that this procedure does not reverse the damage. It is, however, a proven alternative to the laminectomy, performed for so many years, which does not relieve the compressive abnormality, adds to instability, and is to be condemned in these fractures and fracture-dislocations.

In certain burst fractures that have remained untreated for longer than 3 to 4 weeks, it becomes impossible to obtain a satisfactory reduction by posterior Harrington distraction rods alone. In these instances excision of the vertebral body anteriorly is necessary, removing the retropulsed bony plug. The gap can then be spanned by an iliac crest or fibular strut graft (Fig. 69-29). At a second stage a Harrington compression system is applied posteriorly.

Late deformities of kyphosis and spinal canal stenosis caused by fractures and fracture-dislocations are best treated with a first-stage anterior dorsal or dorsolumbar decompression and fusion, followed in 2 weeks by a second-stage posterior Harrington compression instrumentation and fusion.

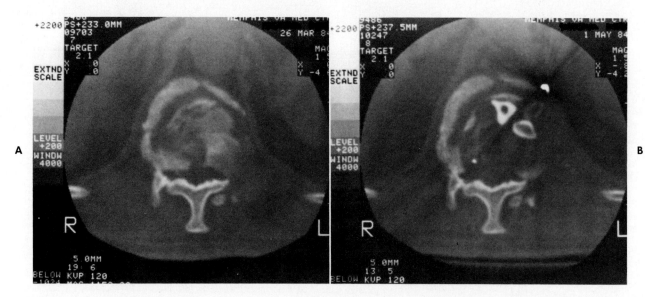

Fig. 69-29. A, Preoperative computed tomographic scan indicating severe spinal stenosis in patient with fracture of L1. **B,** Postoperative scan of same patient after anterior vertebral body excision and fibular strut graft. Note excellent decompression of spinal canal obtained by vertebral body corpectomy.

TECHNIQUE OF OPEN REDUCTION OF PURE DISLOCATION. Through a longitudinal incision, 12.5 cm long, centered over the area of the dislocation, expose the spinous processes. Separate the muscles subperiosteally from the spinous processes and laminae and remove the extravasated blood. If necessary, excise the proximal spinous process at its base for better access to the superior articular facets. In a patient with complete separation of the articular facets and a rotational and lateral deformity, Rogers reduces the dislocation by the following method. After the articular facets are freed, the spine is carefully flexed by lowering the ends of the operating table. The vertebra is then rotated into alignment with a periosteal elevator, and the dislocation is reduced by hyperextension.

If the articular facets are overlapped, Munro and Irwin use the following procedure. One of the superior articular facets of the distal vertebra is removed; then an assistant attempts reduction by hyperextension of the spine. Should this fail, the facet on the opposite side is removed. (For such a patient, it would seem advisable to augment this procedure by wiring and limited fusion.) Exploration of the spinal canal is performed to be certain that no fragments of bone or extruded intervertebral disc material is pressing on the cord. The dislocation can be held reduced by simple spinous process wiring if the articular facets are intact. Another alternative is to apply the Harrington compression system to the involved level.

AFTERTREATMENT. The patient is placed in a regular hospital bed and is allowed to turn from side-to-side but not to sit up. Depending on the level of cord damage, either a Jewett brace or an axillary high Risser cast is applied. Early ambulation and rehabilitation are encouraged. External support is maintained for a minimum of 20 weeks.

TECHNIQUE OF HARRINGTON DISTRACTION RODS. Place the patient prone on the spinal frame or operating table with chest rolls. Perform routine sterile skin preparation and draping. Make a longitudinal incision to the dermis, centered over the spinous processes at the level of injury. Inject this line with a solution of 1:500,000 epinephrine and saline to minimize bleeding. Deepen the incision and expose six spinous processes, two above and two below the level of injury. By sharp dissection, remove the muscles from the spinous processes and laminae, maintaining meticulous hemostasis and a dry field. Preserve the facet joint capsules while proceeding laterally and maintain exposure with self-retaining Weitlaner retractors. Identify the blood clot that reveals the area of ruptured interspinal and flaval ligaments. Remove the hematoma so that the neural elements are visible, and record the extent of injury. Reduce pure dislocations by the method of Rogers and stabilize the vertebrae with a no 18 wire fixation about the spinous processes. The Harrington compression system may be used as an alternative. In the case of a fracture-dislocation, introduce a Harrington distraction system. Place two No. 1252 hooks in the facet joints in the second vertebra above and two No. 1254 hooks beneath the laminae in the second vertebra below the lesion. If one side of the lamina or one side of the vertebral body seems to be most involved, the first distraction rod is placed on the opposite side. If one is concerned about the presence of an anterior bony fragment, a small laminotomy can be made. Then, while the fracture is reduced, inspect the spinal canal. Insert the opposite rod, taking care that no further damage is done to the contents of the spinal canal. Now distract the rods until quite snug. Take a cross-table lateral roentgenogram to assess the alignment and reduction. Procure an autogenous iliac bone graft while the roentgenogram is being developed. Perform a posterior and posterolateral fusion, spanning from hook-to-hook of the instrumentation, or limit it to the area of ligamentous injury. In the latter case the rods must be removed after 1 year or at the time of solid fusion.

In the special instance of a burst fracture with a retropulsed bony plug, one cannot rely completely on reduction of the main fracture with the distracton rods to reduce the plug. In many cases this will occur, but one must be certain of this at the time of surgery. After the first distraction rod is applied, the bony plug can be palpated through a small laminotomy with a neurosurgical ball hook. If it is found to still be retropulsed into the canal, then a posterolateral decompression should be performed (see below). If the fracture is in the lumbar spine in the area of lordosis, the Harrington rods must be contoured into lordosis to obtain maximum reduction, and the use of square-ended rods is necessary to prevent their rotation and a subsequent scoliosis deformity.

AFTERTREATMENT. The patient is kept flat in bed and is turned with a logroll technique. At 5 to 7 days a Risser cast is applied up to the axillae if skin sensation is normal beneath the cast, and ambulation is begun. If sensation is abnormal, a Jewett brace or bivalved polypropylene body jacket is used. External support is maintained for a minimum of 20 weeks. Early ambulation and rehabilitation are encouraged.

TECHNIQUE (ERICKSON, LEIDER, AND BROWN). When the retropulsed bony fragment is not reduced with the main fracture reduction, a posterolateral decompression is needed. Insert the Harrington distraction rod on the side with the least bony damage. If the bony fragment is not reduced, remove the lateral lamina, facet, and pedicle at the level that will allow lateral exposure of the area of spinal deformity. This is done with a ronguer and air drill (Fig. 69-30). Identify the exiting nerve root, and expose the lateral dural sac in the area of the fracture, similar to a costotransversectomy approach. Remove any obviously loose bony or disc fragments from within the canal. Most often, however, the anterior deformity is caused by a retropulsed comminuted burst fracture of the vertebral body. In this instance enter directly into the vertebral body, lateral to the dural sac, and undermine the body beneath the sac, leaving only a thin cortical shell (Fig. 69-31). Then fracture the cortical shell anteriorly away from the dural sac, accomplishing the decompression without retraction of the dura. Determine the adequacy of decompression by passing a curved dissector or ball hook beneath the dural sac to the opposite side of the spinal canal. Achieve hemostasis with Gelfoam pledgets or bone wax. Insert the second Harrington rod as in the distraction technique just described.

AFTERTREATMENT. The care after surgery is the same as that described for Harrington distraction rod fixation (see above).

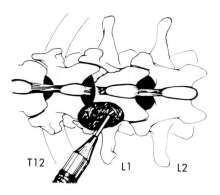

Fig. 69-30. Initiation of lateral decompression. (From Erickson, D.L., Leider, L.C., Jr., and Brown, W.E.: Spine **2:**53, 1977.)

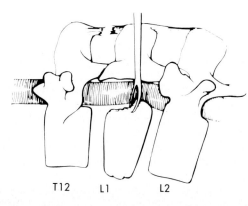

Fig. 69-31. Removal of retropulsed portion of vertebral body. (From Erickson, D.L., Leider, L.C., and Brown, W.E.: Spine **2:**53, 1977.)

Anterior vertebral body excision for burst fractures

Anterior vertebral body excision and grafting, as already mentioned, may be necessary in certain burst fractures untreated for 3 or 4 weeks or longer. In these instances a satisfactory reduction is impossible by use of the Harrington distraction rods alone; the vertebral body along with the retropulsed bony fragments is excised, and the gap is spanned by an iliac crest or fibular strut graft. Then posterior Harrington rod fixation and usually a posterior fusion are carried out later.

TECHNIQUE OF ANTERIOR VERTEBRAL BODY EXCISION. Approach the spine anteriorly through a retroperitoneal or retropleural approach (Chapter 68). Identify the fractured vertebra and excise the intervertebral discs above and below. Next remove the bulk of the fractured vertebral body using a rongeur and osteotome or if necessary a small power burr. It is best to remove most of the vertebral body before removing the posterior cortex, which exposes the dura. If decompression of the posterior cortex is begun on the side of the body opposite the surgeon, troublesome bulging of the dura into the space created by removing the vertebral body will be minimized and the surgeon's view will be blocked less. Control bleeding from the bone with

bone wax and epidural bleeding with Gelfoam. After the decompression has been completed, cut slots into the end plates of the vertebral bodies above and below the defect: undercut the ends of the slots about 1 cm to allow the graft to be keyed in place. Place Gelfoam over the dura for protection and keep all bone grafts anterior and away from the dura itself. Next obtain a bicortical iliac graft or a fibular graft, whichever is preferable. Undercut the ends of the graft and key it into place to prevent it from dislodging. Do not place any bone deep to the graft in the area of decompression. Finally obtain hemostasis and close the wound in a routine manner over suction drains.

AFTERTREATMENT. The patient is kept at bed rest until it is certain that wound infection or other complications are absent. At 7 to 10 days a Risser cast is applied, and if a posterior stabilization has been performed the cast is worn for 6 months. If posterior stability is questionable and the posterior elements have not been stabilized, the cast is worn for 12 months.

RESIDUALS OF SPINAL CORD INJURY

The paralyzed individual undergoes mixed psychologic as well as physical trauma. The reality of being paralyzed is difficult to accept, but overcoming the trauma of knowing there will be no recovery is the greatest difficulty. The usual sequence of emotions includes depression, aggression, passivity, denial, and dependence. Well-planned rehabilitation is a vital part of these patients' total care, with the aim of improving self-worth and starting a new vocation.

Pain may further complicate the already devastated patient and deserves aggressive treatment. It may originate from the site of trauma, from damaged nerve roots, or from below the level of injury, alone or in combination as outlined by Davis. At the site of trauma, tissues heal and pain usually diminishes over weeks to months. Instability of the vertebral column responds to surgical fusion. Intractable pain may respond to transcutaneous nerve stimulation or rhizotomy. Pain emanating from damaged nerve roots is sharp, shooting, aching, burning, tingling, or cramping; it radiates into dermatomal areas. A transitional zone exists between sensation and anesthesia. Extradural pressure should be investigated by myelography. Considerable pain will be relieved by appropriate decompressive procedures combined with fusion as indicated.

Extensive and severe intractable pain in the cauda equina area is the most difficult management problem and demands a thorough physical, psychologic, and social evaluation. The pain may indicate a pathologic process of the genitourinary, gastrointestinal, or musculoskeletal system. The possibility of the patient's somatization of anxieties must be investigated. After management of proven pathologic or psychologic problems, treatment may consist of transcutaneous nerve stimulation, carbamazepine, or phenytoin. These nonoperative methods of pain control have enjoyed greater success than operative rhizotomy or cordotomy. Spinal cord dysesthesias below the level of injury occur in 82% to 94% of these patients and include numbness, tingling, burning, or aching. When intense, these sensations have been referred to as phantom or central pain; a sympathetic pathway is implicated. Treatment is the same as for radicular pain; surgical treatment is strongly contraindicated.

Pathologic processes must be differentiated from emotional problems so that proper treatment programs can be selected. Davis emphasizes that excessive spasticity should be recognized as a substitute symptom for pain and can indicate infections, renal calculi, pressure sores, or other pain-producing conditions; it should not be regarded as a normal state.

In a detailed review of 64 juvenile patients with spinal cord injury. Campbell and Bonnett noted spinal deformity in 91%. The more cephalad the injury, the greater the chance of deformity. Increasing spinal deformity results in pelvic obliquity and loss of sitting balance. In young children, orthotic management is preferred as long as the spine remains supple. Once fixation of the spinal deformity begins, surgical stabilization to the pelvis is indicated (see the discussion of neuromuscular scoliosis).

REFERENCES

Allen, B.L., Jr., Ferguson, R.L., Lehmann, R., and O'Brian, R.P.: Mechanistic classification of closed indirect fractures and dislocations of the lower cervical spine, Spine 7:1, 1982.

Allen, W.E., III, D'Angelo, C.M, and Kies, E.L.: Correlation of microangiographic and electrophysiologic changes in experimental spinal cord trauma, Radiology 111:107, 1974.

Anden, U., Lake, A., and Norwall, A.: The role of the anterior longitudinal ligament and Harrington rod fixation of unstable thoracolumbar spinal fractures, Spine 5:23, 1980.

Anderson, L.D., and D'Alonzo, R.T.: Fractures of the odontoid process of the axis, J. Bone Joint Surg. 56-A:1663, 1974.

Aronson, N., Feltzer, D.L., and Bagan, M.: Anterior cervical fusion by Smith-Robinson approach, J. Neurosurg. 29:397, 1968.

Aufdermaur, M.: Spinal injuries in juveniles: necropsy findings in twelve cases, J. Bone Joint Surg. 56-B:513, 1974.

Bailey, R.W., and Badgley, C.E.: Stabilization of the cervical spine by anterior fusion, J. Bone Joint Surg. 42-A:565, 1960.

Beatson, T.R.: Fractures and dislocations of the cervical spine, J. Bone Joint surg. 45-B:21, 1963.

Bedbrook, G.M.: Treatment of thoracolumbar dislocation and fractures with paraplegia, Clin. Orthop. 112:27, 1975.

Bick, E.M.: Source book of orthopaedics, Baltimore, 1948, The Williams & Wilkins Co.

Blount, W.P.: Fractures in children, Baltimore, 1954, The Williams & Wilkins Co.

Bohlman, H.H.: Pathology and current treatment concepts of acute spine injuries. In American Academy of Orthopaedic Surgeons: Instructional course lectures, vol. 21, St. Louis, 1972, The C.V. Mosby Co.

Bohlman, H.H.: Complications of treatment of fractures and dislocations of the cervical spine. In Epps, C.H., editor: Complications in orthopaedic surgery, Philadelphia, 1978, J.B. Lippincott Co.

Bohlman, H.H.: Acute fractures and dislocations of the cervical spine, J. Bone Joint Surg. 61-A:1119, 1979.

Bors, E.: Phantom limbs of patients with spinal cord injury, Arch. Neurol. Psychiat. 66:610, 1951.

Bosch, A., Stauffer, E.S., and Nickel, V.L.: Incomplete traumatic quadriplegia: a ten-year review, JAMA 216:473, 1971.

Braakman, R., and Vinken, P.J.: Old luxations of the lower cervical spine, J. Bone Joint Surg. 50-B:52, 1968.

Bradford, D.S., Akbarnia, B.A., Winter, R.D., and Seljeskog, E.C.: Surgical stabilization of fractures and fracture-dislocations of the thoracic spine, Spine 2:185, 1977.

Brashear, H.R., Jr., Venters, G.C., and Preston, E.T.: Fractures of the neural arch of the axis: a report of 29 cases, J. Bone Joint Surg. 59-A:879, 1975.

Brav, E.A., Miller, J.A., and Bouzard, W.C.: Traumatic dislocation of the cervical spine: Army experience and results, J. Trauma 3:569, 1963.

Brooks, A.L., and Jenkins, E.B.: Atlanto-axial arthordesis by the wedge compression method, J. Bone Joint Surg. 60-A:279, 1978.

Bryant, C.E., and Sullivan, J.A.: Management of thoracic and lumbar spine fractures with Harrington distraction rods supplemented with segmental wiring, Spine 8:532, 1983.

Burke, D.C.: Hyperextension injuries of the spine, J. Bone Joint Surg. 53-B:3, 1971.

Burke, D.C., and Murray, D.D.: The management of thoracic and thoracolumbar injuries of the spine with neurological involvement, J. Bone Joint Surg. 58-B:72, 1976.

Callahan, R.A., et al.: Cervical facet fusion for control of instability following laminectomy, J. Bone Joint Surg. 59-A:991, 1977.

Campbell, J., and Bonnett, C.: Spinal cord injury in children, Clin. Orthop. 112:114, 1975.

Cattell, H.S., and Filtzer, D.L.: Pseudosubluxation and other normal variations of the cervical spine in children: a study of 160 children, J. Bone Joint Surg. 47-A:1295, 1965.

Clark, W.K.: Spinal cord decompression in spinal cord injury, Clin. Orthop. 154:9, 1981.

Cloward, R.B.: New method of diagnosis and treatment of cervical disc disease, Clin. Neurosurg. 8:93, 1962.

Cone, W., and Turner, W.G.: The treatment of fracture-dislocation of the cervical vertebrae by skeletal traction and fusion, J. Bone Joint Surg. 19:584, 1937.

Convery, F.R., Minteer, M.A., Smith, R.W., and Emerson, S.M.: Fracture-dislocation of the dorsal-lumbar spine, Spine 3:160, 1978.

Conwell, H.E., and Reynolds, F.C.: Key and Conwell's management of fractures, dislocations, and sprains, ed. 7, St. Louis, 1961, The C.V. Mosby Co.

Cornish, B.L.: Traumatic spondylolisthesis of the axis, J. Bone Joint Surg. 50-B:31, 1968.

Crutchfield, W.G.: Skeletal traction for dislocation of the cervical spine, South. Surgeon 2:156, 1933.

Crutchfield, W.G.: Fracture-dislocations of the cervical spine, Am. J. Surg. 38:592, 1937.

Crutchfield, W.G.: Treatment of injuries of the cervical spine, J. Bone Joint Surg. 20:696, 1938.

Crutchfield, W.G.: Skeletal traction in the treatment of injuries to the cervical spine, JAMA 155:29, 1954.

Davies, W.E., Morris, J.H., and Hill, V.: An analysis of conservative (nonsurgical) management of thoracolumbar fractures and fracture dislocations with neural damage, J. Bone Joint Surg. 62-A:1324, 1980.

Davis, L.: Treatment of spinal cord injuries, Arch. Surg. 69:488, 1954.

Davis, L., and Martin, J.: Studies upon spinal cord injuries: Part II. The nature and treatment of pain, J. Neurosurg. 4:483, 1947.

Davis, R.: Pain and suffering following spinal cord injury, Clin. Orthop. 112:76, 1975.

Davis, R.: Spasticity following spinal cord injury, Clin. Orthop. 112:66, 1975.

De La Torre, J.C.: Spinal cord injury: review of basic and applied research, Spine 6:315, 1981.

Dickson, J.H., Harrington, P.R., and Erwin, W.D.: Harrington instrumentation in the fractured, unstable thoracic and lumbar spine, Texas Med 69:91, 1973.

Dickson, J.H., Harrington, P.R., and Erwin, W.D.: Results of reduction and stabilization of the severely fractured thoracic and lumbar spine, J. Bone Joint Surg. 60-A:799, 1978.

Dorr, L.D., Harvey, J.P., and Nickel, V.L.: Clinical review of the early stability of spine injuries, Spine 7:545, 1982.

Dunbar, H.S., and Ray, B.S.: Chronic atlanto-axial dislocations with late neurologic manifestations, Surg. Gynecol. Obstet. 113:757, 1961.

Durbin, F.C.: Fracture-dislocations of the cervical spine, J. Bone Joint Surg. 39-B:23, 1957.

Eastwood W.J., and Jefferson, G.: Discussion on fractures and dislocation of the cervical vertebrae, Proc. R. Soc. Med. 33:651, 1939.

Erickson, D.L., Leider, L.C., Jr., and Brown, W.E.: One-stage decompression-stabilization for thoraco-lumbar fractures, Spine 2:53, 1977.

Evans, D.K.: Reduction of cervical dislocations, J. Bone Joint Surg. 43-B:552, 1961.

Evans, D.K.: Anterior cervical subluxation, J. Bone Joint Surg. 58-B:318, 1976.

Fielding, J.W.: Selected observations on the cervical spine in the child. In Ahstrom, J.P., Jr., editor: Current practice in orthopaedic surgery, vol. 5, St. Louis, 1973, The C.V. Mosby Co.

Fielding, J.W., Cochran, G.V.B., Lawsing, J.F., III, and Hohl, M.: Tears of the transverse ligament of the atlas: a clinical and biomechanical study, J. Bone Joint Surg. 56-A:1683, 1974.

Fielding, J.W., and Griffin, P.P.: Os odontoideum: an acquired lesion, J. Bone Joint Surg. 56-A:187, 1974.

Fielding, J.W., and Hawkins, R.J.: Atlanto-axial rotatory fixation: fixed rotatory subluxation of the atlanto-axial joint, J. Bone Joint Surg. 59-A:37, 1977.

Fielding, J.W., Hawkins, R.J., and Ratzan, S.A.: Spine fusion for atlanto-axial instability, J. Bone Joint Surg. 58-A:400, 1976.

Finerman, G.A.M., Sakai, D., and Weingarten, S.: Atlanto-axial dislocation with spinal cord compression in a mongoloid child: a case report, J. Bone Joint Surg. 58-A:408, 1976.

Flesch, J.R., Leider, L.L., Erickson, D., Chou, S.N., and Bradford, D.S.: Harrington instrumentation and spine fusion for unstable fractures and fracture dislocations of the thoracic and lumbar spine, J. Bone Joint Surg. 59-A:143, 1977.

Forsyth, H.F., Alexander, E., Jr., Davis, D., Jr., and Underdal, R.: The advantages of early spine fusion in the treatment of fracture-dislocation of the cervical spine, J. Bone Joint Surg. 41-A:17, 1959.

Fountain, S.S., Hamilton, R.D., and Jameson, R.M.: Transverse fractures of the sacrum; a report of six cases, J. Bone Joint Surg. 59-A:486, 1977.

Frankel, H.L., et al.: The value of postural reduction in the initial management of closed injuries of the spine with paraplegia and tetraplegia: Part I. Paraplegia 7:179, 1969.

Freeman, L.W., and Heimburger, R.F.: Surgical relief of pain in paraplegic patients, Arch. Surg. 55:433, 1947.

Freiberger, R.H., Wilson, P.D., Jr., and Nicholas, J.A.: Acquired absence of the odontoid process: a case report, J. Bone Joint Surg. 47-A:1231, 1965.

Fried, L.C.: Atlanto-axial fracture-dislocations: failure of posterior C.1 to C.2 fusion, J. Bone Joint Surg. 55-B:490, 1973.

Gallie, W.E.: Fractures and dislocations of the cervical spine, Am. J. Surg. 46:495, 1939.

Green, B.A., Callahan, R.A., Klore, K.J., and De La Torre, J.: Acute spinal cord injury: current concepts, Clin. Orthop. 154:125, 1981.

Griswold, D.M., Albright, J.A., Schiffman, E., Johnson, R., and Southwick, W.O.: Atlanto-axial fusion for instability, J. Bone Joint Surg. 60-A:285, 1978.

Guttmann, L.: The treatment and rehabilitation of patients with injuries of the spinal cord. In Cope, Z., editor: Medical history of the second world war: surgery, London, 1953, His Majesty's Stationery Office.

Guttmann, L.: A new turning-tilting bed, Paraplegia 3:193, 1965.

Guttmann, L.: Spinal deformities in traumatic paraplegics and tetraplegics following surgical procedures, Paraplegia 7:38, 1969.

Haralson, R.H., and Boyd, H.B.: Posterior dislocation of the atlas on the axis without fracture: report of a case, J. Bone Joint Surg. 51-A:561, 1969.

Hawkins, R.J., Fielding, J.W., and Thompson, W.J.: Os odontoideum: congenital or acquired: a case report, J. Bone Joint Surg. 58-A:413, 1976.

Herzeberger, E.E., et al.: Anterior interbody fusion in the treatment of certain disorders of the cervical spine, Clin. Orthop. 24:83, 1962.

Heyl, H.L.: Some practical aspects in the rehabilitation of paraplegics, J. Neurosurg. 13:184, 1956.

Holdsworth, F.W.: Traumatic paraplegia. In Platt, H., editor: Modern trends in orthopaedics (second series), New York, 1956, Paul B. Hoeber, Inc.

Holdsworth, F.W.: Fractures, dislocations, and fracture-dislocations of the spine, J. Bone Joint Surg. 45-B:6, 1963.

Holdsworth, F.W.: Fractures, dislocations, and fracture-dislocations of the spine, J. Bone Joint Surg. 52-A:1534, 1970.

Holmes, G.: Pain of central origin. In Contributions to medical and biological research, vol. 1, New York, 1919, Paul B. Hoeber Medical Books.

Holmes, J.C., and Hall, J.E.: Fusion for instability and potential instability of the cervical spine in children and adolescents, Orthop. Clin. North Am. 9:923, 1978.

Horal, J., Nachemson, A., and Scheller, S.: Clinical and radiological long term follow-up of vertebral fractures in children, Acta Orthop. Scand. 43:491, 1972.

Horwitz, M.T.: Structural deformities of the spine following bilateral laminectomy, Am. J. Roentgen. 46:836, 1941.

Hubbard, D.D.: Injuries of the spine in children and adolescents, Clin. Orthop. 100:56, 1974.

Jacobs, B.: Cervical fractures and dislocations (C3-7), Clin. Orthop. 109:18, 1975.

Jacobs, R.R., Asher, M.A., and Snider, R.K.: Thoracolumbar spinal injuries: a comparative study of recumbent and operative treatment in 100 patients, Spine 5:463, 1980.

Jacobs, R.R., Nordwall, A., and Nachemson, A.: Reduction, stability and strength provided by internal fixation systems for thoracolumbar spinal injuries, Clin. Orthop. 171:300, 1982.

Jefferson, G.: Fracture of the atlas vertebra: report of four cases and a review of those previously recorded, Br. J. Surg. 7:407, 1920.

Johnson, R.M., Hart, D.L., Simmons, E.F., Ramsby, G.R., and Southwick, W.O.: Cervical orthoses: a study comparing their effectiveness in restricting cervical motion in normal subjects, J. Bone Joint Surg. 59-A:332, 1977.

Johnson, J.R., Leatherman, K.D., and Holt, R.T.: Anterior decompression of the spinal cord for neurological deficit, Spine 8:396, 1983.

Johnson, R.M., Owen, J.R., Hart, D.L., and Callahan, R.A.: Cervical orthoses: a guide to their selection and use, Clin. Orthop. 154:34, 1981.

Kahn, E.A.: On spinal-cord injuries (editorial), J. Bone Joint Surg. 41-A:6, 1959.

Kahn, E.A., and Yglesias, L.: Progressive atlantoaxial dislocation, JAMA 105:348, 1935.

Kaufer, H., and Hayes, J.T.: Lumbar fracture-dislocation: a study of twenty-one cases, J. Bone Joint Surg. 48-A:712, 1966.

Kelly, R.P., and Whitesides, T.E., Jr.: Treatment of lumbodorsal fracture-dislocations, Ann. Surg. 167:705, 1968.

Kostuik, J.P.: Indications of the use of halo immobilization, Clin. Orthop. 154:46, 1981.

Kostuik, J.P.: Anterior spinal cord decompression for lesions of the thoracic and lumbar spine: techniques, new methods of internal fixation, results, Spine 8:512, 1983.

Kraus, D.R., and Stauffer, E.S.: Spinal cord injury as a complication of elective anterior cervical fusion, Clin. Orthop. 112:130, 1975.

Laborde, J.M., Bahniuk, E., Bohlman, H.H., and Samson, B.: Comparison of fixation of spinal fractures, Clin. Orthop. 152:305, 1980.

Lewis, J., and McKibbin, B.: The treatment of unstable fracture-dislocations of the thoraco-lumbar spine accompanied by paraplegia, J. Bone Joint Surg. 56-B:603, 1974.

Lindahl, S., Willen, J., Nordwall, A., and Irstam, I.: The crush-cleavage fracture: a "new" thoracolumbar unstable fracture, Spine 8:559, 1983.

Lipscomb, P.R.: Cervico-occipital fusion for congenital and post-traumatic anomalies of the atlas and axis, J. Bone Joint Surg. 39-A:1289, 1957.

Lipson, S.J.: Fractures of the atlas associated with fracture of the odontoid process and transverse ligament ruptures, J. Bone Joint Surg. 59-A:940, 1977.

Luque, E.R., Cassis, N., and Ramirez-Weilla, G.: Segmental spinal instrumentation in the treatment of fractures of the thoracolumbar spine, Spine 7:312, 1982.

Macnab, I.: Acceleration injuries of the cervical spine, J. Bone Joint Surg. 36-A:1797, 1964.

Malcolm, B.W., Bradford, D.S., Winter, R.B., and Chou, S.N.: Post-traumatic kyphosis: a review of 48 surgically treated patients, J. Bone Joint Surg. 63-A:891, 1981.

Marar, B.C.: Hyperextension injuries of the cervical spine: the pathogenesis of damage to the spinal cord, J. Bone Joint Surg. 56-A:1655, 1974.

Marar, B.C.: Fracture of the axis arch: "hangman's fracture" of the cervical spine, Clin. Orthop. 106:155, 1975.

Marar, B.C., and Balachandran, N.: Non-traumatic atlanto-axial dislocation in children, Clin. Orthop. 92:220, 1973.

McAfee, P.C., Yuan, H.A., and Lasada, N.A.: The unstable burst fracture, Spine 7:365, 1982.

McGraw, R.W., and Rusch, R.M.: Atlanto-axial arthrodesis, J. Bone Joint Surg. 55-B:482, 1973.

McPhee, I.B.: Spinal fractures and dislocations in children and adolescents, Spine 6:533, 1981.

Meijers, K.A.E., van Beusekom, G.T., Luyendijk, W., and Duijfjes, F.: Dislocation of the cervical spine with cord compression in rheumatoid arthritis, J. Bone Joint Surg. 56-B:668, 1974.

Meyer, P.R.: Complications of treatment of fractures and dislocations of the dorsolumbar spine. In Epps, C.H., editor: Complications in orthopaedic surgery, Philadelphia, 1978, J.B. Lippincott Co.

Morgan, F.H., Wharton, W., and Austin, G.N.: The results of laminectomy in patients with incomplete spinal cord injuries, Paraplegia **9**:14, 1971.

Munro, A.H.G., and Irwin, C.G.: Interlocked articular processes complicating fracture-dislocation of the spine, Br. J. Surg. **25**:621, 1938.

Munro, D.: Treatment of fractures and dislocations of the cervical spine, complicated by cervical-cord and root injuries: a comparative study of fusion vs. nonfusion therapy, N. Engl. J. Med. **264**:573, 1961.

Nagel, D.A., Koogle, T.A., Piziali, R.L., and Perkash, I.: Stability of the upper lumbar spine following progressive disruptions in the application of individual internal and external fixation devices, J. Bone Joint Surg. **63-A**:62, 1981.

Nickel, V.L., Perry, J., Garrett, A., and Heppenstall, M.: The halo: a spinal skeletal traction fixation device, J. Bone Joint Surg. **50-A**:1400, 1968.

Norton, W.L.: Fractures and dislocations of the cervical spine, J. Bone Joint Surg. **44-A**:115, 1962.

O'Brien, P.J., Schweigel, J.F., and Thompson, W.J.: Dislocation of the lower cervical spine, J. Trauma **22**:710, 1982.

Osebold, W.R., Weinstein, S.L., and Sprague, B.L.: Thoracolumbar spine fractures: results of treatment, Spine **6**:13, 1981.

Perret, G., and Greene, J.: Anterior interbody fusion in the treatment of cervical fracture dislocation, Arch. Surg. **96**:530, 1968.

Perry, J., and Nickels, V.L.: Total cervical-spine fusion for neck paralysis, J. Bone Joint Surg. **41-A**:37, 1959.

Pierce, D.S.: Surgery of the cervical spine. In American Academy of Orthopaedic Surgeons: Instructional course lectures, vol. 21, St. Louis, 1972, The C.V. mosby Co.

Pinzar, M.S., et al.: Measurement of internal fixation device, a report in experimentally produced fractures of the dorsolumbar spine, Orthopaedics **2**:28, 1979.

Pollock, L.J., et al: Pain below the level of injury of the spinal cord, Arch. Neurol. Psychiat. **65**:319, 1951.

Post, M.J.D., et al.: Value of computed tomography in spinal trauma, Spine **7**:417, 1982.

Purcell, G.A., Markolf, K.L., and Dawson, E.G.: Twelfth thoracic-first lumbar vertebral mechanical stability of fractures after Harrington rod instrumentation, J. Bone Joint Surg. **63-A**:71, 1981.

Ramsey, R., and Doppman, J.L.: The effect of epidural masses on spinal cord blood flow: an experimental study in monkeys, Radiology **107**:99, 1973.

Ransohoff, J.: Discussion of relief of myelopathic pain by percutaneous cervical cordotomy. In Proceedings of the Spinal Cord Injury Conference, vol. 17, New York, 1969, Bronx Veterans Administration Hospital.

Reich, R.S.: Posterior dislocation of the first cervical vertebra with fracture of the odontoid process, Surgery **3**:416, 1938.

Ricciardi, J.E., Kaufer, H., and Louis, D.S.: Acquired os odontoideum following acute ligament injury: report of a case, J. Bone Joint Surg. **58-A**:410, 1976.

Riggins, R.S., and Kraus, J.F.: The risk of neurologic damage with fractures of the vertebrae, J. Trauma **17**:126, 1977.

Roberts, A., and Wickstrom, J.: Prognosis of odontoid fractures, Acta Orthop. Scand. **44**:21, 1973.

Roberts, J.B., and Curtiss, P.H., Jr.: Stability of the thoracic and lumbar spine in traumatic paraplegia following fracture or fracture-dislocation, J. Bone Joint Surg. **52-A**:1115, 1970.

Robinson, R.A.: Fusions of the cervical spine (editorial), J. Bone Joint Surg. **41-A**:1, 1959.

Robinson, R.A.: Anterior and posterior cervical spine fusions, Clin. Orthop. **35**:34, 1964.

Robinson, R.A., and Southwick, W.O.: Surgical approaches to the cervical spine. In American Academy of Orthopaedic Surgeons: Instructional course lectures, vol. 17, St. Louis, 1960, The C.V. Mosby Co.

Robinson, R.A., and Southwick, W.O.: Indications and technics for early stabilization of the neck in some fracture dislocations of the cervical spine, South. Med. J. **53**:565, 1960.

Robinson, R.A., Walker, A.E., Ferlic, D.C., and Wiecking, D.K.: The results of anterior interbody fusion of the cervical spine, J. Bone Joint Surg. **44-A**:1569, 1962.

Rogers, W.A.: Cord injury during reduction of thoracic and lumbar vertebral-body fracture and dislocation, J. Bone Joint Surg. **20**:689, 1938.

Rogers, W.A.: Treatment of fracture-dislocation of the cervical spine, J. Bone Joint Surg. **24**:245, 1942.

Rogers, W.A.: Fractures and dislocations of the cervical spine: an end-result study, J. Bone Joint Surg. **39-A**:341, 1957.

Rosomoff, H.L.: Discussion of relief of myelopathic pain by percutaneous cervical cordotomy. In Proceedings of the Spinal Cord Injury Conference, vol. 17, New York, 1969, Bronx Veterans Administration Hospital.

Rosomoff, H.L.: Percutaneous radiofrequency cervical cordotomy for intractable pain. In Bonica, J.J., editor: International symposium on pain. In Advances in neurology, vol. 4, New York, 1974, Raven Press.

Roth, D.A.: Cervical analgesic discography: a new test for the definitive diagnosis of the painful-disk syndrome, JAMA **235**:1713, 1976.

Schatzker, J., Rorabeck, C.H., and Waddell, J.P.: Fractures of the dens [odontoid process]: an analysis of thirty-seven cases, J. Bone Joint Surg. **53-B**:392, 1971.

Schlesinger, E.B., and Taveras, J.M.: Lesions of the odontoid and their management, Am. J. Surg. **95**:641, 1958.

Schlicke, L.H., and Callahan, R.A.: A rational approach to burst fractures of the atlas, Clin. Orthop. **154**:18, 1981.

Schneider, R.C., and Kahn, E.A.: Chronic neurological sequelae of acute trauma to the spine and spinal cord: Part I. The significance of the acute-flexion or ''tear-drop'' fracture-dislocation of the cervical spine, J. Bone Joint Surg. **38-A**:985, 1956.

Schneider, R.C., and Kahn, E.A.: Chronic neurological sequelae of acute trauma to the spine and spinal cord: Part II. The syndrome of chronic anterior spinal cord injury or compression: herniated intervertebral discs, J. Bone Joint surg. **41-A**:449, 1959.

Seimon, L.P.: Fracture of the odontoid process in young children, J. Bone Joint Surg. **59-A**:943, 1977.

Sherk, H.H., Schut, L., and Lane, J.M.: Fractures and dislocations of the cervical spine in children, Orthop. Clin. North Am. **7**:593, 1976.

Smith, W.S., and Kaufer, H.: Patterns and mechanisms of lumbar injuries associated with lap seat belts, J. Bone Joint Surg. **51-A**:239, 1969.

Soref, J., Axdorph, G., Bylund, P., Odien, I., and Olerud, S.: Treatment of patients with unstable fractures of the thoracic and lumbar spine: a follow-up of surgical and conservative treatment, Acta Orthop. Scand. **53**:369, 1982.

Southwick, W.O.: Management of fractures of the dens (odontoid process), J. Bone Joint surg. **62-A**:482, 1980.

Speed, K.: A textbook of fractures and dislocations, Philadelphia, 1928, Lea & Febiger.

Spence, K.F., Jr., Decker, S., and Sell, K.W.: Bursting atlantal fracture associated with rupture of the transverse ligament, J. Bone and Joint Surg. **52-A**:543, 1970.

Stanger, J.K.: Fracture-dislocation of the thoracolumbar spine, J. Bone Joint Surg. **29**:107, 1947.

Stauffer, E.S.: Spinal injuries in the multiply injured patient: Part II. Postacute care and rehabilitation, Orthop. Clin. North Am. **1**:137, 1970.

Stauffer, E.S.: Diagnosis and prognosis of acute cervical spinal cord injury, Clin. Orthop. **112**:9, 1975.

Stauffer, E.S., and Kelly, E.G.: Fracture-dislocations of the cervical spine: instability and recurrent deformity following treatment by anterior interbody fusion, J. Bone Joint Surg. **59-A**:45, 1977.

Stauffer, E.S., and Neil, J.L.: Biomechanical analysis of structural stability of internal fixation in fractures of the thoracolumbar spine, Clin. Orthop. **112**:159, 1975.

Torg, J.S., et al.: Spinal injury at the level of the third and fourth cervical vertebrae from football, J. Bone Joint Surg. **59-A**:1015, 1977.

Watson, D., and Maguire, W.B.: Cervical facets locked unilaterally, Med. J. Aust. **1**:444, 1964.

Watson-Jones, R.: Fractures and joint injuries, ed. 4, Baltimore, vol. 1, 1952, and vol. 2, 1955, The Williams & Wilkins Co.

Webb, J.K., Broughton, R.B.K., McSweeney, T., and Park, W.M.: Hidden flexion injury of the cervical spine, J. Bone Joint Surg. **58-B**:322, 1976.

Weir, D.C.: Roentgenographic signs of cervical injury, Clin. Orthop. **109**:9, 1975.

White, A.A., III, Johnson, R.M., Panjabi, M.M., and Southwick, W.O.: Biomechanical analysis of clinical stability in the cervical spine, Clin. Orthop. **109**:89, 1975.

White, A.A., III, Panjabi, M.M., Posner, I., Edwards, W.T., and Hayes, W.C.: Spine stability: evaluation and treatment. In American Academy of Orthopaedic Surgeons: Instructional course lectures, vol. 30, St. Louis, 1981, The C.V. Mosby Co.

White, A.A., Southwick, W.O., and Panjabi, M.M.: Clinical instability in the lower cervical spine: a review of past and current concepts, Spine **1:**15, 1976.

White, R.R., Newberg, A., and Seligson, D.: Computerized tomographic assessment of the traumatized dorsolumbar spine before and after Harrington instrumentation, Clin. Orthop. **146:**149, 1980.

Whitesides, T.E., Jr., and Shah, S.G.A.: On the management of unstable fractures of the thoracolumbar spine: rationale for use of anterior decompression and fusion and posterior stabilization, Spine **1:**99, 1976.

Willard, D., and Nicholson, J.T.: Dislocation of the first cervical vertebra, Ann. Surg. **113:**464, 1941.

Yosipovitch, Z., Robin, G.C., and Makin, M.: Open reduction of unstable thoracolumbar spinal injuries and fixation with Harrington rods, J. Bone Joint Surg. **59-A:**1003, 1977.

Young, R., and Thomasson, E.H.: Step-by-step procedure for applying halo ring, Orthop. Rev. **3**(6): 62, 1974.

CHAPTER 70

Arthrodesis of spine

Allen S. Edmonson

Although it is difficult to separate discussions of fractures and arthrodesis, we have attempted to do so. This section discusses various techniques of arthrodesis useful in both traumatic and nontraumatic disorders of the spine.

CERVICAL SPINE
Anterior arthrodesis of cervical spine

Anterior cervical discectomy and interbody fusion have gained wide acceptance by both neurosurgeons and orthopaedic surgeons in the management of refractory symptoms of cervical disc disease. The literature attests to a low incidence of major complications and postoperative morbidity and a high degree of success in relieving these symptoms. The fundamental difference in the many techniques is whether surgery is limited to simple discectomy and interbody fusion or whether an attempt is made to enter the spinal canal to remove osteophytes or otherwise decompress the spinal cord and nerve roots. The procedures of Robinson and Smith, Bailey and Badgley, and Dereymaker and Mulier are similar in that they limit surgery to simple discectomy and interbody fusion. The technique is thus reserved for discogenic and radicular pain syndromes that are not accompanied by significant objective signs of neurologic involvement. They also performed a posterior decompression operation or a drill and dowel technique if the patient had definite cervical nerve root or cord compression signs.

Extreme care must be exercised in anterior fusion of the cervical spine. Kraus and E.S. Stauffer reported 10 patients with spinal cord injury. An incomplete spinal cord injury was present in three patients, including two incomplete quadriplegias of the anterior cervical cord type and one incomplete quadriplegia of the Brown-Séquard type. Seven patients were reviewed from the literature and personal communications. The causes were identified in four of the last six patients as: (1) operation of a drill without the protection of the drill guard, which allowed the drill to enter the spinal canal, and (2) displacement of a dowel bone graft into the spinal canal, either during surgery or postoperatively, which damaged the cervical cord. One of the other two patients sustained a transient postoperative transverse myelitis attributed to the use of electrocoagulation on the posterior longitudinal ligament. The final patient mentioned in a medical liability report was not definite, but posterior displacement of the bone plug was implicated. All of these fusions had been performed by the drill and dowel method.

Aronson et al. have shown that anterior discectomy and interbody fusion have a much wider application producing excellent results in virtually all forms of cervical disc disease and spondylosis, regardless of the objective neurologic signs. Despite subtle differences in surgical technique, the intent of their surgery is still discectomy and interbody fusion with no attempt to remove osteophytes. The extent to which the posterior and posterolateral osteophytes with spondylosis contribute to the symptoms of cervical disc disease and the indications for removing them have not been determined. One is always impressed with the frequent discrepancy between the degree of bony spurring or other roentgenographic changes and the symptoms present. Also the level of neurologic involvement does not always coincide with the site of the greatest roentgenographic findings. Nugent aptly summarized these inconsistencies and attributed them to the fact that spondylosis is a complex disease with many factors involved, including vascular, connective tissue, and mechanical factors. The symptoms of the degenerative processes are related to the interplay of multiple aspects of the disease process and not solely to the amount of bony spurs present. Observation of patients who have had fusions shows that a significant percentage of the osteophytes will be spontaneously absorbed postoperatively in the presence of a stable interbody fusion. DePalma and Rothman concurred with this observation and noted that in the presence of a stable fusion the results were not influenced by the subsequent fate of these osteophytes. Aronson et al. have therefore demonstrated

3143

an important factor, namely, stabilization of the disc space as the sole procedure, thereby avoiding the hazard of entering the spinal canal routinely.

GENERAL COMPLICATIONS

Macnab has summarized the complications of anterior cervical fusion extremely well. For every anatomic structure present in the neck, there is a possibility of a surgical error; however, he points out that poor results also occur because of poor indications and surgical technique.

1. The *wrong patient* may be operated on, since the neck is a common target for psychogenic pain. Careful preoperative evaluation is essential to rule out a hysterical personality or a chronic anxiety state. A careful pain study is essential, including thiopental (Pentothal) narcosis or discography. Disc degeneration may be a multifocal disease as in the cervical and lumbar spine. Even if an examination seems to point to a single level, it is possible that within a short time other segments will become symptomatic and surgery will be of no long-term benefit. With multicentric disc degeneration results have not been gratifying. Best results are obtained with a single-segment discectomy and fusion for definite nerve root impairment or for localized disc disease without root compression. Fusions of more than two segments produce fair or poor results; improvement, not cure, is the best possible result.

2. The operation can be done at the *wrong level* if an incorrect vertebral count is made at surgery. Use of a check film with a metal marker is mandatory, and the first or second cervical vertebra must always be shown on this check film. The marker needle should be directed cranially so that the tip butts the vertebra above and avoids the theca. Roentgenographic analysis of the level may be insufficient, and the true level may only be found clinically by reproducing the pain on discography, which is more accurate than myelography. Reproduction of the clinical pain pattern on discography is best achieved by injecting a small quantity of local anesthetic.

3. The operation may be performed in the *wrong way;* for example, the recurrent laryngeal nerve, esophagus, or pharynx may be injured by retractors. Sympathetic nervous system injuries are avoided by dissecting in the correct planes. Keeping the dissection medial to the carotid avoids the sympathetic nervous system. An approach from the left is less likely to damage the recurrent laryngeal nerve. In an approach from the right the recurrent laryngeal nerve is in jeopardy from C6 downward, and it should be specifically identified and protected. This nerve enters the groove between the trachea and the esophagus at the point where the inferior thyroid artery enters the lower pole of the thyroid.

Curets may tear the dura and must be used with extreme caution in removing the posterior disc fragments.

The neurocentral facet should be removed with a right-angled curet kept in contact with the bone and placed medially to avoid the venous plexus and vertebral artery. An osteophyte compressing the vertebral artery is best removed through a large intervertebral exposure with a thin antral punch.

Osteotomes must be very sharp or have a shoulder guard to prevent injury to the cervical cord. Blunt osteotomes are more likely to cause injury. Grafts must be accurately measured and tightly fitted under compression.

4. The operation may be done at the *wrong time*. Timing of an operation is important, surgery should not be delayed if root conduction is significantly impaired. In patients in whom the clinical findings are purely subjective, the thought is usually given to delay of surgery until any possible litigation is settled. However, this may lead to chronic pain patterns difficult to eradicate. If such a patient has been significantly disabled for more than a year and has shown no improvement over the past 6 months, Macnab advises a thiopental pain study and discography. If a significant physiogenic basis for the pain is demonstrated, prompt anterior cervical fusion should be carried out without awaiting the results of litigation.

POSTOPERATIVE COMPLICATIONS

All anterior surgical wounds are best drained to avoid the hazards of a retropharyngeal hematoma. The latter can produce obstruction of the airway with its subsequent complications.

Extrusion of a graft is most commonly seen in the treatment of fracture-dislocations of the neck with posterior instability. This is not as commonly seen in fusions for disc degeneration with posterior stability of the ligamentous structures. A rectangular graft has more firm fixation than a circular Cloward graft. Unless the graft extrudes more than 50% of its width or unless it causes dysphagia, another operation is not indicated. The extruded portion will be absorbed and the graft will ossify, but the recovery time is protracted. Whitehill et al. reported a late esophageal perforation from a corticocancellous strut graft from the iliac crest. The first symptoms of dsyphagia occurred 2½ months after the surgery and an "inferior osseous spike" on the graft apparently eroded into the esophagus.

Collapse of a vertebral body is seen on occasions with the dowel technique, which jeopardizes the vertebral blood supply. This is caused by excessive thinning of the vertebral body at its midpoint.

Nonunion of an anterior cervical fusion is unusual. It is most likely to occur in a three-segment fusion and is best treated by posterior cervical fusion.

When anterior cervical arthrodesis is being performed for traumatic disorders with resultant instability from ligamentous tears or posterior element fractures, postoperative treatment must be planned to accommodate this added factor. The aftertreatment described here usually applies to arthrodesis for "stable" degenerative or other nontraumatic conditions. When cervical instability is present, the standard aftertreatment of 6 weeks in skeletal traction followed by a rigid brace has more recently yielded to early walking in a halo-cast or more often a halo-vest.

TYPES OF ANTERIOR ARTHRODESIS OF CERVICAL SPINE

Of the three commonly used techniques for anterior cervical spine fusion—those of Robinson and Smith, Bailey and Badgley, and Cloward—White and Hirsch found the Robinson and Smith configuration to be the strongest in compressive loading. This was followed by the Bailey and Badgley and the Cloward configurations in that order. These grafts could all bear loads of 2½ to 5 times the body

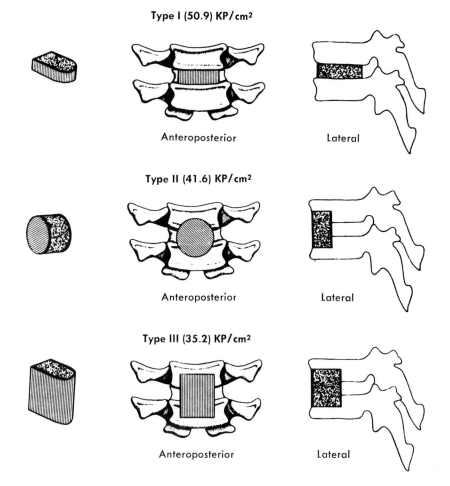

Type I (50.9) KP/cm²

Anteroposterior   Lateral

Type II (41.6) KP/cm²

Anteroposterior   Lateral

Type III (35.2) KP/cm²

Anteroposterior   Lateral

Fig. 70-1. Types (configurations) of grafts used in anterior arthrodesis of cervical spine. *Type I,* Robinson and Smith; *Type II,* Cloward; *Type III,* Bailey and Badgley. Numbers are means for load-bearing capacity for each. (From White, A.A., III, et al.: Clin. Orthop. **91:**21, 1973.)

weight, much more than the loads the cervical spine is normally expected to bear. Thus the limiting factor was not the graft itself but the graft vertebral construction (Fig. 70-1). The major load on the vertebrae in vivo is that of axial compression, but Simmons, and Bhalla and Butt have directed attention to the rotary displacement taking place in the spine and its relationship to the various constructions of the bone grafts. The strong configuration of the Robinson and Smith arthrodesis is the result of leaving intact the cortical shell of the vertebral body. Since it has been shown that 40% to 75% of the strength of the vertebra comes from the cortical bone, preserving the end plate is of great importance, as it prevents collapse into the cancellous portion of the body with subsequent displacement.

Bailey and Badgley, Robinson et al., Simmons et al. Macnab, and others have fused the cervical spine anteriorly for instability after extensive laminectomy, fractured posterior arch elements, certain fracture-dislocations, and destructive lesions. Robinson et al., Williams, Allen, and Harkess, and many others have combined excision of cervical intervertebral discs with anterior fusion. The various approaches to the anterior aspect of the cervical spine are described beginning on p. 3093.

TECHNIQUE (BAILEY AND BADGLEY). This technique is altered as the specific pathologic problem demands. The operation is done with the patient on a Stryker frame, Foster bed, or operating table with skull-tong traction in place. Endotracheal anesthesia is used.

Place a folded towel beneath the interscapular region to hold the neck in moderate extension. Rotate the patient's head about 15 degrees to the left and approach the cervical spine anteriorly from the right (p. 3099). When the prevertebral fascia is reached but before it is incised, insert a drill as a marker in one of the vertebral bodies and identify it with a lateral roentgenogram. After this orientation, incise the prevertebral fascia longitudinally in the exact midline. Place heavy silk sutures in the fascia to facilitate retraction and later to use in closure. Mobilize it from the anterior surfaces of the vertebral bodies and control bleeding from the bone with electrocautery or bone wax. Identify the vertebrae to be fused and cut a trough in the anterior aspect of the vertebral bodies about 1.2 cm wide and 4.7 mm deep from near the top of the upper vertebra to near the bottom of the lower one. A small power saw or drill is less traumatic than an osteotome and a mallet. Clean out the intervertebral disc spaces with a rongeur and

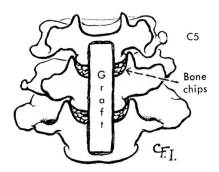

Fig. 70-2. Anterior fusion of cervical spine. Trough has been cut in anterior aspect of vertebral bodies, intervertebral disc spaces have been cleared and filled with iliac bone chips, and iliac graft has been mortised into trough. (Redrawn from Bailey, R.W., and Badgley, C.E.: J. Bone Joint Surg. **42-A:**565, 1960.)

remove the cartilaginous plates on the inferior and superior aspects of the bodies to be fused. Obtain and gently pack chips of cancellous iliac bone into the cleaned intervertebral disc spaces, trim an iliac graft to fit, and mortise it into the trough in the vertebrae (Fig. 70-2). Now decrease the extension of the cervical spine by raising the traction, thus wedging the graft more securely in the trough. The graft must not project further anteriorly than the anterior surface of the vertebral bodies.

When the graft is properly seated, tie the sutures previously placed in the prevertebral fascia; the fascia maintains the graft in its bed. Place a large Penrose drain or suction drainage tubes in the retropharyngeal space and bring it out through the lower portion of the incision. Close the wound in layers with interrupted sutures.

AFTERTREATMENT. Traction is maintained on a Stryker frame or Foster bed. The drain is advanced in 24 hours and is removed after 48 hours. After 6 weeks in traction, the patient is allowed to get up with the neck immobilized in a Taylor back brace with an attached Forrester collar. The brace is worn until fusion is complete, usually for 4 to 6 months.

A halo-cast or a halo-vest is more frequently used not than 6 weeks of traction. This allows much earlier ambulation and consequently much earlier hospital discharge. Provided that the halo-cast or halo-vest is properly supervised and maintained, the results should be equally satisfactory. We usually keep a halo-cast or halo-vest in place for about 3 months, using a brace and then a cervical collar during the next 4 to 6 weeks as immobilization is gradually decreased and as rehabilitation progresses.

Fielding, Lusskin, and Batista have found the method of Bailey and Badgley satisfactory in fusing several segments for instability after multiple laminectomies; in this situation in children, Cattell and Clark have used a strut graft of tibial bone as described by Robinson.

Robinson et al. have arthodesed the cervical spine anteriorly for intervertebral disc degeneration by excising the disc and the cartilaginous plates from the selected disc space or spaces and inserting blocks of iliac bone.

TECHNIQUE (ROBINSON ET AL.). Place the patient on the operating table and replace part of the mattress by a cassette holder that extends from the spines of the scapulae to

above the head and by a pneumatic roll between the neck and the cassette holder. Adjust the roll to permit moderate extension of the neck. When anesthesia is well established by the endotracheal method, apply a head halter, and by means of an outrigger at the head of the table apply 5 pounds (2.2 kg) of traction.

Rotate the patient's head to the right and approach the cervical spine anteriorly from the left through one of several incisions (p. 3094). Continue the approach until the exact midline of the spine has been reached. Then in the midline incise vertically and retract the alar and prevertebral fasciae. The anterior longitudinal ligament and any osteoarthritic spurs are then visible. Insert a needle into one disc and identify its level by a lateral roentgenogram. Test the resiliency of the various discs by palpation with a finger or the tip of a forceps; also test their consistency by penetrating each with a needle. Then examine each suspicious disc by discography.

Having selected the disc space or spaces to be cleared and replaced by bone, proceed with the fusion. At the front of the disc space make a rectangular window in the anterior longitudinal ligament and the anulus about 1.5 cm wide. Then with a small curet loosen the disc material and remove it with a pituitary rongeur. Also remove the cartilaginous plate from the subchondral bone above and below the space back to the posterior part of the anulus and the posterior longitudinal ligament. After proper preparation the space created measures about $1.5 \times 1.5 \times 0.6$ to 0.8 cm. Trim sparingly any bony spurs along the superior and inferior edges of the space but never enough to remove the normal ridge of cortical bone from the anterior part of the vertebral bodies. Now drill a few holes into the underlying cancellous bone of the vertebrae if there is no bleeding after excision of the cartilaginous plates.

Shape a 1.5 cm long iliac graft so that its cancellous part will lie against the subchondral bone above and below the space while its cortical part will form the support between the vertebrae (Fig. 70-3). Then apply 15 additional pounds (6.7 kg) of traction and hyperextend the head and neck. Insert the graft and carefully tamp it into place with a bone punch and mallet. Countersink the graft just posterior to the anterior margins of the vertebral bodies; it should be firmly fixed even before the traction is removed. Repeat the procedure at each disc space as necessary. Now suture the alar and prevertebral fasciae and close the wound.

Bloom and Raney have recommended reversing the orientation of the iliac graft as it is inserted so that the rounded cortical edge of the iliac cortex is placed posteriorly and the cancellous edge is anterior. They claim that protruding portions of the graft can be trimmed off easily with a rongeur without sacrificing the cortical portion and decreasing the strength of the graft.

AFTERTREATMENT. The patient is placed supine in bed with sandbags on each side of the head for about 24 hours and in 1 or 2 days is allowed out of bed. In about 4 days a neck brace is fitted and is worn during the day for 3 months.

• • •

The cervical arthrodesis with discectomy described by Simmons et al. has produced excellent results in 80.8% of

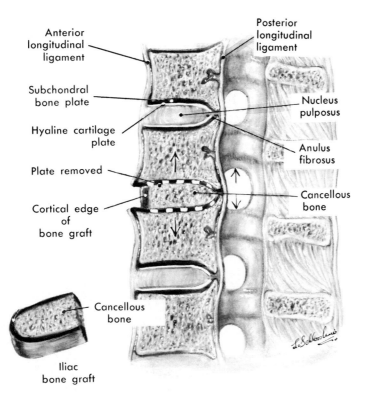

Anterior
longitudinal
ligament

Subchondral
bone plate

Hyaline cartilage
plate

Plate removed

Cortical edge
of
bone graft

Cancellous
bone

Iliac
bone graft

Posterior
longitudinal
ligament

Nucleus
pulposus

Anulus
fibrosus

Cancellous
bone

Fig. 70-3. Technique of Robinson et al. for anterior fusion of cervical spine (see text). (Modified from Robinson, R.A., et al.: J. Bone Joint Surg. **44-A:**1569, 1962.)

their patients. Our major experience with this technique has been with trauma, but it does provide a stable configuration.

TECHNIQUE (SIMMONS ET AL.). Use endotracheal anesthesia. Place the patient on the operating table and strap the ankles to the table. Apply a sterile head halter and drape the patient. Using a right-sided approach, make a transverse skin incision along the line of the skin creases. Divide the platysma transversely, retract the strap muscles and viscera medially, and retract the sternocleidomastoid muscle and great vessels laterally. Insert a needle in the exposed disc and obtain roentgenographic proof of the exact level. Remove a keystone square or rectangle of tissue, beveling it upward into the vertebra above and downward into the vertebra below using special osteotomes and chisels of Simmons' design, with a depth of 1.2 cm each and with widths of 1.27, 1.1, and 0.95 cm (Fig. 70-4, *A*). Exercise care to avoid outward progression of the chisel while keeping the cut in the true anteroposterior plane. Remove a 1.27 cm square of tissue for the one-level fusion in most patients. When this material is completely removed with rongeurs and by curettage, remove the disc from posteriorly to anteriorly. At the final stage of cleansing of this space ask the anesthetist to apply strong head halter traction, which opens the disc space and allows cleaning to be carried out well to the neurocentral joints. Deepen the trough to the posterior cortex of the vertebrae. Next carefully cut the corners squarely. Measure the length of the rectangle while forceful traction is placed on the head halter to allow opening of the space at least 3 mm. Obtain a

rectangular graft from the iliac crest and shape it to fit the trough. Bevel the ends upward and downward to approximately 14 to 18 degrees. Now distract the neck fully by forceful traction and place the graft into the defect. Release the traction; the graft is thus locked firmly into position, maintaining fixed distraction and immobilization (Fig. 70-4, *B*). In a two-level fusion extend the trough and graft through the intervening vertebra into the one above and below.

AFTERTREATMENT. Early mobilization is allowed in a brace until union is achieved. Since grafting under distraction is quite stable, postoperative pain is much less than pain after other types of cervical spine arthrodesis.

Anterior occipitocervical arthrodesis by extrapharyngeal exposure

Rarely an anterior occipitocervical fusion is required for a grossly unstable cervical spine when posterior fusion is not feasible because of a previous extensive laminectomy. It was used by de Andrade and Macnab in patients who had had extensive laminectomies for rheumatoid arthritis, traumatic quadriparesis, neoplastic metastasis to the spine, and congenital abnormalities. This operation is a cranial extension of the approach described by Robinson and Smith and by Bailey and Badgley; it permits access to the base of the occiput and the anterior aspect of all the cervical vertebrae.

TECHNIQUE (DE ANDRADE AND MACNAB). Maintain initial spinal stability by applying a cranial halo with the patient on a turning frame. Keep the patient on the frame and

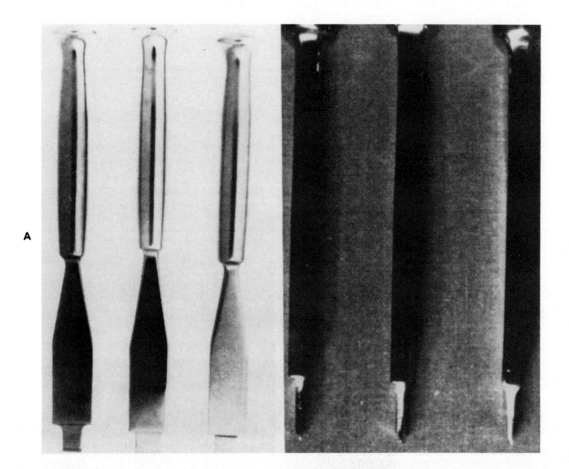

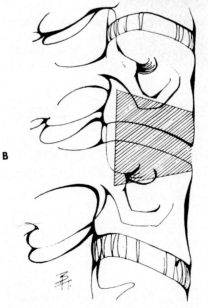

Fig. 70-4. A, Special osteotomes and chisels of Simmons et al. **B,** Placement of keystone graft shown in lined area. (From Simmons, E.H., Bhalla, S.K., and Butt, W.P.: J. Bone Joint Surg. **51-B:**225, 1969.)

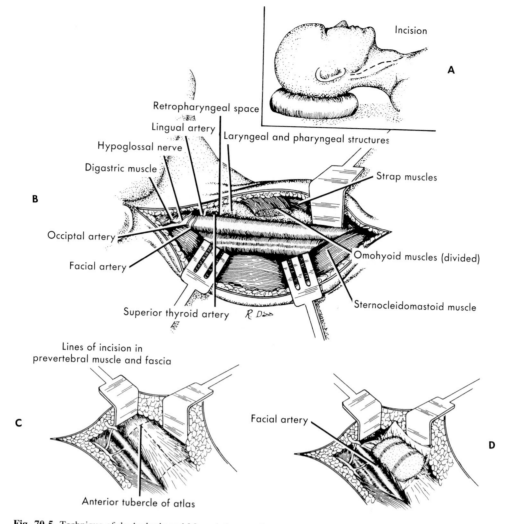

Fig. 70-5. Technique of de Andrade and Macnab for anterior occipitocervical arthrodesis (see text). (Redrawn from de Andrade, J.R., and Macnab, I.: J. Bone Joint Surg. **51-A:**1621, 1969.)

maintain the traction throughout the operation. Make the exposure from the right side with an incision coursing along the anterior border of the sternocleidomastoid muscle from above the angle of the mandible to below the cricoid cartilage (Fig. 70-5). Divide the platysma and deep cervical fascia in line with the incision and expose the anterior border of the sternocleidomastoid. Take care not to injure the spinal accessory nerve as it enters the anterior aspect of the sternocleidomastoid at the level of the transverse process of the atlas. Retract the sternocleidomastoid laterally and the pretracheal strap muscles anteriorly and palpate the carotid artery in its sheath. Expose the latter. Divide the omohyoid muscle as it crosses at the level of the cricoid cartilage. Identify the digastric muscle and hypoglossal nerve at the cranial end of the wound. Bluntly dissect the retropharyngeal space and enter it at the level of the thyroid cartilage. Now divide the superior thyroid, lingual, and facial arteries and veins to gain access to the retropharyngeal space in the upper part of the wound. Continue blunt dissection in the retropharyngeal space and palpate the anterior arch of the atlas and the anterior tu-

bercle in the midline. Continue above this with the exploring finger and enter the hollow at the base of the occiput. Dissection cannot be carried further cephalad because of the pharyngeal tubercle, to which the pharynx is attached. Insert a broad right-angled retractor under the pharynx and displace it anterosuperiorly. Use intermittent traction on the pharyngeal and laryngeal branches of the vagus nerve during this maneuver to minimize temporary hoarseness and inability to sing high notes. The anterior aspect of the upper cervical spine and the base of the occiput are now exposed. Coagulate the profuse plexus of veins under the anterior border of the longus colli. Separate the muscles from the anterior aspect of the spine by incising the anterior longitudinal ligament vertically and transversely and expose the anterior arch of C1 and the bodies of C2 and C3. The working space is approximately 4 cm, since the hypoglossal nerve exits from the skull through the anterior condyloid foramen about 2 cm lateral to the midline. Roughen the anterior surface of the base of the occiput and upper cervical vertebrae with a curet. Obtain from the iliac crest slivers of fresh autogenous cancellous bone and place

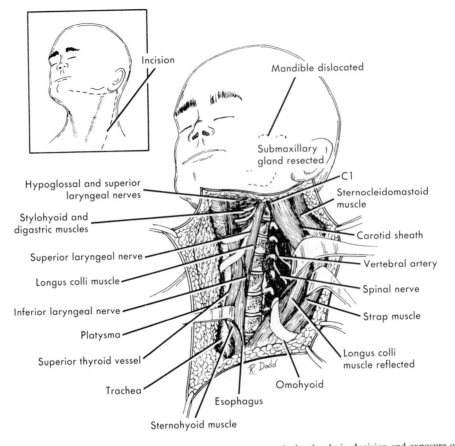

Incision

Mandible dislocated

Submaxillary
gland resected

C1

Hypoglossal and superior
laryngeal nerves

Sternocleidomastoid
muscle

Stylohyoid and
digastric muscles

Carotid sheath

Superior laryngeal nerve

Vertebral artery

Longus colli muscle

Spinal nerve

Inferior laryngeal nerve

Strap muscle

Platysma

Longus colli
muscle reflected

Superior thyroid vessel

Trachea

Omohyoid

Esophagus

Sternohyoid muscle

R. Dodd

Fig. 70-6. Technique of Robinson and Riley for anterior upper cervical arthrodesis. Incision and exposure of cervical spine. (Redrawn from Robinson, R.A., and Riley, L.H., Jr.: Clin. Orthop. **109**:78, 1975.)

them on the anterior surface of the vertebrae to be fused. Make the slivers no thicker than 4.2 mm to prevent excessive bulging into the pharynx. Close the wound by suturing the platysma and skin only with a suction drain left in the retropharyngeal space for 48 hours.

AFTERTREATMENT. The patient is kept on a turning frame and traction is maintained for 6 weeks. A tracheostomy set must be kept by the bedside in case upper airway obstruction occurs. For earlier ambulation a halo-cast or halo-vest (Chapter 71) may be applied; the halo is removed 16 weeks after the operation. Consolidation of the graft should occur by this time.

Anterior upper cervical arthrodesis

TECHNIQUE (ROBINSON AND RILEY). Perform a tracheostomy and maintain anesthesia via this route. Begin the incision just to the left of the midline in the submandibular region. Carry it posteriorly to the angle of the mandible, then gently curve it lateral to the posterior border of the sternocleidomastoid muscle to the base of the neck, finally curve it anteriorly and inferiorly across the clavicle, and end it in the suprasternal space (Fig. 70-6). Develop the incision through the platysma muscle and retract the muscle flap so outlined medially to expose the sternocleidomastoid and strap muscles, the pharynx, the thyroid gland, the edge of the mandible, and the submaxillary triangle.

Identify the anterior surface of the lower cervical spine by retracting the sternocleidomastoid muscle and carotid sheath laterally and transecting the tendinous portion of the omohyoid muscle. Incise the prevertebral fascia in the midline and retract the thyroid gland, esophagus, and trachea medially. Now note that the continuation of this plane superiorly is impeded by the superior thyroid artery, the superior laryngeal neurovascular bundle, the hypoglossal nerve, the stylohyoid muscle, and the digastric muscle. Ligate and divide the superior thyroid artery. Divide and reflect the stylohyoid muscle and digastric muscle; identify and protect the superior laryngeal and hypoglossal nerves. Retract the larynx and the pharynx medially and the external carotid artery laterally, and identify the floor of the submaxillary triangle. Maintain superior retraction so that the base of the skull and the anterior arch of the first cervical vertebra are visible. To gain additional exposure, excise the submaxillary gland and dislocate the temporomandibular joint anteriorly by rotating the mandible superiorly and toward the right. The anterior arch of the first cervical vertebra, the odontoid process, and both vertebral arteries are now visible. Cut a trough in the anterior aspect of the second and third vertebral bodies to the level of the posterior cortex of the odontoid process. Remove cancellous bone from the odontoid process with a small curet and convert it to a hollow shell (Fig. 70-7). Shape a bone graft

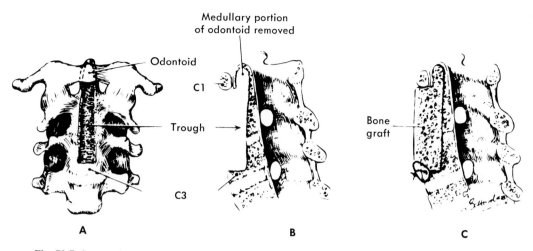

Fig. 70-7. Same technique as Fig. 70-6. Insertion of grafts into upper cervical spine. (From Robinson, R.A., and Riley, L.H., Jr.: Clin. Orthop. **109**:78, 1975.)

removed from the anterior iliac crest to the dimensions of the previsouly constructed trough. Shape the superior end of the graft to resemble a saddle and fit one protrusion into the odontoid process and the other protrusion abutting the anterior arch of the first cervical vertebra. With the saddle supporting the anterior cortex of the odontoid and the inferior portion of the anterior arch of the first cervical vertebra, secure the inferior end of the graft with a loop of wire or heavy suture material through the cortex of the inferior vertebral body. If a twisted wire loop has been placed, use a small amount of methylmethacrylate bone cement to cover its sharp edges and avoid wire protrusion into the posterior pharynx.

AFTERTREATMENT. The aftertreatment is the same as described for the Bailey and Badgley technique (p. 3146).

Fibular strut graft in cervical spine arthrodesis

TECHNIQUE (WHITECLOUD AND LAROCCA). Use the surgical approach of Robinson. Make a trough in the anterior aspect of the vertebral column, initially with a rongeur and then with a dental burr. Perform a partial vertebrectomy when long tract signs call for decompression. Use a full segment of the fibula, placing it into prepared notches in the vertebrae at both ends of the segment to be spanned. Make notches of equal length in the superior end, but make the posterior extension of the inferior notch slightly shorter than the anterior one to allow for easier graft insertion. Prepare the end plates of the superior and inferior vertebrae to accept the graft, which produces a hole within the body itself. Preserve the anterior portion of the vertebral cortex to prevent graft displacement. Increase the traction weight on the head and insert the graft into the superior vertebra. Use an impactor to sink the inferior portion of the graft into the trough and pull distally, locking it into place. Two thirds of the graft then comes to lie posterior to the anterior aspect of the vertebral column. Check the graft position by roentgenogram and close the wound over the drains.

AFTERTREATMENT. Initial immobilization is continued by skeletal traction, a plastic collar, a Philadelphia brace, or a cervicodorsal brace. The time required for fusion will understandably be longer with cortical bone than with a corticocancellous bone graft. Whitecloud and LaRocca kept their patients immobilized in a hard cervical collar, Philadelphia brace, or cervicodorsal brace for an average of 15 weeks. They concluded that this is too short a time; perhaps, like the canine fibular transplantation studied by Enneking et al., the graft may require a year for incorporation in humans. Therefore prolonged immobilization is necessary.

Posterior arthrodesis of cervical spine

The techniques of posterior arthrodesis of the cervical spine are discussed in the section on fractures, dislocations, and fracture-dislocations of the cervical spine (p. 3119).

DORSAL AND LUMBAR SPINE

The indications for arthrodesis of the spine are now considerably different from in the days of Hibbs and Albee. Fusion of the lumbosacral region for degenerative, traumatic, and congenital lesions is now more common. Indications for and techniques of spinal fusion and care after surgery vary from one orthopaedic center to another. Many orthopaedists prefer posterior arthrodesis, usually some modification of the Hibbs procedure with the addition of a large quantity of autogenous iliac bone. Internal fixation is frequently used with posterior arthrodesis. Posterolateral or intertransverse process fusions are used frequently, either alone or in combination with a posterior fusion and with or without posterior internal fixation. Interbody fusions from an anterior or a posterolateral approach are preferred by other orthopaedic surgeons. For routine spinal fusion, we usually prefer: (1) a modified Hibbs procedure, usually combined in the thoracic and thoracolumbar spines with internal fixation and always supplemented with a great deal of autogenous iliac bone; (2) a modified Hibbs posterior fusion combined with a posterolateral fusion; or (3) a bilateral posterolateral fusion. Anterior interbody fusions are usually reserved for patients who do not have sufficient bone structure remaining for posterior fusion or who have some other unusual problem.

Posterior arthrodeses of the spine are generally based on the principles originated by Hibbs in 1911. In the Hibbs operation fusion of the neural arches is induced by overlapping numerous small osseous flaps from contiguous laminae, spinous processes, and articular facets. In the thoracic spine the arthrodesis is generally extended laterally out to the tips of the transverse processes so that the posterior cortex and cancellous bone of these portions of the vertebrae are used to widen the fusion mass. Accurate identification of a specific verterbral level is always difficult except when the sacrum can be exposed and thus identified. At any other level, despite the fact that identification of a given vertebra is frequently possible because of the anatomic peculiarities of spinous processes, laminae, and articular facets, it is almost always advisable to make marker roentgenograms at surgery. Marker films are occasionally made before surgery using a metal marker on the skin or a scratch on the skin to identify the level. We recommend a much better method consisting of the roentgenographic identification of a marker of adequate size clamped to or inserted into a spinous process within the operative field. The closer to the base of the spinous process the marker can be inserted, the more accurate and easier is the identification. Anteroposterior roentgenograms on the operating table to compare with good quality preoperative roentgenograms are usually sufficient to allow accurate identification of the vertebral level.

Bone grafts in posterior fusion of spine

Autogenous bone grafts from the ilium are generally preferable to other types of grafts. Cancellous iliac bone will be incorporated into the fusion mass more rapidly than cortical tibial bone. Fresh autogenous grafts are preferable to bone bank grafts.

TECHNIQUE FOR OBTAINING ILIAC GRAFTS. This technique is discussed on p. 17.

Hibbs fusion of spine

By the Hibbs technique fusion is attempted at four different points—the laminae and articular processes on each side. The procedure has been modified slightly over the years; at the New York Orthopaedic Hospital it is performed as follows.

TECHNIQUE (HIBBS*). Incise the skin and subcutaneous tissues in the midline along the spinous processes and attach towels to the skin edges with Michel clips or use an adhesive plastic drape. Divide the deep fascia and supraspinous ligament in line with the skin incision. With a Kermission or Cobb elevator, remove the supraspinous ligament from the tips of the spines. Next strip the periosteum from the sides of the spines and the dorsal surface of the laminae with a curved elevator. Control bleeding with long thin sponge packs (Hibbs sponges). Incise the interspinous ligaments in the direction of their length, making a continuous longitidunal exposure. Now elevate the muscles from the ligamentum flavum and expose the

---

*As described by Howorth.

fossa distal to the lateral articulation. Excise the fat pad in the fossa with a scalpel or curet. Thoroughly denude the spinous processes of periosteum and ligament with elevator and curet, split them longtiudinally and transversely with an osteotome, and remove them with the Hibbs biting forceps. Using a thick chisel elevator, strip away the capsules of the lateral articulations. Free with a curet the posterior layer (about two thirds) of the ligamentum flavum from the margins of the distal and proximal laminae in succession and peel it off the anterior layer; leave the latter to cover the dura. Excise the articular cartilage and cortical bone from the lateral articulations with special thin osteotomes, either straight or angled at 30, 45, or 60 degrees as required. (A. DeF. Smith emphasized that the lateral articulations of the vertebra above the area of fusion must not be disturbed, for this may cause pain later. However, it is important to include the lateral articulations within the fusion area, for if they are not obliterated, the entire fusion is jeopardized. After curretting the lateral articulations in the fusion area, he narrowed the remaining defect by making small cuts into the articular processes parallel with the joint line so that these thin slices of bone separate slightly and fill the space. This, he believed, is preferable to packing the joint spaces with cancellous bone chips.)

Using a gouge, cut chips from the fossa below each lateral articulation and turn them into the gap left by the removal of the articular cartilage or insert a fragment of spinous process into the gap. Denude the fossa of cortical bone and pack it fully with chips. Also with a gouge remove chips from the laminae and place them in the interlaminal space in contact with raw bone on each side. Use fragments from the spinous processes to bridge the laminae. Use also additional bone from the ilium near the posterosuperior spine or from the spinous processes beyond the fusion area. When large or extensive grafts are taken from the posterior ilium, postoperative pain or sensitivity of the area may be marked. Care should be taken to avoid injury to the cluneal nerves with subsequent neuroma formation. Bone from the bone bank may be used, especially if the bone available locally is scant because of spina bifida. The bone grafts should not extend beyond the laminae of the end vertebrae, for the projecting ends of the grafts may cause irritation and pain. If the nucleus pulposus is to be removed, the chips are cut before exposure of the nucleus and are kept until needed. The remaining layer of the ligamentum flavum is freed as a flap with its base at the midline, is retracted for exposure of the nerve root and nucleus, and after removal of the nucleus is replaced to protect the dura.

Suture the periosteum, ligaments, and muscles snugly over the chips with interrupted sutures. Then suture the subcutaneous tissue carefully to eliminate dead space, and close the skin either with a subcuticular suture or nonabsorbable skin suture technique.

At this clinic we routinely use an adhesive plastic film material to isolate the skin surface from the wound rather than attaching towels to skin edges with Michel clips. Michel clips have an unfortunate tendency to become displaced and may get lost within the wound. We also routinely use modified Cobb elevators, which when sharp are quite efficient in stripping away the capsules of the lateral articulations.

Modified Hibbs technique supplemented by chip or sliver grafts

The technique of Henry and Geist is said to be suitable for patients of any age (Fig. 70-8). At this clinic inclusion of the posterior articulations in the fusion is considered to be quite important. Consequently, we now rarely use this technique.

TECHNIQUE (HENRY AND GEIST, MODIFIED). Through a midline incision expose the designated spinous processes and dissect the soft tissues from the processes and laminae. With a gouge gently remove thin shavings from the bone until raw cancellous bone is visible and the facets are destroyed. Chip off the spines at their bases and save them. Cut the spinous processes obliquely at each end of the wound to eliminate disfiguring projections.

Remove posterior iliac cancellous bone chips and cut them and the spinous processes into chips. Distribute the

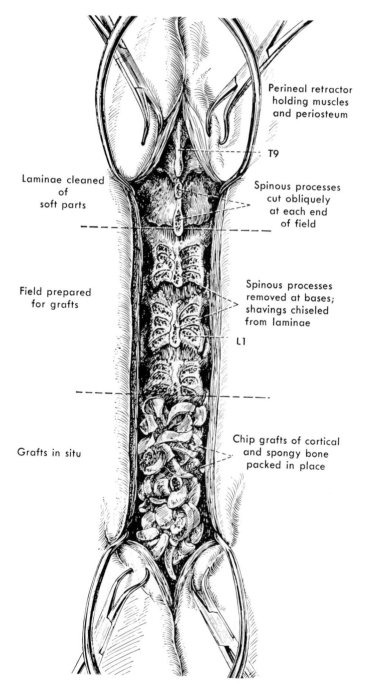

Perineal retractor holding muscles and periosteum

T9

Laminae cleaned of soft parts

Spinous processes cut obliquely at each end of field

Field prepared for grafts

Spinous processes removed at bases; shavings chiseled from laminae

L1

Grafts in situ

Chip grafts of cortical and spongy bone packed in place

Fig. 70-8. Henry and Geist technique of spine fusion. (From Henry, M.O., and Geist, E.S.: J. Bone Joint Surg. **15**:622, 1933.)

chips up and down the graft bed and press them into contact with the laminae and with each other.

AFTERTREATMENT. We routinely use closed wound suction for 12 to 36 hours, with removal mandatory by 48 hours. Depending on the level of the arthrodesis, the age of the patient, and the presence or absence of internal fixation, we attempt to walk the patient at 7 to 10 days. Skin sutures may be removed early, after several days, and replaced with adhesive strips if a Risser type of well-molded cast is to be applied. If not, they remain in place for up to 2 weeks. More appropriate postoperative immobilization for older adults include lower back braces, prefabricated plastic jackets, and custom-made, bivalved, plastic jackets. For obese patients, all types of external fixation or support will likely be inadequate and limitation of activity may be the only reasonable alternative.

Clothespin (H or prop) graft in spinal fusion

In 1931 Gibson, in an attempt to obtain firmer fixation in fusion of the spine, devised a tibial graft with clefts at each end that grasped the spinous processes of the proximal and distal ends of the fusion area, the intervening spinous processes being resected. This procedure is not used often, except for a modification by Bosworth using a double clothespin graft from the ilium reinforced by strips of cancellous bone (Fig. 70-9). When the patient stands and walks postoperatively, it is likely that this mechanical effect is rapidly lost. Regen, Moore, and others, including us, have used variations of the clothespin graft, particu-larly in lumbosacral fusions. By flexing the lumbosacral spine when the graft is inserted, it is possible to partially reduce the lumbar lordosis, to wedge open the lumbosacral joint, to restore the lumbosacral articular facets to a more normal relationship, and to spread the intervertebral foramina.

If the spinous process of the sacrum is underdeveloped or absent, the lower end of the graft is simply beveled to lie snugly in a bed on the dorsum of the sacrum. In the presence of spina bifida of one or more of the sacral segments, the lower end of the graft is fashioned as a double strut and is placed in grooves cut transversely in the region of the articular facets of the first sacral vertebra.

When the spine is fused with a clothespin graft, it is important that the laminae be denuded of cortical bone and that cancellous bone be packed across the laminae and about the graft, as in a Hibbs or modified Hibbs operation.

Internal fixation in spinal fusion

Many surgeons have used various types of internal fixation in spinal fusion. The object is to immobilize the joints during fusion and thus hasten consolidation and reduce pain and disability after surgery. For many years several of us at this clinic have fixed the spinous processes of the lumbar spine with heavy wire loops as described by Rogers for fracture-dislocation of the cervical spine (p. 3126). The wire helps stabilize the grafts as well as the vertebrae.

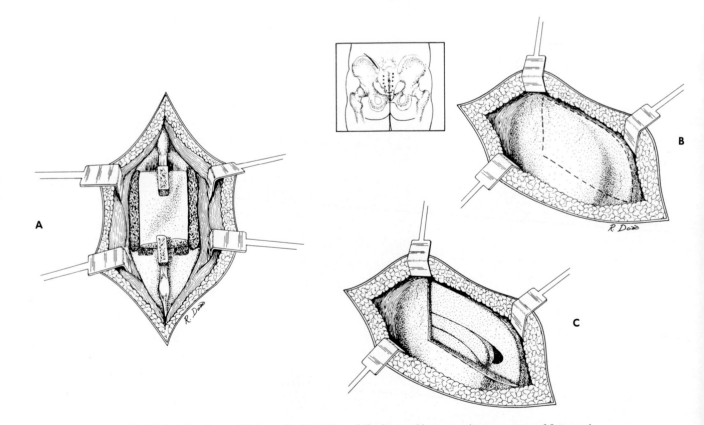

Fig. 70-9. A, Lumbosacral fusion, with clothespin graft firmly seated between spinous processes of first sacral and fifth lumbar vertebrae. **B,** Graft fashioned from segment of posterior crest of ilium. **C,** Reinforcing cancellous iliac grafts. (Redrawn from Bosworth, D.M.: Am. J. Surg. **67:**61, 1945.)

In 1949 McBride reported a method of fixing the articular facets with bone blocks. Later he used cylindrical bone grafts to transfix the facets, particularly at the lumbosacral joint. Still later he elevated subperiosteally the soft tissue attachments to the spinous processes and laminae, removed the spinous processes of L4, L5, and S1 at their bases, and with special trephine cutting tools, cut mortise bone grafts from them. If one object of the operation is exploration for a ruptured disc, this is done next. The laminae are then spread forcibly with laminae distractors, and again using special trephine cutting tools, a round hole is made across each facet joint into the underlying pedicle. The bone grafts are then impacted firmly across each joint into the pedicle, and the distractors are removed.

Overton has also fixed the articular facets with bone grafts, but in addition he uses H grafts between the spinous processes and adds bone chips about the fusion area. Of 187 patients treated by his method, 174 or 93% obtained solid fusion as judged by roentgenograms.

TECHNIQUE (OVERTON). Expose the lower spine through a midline longitudinal incision. Expose subperiosteally the spinous processes, laminae, and apophyseal joints. Remove the interspinous ligament, the ligamenta flava, and the inferior portion of the capsules of the articular facets.

This allows distraction of the laminae. Repeat this procedure between all vertebrae that are to be arthrodesed. Cut notches on the inferior surface of the base of the upper spinous process and on the superior surface of the lower one to allow locking of the H graft. Turn up the posterior cortex of the sacrum if further locking of the lower end of the graft is necessary. If more than two vertebrae are to be fused, remove the intervening spinous process. Now with an interspinous separator distract the spinous processes and laminae enough to correct lordosis to the normal angle or until the normal space of the intervertebral foramina is restored. Turn up bone chips from the laminae and place them across the interlaminar spaces and add chips from the spinous process.

Through the same incision, or if necessary another one, obtain a large single bone graft from the ilium. Now drill a small hole through the inferior and superior facets of each joint into the pedicle. Enlarge the holes with hand reamers as much as is tolerated by the pedicle (Fig. 70-10). Now fashion dowel grafts from the iliac graft and drive these across each apophyseal joint. Add bone chips from the ilium across the interlaminar spaces. Cut the remaining iliac graft in the shape of an H and wedge it between the spinous processes above and below. Remove the interspinous separator and close the wound in layers.

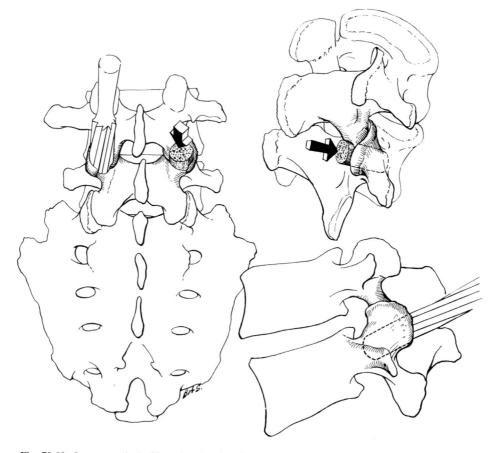

Fig. 70-10. Overton method of inserting dowel grafts across apophyseal joints. *Left* and *lower right,* reamer has been passed through inferior and superior facets of joint. *Left* and *upper right,* grafts of iliac bone have been driven across joint. (From Overton, L.M.: Am. Surg. **25:**771, 1959.)

Treatment after posterior arthrodesis

Opinions vary as to the proper treatment after spinal fusion. Usually the patient is placed on a firm bed with soft mattress pad. No one knows for sure how long bed rest or the use of any external support should be continued; certainly this will vary somewhat with the pathologic condition and the location and extent of the fusion. We once believed that absolute bed rest should be maintained for at least 6 and preferably 8 weeks after lumbosacral fusion, even when screws had been inserted through the lateral articulations, wires or plates had been applied to the spinous processes, or clothespin or distraction grafts had been inserted between the spinous processes. Yet many others have allowed walking in a light support soon after surgery. At this clinic, treatment now depends somewhat on the pathologic condition and the technique of fusion, but more on the preference of the various surgeons. Most of our surgeons now allow the patient to walk in 1 to 2 weeks. If the lumbosacral area is fused, the postoperative immobilization should be in a well-molded body cast or plastic jacket applied 7 to 14 days after fusion. Some of our surgeons use an extension down to the knee on one side. The most important single project at the time of surgery is the preparation of an extensive fresh cancellous bed to receive the grafts. This means denuding the facets, pars interarticulares, laminae, and spinous processes completely. Walking is not allowed until after cast application in those patients with internal fixation or a prop graft, whereas those with a lateral transverse process fusion may walk before cast application. At 2 to 4 months most surgeons apply a rigid lower back brace that is worn until consolidation of the fusion mass is complete as seen in anteroposterior, oblique, and lateral roentgenograms.

Anteroposterior roentgenograms made supine in right and left bending positions and lateral roentgengrams made in flexion and extension are necessary between 6 and 12 months postoperatively to confirm consolidation of the fusion mass.

Pseudarthrosis after spinal fusion

The frequency of pseudarthrosis after spinal arthrodesis should be remembered from the time the operation is proposed until the fusion mass is solid. A frank discussion of this problem with each patient before operation is important.

In a study of lumbosacral spine fusions performed on 594 patients, Cleveland et al. found pseudarthrosis in 119, an incidence of 20%. When calculated on the basis of the number of intervertebral spaces fused, the incidence was 12.1%. There was a definite relationship between the extent of fusion and the incidence of pseudarthrosis. When the fifth lumbar vertebra was fused to the sacrum, the pseudarthrosis rate was 3.4%, when the fourth lumbar vertebra was included, the rate was 17.4%; and when the fusion extended up to the third or second lumbar vertebra, one third of the patients showed one or more pseudarthroses. Bosworth, as a matter of fact, recommended that in the lumbosacral region arthrodesis should extend only from the fourth lumbar vertebra to the sacrum as a maximum at one stage, unless the situation at the time of surgery requires more extensive fusion. Other segments to be included in the final fusion area are added later. Ralston and Thompson, in a study of 1096 patients after spine fusion, found an overall pseudarthrosis rate of 16.6%. Prothero, Parkes, and Stinchfield, in a review of 430 fusions, found a rate of 15.1%; as in the study of Cleveland et al., the rate varied with the extent of the fusion: when the fifth lumbar vertebra was fused to the sacrum, the rate was 8.3%; when the fourth lumbar vertebra was included, the rate was 15.8%; and when the fusion extended to the third lumbar vertebra, the rate was 26.6%. In contrast, DePalma and Rothman, in a review of 448 patients 5 to 17 years after spinal fusion, found an overall pseudarthrosis rate of only 8.7%.

It has been estimated that 50% of patients with pseudarthrosis have no symptoms. Bosworth, in a review of 101 patients with pseudarthrosis, found 43 who had no pain. DePalma and Rothman matched 39 patients with pseudarthrosis against 39 otherwise similar patients without pseudarthrosis. The results were a little better when the fusions were solid but the difference was not marked. In each group some patients had pain and some did not. We have presumed that any persistent pain after spinal fusion is caused by a pseudarthrosis when present. Yet in some instances pain has continued after a successful repair. Even so, repair of any pseudarthrosis is indicated when disabling pain persists; certainly repair is contraindicated when pain is slight or absent.

The following findings are helpful in making a diagnosis of pseudarthrosis: (1) sharply localized pain and tenderness over the fusion area, (2) progression of the deformity or disease, (3) localized motion in the fusion mass, as found in biplane bending roentgenograms, and (4) motion in the fusion mass found on exploration. Cobb and others have pointed out that exploration is the only way one can be absolutely certain that a fusion mass is completely solid.

PSEUDARTHROSIS REPAIR

TECHNIQUE (RALSTON AND W.A.L. THOMPSON). Expose the entire fusion plate subperiosteally through the old incision; should the defect be wide and filled with dense fibrous tissue, subperiosteal stripping in that area may be difficult. On the other hand, a narrow defect is often difficult to locate, for the surface of the plate is usually irregular, and the line of pseudarthrosis may be sinuous in both coronal and sagittal planes. Thoroughly clean the fibrous tissue from the fusion mass in the vicinity of the pseudarthrosis. The adjacent superior and inferior borders of the fusion mass on either side of the pseudarthrosis will usually be seen to move when pressure is applied with a blunt instrument. As the defect is followed across the fusion mass, it will be found to extend into the lateral articulations on each side. Carefully explore these articulations and excise all fibrous tissue and any remaining articular cartilage down to bleeding bone. Should the defect be wide, excise the fibrous tissue that fills it to a depth of 3.0 to 6.0 mm across the entire mass and protect the underlying spinal dura. Thoroughly freshen the exposed edges of the defect. When the defect is narrow and motion is minimal, limit the excision of the interposed soft tissue to avoid loss of fixation. Now fashion a trough 6.0 mm wide and 6.0 mm deep on each side of the midline, extending longitudinally both well above and below the defect. "Fish scale" the entire fusion mass on both sides of the defect, the bases of the bone chips raised being away from the defect. Now obtain both strip and chip bone grafts either from the fusion mass above or below or from the ilium, preferably the latter. Pack these grafts tightly into the lateral articulations, into the pseudarthrosis defect, and into the longitudinal troughs. Then place small grafts across the pseudarthrosis line and wedge the edge of each transplant beneath the fish-scaled cortical bone chips. Use all remaining graft material to pack neatly in and about the grafts.

• • •

Cleveland, Bosworth, and F.R. Thompson have described a somewhat different method of repair, planned particularly for the more difficult pseudarthroses. The operation is unilateral; the paraspinal muscles and the underlying bony masses on the opposite side remain intact for such stability as they may afford.

TECHNIQUE (CLEVELAND, BOSWORTH, AND F.R. THOMPSON). Through the old midline incision denude and cut down to bleeding bone the laminae, the lateral margins of the articular facets, and the bases of the transverse processes on one side of the spine (Fig. 70-11). Remove grafts from the outer cortex of the ilium and place a thin wide graft on edge over the transverse processes and the posterior surfaces of the articular facets. Then place strips of bone over the posterior elements of the involved vertebrae, filling the area between the larger graft and the midline.

AFTERTREATMENT. The patient is immobilized in a body cast or a double plaster spica incorporating both thighs down to the knees for 8 to 12 weeks. The cast is then removed and anteroposterior, lateral, and oblique roentgenograms are made. If it appears that satisfactory bony repair of the pseudarthrosis has been obtained, the patient is allowed up in a body brace or a plaster jacket. If there is suggestion of failure, 4 weeks further immobilization is necessary. Should failure then be definite as determined by

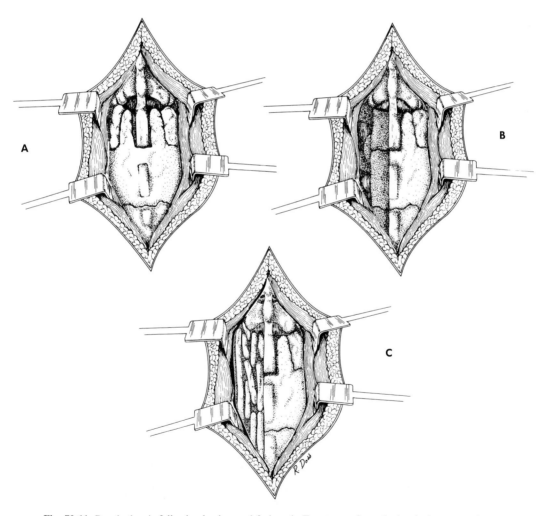

Fig. 70-11. Pseudarthrosis following lumbosacral fusion. **A,** Two types of pseudarthrosis shown: usual transverse type and type that occurs at end of clothespin graft. **B,** Pseudarthrosis repaired on one side only. Opposite half of fusion plate not exposed, being left intact for support. Transverse processes and articular facets exposed, and old fusion mass denuded. Pseudarthrosis cleaned out and packed with cancellous bone. **C,** Wide iliac strip graft placed vertically on transverse processes lateral to facets and in contact with them. Solid sheet of iliac strip grafts then carefully placed over fusion mass on one side only. (Redrawn from Cleveland, M., Bosworth, D.M., and Thompson, F.R.: J. Bone Joint Surg. **30-A:**302, 1948.)

bending roentgenograms, another attempt at repair is advised.

Posterolateral or intertransverse fusions

In 1948 Cleveland, Bosworth, and F.R. Thompson described a technique for repair of pseudarthrosis after spine fusion in which grafts are placed posteriorly on one side over the laminae, lateral margins of the articular facets, and base of the transverse processes (Fig. 70-11). In 1953, 1959, and 1964 Watkins described what he called a posterolateral fusion of the lumbar and lumbosacral spine in which the facets, pars interarticularis, and bases of the transverse processes are fused with chip grafts, and a large graft is placed posteriorly on the transverse processes. When the lumbosacral joint is included, the grafts extend to the posterior aspect of the first sacral segment.

We, like many others, use this operation and its modifications in patients with pseudarthrosis, laminal defects either congenital or surgical, or spondylolisthesis and in postlaminectomy patients with chronic pain of instability. The operation may be unilateral or bilateral, covering one or more joints depending on the stability of the area to be fused. The large instruments designed by McElroy (Fig. 70-12) are useful here.

TECHNIQUE (WATKINS). Make a longitudinal skin incision along the lateral border of the paraspinal muscles, curving it medially at the distal end across the posterior crest of the ilium (Fig. 70-13, *A*). Divide the lumbothoracic fascia and establish the plane of cleavage between the border of the paraspinal muscles and the fascia overlying the trans-

versus abdominis muscle. The tips of the transverse processes can now be palpated in the depths of the wound (Fig. 70-13, *B*). Release the iliac attachment of the muscles with an osteotome, taking a thin layer of ilium. Continue the exposure of the posterior crest of the ilium by subperiosteal dissection and remove the crest almost flush with the sacroiliac joint, taking enough bone to provide one or two grafts. Removal of the iliac crest increases exposure of the spine. Retract the sacrospinalis muscle toward the midline and denude the transverse processes of their dorsal muscle and ligamentous attachments; expose the articular facets by excising the joint capsule. Remove the cartilage from the facets with an osteotome, and level the area down to allow the graft to fit snugly against the facets, pars interarticularis, and base of the transverse process at each level. Comminute the facets with a small gouge or osteotome and turn bone chips up and down from the facet area, upper sacral area, and transverse processes. Now split the resected iliac crest longitudinally into two grafts. Shape one to fit into the prepared bed and impact it firmly in place with its cut surface against the spine (Fig. 70-13, *C*). Preserve the remaining graft for use on the opposite side with or without additional bone from the other iliac crest. Now pack additional ribbons and chips of cancellous bone from the ilium about the graft. Allow the paraspinal muscles to fall in position over the fusion area and close the wound.

AFTERTREATMENT. Aftertreatment is the same as for posterior arthrodesis (p. 3156). Fig. 70-14 shows an excellent result after posterolateral fusion for spondylolisthesis.

• • •

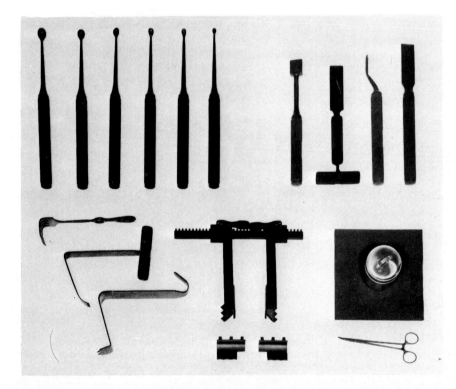

Fig. 70-12. McElroy black glareproof instruments for posterolateral fusion of spine. *Top,* curets and periosteal elevators. *Bottom,* retractors, self-retaining retractor, and container for bone grafts. (Courtesy Richards Medical Co., Memphis, Tenn.)

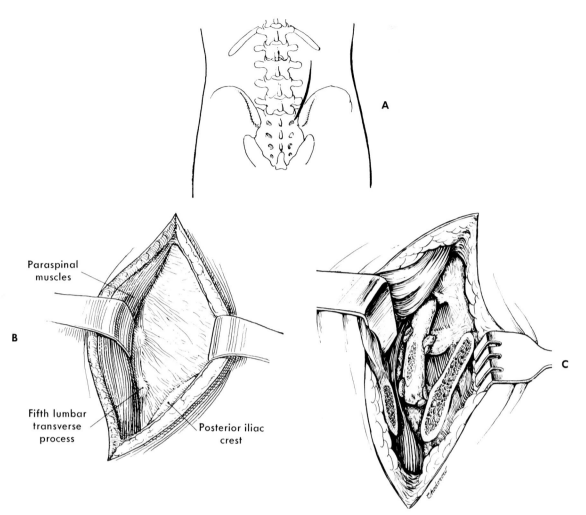

Paraspinal muscles

Fifth lumbar transverse process

Posterior iliac crest

Fig. 70-13. Watkins posterolateral fusion. **A,** Incision. **B,** Lumbothoracic fascia has been incised, paraspinal muscles have been retracted medially, and tips of transverse processes are now palpable. **C,** Split iliac crest and smaller grafts have been placed against spine. (**A** and **B** from Watkins, M.B.: J. Bone Joint Surg. **35-A:**1014, 1953; **C** from Watkins, M.B.: Clin. Orthop. **35:**80, 1964.)

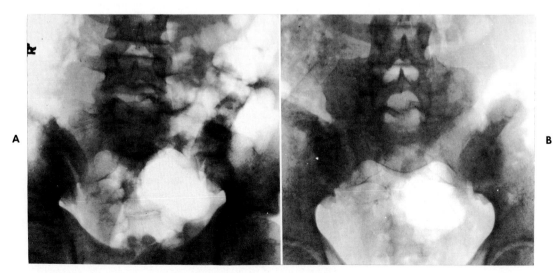

Fig. 70-14. Bilateral posterolateral fusion for moderate spondylolisthesis in 14-year-old boy. **A,** Before surgery. **B,** Solid fusion 17 months after surgery; all symptoms were relieved.

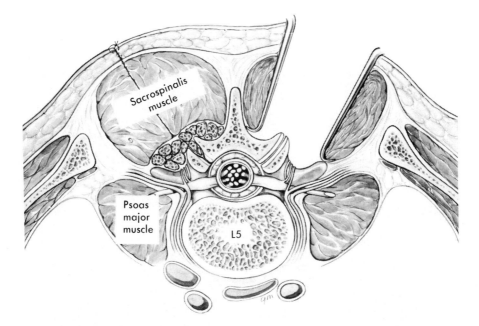

Fig. 70-15. Technique of posterolateral fusion in which sacrospinalis muscle is split longitudinally and laminae, articular facets, and transverse processes are all included in fusion. (Modified from Wiltse, L.L., et al.: J. Bone Joint Surg. **50-A:**921, 1968.)

Wiltse in 1961, Truchly and Thompson in 1962, Rombold in 1966, and Wiltse et al. in 1968 described modifications of the Watkins technique. The latter split the sacrospinalis muscle longitudinally and include the laminae as well as the articular facets and transverse processes in the fusion (Figs. 70-15 and 70-16). Some members of our staff combine a modified Hibbs fusion with a posterolateral fusion using a midline approach in routine lumbar and lumbosacral fusions (Fig. 70-17); they add many chip grafts obtained from the ilium. DePalma and Prabhakar also have combined posterior and posterolateral fusions.

Adkins has used an intertransverse or alartransverse fusion in which tibial grafts are inserted between the transverse processes of L4 and L5 and between that of L5 and the ala of the sacrum on one or both sides.

TECHNIQUE (ADKINS). Dissect the erector spinae muscles laterally from the pedicles, exposing the transverse processes and ala of the sacrum. This is easier when the facets have been removed, but if these are intact, exposure can be obtained without disturbing them. Cut a groove in the upper or lower border of each transverse process with a sharp gouge or forceps. Take care not to fracture the transverse process. In the ala of the sacrum first make parallel cuts in its posterosuperior border with an osteotome, then drive a gouge across the ends of these cuts, and lever the intervening bone out of the slot so made. For fusions of the fourth to the fifth lumbar vertebrae cut a tibial graft with V-shaped ends; insert it obliquely between the transverse processes and then rotate it into position so that it causes slight distraction of the processes and becomes firmly impacted between them. For the lumbosacral joint cut the graft V-shaped at its upper end and straight but slightly oblique at its lower end. Insert one arm of the V

in front of the transverse process and punch the lower end into the slot in the sacrum. If only one side is grafted, arrange the patient so that there is a slight convex curve of the spine on the operated side; thus firm impaction occurs when the spine is straightened. Bilateral grafts are preferred. The grafts should be placed as far laterally as possible to avoid the nerve roots and to gain maximum stability.

AFTERTREATMENT. Aftertreatment is the same as for posterior arthrodesis (p. 1356).

• • •

Bosworth has described a circumduction arthrodesis of the spine in which the fusion begins at the spine above the defect and extends laterally on ribs or transverse processes and returns to the spine below the defect. Some of his patients required multiple procedures, but effective immobilization was obtained in patients with posterior midline infection or who had had wide laminectomy and facetectomy. The reader is referred to his works for details of technique.

Anterior arthrodesis

Sacks, Wiltberger, Harmon, Hoover, Hodgson and Wong, and others have arthrodesed the lumbar and lumbosacral areas anteriorly for spondylolisthesis, deranged intervertebral discs, and other affections. Except in tuberculosis, tumors, kyphosis, scoliosis, or some problem such as a difficult, failed posterior arthrodesis or gross instability after extensive laminectomy, we rarely arthrodese the dorsal and lumbar areas in this manner. The approaches and techniques used in tuberculosis by Hodgson et al. (p. 3333) should be applicable in most instances.

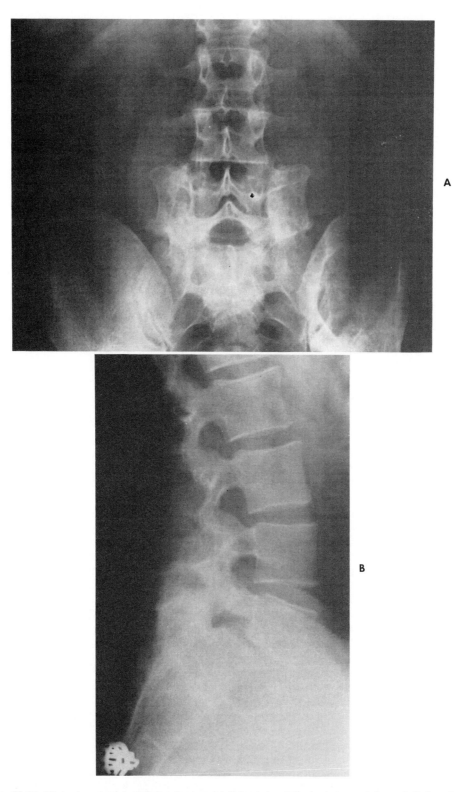

Fig. 70-16. Bilateral posterolateral fusion for spondylolisthesis in adult. **A,** Anteroposterior and, **B,** lateral roentgenograms 6 months after surgery.

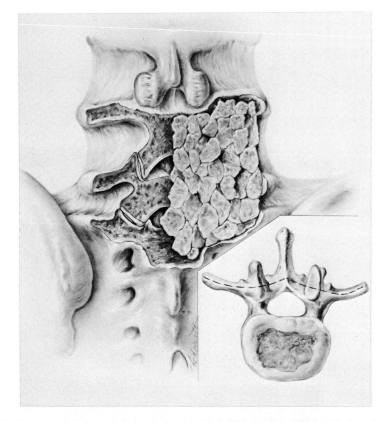

Fig. 70-17. Slocum technique combining posterior (modified Hibbs) and posterolateral fusions. Midline incision is used. *Inset,* All bone posterior to *broken line* is removed. (From Wiltse, L.L.: Clin. Orthop. **21:**156, 1961.)

ANTERIOR DISC EXCISION AND INTERBODY FUSION

The rationale of management of lower back pain must depend on accurate diagnosis. The pain syndromes in this area are many, and diagnostic pitfalls are ever present. Treatment varies according to the physical and emotional profile of the patient and the experience of the surgeon involved. Hemilaminectomy and decompression of nerve roots still constitute the most widely used surgical procedure for unremitting lower back pain. With continued instability of the anterior and posterior elements, supplemental posterior or posterolateral fusion usually proves satisfactory. Rothman has found only a 5% decrease in residual back pain and sciatica when disc excision is combined with spinal fusion, but this was not statistically significant. There was also no difference in postoperative evaluation between patients with solid fusion and those with pseudarthrosis.

There remains a group of patients for whom the aforementioned standard surgical procedures have been unsuccessful. R.N. Stauffer and Coventry have emphasized the causes of persistent symptoms following disc surgery:

1. Mistaken original diagnosis
2. Recurrent herniation of disc material (incomplete removal)
3. Herniation of disc at another level
4. Bony compression of nerve root
5. Perineural adhesions
6. Instability of vertebral segments
7. Psychoneurosis

In this group improved diagnostic accuracy can be obtained with the use of electromyography, a repeat myelogram, or discography and a psychologic profile assessment. Finally, differential spinal anesthesia is helpful in discriminating between the various types of pain. Computerized tomographic scanning adds an exciting new tool in the assessment of these patients.

Only following failure of the usual posterior methods does anterior intervertebral disc excision and interbody spinal fusion find primary use. Goldner et al. used this criterion and found moderate or complete relief of lower back pain in 78% of patients and complete or moderate relief of lower extremity pain in 85%; no patients had pain worse than before surgery. The Mayo Clinic, on the other hand, reported an overall satisfactory result of 36%, the difference attributed chiefly to interpretation of clinical factors and patient type. They also recommended its use primarily as a salvage procedure.

Sacks, polling 15 surgeons in nine different countries, found variations of opinion, no adequate follow-up, and therefore inconclusive long-term results. Conversely, Freebody et al. have performed 466 operations, the first 243 (1956 to 1967) showing 90% satisfactory results. Their indications include (1) instability causing backache and sciatica, (2) spondylolisthesis of all types, (3) pain following

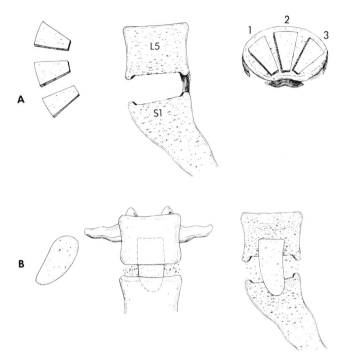

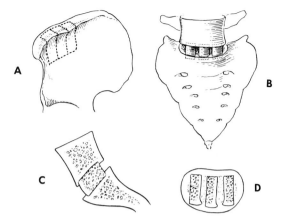

Fig. 70-19. Technique of Goldner et al. for anterior interbody fusion of lumbosacral joint. (From Goldner, J.L., et al.: Orthop. Clin. North Am. **2**:543, 1971.)

Fig. 70-18. Freebody technique for anterior interbody fusion in lower lumbar spine. **A,** Technique for degenerative disease. **B,** Technique for spondylolisthesis. (From Sacks, S.: Orthop. Clin. North Am. **6**:272, 1975.)

multiple posterior explorations, and (4) failed posterior fusions. They use three iliac wedge grafts for degenerative disease and a block graft for spondylolisthesis (Fig. 70-18).

Flynn and Hoque in Florida, Fujimake, Crock, and Bedbrook in Australia, and van Rens and van Horn in the Netherlands have reported a total of 435 patients on whom anterior interbody fusion was done. Flynn and Hoque and van Rens and van Horn had no male patients with retrograde ejaculation and both suggested that the incidence of this complication may be exaggerated.

TECHNIQUE (GOLDNER ET AL.). Administer general anesthesia and place the patient in the Trendelenburg position. Develop the retroperitoneal approach to the vertebral bodies and identify the psoas muscle, the iliac artery and vein, and the left ureter. If more than three interspaces are to be fused, retract the ureter toward the left. Identify the sacral promontory by palpation. Inject saline solution under the prevertebral fascia over the lumbar vertebra and lift the sympathetic chain for easier dissection. Expose the lumbosacral disc space by retracting the left iliac artery and vein to the left. In exposure of the fourth lumbar interspace, displace the left artery and vein and ureter to the right side. Elevate the anterior longitudinal ligament as a flap with the base toward the left. Tag the flap with sutures and retract it to give additional protection to the vessels. Separate the intervertebral disc and anulus from the cartilaginous end plates of the vertebrae with a thin osteotome and remove them with pituitary rongeurs and large curets. Clean the space thoroughly back to the posterior longitudinal ligament without removing bone, thereby keeping

bleeding to a minimum until the site is ready for grafting. Finally remove the end plates from the vertebral bodies with an osteotome until bleeding bone is encountered. Cut shallow notches in the opposing surfaces of the vertebrae and measure the dimensions of the notchs carefully with a caliper. Cut grafts from the iliac wing, making them larger than the notchs for later firm impaction (Fig. 70-19). Hyperextend the spin, insert multiple grafts, and relieve the hyperextension. Electrocautery is useful in obtaining hemostasis, but take care not to coagulate the sympathetic fibers over the anterior aspect of the lumbosacral joint. Use of silver clips in this area is preferred. After completion of the fusion, close all layers with absorbable sutures. Estimate the amount of blood lost and replace it.

AFTERTREATMENT. Nasogastric suction may be necessary for gastric decompression for about 36 hours. Attention must be paid to mobilization of the lower extremities to prevent dependency and blood pooling. In-bed exercises with straight leg raising are started on the third postoperative day and continued indefinitely. By the fifth postoperative day the patient is allowed to sit and walk with a low back corset used for postoperative immobilization. Postoperative roentgenograms are made before discharge from the hospital to serve as a baseline for judging graft appearance. Three months later flexion and extension roentgenograms are made in the standing position to provide information about the success of arthrodesis. Roentgenograms are then repeated at 6 and 12 months after surgery, with the solid fusion not confirmed until 1 year after surgery. Laminagrams may be useful in evaluating suspected pseudarthrosis.

REFERENCES
Arthrodesis

Adkins, E.W.O.: Lumbo-sacral arthrodesis after laminectomy, J. Bone Joint Surg. **37-B**:208, 1955.

Albee, F.H.: Transplantation of a portion of the tibia into the spine for Pott's disease: a preliminary report, JAMA **57**:885, 1911.

Albee, F.H.: A report of bone transplantation and osteoplasty in the treatment of Pott's disease of spine, NY Med. J. **95**:469, 1912.

Allison, N.: Fusion of the spinal column, Surg. Gynecol. Obstet. **46**:826, 1928.

Aronson, N., Bagan, M., and Feltzer, D.L.: Results of using the Smith-Robinson approach for herniated and extruded cervical discs. J. Neurosurg. **32:**721, 1970.

Aronson, N., Feltzer, D.L., and Bagan, M.: Anterior fusion by Smith-Robinson approach, J. Neurosurg. **29:**397, 1968.

Bailey, R.W., and Badgley, C.E.: Stabilization of the cervical spine by anterior fusion, J. Bone Joint Surg. **42-A:**565, 1960.

Baker, L.D., and Hoyt, W.A., Jr.: The use of interfacet Vitallium screws in the Hibbs fusion, South. Med. J. **41:**419, 1948.

Barr, J.S.: Pseudarthrosis in the lumbosacral spine (discussion of paper by Cleveland, M., Bosworth, D.M., and Thompson, F.R., J. Bone Joint Surg. **30-A:**302, 1948), J. Bone Joint Surg. **30-A:**311, 1948.

Beller, H.E., and Kirsh, D.: Spondylolysis and spondylolisthesis following low back fusions, South. Med. J. **57:**783, 1964.

Bloom, M.H., and Raney, F.L., Jr.: Anterior intervertebral fusion of the cervical spine: a technical note, J. Bone Joint Surg. **63-A:**842, 1981.

Bosworth, D.M.: Clothespin graft of the spine for spondylolisthesis and laminal defects, Am. J. Surg. **67:**61, 1945.

Bosworth, D.M.: Techniques of spinal fusion: pseudarthrosis and method of repair. In American Academy of Orthopaedic Surgeons: Instructional course lectures, vol. 5, Ann Arbor, 1948, J.W. Edwards.

Bosworth, D.M.: Technique of spinal fusion in the lumbosacral region by the double clothespin graft (distraction graft; ''H'' graft) and results. In American Academy of Orthopaedic Surgeons: Instructional course lectures, vol. 9, Ann Arbor, 1952, J.W. Edwards.

Bosworth, D.M.: Circumduction fusion of the spine, J. Bone Joint Surg. **38-A:**263, 1956.

Bosworth, D.M.: Surgery of the spine. In American Academy of Orthopaedic Surgeons: Instructional course lectures, vol. 14, Ann Arbor, 1957, J.W. Edwards.

Bosworth, D.M., Wright, H.A., Fielding, J.W., and Goodrich, E.R.: A study in the use of bank bone for spine fusion in tuberculosis, J. Bone Joint Surg. **35-A:**329, 1953.

Boucher, H.H.: A method of spinal fusion, J. Bone Joint Surg. **41-B:**248, 1959.

Breck, L.W., and Basom, W.C.: The flexion treatment for low-back pain: indications, outline of conservative management, and a new spine-fusion procedure, J. Bone Joint Surg. **25:**58, 1943.

Briggs, J.R., and Freehafer, A.A.: Fusion of the Charcot spine: report of 3 cases, Clin. Orthop. **53:**83, 1967.

Brooks, A.L., and Jenkins, E.B.: Atlanto-axial arthrodesis by the wedge compression method, J. Bone Joint Surg. **60-A:**279, 1978.

Callahan, R.A., et al.: Cervical facet fusion for control of instability following laminectomy, J. Bone Joint Surg. **59-A:**991, 1977.

Campbell, W.C.: Operative measures in the treatment of affections of the lumbosacral and sacroiliac articulation, Surg. Gynecol. Obstet. **51:**381, 1930.

Cattell, H.S., and Clark, G.L., Jr.: Cervical kyphosis and instability following multiple laminectomies in children, J. Bone Joint Surg. **49-A:**713, 1967.

Cleveland, M.: Technique of spine fusion for tuberculosis involving vertebrae. In American Academy of Orthopaedic Surgeons: Instructional course lectures, vol. 9, Ann Arbor, 1952, J.W. Edwards.

Cleveland, M., Bosworth, D.M., and Thompson, F.R.: Pseudarthrosis in the lumbosacral spine, J. Bone Joint Surg. **30-A:**302, 1948.

Cleveland, M., Bosworth, D.M., Fielding, J.W., and Smyrnis, P.: Fusion of the spine for tuberculosis in children: a long-range follow-up study, J. Bone Joint Surg. **40-A:**91, 1958.

Cloward, R.B.: The treatment of ruptured lumbar intervertebral discs by vertebral body fusion: I. Indications, operative technique, after care, J. Neurosurg. **10:**154, 1953.

Cloward, R.B.: Vertebral body fusion for ruptured cervical discs: description of instruments and operative technic, Am. J. Surg. **98:**722, 1959.

Cloward, R.B.: Lesions of the intervertebral disks and their treatment by interbody fusion methods: the painful disk, Clin. Orthop. **27:**51, 1963.

Cobb, J.R.: Technique, after-treatment, and results of spine fusion for scoliosis. In American Academy of Orthopaedic Surgeons: Instructional course lectures, vol. 9, Ann Arbor, 1952, J.W. Edwards.

Connor, A.C., Rooney, J.A., and Carroll, J.P.: Anterior lumbar fusion: a technique combining intervertebral and intravertebral body fixation, Surg. Clin. North Am. **47:**231, 1967.

Crock, H.V.: Observations on the management of failed spinal operations, J. Bone Joint Surg. **58-B:**193, 1976.

Curran, J.P., and McGaw, W.H.: Posterolateral spinal fusion with pedicle grafts, Clin. Orthop. **59:**125, 1968.

de Andrade, J.R., and Macnab, I.: Anterior occipito-cervical fusion using an extra-pharyngeal exposure, J. Bone Joint Surg. **51-A:**1621, 1969.

DePalma, A.F., and Prabhakar, M.: Posterior-posterobilateral fusion of the lumbosacral spine, Clin. Orthop. **47:**165, 1966.

DePalma, A.F., and Rothman, R.H.: The nature of pseudarthrosis, Clin. Orthop. **59:**113, 1968.

DePalma, A.F., and Rothman, R.H.: The intervertebral disc, Philadelphia, 1970, W.B. Saunders Co.

DePalma, A.F., Rothman, R.H., Lewinnek, G.E., and Canale, S.T.: Anterior interbody fusion for severe cervical disc degeneration, Surg. Gynecol. Obstet. **134:**755, 1972.

Dereymacker, A., and Mulier, J.: La fusion vertebrale par voie ventrale dans la discopathie cervicale, Rev. Neurol. **19:**597, 1958.

Dommisse, G.F.: Lumbo-sacral interbody spinal fusion, J. Bone Joint Surg. **41-B:**87, 1959.

Dunn, E.J.: Techniques of fusion in treatment of fractures and dislocations of cervical spine, Orthop. Rev. **2:**17, April 1973.

Enneking, W.F., Burchardt, H., Puhl, J., and Protrowski, G.: Physical and biological aspects of repair in dog cortical-bone transplants, J. Bone Joint Surg. **57-A:**237, 1975.

Fang, H.S.Y., Ong, G.B., and Hodgson, A.R.: Anterior spinal fusion, the operative approaches, Clin. Orthop. **35:**16, 1964.

Fielding, J.W., Hawkins, R.J., and Ratzan, S.A.: Spine fusion for atlanto-axial instability, J. Bone Joint Surg. **58-A:**400, 1976.

Fielding, J.W., Lusskin, R., and Batista, A.: Multiple segment anterior cervical spinal fusion, Clin. Orthop. **54:**29, 1967.

Flesch, J.R., Leider, L.L., Erickson, D.L., Chou, S.N., and Bradford, D.S.: Harrington instrumentation and spine fusion for unstable fractures and fracture-dislocations of the thoracic and lumbar spine, J. Bone Joint Surg. **59-A:**143, 1977.

Flynn, J.C., and Hoque, A.: Anterior fusion of the lumbar spine: end-result study with long-term follow-up, J. Bone Joint Surg. **61-A:**1143, 1979.

Freebody, D., Bendall, R., and Taylor, R.D.: Anterior transperitoneal lumbar fusion, J. Bone Joint Surg. **53-B:**617, 1971.

Fujimake, A., Crock, H.V., and Bedbrook, G.M.: The results of 150 anterior lumbar interbody fusion operations performed by two surgeons in Australia, Clin. Orthop. **165:**164, 1982.

Gibson, A.: A modified technique for spinal fusion, Surg. Gynecol. Obstet. **53:**365, 1931.

Goldner, J.L., Urbaniak, J.R., and McCollum, D.E.: Anterior disc excision and interbody spinal fusion for chronic low back pain, Orthop. Clin. North Am. **2:**543, 1971.

Green, P.W.B.: Anterior cervical fusion: a review of thirty-three patients with cervical disc degeneration, J. Bone Joint Surg. **59-B:**236, 1977.

Griswold, D.M., Albright, J.A., Schiffman, E., Johnson, R., and Southwick, W.O.: Atlanto-axial fusion for instability, J. Bone Joint Surg. **60-A:**285, 1978.

Hallock, H., Francis, K.C., and Jones, J.B.: Spine fusion in young children: a long-term end-result study with particular reference to growth effects, J. Bone Joint Surg. **39-A:**481, 1957.

Hallock, H., and Jones, J.B.: Tuberculosis of the spine: an end-result study of the effects of the spine fusion operation in a large number of patients, J. Bone Joint Surg. **36-A:**219, 1954.

Harmon, P.H.: Subtotal anterior lumbar disc excision and vertebral body fusion: III. Application to complicated and recurrent multilevel degenerations, Am. J. Surg. **97:**649, 1959.

Harmon, P.H.: Anterior extraperitoneal lumbar disc excision and vertebral body fusion, Clin. Orthop. **18:**169, 1960.

Harmon, P.H.: Anterior excision and vertebral body fusion operation for intervertebral disk syndromes of the lower lumbar spine: three-to-five-year results in 244 cases, Clin. Orthop. **26:**107, 1963.

Henderson, M.S.: Operative fusion for tuberculosis of the spine, JAMA **92:**45, 1929.

Henry, M.O., and Geist, E.S.: Spinal fusion by simplified technique, J. Bone Joint Surg. **15:**622, 1933.

Hibbs, R.A.: An operation for progressive spinal deformities, NY Med. J. **93:**1013, 1911.

Hibbs, R.A.: A further consideration of an operation for Pott's disease of the spine, Ann. Surg. **55:**682, 1912.

Hibbs, R.A.: An operation for Pott's disease of the spine, JAMA **59:**133, 1912.

Hibbs, R.A., and Risser, J.C.: Treatment of vertebral tuberculosis by the spine fusion operation: a report of 286 cases, J. Bone Joint Surg. **10:**805, 1928.

Hodgson, A.R., and Wong, S.K.: A description of a technic and evaluation of results in anterior spinal fusion for deranged intervertebral disk and spondylolisthesis, Clin. Orthop. **56:**133, 1968.

Hoover, N.W.: Methods of lumbar fusion, J. Bone Joint Surg. **50-A:**194, 1968.

Howorth, M.B.: Evolution of spinal fusion, Ann. Surg. **117:**278, 1943.

Jaslow, I.A.: Intercorporal bone graft in spinal fusion after disc removal, Surg. Gynecol. Obstet. **82:**215, 1946.

Johnson, J.T.H., and Robinson, R.A.: Anterior strut grafts for severe kyphosis: results of 3 cases with a preceding progressive paraplegia, Clin. Orthop. **56:**25, 1968.

Johnson, J.T., and Southwick, W.O.: Bone growth after spine fusion: a clinical survey, J. Bone Joint Surg. **42-A:**1396, 1960.

Kestler, O.C.: Overgrowth (hypertrophy) of lumbosacral grafts, causing a complete block, Bull. Hosp. Joint Dis. **27:**51, 1966.

King, D.: Internal fixation for lumbosacral fusion, Am. J. Surg. **66:**357, 1944.

Kite, J.H.: Nonoperative versus operative treatment of tuberculosis of the spine in children: review of 50 consecutive cases treated by each method, South. Med. J. **26:**918, 1933.

Kraus, D.R., and Stauffer, E.S.: Spinal cord injury as a complication of elective anterior cervical fusion, Clin. Orthop. **112:**130, 1975.

Macnab, I.: The blood supply of the lumbar spine and its application to the technique of intertransverse lumbar fusion, J. Bone Joint Surg. **53-B:**628, 1971.

Macnab, I.: Complications of anterior cervical fusion, Orthop. Rev. **1:**29, September 1972.

McBride, E.D.: A mortised transfacet bone block for lumbosacral fusion, J. Bone Joint Surg. **31-A:**385, 1949.

McBride, E.D., and Shorbe, H.B.: Lumbosacral fusion: the mortised transfacet method by use of the vibrating electric saw for circular bone blocks, Clin. Orthop. **12:**268, 1958.

Mercer, W.: Spondylolisthesis: with a description of a new method of operative treatment and notes of ten cases, Edinburgh Med. J. **43:**545, 1936.

Moore, A.T.: The unstable spine: discogenetic syndrome treatment with self-locking prop bone graft, Int. Surg. **8:**64, 1945; correction **8:**179, 1945.

Moore, A.T.: Multiprop and interbody spinal fusion, Spectator Letter (mimeographed), September 1959.

Newman, P.H.: Surgical treatment for derangement of the lumbar spine, J. Bone Joint Surg. **55-B:**7, 1973.

Norrell, H., and Wilson, C.B.: Early anterior fusion for injuries of the cervical portion of the spine, JAMA **214:**525, 1970.

Nugent, G.R.: Clinicopathologic correlations in cervical spondylosis, Neurology (Minneap.) **9:**273, 1959.

Overton, L.M.: An improved technic for arthrodesis of the lumbosacral spine, Am. J. Surg. **80:**559, 1950.

Overton, L.M.: Arthrodesis of the lumbosacral spine, Clin. Orthop. **5:**97, 1955.

Overton, L.M.: Lumbosacral arthrodesis: an evaluation of its present status, Am. Surg. **25:**771, 1959.

Pennal, G.F., McDonald, G.A., and Dale, G.G.: A method of spinal fusion using internal fixation, Clin. Orthop. **35:**86, 1964.

Petter, C.K.: Rib-splinter graft in spinal fusion for vertebral tuberculosis, J. Bone Joint Surg. **19:**413, 1937.

Pierce, D.S.: Long-term management of thoracolumbar fractures and fracture dislocations. In American Academy of Orthopaedic Surgeons: Instructional course lectures, vol. 21, St. Louis, 1972, The C.V. Mosby Co.

Prothero, S.R., Parkes, J.C., and Stinchfield, F.E.: Complications after low-back fusion in 1000 patients: a comparison of two series one decade apart, J. Bone Joint Surg. **48-A:**57, 1966.

Ralston, E.L., and Thompson, W.A.L.: The diagnosis and repair of pseudarthrosis of the spine, Surg. Gynecol. Obstet. **89:**37, 1949.

Regen, E.M.: Pseudarthrosis in the lumbosacral spine (discussion of paper by Cleveland, M., Bosworth, D.M., and Thompson, F.R., J. Bone Joint Surg. **30-A:**302, 1948), J. Bone Joint Surg. **30-A:**311, 1948.

Rennie, W., and Mitchell, N.: Flexion distraction fractures of the thoracolumbar spine, J. Bone Joint Surgery. **55-A:**386, 1973.

Riley, L.H., Jr.: Cervical disc surgery: its role and indications, Orthop. Clin. North Am. **2:**443, 1971.

Roaf, R., Kirkaldy-Willis, W.H., and Cathro, A.J.M.: Surgical treatment of bone and joint tuberculosis, Edinburgh, 1959, E. & S. Livingstone, Ltd.

Robinson, R.A.: Anterior and posterior cervical spine fusions, Clin. Orthop. **35:**34, 1964.

Robinson, R.A., and Smith, G.W.: Anterolateral cervical disc removal and interbody fusion for cervical disc syndrome (abstract), Bull. Johns Hopkins Hosp. **96:**223, 1955.

Robinson, R.A., Walker, E.A., Ferlic, D.C., and Wiecking, D.K.: The results of anterior interbody fusion of the cervical spine, J. Bone Joint Surg. **44-A:**1569, 1962.

Rombold, C.: Treatment of spondylolisthesis by posterolateral fusion, resection of the pars interarticularis, and prompt mobilization of the patient: an end-result study of seventy-three patients, J. Bone Joint Surg. **48-A:**1282, 1966.

Rothman, R.H.: New developments in lumbar disk surgery, Orthop. Rev. **4:**23, March 1975.

Rothman, R.H., and Booth, R.: Failures of spinal fusion, Orthop. Clin. North Am. **6:**299, 1975.

Roy, L., and Gibson, D.A.: Cervical spine fusions in children, Clin. Orthop. **73:**146, 1970.

Sacks, S.: Anterior interbody fusion of the lumbar spine, J. Bone Joint Surg. **47-B:**211, 1965.

Sacks, S.: Anterior interbody fusion of the lumbar spine: indications and results in 200 cases, Clin. Orthop. **44:**163, 1966.

Sacks, S.: Present status of anterior interbody fusion in the lower lumbar spine, Orthop. Clin. North Am. **6:**275, 1975.

Schmidt, A.C., Flatley, T.J., and Place, J.S.: Lumbar fusion using facet inlay grafts, South. Med. J. **68:**209, 1975.

Sim, F.H., Svien, H.J., Bickel, W.H., and Janes, J.M.: Swan-neck deformity following extensive cervical laminectomy: a review of twenty-one cases, J. Bone Joint Surg. **56-A:**564, 1974.

Simeone, F.A.: The modern treatment of thoracic disc disease, Orthop. Clin. North Am. **2:**453, 1971.

Simmons, E.H., and Bhalla, S.K., and Butt, W.P.: Anterior cervical discectomy and fusion: a clinical and biomechanical study with eight-year follow-up, J. Bone Joint Surg. **51-B:**225, 1969.

Smith, A.D.: Lumbosacral fusion by the Hibbs technique. In American Academy of Orthopaedic Surgeons: Instructional course lectures, vol. 9, Ann Arbor, 1952, J.W. Edwards.

Smith, A.D.: Tuberculosis of the spine: results in 70 cases treated at the New York Orthopaedic Hospital from 1945 to 1960, Clin. Orthop. **58:**171, 1968.

Smith, G.W., and Robinson, R.A.: The treatment of certain cervical-spine disorders by anterior removal of the intervertebral disc and interbody fusion, J. Bone Joint Surg. **40-A:**607, 1958.

Sorrel, E.: The indications for, and results of, osteosynthesis in the treatment of Pott's disease, Int. Abstr. Surg. **50:**357, 1930. (Abstracted from J. Chir. **34:**439, 1929.)

Speed, K.: Spondylolisthesis: treatment by anterior bone graft, Arch. Surg. **37:**175, 1938.

Stauffer, R.N., and Coventry, M.B.: A rational approach to failures of lumbar disc surgery: the orthopedist's approach, Orthop. Clin. North Am. **2:**533, 1971.

Stauffer, R.N., and Coventry, M.B.: Anterior interbody lumbar spine fusion: analysis of Mayo Clinic Series, J. Bone Joint Surg. **54-A:**756, 1972.

Stauffer, R.N., and Coventry, M.B.: Posterolateral lumbar-spine fusion: analysis of Mayo Clinic series, J. Bone Joint Surg. **54-A:**1195, 1972.

Stinchfield, F.E., and Sinton, W.A.: Criteria for spine fusion with use of "H" bone graft following disc removal: results in 100 cases, Arch. Surg. **65:**542, 1952.

Thompson, W.A.L., and Ralson, E.L.: Pseudarthrosis following spine fusion, J. Bone Joint Surg. **31-A:**400, 1949.

Toumey, J.W.: Internal fixation in fusion of the lumbosacral joint. Lahey Clin. Bull. **3:**188, 1943.

Truchly, G., and Thompson, W.A.L.: Posterolateral fusion of the lumbosacral spine, J. Bone Joint Surg. **44-A:**505, 1962.

van Rens, Th.J.G., and van Horn, J.R.: Long-term results in lumbosacral interbody fusion for spondylolisthesis, Acta Orthop. Scand. **53:**383, 1982.

Verbiest, H.: Anterolateral operations for fractures and dislocations in the middle and lower parts of the cervical spine: report of a series of forty-seven cases, J. Bone Joint Surg. **51-A:**1489, 1969.

Wagoner, G.: A technique for lessening hemorrhage in operations on the spine, J. Bone Joint Surg. **19**:469, 1937.

Watkins, M.B.: Posterolateral fusion of the lumbar and lumbosacral spine, J. Bone Joint Surg. **35-A**:1004, 1953.

Watkins, M.B.: Posterolateral bone-grafting for fusion of the lumbar and lumbosacral spine, J. Bone Joint Surg. **41-A**:388, 1959.

Watkins, M.B.: Posterolateral fusion in pseudarthrosis and posterior element defects of the lumbosacral spine, Clin. Orthop. **35**:80, 1964.

Webb, J.K., et al: Hidden flexion injury of the cervical spine, J. Bone Joint Surg. **58-B**:322, 1976.

Weiss, M.: Dynamic spine alloplasty (spring-loading corrective devices) after fracture and spinal cord injury, Clin. Orthop. **112**:150, 1975.

Weiss, M., and Bentkowski, Z.: Biomechanical study in dynamic spondylodesis of the spine, Clin. Orthop. **103**:199, 1974.

White, A.A., III, and Hirsch, C.: An experimental study of the immediate load bearing capacity of some commonly used iliac bone grafts, Acta Orthop. Scand. **42**:482, 1971.

White, A.A., III, Southwich, W.O., Deponte, R.J., Gainor, J.W., and Hardy, R.: Relief of pain by anterior cervical-spine fusion for spondylosis: a report of sixty-five patients, J. Bone Joint Surg. **55-A**:525, 1973.

White, A.A., III, et al.: An experimental study of the immediate load bearing capacity of three surgical constructions for anterior spine fusions, Clin. Orthop. **91**:21, 1973.

Whitecloud, T.S., III, and LaRocca, H.: Fibular strut graft in reconstructive surgery of the cervical spine, Spine **1**:33, 1976.

Whitehill, R., Sirna, E.C., Young, D.C., and Cantrell, R.W.: Late esophageal perforation from an autogenous bone graft: report of a case, J. Bone Joint Surg. **67-A**:644, 1985.

Williams, J.L., Allen, M.B., Jr., and Harkess, J.W.: Late results of cervical discectomy and interbody fusion: some factors influencing the results, J.Bone Joint Surg. **50-A**:277, 1968.

Williams, P.C.: Lesions of the lumbosacral spine: chronic traumatic (postural) destruction of the lumbosacral intervertebral disc, J. Bone Joint Surg. **19**:690, 1937.

Wilson, P.D., and Straub, L.R.: Lumbosacral fusion with metallic plate fixation. In American Academy of Orthopaedic Surgeons: Instructional course lectures, vol. 9, Ann Arbor, 1952, J.W.Edwards.

Wiltberger, B.R.: The dowel intervertebral-body fusion as used in lumbar-disc surgery, J. Bone Joint Surg. **39-A**:284, 1957.

Wiltberger, B.R.: Intervertebral body fusion by the use of posterior bone dowel, Clin. Orthop. **35**:69, 1964.

Wiltse, L.L.: Spondylolisthesis in children, Clin. Orthop. **21**:156, 1961.

Wiltse, L.L., Bateman, J.G., Hutchinson, R.H., and Nelson, W.E.: The paraspinal sacrospinalis-splitting approach to the lumbar spine, J. Bone Joint Surg. **50-A**:919, 1968.

Young, M.H.: Long-term consequences of stable fractures of the thoracic and lumbar vertebral bodies, J. Bone Joint Surg. **55-B**:295, 1973.

Yosipovitch, Z., Robin, G.C., and Makin, M.: Open reduction of unstable thoracolumbar spinal injuries and fixation with Harrington rods, J. Bone Joint Surg. **59-A**:1003, 1977.

CHAPTER 71

Scoliosis

Allen S. Edmonson

Scoliosis is a lateral curvature of the spine. Structural curves are those in which lateral bending of the spine is asymmetric or the involved vertebrae are fixed in a rotated position, or both. These, then, are curves that the patient either cannot correct or can but cannot keep corrected. Lateral bending is asymmetric when the long gentle curve formed by the entire spine on bending to each side is asymmetric in some way, either in regard to the areas that bend or to the degree of bending (Fig. 71-1). Nonstructural curves, in contrast, are those in which intrinsic changes in the spine or its supporting structures are absent. In these curves, then, lateral bending is symmetric and the involved vertebrae are not fixed in a rotated position. Generally a nonstructural curve requires no treatment or any necessary treatment is directed toward its cause, which is not located in the spine itself.

According to its cause, scoliosis is of two main types: (1) that of unknown cause, idiopathic, and (2) that of known cause. Several geneologic studies with emphasis on heredity or genetic transmission of scoliosis made in both Great Britain and the United States support the hypothesis that idiopathic scoliosis is genetic with a mode of inheritance that is complex. Recent studies suggest a neurologic developmental delay in the brain stem. In about 75% to 80% of patients scoliosis is idiopathic. In the remainder it is caused by such conditions as congenital skeletal abnormalities, both vertebral and extravertebral, neuromuscular diseases, neurofibromatosis, arthrogryposis, trauma, irritative phenomena caused by nerve root compression or spinal cord tumors, and miscellaneous affections. Obviously the prognosis and treatment of scoliosis vary with the cause.

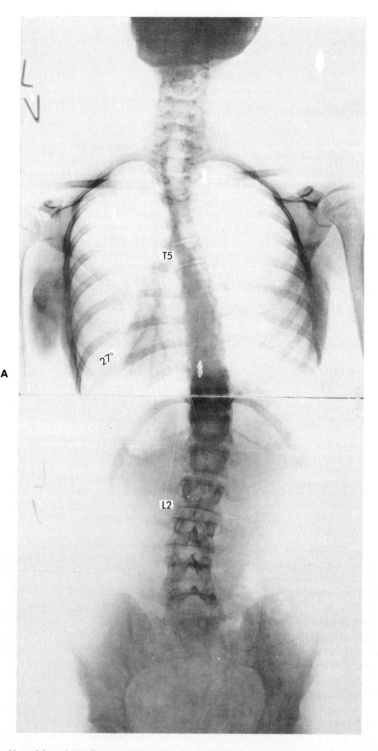

Fig. 71-1. Use of lateral bending roentgenograms to determine whether curve is structural (primary). **A,** Idiopathic thoracolumbar curve in girl 14 years of age, extending from T5 through L2 and measuring 27 degrees while standing. Rotation is minimal.

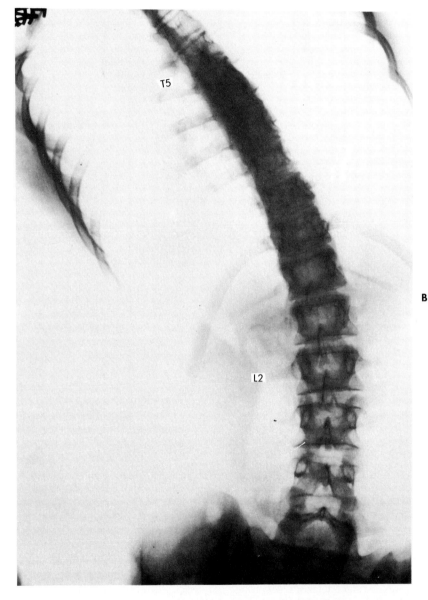

Fig. 71-1, cont'd. B, On bending to left there is long smooth continuous curve from T1 through L5.

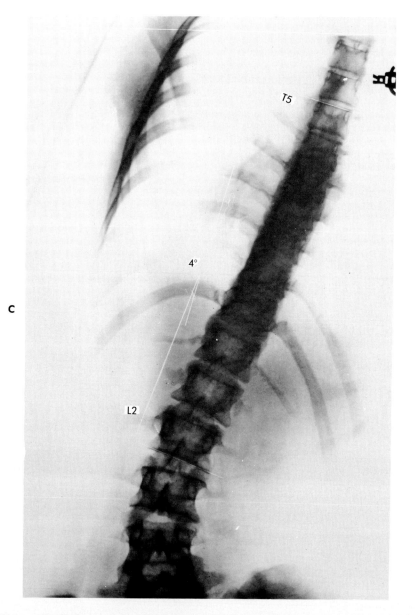

Fig. 71-1, cont'd. C, On bending to right there is a residual curve of 4 degrees. Therefore lateral bending is asymmetric. Use of lateral bending roentgenograms is most reliable way of demonstrating whether scoliotic curves are structural.

IDIOPATHIC SCOLIOSIS

Idiopathic scoliosis is the most common of all types and is divided into infantile, juvenile, and adolescent according to the age of the patient when it is first diagnosed. The last group is our largest responsibility, and the infantile form is rarer here than in Europe. Research and the accumulation of more clinical information now make it more than probable that scoliosis is a genetic disease. The inheritance pattern has not been established, but studies have confirmed the long suspected fact that many of the predecessors of patients with scoliosis seeking treatment have had unrecognized scoliosis. Just how the variation in the age of onset of the curve (any time from infancy to adolescence) can be explained genetically is another problem under study. Metabolic abnormalities have not been discovered in the many studies of children with scoliosis. Vanderpool, James, and Wynne-Davies of Edinburgh studied scoliosis developing in patients over 50 years of age and attributed it to metabolic diseases such as osteoporosis and osteomalacia; scoliosis of this type is in no way related to idiopathic scoliosis of childhood. Enneking and Harrington in studying several hundred specimens of articular processes in normal and scoliotic children found that impaired chondrogenesis, premature cessation of osteogenesis, increased subchondral maturation, and degenerative changes in the articular surfaces were not related to the severity of the deformity and were seen more often on the convex side of the curve rather than on the concave side. They concluded that the deformities seen in the posterior elements of the spine in scoliosis are not caused by asymmetric enchondral growth; furthermore, they postulated that idiopathic scoliosis is produced by an extraosseous cause and that the changes in bone and cartilage are secondary adaptations. It seems apparent at present that while the exact mechanism of the production of the curves is unknown, idiopathic scoliosis is most likely of genetic origin.

Routine evaluation of schoolchildren aged 10 to 14 years has shown an incidence of scoliosis of up to 12% with the incidence lower in most evaluations. Most of these patients have small curves (under 15 degrees), and at a younger age the incidence is equal in boys and girls. Beyond 10 or 11 years of age 80% of patients with a significant curve (greater than 20 degrees) are female and 20% are male. The findings of a feminine predominance may argue for hormonal influences rather than genetic ones. School screening in South Africa has revealed an incidence of 2% in blacks and 6% in whites. Brace treatment regardless of the brace type is usually effective only in preventing increases in spinal curvatures. Their main value remains in small curves detected early.

The generally accepted pattern of change in idiopathic scoliosis is that while relatively mild curves seem to increase little with growth, most do increase considerably. Some curves increase steadily but in most the increase varies with growth; they often increase markedly during spurts of growth, especially in adolescents. For many years the most common treatment consisted of the periodic observation of patients until the curves became severe enough to justify surgery and then correction of the curves and spinal fusion.

The use of bracing for the nonsurgical treatment of idiopathic scoliosis by Blount, by Moe, and by others has been effective enough to alter the treatment in skeletally immature patients. We have found that an efficient Milwaukee brace, conscientiously worn, will halt the increase in most mild or moderate curves. Furthermore, when the brace is worn to skeletal maturity, we have obtained an average decrease in curves of 6 degrees or about 20% of the curve present before application of the brace. Occasionally a Milwaukee brace produces spectacular improvement. We believe that treatment consisting only of observation of an increasing curve until the patient is mature or the curve becomes severe enough to justify fusion is rarely if ever realistic.

Employing the guides formulated by Lonstein et al., we have attempted to apply brace treatment appropriately, using such factors as skeletal age, menstrual history, and iliac epiphyses, along with an evaluation of cosmetic deformity or structural change that is both subjective and objective. The ''probability of progression'' factors from Lonstein et al. provide numeric values to add to common sense judgments on which we have relied in the past. We still use the 20-degree level as a rule to consider bracing. Recently surface electrical stimulation has been widely used to replace bracing. We believe that Milwaukee or Boston types of underarm braces are more reliable and predictable than surface electrical stimulation, according to published reports. Despite the reports of Ponseti and Nachemson, our experience agrees with that of Moe et al. in that we see many adults with painful scoliosis in whom operative treatment has resulted in relief. Adults with

curves of 60 degrees or more stand a greater risk of an increasing curvature. Kostiuk et al. found that of 107 adults with scoliosis that was treated surgically 63% sought help because of pain and 55% because of progressive deformity.

Various methods of decreasing or correcting the curves in scoliosis have been devised, and some are discussed later in this chapter. We know of no surgical treatment of scoliosis in which permanent correction has been demonstrated unless spinal fusion of some type has been included in the operation. Harrington instrumentation and segmental instrumentation, are established methods of assisting in the correction of curves and of providing internal fixation, but they must be combined with spinal fusion.

There is little if any evidence that structural scoliosis can be decreased or its increase halted by exercises alone.

CONSIDERATIONS FOR TREATMENT
Primary and secondary curves in scoliosis

In scoliosis structural and secondary lateral curves are different in several ways. In all patients an attempt should be made to identify the structural curve or curves because they are important in prognosis, and when indicated, in deciding in which area of the spine the curve or curves should be corrected and a fusion performed.

Characteristically structural curves deform and develop structural changes simultaneously and do not tend to correct themselves spontaneously or to retain any correction secured mechanically. On the other hand, secondary curves develop structural changes more slowly, tend to retain much longer the ability to correct themselves spontaneously, and can retain correction secured mechanically. Because secondary curves of long duration do develop structural changes, they may be difficult to distinguish from original structural curves. According to Cobb, any abnormal wedging, angulation, rotation, or position of vertebrae in a lateral spinal curve is a sign of structural change.

As a rule, an original structural curve or curves may be distinguished from secondary ones by the following criteria:

1. The vertebrae in the structural curve are usually displaced from the midline to the side of the convexity of this curve, whereas in a secondary curve they are usually displaced to the side of the concavity of the secondary curve.

2. When there are three curves, the middle one is usually structural.

3. When there are four curves, the two middle ones are usually structural.

4. The greater curve, or the one toward which the trunk is shifted, is the structural curve.

5. The curve that is least flexible and thus least correctable is the structural curve; this is determined by the lateral bending test described by Schmidt. In this test anteroposterior roentgenograms of the spine are made to show how much the structural and secondary curves can be passively corrected before spinal fusion, as is discussed later; in other words, they show the severity of structural change in each curve. The roentgenograms are made with the patient supine and the trunk bent laterally with maximum force, even to the point of discomfort, first to the right and then to the left (Fig. 71-1). It is important that the pelvis and shoulders be kept flat on the cassette or table. The roent-

genograms should include the spine from the first sacral vertebra and the iliac crests inferiorly to and including most of the cervical spine superiorly, even if two large roentgenograms must be made while the trunk is bent in each direction.

If the head is to be balanced above the pelvis when the patient is erect, any curve or curves of the spine in one direction require a curve or curves in the opposite direction. The formation of this curve or curves in the opposite direction is called compensation. Thus in a structural thoracolumbar curve of 40 degrees convex to the right there must be secondary curves convex to the left the sum of whose angles totals 40 degrees if compensation is to be complete. If the angles of the secondary curves total less than 40 degrees, the curve is called decompensated, and if the total is more than 40 degrees, the curve is said to be overcompensated. These secondary curves develop both above and below the structural curve or curves. However, because the lumbar spine is more mobile and more efficient mechanically, it always provides a maximum secondary curve that is as low in the lumbar spine as possible.

Natural history of idiopathic scoliosis

In deciding if and when idiopathic scoliosis should be corrected and the spine fused, a knowledge of the natural history of the disease is important. Ponseti and Friedman in 1950 and James in 1954 made extensive studies that are helpful; the conclusions from these two studies are essentially the same. Collis and Ponseti in 1969 increased this knowledge by studying a second time about one half of the patients included in the 1950 study.

Ponseti and Friedman reviewed 394 patients with idiopathic scoliosis in whom surgery had not been performed; of these, 335 were observed to maturity. Patients with mild scoliosis were excluded. Collis and Ponseti about 20 years later reported a long-term study of 195 of these same patients. They found that these patients had been living what they described as relatively normal lives with little difficulty caused by the scoliosis. More than 50%, however, believed that their deformity was apparent to others even when they were dressed. The most common symptom was dull backache after unusual activity. The frequency of backache was as follows: about one third never or very rarely had it, about one third had it occasionally, and about one third had it frequently or daily. They could find no correlation between the severity of any backache and the type or severity of the scoliosis. Forty-five percent had vital capacities of less than 85% of the predicted normal. Collis and Ponseti found an average increase in the curves of 15 degrees between the time of complete ossification of the epiphyses of the iliac crests and the time of the study more than 20 years later. The increase was 15 degrees or more in 26% and more than 25 degrees in 8% of 61 patients even after fusion of the epiphyses of the iliac crests. They considered this as evidence against the hypothesis that idiopathic scoliosis results from asymmetric growth of the vertebrae. They found some correlation between the type and severity of the curves and whether the curves tended to increase after maturity.

Nilsonne and Lundgren studied untreated scoliosis as much as 50 years after diagnosis. They found that most patients had a reduced work capacity: 76% were unmarried; 90% had pain in the back, and many used back supports; and 47% of those living were disabled. The mean age at death was 46.6 years. Nachemson reported on 130 untreated scoliotic adults and found a mortality rate twice that of normal, a decreased ability for ordinary work, and pain as a relatively constant symptom.

In idiopathic scoliosis most of the characteristic features of the primary curve or curves are present at the onset of deformity and rarely change. As a primary curve increases, one or two vertebrae may be added to it, but its apex, its location, and the direction of rotation of the vertebrae it includes remain unchanged. The curves were found by Ponseti and Friedman to form five main patterns that behaved differently.

Weinstein and Ponsetti in 1983 again studied untreated scoliosis, and the reader is encouraged to use this study.

SINGLE MAJOR LUMBAR CURVE

In the study of Ponseti and Friedman 23.6% of the patients had this curve, which was described as the most benign and the least deforming of all curves (Fig. 71-2). It was first noticed at the average age of 13.25 years and "ceased to increase at the average of 14.5 years." It usually contained five vertebrae, T11 to L3, with the apex at L1 or L2; its average angle at maturity while standing was 36.8 degrees. In the study of Collis and Ponseti the average increase in this curve was 9 degrees after skeletal maturity, with curves greater than 31 degrees increasing an average of 18 degrees, but curves of less than 31 degrees not increasing. Mild degenerative arthritic changes were found in about 20% of the patients, but no correlation between the severity of the curve and the frequency of back symptoms was found. Eight of 52 patients had daily backache, but patients with lumbar curves noted no more backache than patients of the group as a whole.

SINGLE MAJOR THORACOLUMBAR CURVE

In the study of Ponseti and Friedman this curve was found in 16% of patients, usually included six to eight vertebrae, and extended from T6 or T7 to L1 or L2. Its apex was at T11 or T12. The study of Collis and Ponseti included 24 patients with such curves, many of which were severe. The curves had increased an average of 17 degrees after skeletal maturity. Only 5 patients had decreased vital capacities and 4 of these had curves greater than 60 degrees. In our experience curves of this type produce more cosmetically objectionable deformities than thoracic or lumbar curves of the same magnitude, especially when the curves are long.

COMBINED THORACIC AND LUMBAR CURVES (DOUBLE MAJOR CURVE)

In the study of Ponseti and Friedman this pattern was found in 37% of patients, the two curves being present from onset and essentially equal. The thoracic curve was usually to the right and included five or six vertebrae from T5 or T6 to T10 or T11. Its apex was at T7 or T8. The lumbar curve was usually to the left and included five or six vertebrae from T10 or T11 to L3 or L4. Its apex was at L1 or L2. Often a neutral or unrotated vertebra was common to the adjacent ends of the curves. The prognosis

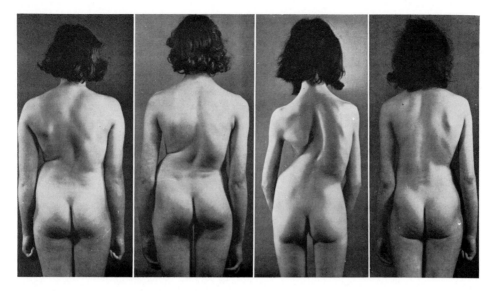

Fig. 71-2. Scoliosis. Deformity varies with pattern of curve. In each patient shown, angle of primary curve or curves is 70 degrees, but pattern of curve is different. *Left to right:* lumbar, thoracolumbar, thoracic, and combined thoracic and lumbar curves. (From James, J.I.P.: J. Bone Joint Surg. **36-B**:36, 1954.)

as to cosmesis in this pattern, first noticed at the average age of 12.3 years, was good, since the trunk usually remained well aligned when the curves increased simultaneously. The study of Collis and Ponseti more than 20 years after skeletal maturity supported this favorable cosmetic prognosis. After ossification of the epiphyses of the iliac crests was complete, the lumbar curves increased an average of only 9 degrees and the thoracic curves of only 11 degrees; after fusion of these epiphyses, the lumbar curves increased an average of only 7 degrees and the thoracic curves of only 9 degrees. Deformity of the back and decrease in the vital capacity were less severe than in single thoracic curves.

SINGLE MAJOR THORACIC CURVE

In the study of Ponseti and Friedman this curve was found in 22% of patients and its onset was earlier than that of any other curve (average age of 11.1 years). It usually included six vertebrae from T5 or T6 to T11 or T12 and had its apex at T8 or T9. Because of the thoracic location of this curve, rotation of the involved vertebrae was usually marked. The curve produced prominence of the ribs on its convex side and depression of the ribs on its concave side and elevation of one shoulder, resulting in an unpleasant deformity (Fig. 71-2). The prognosis was poor when the curve was first noticed before the age of 12 years, presumably because the remaining growth potential was great. In the study of Collis and Ponseti made about 20 years later, curves measuring 60 degrees to 80 degrees when ossification of the epiphyses of the iliac crests was complete were found to increase an average of 28 degrees. Curves of less than 60 degrees or of more than 80 degrees tended to increase less. Only 27% of the curves were less than 75 degrees. Backache was less common in patients with this curve than in the group as a whole. Mild osteoarthritic changes were seen in the roentgenograms in 71% of the patients, and the most severe cardiopulmonary symptoms were found in patients with this curve. The severity of the

pulmonary symptoms and of the decrease in the vital capacity correlated well with the severity of the curves, especially in curves greater than 80 degrees.

CERVICOTHORACIC CURVE

There were only five patients with this curve in the entire series of Ponseti and Friedman. While the curve never seemed to become large, the deformity was unsightly because of the elevated shoulder and deformed thorax, which could be but poorly disguised by clothing. The apex usually was at T3 with the curve extending from C7 or T1 to T4 or T5. The curve was usually less flexible. Correction and fusion of this curve when indicated is usually for cosmetic reasons and is usually indicated early for severe deformity.

DOUBLE MAJOR THORACIC CURVES

This pattern was not included in the studies just discussed but was described by Moe. It consists of a short upper thoracic curve often extending from T1 to T5 or T6 with considerable rotation of the vertebrae and other structural changes in combination with a lower thoracic curve extending from T6 to T12 or L1. The upper curve is usually to the left and the lower is usually to the right (Fig. 71-3). The appearance of patients with this curve is usually better than when a single thoracic curve is present, but because of asymmetry of the neckline produced by the upper curve, this pattern is more deforming than combined dorsal and lumbar curves. In double thoracic curves the fact that the upper curve is highly structural can be overlooked if the roentgenograms, especially the bending films, do not include the lower part of the cervical spine. If only the lower thoracic curve is corrected and fused using the Harrington instruments, the upper curve may not be flexible enough to allow an erect posture. Consequently both curves should usually be corrected and fused.

Winter et al. reported a rare group of patients who appeared emaciated, whose histories indicated a normal appetite but failure to gain weight, and who were found to have scoliosis with an exaggerated thoracic lordosis. These rare patients do not benefit from the Milwaukee brace but should undergo posterior Harrington distraction instrumentation and fusion. Contoured rods combined with segmental wiring can be beneficial in reducing or reversing the lordotic thoracic spine. We usually use the Drummond type of segmental wiring to minimize risks. A direct relationship can be found between the amount of correction of the lordosis and the improvement in respiratory function. Rapid mobilization of these patients with an active pulmonary exercise program yields good results.

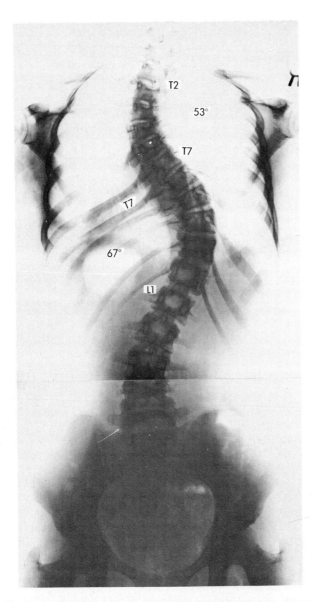

Fig. 71-3. Idiopathic scoliosis with double thoracic curves in girl 14 years of age. Primary or structural upper thoracic curve extends from T2 through T7 and measures 53 degrees, and primary or structural lower thoracic curve extends from T7 through L1 and measures 67 degrees. Shoulders and pelvis are level and patient is less deformed than in single thoracic curve.

Examination of patient

The original examination of the patient should include a thorough general physical examination, a neurologic examination, an examination of the back, and roentgenograms of the spine.

After the general physical examination the back should be examined carefully, and the characteristics of the deformity should be recorded. Furthermore, the height of the patient while standing and while sitting should be measured and recorded; in following the patient later these measurements are used to determine clinically whether the total height increases or decreases and whether any change is due principally to growth of the lower extremities or to an increase or decrease in the height of the trunk. It is encouraging to find that the patient's height while sitting has increased during a period when roentgenograms of the spine show no increase in the scoliosis. Next a thorough neurologic examination should be performed because occasionally an intraspinal neoplasm or other neurologic disorder may be the cause of scoliosis. An intraspinal neoplasm usually produces detectable neurologic signs and frequently an increase in the distances between the pedicles or erosion of one or more pedicles; thus the anteroposterior roentgenograms should be examined carefully for these changes. However, Bucy and Heimburger have pointed out that for an intraspinal neoplasm to produce a deformity of the spine, the patient must be young and the tumor must grow slowly; obviously these criteria are rarely fulfilled. We have seen scoliosis in adolescents caused by benign tumors of the vertebrae such as osteoid osteomas or eosinphilic granulomas. Both of these lesions are painful and can be discovered by careful study.

Posteroanterior roentgenograms of the spine, including distally the iliac crests and proximally most of the cervical spine, should be made with the patient standing. Supine or horizontal posteroanterior roentgenograms may be made. Usually we prefer instead right and left bending films of the spine made as described by Schmidt (p. 3171), but as a rule, make these only when evaluation for surgery is appropriate. A standing lateral roentgenogram of the spine and a spot lateral roentgenogram of the lumbosacral joint should also be made during the initial examination. Any spondylolisthesis in the lumbosacral area should not be overlooked because it may be the cause of any symptoms and may determine the treatment necessary. In the posteroanterior roentgenogram made with the patient standing, any significant discrepancy in the leg length can be determined by observing the comparative levels of the iliac crests and the femoral heads. The angle of the primary or structural curve or curves on the right and left lateral bending films gives a reasonably accurate estimate of the flexibility or correctability of the curves, important also in selecting treatment. In the standing lateral roentgenogram a search should be made for anomalies such as epiphysitis, neoplastic or infectious lesions, and congenital anomalies such as hemivertebrae or fusion between vertebrae that can be seen only in this view. We believe that one roentgenogram made with the patient standing and no oftener than every 4 to 6 months is sufficient for most clinical follow-up evaluations. Gonad shielding for all roentgenograms is the rule. Posteroanterior views reduce radiation to breast areas. Complete breast shielding has been difficult to accomplish routinely without blocking out the spinal image. Certainly if the scoliosis is increasing or if for any other reason a change in treatment is being considered, then any additional roentgenograms should be made as indicated. It is important to avoid making several roentgenograms routinely as a ''scoliosis series'' and to order only the individual film or films actually necessary for reevaluation of the patient.

An anteroposterior roentgenogram of the hand and wrist should be made and used with one of the standard atlases to determine the skeletal age. Because the skeletal age may deviate considerably from the chronologic age, the skeletal age should be used in evaluating the patient for treatment. Additional signs of maturation to be used are ossification of the vertebral ring epiphipees, iliac epiphysis excursion, physiologic signs of breast development or pubic hair appearance, cessation of increasing height, and chronologic age.

Finally photographs of the patient may be made to provide an objective record of the posture and deformity and should be repeated at intervals later to record any increase in deformity or any decrease in deformity after treatment. They should be made of the front and back while standing and, because asymmetry or deformity of the thorax is usually most apparent when the spine is flexed, also of the back and side while the patient is bending forward.

Measurement of curves

The methods of measuring curves attributed to Cobb and to Ferguson have both been widely used. They are fundamentally different and cannot be used interchangeably. For this reason a single method, the one attributed to Cobb, has been recommended by the Terminology Committee of the Scoliosis Research Society to permit comparison of patients and results of treatment of different surgeons. Consequently we have used the Cobb method, employing usually as references the end plates of the end vertebrae, but when these are not visible on the roentgenograms, employing instead the pedicles of these vertebrae.

COBB METHOD

This method consists of three steps: (1) locating the superior end vertebra, (2) locating the inferior end vertebra, and (3) drawing intersecting perpendiculars from the superior surface of the superior end vertebra and from the inferior surface of the inferior end vertebra. The angle of deviation of these perpendiculars from a straight line is the angle of the curve. The end vertebrae of the curve are the ones that tilt the most into the concavity of the curve being measured. Generally, as one moves away from the apex of the curve being measured, the next intervertebral space inferior to the inferior end vertebra or superior to the superior end vertebra is wider on the concave side of the curve being measured. Within the curve being measured the intervertebral spaces are usually wider on the convex side and narrower on the concave side. When significantly wedged, the vertebrae themselves rather than the intervertebral spaces may be wider on the convex side of the curve and narrower on the concave side.

FERGUSON METHOD

The first step in measuring a curve by the Ferguson method is to locate the superior and inferior end vertebrae as just described. Then the centers of the bodies of the superior and inferior end vertebrae and of the vertebra at the apex of the curve are located. Next two lines are drawn, one from the center of the vertebra at the apex of the curve to the center of the inferior end vertebra and one from the center of the vertebra at the apex to the center of the superior end vertebra. The angle of deviation of these two lines from a straight line is the angle of the curve.

SURGICAL TREATMENT OF SCOLIOSIS
Considerations for correction of curves and for spinal fusion

The normal thoracic spine is relatively inflexible, and in scoliosis it is even more so because of secondary changes in the ribs and other supporting structures. Casts used in correcting curves were less efficient in the thoracic spine than in the lumbar. Significant correction of a high thoracic curve was often complicated by traction neuritis of the cervical or brachial plexus if a turnbuckle cast was used. High thoracic curves cause severe deformities such as elevation of the shoulder, prominence of the scapula, and projection of the ribs or razorback deformity, all on the convex side of the curve (Fig. 71-2). Therefore surgery is indicated earlier than in lower thoracic curves, although the fundamental indications for surgery must be considered in each specific patient. In general then, the higher the curve in the thoracic spine, the more severe is the deformity, the more difficult it is to correct, and the earlier surgery is indicated. Conversely the lower the curve in the thoracic spine, the greater is the compensation by secondary curves, the less is the deformity, the more easily the curve can be corrected, and the later surgery is indicated.

In lumbar scoliosis there is less deformity. Although rotation of the spine may cause the lumbar muscles to bulge unilaterally, this bulge never approaches the severe prominence (razorback deformity) produced by the same amount of rotation of the thoracic spine. The lumbar spine is much more flexible and from a mechanical standpoint more easily controlled by apparatus designed to correct the scoliosis. Tilting of the fifth lumbar vertebra, whether developmental or paralytic, exerts either an exaggerative or corrective influence on the primary lumbar curve and must always be considered in treatment.

Considerations of cardiopulmonary function

Patients with severe deformity of the thorax have a high incidence of chronic pulmonary disease, have frequent late cardiac failure, and tend to die prematurely. Many studies have been made of the cardiopulmonary function of patients with idiopathic and paralytic scoliosis. Although the findings of many of the studies do not necessarily reinforce those of the others, several general statements can be made from these findings. Using ordinary pulmonary function studies with spirometry, a measurable decrease in pulmonary function can be found in almost all patients with significant scoliosis. According to pulmonary physiologists, most of this decrease in function is caused by restrictive lung disease and is most readily demonstrated in the vital capacity. Although the severity of the curve or of the thoracic deformity does not correlate exactly with the decrease in the vital capacity, it is generally agreed that the more severe the curve or deformity, the more severe is the decrease in the vital capacity. Opinions vary concerning the effect on the vital capacity of the usual methods of treating scoliosis. It seems apparent that the application of a Risser localizer or any other type of corrective cast decreases the vital capacity immediately. The Milwaukee brace is said to be less harmful in this respect and the halo traction device is said not to decrease significantly the vital capacity. This harmful effect of immobilization with casts is only temporary, however, because in the reports of Gazioglu et al. and of Makley et al. the vital capacity definitely improved above the level present before surgery when the patient was examined several months after having resumed normal activities without any restrictive or corrective devices. In the study of Makley et al. the vital capacity definitely increased, but since vital capacity is often measured as a percent of normal related to the height of the patient, when the height increases after surgery the expected normal also increases and any actual increase in the vital capacity may be lost in the computation. Johnson and Westgate demonstrated that the vital capacity was best estimated on the nondeformed height, especially with curves greater than 60 degrees. The nondeformed height was obtained by dividing the arm span by 1.03 in men and 1.01 in women. Using the regression equations of Cook and Hamann, the predicted vital capacity of preoperative patients could be obtained. A vital capacity of 100% to 80% was considered normal; 80% to 60% mild restriction; 60% to 40% moderate restriction; and less than 40% severe restriction. Westgate and Moe reported that correction and fusion using the Harrington instrumentation do not improve the average vital capacity or maximum breathing capacity but may improve arterial oxygen saturation. Even if the importance of these findings is minimized, it does seem obvious that correction and fusion of a spinal curve, either idiopathic or paralytic, at least prevent further deterioration of pulmonary function because they decrease the thoracic deformity or prevent it from increasing.

In the evaluation before surgery, pulmonary function studies are usually indicated in patients with paralytic scoliosis or with idiopathic or congenital scoliosis when the curves are severe or are associated with a significant kyphosis. All adults should have thorough cardiopulmonary function studies before surgery. We do not routinely obtain special pulmonary function studies in patients with idiopathic curves of less than 50 or 60 degrees as measured by the Cobb method unless warranted by some special circumstance. Garrett, Perry, and Nickel advocated a policy requiring a tracheostomy before surgery in any patient with paralytic scoliosis whose vital capacity is less than 30% of the predicted normal. We have in general used this policy but have found that the indications for tracheostomy can be safely narrowed if the patient spends several days after surgery in an adequately staffed intensive care unit in which respiratory functions can be constantly supervised and in which mechanical aids for respiration are readily available.

Indications for correction of curves and for spinal fusion

Nonsurgical treatment of scoliosis is possibly more important than surgical treatment, but one must be able during nonsurgical treatment to recognize the indications for surgery so that treatment may be changed accordingly. The indications are not always definite, but the following are the chief ones.

1. *An increasing curve in a growing child.* The spine can be safely fused in a young child. Solid fusion of the spine causes longitudinal growth in the fused area to cease or at least to be severely retarded. But the lengthening of the spine brought about by correcting the curve or curves usually exceeds the loss of longitudinal growth caused by any fusion. And as Blount has said, a moderately short but straight trunk is better than a very short and crooked one. When the scoliosis is not severe and is either not increasing or is being controlled by bracing or other conservative means, consideration may be given to postponing surgical treatment in the young child possibly up to adolescence in deference to trunk growth. This suggestion must not be used to justify withholding surgery when deformity is increasing. It is highly preferable, however, to postpone fusion as long as possible, with the important provision that the scoliosis is not increasing or is increasing very slowly and is being controlled by bracing or other conservative means. It has been generally believed that when growth of the spine is complete, the scoliosis almost always ceases to increase. Risser pointed out a valuable sign in determining when growth of the spine has ceased in an individual patient. He found that the epiphyses of the iliac crests gradually ossify from aneriorly to posteriorly and that growth of the spine continues until this ossification reaches the posterosuperior iliac spines and turns medially and inferiorly toward the sacroiliac joints. He and others have stated that growth of the spine then usually ceases, and an increase in idiopathic scoliosis is unlikely. But recently in many patients with idiopathic scoliosis being treated conservatively, curves have been found to increase for a year or more after ossification of the epiphyses of the iliac crests is complete. Therefore some surgeons have proposed that the time of fusion rather than the time of completion of ossification of these epiphyses is a more reliable sign. There are indications that the time of fusion of the ring epiphyses to the vertebral bodies is more significant in this regard. Establishing the skeletal age by studying roentgenograms of the hand and wrist is another method of determining when the skeleton is mature. A skeletal age of 16 years in a female and 18 years in a male is a reasonably conservative indication of skeletal maturity. The relationship between the time when curves cease to increase and the appearance of the several signs used in determining skeletal maturation seems to vary considerably. While completion of ossification of the ring epiphyses of the vertebral bodies is probably the most important single sign of the maturing skeleton, no one sign can be used alone as a definite indication that a curve will not increase in an individual patient.

2. *A severe deformity with asymmetry of the trunk in an adolescent, regardless of whether growth of the spine has ceased.*

3. *In older patients pain that cannot be controlled by conservative measures.*The amount of correction obtainable is often small and the chief aim of treatment should be to produce a solid fusion. Pain in young children or adolescents with scoliosis requires extensive investigation for a cause of pain and curvature other than idiopathic scoliosis.

Patient orientation

An essential part of a successful spinal fusion and instrumentation is patient orientation. We agree with Harrington that successful surgery includes (1) spending time with patients to gain their confidence and allay hidden fears and (2) showing the patients examples of the expected results and names of other patients with whom they may confer and explaining the use of instrumentation and its limitations as well as benefits.

Correction of curves

The first aim in the treatment of scoliosis is to restore the symmetry of the trunk by centering the first thoracic vertebra above the sacrum and at the same time keeping the pelvis and shoulders level. The second and equally important aim is to straighten the structural curves enough, primarily in the thoracic area, to halt the deterioration in pulmonary function and to minimize the unsightly deformity of the thorax. Right and left bending roentgenograms and a standing anteroposterior roentgenogram of the entire spine are made to determine which curves are primary or structural, which are secondary, and which should be included in the fusion. As already stated, any structural changes in a curve produce asymmetry in the side bending roentgenograms (Fig. 71-1). As a general rule, unless the curves are relatively mild, all thoracic structural curves should be included in the fusion. In combined double major curves of equal size on the standing roentgenogram and involving the dorsal and lumbar areas, the thoracic curve is often highly structural and the lumbar curve is only mildly so and will correct almost completely on side bending against the curve. In these instances, especially when the Harrington instruments are used, fusing only the thoracic curve may be possible because the lumbar curve will usually accommodate itself to the angle of the residual thoracic curve after fusion. If the patient is immature, and therefore it is known that growth will continue, one must continue to observe the lumbar curve for any increase until maturity.

Cobb, who used primarily a turnbuckle cast to correct the curves, described a method to determine how much the secondary curves might be expected to correct spontaneously after spinal fusion and how much the primary curve or curves should be corrected before fusion. A description of this method follows. In a patient with a structural thoracic curve, to determine the spontaneous correction possible in the lumbar secondary curve an anteroposterior roentgenogram of the lumbar spine is made while the patient sits with the buttock elevated 3 to 4 inches (7.5 to 10 cm) on the convex side of the lumbar curve. Next to determine the spontaneous correction possible in the upper secondary curve the patient is placed supine, and an anteroposterior roentgenogram of the cervical and dorsal spine is made while the patient is bent toward the convex side of the upper curve. The sum of the residual angles of the secondary curves is the total residual curvature of the spine in one direction caused by the secondary curves. Since for the spine to be completely compensated there must be an equal residual curvature in the opposite direction, the primary curve must not be corrected to an angle less than the sum of the residual angles of the secondary curves.

Cobb found that if the total residual curvature caused by the secondary curves is 0 degrees, then the primary or structural thoracic curve may be corrected completely. On the other hand, if this total is greater than the primary curve, then no correction of the primary curve is possible. If this total is only 20 degrees to 30 degrees less than the primary curve, then little correction of the primary curve is possible. Before spinal fusion Cobb recommended that a composite film composed of sections of three roentgenograms be assembled; the lumbar section from the film made with the patient sitting and one buttock elevated (as described above) to show the lumbar curve, the upper dorsal section from the film made with the cervical and dorsal spine bent toward the side of the upper dorsal convexity (as described above) to show the upper dorsal curve, and a section from a roentgenogram made through the turnbuckle cast after the curve has been corrected to show the primary curve. These three sections are fixed together and are studied as follows. If the first dorsal vertebra is over the sacrum, then the primary curve has been corrected the right amount; if it is displaced to the concave side of the primary curve, then it has been undercorrected; if it is displaced to the convex side of the primary curve, then it has been overcorrected.

It must be pointed out that when the Harrington instruments are used, how much the primary curve will be corrected at surgery is inaccurately determined before surgery by the method just discussed, but one can expect a 50% to 60% improvement. In the instrumented area, however, including one or two vertebrae superior to the superior end vertebra and one or two inferior to the inferior end vertebra is common practice. When this is done, unless a significantly structural curve has been overlooked, overcorrection of the primary curve is extremely rare. The structural curve most likely to be overlooked is the high curve in the double thoracic pattern described by Moe (p. 3173); usually this curve must also be corrected and fused.

TURNBUCKLE CAST TECHNIQUE (RISSER). Place the patient supine on a horizontal canvas strap attached to a rectangular frame as shown in Fig. 71-4, which also shows the localizers in place, as is described in the technique below. To the head and pelvis apply moderate traction; pull distally on the pelvis on the convex side of the curve to be corrected and deviate the head toward the concave side; in this manner the secondary curves are decreased, and the spine tends to assume the shape of one long C. Pad all bony prominences well and place two or three layers of removable felt under the proposed location of the anterior hinge; these latter pads will be removed later to allow space for correction of the chest deformity as the spine is

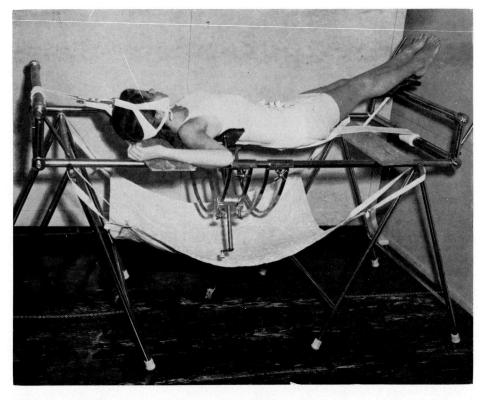

Fig. 71-4. Application of Risser localizer cast (see text). (From Risser, J.C.: In American Academy of Orthopaedic Surgeons: Instructional course lectures, vol. 10, Ann Arbor, 1953, J.W. Edwards.)

bent. Now apply a body cast that includes a headpiece and extends distally to above the knee on the convex side of the curve to be corrected; reinforce the cast over this hip with basswood struts. Incorporate metal hinges in the anterior and posterior aspects of the cast, placed eccentrically toward the convex side of the curve. Thus traction will be applied to the spine as it is bent laterally; if the hinges are placed in the center of the cast anteriorly and posteriorly, maximum bending of the spine is possible but little if any traction. Allow the cast to dry for 3 to 5 days and then at the level of the hinges cut it on its concave side and extend the cut anteriorly and posteriorly to the hinges. Now insert over the cut edges of the cast on its concave side turnbuckle lugs made of two pieces of plumber's tape riveted together to form a right angle. Attach a turnbuckle to these lugs. Then from the opposite side of the cast remove a large elliptical window between the hinges to allow lateral bending in that direction. Turn the turnbuckle each morning; if the patient is uncomfortable, then decrease the pressure by one half in the afternoon. Eliminate any pressure points that develop deep to the hinges and at the edges of the window. At intervals check by roentgenograms how much the curve has been corrected. When the roentgenograms show that the hinges are on the convex side of the correcting curve, then no further correction can be obtained by traction, and the only other correction possible will be obtained by bending the curve at its ends.

When the curve has been corrected as much as desired, reinforce the sides of the cast with plaster and basswood

struts and remove the turnbuckle and lugs. Cut a large window in the back of the cast over the proposed area of fusion.

We have used the Cobb attachments for the Albee-Compere fracture table (Fig. 71-5) or the Risser table when applying a Risser turnbuckle cast. According to Risser, this cast can exert a more powerful force in correcting scoliosis than any other. Yet it has some disadvantages: (1) the patient is bent laterally so much that he cannot walk and thus must remain in bed; and (2) in it, the ends of the spine are held severely bent laterally. Thus when this cast is used, the roentgenograms must be carefully studied, and the length and location of the fusion must be carefully planned, for otherwise the fusion may be insufficient because it is too short, or it may result in decompensation because it is too long or improperly located and fixes a secondary curve in an undesirable position.

The success of spinal instrumentation has largely eliminated the use of the turnbuckle cast.

LOCALIZER CAST TECHNIQUE (RISSER). Risser developed another method of correcting and immobilizing a scoliotic curve. The correction is obtained by applying pressure localized posterolaterally at a point level with the apex of the curve while traction is exerted on the head and pelvis. Thus the apex of the curve is forced laterally between the ends of the curve, which are relatively fixed by the traction. Risser used this jacket almost exclusively because it corrects the curve as well as the turnbuckle cast does and corrects angulation of the ribs even better. There are sev-

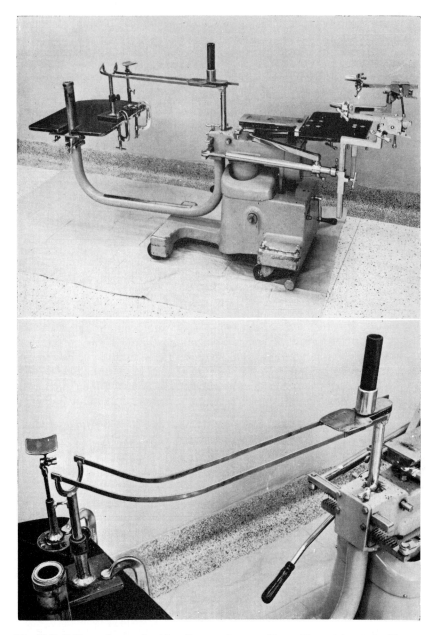

Fig. 71-5. Cobb attachments for Albee-Compere fracture table used in applying turnbuckle cast.

eral advantages of this type of cast. The patient can walk. The patient's position in the cast is not changed by manipulation of the cast as in a turnbuckle or other sectioned cast. The secondary curves are not immobilized in increased angulation, and the spine is "in more or less compensation." When the cast has been applied and does not satisfactorily correct the curve, both Risser and Moe recommend that it be wedged, while fresh, level with the apex of the curve. When the alignment of the body and compensation of the spine are carefully watched, this cast is especially useful in the long fusion usually recommended for the collapsing type of scoliosis caused by poliomyelitis; thus the primary and secondary curves can all be fused in satisfactory alignment.

Place the patient supine on a canvas strap tied to the rectangular plaster frame (Fig. 71-4). Stretch stockinette over him from the head to the knees. Suspend beneath the frame a metallic half circle carrying a movable jack with a metal plate that can be directed toward the apex of the angulation of the ribs. Protect the area of angulation by a heavy piece of felt covered with a previously made contoured square of plaster that rests on the plate. Turn the jack to press the plate in an anterolateral direction on the angulation of the ribs and thus correct both the posterior and the lateral angulation of the spine. If there is a double primary curve or structural changes in a lumbar secondary curve, a second jack may be applied laterally against the transverse processes at the apex of the lumbar curve, and thus the apparatus will correct both curves at the same time. Now apply the plaster cast in sections. First apply a plaster girdle over felt padding and the stockinette that has already been applied. Mold the plaster snugly and carefully around the iliac crests, the anterosuperior iliac spines, the sacrum, and the symphysis pubis. After this section has hardened, apply traction to the head with a halter and to the pelvis with a pelvic belt attached over the plaster girdle. Then gradually increase the longitudinal traction and the pressure with the jack. Beginning with a well-molded neck and shoulder part, which includes the chin and the occiput, finish incorporating the entire trunk with plaster applied snugly over felt padding to maintain the corrected position. After the cast has hardened, trim it to relieve any excess pressure at the site of the localizer or on the point of the chin. At the bottom trim the cast to the groin, leaving it relatively low over the buttocks. Then cut a window over the abdomen so that the upper abdomen, lower costal margin, and the xiphoid process are free.

Spinal fusion may be carried out through a large window cut in the posterior part of the cast and then replaced after surgery. Or the cast may be bivalved and removed before surgery so that fusion may be more easily and safely performed. If so, the bivalved cast is taped in place when the patient has recovered from the anesthetic.

The success of spinal instrumentation has largely eliminated the use of the Risser localizer cast also. Risser-type casts are widely used as external immobilization and to protect spinal instrumentation. When applied for this purpose, they are not corrective and no localizers are used. They usually are applied in one piece and most frequently at underarm level, restricting the cervical or shoulder strap heights for surgery high in the spine.

MODIFIED COTREL (EDF) CAST TECHNIQUE (MOE). Moe has used the Risser table or the Risser attachments for the Bell table to apply casts patterned after those used by Cotrel in France. The cast is applied in one piece using two fabric slings looped around the waist superior to the iliac crests and crossed anteriorly and posteriorly so that as distal traction is applied to the slings and thus to the pelvis, the waistline is molded well proximal to the iliac crests. A disposable halter is used for head traction. The fabric slings are placed between the two layers of stockinette so that they will not adhere to the plaster and can be removed after the cast is applied. Cotrel applies the cast over the two layers of stockinette only. Moe usually applies in addition thin felt padding around the neck, shoulder, and pelvis. When the cast is used to correct curves before surgery, Moe recommends that a heavy layer of felt or other padding be applied to the entire anterior aspect of the pelvic and shoulder girdles so that pressure on localized areas of the skin will be minimal during the several hours the patient is prone on the operating table.

Place the patient supine on a Risser or Bell table. Apply the two layers of stockinette, the fabric slings for pelvic traction, a halter for head traction, and any padding desired. Then apply strong pelvic and head traction and apply rapidly a cast similar to the Risser localizer cast. Next place a canvas strap 15 to 20 cm wide transversely across the table beneath the patient's back at the level of the axillae; attach it to the table frame on the side of the body

opposite the rib prominence, apply it smoothly around the thorax over the rib prominence, and turn it 90 degrees to rise vertically to the overhead winch of the Bell table or to the overhead attachment of the Risser table. Just before the plaster dries tighten the strap securely against the outside of the cast for corrective molding. After the cast has dried remove the halter and the pelvic traction straps and trim the cast as desired over the abdomen and chest, and window it posteriorly if it is to be left in place during surgery. We have used this technique and find it superior to many other casts in correcting deformity, especially of the ribs. This cast is usually also applied after surgery to protect spinal instrumentation.

MILWAUKEE BRACE (BLOUNT AND SCHMIDT)

This brace was developed and used as a means of simultaneously supporting and correcting postoperative scoliosis without instrumentation and without the use of a cast. It is now used more widely for the nonsurgical treatment of scoliosis than for external fixation after spinal fusion. In our opinion this brace does not immobilize the spine sufficiently after surgery without spinal instrumentation and using a cast is preferable. The brace has been used successfully after instrumentation and fusion; nevertheless, in this situation we recommend the use of a plaster cast that is more efficient and that cannot be removed by an uncooperative patient or family.

DISTRACTION TECHNIQUES

The early assumption that the spinal cord moved up and down with vertebral motion has been replaced by evidence that the cord actually changes length as it accommodates the difference in vertebral positions. These length changes have been shown to be an accordian-like response of the fibers within the spinal cord. The neural canal, being posterior to the vertebral body mass, is therefore lengthened when the spine flexes and shortened when it extends. In the lengthened position the fibers of the spinal cord were shown to be in a linear pattern with long and slender blood vessels. When the spine is extended and the cord shortens, the fibers assume a parallel, wavy form with the blood vessels tortuous and broad. The cervical portion of the spinal cord lengthens 25 mm between the extremes of full flexion and extension with an average of 3.6 mm per segment. In the lumbar area the length changes average 15 mm or 3 mm per segment. The least extensible portion of the spine, which is of greatest concern to the surgeon in the treatment of scoliosis, is the thoracic region. Here there is only a 10 mm difference in length of the cord, or an average of 0.8 mm per segment. The studies of Brieg have shown that as the cord is stretched over a mass, such as a protruding disc, the fluidity of the spinal cord tends to distribute the tension so that the degree of damage is not as great as would otherwise be anticipated. These findings, then, dictate a caution to the surgeon treating scoliosis to take care in altering the length of the thoracic portion of the spine.

Halo-femoral distraction

Perry and Nickel in 1959 introduced an excellent halo device (Fig. 71-6) that enjoys widespread use; the device

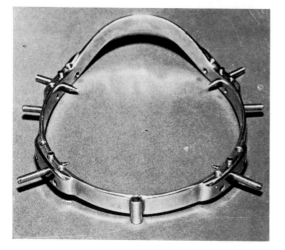

Fig. 71-6. Halo (anterior view) for stabilizing head and neck. (From Perry, J., and Nickel, V.L.: J. Bone Joint Surg. **41-A**:37, 1959.)

provides stable fixation while remaining quite comfortable. Moe reported his results of the combination of this device with femoral pins for correcting spinal deformity.

Halo-femoral distraction has been rarely used since spinal instrumentation and spinal cord monitoring have been developed more extensively. The need for supplemental correction of severe stiff curves and for functional monitoring of an unanesthetized patient has greatly diminished.

The halo may be used as follows:
1. Cervical spine stabilization
   a. Severe cervical muscle paralysis
   b. Cervical fractures
   c. Cervical spine deformity in rheumatoid arthritis
   d. Extensive cervical laminectomy
2. Correction of more distal spine deformities
   a. Halo-femoral traction
   b. Halo-pelvic traction

TECHNIQUE OF HALO APPLICATION. The halo and pins are sterilized. A thorough shampoo of the hair is all that is needed before application. With the hair wet, pin insertion is easier without entangling the hair. Skin preparation can include shaving only in the immediate areas of pin insertion. Smaller children should have general anesthesia, but local anesthesia is routinely used in older patients. Not only the skin but also the periosteum must be thoroughly infiltrated with the local anesthetic when this means is chosen. Preselecting the pin sites through the halo will keep the area of infiltration to a small skin wheal.

The halo must be at or below the maximum diameter of the skull. The front pins should be centered in the groove at the upper margin of the eyebrows between the supraciliary ridge and the frontal prominences. The halo then extends about ⅛ inch (3.2 mm) above the ear, care being taken not to allow the halo to touch the pinnae, which would result in skin necrosis. A bit more distance is allowed between the skull and halo posteriorly and anteriorly. Anteriorly the most medial halo channel is usually chosen for pin insertion. Although some prefer keeping the

pin insertions within the hairline, this requires a more posterior location in the temporalis muscle, a site more likely to produce a pin reaction from the action of the temporalis muscle during chewing and also more likely to be painful. The bone is also thinner in this area. Involvement of the temporalis artery must also be avoided. Posteriorly the central channels are usually the best site for the pins.

With an assistant or positioning device holding the halo in the appropriate position, introduce the pins and tighten two diagonally opposed pins simultaneously. Continue this until the four pins just engage the bone. Then continue tightening diagonally located pairs of pins with a torque screwdriver to about 5½ inch-pounds for adults. Using only the fingertips and not the palm on a short screwdriver will give a final tension of about 5½ inch-pounds. We have used 3.5 to 4 inch-pounds for halos on small children. Alternate tightening of the pins prevents migration of the halo to an asymmetric position. After all pins are tightened to 5½ inch-pounds, unscrew each about one-quarter turn. This will allow the rotary stretch of the skin to return to a relaxed position, preventing any skin necrosis. Finally secure the pins to the halo with a locknut.

AFTERTREATMENT. The halo pins may be cleansed at the pin-skin interface with hydrogen peroxide daily, but we usually recommend only daily inspection and application of a small amount of Betadine ointment. They should not be tightened daily as has been the habit with the use of tongs because the pins rarely enter the skull more than 2 mm, but rather act as a wedge forcing the halo from the skull. In more muscular patients attempts to move the head within the halo may result in pin loosening caused by erosion and accompanied by an inflammatory process. When used with a cast that extends down around the pelvis, apparently little stress on the pins occurs and loosening is rarely a problem. When attached to one of the commercially available plastic halo-vests, loosening of the skull pins is more frequent, and we usually check these every 2 to 3 weeks for tension. The indications for changing the pins are serous drainage, inflammation, or a clicking sensation. The pins should otherwise be undisturbed. If a pin must be replaced, this is achieved by inserting a new sterilized pin into an adjacent hole before removal of the offending pin. Three pins alone will not long hold a halo. O'Brien et al. recommend (1) that slipping of the skull halo be prevented by routine tightening of the skull pins 1 week after their fitting and (2) that 6 pins be used when treatment is to be prolonged.

Halo removal is painless if performed carefully. All traction should be removed from the halo and the pins removed in reverse of the order in which they were applied. External nuts are removed and then diagonal pairs of pins are loosened and removed. It is important than an assistant stabilize the halo while the pins are removed to prevent pain as the number of holding pins decreases. The pin sites will promptly close and heal with small scars that are usually cosmetically acceptable.

TECHNIQUE OF FEMORAL PIN INSERTION. Prepare both knee areas thoroughly and drape them in a sterile field. Introduce a large, smooth Steinmann pin through a stab wound into each distal diaphyseal area well above the epiphysis.

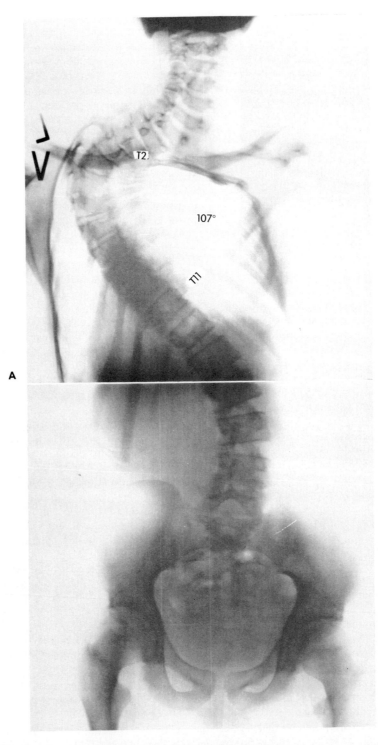

Fig. 71-7. Treatment of severe paralytic scoliosis by halo-femoral distraction and Harrington instrumentation. **A,** Left thoracic curve extending from T2 through T11 and measuring 107 degrees while standing in boy 15 years of age whose skeletal age was 14½ years. Lateral bending roentgenogram to left showed that curve corrected to 70 degrees. Pulmonary function study showed vital capacity of 67% of predicted normal and maximum breathing capacity of 65%. Because of poor pulmonary function and location, severity, and rigidity of curve, halo-femoral distraction was selected for correcting curve.

The addition of a plaster cuff incorporating the pin will prevent medial or lateral migration and decrease pin tract infections.

AFTERTREATMENT. Traction is begun with about 6 kg on the head and 3 kg on each leg. Weights are gradually and equally added to a total of 12 kg on each end. Periods of traction exceeding 10 days have not added improved angular corrections. In pelvic obliquity most of the lower extremity weight can be placed on the high-side limb.

Rather than confine the patient to bed, a halo wheelchair may be substituted as designed by Stagnara. Winter has used this technique with the patient spending days in the chair and nights back in halo-femoral traction in bed.

Letts, Palakar, and Bobechko studied 10 patients with an average curve of 81 degrees. Halo-femoral traction was used over a 2- to 3-week period with 1.8 kg added per day to a maximum total of 18.1 kg. They showed an average improvement of 34 degrees (41%), mostly within the first week. Subsequent Harrington instrumentation added 13.5 degrees (16%) for a total of 47 degrees (57%) correction. They recommend preliminary traction for curves greater than 65 degrees, but not for more than 10 days (Fig. 71-7). Nachemson and Nordwall believe that only the more severe but still flexible curves greater than 90 degrees in patients over 20 years of age need treatment by their two-stage procedure; rigid curves of more than 90 degrees would be treated with halo-pelvic or halo-femoral traction preoperatively.

Halo-pelvic distraction

DeWald and Ray first reported the pelvic halo in 1970; it was designed for use in patients with severe pulmonary restriction, pressure sores from a cast, soft tissue contractures, or inability to control pelvic tilt and rotation (Fig.

Text continues on page 3187.

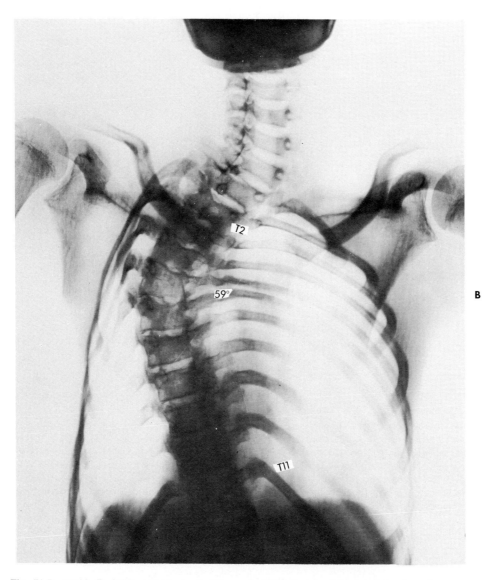

B

Fig. 71-7, cont'd. B, While patient was in 15 pounds (6.8 kg) each of head and distal traction, curve corrected to 59 degrees.

Continued.

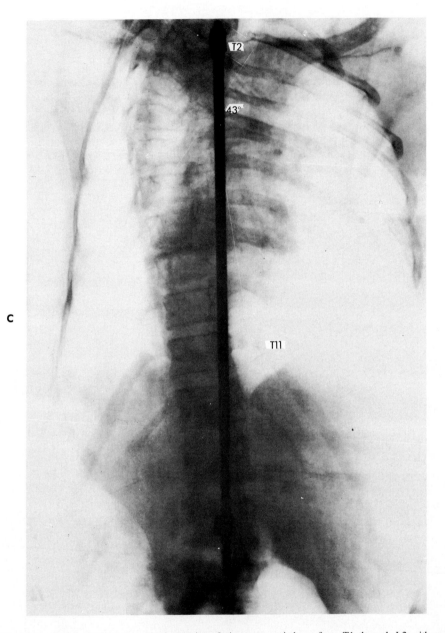

Fig. 71-7, cont'd. C, After 3 weeks in traction, fusion was carried out from T1 through L2 with use of autogenous bone from right ilium and Harrington distraction rod extending from T2 through L2. Rod was inserted upside down deliberately so that its end, which projects past hook, would not produce conspicuous prominence at base of neck. This is especially desirable when superior hook is to be inserted at either T1 or T2 in patient with poliomyelitis whose soft tissues are markedly wasted. Curve was corrected to 43 degrees and plaster cast was applied immediately after surgery. When cast was changed 6 months after surgery, curve measured 44 degrees (roentgenogram not shown).

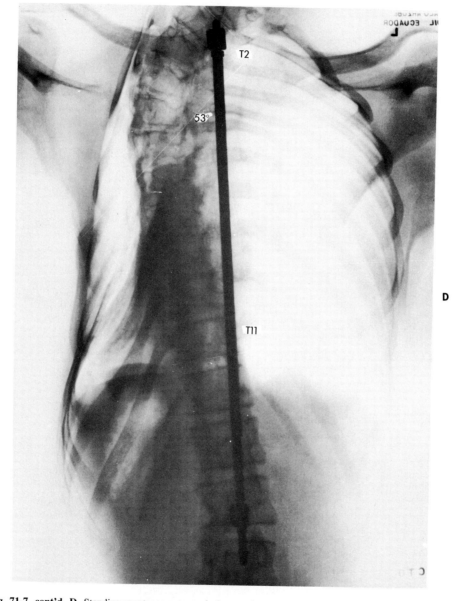

Fig. 71-7, cont'd. D, Standing roentgenogram made 1 year after surgery. Curve measures 53 degrees. In our experience this much loss of correction is not unusual in severe paralytic curves. In idiopathic scoliosis when 10 degrees of correction are lost before removal of cast, pseudarthrosis is often present.

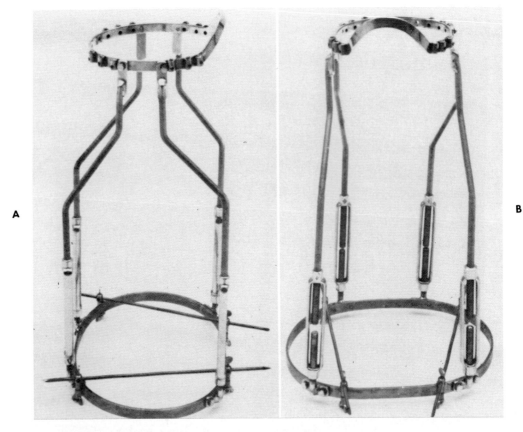

Fig. 71-8. Halo-pelvic distraction apparatus. **A,** Lateral view. **B,** Anterior view. (From Dewald, R.L., and Ray, R.D.: J. Bone Joint Surg. **52-A:**233, 1970.)

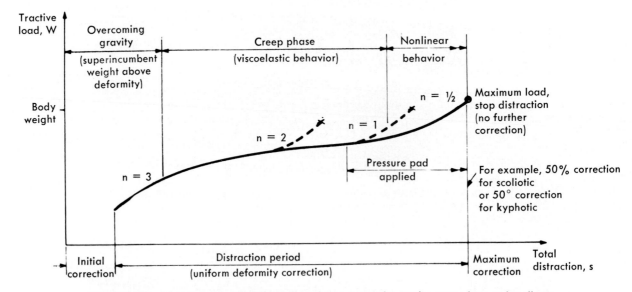

Fig. 71-9. Halo-pelvic distraction divided into three phases: overcoming gravity, creep phase, and nonlinear behavior. n, Rate of distraction in terms per day; t, time in days from beginning of distraction period; W, applied distractive force; s, total increase in length between skull and pelvis. (From Clark, J.A., et al.: Clin. Orthop. **110:**90, 1975.)

71-8). Halo-pelvic distraction is now rarely used. Segmental spinal instrumentation and other internal spinal fixation devices have largely displaced it. The pelvic halo provides gradual and controlled forces that are excellent in treating severe, rigid spinal deformities, and it allows unrestricted respiratory excursions, ambulation, and easy access for spinal surgery. The complications include skin intolerance with pin tract infections, bowel perforation, nerve palsy and paraplegia, hip subluxation, and degenerative cervical arthritis. Furthermore, the areas for obtaining grafts are poorly accessible.

Clark et al. have emphasized that the deformed spine is a nonhomogenous, viscoelastic structure composed of many component parts and exhibiting the biomechanical properties of elasticity and plasticity. Biologic materials have a complex behavior under load. Under consideration are the duration of the applied load, the deformation of strain rate, the rate of application of the load, and yielding that produces permanent deformation or plastic strain. As pointed out by Nachemson and Elfström, these factors have a bearing on the application of externally applied means for correction of deformity. These biomechanical properties are further affected by the cause of the spine deformity, its clinical behavior, and any surgical intervention. During the creep phase of distraction there is a time-dependent relaxation of structures resisting correction of deformity during distraction (Fig. 71-9). The gradient and length of this creep phase are a function of the rigidity of the curve, the angle, and the level of deformity. This explains the great variation from deformity to deformity. Collagen fibers are the extension limiting constituent, the ligaments stiffening abruptly after 30% to 60% strain. The stress-strain relationship in nerves is influenced greatly by the rate of application of the load, with slow stretching producing a greater increase in length without disturbance of function. The turnbuckles originally used on the four uprights have been modified by other investigators and in the system of O'Brien et al. have been replaced by a spring scale to measure distraction forces.

Kalamchi et al. reported on 150 consecutive patients treated with the halo-pelvic device and emphasized that it must be reserved for spinal deformity in which all other means of surgical correction will not yield a satisfactory result. Their indications for use of the device are about the same as those of O'Brien et al. listed below.

O'Brien, Yau, and Hodgson have also had extensive experience with the use of halo-pelvic traction in Hong Kong. Their indications for halo-pelvic traction include: (1) kyphosis; (2) severe scoliosis (over 100 degrees and rigid) with associated problems such as pelvic obliquity, respiratory insufficiency or marked kyphotic elements; (3) salvage procedure following failed spinal surgery; and (4) unstable spine secondary to laminectomy, malignancy, or trauma.

They have recommended the following procedures for preoperative assessment.

1. Myelography in all patients to rule out any intraspinal pathology causing cord compression such as in kyphotic deformities of any cause or diastematomyelia.

2. Tomograms of the deformity to show the presence of any spontaneous fusion, which would require osteotomies before any traction.
3. Lateral roentgenograms of the cervical spine to provide a baseline for comparison with subsequent films of the neck during distraction.
4. Intravenous pyelograms to discover any urinary tract abnormalities, which are present in 20% of patients with congenital deformities.
5. Bending films to define the flexibility of the curve.
6. Respiratory function studies to be used as a baseline for evaluation.

O'Brien et al. emphasize that following application of the halo and pelvic hoop for a kyphotic deformity, a primary anterior osteotomy or excision of a vertebral body should be accomplished. If the spine is not "springy" at the conclusion of this procedure or if a spontaneous fusion is present in this area, a posterior osteotomy must be done. Distraction then can begin with maximum protection of neural structures. Following the period of distraction, when the maximum correction has been reached, the chest is reopened and anterior strut grafting is carried out. Following recovery from this stage of the procedure a posterior fusion is also added as the final stage. The halo-pelvic distraction apparatus can then be maintained for a time and is finally replaced by a properly applied and fitted plaster cast.

O'Brien et al. also recommend that psychologic aspects of treatment be given consideration by letting prospective patients see and talk with those presently under treatment. This demonstrates that they may be ambulatory and that their deformities can be helped by the treatment.

APPLICATION OF PELVIC HALO (O'BRIEN ET AL.). General anesthesia is used. They emphasize that the pelvic pins should enter a point on the iliac crest anteriorly opposite the rough gluteal tubercle and emerge posteriorly just medial to the posterosuperior iliac spine; they believe that this placement is responsible for the few pin tract infections in a large group of patients so treated (Fig. 71-10). Fitting of the drilling jig is likewise important to ensure the proper path of the penetrating and self-tapping pelvic pin introduced with a carpenter's brace (Fig. 71-11).

AFTERTREATMENT. Postoperatively the patient should have no more than minor discomfort from either the skull halo or the pelvic halo. Continuing severe pain indicates something wrong, especially in regard to the pelvic halo. After several days the extension bars are fitted between the cranial halo and the pelvic halo with the patient awake (Fig. 71-12). O'Brien et al. use large spring balances with an upward distracting force of 20 to 30 pounds (9 to 13.5 kg) (Fig. 71-13). The protruding pins in the pelvic region are covered with dry dressings; if drainage begins, appropriate antibiotics are given. Distraction is increased at the rate of 2 or 3 mm per day. If neck pain develops, the distraction is discontinued for several days. A daily neurologic examination of the patient is essential and a clinical examination of those nerves most prone to injury is carefully performed each day. This evaluation includes not only the lower extremities but the upper extremities and cranial nerves as well. To evaluate any overdistraction of the

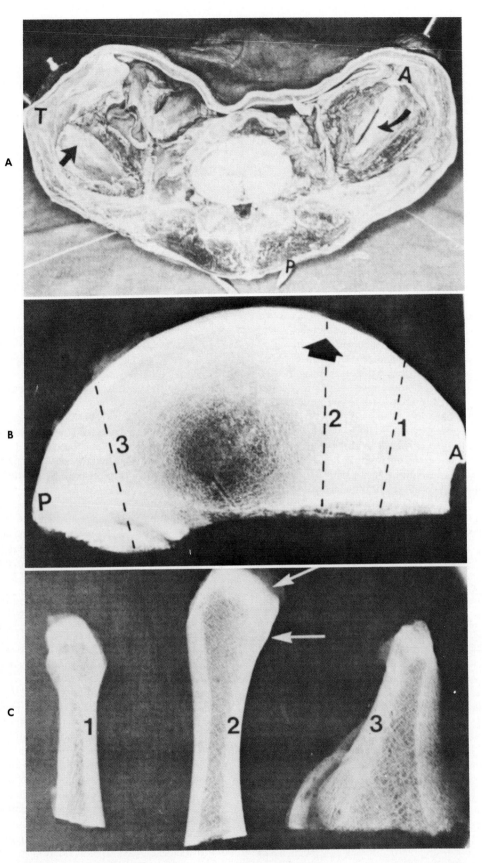

Fig. 71-10. Placement of pelvic pin. **A,** Pin is inserted as at *T* on left to keep it intraosseous. **B,** Pin is inserted at *2,* area of roughened tubercle of iliac crest. **C,** Pin is inserted at *2,* cross section of area *2* in **B.** (From O'Brien, J.P.: Acta. Orthop. Scand. Suppl. No. 163, 1975.)

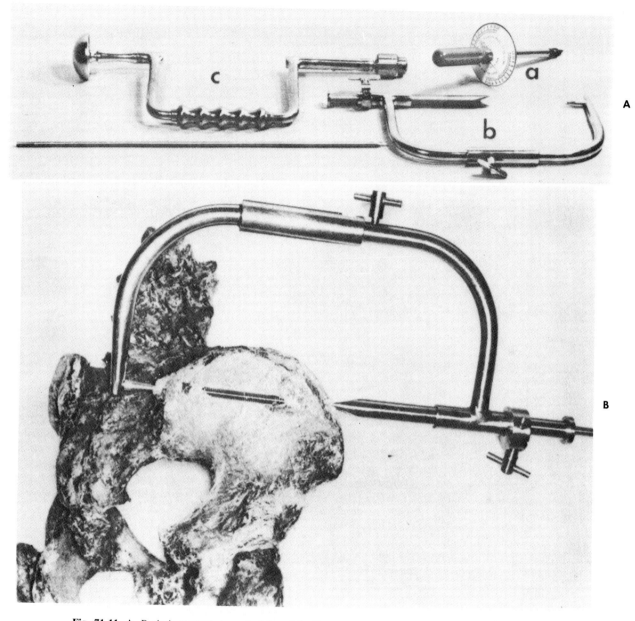

Fig. 71-11. A, Basic instruments to apply halo-pelvic distraction. *a,* Torque screwdriver; *b,* drilling jig; *c,* carpenter's brace. **B,** Use of drilling jig to insert pelvic pin. (**A** from O'Brien, J.P.: Acta Orthop. Scand. Suppl. No. 163, 1975; **B** from O'Brien, J.P., et al.: Clin. Orthop. **93:**179, 1973.)

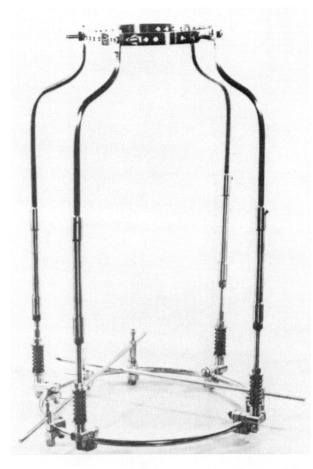

Fig. 71-12. Halo-pelvic apparatus. (From O'Brien, J.P.: Acta Orthop. Scand. Suppl. No. 163, 1975.)

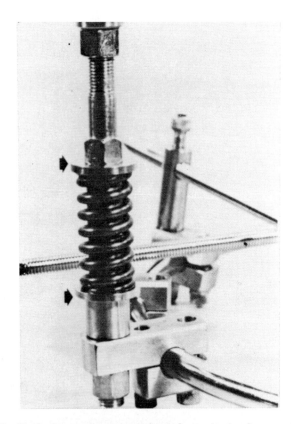

Fig. 71-13. Compression spring at base of extension bar for measuring forces. (From O'Brien, J.P.: Acta Orthop. Scand. Suppl. No. 163, 1975.)

neck, especially at the occipital and atlantoaxial joints, a lateral view of the cervical spine is included each time roentgenograms of the deformed spine are made.

In a study of 104 patients treated by O'Brien et al. the average time in the halo-pelvic apparatus was 7½ months. The average correction of deformity included tuberculous kyphosis, 31%; paralytic scoliosis, 51%; idiopathic scoliosis, 42%; congenital kyphoscoliosis, 26%; and neurofibromatous kyphoscoliosis, 43%. The most common significant complication of halo-pelvic distraction is in the cervical spine; degenerative changes in the posterior joints were found in 34% and avascular necrosis of the upper pole of the odontoid in 17% of patients. Cranial nerve neurapraxias occurred in 7% of the patients and brachial plexus palsy in 3%. The halo-pelvic apparatus is therefore not a casual alternative treatment for spinal deformities but rather must always be a part of a carefully planned approach in the management of severe spinal curvatures.

Halo cast

Combining the cranial halo with a Risser cast has provided ambulatory treatment of cervical fractures and after cervicothoracic fusions. The neckpiece of the cast is replaced by well-padded shoulder straps that support the halo uprights (Fig. 71-14, *A*). A halo yoke described by Houtkin and Levine was a major modification over the large overhead assembly present on the initial halo cast assemblies. Anderson and Bradford presented a new low-profile halo assembly, which is simple in design and has a wide margin of adjustability, an improved cosmetic acceptance, and a low cost (Fig. 71-14, *B*). Several modifications are now available.

Halo vest

Semirigid plastic vests with shoulder straps and metal attachments for a skull halo are commercially available from several sources. They are fitted from measurements and are usually lined with synthetic plastic "sheepskin." Indications include cervicothoracic and cervical fusion and injuries. They do not provide immobilization as secure as a halo cast that includes the pelvis for support and potentially they are only as secure as the patient allows. All straps and adjustments are accessible and can be loosened.

SPINAL FUSION
Determination of fusion area

The minimum fusion area is said to include every vertebra in the primary curve. In idiopathic scoliosis the min-

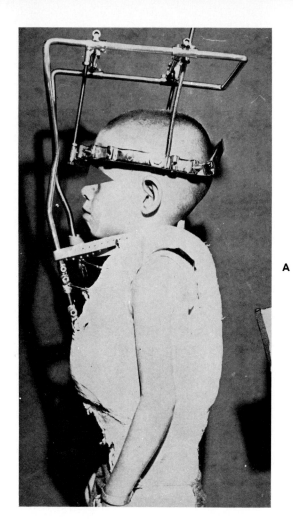

A

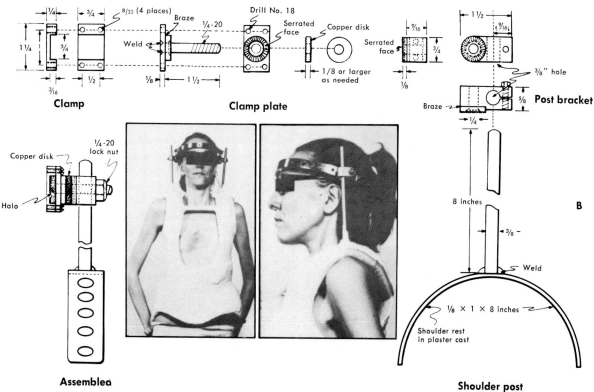

Clamp **Clamp plate** **Post bracket**

Assembled **Shoulder post**

Material: stainless steel except where noted

Fig. 71-14. A, Halo attached to patient and to body cast. **B,** Low-profile halo assembly. (**A** from Garrett, A.L., et al.: J. Bone Joint Surg. **43-A:**474, 1961; **B** from Anderson, S., and Bradford, D.S.: Clin. Orthop. **103:**72, 1974.)

imum fusion area should also include all vertebrae that are rotated in the same direction as those in the primary curve (Fig. 71-15). Even with this additional stipulation, fusing only the minimum fusion area is rarely recommended. Such a fusion might be satisfactory in a congenital curve or in a progressive idiopathic curve in a very young child in whom keeping the length of the fusion as short as possible is desirable to minimize the loss in height of the trunk. But even then, a brace will probably be necessary to control the unfused areas of the spine. The maximum fusion area has traditionally been described as the area of the spine that includes the one or more structural curves with the addition of enough vertebrae at each end so that the end vertebrae will be parallel to each other and transverse to the long axis of the trunk. A fusion area of this type is usually best suited for paralytic scoliosis in which both stabilizing the trunk and treating the deformity are desirable. When one considers the minimum and maximum fusion areas as just described, the area of fusion usually recommended includes the minimum area (all the primary curves plus the vertebrae at each end that are rotated in the same direction as those in the curve) with the addition of at least one vertebra at each end.

Side bending roentgenograms are especially important in selection of the fusion area (Fig. 71-1). For example, in a right thoracic, left lumbar pattern there is usually a large structural thoracic component with the lumbar curve having a large flexible component. In this case thoracic fusion

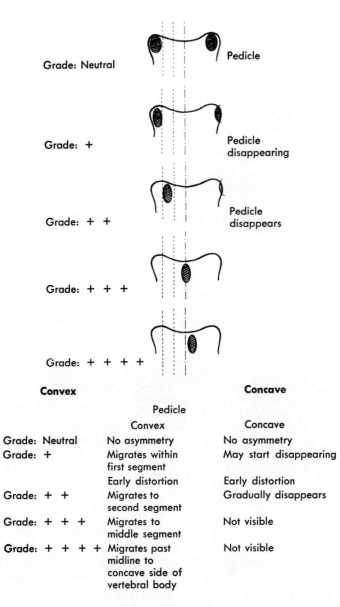

Grade: Neutral	Pedicle
Grade: +	Pedicle disappearing
Grade: + +	Pedicle disappears
Grade: + + +	
Grade: + + + +	

Convex **Concave**

	Pedicle	
	Convex	Concave
Grade: Neutral	No asymmetry	No asymmetry
Grade: +	Migrates within first segment	May start disappearing
	Early distortion	Early distortion
Grade: + +	Migrates to second segment	Gradually disappears
Grade: + + +	Migrates to middle segment	Not visible
Grade: + + + +	Migrates past midline to concave side of vertebral body	Not visible

Fig. 71-15. Pedicle method of determining vertebral rotation. Vertebral body is divided into 6 segments and grades from 0 to 4+ are assigned, depending on location of pedicle within segments. Because pedicle on concave side disappears early in rotation, pedicle on convex side easily visible through wide range of rotation is used as standard. (From Nash, C.L., Jr., and Moe, J.H.: J. Bone Joint Surg. **51-A**:223, 1969.)

alone is often possible as the lumber flexibility will allow it to balance and compensate for a surgically corrected curve.

Vertebral rotation, as already mentioned, must be analyzed and the basic principle followed that fusion must extend from neutral to neutral vertebrae. The exceptions to this must be determined from cast-corrected films or bending films. Also, in the lumbar region fusion need not extend to the sacrum if L-4 and L-5 are rotated. One segment below the end vertebra is sufficient at this lower level, since the extended rotation is less important as the curve approaches the sacrum. The penalty for lack of careful evaluation of the extent of fusion will be lengthening of the curve with loss of correction and usually an unacceptable cosmetic effect.

General considerations

The most careful study of roentgenograms to determine the exact location and extent of the fusion area is obviously of little value unless during the operation the vertebrae in the operative field can be identified precisely. The sacrum is an unmistakable anatomic landmark, but the contour of the various individual vertebrae are not sufficiently characteristic for exact identification. A method frequently used to identify vertebrae is to make a marker film. A small amount of a solution of sterile methylene blue is injected into the periosteum and bone of the spinous process of one or more vertebrae within the fusion area before surgery. A small radiopaque object such as a short piece of heavy wire is then strapped to the skin over the point of injection and an anteroposterior roentgenogram is made to identify the spinous process so marked. The use of superficial marks or scratches on the skin or the injection of dye into the soft tissues before making the marker film has not been reliable in identifying vertebrae. The simplest and most reliable method of establishing a landmark and the one we use consists of pausing briefly to make a marker roentgenogram when the spine has been exposed enough that the spinous processes are accessible. Before the patient is placed on the table, a cassette holder is properly positioned beneath him. Then during the operation a metal marker, usually an instrument, is attached to the spinous process of a vertebra in the fusion area, the operative field is covered by a sterile drape, and a roentgenogram is made using a film placed in the cassette holder. In identifying the vertebra it must be remembered that the spinous processes, especially in the thoracic area, droop inferiorly, usually as far as the body of the next vertebra inferior to the one in question.

The skin incision is best made in a straight line from a level one vertebra superior to the proposed fusion area to a level one vertebra inferior to it. A straight scar improves the appearance of the back, but a curved one over the spinous processes draws attention to any residual curve. When autogenous iliac bone is to be added to the fusion area, it is usually obtained through a vertical incision made just lateral to the posterosuperior iliac spine, avoiding cluneal nerve injury. It need not be made when the level of fusion is in the lower lumbar or in the lubosacral area because the posterior part of the ilium can be reached by dissecting from the midline incision laterally just superficial to the fascia and deep to the subcutaneous tissue.

The exact techniques of fusion used by various orthopaedic surgeons experienced in the surgical treatment of scoliosis vary in detail, but all aim at forming a fusion plate that is as substantial as possible. Harrington and Dickson made a thorough study of 578 patients with idiopathic scoliosis treated by one of eight methods. Differences among the methods included varying the instrumentation, the use or nonuse of extra autogenous iliac bone grafts, varying the type of cast, and varying the time of ambulation. During this 11-year study, each of the eight groups illustrated a step in the evolution of the design of instrumentation and the change in spinal fusion procedure or postoperative management. They concluded that (1) the spine can be satisfactorily corrected with the Harrington distraction and compression systems providing the maximum correction, (2) the correction is maintained, with a loss of 6% (2.5 degrees), (3) a robust well-developed fusion results from a facet block fusion in the thoracic region with a lateral gutter extension widening the base of the fusion mass in the lumbar region and using autogenous iliac supplemental bone grafts, and (4) external immobilization with a well-molded body cast is necessary for a minimum of 9 months after surgery. Gradual ambulation within days of the fusion, reaching a near normal level by 3 months, promotes early fusion and a robust fusion mass.

Most surgeons, in addition to using all bone available in the fusion area, add other grafts, preferably of autogenous bone and usually from the posterior ilium. When the spinal fusion is performed through a window in the cast, now rarely done, autogenous iliac grafts can usually be obtained satisfactorily if the window in either a turnbuckle or localizer cast is enlarged over the ilium on the convex side of the curve to be fused. When necessary, additional grafts may be obtained by resecting one or more segments of any prominent ribs. We dislike removing grafts from the patient's tibia. A large defect in the bone and the osteoporosis of disuse may cause the tibia to be fractured, especially since when the patient is first allowed up, the lack of normal agility and the weight of the plaster cast increase the stresses that the bone must withstand.

With modern techniques of anesthesia and blood replacement, carrying out spinal fusions in two or more stages as was so often done in the past is now rarely necessary. If such a staged procedure is necessary, the principle of fusing the apex of the curve during the first stage and then both ends of the curve during the second stage should be followed so that the fusion areas do not overlap at the point of maximum stress. Endotracheal anesthesia, usually with either controlled or assisted respiration, is essential. Equipment for warming blood before transfusion should be used so that rapid replacement of lost blood with refrigerated blood is unnecessary. Access to one or preferably two veins large enough for intravenous infusions should be maintained throughout the operation and the period immediately after surgery. In larger children and adolescents we avoid the veins of the legs for infusions because of the risk of thrombophlebitis in these age groups. All sponges should be weighed and all liquid blood removed by suction from the operative field should be carefully measured. A timesaving and accurate method of

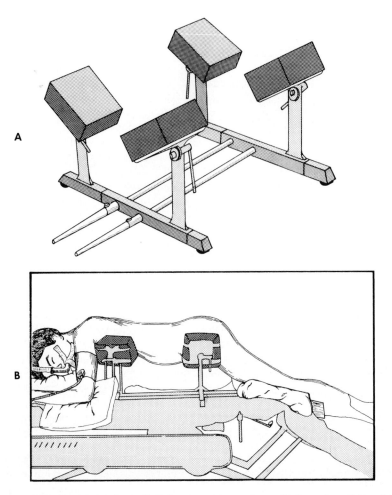

Fig. 71-16. A, Scoliosis operating frame. **B,** Patient in position on frame. (Redrawn from Relton, J.E.S., and Hall, J.E.: J. Bone Joint Surg. **49-B:**327, 1967.)

measuring the blood loss is to use 1000 ml graduated cylinders as the primary trap bottles in the suction system. The amount of liquid blood suctioned away can then be read directly from the trap bottle. For smaller children in whom accurate blood loss determinations are even more important, smaller and therefore more accurately graduated cylinders can be used. By using appropriate self-retaining retractors and an electrocautery with large bayonet forceps as one of the electrodes, spinal fusions can be carried out quite satisfactorily with one assistant who can operate the suction and the electrocautery. Meticulous attention to details of hemostasis will reduce blood loss to less than 1000 ml in most uncomplicated cases.

Autotransfusions of stored blood or of washed red cells obtained from wound suction have been used to help avoid or minimize the use of homologous blood transfusions.

Spinal surgery requires extensive dissection and the possibilities of severe blood loss. Relton and Hall first emphasized the role of intraabdominal pressure and designed an apparatus to reduce blood loss (Fig. 71-16). The use of this frame has been beneficial for us as well as other spine surgeons. Modifications of this frame have been reported by Mouradian and Simmons.

The gouges, osteotomes, curets, and other instruments used in the operations should have large long handles so that they may be controlled with both hands. Their edges should be sharp so that forceful use of a mallet can be minimized. A few very small gouges should be available for use in children below the age of 6 years.

Techniques of fusion

The importance of the technique of fusion in scoliosis is difficult to evaluate because many different techniques have been successful. The classic Hibbs technique has been replaced at our clinic by a modification of the intraarticular fusion of the lateral articulations described by Moe and the meticulous dissection around the transverse processes recommended by Goldstein. Improved operative techniques over the past 20 years have made it possible to correct a curvature between 50% to 60% with an infection rate of 1% or less and a pseudarthrosis rate of 2% or less. The higher fusion rate has resulted from ensuring complete facet joint excision, replacement with autogenous iliac bone, thorough decortication of the entire laminal area, and addition of further autogenous iliac bone. A few examples of the techniques used in this country are described here; some methods are of historical interest and others are

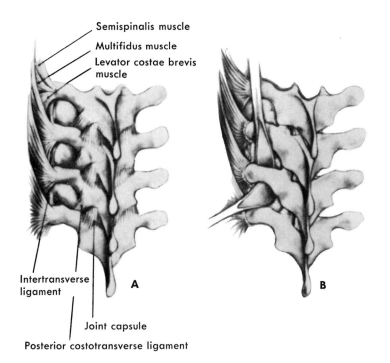

Semispinalis muscle
Multifidus muscle
Levator costae brevis muscle

Intertransverse ligament

A

B

Joint capsule

Posterior costotransverse ligament

Fig. 71-17. In Goldstein technique muscles and ligaments are stripped from transverse processes in thoracic area with Cobb elevator. **A,** Muscle attachments and ligaments usually seen during exposure of thoracic spine for fusion. **B,** After reflection of all soft tissue structures from laminae, lateral articulations, and transverse processes. (Modified from Goldstein, L.A., and Dickerson, R.B.: Atlas of orthopedic surgery, St. Louis, 1969, The C.V. Mosby Co.)

current; all seek to lower the pseudarthrosis rate and improve angular correction.

TECHNIQUE (COBB). Cobb preferred and used most often the Hibbs technique, which is essentially an extraarticular fusion to which autogenous iliac grafts are added. He described his method in great detail (1958), and his description is recommended. The operation is performed through a window cut in the back of the turnbuckle cast; a marker film made before surgery is essential. After the spine has been exposed, turn long spicules of bone from the spinous processes, laminae, and pedicles across the adjacent intervertebral spaces to lock under laterally bent spicules on the laminae and pedicles of the adjacent vertebrae. Use all bone available in the area to create as many spicules as possible still attached at their bases. However, Cobb recommended leaving intact the superior half of the spinous process of the superior vertebra of the fusion area and the inferior half of the spinous process of the inferior one so that the interspinous ligaments can become attached better, thus resulting in a more normal relationship between the superior and inferior ends of the fusion mass and the adjacent vertebrae. Cobb believed that the time necessary to carry out intraarticular fusion can be better used in obtaining more spicules of bone for bridging the intervertebral spaces. However, he stated that intraarticular fusion may be preferable in the lumbar area but not in the cervical area. He often used cancellous homogenous bone to shorten the operating time and to minimize shock. His results were excellent.

TECHNIQUE (GOLDSTEIN). At the sites of incision, infiltrate the skin and subcutaneous tissue with a 1:500,000 solution

of epinephrine in saline unless this is contraindicated by the anesthetic agent being used. Next expose the ilium widely through an incision parallel to the posterior two thirds of the iliac crest and obtain cortical and cancellous bone for grafting. Remove the cortex in strips with a gouge or an osteotome and the cancellous bone in strips from the entire exposed surface with a sharp hand gouge. Cut the cortical strips into thin slivers and save the cancellous strips intact. Close the incision over the ilium in layers. Then expose the spine subperiosteally, including the transverse processes in the thoracic area and the lateral articulations in the lumbar area. In the thoracic area carefully strip with a Cobb elevator all of the ligamentous attachments from the transverse processes, including the posterior costotransverse ligaments on the concave side of the curve (Fig. 71-17). In the lumbar area meticulously clean the posterior cortical surface of the spine and remove the capsules of the lateral articulations. Control bleeding with electrocautery and with self-retaining retractors. Thus the operative field is widely exposed with the soft tissues under tension. Using a sharp gouge with both hands, apply firm pressure to the spine and with a twisting motion carefully decorticate it (Fig. 71-18). Have several sharp gouges available and use a mallet only in older adolescents or adults with harder bone. In the lumbar area resect the posterior part of the lateral articulations while decorticating the laminae. In the thoracic area remove the inferior edges of the inferior articular processes, the adjacent bases of the superior articular processes, and the exposed cartilaginous surfaces while decorticating the laminae. Lay the strips of bone thus obtained and some of the bone grafts obtained

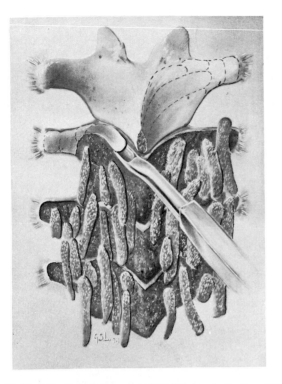

Fig. 71-18. Goldstein technique of spinal fusion (see text). (From Goldstein, L.A.: J. Bone Joint Surg. **41-A:**321, 1959.)

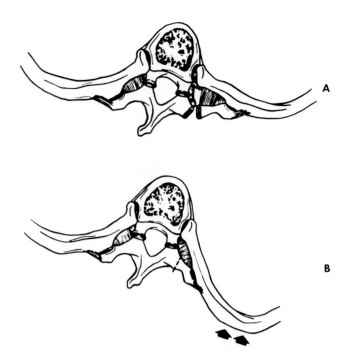

Fig. 71-19. Osteotomy for convex rib hump through transverse process. **A,** Correction after osteotomy and cast application. **B,** Deformity before surgery. (From Goldstein, L.A.: Clin. Orthop. **93:**131, 1973.)

from the ilium along the lateral edges of the spine, covering the intertransverse spaces, the lateral articulations, and the interlaminar areas. Then distribute the rest of the grafts along the fusion area, making the fusion mass slightly thicker on the concave than on the convex side of the curve. Insert the cancellous grafts first and the cortical grafts last. When using the Harrington instruments, prepare the insertion sites for the distraction hooks before starting the decortication. Then remove the spinous processes from the vertebrae and decorticate the laminae and transverse processes on the concave side of the curve only, but lay the bone chips aside. Next insert the distraction hooks, attach the distraction rod, and correct the curve as much as possible. If a compression rod assembly is also used, attach it and then decorticate the medial part of the laminae on the convex side of the curve and all of the laminae and transverse processes that are not used for hook attachments. For rib hump reduction when not using the compression system, perform an osteotomy of the convex transverse processes (Fig. 71-19). Finally insert the bone grafts. The fusion must include all vertebrae on which a purchase has been made by either distraction or compression hooks.

AFTERTREATMENT. If the curves have been corrected by a cast only, a new localizer cast is applied 12 to 20 days after surgery and the patient is discharged home to remain in bed for a total of 6 months. If the correction obtained is not being lost and an anteroposterior and two oblique roentgenograms of the fusion area show no evidence of a pseudarthrosis, then a new Risser localizer cast is applied and the patient is allowed to walk. This cast is worn for 3

or 4 months. Thus the average total time a cast is worn is 9 or 10 months. Originally, if Harrington instrumentation was used, patients with thoracic fusions were kept in bed for 3 months and patients with both thoracic and lumbar curves or thoracolumbar curves were kept in bed for 4 months. The localizer cast was worn for an additional month while the patient began to walk. Then a "double shoulder strap cast" was applied and was worn for 2 to 4 months. Thus the average total time of cast immobilization was about 8 months. Early ambulation can produce results equal to or better than those obtained with 3 to 6 months of bed rest. This is the result of secure spinal instrumentation combined with a well-fitted cast. Loss of as little as 5 degrees of correction can be achieved, and the arthrodesis appears to be stronger with vertical loading. The psychologic benefits for the child are immeasurable.

TECHNIQUE (MOE). Position the patient prone on a four-poster frame. Make a straight incision along the spine through the dermis only and inject an epinephrine solution (1:500,000) (Fig. 71-20). Continue the incision deeper and keep the skin margins forcibly retracted with Weitlaner retractors. Cauterize small vessels as they are encountered. Continue this incision down to the supraspinous ligament overlying the spinous process at each level. Then expose the spine subperiosteally by an incision in the middle of the cap of the spinous process and continue subperiosteal dissection laterally down the lamina to the tips of the transverse processes in the thoracic area and beyond the lateral articulations in the lumbar area (Fig. 71-21). At this time mark several spinous processes with an instrument, pack the wound, and obtain a localizing roentgeno-

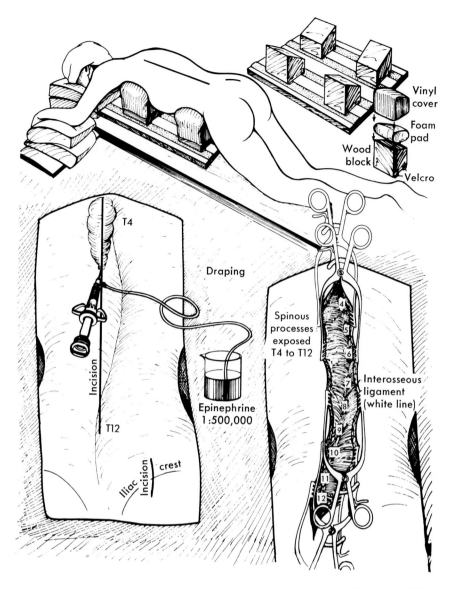

Fig. 71-20. Moe technique. Positioning of patient and skin incision (see text). (From Moe, J.H., et al.: Scoliosis and other spinal deformities, Philadelphia, 1978, W.B. Saunders Co.)

gram. While the roentgenogram is being developed, reopen the wound and continue subperiosteal exposure of the entire area to be fused, maintaining the retractors tight at all times. With a curet and a small pituitary rongeur completely clean the lateral articulations of all ligaments in the thoracic and lumbar areas (Fig. 71-22). If Harrington instrumentation is being carried out, prepare the hook sites and insert the hooks to be sure they are securely seated (Fig. 71-23). If a compression assembly is to be used also, apply it at this time (Fig. 71-24). A facet joint fusion is now carried out by a variety of techniques. In the thoracic area treat each lateral articulation as follows: elevate two hinge fragments of bone from the adjacent transverse processes, moving them laterally to fill the intertransverse area. This gains access to the superior articular process and its cartilage, which is thoroughly removed. Insert into the articulation a small block of bone cut from the transverse

or spinous process or ilium (Fig. 71-25). The similar technique of Hall can be used if desired (Fig. 71-26). In the lumbar area use a small osteotome to cut away the joint surfaces and reach the floor of the joint. Curet the latter free of all cartilage and firmly impact a block of cancellous bone into the defect created (Fig. 71-27). Next turn down multiple flaps of bone as thick as possible, crossing them over the spaces between the lamina and transverse processes. If a preoperative cast has not been used, a Harrington outrigger may be inserted, as shown in Fig. 71-28. Carefully controlled distraction must be used since this has great potential force. It is our preference to insert the distraction rod and correct the curve until the rod bows slightly. We then complete the decortication (Fig. 71-29) and add a large amount of autogenous iliac bone to the fusion, concentrating on the thoracolumbar and lumbar areas. Additional bone is also concentrated on the concave

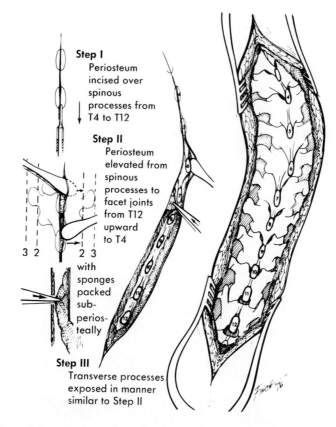

Step I
Periosteum incised over spinous processes from T4 to T12

Step II
Periosteum elevated from spinous processes to facet joints from T12 upward to T4

3 2   2 3

with sponges packed sub-periosteally

Step III
Transverse processes exposed in manner similar to Step II

Fig. 71-21. Moe technique. Exposure of posterior elements from T4 to T12 (see text). (From Moe, J.H., et al.: Scoliosis and other spinal deformities, Philadelphia, 1978, W.B. Saunders Co.)

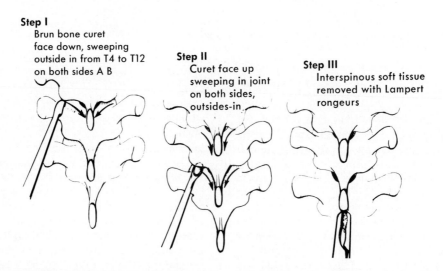

Step I
Brun bone curet face down, sweeping outside in from T4 to T12 on both sides A B

Step II
Curet face up sweeping in joint on both sides, outsides-in

Step III
Interspinous soft tissue removed with Lampert rongeurs

Fig. 71-22. Moe technique. Removal of soft tissue from bone (see text). (From Moe, J.H., et al.: Scoliosis and other spinal deformities, Philadelphia, 1978, W.B. Saunders Co.)

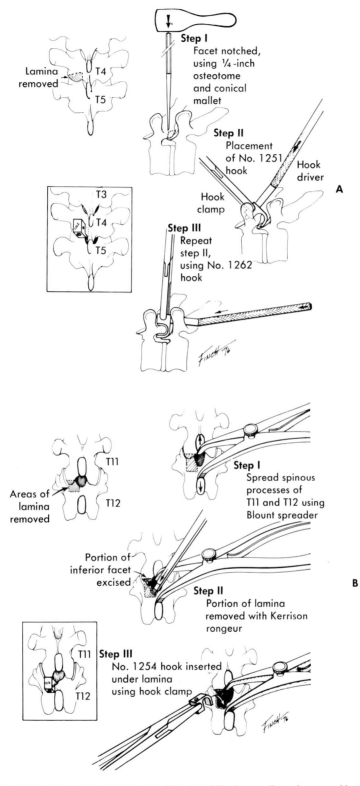

Fig. 71-23. Preparation of bone for insertion of hooks of Harrington distraction assembly (see text). **A,** Preparation for upper hook (T4 and T5). **B,** Preparation for lower hook (T11 and T12). (From Moe, J.H., et al.: Scoliosis and other spinal deformities, Philadelphia, 1978, W.B. Saunders Co.)

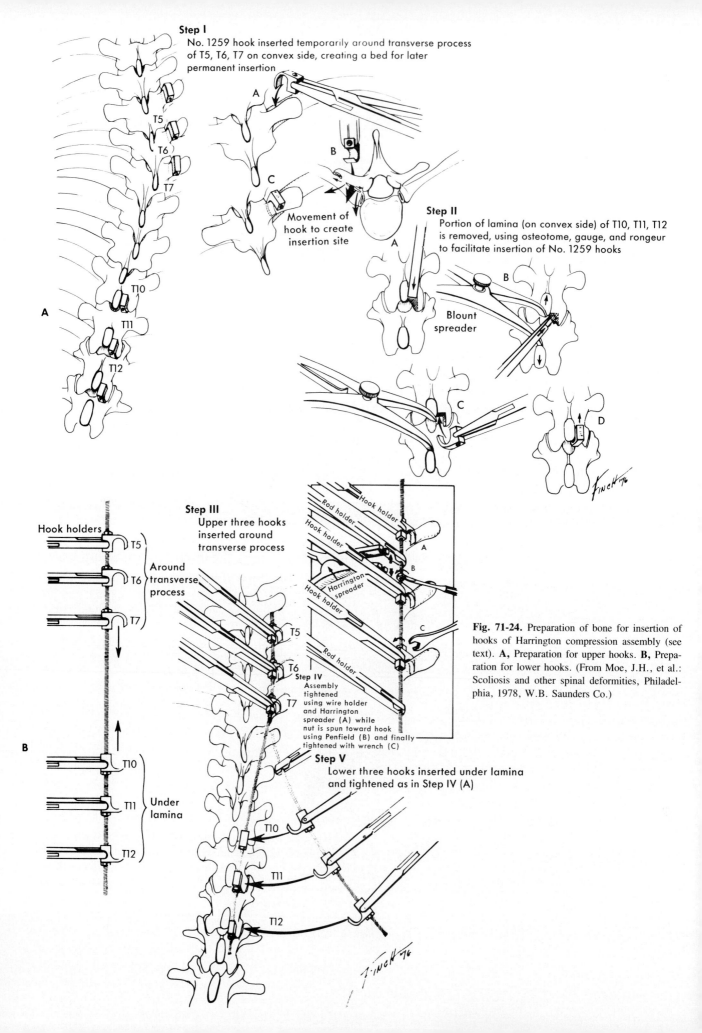

Step I
No. 1259 hook inserted temporarily around transverse process of T5, T6, T7 on convex side, creating a bed for later permanent insertion

A

B

C
Movement of hook to create insertion site

Step II
Portion of lamina (on convex side) of T10, T11, T12 is removed, using osteotome, gauge, and rongeur to facilitate insertion of No. 1259 hooks

A

B
Blount spreader

C

D

A

T5

T6

T7

T10

T11

T12

Hook holders

Step III
Upper three hooks inserted around transverse process

Around transverse process

Under lamina

B

T5

T6

T7

T10

T11

T12

Rod holder

Hook holder

Hook holder

A

B

Hook holder

Harrington spreader

Hook holder

C

Rod holder

Step IV
Assembly tightened using wire holder and Harrington spreader (A) while nut is spun toward hook using Penfield (B) and finally tightened with wrench (C)

Step V
Lower three hooks inserted under lamina and tightened as in Step IV (A)

T10

T11

T12

T7

Fig. 71-24. Preparation of bone for insertion of hooks of Harrington compression assembly (see text). **A,** Preparation for upper hooks. **B,** Preparation for lower hooks. (From Moe, J.H., et al.: Scoliosis and other spinal deformities, Philadelphia, 1978, W.B. Saunders Co.)

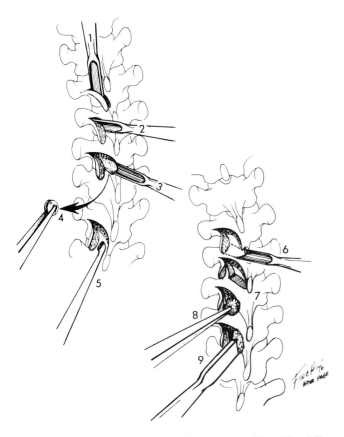

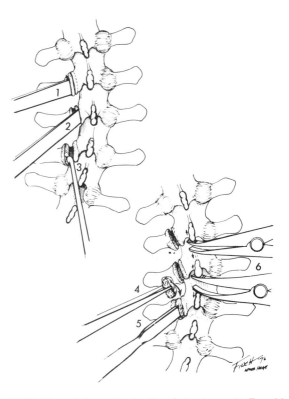

Fig. 71-25. Moe technique of facet fusion (see text). (From Moe, J.H., et al.: Scoliosis and other spinal deformities, Philadelphia, 1978, W.B. Saunders Co.)

Fig. 71-27. Moe technique of lumbar facet fusion (see text). (From Moe, J.H., et al.: Scoliosis and other spinal deformities, Philadelphia, 1978, W.B. Saunders Co.)

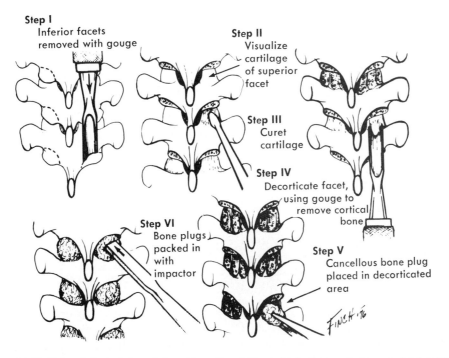

Step I
Inferior facets removed with gouge

Step II
Visualize cartilage of superior facet

Step III
Curet cartilage

Step IV
Decorticate facet, using gouge to remove cortical bone

Step V
Cancellous bone plug placed in decorticated area

Step VI
Bone plugs packed in with impactor

Fig. 71-26. Hall technique of facet fusion. (From Moe, J.H., et al.: Scoliosis and other spinal deformities, Philadelphia, 1978, W.B. Saunders Co.)

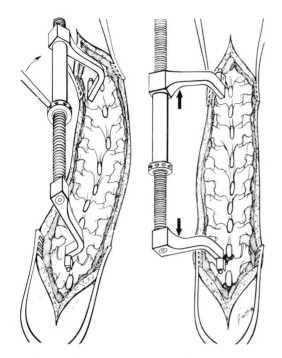

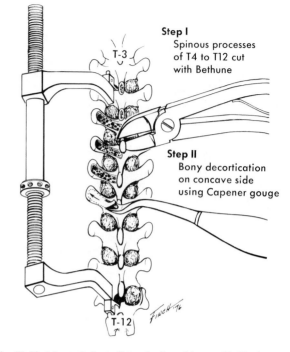

Fig. 71-28. Harrington outrigger for straightening spine (see text). (From Moe, J.H., et al.: Scoliosis and other spinal deformities, Philadelphia, 1978, W.B. Saunders Co.)

Fig. 71-29. Moe technique. Decortication of bone with Harrington outrigger in place. (From Moe, J.H., et al.: Scoliosis and other spinal deformities, Philadelphia, 1978, W.B. Saunders Co.)

side of the curves. Moe has osteotomized the bases of the transverse processes on the convex side of the curve in the absence of compression instrumentation (Fig. 71-30, *Inset*). As also recommended by Goldstein and by Cotrel of France, this technique reportedly allows more correction of the rib hump deformity with the use of the derotation strap at the time of postoperative casting. Immediately prior to closure secure a washer or a No. 18 wire about the upper end of the distraction rod against the upper hook and flatten the compression assembly threads with an instrument near the nut. Close the wound in three layers using a subcuticular suture for improved cosmesis.

AFTERTREATMENT. If spinal instrumentation has not been carried out, the patient may be kept supine in a cast for 3 to 6 months before the first cast change. With the use of secure instrumentation, a cast is applied after 1 week using a Risser-Cotrel technique and ambulation is allowed immediately. The cast is worn for 4 to 5 months. At that time it is changed and right and left oblique and anteroposterior roentgenograms are taken with the patient out of the cast to determine union. If the correction of the curves is being lost or if a pseudarthrosis can be seen on the roentgenograms, the fusion area is explored immediately and is repaired. If Harrington instrumentation has been carried out and the instruments are thought to be stable with strong purchases on bone, Moe has allowed early walking. Currently the cast preferred by him is similar to a Risser localizer cast but uses the principles developed by Cotrel.

Leider et al., in a study of 106 consecutive patients 12 to 20 years old, found that early ambulation after posterior instrumentation and fusion decreased the morbidity and

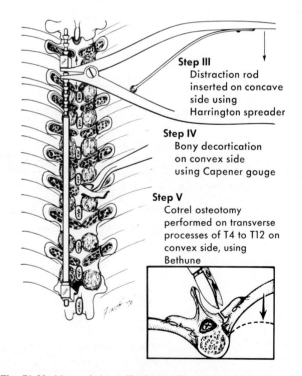

Fig. 71-30. Moe technique. Harrington distraction rod is inserted. Decortication is done on convex side of spine and Cotrel osteotomies *(Inset)* to correct rib hump are performed. (From Moe, J.H., et al.: Scoliosis and other spinal deformities, Philadelphia, 1978, W.B. Saunders Co.)

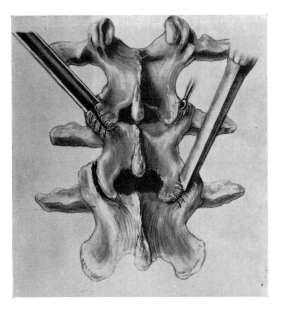

Fig. 71-31. Risser technique for intraarticular fusion in lumbar area (see text). (From Moe, J.H.: South. Med. J. **50**:79, 1957.)

was quite beneficial psychologically. These patients had fusion in an adequately prepared preoperative cast using Harrington instrumentation and autogenous iliac bone grafting. In 7 to 10 days a Risser-Cotrel cast was applied over double stockinette, emphasizing proper molding about the iliac crests and over the apex of the curve. The patients were allowed to walk within 10 days and had a cast change in 4 to 5 months, with a total cast time of 9 months. The loss of correction compared favorably with earlier methods, with a loss of only 5 degrees and a pseudarthrosis rate of 4.7%. A loss greater than 5 degrees indicates poor casting methods, and a change into a new, good cast is mandatory.

TECHNIQUE (RISSER). Correct the scoliosis by a localizer cast. Bivalve the cast and perform the fusion with the patient out of it. Expose the fusion area subperiosteally. In the dorsal area elevate the posterior half of the lateral facet, curet the lateral joint, and raise a flap of bone from the base of the transverse process and turn it into the joint. In the lumbar area carefully curet the articular facets, make longitudinal and transverse cuts across the facets into the joints, and then impact the resulting fragments of bone into the joints (Fig. 71-31). Next carry out a Hibbs fusion and add to the fusion area autogenous iliac bone.

AFTERTREATMENT. When the patient has recovered from the anesthetic, the bivalved localizer cast is reapplied. At 7 to 10 days the cast and sutures are removed, and a new localizer cast is applied. The patient is then allowed to be up and to walk. According to Risser, a loss of 2 to 3 degrees of correction with the patient standing and in the cast is acceptable; if greater loss occurs, the cast is inadequate. The cast is changed at intervals of 3 to 4 months until the fusion is mature. According to Risser, because each localizer cast is a corrective one, the correction is less frequently lost than when other casts are used.

Risser and Norquist report that of 177 patients treated

with a turnbuckle cast and fusion, the correction was maintained in 41%, and of 62 treated with a localizer cast and fusion, the correction was maintained in 68% even though walking was allowed early. We have adopted early ambulation following spinal fusion in uncomplicated idiopathic curves; results have been equal to those reported, and we have found the psychophysiologic benefits tremendous.

Harrington instrumentation and fusion

In 1972 Harrington reviewed 1055 patients with curves ranging from 35 to 170 degrees; there were 37 different causes, and ages of the patients ranged from 4 to 63 years. The minimum follow-up was 3 years. He drew the following conclusions:

1. The scoliotic spine is structurally unsound in a growing child when the factor is 3 or more, and curvature will progress at an unpredictable rate. The factor is obtained by dividing the number of degrees of curvature by the Cobb method by the number of vertebrae in the curve.
2. The scoliotic spine in the mature patient is structurally unsound when the curve has reached a factor of 5. After maturity progression can be expected in all patients when the factor is 7. Progression or degeneration of the spine proceeds at an unpredictable rate but generally follows that rate cited by Risser of 1 degree per year.
3. When the major curve is located in the thoracic segment of the spine, the structurally unsound and deformed spine will cause cardiopulmonary compromise and can lead to shortening of the expected life span.
4. When the major curve is in the lower segment of the spine, the symptoms are primarily pain and fatigue with a diminished work capacity. Terminal disabilities may be moderate or severe, with the possibility of paraplegia.
5. A structurally unsound, deformed spine with a kyphotic component will lead to increased deformity and with the passage of time may produce a paraplegia.
6. The cosmetic effects to be gained by instrumentation of the scoliotic spine must be considered to be secondary, for although they are gratifying to both the patient and the surgeon, this aspect should not take precedence in the surgeon's judgment.

Instrumentation is a metallic system designed to apply forces of distraction and compression over several segments of the spine in the area of the posterior elements. The instruments hold the correction obtained for a reasonable length of time until the fusion can develop and take over stabilization of the original correction. Although the major force is provided by the distraction system, the contribution of the compression system is integral to the effectiveness of the total system. To dispense with the compression mechanism altogether amounts to an infraction on the correcting and holding potential of the total system. From 80 to 100 pounds (36.3 to 45.4 kg) is the safe range of force applied to a distraction hook; force on the compression hook is rarely more than 25 pounds (11.3 kg).

The general rule is that hooks should be one vertebra

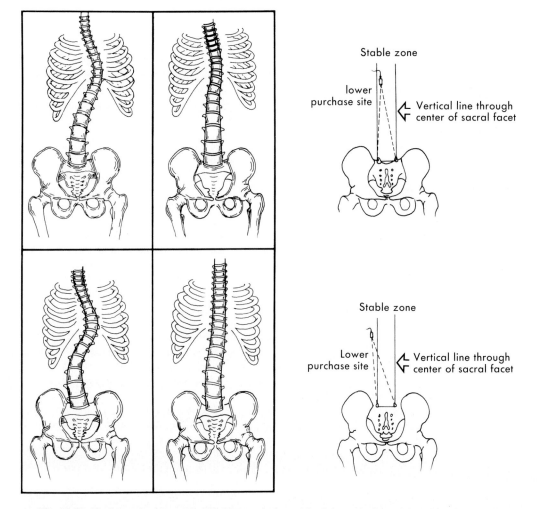

Fig. 71-32. Harrington instrumentation. Stable zone is formed by lines vertically projected from S1 articulations. Lower hook must fall within this zone. (Redrawn from Harrington, P.R.: Orthop. Clin. North Am. **3:**49, 1972.)

above the vertebra at the top end of the major curve and two vertebrae below the vertebra at the lower end. If the centroid of function of the lower hook does not fall within the stable zone, as illustrated in Fig. 71-32, the instrumentation must be supplemented. This can be done in three ways: by overlapping distraction rods, by a dollar sign application, or by adding a sacral bar. The sacral bar is used only in paralytic scoliosis and never in idiopathic curves. Harrington therefore recommends the following basic rules:

1. With primary thoracic and primary thoracolumbar curves, hooks should be placed one vertebra above the top vertebra and two vertebrae below the lowest vertebra of the curve.
2. With a double primary curve, the dollar sign application should be used.
3. With a primary lumbar curve, hooks should be placed one vertebra above the top end vertebra and at the lower end vertebra (Fig. 71-33).

Seating of a hook requires utmost care to prevent instrument failure, such as lateral rotation. This is prevented in three ways: (1) the distraction hook should be seated in the pedicle at the prescribed angle; (2) the keel of the No.

1252 hook will prevent rotation and lateral slipping; and (3) the whole shoe of a No. 1253 hook can be introduced into the spinal canal with no harmful effect (Figs. 71-34 and 71-35). The lower hook is always placed in the spinal canal. Although Harrington recommends that L5 should not be instrumented because of its lordotic posture, we have not found disengagement to be a factor at this level (Fig. 71-36). The compression hooks (No. 1259) are always seated on the convex side of the curve at the base of the transverse processes in the thoracic area (Fig. 71-37) and at the lamina of the lumbar vertebra. Ease of entry of these hooks can be aided by preforming a hole in the soft tissues with a sharp No. 1259 hook on a hook holder.

The sequence of application should be compression first, followed by distraction. The application of the forces then, both distraction and compression, should never be rapid. Force should continue until the first plateau of resistance is encountered. At this juncture it is our habit to obtain the bone grafts and allow fatigue of the resisting structures. Additional correction can then be obtained with attention being paid to the purchase sites of the distraction hooks for any crushing of bone. The apical hooks of the compression system are compressed first, moving sequentially toward

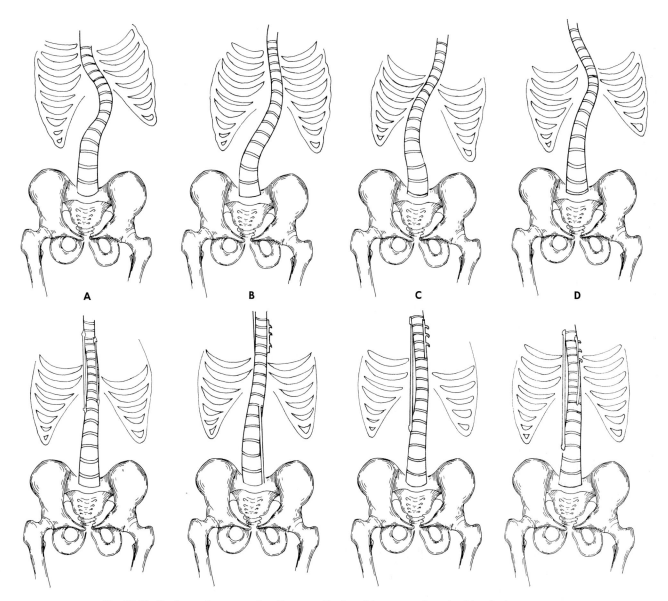

Fig. 71-33. Harrington instrumentation. Proper application of instruments in each of four basic curve types. **A,** Primary thoracic. **B,** Double primary. **C,** Primary lumbar. **D,** Thoracolumbar. (Redrawn from Harrington, P.R.: Orthop. Clin. North Am. **3:**49, 1972.)

the respective ends of the rod. Force should be continued as long as there is correction toward the concave side but discontinued immediately if lordosis begins. Although a distraction system has been used alone, Harrington warns that this weakens the correcting and holding potential of the instrumentation and reduces the correction from about 64% to 51%. It must be reemphasized that correction of the deformity must be accomplished by small, gradual increments in force. He has found that 1.4 mm of erosion at a distraction hook will equal a 6 to 8 degree loss in correction. Therefore this must be carefully observed periodically during the application of force.

All instrumented spines must have an accompanying posterior spinal fusion extending at least from the superior to the inferior hook (Fig. 71-38). Harrington varied the type of fusion, the type of external immobilization, and the time from surgery to ambulation, and made the following recommendations:

1. Complete decortication of the fusion site is mandatory.
2. Eradication of all facets within the extent of the fusion is mandatory.
3. A broad lateral gutter fusion at the base of the operative site is superior.
4. Supplementary bone is mandatory; the autogenous iliac source provides superior material.
5. Supplementary bone should be laid down in a linear fashion, primarily on the concave side and with a broad base.
6. A gradual controlled gravity loading program over a 6-month period after surgery is of definite benefit in maturation of the fusion mass (Fig. 71-39).

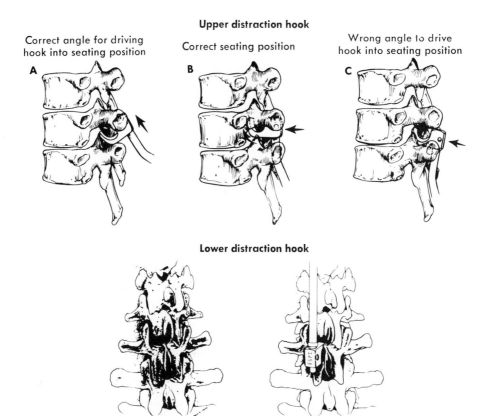

Upper distraction hook

A Correct angle for driving hook into seating position

B Correct seating position

C Wrong angle to drive hook into seating position

Lower distraction hook

Fig. 71-34. Intricate details of upper and lower distraction hook placement. (From Harrington, P.R.: Orthop. Clin. North Am. **3:**49, 1972.)

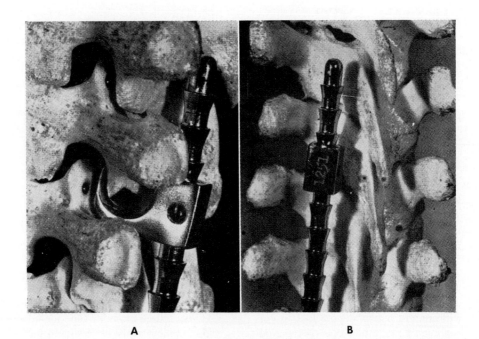

A   B

Fig. 71-35. Upper distraction hook. **A,** Lateral view of several dorsal vertebrae showing relation of upper distraction hook, ratchet rod, and articular process where it is engaged. Notch of hook is inserted into margin of inferior articular process at black area shown here. **B,** Posterior view showing upper distraction hook and ratchet rod in place. (From Harrington, P.R.: J. Bone Joint Surg. **44-A:**591, 1962.)

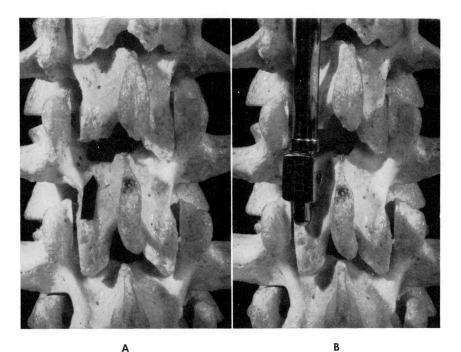

A   B

Fig. 71-36. Lower distraction hook. **A,** Posterior view of several lumbar vertebrae showing point of placement of hook; arrow points to notch prepared in superior laminal ridge. Note that inferior facet of vertebra above has been resected to make room for preparing notch and placing hook. **B,** Posterior view showing lower distraction hook and distraction rod in place. Thorough knowledge of anatomy of region is necessary in preparing notch and placing hook; no meningitis or cord symptoms should ever follow this procedure. (Courtesy Dr. Paul R. Harrington.)

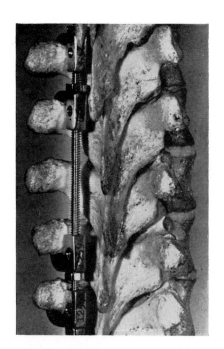

Fig. 71-37. Compression assembly with four hooks properly placed on base of transverse process of four dorsal vertebrae. (From Harrington, P.R.: J. Bone Joint Surg. **44-A:**591, 1962.)

Adequate instrumentation operates as an elastic module that makes it possible to promote a transformation of the fusion mass. These undulating forces, rather than sustained ones, prevent necrosis at the hook purchase site.

The most common fracture of instrumentation is that of the distraction rod, which occurs in about 15% of cases. This occurs at the first ratchet junction, and usually between the eighteenth and thirty-sixth months after implant. If this causes no symptoms, periodic observation (every 3 to 6 months) should be made, asking the questions, Does the rod show progressive overlap? Has the curvature increased? If the answers to these questions are in the affirmative, pseudarthrosis is to be be expected, and exploration of the spine with new instrumentation and fusion should be carried out. In the majority of cases, if this does not occur and the curve remains stable, continued observation without reoperation is indicated.

The compression assembly was not for a time used routinely by many surgeons who used the Harrington method because it was common practice to protect the spine after surgery with plaster casts until the fusion mass was solid. The technique of Harrington instrumentation has been modified frequently because the instruments are now widely used both to correct curves primarily (or to increase any correction already obtained) and to internally fix the corrected curves during spinal fusion. Our modified technique for Harrington instrumentation and spinal fusion is described here.

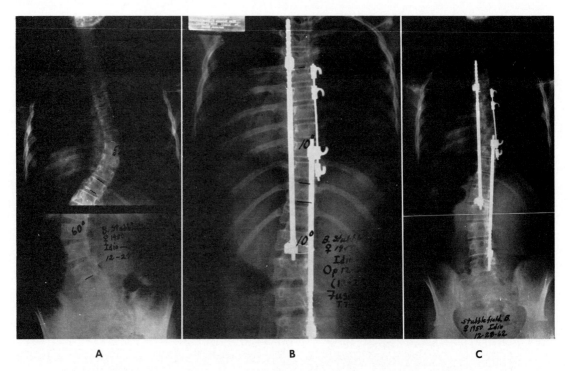

A   B   C

Fig. 71-38. Harrington treatment by instrumentation and fusion. **A,** Spine of 11-year-old girl with idiopathic scoliosis with right dorsal primary curve of 55 degrees and left lumbar one of 60 degrees. **B,** Spine after curves have been corrected to 10 degrees each by instrumentation; spine has been fused by Moe technique. **C,** Spine 2 years after fusion. Note that ossification of iliac epiphyses is complete. About 5 degrees of correction have been lost, but spine is stable and patient is free of discomfort. Removing instruments at 5 years after surgery is planned. (Courtesy Dr. Paul R. Harrington.)

TECHNIQUE (HARRINGTON, MODIFIED). Although Moe and others originally operated through a large window cut in the posterior aspect of the cast, almost all routinely carry out scoliosis surgery with patients out of the cast. The preparation of the skin and the sterile draping are more efficient in the absence of a cast and the advantage to the anesthesiologist and the surgeon of having the entire thorax free for any examination and emergency treatment necessary during surgery is also to be considered. The advantage of having the patient in a cast during surgery is that the curve or curves are then partially corrected and the Harrington instrumentation is usually somewhat easier; furthermore, the support of the spine after the instrumentation is uninterrupted.

Endoctracheal anesthesia with controlled or assisted respiration is always used. One or more veins must be made accessible to ensure that fluids and blood can be administered. The blood sucked from the wound must be measured accurately and the wet sponges must be carefully weighed. We use graduated cylinders for the trap bottles in the wound suction system. Any fluid used for irrigating the wound must be carefully measured and subtracted from the total fluid in the bottle. The blood content of the sponges discarded during surgery is calculated by weight as the operation progresses. The amount of blood typed and crossmatched before surgery should be about twice the anticipated requirement. For the average adolescent we routinely have available 2000 ml because the average

blood loss is between 500 and 1200 ml. Obviously having to discontinue an operation because not enough blood is available for transfusion is always unfortunate. The problem is lessened by meticulous attention to hemostasis and dissection.

Place the patient prone on the operating frame so that the abdomen is relatively free of pressure. In placing the supports at the pelvis, avoid pressure on the femoral vessels. Do not elevate or abduct the arms at the shoulder more than 90 degrees because brachial plexus palsies are much more common when these positions are more extreme. Prepare the skin thoroughly, including the entire back and the base of the neck, and drape out a wide area, including the entire thoracic and lumbar parts of the spine and the posterior aspect of both iliac crests. Draping out both iliac crests rather than only one is preferable because if any bone grafts are lost or dropped or if the quantity of bone from one ilium is insufficient for a heavy fusion mass, the other ilium is immediately available. After the drapes have been applied, cover the entire field with a large piece of transparent adherent plastic material that is commercially available.

Now make a straight skin incision over the spine or if the curve is extremely flexible and marked correction of it is anticipated, a slightly curved one to follow the scoliotic curve. Make the incision only partially through the skin at first and infiltrate the skin and subcutaneous tissues with a 1:500,000 solution of epinephrine in saline. The anes-

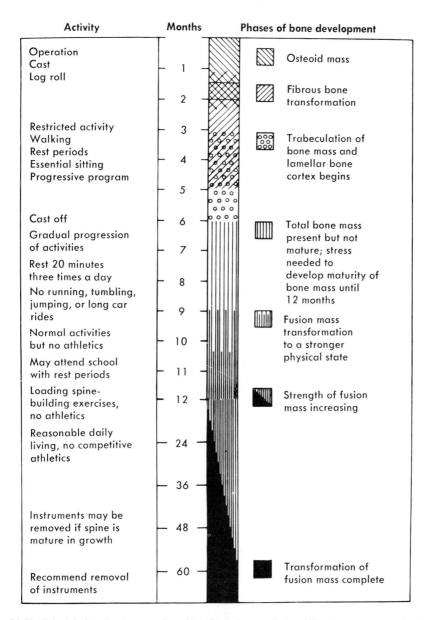

| Activity | Months | Phases of bone development |

Fig. 71-39. Spinal fusion development timetable. Gradual controlled mobilization program results in same fusion mass at 6 months that would be attained after 12 to 18 months without early mobilization. (From Harrington, P.R.: Orthop. Clin. North Am. **3:**49, 1972.)

thetic agent must be suitably chosen in advance even if a small amount of epinephrine is to be used in this way. This superficial infiltration saves both time and blood in the early stages of the operation. Now carry the dissection directly down to the lumbodorsal fascia and use several self-retaining retractors to keep tension on the soft tissues until the most superficial part of the supraspinous ligament is reached. Follow the contour of the curve and locate and identify the tips of the spinous processes. Then carry the sharp dissection directly to the tip of each spinous process and in the midline split the cartilage cap of each in immature patients or the periosteum in more mature patients in whom the cartilage cap is no longer present. Then connect the incisions over the tips of these processes by splitting the supraspinous ligament, keeping in the midline as

accurately as possible because the tissues are less vascular here. Then with a Cobb elevator split and separate the cartilage caps or the periosteum directly over the spinous processes and start the subperiosteal dissection down each side of each individual process. By using the Cobb elevator and dissecting from inferiorly to superiorly the subperiosteal dissection and the separation of the interspinous ligaments and the muscles from the midline are made easier. As the soft tissues are separated laterally on each side, lower the self-retaining retractors progressively deeper into the wound and spread them widely against the soft tissues to increase the exposure and to minimize bleeding. Bleeding is controlled by the assistant with the suction tube and with an electrocautery to which a large or medium-sized bayonet forceps is attached. At this point in the operation have an anteroposterior roentgenogram of the spine made after attaching a metal marker to the most inferior spinous process in the wound. This spinous process is selected because the lower thoracic and the lumbar vertebrae are the most easily identified. This marker film is important because the exact location of the fusion area must be determined. An error of one or two vertebral levels in placing the hooks can seriously affect the efficiency of the instrumentation and the correction of the curve. Now with the Cobb elevators reflect the soft tissues and strip the many ligamentous and muscular attachments from the posterior elements of the spine as close to bone as possible, leaving little soft tissue on the area to be fused. Carry the dissection laterally to the tips of the transverse processes in the thoracic area and beyond the lateral articulations in the lumbar area. Usually at least one segmental artery is encountered near the lateral articulations between the bases of adjacent transverse processes in the thoracic area. Prompt cauterization at each level is vital in minimizing total blood loss. When the entire exposure has been completed and the soft tissues have been retracted and held under tension by several self-retaining retractors, use sharp curets of several sizes to clean the remaining soft tissue from the exposed bone. Take special care to remove the capsular tissue from the lateral articulations in the thoracic area. Meticulous removal of the soft tissue is quite important in obtaining a successful fusion.

After bleeding from the soft tissues has been controlled by the electrocautery and the occasional bleeding from the bone has been controlled by small bits of bone wax, choose sites for placement of the distraction hooks on the concave side of the curve. Insert the most superior hook into the lateral articulation inferior to the most superior vertebra in the fusion area; insert it under the lamina of this vertebra directly into the joint (Fig. 71-35). This vertebra will then be included in the fusion area. Using the hook inserter, insert a sharp-edged plain large Harrington hook (No. 1251) without excessive force, making sure that the blade of the hook actually goes between the two joint surfaces and not within the medulla of the lamina of the vertebra above. When the location for the hook has been established, withdraw this hook and insert a large dull flanged hook (No. 1262) in its place. The vertical flange is designed to prevent the blade in the hook from slipping laterally out of the joint or the unlikely possibility of its slipping medially toward the spinal canal. Once the hook is fully seated, check its stability by forcing it superiorly with the inserter to be sure that an adequate distractive force can be applied to it. If the stability of the hook is doubtful, consider placing the hook in a different joint, usually the next one superiorly. The most inferior distraction hook is usually placed in a lumbar vertebra. We have occasionally placed this hook in the lamina of T12 when the posterior elements of this vertebra were similar to those of a lumbar vertebra; do not place the hook through the lamina of a thoracic vertebra. On the selected lumbar vertebra insert a dull hook (No. 1254 or 1253 if there is enough space) under the lamina after curettage of the ligamentum flavum and cutting away portions of the lamina laterally in addition to the caudalmost portion of the inferior articular process of the superior vertebra. Do this

carefully with a Kerrison rongeur as illustrated in Fig. 71-23, *B*.

Now check the stability of this hook by manual force before attempting to use the hook for distraction. Again if the stability is doubtful, the next vertebra inferiorly can generally be used without any serious problem. Then select a distraction rod of suitable length and insert its notched end through the superior hook while holding the hook in place with a hook holder. Then while the superior hook and hook holder are held by an assistant, grasp the inferior hook with a hook holder and feed the inferior end of the rod into the eye of that hook. Next fit the spreader or distractor between the superior hook and the notch in the rod just inferior to it and by repeated spreading of the instrument force the superior hook up the notched part of the rod. Thus the distance between the hooks at each end of the rod is increased with each successive click of the instrument. Proceed carefully with the distraction while observing the stability of both hooks. As the distraction becomes more difficult and the instruments tighten, any evidence of fracture or tearing of the posterior elements indicates that the distraction should be stopped and the correction obtained at that point should be accepted. The correction obtainable varies considerably depending on the age and maturity of the patient and the hardness of the bone. When the bone is mature, usually the distraction can be continued until the rod begins to bow. It must always be remembered that considerably more force can be exerted with the Harrington distractor than can be tolerated by any of the posterior elements.

Now apply the compression rod assembly using the smaller threaded rod ($\frac{5}{16}$ inch or 8.0 mm) and the No. 1259 hooks. Cut the costotransverse ligaments using a sharp No. 1259 hook introduced beneath the transverse process with a hook holder. Direct this caudad on all vertebrae above the apex of the curve and cephalad below. Caudal to T11 the transverse processes are inadequate; place the hooks under the lamina. Grasp the assembly with hook holders. Beginning cranially, place all of the hooks beneath the transverse processes and laminae, and begin the tightening using the spreader between the rod and hook holders. The wrench can also be used to tighten the nuts (Fig. 71-24, *B*). This device produces lordosis and tightening should cease when it begins to occur.

Now pack the wound with sponges and obtain additional bone for the fusion mass from the posterior iliac crest. Incise the skin over the crest and infiltrate it with epinephrine as already described for the midline incision. Incise the lateral edge of the epiphysis of the crest or the periosteum along the lateral edge of the crest and expose the external surface of the ilium subperiosteally from a point inferior to the posterosuperior iliac spine laterally and anteriorly. With sharp gouges remove strips of cortical and cancellous bone from the large exposed area of the iliac wing down to but not including the inner cortex. Take care not to tear or cut the branch of the gluteal artery in the depths of the wound adjacent to the sciatic notch or to extend the dissection into either the hip joint capsule or the sciatic nerve. After all available bone has been removed, suture the periosteum or the edge of the epiphysis to the soft tissues over the iliac crest, being careful that the gluteal muscles and consequently the buttock is not displaced laterally; pull the large gluteal flap medially with each suture. If necessary place a plastic tube for suction drainage in the iliac wound; this may not be necessary if bleeding from the bone is only slight. While the grafts are being cut into small slivers, expose the spine again with several self-retaining retractors and begin the decortication. Carry out a Moe type of intraarticular fusion of the lateral articulations (p. 3196) combined with the meticulous decortication of the laminae and transverse processes recommended by Goldstein (p. 3195). The distraction rod on the concave side of the curve will be in the way, but we have not found that it prevents us from performing an adequate intraarticular fusion. The advantage of not having to carry out the distraction in the face of active bleeding from decortication more than outweighs the disadvantage of having the rod in the way. As the decortication continues, bleeding may be brisk. Systematic and continuous decortication minimizes time to completion and thereby can decrease the blood loss at this stage of the procedure.

After the decortication and the intraarticular fusion are complete, insert the bone grafts obtained from the ilium; pack them between the transverse processes on the concave side of the curve in the thoracic area and between the lateral articulations in the lumbar area. Always pack more bone on the concave side of the curve; pack bone beneath the rod but usually not lateral to it. Make the fusion mass heaviest in the lumbar and thoracolumbar areas. Next insert a plastic tube for suction drainage into the depths of the wound and close the wound with a running No. 0 or 1 chromic suture at the level of the cartilge caps or the supraspinous ligament; make this closure tight. Then carefully approximate the subcutaneous tissue to eliminate dead spaces between the skin and the fascia over the spinal musculature: hematomas in dead spaces may have been important in the infections that we have seen. Next approximate the skin edges with a subcuticular absorbable suture and secure the skin edges with skin staples. Replace blood as dictated by the amount lost, preoperative hematocrit, and general condition of the patient.

AFTERTREATMENT. At 48 hours the dressing is changed and the suction drainage tube is removed. On the fifth to seventh day a Risser type of cast is applied under moderate traction. Alternatively, a molded plastic body jacket that can be removed for showering is used. This removable jacket is appropriate for adults and responsible teenagers. Ambulation is allowed immediately if no soft bone or instrumentation problems exist. At 4 to 5 months the cast is removed and horizontal anteroposterior and right and left oblique roentgenograms of the fusion area are made. If the fusion mass is intact and appears to be maturing satisfactorily, a new snug Risser cast is applied. If the fusion is below T5, the cast may be only axillary high. We usually protect the fusion mass for a total of 9 or 10 months.

PARTIAL DISCECTOMY

Schultz and Hirsch have shown experimentally that in cadaver spines the stiffness in lateral bending of a typical thoracic spine motion segment is in the order of 20 kpcm per degree. This would mean that a curve of 60 degrees over six vertebral levels would require a corrective mo-

ment on the order of 200 kpcm. The present methods of correction do not produce moments of this magnitude. It further has been shown that the intervertebral disc and longitudinal ligaments contribute 80% to 90% of the stiffness of the motion segment in lateral bending. The surgical attack on intervertebral discs does significantly decrease resistance to correction as exemplified by the Dwyer procedure. Similarly, partial discectomy allows better correction with Harrington instrumentation when lateral deviations are great or enables one to improve correction when lateral corrective forces are used such as in casting. Moreover, greater derotations are possible with partial discectomy in conjunction with lateral force correcting procedures.

SEGMENTAL SPINAL INSTRUMENTATION

Eduardo Luque of Mexico City in 1973 reported the use of multiple wires passed beneath the laminae on each side of each spinous process to mechanically straighten or contour the spine by twisting the wires around long round rods laid along each posterior laminar surface. Contouring the two rods allows the spine to be pulled over to the corrected position as the wires are tightened. Internal fixation is more rigid than with the Harrington instrumentation, and arthrodesis seems to be enhanced. The internal fixation provided has been efficient enough to convince many spine surgeons that external immobilization is not needed postoperatively. Neurologic complications, apparently from passage or manipulation of the wires in the spinal canal, have been reported frequently enough that the procedure should be used in neurologically normal patients only by experienced spine surgeons in medical centers where spinal cord monitoring can be carried out.

Drummond et al. in 1984 reported segmental spinal instrumentation or wiring in which the wires are passed transversely through a small steel button and then through the base of the spinous process to be twisted and tightened around rods laid on the laminae as with the Luque technique. Thus the spinal canal is not invaded by the wires and neurologic complications are minimal. As a rule we use Drummond wiring for neurologically intact patients and Luque wiring for patients with neuromuscular scoliosis and for patients with complete neurologic deficits.

DWYER INSTRUMENTATION

For most patients with spinal deformity surgery from the posterior approach is preferred, but for some patients posterior surgery is impossible or alone is insufficient. In 1964 Dwyer, in cooperation with Newton, developed instrumentation for correction and fixation through an anterior approach. Dwyer instrumentation uses large metal staples of several sizes that fit over the vertebral bodies and are attached to each body with a large screw. The screws have a large head with a hole for passage of a cable that is tightened at each level and then fixed by crimping the screw head.

By placing the staples more anteriorly, lordosis can be corrected. By placing the staples and screws in the same location in each vertebral body regardless of the position of the body, rotation can also be corrected as the curve straightens. Kyphosis will be made worse by Dwyer instrumentation.

The indications for the Dwyer procedure are limited. The Dwyer procedure is a valuable adjunct to treatment of selected spinal deformities, but most deformities can be treated properly with posterior instrumentation. At present, the indications for the Dwyer procedure are (1) lumbar curves in patients with deficient posterior elements such as in myelomeningocele, (2) thoracolumbar curves with extreme lordosis, and (3) rigid thoracolumbar paralytic curves for which a combined anteroposterior fusion in two stages is required. An absolute contraindication to the Dwyer procedure is kyphosis in the area to be treated. The Dwyer apparatus is not recommended for children less than 10 years of age because of the small size of the vertebral bodies. It is also not recommended for adults with extremely osteoporotic bone. There are several advantages of Dwyer instrumentation, anterior correction, and fusion:

1. Because the discs are large, their removal results in marked mobilization with increased correction and sound fixation of the curve obtained at every level.
2. Excellent correction of lordosis is obtained.
3. Correction of rotation along with the curve is possible by placing the screw and staple in the same relative position in each vertebral body.

The Dwyer procedure also has disadvantages:

1. The procedure is time consuming.
2. Instrumentation of the sacrum is difficult, and therefore correction of pelvic obliquity is difficult.
3. Instrumentation above the T6 level is difficult.

Complications of the Dwyer procedure include those common to any major anterior surgical exposure of the spine: pneumothorax, hemothorax, aspiration pneumonia, and paralytic ileus. In addition to these there is the possibility of mechanical damage to the spinal cord by a screw or vascular damage to the cord from the extensive exposure with division of multiple segmental arteries. The latter, while possible theoretically, may or may not have occurred clinically. In addition, cable breakage and loss of fixation at one level are common, and even with an intact apparatus, solid interbody fusion does not always occur. With the Dwyer procedure alone for rigid paralytic curves, the group at Rancho Los Amigos Hospital has noted a pseudarthrosis rate of over 50% and consequently recommends that the anterior Dwyer fusion be supplemented by a posterior fusion.

TECHNIQUE (DWYER). Position the patient with the convex aspect of the curve uppermost. Approach the thoracic and thoracolumbar spines anteriorly as indicated (p. 3098 and p. 3099). The exposure gains access to the spine anteriorly and is followed by a disc excision in two stages. First remove the anulus along with the nucleus pulposus and leave only the posterior anulus. Next remove the cartilage end plates as completely as possible. At this stage the first major bleeding is encountered; minimize it by packing the spaces to slow the oozing from the cancellous bone (Fig. 71-40, A).

Instrumentation proceeds from above downward on the convex side of the curve except in rare circumstances (Fig. 71-40, B). Incise the anulus of the intact disc of the uppermost body to allow the flange of the staple to grip just over the end plate. During placement of the screws, check and recheck the direction to avoid penetration of the pos-

terior cortex and the spinal canal (Fig. 71-40, A). The ideally placed screw runs horizontally across the body, just engaging the opposite cortex and lying safely in front of the neural foramen.

After the first two plates and screws have been placed, insert rib chips into the disc space. Introduce the cable through the two screws and tension it. When correction is obtained, crimp the screw head onto the cable and deal with the succeeding spaces in the same manner. Crimp an extra collar on the cable below the final screw. At the conclusion, cover the cables and screws by suturing over the pleura or the psoas muscle in the thoracic or lumbar area, respectively (Fig. 71-40, C).

AFTERTREATMENT. At the end of 2 weeks a plaster jacket is applied and ambulation is allowed. Dwyer's only known failure to obtain good fusion occurred in the absence of plaster immobilization. Dwyer gave antibiotics until 2 weeks after the temperature was normal. The aftertreatment is then as described for the Harrington technique (p. 3211).

ZIELKE INSTRUMENTATION

Zielke of Germany modified Dwyer's principles by using a solid, flexible rod instead of a cable. Experienced spine surgeons in medical centers have successfully used this type of anterior instrumentation, which can be used in kyphotic areas of the spine and is recommended for its derotating ability.

COMPLICATIONS OF TREATMENT

The operative treatment of scoliosis is formidable, and many significant complications are possible during this treatment. These complications may occur in any stage of treatment from the time of application of a corrective cast until the convalescence after surgery is complete. They should be prevented, of course, if at all possible.

Complications in cast

In the cast pressure sores may develop over any improperly padded bony prominence. Any complaint of localized pain under the cast should be investigated immediately, and usually a part of the cast should be removed and repadded or the entire cast should be removed and reapplied. Moe recommends making a cruciate cut in the cast over the painful area and carefully bending out the plaster at the edges. Brachial plexus palsies were much more common when turnbuckle casts were usually used than now when the Risser or similar casts are used. Single nerve palsies are still occasionally produced by localized pressure at the edge of the cast. Meticulous technique in applying casts will minimize or almost eliminate pressure sores and nerve palsies.

Compression of the duodenum in its third portion by the superior mesenteric artery was described by Rokitansky more than 100 years ago. This condition may appear in two forms: the acute form and the chronic form, designated Wilkie's syndrome. The condition has been observed in various pathologic states. The cast syndrome described by Dorph in 1950 is an acute form of this syndrome. The syndrome consists of vascular compression of the duodenum leading to acute duodenal obstruction and gastric dilatation. Pernicious and often projectile vomiting ensue

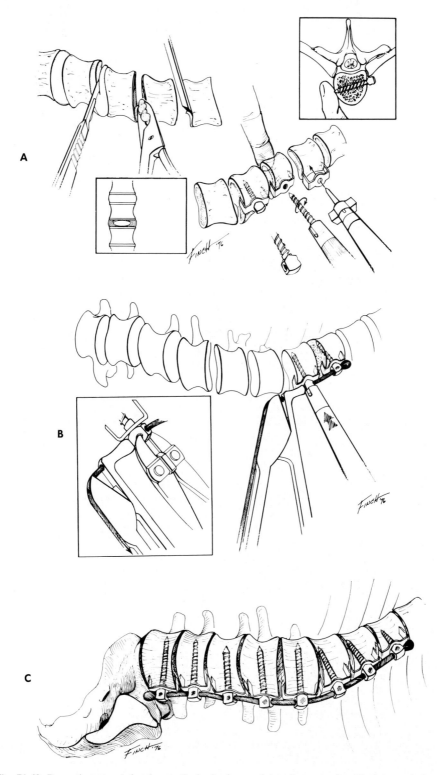

Fig. 71-40. Dwyer instrumentation (see text). **A,** Anulus, nucleus pulposus, and cartilaginous end plates are removed at each level and instrumentation is begun. **B,** Instrumentation proceeds from above downward to convex side of curve. **C,** Instrumentation has proceeded to L5. Two reinforcing collars are applied at end of cable to cover it. (**A** to **C** from Moe, J.H., et al.: Scoliosis and other spinal deformities, Philadelphia, 1978, W.B. Saunders Co.)

Continued.

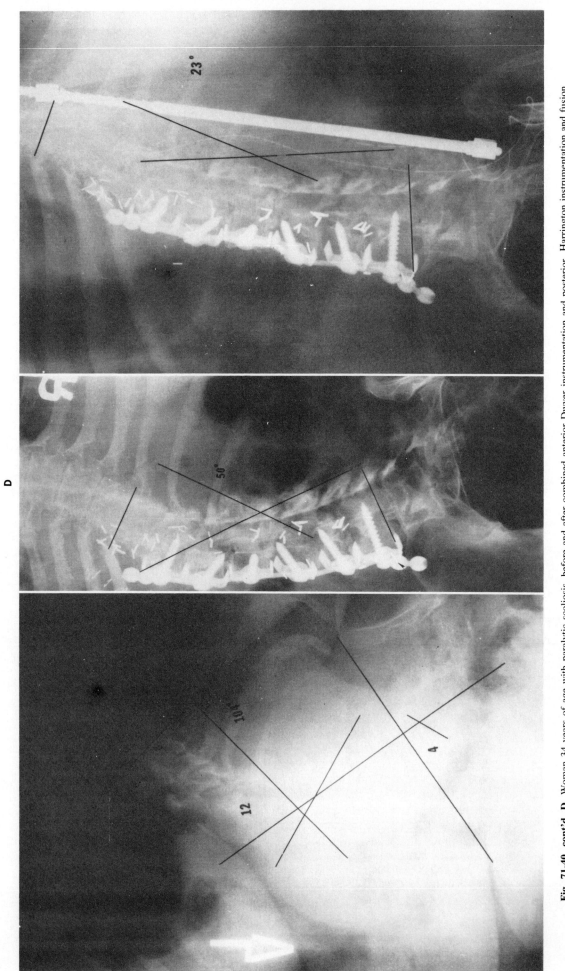

Fig. 71-40, cont'd. D, Woman 34 years of age with paralytic scoliosis before and after combined anterior Dwyer instrumentation and posterior Harrington instrumentation and fusion.

and a potentially dangerous situation exists. A high index of suspicion must be maintained in those individuals with vomiting, abdominal distention, and mild pain. Since this is a partial obstruction, flatus will continue to be passed and symptoms may be intermittent. Diagnosis is based on the radiologic findings of a dilated duodenum. Contrast studies will show a linear obstruction at the level where the superior mesenteric vessels cross the duodenum. A lateral decubitus examination of the abdomen with the patient's right side up will reveal a dilated duodenal loop with a long air fluid level. When combined with the appropriate history and physical findings, this is virtually a pathognomonic sign. The treatment should consist of prompt removal of the cast if present, combined with early nasogastric suction. Other measures should be position changes, particularly to a prone position, restriction to a liquid diet, and ambulation if possible. General surgical consultation should be sought early since those facing prolonged immobilization may require surgery.

Evarts, Winter, and Hall reported on 30 patients from the literature and from their own experience with vascular compression of the duodenum properly termed a superior mesenteric artery syndrome. Eighteen of these cases had occurred with correction of the scoliosis operatively; 12 occurred with the application of body casts only. It is emphasized that with correction of the curvature an increase in the angle of the superior mesenteric artery with the aorta results in compression of the duodenum and symptoms of partial intestinal obstruction.

We have seen this syndrome develop in a patient in whom the course had been uneventful during the correction of scoliosis by a cast followed by Harrington instrumentation and rest in bed in a Risser cast for 6 months. Yet 2 years later after a spica cast was applied after reconstructive surgery on a hip, the typical syndrome developed.

Complications of skeletal traction

Skeletal traction is a safe method for correcting many types of spinal curves when carefully supervised. Halo-femoral traction is not recommended for congenital kyphosis, and for any other type of pure kyphosis it must be considered dangerous. Moe has been a pioneer in the use of this traction and has stated that forces of more than 25 to 35 pounds (11.3 to 15.9 kg) are not helpful even in older patients and that probably a force of 20 pounds (9 kg) is sufficient. We have used 15 to 25 pounds (16.8 to 11.3 kg) without neurologic complications. Temporary palsies of the extraocular muscles and of the brachial plexus have been reported when the traction was too forceful. One patient of ours, a male 18 years of age, developed severe hypertension while in halo-femoral traction. When the traction was discontinued, the hypertension subsided and we were unable to find any other cause for the hypertension. When the weights are added in small increments and the patient is observed carefully, we believe that skeletal traction is probaby the safest method for correcting congenital scoliosis and very long or stiff curves of any type. Infections around the halo pins are rare and usually can be avoided by meticulous skin care and by moving pins to new locations when necessary. We have had no experience with the halo-pelvic traction. Skeletal traction, both the halo-femoral and halo-pelvic types, are now rarely used as modern internal corrective devices become more efficient.

Complications during surgery

Other complications were included in the discussions of operative techniques, but neurologic sequelae remain the most feared and intangible. Because of this situation, spinal cord monitoring is not only being used clinically as a routine but also is being investigated in many centers. The widely used ''wake-up'' test of Stagnara is practiced clinically but must be repeated 20 or 30 minutes after the first negative test for further assurance of preserved neurologic function. The definitive test is the ''wake-up'' in the operating room with demonstration of function. For many years this was the only test we used and we did not move the patient from the surgical suite until function was clearly demonstrated. Reporting 124 patients in 1973, Stagnara described a method of anesthesia to sufficiently dissociate pain and consciousness while permitting spontaneous motion on command after instrumentation. By observing motion of the hands and feet the surgeon can establish the neurologic function distal to the spinal surgery. If motor power does not clearly appear in the lower extremities but does so in the hands, instrumentation is immediately removed and the request repeated. The success depends on careful and controlled anesthesia. On the other hand, Engler et al. point out the real hazards in arousing a prone, intubated patient from anesthesia:

1. Raising the head may cause accidental extubation, which could be disastrous; reintubation is difficult with the patient prone.
2. A sudden deep inhalation while awakening could possibly lead to air embolism through aspiration of air into the open vessels of the wound.
3. A violent movement could dislodge the spine instrumentation or intravenous tubing or could result in laminar fractures.

SPINAL CORD MONITORING

Research and development of techniques to detect intraoperative neurologic complications during spinal surgery have been active in past years. The ''wake-up'' test described by Vauzell, Stagnara, and Jouvinroux has been widely used to functionally test spinal cord conductivity by lightening anesthesia during surgery so that the patient becomes alert enough to move actively both upper and lower extremities in response to commands. As Brown and Nash have pointed out, this test documents only that spinal cord function has not suffered a major compromise at the time the test is performed. Therefore the time the test is performed during the surgical procedure is quite critical. Because of this, multiple wake-up tests have been performed by spine surgeons to increase the safety factor. It is widely accepted that the earliest recognition of compromise of spinal cord function probably allows the best possibility of its reversal. Difficulties of significant magnitude with performance of the wake-up test have led surgeons to delay stressful portions of the surgical procedure to as late a stage of the operation as possible and then to rely on immediate waking of the patient in the operating room for functional tests at the completion of the procedure. Thus, if a functional deficit develops sterile equipment is immediately accessible so that mechanical reversal such as rod removal, decompression, and so forth can be accomplished promptly. Intraoperative difficulties such as uncontrolled, violent activity and removal of endotracheal tubes during wake-up tests can occur even with experienced and highly competent anesthesia personnel.

To enhance the safety of spinal surgery, electrical monitoring of spinal cord function has evolved as researchers have approached the problem from at least three slightly different directions. Stimulation of a peripheral nerve produces an evoked response or electrical potential that with sophisticated electronic equipment can be detected proximally in the spinal cord itself, in the vertebrae proximally at spinal cord level, and from the cerebral cortex. These spinal evoked potentials from the cord and cortical evoked potentials from the brain are frequently referred to as somatosensory evoked potentials. It is generally accepted that these potentials and their transmissions effectively reflect function of the dorsal columns; the degree to which they reflect anterior cord function is not yet well established.

Researchers have used (1) direct dural recording, (2) vertebral body recording in developing techniques to monitor spinal evoked potentials, and (3) cerebral cortex recording through needle electrodes in the scalp to monitor cortical evoked potentials. Dural recordings are necessarily invasive and thus are ordinarily feasible only during open spinal surgery. Vertebral body recordings are also invasive during surgery, but can be recorded with percutaneous electrodes well proximal to the surgical field. These techniques to monitor spinal evoked potentials have the advantage of being relatively unaffected by anesthetic agents and commonly used drugs. Scalp recordings of cortical evoked responses have the advantage of being essentially noninvasive and thus can be used preoperatively and postoperatively. This feature can be vitally important perioperatively to evaluate positioning of the patient on supportive equipment or in skeletal traction in the operating room. The greatest disadvantage of monitoring by cortical evoked response is its sensitivity to anesthetic agents, especially halothane. Equipment and technical assistance must routinely be better than adequate to consistently effect dependable cortical monitoring. The most dependable setup in our experience has used surface stimulation of both median and tibial nerves and recordings from percutaneous spinal electrodes at C2, in addition to scalp electrodes for cortical readings. With both upper and lower extremity stimuli and both spinal and cortical evoked potentials available to monitor, technical and equipment malfunction can be more easily identified. Conversely, apparent spinal cord malfunctions can be verified as being organic with considerable confidence.

Aside from evaluating evoked potentials with a normal wave pattern and normal latency and the opposite, an absent wave, interpretation of recordings obviously is critical and requires both skill and experience. As previously mentioned, cortical evoked responses can be somewhat prone to artifactual distortion, some of which occasionally defies explanation. Reports both clinical and laboratory suggest that increases in latency and decreases in amplitude are significant signs of change in evoked potentials and may be evidence of deterioration in spinal cord function. Decreases in amplitude of up to 50% when sustained only temporarily have rarely if ever been associated with neurologic deficit, while decreases in amplitude of over 50%, especially when sustained, have on occasion been an indication of impaired function that was clinically evident at the completion of the operation. Wilber, Thompson, Shaffer, Brown, and Nash consider that more than 50% decrease in peak-to-peak amplitude of the primary complex or an increase of more than 3 mm in the peak latency associated with the complex are abnormal findings indicative of possible neurologic injury. Statements of principle more conclusive than this are probably not warranted, given the current state of the art. We conclude that (1) spinal cord monitoring even in expert hands can indicate that spinal cord function is impaired but does not with certainty develop this information before irreversible spinal cord pathology and (2) regardless of monitoring findings, movement by the patient on command is the ultimate test of neurologic function and obviously must be basic to clinical decision making when monitoring findings are uncertain or confusing.

When competently performed, spinal cord monitoring, by demonstrating changes in evoked potentials, may provide some measure of early warning of spinal cord pathology and therefore add one more safety factor to those already available for spinal surgery.

Complications immediately after surgery

Ileus is a common complication after spinal fusion in scoliosis. We prefer to withhold oral feedings until the bowel sounds return, usually in 36 to 72 hours after surgery. Until then intravenous fluids must be administered.

Atelectasis is a common cause of a fever after surgery. Frequent turning of the patient and deep breathing and coughing will usually control or prevent serious atelectasis. The use of inhalation therapy with intermittent positive pressure breathing may be beneficial in cooperative patients, but inflation of the stomach during this type of breathing must be avoided. Incentive spirometry is now commonly used instead.

A deep *wound infection* after a scoliosis fusion is a major complication but is rarely disastrous. The tissues in the area of fusion are vascular and both the posterior elements of the spine and the autogenous cancellous bone grafts seem to be extremely resistant to most infections. The extensive operating dissection, the lengthy time required for the operation, the use of metallic implants, and the closure of the wound over freely bleeding bone are all factors common to most surgery for scoliosis and theoretically make infection more likely. Also, infection rates are higher (1) in myelodysplasia, (2) with urinary tract infections, and (3) with increased traffic in the operating room. Among the general factors important in preventing infection in the operating room are careful control of the circulating air and of the circulating personnel, frequent evaluation of the equipment used for sterilizing instruments and linen, and proper development of the surgical technique. In the surgical technique, the skin must be carefully prepared both on the ward and in the operating room, the drapes must be carefully applied, and the wound must be carefully closed to avoid leaving dead spaces, especially in the subcutaneous tissues. Suction drainage and careful closure of the subcutaneous tissues and the skin help prevent subcutaneous hematomas or seromas. Certainly hematomas are always present around the fusion mass but in the wound infections with which we have had experience, a large hematoma has always been found between the skin and the deep fascia overlying the spinal muscles. We always use suction drainage with one tube in the fusion area and at 48 hours remove the tube and dress the wound. Although we have not used them routinely, reports have shown decreased infection rates with the use of prophylactic antibiotics.

Moe has reported two types of wound infections after surgery. The first type is quite obvious in that sepsis with a high fever develops, usually within 2 to 5 days after surgery, and the wound almost always appears infected. In the second type the temperature is elevated only slightly or moderately and the wound appears relatively normal. Diagnosis of wound sepsis may be difficult. Patients often have a postoperative temperature elevation of up to 102° F daily. This should gradually decline over the first 4 days. Any spike of temperature above 102° F should raise strong suspicion of a deep wound infection, especially if a steady improvement in the general condition is not seen. The appearance of the wound is usually deceiving, with no significant swelling, erythema, or tenderness. Moe et al. recommend prompt aspiration of the wound in several sites. Cultures should be submitted, but results should not be awaited, and reoperation should be planned immediately.

The treatment of such an established infection requires that the patient be given an antibiotic for a penicillin-resistant *Staphylococcus aureus* since this is the most common offending organism. With additional blood transfusions available, the patient is operated on under general anesthesia; all infected necrotic tissue is removed by careful debridement. The bone grafts and instrumentation are left in place, and the wounds are closed over two plastic ingress-egress tubes. Antibiotic wound irrigation is carried out for about 5 days and is discontinued when the patient is afebrile and laboratory evidence of infection is decreasing. Intravenous antibiotics are administered for approximately 10 days with oral administration continued for a minimum of 6 weeks.

Most fusion masses become solid even after an infection but occasionally a draining sinus persists until the instruments are removed. After removal of the instruments the wound should be closed and should again be irrigated.

Another treatment for deep wound infections in which the Harrington instruments or other devices have been implanted is the time-honored technique of opening the wound widely and allowing it to close secondarily. This treatment may be satisfactory but the morbidity is much greater than in the treatment just described and the cosmetic result less desirable. Regardless of the treatment used it is essential, as pointed out by Moe, that procrastination be avoided. According to him, exploring a suspicious but clean wound is better than procrastinating in the exploration of an infected wound.

Late complications

The most common complications that develop late are pseudarthrosis and recurrence of the deformity. A pseudarthrosis represents a failure of the operation to fully accomplish its purpose (Fig. 71-41). Recurrence of the deformity is usually caused by one or more pseudarthroses but can be caused instead by bending of the fusion mass, traumatic fracture of the fusion mass, or the addition to the curve of one or more adjacent vertebrae superior or inferior to the fusion so that the curve is lengthened (Fig. 71-42). The frequency of these last three causes can be decreased by good judgment in evaluating the maturity of the fusion mass and by locating correctly the fusion area at the time of surgery and including all vertebrae in the fusion that are rotated in the same direction as are the vertebrae in the curve. Rotation is determined by the shadows of the pedicles on the roentgenograms (Fig. 71-15). An additional safeguard against the addition of more vertebrae to the curve is to include in the fusion one unrotated vertebra at each end of the curve.

Improvements in the treatment of scoliosis have produced a steady decrease in the rate of pseudarthrosis. The protection of the fusion mass after surgery, the development of both corrective and internal fixation devices, and the development of better surgical technique including meticulous removal of the soft tissues, intraarticular fusion of the lateral articulations, and the addition of much autogenous cancellous bone to the fusion mass have all been helpful. The intelligent use of the Harrington and other instruments for internal fixation has probably been one of the most important factors in preventing pseudarthroses.

A spinal fusion for scoliosis is usually considered successful if the correction obtained is not lost. A loss of correction then is the only indication for repair of a suspected pseudarthrosis. Late breakage of internal fixation devices usually is presumptive evidence that the fusion is not solid. If there is no significant loss of correction, however, this is not a definite indication for reoperation. Pain or other symptoms caused by pseudarthroses in the absence of demonstrable loss of correction must be extremely rare. In years past scoliosis fusions were explored routinely in several centers during the first 6 months after surgery. Although an extremely high incidence of defects in the fusion mass was reported by surgeons at these centers, we believe that exploration is indicated only if correction is being lost. A pseudarthrosis can frequently be demonstrated on anteroposterior and right and left oblique roentgenograms of good quality. But if the correction is being maintained, then the fusion mass is functioning successfully and a diagnosis of pseudarthrosis is of no practical significance.

The finding roentgenographically of a wedged or "open" interspace, an unfused lateral articulation, or a defect in the fusion mass is helpful in locating a pseudarthrosis. At exploration the cortex is usually smooth and firm over the mature and intact areas of the fusion mass and the soft tissues strip away easily. Conversely, at a pseudarthrosis the soft tissues are usually adherent and are continuous into the defect. Then locating the pseudarthrosis is usually easy. However, a narrow pseudarthrosis may be extremely difficult to locate, especially if motion

Text continued on page 3223.

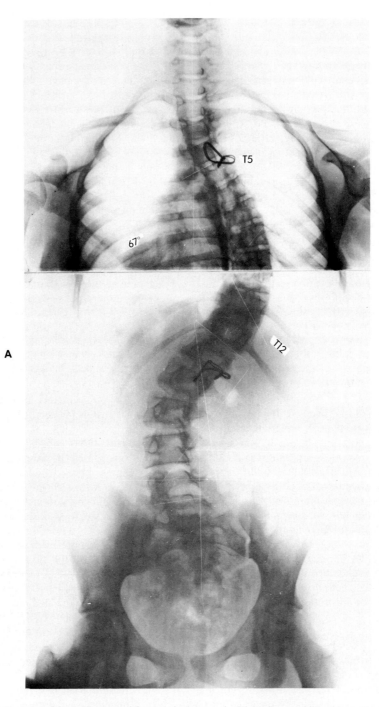

Fig. 71-41. Loss of correction caused by pseudarthroses. **A,** Right thoracic idiopathic scoliosis. Original thoracic curve extended from T5 through T12 and measured 75 degrees while patient was standing. When patient was 12⅔ years of age, fusion from T4 through L1 was carried out elsewhere. Curve had been corrected before surgery to 30 degrees. She was immobilized in cast in bed for about 4 months and was then allowed to walk. Curve increased to 67 degrees. Pseudarthroses were seen on bending roentgenograms and on one oblique roentgenogram.

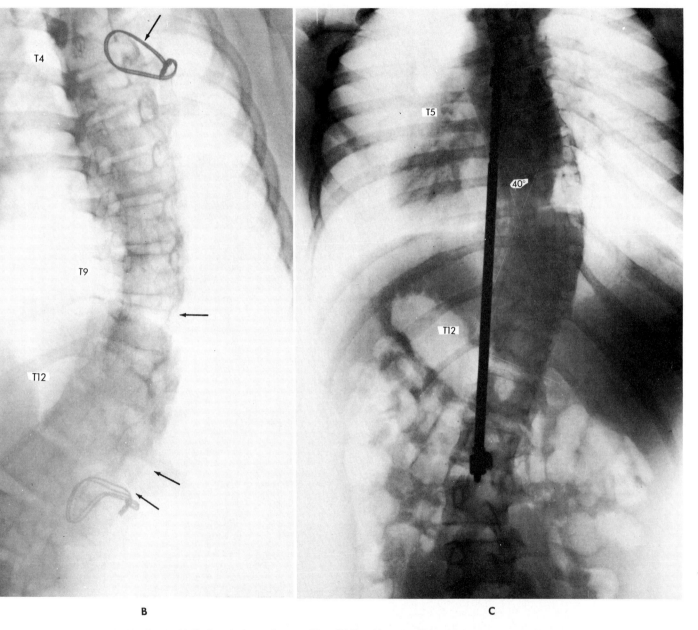

Fig. 71-41, cont'd. B, Pseudarthroses between T9 and T10 and between T12 and L1 on convex side of curve. At surgery additional pseudarthroses were found between T11 and T12 and between T4 and T5. **C,** After additional surgery. Fusion mass was explored from T4 to L2 and all of pseudarthroses were cleared of fibrous tissue to increase movement in them. Even so, curve of 40 degrees remained. One or two osteotomies through fusion mass probably would have allowed additional correction.

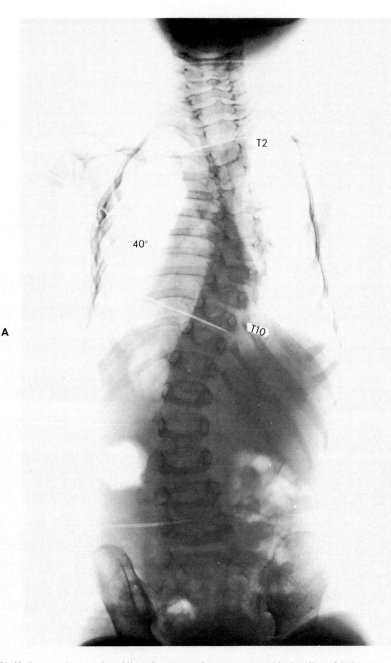

Fig. 71-42. Increase in curve by adding of more vertebrae to curve and by bending of fusion mass after fusion in young child. **A,** Paralytic scoliosis with curve extending from T2 through T10 and measuring 40 degrees in boy 2 years of age who contracted poliomyelitis at age of 3 months, with severe involvement of trunk and upper extremities. Because of severe paralysis and steady increase in curve, spinal fusion was performed at age of 2½ years. As was then our custom, Milwaukee brace was used for correction before surgery and for immobilization after surgery.

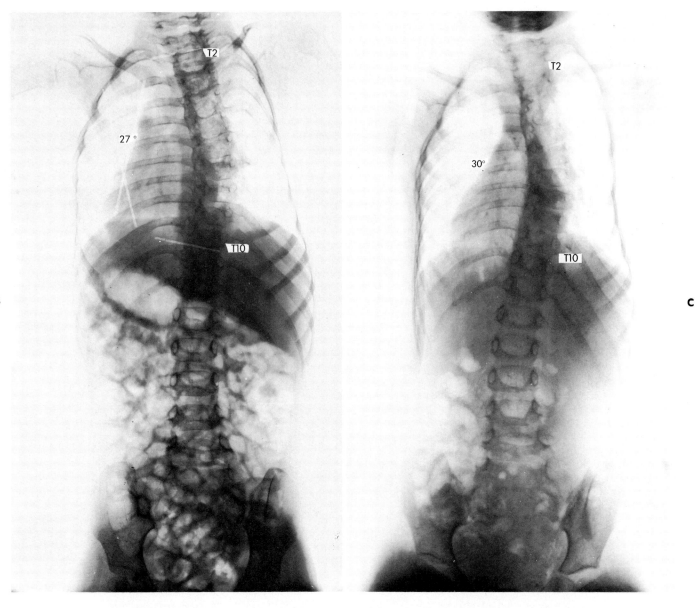

Fig. 71-42, cont'd. B, Curve was corrected to 27 degrees before surgery. **C,** At 6 months patient was allowed to walk in brace and at 1 year brace was removed. Age was then 3½ years and curve from T2 through T10 measured 30 degrees. Spine was compensated and curve did not extend past T10, although T11 was then neutral. Notice that in **A** T11 was rotated to concavity of curve. *Continued.*

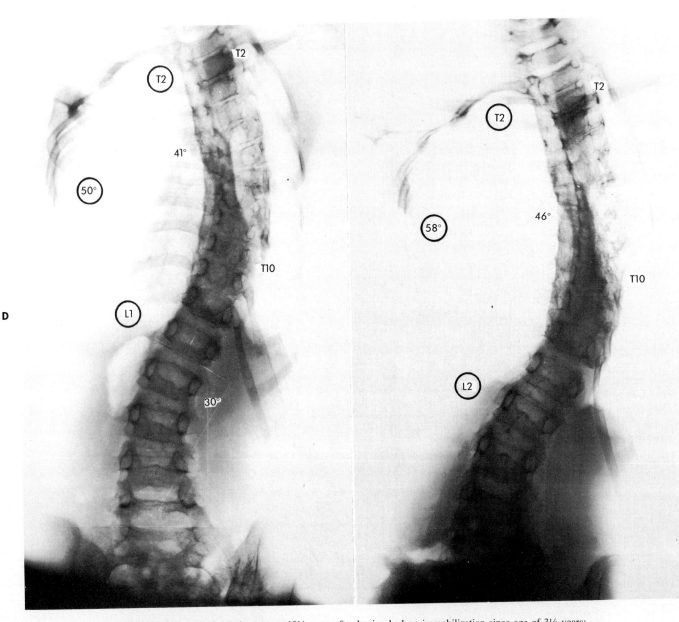

Fig. 71-42, cont'd. D, Patient at age 10½ years after having had no immobilization since age of 3½ years; curve extending from T2 through T10 now measures 41 degrees, even though graft was solid. Fusion mass showed no angulations and all interspaces covered by it were uniformly narrowed. We agree with Moe that, if unprotected, fusion mass can bend in young child, especially in paralytic scoliosis. Notice that T12 and L1 have been added to primary curve. Notice also that T12, which was stripped of soft tissues but was not included in fusion area, has spontaneously fused to inferior end of fusion mass. New curve extending from T2 through L1 then measured 50 degrees. **E,** Patient at age 13; L2 has also been added to curve. Not only is L2 rotated but interspace between L1 and L2 that was open on concave side of primary curve originally is now open slightly on convex side. Original curve in fusion area, T2 through T10, now measures 46 degrees, indicating more bending of graft. We believe that best treatment for this patient now would be to extend fusion through L3, using Risser cast and Harrington distraction rod if suitable purchase could be obtained in superior end of fusion area. Osteotomies of fusion mass would probably allow more correction. Alternative treatment would be wearing of Milwaukee brace until maturity. In summary, this patient demonstrates two of complications possible after spinal fusion for scoliosis in very young child: (1) adding of vertebrae to primary curve and (2) bending of fusion mass.

in it is only slight. In this instance decorticating the fusion mass in suspicious areas is indicated. Futhermore, a search should always be made for several pseudarthroses. When the one or more present have been identified, they are cleared of fibrous tissue and the curves are again corrected by instrumentation. When the loss of correction has been significant, osteotomy of one or more intact areas of the fusion mass is sometimes justified to obtain additional correction. In patients in whom most or all of the correction has been lost and the spine is explored late, a solid fusion mass is often found and several osteotomies may be indicated to permit correction of the curve. These osteotomies and any pseudarthroses are treated as ordinary joints to be fused and their edges are freshened and decorticated. If the fusion mass is thick and of good quality, it may be decorticated throughout to obtain additional bone for grafting. If necessary, fresh autogenous iliac bone is added. We have used halo-femoral traction to regain correction after multiple osteotomies, but instrumentation can be used as well if spinal cord function is monitored. The same criteria are used in judging the maturity of the fusion mass after repair of a pseudarthrosis as after the original fusion. After this repair, however, the period of immobilization is usually shorter than after a primary correction and fusion. This is especially true when the pseudarthrosis is discovered and repaired during convalescence before the fusion mass is completely mature. According to most reports, pseudoarthroses are most common at the thoracolumbar junction, in the lumbar area, and at the extreme ends of the fusion mass. Cobb pointed out that the success of any fusion depends on good surgical technique, the use of a large mass of good bone in the fusion area, sufficient immobilization for a time long enough to permit the fusion mass to mature, and good bone metabolism. A heavier fusion mass than usual is generally necessary to maintain correction when the deformity has been severe, especially in patients with neurofibromatosis when the deformity includes a kyphosis.

PARAPLEGIA SECONDARY TO SCOLIOSIS

The development of paraplegia in a patient with scoliosis is rarely if ever caused by the scoliotic deformity alone. A progressive neurologic deficit or paraplegia is most common in congenital scoliosis but is usually caused by some other anomaly such as diastematomyelia, and treating the scoliosis alone will probably not be helpful. Furthermore, measures to correct the curve may be extremely dangerous and may cause a marked increase in the neurologic deficit. In congenital scoliosis associated with congenital kyphosis, paraplegia may be caused by pressure on the anterior aspect of the cord by the vertebral body or fragment of a body at the apex of the curve. Laminectomy is not beneficial and usually should not be attempted. Rather, anterior decompression by removing the offending bone and anterior interbody fusion are indicated. Then a posterior fusion in which attempts are made to correct the deformity superior and inferior to the apex of the curve may be necessary later. The same combination of scoliosis and kyphosis is common in neurofibromatosis and is treated similarly. We have not seen paraplegia in progressive idiopathic or progressive paralytic scoliosis unless either an angular kyphosis or some other pathology is present in addition to the scoliosis.

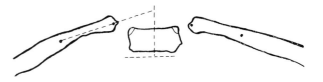

Fig. 71-43. Construction of rib vertebra (RV) angle (see text). (From Mehta, M.H.: J. Bone Joint Surg. **54-B:**230, 1972.)

INFANTILE IDIOPATHIC SCOLIOSIS

Infantile idiopathic scoliosis is defined by James as a structural curve developing before the age of 3 years in which rotation of the vertebral bodies is fixed even during forward bending. Although many curves fulfilling these criteria have been seen in Great Britain, only a few have been reported in the United States. Two types are recognized: progressive infantile idiopathic scoliosis, which usually progresses rapidly, and resolving infantile idiopathic scoliosis, also known as structural resolving scoliosis, which resolves spontaneously within a few years whether treated or not. The resolving type is said to constitute 70% to 90% of the group. Both types usually occur in boys and the curves are usually thoracic and to the left. The most severe structural curve James has seen resolve spontaneously measured 37 degrees by the Cobb method. Unfortunately, when a curve is mild no absolute criteria are available for differentiating the two types. According to James, when compensatory or secondary curves have developed or when the curve measures more than 37 degrees by the Cobb method when first seen, the scoliosis will probably be progressive. Conversely if the curve measures only 10 to 15 degrees when first seen, it probably will resolve because progressive curves are usually more severe than this before the scoliosis is discovered. Whether a given curve is progressive can be determined by observing it for only a few months. Mehta has developed a method for differentiating resolving from progressive curves in infantile idiopathic scoliosis. Her judgment is based on the development of the rib-vertebral (RV) angle. This angle is formed between each side of the apical thoracic vertebra and its corresponding rib (Fig. 71-43). The rib-vertebral angle difference (RVAD) is the difference between the values of the RV angles on the concave and convex sides of the curve at any given level. A line is drawn perpendicular to the middle of either the upper or the lower surface of the body of the selected vertebra and is called the datum line. Another line is drawn from the midpoint of the head of the rib to the midpoint of the neck just medial to the region where the neck widens into the shaft of the rib. This rib line is extended medially to intersect the datum line, forming the RV angle. It was found that the RVAD was consistently greater in progressive curves. Any curve with an initial RVAD of 20 degrees or more is regarded as potentially progressive until proved otherwise.

Wynne-Davies noted plagiocephaly in 97 children developing curves in the first 6 months of life with the flat side of the head on the concave side of the curve. She thought that the cause must be multifactorial.

Lloyd-Roberts and Pilcher reported a male infant with a left thoracic curve that progressed from 8 to 35 degrees before beginning to resolve spontaneously at the age of 14 months. They suggested that intrauterine molding may be a cause of structural infantile idiopathic scoliosis.

TREATMENT. For infantile curves measuring more than 37 to 40 degrees James recommended a succession of plaster body jackets until the age of 3 or 3½ years when a Milwaukee brace can be fitted. Walker reported a series of 49 patients treated in the Denis Browne "bucket" or "tray" and found no difference in the percentage of infants whose curves became progressive when compared with untreated infants. Several types of splints, straps, and other devices have been suggested for very young infants but with questionable evidence that they are beneficial. Plastic underarm body jackets, both prefabricated and custom-made, are frequently fitted but results in our hands have not been uniform.

Curves of less than 20 degrees can be observed every 3 months unless the RV angle suggests a progressive curve; then treatment is instituted immediately. Once a Milwaukee brace can be fitted satisfactorily, progression of many infantile curves can be prevented and often a significant improvement can be obtained during the period of growth. Frequently an efficient brace maker can make a satisfactory Milwaukee brace for a child under 3 years of age. If a child is seen late and the curve is severe or if the curve increases despite the use of a Milwaukee brace, a relatively short fusion including only the structural or primary curve is probably the best treatment. Then the spine must be controlled by a Milwaukee brace until growth is complete. After the brace has been worn constantly for several years, using it only part of the time is often sufficient. According to James, all patients with progressive infantile idiopathic scoliosis will require surgery by the age of 10 years even when treated in a Milwaukee brace. For these patients he recommends a fusion long enough to include the entire primary or structural curve and all vertebrae rotated in the same direction as those in the primary curve and possibily one more at each end to prevent more vertebrae from being added to the curve during growth. But results with the Milwaukee brace have recently been good enough to suggest that fusion at the age of 10 years may not always be necessary and that a good result can be obtained by using the brace into adolescence. James has pointed out, however, that if the curve is severe and is not decreasing significantly in the Milwaukee brace, it will be very stiff and very difficult to correct by the time the skeleton is mature at the end of adolescence. Morel of Berck-Plage has observed success with serial EDF casts applied every 2 to 3 months until curves are less than 10 degrees. At that value a plastic corset or a Milwaukee brace is used. Further analysis may provide a valuable treatment regimen.

ADULT SCOLIOSIS

The management of scoliosis in adults remains controversial. Although Nachemson in Sweden contends that the incidence of pain in scoliosis is no greater than in the general population, it has been the experience of Kostuik et al. that pain can often be severe and incapacitating and does constitute a major surgical problem. Although Ponseti found a death rate similar to that of the normal population, Nachemson found the morbidity and mortality higher in his series in Sweden. It has also been noted that curves

may increase after the end of growth, the greatest increase occurring in curves measuring over 60 degrees and that progression of 1 degree per year may occur. The recent study of Weinstein and Ponsetti on curve progression after skeletal maturity adds specificity to the prognosis.

Ponder et al. studied 132 patients older than 20 years undergoing Harrington instrumentation and fusion. Seventy percent of these patients underwent surgery for back pain; this is similar to the findings of Dawson et al. that 71% had pain and of Kostuik that 62% underwent surgery for pain and 55% for progression of the curve. Studies by Sicard et al. and Stagnara of 70 and 50 patients, respectively, showed surgery also primarily performed for pain. The average correction obtained was only 48%, but the mechanical symptoms of fatigue were consistently relieved. Seventy percent still had some low back pain, and it was emphasized that surgical correction of adult idiopathic scoliosis does not render the patient normal in any sense of the word.

Kostuik found that the blood loss compared favorably with most reported adolescent groups while Sicard et al. and Stagnara found it higher. The correction achieved was 40% and pain was relieved in 62% of patients. Complications included a 10% pseudoarthrosis rate in all the groups, ranging from 7% in the idiopathic group to 23% in those with previous adolescent spine surgery.

In summary, surgical treatment for adult scoliosis is recommended for pain, progression of deformity, or a combination of both. The surgical exposure is more difficult and the postoperative care more demanding than in younger patients. Mortality and morbidity are correspondingly greater, and patients with failed or unsatisfactory fusions present a more difficult problem.

SCOLIOSIS OF KNOWN CAUSE
Neuromuscular scoliosis

Neuromuscular scoliosis may be secondary to an array of underlying disorders, and patients have varying sensory abnormalities, asymmetric or symmetric paralysis, and progressive or nonprogressive disease. However, common to all is a paralytic state resulting in lumb and spinal deformities. An abbreviated classification is as follows:

A. Neuropathic
   1. Spinal cord injury
   2. Poliomyelitis
   3. Progressive neurologic disorders
   4. Syringomyelia
   5. Myelomeningocele
   6. Cerebral palsy
B. Myopathic
   1. Arthrogryposis
   2. Muscular dystrophy
C. Neurofibromatosis
D. Miscellaneous

O'Brien and Yau and others emphasize the different problems in paralytic and idiopathic scoliosis. First, as J.I.P. James indicates, paralytic curves are longer. Second, pelvic obliquity often exists with muscle imbalance affecting the ultimate fusion mass. Third, the pseudarthrosis rate is higher and approaches 20% as reported by Winter or 50% as reported by Bonnett. Pelvic obliquity results in pressure sores on the ischium on the low side of the pelvis with hip subluxation on the high side as the severity of the deformity increases. Regular follow-up is essential to prevent these severe sequelae and should be combined with appropriately timed treatment.

In paralytic scoliosis the aim of surgery is not only correction of the curves and prevention of their recurrence but also secure stabilization of the weakened trunk as well. Consequently the indications for fusion and the determination of the fusion area are different from those in idiopathic scoliosis.

Blount et al. once advised fusion from D1 to L3 or L4 in two or three posterior stages for severe paralysis of the trunk. Bonnett et al., reporting the Rancho Los Amigos experience with paralytic scoliosis in 351 patients, provided the following indications for surgery:
1. A collapsing and unstable paralytic deformity
2. Progressive increase in the scoliosis
3. Decreasing cardiorespiratory function
4. Decreased independence necessitating the use of hands for more stable sitting
5. Back pain or loss of sitting balance coincident with increasing pelvic obliquity.

As experience at Rancho Los Amigos and elsewhere increased and technologic advances appeared, the results improved. This occurred because of improved skeletal fixation. It has been found that the Dwyer anterior operation is excellent for improving the percentage of correction but is inadequate in that the fusion mass is too short. The Harrington posterior distraction rod allows greater correction above and below the apex of the curve. The combined anterior and posterior approach therefore permits improved correction and a decrease in the rate of pseudarthrosis. Posterior segmental instrumentation (p. 3211) generally and with extension to the pelvis as performed by Allen et al. has become the most widely used method of stabilization and correction for neuromuscular deformity.

An unacceptable curve that increases despite conservative treatment should be corrected and fused regardless of the patient's age. However, if an increase in the curve can be prevented with an orthosis, it is preferable to wait until the patient is 10 years of age or older. Moe has stated that high cervicodorsal curves should not be treated conservatively but should be fused early because in them irreversible structural changes soon develop, and because even when moderate they produce severe deformity. Garrett, Perry, and Nickel have had much experience in treating severe instability of the neck and trunk caused by paralysis of the muscles that control them. To them, even in the absence of scoliosis, instability itself is an indication for fusion. They devised a halo (Fig. 71-6) that is attached to a body cast (Fig. 71-14, *A*) to stabilize the head and neck during and after fusion of the cervical spine. They point out that the ease with which a patient can balance his head and trunk determines to a great extent how much he can develop the muscles of his extremities. If less energy is required to maintain erect posture, the demands of respiratory function are decreased, fatigue is decreased, and the patient's efforts can be better directed toward productive activity. Therefore stabilizing the paralyzed trunk is the first consideration in treatment. They also recommended that tracheotomy be made routinely before any fusion operation in patients with severe respiratory embarrassment

and that often respiratory aids be used afterward. With better pulmonary medicine and critical care units, tracheotomies are rarely mandatory.

To stabilize the trunk effectively in a patient with paralytic scoliosis or with an unstable spine, a much longer fusion is necessary than is usually indicated in one with idiopathic scoliosis. While in idiopathic scoliosis only the primary curve need necessarily be fused, in paralytic scoliosis the area including the primary and both secondary curves must often be fused. This area generally extends from a horizontal vertebra in the upper spine to a horizontal vertebra in the lower. As already mentioned, Blount et al. have recommended that a severely paralyzed trunk be stabilized by fusion from D1 to L3 or L4. Of course, the spine must be compensated (the head centered over the pelvis) by the fusion or the instrumentation procedure.

The paralytic patient presents additional problems to the unwary such as (1) significant pulmonary function deficits caused by intercostal paralysis, (2) more osteoporotic bone and the possibility of instrument failure, (3) atrophic pelvis with insufficient bone for grafting, (4) an increased blood loss in a patient with an initially smaller blood volume, (5) prolonged postoperative immobilization, (6) more postoperative pulmonary complications, and (7) immobilization pressure sores, especially in those with altered skin sensation. Suffice it to say that a more complicated course is to be expected and appropriate measures must be taken to prepare for and manage any eventuality.

The consensus is therefore that nonoperative treatment may be entirely futile and that superior results occur with operative management. Procedures that provide segmental instrumentation, such as Luque instrumentation with intralaminar wiring, are usually efficient in correction and fusion of neuromuscular scoliosis (p. 3211). Surgery most often is performed later than is ideal.

A progressive kyphosis is managed as discussed in the section on kyphosis (p. 3237).

SPINAL CORD INJURY

Of 104 children with spinal cord injury reviewed by Kilfoyle et al. 97 developed spinal curvature and pelvic obliquity; lordosis was most common, scoliosis second, and kyphosis least common. Early surgical treatment was "considered an expression of conservatism." Bonnett et al. reported 57 to 123 patients with significant spinal deformity and stressed the progression of deformity in the growing child. Total care of the cord-injured child was emphasized. Milwaukee braces and plastic orthoses are of limited value in the presence of anesthetic skin. Surgical stabilization is needed in virtually all children before the growth spurt. Internal stabilization is of utmost importance, and segmental wiring techniques that allow mobilization without external support are highly suitable for these patients with anesthetic skin and frequently diminished respiratory ability. Combined anterior and posterior procedures are effective.

POLIOMYELITIS

Curves in poliomyelitis may affect any part of the spine including the neck, may resemble the idiopathic type or be the long **C** type, and may have the many features of other paralytic curves. Nonoperative treatment is primarily for delaying fusion until the optimal age. The surgical management follows the same principles mentioned previously, but it must be emphasized that a *long* fusion is necessary to result in a balanced spine. Halo-femoral traction may produce additional osteoporosis and can be avoided in flexible curves. Postoperative immobilization may include a Risser-Cotrel cast, halo cast, or plastic orthosis as the curve and other factors dictate. Again, segmental instrumentation techniques are usually efficient in management of this type of paralytic scoliosis even though skin sensation is intact.

PROGRESSIVE NEUROLOGIC DISORDERS

Hensinger and MacEwen point out that these conditions carry a significant risk of serious spinal deformity as with paralytic scoliosis following poliomyelitis. The curves are difficult to control with bracing and do not cease progression at maturation. Increasing spinal curvature leads to loss of ambulation, or for the wheelchair-bound patient, loss of sitting balance. Hardy noted scoliosis in 19% of patients under age 5 years, 58% between 6 and 11 years, and 84% at 12 years and older. Spinal muscular atrophy is a genetically determined neuromuscular disorder characterized by widespread weakness secondary to degeneration of the anterior horn cells of the spinal cord (see also Chapter 67). This disease has been given many names, including Werdnig-Hoffman's disease, Kugelberg-Welander's disease, Oppenheim's disease, amyotonia congenita, proximal spinal muscular atrophy, juvenile spinal muscular atrophy, and anterior horn cell disease. Infantile spinal muscular atrophy (Werdnig-Hoffmann's disease) begins in the first year of life and the patient usually dies by the fourth year of life. The juvenile form (Kugelberg-Welander's disease) begins between the ages of 2 and 12 years with the patient surviving into adult life. Intermediate forms exist between these two, and all patients with spinal muscular atrophy have muscle wasting, hypotonia, and loss of deep tendon reflexes. Weakness is more marked proximally than distally. In the report of Hensinger and MacEwen 29 of 50 patients evaluated had a significant scoliosis. They recommended surgery with emphasis on proper preoperative management, including an intensive physical therapy program for general muscle strengthening initially. Special attention must be paid to cardiorespiratory problems, and instructions in pulmonary exercises should also be included. Fusion was by a standard posterior approach with Harrington instrumentation and bone grafting. The children were of small stature with reduced blood volume, and blood loss was of major proportions. This requires that surgery be accomplished with speed and skill. Dorr et al. fused an average of 18 levels and used postoperative support for 17 months.

Postoperatively casts were applied as early as practical, the patients were brought to the upright position with the use of a CircOlectric bed, and they were allowed to walk as soon as possible. Those unable to walk preoperatively were returned to their previous wheelchair activities. Ten months of spinal immobilization with either a cast or plastic orthosis was used.

In Friedreich's ataxia, as in spinal muscular atrophy, bed rest in preoperative traction or during the postoperative period must be kept to a minimum; otherwise a rapid increase in weakness will occur. In contrast, patients with Charcot-Marie-Tooth disease and familial dysautonomia are more like those with poliomyelitis and cerebral palsy and are able to tolerate longer periods of bedrest. Selection of patients with Freidreich's ataxia is influenced by the degree of cardiac involvement since this is the most common cause of death in these patients. Since the mean age of death in Friedreich's ataxia is 36 years, evaluation of a teenager with progressive scoliosis must consider this factor. Patients with familial dysautonomia present many problems in management. Experience in surgery with these patients is quite limited. The surgical treatment is that for a collapsing spine. Pulmonary compromise, if severe, requires tracheostomy or nasotracheal intubation and positive pressure support. Surgery consists of instrumentation with multiple Harrington rods with fusion to the sacrum using alar hooks. Bone bank bone or parental bone should be used in abundance. The patient should be returned to the upright position as soon as possible in a bivalved plastic orthosis that leaves the hips free; support is maintained for 18 months.

Segmental spinal instrumentation techniques such as those of Luque, Drummond, and Allen are most frequently recommended now for these patients so that most if not all external support can be eliminated.

SYRINGOMYELIA

Huebert and MacKinnon reported the presence of scoliosis in 63% of 43 children with synringomyelia. Scoliosis was found in 82% when symptoms of the disease had been noted before the age of 16 years. Syringomyelia is discussed here for two reasons. First, in patients with scoliosis and a neurologic deficit, syringomyelia should be considered in the differential diagnosis. Second, of two patients with severe curves reported by Huebert and MacKinnon, the curve was corrected and fused using the Harrington instruments in one but a spinal fusion after a laminectomy was fatal in the other when a large cyst in the cord ruptured. Obviously, the rate of progression of the neurologic deficit and the prognosis of life should be considered before any extensive operations are considered for patients with this disease. Experience with this condition is limited, but the curve patterns resemble idiopathic and not paralytic scoliosis and hence may be misdiagnosed. In a study by Weber 19 of 51 patients with syringomyelia had scoliosis; the curves were usually thoracic, were more common in males, and correlated with the neurologic level.

MYELOMENINGOCELE

Since advances in neurosurgical and urologic skills have enabled more children with myelomeningocele to survive, there are now more cases of a type of scoliosis that has been the most severe and most difficult form to treat. In response to this challenge capabilities to handle severe deformities have increased; however, the spine problem cannot be handled in isolation and the total child must be cared for in a multidisciplinary setting. (See discussion of myelomeningocele on p. 3023.)

Raycroft and Curtis reported an incidence of spine deformity in 52% of 103 patients without vertebral body abnormalities with myelomeningocele; 41 patients had scoliosis, 30 had lordosis, and 12 had kyphosis; of the 27 with vertebral body abnormalities 100% had a congenital spine deformity. Mackel and Lindseth report a 66% incidence in 82 patients; Banta et al. pointed out an increase in deformity in the higher level lesions in 268 patients, and Shurtleff et al. showed an increased incidence with advancing age.

Nonoperative bracing is difficult but can be effective for several years until fusion is indicated. The surgical treatment must be individualized using the principles of treatment established for other paralytic curves.

Sriram, Bobechko, and Hall reported 33 patients with spina bifida undergoing operative fusion. They had 16 good results, 8 fair, and 9 poor. The surgical procedures varied considerably, but the following observations could be made. Posterior spinal fusion is fraught with many difficulties, primarily because of densely scarred and adherent soft tissue. Spinal exposure is often lengthy and hemorrhagic. The deformity is often rigid and proper correction impossible. The quality of the bone often provides poor seating for Harrington hooks, and the inadequacy of the posterior bone mass provides a poor bed for grafting. Segmental spinal instrumentation and fusion probably are used most commonly now. The infection rate is quite high. Pseudarthrosis can possibly be best managed by anterior procedures such as Dwyer instrumentation and fusion.

Hall, Lindseth, Campbell, and Kalsbeck reported 14 patients with communicating hydrosyringomyelia. They found a compensated hydrocephalus in all of their myelodysplastic patients with developmental scoliosis. The hydrosyringomyelia produced progressive extremity paresis, often with spasticity. After the initial detection of a developmental scoliosis in patients with myelodysplasia, an investigation for hydrosyringomyelia should be instituted. This can be studied with computerized axial tomography, positive contrast shuntogram under fluoroscopy, or radioisotope ventriculography. Treatment of the hydrosyringomyelia is accomplished by ventricular drainage using a standard shunt procedure. This resulted in short-term stabilization in six of their patients; two patients with advanced curves continued to progress. Even advanced neurologic deficits were improved. Arrested hydrocephalus was present in all 14 patients.

CEREBRAL PALSY

Scoliosis is often overlooked in patients with cerebral palsy. Rosenthal et al. examined 50 adolescents and found a 38% incidence, Robson found an incidence of 23% in 152 patients, and Samilson and Bechard found an incidence of 25.6% in 906 patients. The average age in the latter group was 22 years. Of the 232 patients with scoliosis 22 were ambulatory, 41 were sitters, and 169 were bed care patients. There were 58 primary lumbar curves, 104 thoracolumbar curves, 37 thoracic curves, and 33 double primary curves. The most severe curves were thoracolumbar in location. MacEwen reported 100 cerebral palsy patients, most of whom were ambulatory, with a 21% incidence of scoliosis.

Of 294 patients with cerebral palsy seen at Rancho Los Amigos Hospital by Bonnett et al., 42 were considered to have clinically significant lumbar and thoracolumbar scoliosis (31 to 135 degrees). Of these 42 patients 33 were treated by spine surgery, 10 by Harrington instrumentation and posterior spinal fusion, 18 by the Dwyer procedure and anterior fusion, and 5 by a two-stage combined anterior and posterior fusion. They concluded that only the combined procedure appeared to give adequate correction and a low incidence of pseudarthrosis; this was also recommended by Moe et al. They concluded that for severe spastic and progressive scoliosis in a patient with the potential for rehabilitation, surgical treatment is indicated. Improved results are seen in curves of less than 60 degrees at the time of surgery.

MacEwen reported 10 patients with severe and progressive curves treated surgically; 2 required repair of pseudarthroses before a successful fusion was accomplished. Our experience with this type of surgery in cerebral palsy has also been favorable and we agree that to avoid surgery for scoliosis in these patients who already have serious problems in walking and in trunk stability is unreasonable. In fact, scoliosis in cerebral palsy can be treated surgically with reasonable efficiency and safety. The use of segmental instrumentation probably is advantageous.

ARTHROGRYPOSIS MULTIPLEX CONGENITA

In arthrogryposis multiplex congenita any scoliosis is secondary to the abnormality of the muscles and ligaments rather than to any abnormality of bone. That scoliosis may develop should be anticipated from birth, and the spine should be included in each examination. In 1978 Herron, Westin, and Dawson reported on 88 patients with arthrogryposis multiplex congenita, finding scoliosis in 18 patients (20%). The predominate pattern was a thoracolumbar curve associated with pelvic obliquity and lumbar hyperlordosis. The curves were mostly progressive, becoming rigid and fixed at an early age. Significant associated contractures of the hips, dislocation of the hips, or both were present in all but one patient. Boys were affected three times as often as girls. If scoliosis was detected at birth or within the first few years of life, progression of a pelvic obliquity always meant progression of the curve and demanded aggressive treatment. Correction of hip contractures must often be followed by spinal fusion to the sacrum to halt progression of the curve. The postoperative complication rate is high in this group, and appropriate intraoperative and postoperative measures are mandatory. Seibold, Winter, and Moe observed that the scoliosis in this condition is usually of a neuromuscular pattern. They found the Milwaukee brace to be a valuable treatment for mild curves. In larger curves for which surgery is necessary halo-femoral traction can be effective, but it is complicated by associated osteoporosis and halo pin slippage. Spinal fusion was as effective as in idiopathic scoliosis, but the complications included excessive blood loss, infection, and instrument failure. If surgery becomes necessary, it must be remembered that respiratory problems are common in patients with this disease and segmental instrumentation may be best.

MUSCULAR DYSTROPHY

According to Bunch, in muscular dystrophy spinal deformity seldom occurs in ambulatory patients but rather develops after 1 to 3 years of wheelchair existence. Robin and Brief analyzed 27 patients averaging 14.8 years (6 to

26 years) of age and found 24 with spine deformity. The curves were predominantly long thoracolumbar curves with pelvic obliquity, the collapse caused by absence of muscles and not asymmetric muscle activity or contracture. The curves increased with advancing age to a severe deformity. Dubowitz found no scoliosis in patients who were ambulatory or had been in a wheelchair less than 1 year. Beyond 1 year 32 of 50 had scoliosis.

Wilkins and Gibson studied 62 patients with Duchenne muscular dystrophy ranging in age from 7 to 24 years. They identified five major groups each composed of basically the same number of patients. Group I patients had essentially straight spines averaging a curve of about 7 degrees and an average age of 9.9 years. Group II patients had kyphotic spines with average curves of 14.5 degrees and an average age of 11.1 years. Group III patients had kyphoscoliotic spines with average curves of 65 degrees and an average age of 14.6 years. Group IV patients had scoliotic spines without kyphosis with average curves of 82 degrees and with an average age of 16.1 years. Group V patients had extended spines with lateral curves averaging 20 degrees and an average age of 19.3 years. The severity of the deformity increased as the age increased in groups I to IV, but the unique group V patients all had extended spines with little scoliotic deformity. Wilkins and Gibson thought that perhaps an extended spine maintained the facet joints in a locked position and was therefore less prone to develop a scoliotic deformity. They recommended early spinal support to stabilize the pelvis in a level position, providing some extension moment to prevent kyphosis and ultimately severe scoliosis.

Nonoperative treatment is best accomplished using bivalved plastic orthoses when curves exceed 20%. Surgery frequently was rarely done because of the early death of these patients. The decreased morbidity after long segmental spinal instrumentation with minimal or no external support has changed the outlook for these patients, allowing spinal fusion to be done more frequently.

NEUROFIBROMATOSIS

The patterns of the curves in patients with neurofibromatosis vary. Long gentle curves that develop slowly and fail to increase significantly are occasionally seen. Perhaps these curves are caused by involvement of the soft tissues by the disease or by asymmetry of the arms or legs. For these conservative treatment is usually sufficient but the patient must be observed carefully. Roentgenologic findings were delineated by Hunt and Pugh and included the following:

1. The classic sharply angulated curve has five to eight vertebrae with an acute kyphosis in the same area; these vertebrae are typically dystrophic, whereas those in nonkyphotic curves are less so.
2. Ribs at the apical portion of the curve show "penciling."
3. Vertebrae are scalloped, with invaginations on myelography probably caused by meningoceles.
4. Dystrophic vertebrae are less common in patients with more skin manifestations.
5. An idiopathic-type curve or congenital vertebral abnormalities may occur.
6. Enlarged intervertebral foramina may be present.

Chaglassian, Riseborough, and Hall, reporting on 141 patients, found the incidence of scoliosis to be 26%. Other reported series range from 10% reported by James to as high as 58%. Chaglassian et al. found no standard pattern of spinal deformity in neurofibromatosis, but single right thoracic curves were the most common. The traditional short curve considered indicative of neurofibromatosis was not as common as long curves (more than five vertebrae) in this series. These curves showed a higher incidence of progression, but both types did progress. Kyphosis occurred in 19%. The most effective treatment was posterior Harrington instrumentation and fusion. Postoperative complications ran as high as 36%. Severity of progression of the scoliosis was not necessarily related to the severity of the systemic neurofibromatosis and did not depend on the curve length.

Even though actual neurofibromas of the intraspinal, extraspinal, or combined or dumbbell type have been described, biopsies of the spine both anteriorly and posteriorly usually are completely negative. Furthermore, no visible neurofibromatosus tissue in or around the spine has been reported even in extremely severe kyphoscoliosis. Many methods of correction and fusion have been used in this disease. The idiopathic type of curve can be managed like any other idiopathic curve and the congenital form like any other congenital curve. When the kyphosis is severe, anterior spinal fusion with grafts bridging the apex of the kyphos combined with a posterior fusion is necessary. Myelographic studies may be indicated before treatment because intraspinal tumor masses and congenital anomalies have been reported in patients with neurofibromatosis. Even though skeletal traction for correcting a purely kyphotic deformity of the spine is extremely dangerous, we have, as have Moe et al., decreased considerably a severe kyphosis associated with a severe scoliosis without producing neurologic complications.

MISCELLANEOUS CAUSES OF SCOLIOSIS

In a report by Hilal, Marton, and Pollack, 34 patients with diastematomyelia were studied. Fifteen patients had no scoliosis and had an average age of 4 years, 5 months; 7 patients had moderate scoliosis with an average age of 7 years, 7 months; 12 patients had severe scoliosis and an average age of 11 years, 1 month. This suggests that the natural history of the condition is an increasing tendency for scoliosis to develop with age. Scoliosis was also more common in patients with a higher location of the septa within the spinal canal. Guthkelch supports the observation that scoliosis is more frequently associated with spurs in the thoracic region. Herring has reported a case of rapidly progressive scoliosis in multiple epiphyseal dysplasia necessitating spinal instrumentation and fusion. Micheli, Hall, and Watts have reported spinal instability in Larson's syndrome, which consists of multiple congenital anomalies including anterior dislocation of the knees, dislocation of the elbows and hips, and equinovarus deformities of the feet. Associated shortened metacarpals and long, cylindric fingers characterize the hands; the facial features include hypertelorism, prominent forehead, and depressed nasal bridge. Significant spinal anomalies were found in the cervical and thoracic regions. This was characterized by cervical vertebrae that were flattened and hypoplastic, resulting in a midcervical kyphosis. Thoracolumbar scoliosis has also been reported. Sudden deaths that have been reported may have resulted from this cervical instability. It is recommended therefore that careful evaluation of the cervical spine be made and appropriate bracing or early surgical stabilization be considered.

Congenital scoliosis

Congenital scoliosis is a lateral curvature of the spine caused by congenital anomalies of the vertebrae and the adjacent supporting structures. Some type of anomaly must be visible on the roentgenograms of the spine before a diagnosis of congenital scoliosis can be made. Scoliotic curves in the presence of fused ribs are said to be congenital unless proved otherwise; we believe this statement is valid. Fused ribs in the absence of scoliosis are rarely of clinical significance. Many patients with congenital scoliosis have other congenital anomalies. The most serious anomalies of the spine are those involving the neural elements such as diastematomyelia and the many types of spinal dysraphism. Spina bifida with meningomyelocele is often accompanied by other congenital anomalies of the spine such as errors in segmentation and often either congenital scoliosis or congenital kyphosis. Any neurologic abnormality associated with congenital scoliosis makes vigorous treatment of the scoliosis potentially dangerous.

In a study by Winter, Moe, and Eilers of 234 patients with congenital scoliosis, the type of spinal anomaly, except for the unilateral bar, was not found to be significant in the prognosis. They again emphasized that observing patients with congenital scoliosis throughout the period of growth is absolutely essential; neurologic examinations and roentgenograms of the spine are necessary periodically. Characteristically the curves in their patients that progressed did so gradually and continuously during periods of slow growth, frequently no more than 5 degrees a year, and then increased rapidly during spurts of rapid growth, usually in preadolescence. All roentgenograms must be measured carefully and must be compared not only with the most recent roentgenograms but also with the earliest ones available so that very slow increases in the curves can be detected. The unilateral bar (Fig. 71-44), usually caused by failure of segmentation of the posterior elements of two or more vertebrae on one side, is the type of anomaly most likely to cause significant progressive scoliosis. This unilateral failure of segmentation may also involve the vertebral bodies. The study by Winter, Moe, and Eilers indicated that the area in which the spine is anomalous is of prognostic significance. All of the thoracic curves followed to maturity increased. Usually thoracic and thoracolumbar curves increased more than cervicothoracic, lumbar, or miscellaneous curves with multiple anomalies.

Winter in 1973 emphasized the unique nature of congenital scoliosis. The classification of MacEwen has been well accepted:

A. Failure of formation
 1. Partial failure of formation (wedge vertebra)
 2. Complete failure of formation (hemivertebra)
B. Failure of segmentation
 1. Unilateral failure of segmentation (unilateral unsegmented bar)

 2. Bilateral failure of segmentation (block vertebra)
C. Miscellaneous

If one thinks of the balance of growth potentials in the spine, it is clear that if one side is unsegmented and has no growth potential, the opposite side with growth potential will produce a progressive curve. On the other hand, if the spine has a group of miscellaneous anomalies, the growth potential may be approximately the same on the two sides. Therefore the most malicious anomaly is the unilateral unsegmented bar. The second most malicious is multiple hemivertebrae adjacent to one another on the same side of the spine. Single hemivertebrae are less predictable. The greater the curve in terms of degrees and the longer the curve in terms of the number of vertebral segments involved, the more likely is progression to take place.

Careful measurements and comparison of spine films at 6-month intervals must be made, using the Cobb system of measurement. It is then determined whether the curve is progressive; Winter has shown progression to occur at about 5 degrees per year. If the curve is proved to be progressive, prompt treatment must be instituted. All curves must be measured, including the compensatory or secondary ones in the seemingly normal parts of the spine. We measure from each end of the anomalous area as well as from each end of the entire curve generally considered in treatment, that is, from the vertebra maximally tilted at each end. We believe that measuring the anomalous area separately is possibly a more accurate way of determining whether growth is asymmetric or the curve is increasing because more vertebrae are being added to it. Because a congenital kyphosis is often produced by a posterior or posterolateral hemivertebra or other errors in segmentation, lateral roentgenograms of the spine should be made at intervals to detect a kyphos. When a congenital kyphosis increases, an early posterior fusion is mandatory and while the deformity is relatively mild this treatment is usually sufficient. A more severe kyphosis, however, is more difficult to control. Winter, Moe, and Eilers have been unable to obtain a solid fusion or stablize a congenital kyphosis with an angle of more than 60 degrees without combining posterior and anterior fusions.

The physical examination must be thorough, looking for other congenital anomalies and the state of the nervous system. There is a 20% incidence of associated genitourinary anomalies and a 7% incidence of congenital heart disease. Diastematomyelia may occur in approximately 5% of patients. Appropriate evaluation of any associated abnormality must precede definitive care of the spine. Myelography may be used routinely and must be used if there is a suspicion of a diastematomyelia or if any neurologic abnormality exists in the lower extremities. Gillespie et al. reported their experience with 31 patients with congenital scoliosis and intraspinal anomalies, 17 with diastematomyelia, and 14 with a miscellaneous group of developmental tumors. They emphasized the probable high risk of congenital intraspinal anomalies with congenital scoliosis. A significant number of these may have no cutaneous manifestations. Preoperative myelography is clearly advisable in these patients, with neurosurgical management preceding spinal fusion.

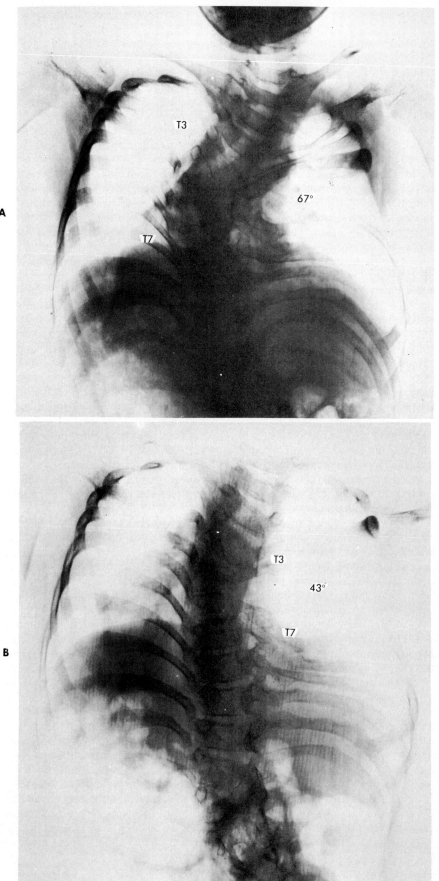

Fig. 71-44. Congential scoliosis with unilateral bar treated by osteotomy and halo-femoral distraction. **A,** Curve in boy 9 years of age extending from T3 through T7 and measuring 67 degrees; bar is on right. At surgery, bar was osteotomized across its center and fusion from T2 through T8 was performed. Halo-femoral distraction was applied in operating room after surgery. **B,** After patient had been in traction 2 weeks, curve had been corrected to 43 degrees. Additional surgery will be necessary to stabilize congenital kyphosis in lumbar spine.

NONOPERATIVE TREATMENT

The Milwaukee brace is the most effective nonoperative treatment. It is used primarily for the more flexible secondary curves below the congenital one. If the brace maintains a curve in an acceptable position, it can be continued. If, however, the curve begins to deteriorate despite faithful brace wearing, fusion is indicated. No attempt should be made to brace curves exceeding 50 degrees.

OPERATIVE TREATMENT

Surgery remains the fundamental treatment for congenital scoliosis since 75% of the curves are progressive and the Milwaukee brace is relatively ineffective. Fusion for congenital scoliosis may be done at very young ages since it is far better to take away the growth on the convex side and prevent progression. We do not routinely use a Milwaukee brace after scoliosis fusions in young patients. The brace may be required, however, in a patient with congenital scoliosis in which the primary curve is not increasing but the secondary curves in the normal part of the spine must be controlled until growth is complete. Without this type of treatment the curves in the previously normal area of the spine sometimes become structural and more than double the angle of the congenital curve.

Fusion in situ. Fusion in situ is appropriate for those curves detected at an early stage with minor deformity. A wide exposure of the area to be fused is gained to the tips of the transverse processes bilaterally by careful subperiosteal dissection. The facet joints are then excised and the cartilage is removed. Preferrably autogenous iliac bone should be placed in the facet joints with the entire area decorticated and additional bone added. The top and bottom of the fused area can be marked with a wire suture or metal clip for postoperative observation. Postoperative immobilization is in a Risser cast and the patient is continued ambulatory.

Cast correction and fusion. Cast correction and fusion are fundamental procedures for congenital scoliosis. Casting can be done either preoperatively or postoperatively. The fusion should always encompass the measured curve with at least one vertebra above and one below, and all vertebrae rotated in the same direction as those in the apex of the curve should be included. The surgical technique is the same as for fusion in situ. Cast application is by maximal correction using longitudinal traction and localizer force. The patient is then kept in bed for 6 months. An ambulatory cast is then applied for an additional 4 months. Recently most children have been ambulated even though some correction may be lost. A Milwaukee brace is usually necessary until at least 12 years of age to prevent bending of the fusion mass and lengthening of the curve, and to control the secondary curves. Pseudarthroses are repaired early if identified on roentgenograms 6 and 9 months after surgery.

Halo-femoral traction and fusion. Halo-femoral traction and fusion are reserved for the more rigid curves for which cast correction is inadequate and a greater degree of correction is desired. As a general rule, the amount of weight used in the traction should not exceed 50% of the total body weight. Weights are added slowly and gradually each day with careful monitoring of the neurologic status. An inability to void would be the first sign of neurologic dysfunction of the cord. Cranial nerve function should be evaluated as well as peripheral nerve function. Any sudden pain, numbness, or weakness should result in all weights being discontinued and only gradually restarted after symptoms have disappeared. Usually a period up to 3 weeks is necessary to gain maximum correction with the slow addition of weights. The patient is operated on in traction with the weights reduced 50%. The weights are gradually brought back up to the preoperative level between 24 and 72 hours postoperatively. Harrington instrumentation should be added only as a stabilizing strut to prevent collapse when the traction is removed and at the time of casting. Any attempt at further correction with Harrington instrumentation may result in paraplegia. Alternatively, a halo cast can be used postoperatively.

Harrington instrumentation and fusion. Harrington instrumentation and fusion are far more dangerous in congenital scoliosis than idiopathic and should be used with spinal cord monitoring. Instrumentation is inserted sometimes as a stabilizing strut only, relying on all correction to have been achieved by halo-femoral or cast correction.

Wedge resection (hemivertebra excision). Wedge resection is used in a small number of cases since it is far better to perform an early fusion to prevent progression. This must be reserved for those with pelvic obliquity uncorrectable by other means or with a fixed lateral translation of the thorax that can not be corrected by other means. The safest level to perform such excision is at the L3 and L4 level below the conus medullaris. Wedge resection in the T4 to T9 area should be viewed with alarm since this is the area of the narrowest spinal canal and the least blood supply to the cord. Hemivertebra excision is best performed as a two-stage procedure as described by Leatherman in which the vertebral body is removed by an anterior exposure initially. Two weeks later a posterior approach and excision of the remainder of the hemivertebra are carried out. The defect can then be closed with a Harrington compression rod. This procedure must always be accompanied by a fusion of the appropriate length. Postoperative care consists of cast immobilization in a supine position for 6 months, followed by an ambulatory cast for another 4 months or until fusion is completely solid.

REFERENCES

Abbott, E.G.: Correction of lateral curvature of the spine, N.Y. Med. J. **95:**833, 1912.

Akbarnia, B.A., and Moe, J.H.: Familial congenital scoliosis with unilateral unsegmented bar: case report of two siblings, J. Bone Joint Surg. **60-A:**259, 1978.

Alexander, J.: Postoperative management of thoracoplasty patients, Am. Rev. Tuberc. **61:**57, 1950.

Allen, B.L., Jr., and Ferguson, R.L.: The Galveston technique for L rod instrumentation of the scoliotic spine, Spine **7:**276, 1982.

Anderson, S., and Bradford, D.S.: Lo-profile halo, Clin. Orthop. **103:**72, 1974.

Arkin, A.M.: Correction of structural changes in scoliosis by corrective plaster jackets and prolonged recumbency, J. Bone Joint Surg. **46-A:**33, 1964.

Armstrong, G.W.D., and Connock, S.H.G.: A transverse loading system applied to a modified Harrington instrumentation, Clin. Orthop. **108:**70, 1975.

Balmer, G.A., and MacEwen, G.D.: The incidence and treatment of scoliosis in cerebral palsy, J. Bone Joint Surg. **52-B:**134, 1970.

Banta, J.V., and Hamada, J.S.: Natural history of the kyphotic deformity in myelomeningocele, J. Bone Joint Surg. 58-A:279, 1960.

Bennett, S.H., Hoye, R.C., and Riggle, G.C.: Intraoperative autotransfusion: preliminary report of a new blood suction device for anticoagulation of autologous blood, Am. J. Surg. 123:257, 1972.

Bloom, M.H., and Raney, F.L., Jr.: Anterior intervertebral fusion of the cervical spine: a technical note, J. Bone Joint Surg. 63-A:842, 1981.

Blount, W.P., and Schmidt, A.C.: The Milwaukee brace (mimeographed privately), 1953.

Blount, W.P., Schmidt, A.C., and Bidwell, R.G.: Making the Milwaukee brace, J. Bone Joint Surg. 40-A:526, 1958.

Blount, W.P., Schmidt, A.C., Keever, E.D., and Leonard, E.T.: The Milwaukee brace in the operative treatment of scoliosis, J. Bone Joint Surg. 40-A:511, 1958.

Bonnett, C.A.: The cord injured child. In Lovell, W.W., and Winter, R.B., editors: Children's orthopaedics, Philadelphia, 1978, J.B. Lippincott Co.

Bonnett, C., Brown, J., and Brooks, H.L.: Anterior spine fusion with Dwyer instrumentation for lumbar scoliosis in cerebral palsy, J. Bone Joint Surg. 55-A:425, 1973.

Bonnett, C., Brown, J.C., and Grow, T.: Thoracolumbar scoliosis in cerebral palsy: results of surgical treatment, J. Bone Joint Surg. 58-A:328, 1976.

Bonnett, C., Perry, J., and Brown, J.: Cord injury and spine deformity in children. Presented at the Scoliosis Research Society, 1972.

Bonnett, C., et al.: Evolution of treatment of paralytic scoliosis at Rancho Los Amigos Hospital, J. Bone Joint Surg. 57-A:206, 1975.

Bradford, D.S.: Neurological complications of Scheuermann's disease, J. Bone Joint Surg. 51-A:657, 1969.

Bradford, D.S., and Moe, J.H.: Scheuermann's juvenile kyphosis: a histologic study, Clin. Ortho. 110:45, 1975.

Bradford, D.S., Moe, J.H., and Winter, R.B.: Kyphosis and postural roundback deformity in children and adolescents, Minn. Med. 56:114, 1973.

Bradford, D.S., Moe, J.H., Montalvo, F.J., and Winter, R.B.: Scheuermann's kyphosis and roundback deformity, results of Milwaukee brace treatment, J. Bone Joint Surg. 56-A:749, 1974.

Bradford, D.S., Moe, J.H., Montalvo, F.J., and Winter, R.B.: Scheuermann's kyphosis: results of surgical treatment in twenty-two patients, J. Bone Joint Surg. 57-A:439, 1975.

Bradford, D.S., Brown, D.M., Moe J.H., Winter, R.B., and Jowsey, J.: Scheuermann's kyphosis: a form of juvenile osteoporosis? Clin. Orthop. 118:10, 1976.

Bradshaw, K., Webb, J.K., and Fraser, A.M.: Clinical evaluation of spinal cord monitoring in scoliosis surgery, Spine 9:636, 1984.

Breig, A.: Biomechanis of the central nervous system: some basic normal and pathologic phenomena concerning spine, discs, and cord, Stockholm, 1960, Almquist and Wiksell (translated by Victor Braxton, Chicago, 1960, Year Book Medical Publishers).

Brown, R.H., and Nash, C.L., Jr.: Current status of spinal cord monitoring, Spine 4:466, 1979.

Bucy, P.C., and Heimburger, R.F.: The neurological aspects of deformities of the spine, Surg. Clin. North Am. 29:163, 1949.

Bunch, W.H.: Muscular dystrophy. In Hardy, J.H., editor: Spinal deformity in neurological and muscular disorders, St. Louis, 1974, The C.V. Mosby Co.

Bunch, W., and Delaney, J.: Scoliosis and acute vascular compression of the duodenum, Surgery 67:901, 1970.

Butte, F.L.: Scoliosis treated by the wedging jacket: selection of the area to be fused, J. Bone Joint Surg. 20:1, 1938.

Chaglassian, J.H., Riseborough, E.J., and Hall, J.E.: Neurofibromatous scoliosis: natural history and results of treatment in thirty-seven cases, J. Bone Joint Surg. 58-A:695, 1976.

Clark, J.A., Hsu, L.C.S., and Yau, A.C.M.C.: Viscoelastic behaviour of deformed spines under correction with halo pelvic distraction, Clin. Orthop. 110:90, 1975.

Cobb, J.R.: The Murk Jansen plaster bed. In Scientific papers, New York, 1939, Hospital for the Ruptured and Crippled.

Cobb, J.R.: The treatment of scoliosis, Conn. Med. J. 7:467, 1943.

Cobb, J.R.: Observations on the treatment of idiopathic scoliosis (unpublished), 1948.

Cobb, J.R.: Outline for the study of scoliosis. In American Academy of Orthopaedic Surgeons: Instructional course lectures, vol. 5, Ann Arbor, 1948, J.W. Edwards.

Cobb, J.R.: Correction of scoliosis. In Poliomyelitis, Second International Poliomyelitis Congress, Philadelphia, 1952, J.B. Lippincott Co.

Cobb, J.R.: Technique, after-treatment, and results of spine fusion for scoliosis. In American Academy of Orthopaedic Surgeons: Instructional course lectures, vol. 9, Ann Arbor, 1952, J.W. Edwards.

Cobb, J.R.: Spine arthrodesis in the treatment of scoliosis, Bull. Hosp. Joint Dis. 19:187, 1958.

Cobb, J.R.: The problem of the primary curve, J. Bone Joint. 42-A:1413, 1960.

Collis, D.K., and Ponseti, I.V.: Long-term follow-up of patients with idiopathic scoliosis not treated surgically, J. Bone Joint Surg. 51-A:425, 1969.

Conner, A.N.: Developmental anomalies and prognosis in infantile idiopathic scoliosis, J. Bone Joint Surg. 51-B:711, 1969.

Cook, C.D., Barrie, H., Deforest, S.A., and Helliesen, P.J.: Pulmonary physiology in children: III. Lung volumes, mechanics of respiration and respiratory muscle strength in scoliosis, J. Pediatr. 25:766, 1960.

Cowell, H.R., and Swickard, J.W.: Autotransfusion in children's orthopaedics, J. Bone Joint Surg. 56-A:908, 1974.

Dawson, E.G., Moe, J.H., and Caron, A.: Surgical measurement of scoliosis in the adult, Scoliosis Research Society, 1972, J. Bone Joint Surg. 55-A:437, 1973.

DeWald, R.L.: New trends in the operative treatment of scoliosis. In Ahstrom, J.P., Jr., editor: Current practices in orthopaedic surgery, vol. 5, St. Louis, 1973, The C.V. Mosby Co.

DeWald, R.L., and Ray, R.D.: Skeletal traction for the treatment of severe scoliosis: the University of Illinois halo-loop apparatus, J. Bone Joint Surg. 52-A:233, 1970.

DeWald, R.L., Mulcahy, T.M., and Schultz, A.B.: Force measurement studies with the halo-loop apparatus in scoliosis, Orthop. Rev. 2:17, December 1973.

Dickson, J.H.: Spinal instrumentation and fusion in adolescent idiopathic scoliosis: indications and surgical techniques, Contemp. Orthop. 4:397, 1982.

Dickson, J.H., and Harrington, P.R.: The evolution of the Harrington instrumentation technique in scoliosis, J. Bone Joint Surg. 55-A:993, 1973.

Dolan J.A., and MacEwen, G.D.: Surgical treatment of scoliosis, Clin. Orthop. 76:125, 1971.

Donaldson, W.F., Jr., and Wissinger, H.A.: The results of surgical exploration of spine fusion performed for scoliosis, Western J. Surg. Obstet. Gynecol. 72:195, 1964.

Dorang, L.A., Klebanoff, G., and Kemmerer, W.T.: Autotransfusion in long-segment spinal fusion: an experimental model to demonstrate the efficacy of salvaging blood contaminated with bone fragments and marrow, Am. J. Surg. 123:686, 1972.

Dorph, M.H.: The cast syndrome, N. Engl. J. Med. 243:440, 1950.

Dorr, J., Brown, J., and Perry, J.: Results of posterior spine fusion in patients with spinal muscle atrophy: a review of 34 cases. Presented at the Scoliosis Research Society, 1972.

Drummond, D.S., Keene, J.S., and Breed, A.: The Wisconsin system: a technique of interspinous segmental spinal instrumentation, Contemp. Orthop. 8:29, 1984.

Drummond, D., et al.: Interspinous process segmental spinal instrumentation, J. Pediatr. Orthop. 4:397, 1984.

Dubowitz, V.: Some clinical observations on childhood muscular dystrophy, Br. J. Clin. Pract. 17:283, 1963.

Dunn, H.K., and Bolstad, K.E.: Fixation of Dwyer screws for the treatment of scoliosis: a postmortem study, J. Bone Joint Surg. 59-A:54, 1977.

Dwork, R.E., Dinken, H., and Hurst, A.: Postthoracoplasty scoliosis, Arch Phys. Med. 32:722, 1951.

Dwyer, A.F.: Experience of anterior correction of scoliosis, Clin. Orthop. 93:191, 1973.

Dwyer, A.F., Newton, N.C., and Sherwood, A.A.: An anterior approach to scoliosis: a preliminary report, Clin. Orthop. 62:192, 1969.

Engler, G.L., et al.: Somatosensory evoked potentials during Harrington instrumentation for scoliosis, J. Bone Joint Surg. 60-A:528, 1978.

Enneking, W.F., and Harrington, P.: Pathological changes in scoliosis, J. Bone Joint Surg. 51-A:165, 1969.

Erwin, W.D., Dickson, J.H., and Harrington, P.R.: The postoperative management of scoliosis patients treated with Harrington instrumentation and fusion, J. Bone Joint Surg. 58-A:479, 1976.

Evarts, C.M.: The cast syndrome: report of a case after spinal fusion for scoliosis, Clin. Orthop. 75:164, 1971.

Evarts, C.M., Winter, R.B., and Hall, J.E.: Vascular compression of the duodenum associated with the treatment of scoliosis: review of the literature and report of eighteen cases, J. Bone Joint Surg. **53-A**:431, 1971.

Ferguson, A.B.: The study and treatment of scoliosis, South. Med. J. **23**:116, 1930.

Ferguson, A.B.: Roentgen interpretations and decisions in scoliosis. In American Academy of Orthopaedic Surgeons: Instructional course lectures, vol. 7, Ann Arbor, 1950, J.W. Edwards.

Ferguson, R.L., and Allen, B.L., Jr.: Segmental spinal instrumentation for routine scoliotic curve, Contemp. Orthop. **2**:450, 1980.

Fielding, J.W., and Waugh, T.: Postoperative correction of scoliosis, JAMA **182**:541, 1962.

Flynn, J.C., and Hoque, A.: Anterior fusion of the lumbar spine: end-result study with long-term follow-up, J. Bone Joint Surg. **61-A**:1143, 1979.

Fujimake, A., Crock, H.V., and Bedbrook, G.M.: The results of 150 anterior lumbar interbody fusion operations performed by two surgeons in Australia, Clin. Orthop. **165**:164, 1982.

Gaines, R., York, D.H., and Watts, C.: Identification of spinal cord pathways responsible for the peroneal-evoked response in the dog, Spine **9**:810, 1984.

Galeazzi, R.: The treatment of scoliosis, J. Bone Joint Surg. **11**:81, 1929.

Gardner, R.C.: Blood loss after spinal instrumentation and fusion in scoliosis (Harrington procedure): results using a radioactive tracer and an electronic blood volume computer: a preliminary report, Clin. Orthop. **71**:182, 1970.

Garrett, A.L., Perry, J., and Nickel, V.L.: Paralytic scoliosis, Clin. Orthop. **21**:117, 1961.

Garrett, A.L., Perry, J., and Nickel, V.L.: Stabilization of the collapsing spine, J. Bone Joint Surg. **43-A**:474, 1961.

Gazioglu, K., Goldstein, L.A., Femi-Pearse, D., and Yu, P.N.: Pulmonary function in idiopathic scoliosis: comparative evaluation before and after orthopaedic correction, J. Bone Joint Surg. **50-A**:1391, 1968.

Gillespie, R., et al.: Intraspinal anomalies in congenital scoliosis, Clin. Orthop. **93**:103, 1973.

Goldstein, L.A.: Results in the treatment of scoliosis with turnbuckle plaster cast correction and fusion, J. Bone Joint Surg. **41-A**:321, 1959.

Goldstein, L.A.: The surgical management of scoliosis, Clin. Orthop. **35**:95, 1964.

Goldstein, L.A.: Surgical management of scoliosis, J. Bone Joint Surg. **48-A**:167, 1966.

Goldstein, L.A.: Treatment of idiopathic scoliosis by Harrington instrumentation and fusion with fresh autogenous iliac bone grafts: results in eighty patients, J. Bone Joint Surg. **51-A**:209, 1969.

Goldstein, L.A., and Evarts, C.M.: Further experiences with the treatment of scoliosis by cast correction and spine fusion with fresh autogenous iliac-bone grafts, J. Bone Joint Surg. **48-A**:962, 1966.

Goldstein, L.A.: The surgical management of scoliosis, Clin. Orthop. **77**:32, 1971.

Goldstein, L.A.: The surgical treatment of idiopathic scoliosis, Clin. Orthop. **93**:131, 1973.

Gollehon, D., Kahanovitz, N., and Happel, L.T.: Temperature effects on feline cortical and spinal evoked potentials, Spine **8**:443, 1983.

Hall, J.E.: The place of the anterior approach to the spine in scoliosis surgery. In Keim, H.A., editor: Postgraduate course on the management and care of the scoliosis patient, pp. 32-34, Nov. 5-7, 1970.

Hall, J.E., Levine, C.R., and Sudhir, K.G.: Intraoperative awakening to monitor spinal cord function during Harrington instrumentation and spine fusion: descriptions of procedure and report of three cases, J. Bone Joint Surg. **60-A**:533, 1978.

Hall, P.V., et al.: Myelodysplasia and developmental scoliosis: a manifestation of syringomyelia, Spine **1**:48, 1976.

Hamel, A.L., and Moe, J.H.: The collapsing spine, Surgery **56**:364, 1964.

Hardy, J.: Neuromuscular scoliosis, J. Bone Joint Surg. **52-A**:407, 1970.

Hardy, J.H., and Gossling, H.R.: Combined halo and sacral bar fixation: a method for immobilization and early ambulation following extensive spine fusion, Clin. Orthop. **75**:205, 1971.

Harrington, P.R.: Treatment of scoliosis. Correction and internal fixation by spine instrumentation, J. Bone Joint Surg. **44-A**:591, 1962.

Harrington, P.R.: The management of scoliosis by spine instrumentation: an evaluation of more than 200 cases, South. Med. J. **56**:1367, 1963.

Harrington, P.R.: Technical details in relation to the successful use of instrumentation in scoliosis, Orthop. Clin. North Am. **3**:49, 1972.

Harrington, P.R.: The history and development of Harrington instrumenation, Clin. Orthop. **93**:110, 1973.

Harrington, P.R., and Dickson, J.H.: An eleven-year clinical investigation of Harrington instrumentation: a preliminary report of 578 cases, Clin. Orthop. **93**:113, 1973.

Hattori, S., Saiki, K., and Kawai, S.: Diagnosis of the level and severity of cord lesion in cervical spondylotic myelopathy: spinal evoked potentials, Spine **4**:478, 1979.

Hensinger, R.N., and MacEwen, G.D.: Spinal deformity associated with heritable neurological conditions: spinal muscular atrophy, Friedreich's ataxia, familial dysautonomia, and Charcot-Marie-Tooth disease, J. Bone Joint Surg. **58-A**:13, 1976.

Herring, J.A.: Rapidly progressive scoliosis in multiple epiphyseal dysplasia: a case report, J. Bone Joint Surg. **58-A**:703, 1976.

Herring, J.A.: The spinal disorders in diastrophic dwarfism, J. Bone Joint Surg. **60-A**:177, 1978.

Herring, J.A., and Wenger, D.R.: Segmental spinal instrumentation: a preliminary report of 40 consecutive cases, Spine **7**:285, 1982.

Herron, L.D., and Dawson, E.G.: Methylmethacrylate as an adjunct in spinal instrumenation, J. Bone Joint Surg. **59-A**:866, 1977.

Herron, L.D., Westin, G.W., and Dawson, E.G.: Scoliosis in arthrogryposis multiplex congenita, J. Bone Joint Surg. **60-A**:293, 1978.

Hibbs, R.A.: A report of fifty-nine cases of scoliosis treated by the fusion operation, J. Bone Joint Surg. **6**:3, 1924.

Hibbs, R.A., Risser, J.C., and Ferguson, A.B.: Scoliosis treated by the fusion operation, J. Bone Joint Surg. **13**:91, 1931.

Houtkin, S., and Levine, D.B.: The halo yoke: a simplified device for attachment of the halo to a body cast, J. Bone Joint Surg. **54-A**:881, 1972.

Hsu, L.C.S., Zucherman, J., Tang, S.C., and Leong, J.C.Y.: Dwyer instrumentation in the treatment of adolescent idiopathic scoliosis, J. Bone Joint Surg. **64-B**:536, 1982.

Huebert, H.T., and MacKinnon, W.B.: Syringomyelia and scoliosis, J. Bone Joint Surg. **51-B**:338, 1969.

Jacobsen, S., Rosenklint, A., and Halkier, E.: Post-pneumonectomy scoliosis, Acta Orthop. Scand. **45**:867, 1974.

James, J.I.P.: Two curve patterns in idiopathic structural scoliosis, J. Bone Joint Surg. **33-B**:399, 1951.

James, J.I.P.: Idiopathic scoliosis: the prognosis, diagnosis, and operative indications related to curve patterns and the age at onset, J. Bone Joint Surg. **36-B**:36, 1954.

James, J.I.P.: Infantile idiopathic scoliosis, Clin. Orthop. **21**:106, 1961.

James, J.I.P., Lloyd-Roberts, G.C., and Pilcher, M.F.: Infantile structural scoliosis, J. Bone Joint Surg. **41-B**:719, 1959.

James, J.I.P.: The management of infants with scoliosis, J. Bone Joint Surg. **57-B**:422, 1975.

Johnson, B.E., and Westgate, H.D.: Methods of predicting vital capacity in patients with thoracic scoliosis, J. Bone Joint Surg. **52-A**:1433, 1970.

Jones, S.J., Edgar, M.A., Ransford, A.O., and Thomas, N.P.: A system for the electrophysiological monitoring of the spinal cord during operations for scoliosis, J. Bone Joint Surg. **65-B**:134, 1983.

Kalamchi, A., Yau, A.C.M.C., O'Brien, J.P., and Hodgson, A.R.: Halo-pelvic distraction apparatus: an analysis of one hundred and fifty consecutive patients, J. Bone Joint Surg. **58-A**:1119, 1976.

Keller, R.B., and Pappas, A.M.: Infection after spinal fusion using internal fixation instrumenation, Orthop. Clin. North Am. **3**:99, 1972.

Kilfoyle, R.M., Foley, J.J., and Norton, P.L.: Spine and pelvic deformity in childhood and adolescent paraplegia: a study of 104 cases, J. Bone Joint Surg. **47-A**:659, 1965.

Kleinberg, S.: A survey of structural scoliosis: the principles of treatment and their application. In American Academy of Orthopaedic Surgeons: Instructional course lectures, vol. 7, Ann Arbor, 1950, J.W. Edwards.

Kleinberg, S.: Scoliosis with paraplegia, J. Bone Joint Surg. **33-A**:225, 1951.

Kleinberg, S.: Scoliosis: pathology, etiology, and treatment, Baltimore, 1951, The Williams & Wilkins Co.

Kleinberg, S., and Kaplan, A.: Scoliosis complicated by paraplegia, J. Bone Joint Surg. **34-A**:162, 1952.

Kojima, Y., Yamamoto, T., Ogino, H., Okada, K., and Ono, K.: Evoked spinal potentials as a monitor of spinal cord viability, Spine **4**:471, 1979.

Kostuik, J.P., Israel, J., and Hall, J.E.: Scoliosis surgery in adults, Clin. Orthop. **93:**225, 1973.

Kuhn, R.A., and Garrett, A.: The halo in the management of cervical spine lesions, Orthop. Rev. **1:**25 December, 1972.

Larson, S.J., Walsh, P.R., Sances, A., Jr., Cusick, J.F., Hemmy, D.C., and Mahler, H.: Evoked potentials in experimental myelopathy, Spine **5:**299, 1980.

Leatherman, K.D.: The management of rigid spinal curves, Clin. Orthop. **93:**215, 1973.

Leider, L.L., Jr., Moe, J.H., and Winter, R.B.: Early ambulation after the surgical treatment of idiopathic scoliosis, J. Bone Joint Surg. **55-A:**1003, 1973.

Letts, R.M., and Bobechko, W.P.: Fusion of the scoliotic spine in young children: effect on prognosis and growth, Clin. Orthop. **101:**136, 1974.

Letts, R.M., Palakar, G., and Bobechko, W.P.: Preoperative skeletal traction in scoliosis, J. Bone Joint Surg. **57-A:**616, 1975.

Levy, W.J., and York, D.H.: Evoked potentials from motor tracts in humans, Neurosurgery **12:**422, 1983.

Lindseth, R.E.: Posterior iliac osteotomy for fixed pelvic obliquity, J. Bone Joint Surg. **60-A:**17, 1978.

Lonstein, J., Winter, R., Moe, J., and Gaines, D.: Wound infection with Harrington instrumentation and spine fusion for scoliosis, Clin. Orthop. **96:**222, 1973.

Loynes, R.D.: Scoliosis after thoracoplasty, J. Bone Joint Surg. **54-B:**484, 1972.

Lueders, H., Gurd, A., Hahn, J., Andrish, J., Weiker, G., and Klem, G.: A new technique for intraoperative monitoring of spinal cord function: multichannel recording of spinal cord and subcortical evoked potentials, Spine **7:**110, 1982.

Luque, E.R.: Anatomy of scoliosis and its correction, Clin. Orthop. **105:**298, 1974.

Luque, E.R.: The anatomic basis and development of segmental spinal instrumentation, Spine **7:**256, 1982.

Luque, E.R.: Segmental spinal instrumentation for correction of scoliosis, Clin. Orthop. **163:**192, 1982.

MacEwen, G.D., Winter, R.B., and Hardy, J.H.: Evaluation of kidney anomalies in congenital scoliosis, J. Bone Joint Surg. **54-A:**1451, 1972.

MacEwen, G.D., Bunnell, W.P., and Sriram, K.: Acute neurological complications in the treatment of scoliosis: a report of the Scoliosis Research Society, J. Bone Joint Surg. **57-A:**404, 1975.

Machida, M., Weinstein, S.L., Yamada, T., and Kimura, J.: Spinal cord monitoring: electrophysiological measures of sensory and motor function during spinal surgery, Spine **10:**407, 1985.

Mackel, J.L., and Lindseth, R.E.: Scoliosis in myelodysplasia, J. Bone Joint Surg. **57-A:**1031, 1975.

Makley, J.T., Herndon, C.H., Inkley, S., Doershuk, C., Matthews, L.W., Post, R.H., and Littell, A.S.: Pulmonary function in paralytic and non-paralytic scoliosis before and after treatment: a study of sixty-three cases, J. Bone Joint Surg. **50-A:**1379, 1968.

Mankin, H.J., Graham, J.J., and Schack, J.: Cardiopulmonary function in mild and moderate idiopathic scoliosis, J. Bone Joint Surg. **46-A:**53, 1964.

May, V.R., Jr., and Mauck, W.R.: Exploration of the spine for pseudarthrosis following spinal fusion in the treatment of scoliosis, Clin. Orthop. **53:**115, 1967.

McCarroll, H.R., and Costen, W.: Attempted treatment of scoliosis by unilateral vertebral epiphyseal arrest, J. Bone Joint Surg. **42-A:**965, 1960.

McKenzie, K.G., and Dewar, F.T.: Scoliosis with paraplegia, J. Bone Joint Surg. **31-B:**162, 1949.

McKittrick, J.E.: Banked autologous blood in elective surgery, Am. J. Surg. **128:**137, 1974.

McMaster, M.J., and James, J.I.P.: Pseudarthrosis after spinal fusion for scoliosis, J. Bone Joint Surg. **58-B:**305, 1976.

Mehta, M.H.: The rib-vertebra angle in the early diagnosis between resolving and progressive infantile scoliosis, J. Bone Joint Surg. **54-B:**230, 1972.

Mehta, M.H.: Radiographic estimation of vertebral rotation in scoliosis, J. Bone Joint Surg. **55-B:**513, 1973.

Meiss, W.C.: Spinal osteotomy following fusion for paralytic scoliosis, J. Bone Joint Surg. **37-A:**73, 1955.

Micheli, L.J., Hall, J.E., and Watts, H.G.: Spinal instability in Larsen's syndrome: report of three cases, J. Bone Joint Surg. **58-A:**562, 1976.

Mir, S.R., et al.: Early ambulation following spinal fusion and Harrington instrumentation in idiopathic scoliosis, Clin. Orthop. **110:**54, 1975.

Moe, J.H.: The management of paralytic scoliosis, South. Med. J. **50:**67, 1957.

Moe, J.H.: A critical analysis of methods of fusion for scoliosis: an evaluation in two hundred and sixty-six patients, J. Bone Joint Surg. **40-A:**529, 1958.

Moe, J.H.: Complications of scoliosis treatment, Clin. Orthop. **53:**21, 1967.

Moe, J.H.: Methods of correction and surgical techniques in scoliosis, Orthop. Clin. North Am. **3:**17, 1972.

Moe, J.H., and Gustilo, R.B.: Treatment of scoliosis: results in 196 patients treated with cast correction and fusion, J. Bone Joint Surg. **46-A:**293, 1964.

Morgan, T.H., and Scott, J.C.: Treatment of infantile idiopathic scoliosis, J. Bone Joint Surg. **38-B:**450, 1956.

Morgenstern, J.M., Hassmann, G.C., and Keim, H.A.: Modifying post-transfusion hepatitis by gamma globulin in spinal surgery, Orthop. Rev. **4:**29, June 1975.

Mouradian, W.H., and Simmons, E.H.: A frame for spinal surgery to reduce intra-abdominal pressure while continuous traction is applied, J. Bone Joint Surg. **59-A:**1098, 1977.

Nach, C.D., and Keim, H.A.: Prophylactic antibiotics in spinal surgery, Orthop. Rev. **2:**27, June 1973.

Nachemson, A.: A long term follow-up study of nontreated scoliosis, Acta Orthop. Scand. **39:**466, 1968.

Nachemson, A.: A long term follow-up study of nontreated scoliosis, J. Bone Joint Surg. **50-A:**203, 1969.

Nachemson, A.L., and Elfström, G.: Intravital wireless telemetry of axial forces in Harrington distraction rods in patients with idiopathic scoliosis, J. Bone Joint Surg. **53-A:**445, 1971.

Nachemson, A., and Nordwall, A.: Effectiveness of preoperative Cotrel traction for correction of idiopathic scoliosis, J. Bone Joint Surg. **59-A:**504, 1977.

Nachlas, I.W., and Borden, J.N.: The cure of experimental scoliosis by directed growth control, J. Bone Joint Surg. **33-A:**24, 1951.

Nasca, R.J.: Segmental spinal instrumentation, South. Med. J. **78:**303, 1985.

Nash, C.L., Jr., Lorig, R.A., Schatzinger, L.A., and Brown, R.H.: Spinal cord monitoring during operative treatment of the spine, Clin. Orthop. **126:**100, 1977.

Nash, C.L., Schatzinger, L., and Lorig, R.: Intraoperative monitoring of spinal cord function during scoliosis spine surgery (abstract), J. Bone Joint Surg. **56-A:**1765, 1974.

Nickel, V.L., Perry, J., Garrett, A., and Heppenstall, M.: The halo: a spinal skeletal traction fixation device, J. Bone Joint surg. **50-A:**1400, 1968.

Nilsonne, U., and Lundgren, K.D.: Long-term prognosis in idiopathic scoliosis, Acta Orthop. Scand. **39:**456, 1968.

Nordwall, A., et al.: Spinal cord monitoring using evoked potentials recorded from vertebral bone in cat, Spine **4:**486, 1979.

O'Brien, J.P.: The halo-pelvic apparatus: a clinical, bio-engineering and anatomical study, Acta Orthop. Scand. Suppl. 163, 1975.

O'Brien, J.P., Dwyer, A.P., and Hodgson, A.R.: Paralytic pelvic obliquity: its prognosis and management and the development of a technique for full correction of the deformity, J. Bone Joint Surg. **57-A:**626, 1975.

O'Brien, J.P., and Yau, A.C.M.C.: Anterior and posterior correction and fusion for paralytic scoliosis, Clin. Orthop. **86:**151, 1972.

O'Brien, J.P., Yau, A.C.M.C., and Hodgson, A.R.: Halo pelvic traction: a technic for severe spinal deformities, Clin. Orthop. **93:**179, 1973.

O'Brien, J.P., Yau, A.C.M.C., Smith, T.K., and Hodgson, A.R.: Halo pelvic traction: a preliminary report on a method of external skeletal fixation for correcting deformities and maintaining fixation of the spine, J. Bone Joint Surg. **53-B:**217, 1971.

Ogilve, J.W., and Millar, E.A.: Comparison of segmental spinal instrumentation devices in the correction of scoliosis, Spine **8:**416, 1983.

Osmond-Clarke, H.: Scoliosis. In Platt, H., editor: Modern trends in orthopaedics, New York, 1950, Paul B. Hoeber, Inc.

Perry, J.: The halo in spinal abnormalities: practical factors and avoidance of complications, Orthop. Clin. North Am. **3:**69, 1972.

Pieron, A.P., and Welply, W.R.: Halo traction, J. Bone Joint Surg. **52-B:**119, 1970.

Piggott, H.: Treatment of scoliosis by posterior fusion, Harrington instrumentation and early walking, J. Bone Joint Surg. **58-B:**58, 1976.

Ponder, R.C., Dickson, J.H., Harrington, P.R., and Erwin, W.D.: Results of Harrington instrumentation and fusion in the adult idiopathic scoliosis patient, J. Bone Joint Surg. **57-A:**797, 1975.

Ponseti, I.V., and Friedman, B.: Changes in the scoliotic spine after fusion, J. Bone Joint Surg. **32-A:**751, 1950.

Ponseti, I.V., and Friedman, B.: Prognosis in idiopathic scoliosis, J. Bone Joint Surg. **32-A:**381, 1950.

Prolo, D.J., Runnels, J.B., and Jameson, R.M.: The injured cervical spine: immediate and long-term immobilization with the halo, JAMA **224:**591, 1973.

Puranik, S.R., Keiser, R.P., and Gilbert, M.G.: Arteriomesenteric duodenal compression in children, Am. J. Surg. **124:**334, 1972.

Ransford, A.O., and Manning, C.W.S.F.: Complications of halo-pelvic distraction for scoliosis, J. Bone Joint Surg. **57-B:**131, 1975.

Rappaport, M., Hall, K., Hopkins, K., Belleza, T., and Fountain, S.: Effects of corrective scoliosis surgery on somatosensory evoked potentials, Spine **7:**404, 1982.

Raycroft, J.F., and Curtis, B.H.: Spinal curvature in myelomeningocele: natural history and etiology. In American Academy of Orthopaedic Surgeons: Symposium on myelomeningocele, St. Louis, 1972, The C.V. Mosby Co.

Reger, S.I., Henry,D.T., Whitehill, R., Wang, G.-J., and Stamp, W.G.: Spinal evoked potentials from the cervical spine, Spine **4:**495, 1979.

Reid, R.L., and Gamon, R.S., Jr.: The cast syndrome, Clin. Orthop. **79:**85, 1971.

Relton, J.E.S., and Hall, J.E.: An operation frame for spinal fusion: a new apparatus designed to reduce haemorrhage during operation, J. Bone Joint Surg. **49-B:**327, 1967.

Renshaw, T.S.: Spinal fusion with segmental instrumentation, Contemp. Orthop. **4:**413, 1982.

Resina, J., and Alves, A.F.: A technique for correction and internal fixation for scoliosis, J. Bone Joint Surg. **59-B:**159, 1977.

Rieth, P.L., Hopkins, W.A., and Dunlap, E.B., Jr.: A new surgical procedure in scoliosis therapy: unilateral vertebral body growth arrest by transpleural approach, Southern Surg. **16:**368, 1950.

Riseborough, E.J.: The anterior approach to the spine for the correction of deformities of the axial skeleton, Clin. Orthop. **93:**207, 1973.

Riseborough, E.J., and Wynne-Davies, R.: A genetic study of idiopathic scoliosis in Boston, Massachusetts, J. Bone Joint Surg. **55-A:**974, 1973.

Risser, J.C.: Acquired scoliosis. In The cyclopedia of medicine, vol. 11, Philadelphia, 1933, F.A. Davis Co.

Risser, J.C.: Important practical facts in the treatment of scoliosis. In American Academy of Orthopaedic Surgeons: Instructional course lectures, vol. 5, Ann Arbor, 1948, J.W. Edwards.

Risser, J.C.: Scoliosis. In American Academy of Orthopaedic Surgeons: Instructional course lectures, vol. 14, Ann Arbor, 1957, J.W. Edwards.

Risser, J.C.: Modern trends in scoliosis, Bull. Hosp. Joint Dis. **19:**166, 1958.

Risser, J.C.: The iliac apophysis: an invaluable sign in the management of scoliosis, Clin. Orthop. **11:**111, 1958.

Risser, J.C.: Plaster body-jackets, Am. J. Orthop. **3:**19, 1961.

Risser, J.C.: Scoliosis: past and present, J. Bone Joint Surg. **46-A:**167, 1964.

Risser, J.C.: Scoliosis treated by cast correction and spine fusion: a long term follow-up study, Clin. Orthop. **116:**86, 1976.

Risser, J.C., and Ferguson, A.B.: Scoliosis: its prognosis, J. Bone Joint Surg. **18:**667, 1936.

Risser, J.C., Lauder, C.H., Norquist, D.M., and Craig, W.A.: Three types of body casts. In American Academy of Orthopaedic Surgeons: Instructional course lectures, vol. 10, Ann Arbor, 1953, J.W. Edwards.

Risser, J.C., and Norquist, D.M.: A follow-up study of the treatment of scoliosis, J. Bone Joint Surg. **40-A:**555, 1958.

Roaf, R.: Vertebral growth and its mechanical control, J. Bone Joint Surg. **42-B:**40, 1960.

Roaf, R.: The treatment of progressive scoliosis by unilateral growth-arrest, J. Bone Joint Surg. **45-B:**637, 1963.

Roaf, R.: Wedge resection for scoliosis, J. Bone Joint Surg. **46-B:**798, 1964.

Roaf, R.: Scoliosis, Baltimore, 1966, The Williams & Wilkins Co.

Robin, G.C., and Brief, L.P.: Scoliosis in childhood muscular dystrophy, J. Bone Joint Surg. **53-A:**466, 1971.

Robins, P.R., Moe, J.H., and Winter, R.B.: Scoliosis in Marfan's syndrome: its characteristics and results of treatment in thirty-five patients, J. Bone Joint Surg. **57-A:**358, 1975.

Robson, P.: The prevalence of scoliosis in adolescents and young adults with cerebral palsy, Dev. Med. Child Neurol. **10:**447, 1968.

Rogala, E.J., Drummond, D.S., and Gurr, J.: Scoliosis: incidence and natural history; a prospective epidemiological study, J. Bone Joint Surg. **60-A:**173, 1978.

Rosenthal, R.K., Levine, D.B., and McCarver, C.L.: The occurence of scoliosis in cerebral palsy, Dev. Med. Child Neurol. **16:**664, 1974.

Roth, A., et al.: Scoliosis and congenital heart disease, Clin. Orthop. **93:**95, 1973.

Ruhlin, C.W., and Albert, S.: Scoliosis complicated by spinal cord involvement, J. Bone Joint Surg. **23:**877, 1941.

Samilson, R.L., and Bechard, R.: Scoliosis in cerebral palsy: incidence, distribution of curve patterns, natural history, and thoughts on etiology. In Ahstrom, J.P., Jr., editor: Current practice in orthopaedic surgery, vol. 5, St. Louis, 1973, The C.V. Mosby Co.

Scheuermann, H.W.: Kyphosis juvenilis (Scheuermann's krankheit), Fortschr. Geb. Rontgenstrahlen **53:**1, 1936.

Schmidt, A.C.: Fundamental principles and treatment of scoliosis. In American Academy of Orthopaedic Surgeons: Instructional course lectures, vol. 16, St. Louis, 1959, The C.V. Mosby Co.

Schmidt, A.C.: Halo-tibial traction combined with the Milwaukee brace, Clin. Orthop. **77:**73, 1971.

Schultz, A.B., and Hirsch, C.: Mechanical analysis of Harrington rod correction of idiopathic scoliosis, J. Bone Joint Surg. **55-A:**983, 1973.

Schultz, A.B., and Hirsch, C.: Mechanical analysis of techniques for improved correction of idiopathic scoliosis, Clin. Orthop. **100:**66, 1974.

Schwentker, E.P., and Gibson, D.A.: The orthopaedic aspects of spinal muscular atrophy, J. Bone Joint Surg. **58-A:**32, 1976.

Scott, J.C., and Morgan, T.H.: The natural history and prognosis of infantile idiopathic scoliosis, J. Bone Joint Surg. **37-B:**400, 1955.

Selig, S., and Arnheim, E.: Scoliosis following empyemia, Arch. Surg. **39:**798, 1939.

Shands, A.R., Jr., Barr, J.S., Colonna, P.C., and Noall, L.: End-result study of the treatment of idiopathic scoliosis; report of the research committee of the American Orthopaedic Association, J. Bone Joint Surg. **23:**963, 1941.

Shifrin, L.Z.: The lateral position for spine fusion and Harrington instrumentation for scoliosis: a brief report, Clin. Orthop. **81:**48, 1971.

Shurtleff, D.B., et al.: Myelodysplasia: the natural history of kyphosis and scoliosis: a preliminary report, Dev. Med. Child Neurol. **37**(Suppl.):126, 1976.

Sicard, A., Lavarde, G., and Chaleil, B.: La greffe vertébrale dans les scolioses de l'adulte, J. Chir. (Paris) **93:**517, 1967.

Sicard, A., Lavarde, G., and Chaleil, B.: Seventy instances of adult scoliosis treated with spinal fusion, Surg. Gynecol. Obstet. **126:**682, 1968.

Siebold, R.M., Winter, R.B., and Moe, J.H.: The treatment of scoliosis in arthrogryposis multiplex congenita, Clin. Orthop. **103:**191, 1974.

Siegel, I.M.: Scoliosis in muscular dystrophy: some comments about diagnosis, observations on prognosis, and suggestions for therapy, Clin. Orthop. **93:**235, 1973.

Smith, A., DeF., Butte, F.L.,and Ferguson, A.B.: Treatment of scoliosis by the wedging jacket and spine fusion: a review of 265 cases, J. Bone Joint Surg. **20:**825, 1938.

Smith, A. deF., von Lackum, W.H., and Wylie, R.: An operation for stapling vertebral bodies in congenital scoliosis, J. Bone Joint Surg. **36-A:**342, 1954.

Sørenson, K.H.: Scheuermann's juvenile kyphosis, Copenhagen, 1964, Munksgaard.

Spielholz, N.I., Benjamin, M.V., Engler, G.L., and Ransohoff, J.: Somatosensory evoked potentials during decompression and stabilization of the spine: methods and findings, Spine **4:**500, 1979.

Sriram, K., Bobechko, W.P., and Hall, J.E.: Surgical management of spinal deformities in spina bifida, J. Bone Joint Surg. **54-B:**666, 1972.

Stagnara, P.: Scoliosis in adults: surgical treatment of severe forms, Excerpta Med. Found. International Congress Series No. 192, 1969.

Stagnara, P.: Utilization of Harrington's device in the treatment of adult kyphoscoliosis above 100 degrees. Fourth International Symposium, 1971, Nijmegen, Stuttgart, 1973, Georg Thieme Verlag.

Stagnara, P., Fleury, D., Pauchet, R., Mazoyer, D., Biot, B., Vauzelle, C., and Jouvinroux, P.: Scolioses majeures de l'adulte superieures a 100° -183 castraites chirurgicalement, Rev. Chir. Orthop. **61**:101, 1975.

Stagnara, P., Jouvinroux, P., Peloux, J., Pauchet, R., Mazoyer, D., and Callay, C.: Cyphoscolioses essentielles de l'adulte: formes sévères de plus de 100°: redressement partial et arthordése, XI SICOT Congress, 206, Mexico City, 1969.

Stauffer, E.S., and Mankin, H.J.: Scoliosis after thoracoplasty: a study of thirty patients, J. Bone Joint Surg. **48-A**:339, 1966.

Steel, H.H.: Rib resection and spine fusion in correction of convex deformity in scoliosis, J. Bone Joint Surg. **65-A**:920, 1983.

Sullivan, J.A., and Conner, S.B.: Comparison of Harrington instrumentation and segmental spinal instrumentation in the management of neuromuscular spinal deformity, Spine **7**:299, 1982.

Taddonio, R.F.: Segmental spinal instrumentation in the management of neuromuscular spinal deformity, Spine **7**:305, 1982.

Tambornino, J.M., Armbrust, E.N., and Moe, J.H.: Harrington instrumentation in correction of scoliosis: a comparison with cast correction, J. Bone Joint Surg. **46-A**:313, 1964.

Thompson, W.A.L., and Ralston, E.L.: Pseudarthrosis following spine fusion, J. Bone Joint Surg. **31-A**:400, 1949.

Thulbourne, T., and Gillespie, R.: The rib hump in idiopathic scoliosis: measurement, analysis and response to treatment, J. Bone Joint Surg. **58-B**:64, 1976.

Ulrich, H.F.: The operative treatment of scoliosis, Am. J. Surg. **45**:235, 1939.

Van Rens, T.J.G., and Van Horn, J.R.: Long-term results in lumbosacral interbody fusion for spondylolisthesis, Acta Orthop. Scand. **53**:383, 1982.

Vanderpool, D.W., James, J.I.P., and Wynne-Davies, R.: Scoliosis in the elderly, J. Bone Joint Surg. **51-A**:446, 1969.

Vauzelle, C., Stagnara, P., and Jouvinroux, P.: Functional monitoring of spinal cord activity during spinal surgery, Clin. Orthop. **93**:173, 1973.

Vauzell, C., Stagnara, P., and Jouvinroux, P.: Functional monitoring of spinal activity during spinal surgery, J. Bone Joint Surg. **55-A**:441, 1973.

Vom Saal, F.: Management of scoliosis, Am. J. Surg. **52**:433, 1941.

Von Lackum, W.H.: The surgical treatment of scoliosis. In American Academy of Orthopaedic Surgeons: Instructional course lectures, vol. 5, Ann Arbor, 1948, J.W. Edwards.

Von Lackum, W.H.: The surgical treatment of scoliosis. In Bancroft, F.W., and Marble, H.C.: Surgical treatment of the motor-skeletal system, ed. 2, Philadelphia, 1951, J.B. Lippincott Co.

Von Lackum, W.H.: Surgical scoliosis, Surg. Clin. North Am. **31**:345, 1951.

Von Lackum, W.H., and Miller, J.P.: Critical observations of the results in the operative treatment of scoliosis, J. Bone Joint Surg. **31-A**:102, 1949.

Walker, G.F.: An evaluation of an external splint for idiopathic structural scoliosis in infancy, J. Bone Joint Surg. **47-B**:524, 1965.

Weber, F.A.: The association of syringomyelia and scoliosis, J. Bone Joint Surg. **56-B**:589, 1974.

Weinstein, S.L., and Ponsetti, I.V.: Curve progression in idiopathic scoliosis: long-term follow-up, J. Bone Joint Surg. **65-A**:447, 1983.

Weisl, H.: Unusual complications of skull caliper traction, J. Bone Joint Surg. **54-B**:143, 1972.

Wenger, D.R., Carollo, J.J., and Wilkerson, J.A.: Biomechanics of scoliosis correction by segmental spinal instrumentation, Spine **7**:260, 1982.

Wenger, D.R., et al.: Laboratory testing of segmental spinal instrumentation versus traditional Harrington instrumentation for scoliosis treatment, Spine **7**:265, 1982.

Westgate, H.D., and Moe, J.H.: Pulmonary function in kyphoscoliosis before and after correction of the Harrington instrumentation method, J. Bone Joint Surg. **51-A**:935, 1969.

White, A.A., III, et al.: Relief of pain by anterior cervical-spine fusion for spondylosis: a report of sixty-five patients, J. Bone Joint Surg. **55-A**:525, 1973.

Whitehill, R., Sirna, E.C., Young, D.C., and Cantrell, R.W.: Late esophageal perforation from an autogenous bone graft: report of a case, J. Bone Joint Surg. **67-A**:644, 1985.

Wilber, R.G., Thompson, G.H., Shaffer, J.W., Brown, R.H., and Nash, C.L., Jr.: Postoperative neurologic deficits in segmental spinal instrumentation: a study using spinal cord monitoring, J. Bone Joint Surg. **66-A**:1178, 1984.

Wilkins, K.E., and Gibson, D.A.: The patterns of spinal deformity in Duchenne muscular dystrophy, J. Bone Joint Surg. **58-A**:24, 1976.

Williams, J.M., and Stevens, H.: Recognition of surgically treatable neurologic disorders of childhood. JAMA **151**:455, 1953.

Wilson, R.L., Levine, D.B., and Doherty, J.H.: Surgical treatment of idiopathic scoliosis, Clin. Orthop. **81**:34, 1971.

Wiltse, L.L.: Spondylolisthesis in children, Clin. Orthop. **21**:156, 1961.

Wiltse, L.L.: The etiology of spondylolisthesis, J. Bone Joint surg. **44-A**:539, 1962.

Winter, R.B.: Congenital deformities of the spine, New York, 1983, Thieme-Stratton.

Winter, R.B.: Congenital scoliosis, Clin. Orthop. **93**:75, 1973.

Winter, R.B.: Congenital spine deformity: natural history and treatment, Isr. J. Med. Sci. **9**:719, 1973.

Winter, R.B.: Scoliosis and other spinal deformities, Acta Orthop. Scand. **46**:400, 1975.

Winter, R.B.: Congenital kyphoscoliosis with paralysis following hemivertebra excision, Clin. Orthop. **119**:116, 1976.

Winter, R.B., Haven, J.J., Moe, J.H., and Lagaard, S.M.: Diastematomyelia and congenital spine deformities, J. Bone Joint Surg. **56-A**:27, 1974.

Winter, R.B., Lovell, W.W., and Moe, J.H.: Excessive thoracic lordosis and loss of pulmonary function in patients with idiopathic scoliosis, J. Bone Joint Surg. **57-A**:972, 1974.

Winter, R.B., Moe, J.H., and Eilers, V.E.: Congenital scoliosis: a study of 234 patients treated and untreated. Part I: Natural history, J. Bone Joint Surg. **50-A**:1, 1968.

Winter, R.B., Moe, J.H., and Eilers, V.E.: Congenital scoliosis: a study of 234 patients treated and unteated. Part II: Treatment, J. Bone Joint Surg. **50-A**:15, 1968.

Winter, R.B., Moe, J.H., and Wang, J.F.: Congenital kyphosis, J. Bone Joint Surg. **55-A**:223, 1973.

Winter, R.B., Moe, J.H., MacEwen, G.D., and Peon-Vidales, H.: The Milwaukee brace in the non-operative treatment of congenital scoliosis, Spine **1**:33, 1976.

Wynne-Davies, R.: Familial (idiopathic) scoliosis: a family survery, J. Bone Joint Surg. **50-B;**24, 1968.

Wynne-Davies, R.: Genetic and other factors in the etiology of scoliosis, Ph.D. Thesis, University of Edinburgh.

Wynne-Davies, R.: Infantile idiopathic scoliosis: causative factors, particularly in the first six months of life, J. Bone Joint Surg. **57-B**:138, 1975.

Young, R., and Thomassen, E.H.: Step-by-step procedure by applying halo ring, Orthop. Rev. **3**:62, June 1974.

Zielke, K.: Ventral derotation spondylodesis: preliminary report on 58 cases, Beitr. Orthop. Traumatol. **25**:85, 1978.

Zielke, K.: Derotation spondylodese vorlaufiger ergebnisbericht uder 26 operierte falle, Arch Orthop. Unfallchir. **83**:257, 1976.

Zielke, K.: Ventrale Derotationsspondylodese, Behandlungsergenbnisse bei idiopathischen Lumbalskoliosen, Z. Orthop. **120**:320, 1982.

Zuege, R.C., Blount, W.P., and Dicus, W.T.: Indications for operative treatment of spinal deformities, Wisc. Med. J. **74**:S33, 1975.

Zwerling, M.T., and Riggins, R.S.: Use of the halo apparatus in acute injuries of the cervical spine, Surg. Gynecol. Obstet. **138**:189, 1974.

CHAPTER 72

Kyphosis and spondylolisthesis

Allen S. Edmonson

KYPHOSIS

Scheuermann first noted wedging of vertebral bodies in kyphosis, which is also called Scheuermann's juvenile kyphosis. In 1964 Sorenson suggested that the diagnosis be made if the three central vertebrae are wedged 5 degrees or more. This common disorder is thought to occur in approximately 10% of the population.

Although its true cause remains unknown, there are many theories. Present investigation is centered on endocrine abnormalities, hereditary characteristics, malnutrition, osteoporosis, and mechanical factors. Bradford and Moe investigated the gross and histologic changes in two patients and found that the anterior longitudinal ligament was thickened and bowstrung across the apex of the kyphos. It seemed that disc material had been pushed out anteriorly under this ligament, the bodies had become severely compressed, and the disc space was narrowed. Histologic examination and electron microscopy showed normal bone, cartilage, and discs. The ring apophyses showed no definite avascular necrosis. Protrusion of disc material into the bony spongiosa of the vertebral body was noted. Since Scheuermann's kyphosis is seen in a high percentage of patients with Turner's syndrome and in those with cystic fibrosis, and since these conditions are associated with osteoporosis, it is conceivable that an episode of juvenile osteopenia may be the preliminary event in this disorder.

A normal spine viewed laterally shows a continuous smooth arc from the sacrum to the cervical area when the patient bends forward. However, the kyphotic patient will show a hump or angulation in the middle or lower thoracic area. Tight hamstrings and pectoral muscles are commonly seen in this disorder. Roentgenographic evaluation uses a 2 m standing lateral film taken with the patient's arms horizonal. Vertebral wedging is sought as well as Schmorl's nodules and irregular end plates. A mild scoliotic curve is seen in 30% of these patients. Moe et al. consider a thoracic kyphosis greater than 40 degrees in the growing child to be abnormal.

Lower back and neck pain may result from hyperlordosis in these segments in later years. The deformity can also be psychologically quite important to the patient.

Treatment in adolescents has used serial casts, but in 1965 Moe reported the Milwaukee brace to be of greater benefit. Bradford et al. later studied 194 patients with kyphosis and vertebral body wedging and 29 patients with kyphosis but no wedging deformities. It was found that with kyphosis greater than 35 degrees and with at least one vertebra wedged more than 5 degrees, correction was obtained within 6 to 12 months. The curve correction improved 40% overall, with the wedging improving 41% and the lordosis 36%. If a kyphosis exceeds 65 degrees and the wedging of vertebral bodies is greater than 10 degrees, and if the patient is near or past maturity, the results are much poorer. It is therefore recommended that patients with a kyphosis that is supple and without wedging be placed on exercises and observed. If the kyphosis angle increases or if wedging of vertebral bodies appears, then a Milwaukee brace is indicated. Those patients with vertebral body wedging when first examined must be braced immediately. Surgery should rarely be necessary with this approach. Surgery is reserved for a severe deformity after completion of growth, for severe pain in the kyphotic area that has been unresponsive to long-term rehabilitative efforts, and for those patients with neurologic signs or symptoms. Posterior spinal fusion with Harrington compression assemblies and bone grafting will usually be effective in curves of less than 65 degrees.

Surgical treatment

Bradford et al. reported 22 patients with Scheuermann's kyphosis who underwent posterior Harrington compression instrumentation and fusion. Loss of correction occurred in 16 of these patients; these failures were caused by the presence of severe initial deformity, inadequate length of the fusion, severe wedging of the vertebral bodies, and probably a contracted anterior longitudinal ligament. Taylor et al. also reported posterior Harrington instrumentation and fusion in adolescents. They aimed for less correction than Bradford et al., but generally were working with more flexible spines. Their indications were: (1) relatively severe round-back deformities, (2) immature patients with significant deformities who refused bracing, and (3) skeletally mature patients with significant residual deformity.

Of the 27 patients they reported, severe, persistent back pain was present in four. Preoperative skeletal traction was not recommended in contrast to Bradford's report of posterior instrumentation alone in which some type of traction was used on all of the patients. Taylor et al. modified the insertion of the most superior pair of compression hooks, hooking them over the laminae to prevent their dislodging. In their relatively short 6-month follow-up some improvement in the wedging of the apical vertebrae was noted in some of the less mature patients. They were satisfied with less correction than Bradford et al., but had significantly fewer complications.

In a later report Bradford et al. reported on 24 patients with an average age of 21 years who underwent combined anterior and posterior fusion for kyphosis caused by Scheuermann's disease or round-back deformity. Their indications for combined anterior and posterior fusion include a kyphosis of more than 70 degrees in a patient who is skeletally mature and who has pain that cannot be controlled by conservative means. They also consider as good surgical candidates patients who are physiologically immature but in whom the kyphosis has not been controlled by a brace, as well as patients with early spastic paraparesis caused by a rounded kyphosis. This recommendation does not include patients with neurologic changes secondary to a sharply angular kyphotic component or localized anterior cord compression. Although it is not recommended routinely for cosmesis because of the magnitude of the surgery involved, this is a reasonable indication for operation. Preoperative traction does not appear to be beneficial and is not recommended in this later report. Bradford et al., as well as Taylor et al., reported loss of correction when the posterior fusion and instrumentation were not extended to the lowermost and uppermost vertebrae of the kyphosis. The end vertebra at each end should be the last vertebra from the apex that is tilted maximally into the concavity of the curve. We have made it a practice to add at least one vertebra above and one vertebra below this recommendation. Anteriorly the fusion should include the most rigid apical segment of the curve as identified by comparison of the standing lateral roentgenogram with a supine hyperextension roentgenogram. This usually involves six or seven apical vertebrae that can be conveniently exposed through a single thoracotomy incision with removal of a single rib. Using a combined anterior and posterior approach, Bradford et al. were able to obtain over 50% correction.

TECHNIQUE OF ANTERIOR AND POSTERIOR FUSION. Through an anterior approach excise the entire disc and cartilaginous end plate, leaving only the posterior portion of the anulus and the posterior longitudinal ligament (Fig. 72-1). Do not remove the bony end plate. Loosen or mobilize each joint using a Blount or lamina spreader and then pack each joint temporarily, preferably with Gelfoam or Surgicel to minimize blood loss. When all the desired joints have been cleared, remove the packing as each joint is grafted with short transverse segments of rib or other bone. Autogenous iliac bone or preferably bone strips from the exposed vertebral bodies may be added if the single rib is not sufficient. About 2 weeks later perform the posterior fusion, placing the top No. 1259 hooks as high as T2 or T3 and

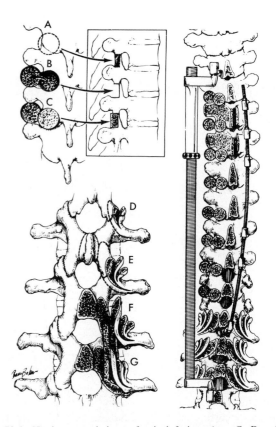

Fig. 72-1. Harrington technique of spinal fusion. *A* to *C,* Doweling method of obliterating concave facets. *D* to *F,* Steps in decortication in lateral gutter fusion. *G,* Note cancellous bone supplement. (From Harrington, P.R., and Dickson, J.H.: Clin. Orthop. **93:**113, 1973.)

engaging the transverse processes, and the lower three hooks engaging the caudal aspect of the appropriate laminae (Fig. 72-2). Use autogenous cancellous bone to supplement the fusion.

Use external immobilization by an underarm Risser cast or a molded plastic jacket for 9 to 12 months or until the fusion is solid.

Congenital kyphosis

In a study of 130 patients, Winter, Moe, and Wang classified congenital kyphosis in three types. In type I vertebral bodies are absent; in type II a failure of vertebral body segmentation is present; and in type III both of these conditions exist (Fig. 72-3). The histories of these patients revealed an average progression of 7 degrees per year. Treatment with a Milwaukee brace has proved to be ineffective, and correction is difficult and perhaps dangerous to obtain. It is recommended that progression be halted by a posterior fusion in patients less than 3 years old. Exploration 6 months after surgery with the addition of more bone grafts is also recommended to develop a large posterior fusion. A spine with a kyphosis of 50 degrees or less of types I and II can be treated by a posterior fusion alone, and type III deformities occasionally require both anterior and posterior fusions. An anterior osteotomy is necessary if correction is sought (Fig. 72-4). In the study of Winter et al. the pseudarthrosis rate was as high as 50% after posterior fusion alone, but it dropped significantly af-

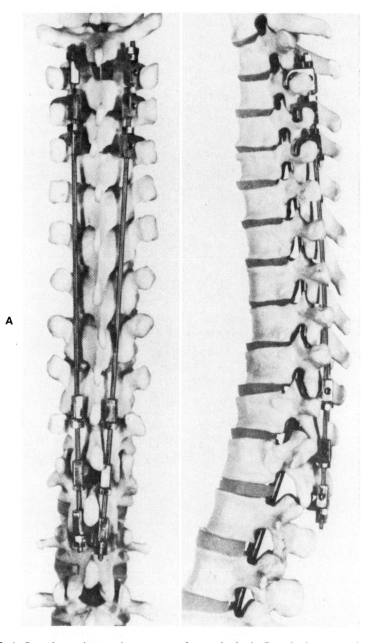

Fig. 72-2. A, Second stage in operative treatment of severe kyphosis. Posterior instrumentation and fusion.

Continued.

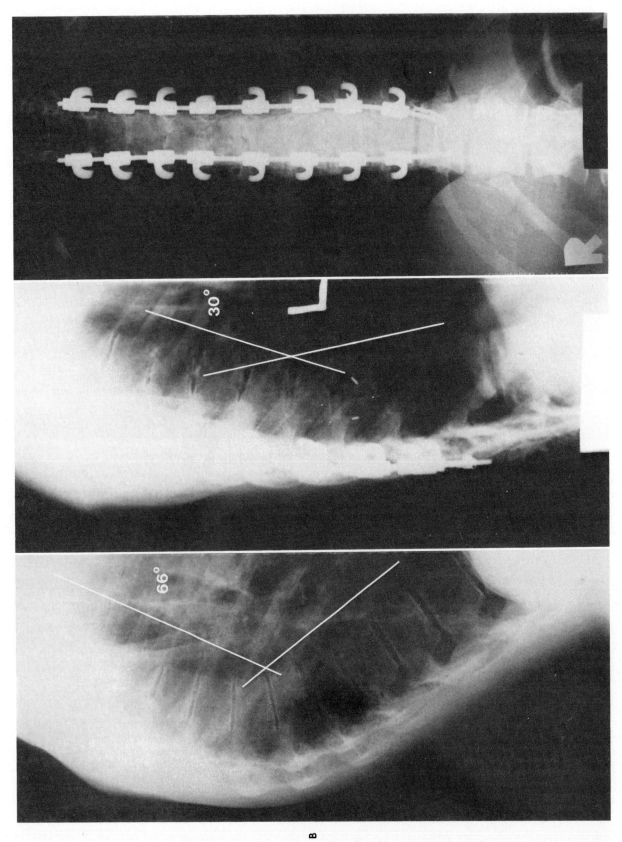

Fig. 72-2, cont'd. B, Woman at 24 years of age before and after anterior discectomy and (**A** from Bradford, D.S., et al.: J. Bone Joint Surg. **57-A**:439, 1975.)

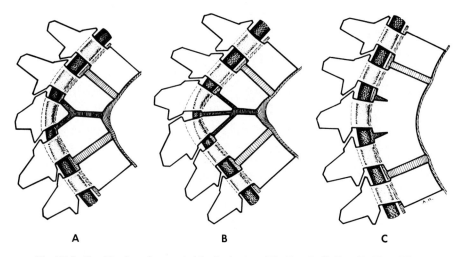

Fig. 72-3. Classification of congenital kyphosis. **A** and **B,** Type I. **C,** Type II. (Type III not shown.) (See text.) (From Winter, R.B., Moe, J.H., and Wang, J.F.: J. Bone Joint Surg. **55-A:**223, 1973.)

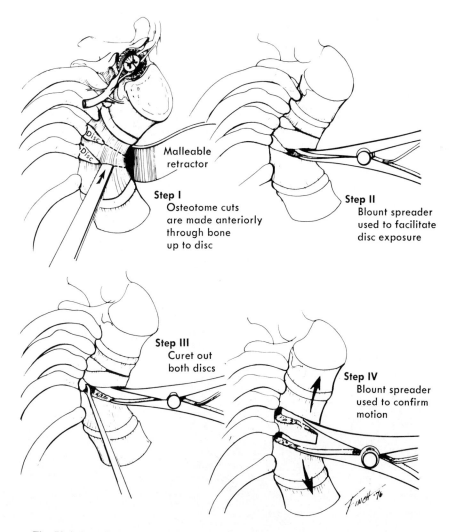

Fig. 72-4. Steps in anterior osteotomy for severe congenital kyphosis. (From Moe, J.H., et al.: Scoliosis and other spinal deformities, Philadelphia, 1978, W.B. Saunders Co.)

ter combined anterior and posterior fusions. Except in quite flexible curves, halo-femoral traction carries a high risk of causing paraplegia, since the spinal cord is stretched tightly over the rigid kyphotic deformity.

Somewhat later, Winter, Moe, and Lonstein reviewed 77 patients operated on for congenital kyphosis with an average age of 5 years and an average kyphosis of 75 degrees. Approximately two thirds had combined anterior and posterior fusions and one third had posterior fusion alone. Combined anterior and posterior fusions produced better correction and better maintenance of correction than posterior fusion alone. They offer the following recommendations.

Posterior arthrodesis alone is adequate for congenital anterior failure of segementation when no correction is needed and for an adolescent or younger patient with mild deformity (less than 55 degrees).

A combination of anterior and posterior arthrodesis is best in all other surgery for congenital kyphosis. Skeletal traction is not recommended for correction because of the risk of neurologic damage. Intraoperative improvement in the deformity was safest in this regard.

Montgomery and Hall, after studying 34 patients treated surgically, made similar recommendations: (1) early posterior fusion for type I lesions and (2) anterior decompression and fusion followed by a staged posterior fusion for curves over 60 degrees and an accompanying neurologic

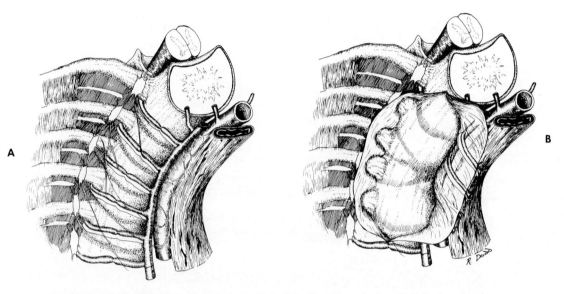

Fig. 72-5. Technique for anterior osteotomy. **A,** Anterolateral exposure of spine. **B,** Reflection of periosteum and anulus fibrosus as single flap. (From Winter, R.B., Moe, J.H., and Wang, J.F.: J. Bone Joint Surg. **55-A:**223, 1973.)

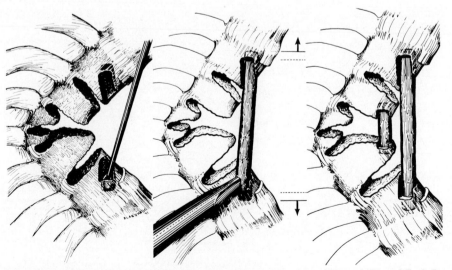

Fig. 72-6. Technique of inserting grafts (see text). (From Winter, R.B., Moe, J.H., and Wang, J.F.: J. Bone Joint Surg. **55-A:**223, 1973.)

deficit. After anterior decompression they used skeletal traction with apparent safety.

Lonstein et al. reviewed 42 patients with kyphosis and neurologic deficits. Except for a few flexible (and noncongenital) kyphoses, anterior decompression and fusion followed by a staged posterior fusion gave the best results. An extensive treatment plan is outlined by them.

For anterior strut grafting of kyphosis, Bradford has reported using a segment of an adjacent rib as a vascularized graft by rotating it on its intact intercostal blood supply. With the vascularized graft, fracture of the strut should be less common and union more rapid than with ordinary strut grafts.

TECHNIQUE (WINTER ET AL.). Expose the spine through an anterior approach appropriate for the vertebral level sought. Ligate the segmental vessels and expose the spine by subperiosteal stripping (Fig. 72-5, *A* and *B*). Divide the thickened anterior longitudinal ligament at one or more levels. Divide one or more vertebral bodies at the foraminal level using gouges first and, progressing posteriorly, curets. Take great care as the area of the posterior longitudinal ligament is reached, for the ligament may be absent. If it is present, resect it to see the dura. Widen this exposure superiorly, inferiorly, and laterally, removing all anteriorly compressing bone. A Blount spreader aids exposure. Once the osteotomy and decompression are complete, insert strut grafts, slotting them into bodies above and below the area of decompression. Hollow out the cancellous bone of each body with a curet. Using rib, fibula, tibia, or iliac crest grafts of sufficient length, insert the upper end in the slot first. Now apply manual pressure from posteriorly against the kyphos and use an impactor to tap the lower end of the graft in place (Fig. 72-6). Place additional grafts in the disc space defects and close the pleura over them if possible.

SPONDYLOLISTHESIS

Spondylolisthesis is generally defined as an anterior or posterior slipping or displacement of one vertebra on another. A unilateral or bilateral defect of the pars interarticularis without displacement of the vertebra is known as spondylolysis or, less frequently, spondyloschisis.

Wiltse, Newman, and Macnab have developed the following classification of spondylolisthesis and spondylolysis:

1. Dysplastic—in this type congenital abnormalities of the upper sacrum or the arch of L5 permit the slipping to occur.
2. Isthmic—the lesion is in the pars interarticularis. Three types can be recognized.
   a. Lytic—fatigue fracture of the pars interarticularis.
   b. Elongated but intact pars interarticularis.
   c. Acute fracture of the pars interarticularis.
3. Degenerative—this lesion results from intersegmental instability of long duration.
4. Traumatic—this type results from fractures in other areas of the bony hook than in pars interarticularis.
5. Pathologic—generalized or localized bone disease is present.

This classification is based on the cause of the defect as descsribed by other authors.

Isthmic spondylolisthesis is characterized by bilateral defects in the pars interarticularis of a vertebra and the resultant anterior displacement of the body of this vertebra and the superincumbent spine on the vertebra below. Only this type of spondylolisthesis is discussed in this chapter. Most frequently the fifth lumbar vertebra is displaced on the sacrum. Rarely a similar anomaly involves the fourth lumbar vertebra and even more rarely other lumbar vertebrae. The cause of the defects is unknown. Repeated minor injuries, a single severe injury, and a stress fracture associated with assuming the upright position in early childhood have all been suggested. Farfan et al. have shown three mechanisms that may result in failure of the neural arch with or without displacement: flexion overload, unbalanced shear forces, and forced rotation. That the defects sometimes tend to occur in families, that they have not been reported in the neonatal period, that they are rarely seen in children under 5 years of age, and that their incidence increases until the late teens seem to indicate a hereditary predisposition to a developmental dysplasia of the vertebrae. The incidence of spondylolisthesis in the general population is about 5% and seems to be about equal in women and men.

Normally the inferior articular facets of the fifth lumbar vertebra prevent the body of this vertebra from being displaced anteriorly on the sacrum. But in isthmic spondylolisthesis the bilateral defects in the pars interarticularis make the neural arch a loose fragment, cause a loss in osseous continuity between the inferior articular facets and the body of the fifth lumbar vertebra, and allow the body of the vertebra to gradually become displaced anteriorly. Gill, Manning, and White have consistently found at the defects fibrocartilaginous masses that they believe cause pressure on the nerve roots. These masses have been found by some surgeons, but their existence is denied by others. Spina bifida occulta is present in about 20% of patients with spondylolisthesis. Standing roentgenograms in spondylolisthesis have been advised by Lowe et al. Twenty-six percent of their group of 50 patients showed increased displacement on standing. Therefore an apparent spondylolysis in recumbent roentgenograms may be revealed as a spondylolisthesis in standing roentgenograms.

The defect in the pars interarticularis may be unilateral or bilateral. When it is bilateral, the fifth lumbar vertebra may or may not become displaced anteriorly; when it is unilateral, it is displaced little if any. In the absence of displacement the presence of the defect or defects is often difficult to demonstrate, and to do so oblique roentgenograms of the lumbosacral area are necessary. Spondylolisthesis, however, is usually easy to see in lateral roentgenograms.

Spondylolisthesis has been classified into grades I, II, III, or IV, depending on the severity of the displacement of the vertebra on the vertebra below. In grade I the displacement is 25% or less of the anteroposterior diameter of the vertebra below; in grade II, between 25% and 50%; in grade III, between 50% and 75%; in grade IV, greater than 75%.

Boxall et al. in 1979 and later Wiltse and Winter have

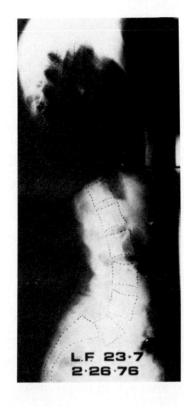

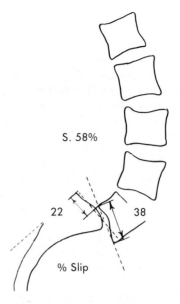

S. 58%

22   38

% Slip

Fig. 72–7. Percentage of slipping calculated by measuring distance from line parallel to posterior portion of first sacral vertebral body to line parallel to posterior portion of body of fifth lumbar vertebra; anteroposterior dimension of fifth lumbar vertebra inferiorly is used to calculate percentage of slipping. (From Boxall, D., et al.: J. Bone Joint Surg. **61-A:**479, 1979.)

Anterior displacement

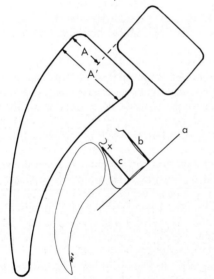

Fig. 72–8. Extent of anterior displacement or slip is expressed as percentage obtained by dividing *A,* amount of displacement (determined by relationship of posterior part of cortex of fifth lumbar vertebra to posterior part of cortex of first sacral vertebra), by *A₁,* maximum anteroposterior diameter of first sacral vertebra, and multiplying by 100. Smaller drawing shows how to determine posteroinferior tip of body of fifth lumbar vertebra, which is often indistinct. Line *a* is drawn parallel to front of body of fifth lumbar vertebra. Line *b* is drawn perpendicular to line *a,* to posterosuperior tip of body of fifth lumbar vertebra. Line *c* is drawn parallel to line *b* and is exactly same length. Point at which line *c* intersects inferior border of body of fifth lumbar vertebra is point *x,* relative constant used in measuring percentage of slip. (From Wiltse, L.L., and Winter, R.B.: J. Bone Joint Surg. **65-A:**768, 1983.)

preferred standard measurement and terminology to describe the anterior displacement of the lumbar vertebra as a percentage of the widest anteroposterior diameter of the body below, usually the first sacral (Fig. 72-7). Wiltse and Winter prefer the term *sagittal rotation* to express the angular relationship of the sacrum and the fifth lumbar vertebra (Fig. 72-8). Boxall et al. earlier used the term *slip angle* to describe the same relationship but measured it differently (Fig. 72-9). Both terms have been subsequently used.

Children may have either the dysplastic or isthmic type of spondylolisthesis. The former is secondary to congenital defects at the lumbosacral joint, and the latter usually results from a fatigue fracture combined with a hereditary element.

Spondylolisthesis in children is characteristically different from that in adults. Periodic follow-up during the patient's growth is necessary to search for further slipping. If severe slipping occurs (75% to 100%), compensatory mechanisms of pelvic flexion with hyperlordosis of the spine above results in a kyphotic deformity at L5 and S1. This abnormal anatomy produces the peculiar gait because of tight hamstrings as described by Phalen and Dickson. Laurent and Einola reported an increase in displacement in 23 of 52 children and adolescents. According to them, displacement is usually slight before the age of 10 years, and progression of displacement is most common between the ages of 10 and 15 years. During adulthood an increase in displacement is rare.

Further slippage will occur in more than 50% of those

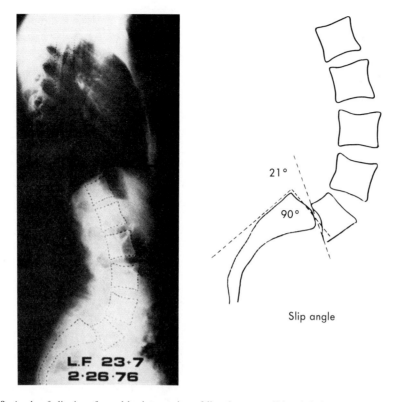

Fig. 72–9. Angle of slipping, formed by intersection of line drawn parallel to inferior aspect of fifth lumbar vertebral body and line drawn perpendicular to posterior aspect of body of first sacral vertebra. (From Boxall, D., et al.: J. Bone Joint Surg. **61-A:**479, 1979.)

with a trapezoid-shaped L5 and a dome-shaped upper sacrum. Therefore those patients with the dysplastic type are more likely to need surgical stabilization. When slippage exceeds 25% and the child is symptomatic, or with slippage of 50% or more in the growing child regardless of symptoms, fusion should be performed. A bilateral lateral fusion from L4 to the sacrum is best for slippages exceeding 50%.

Reduction of severe spondylolisthesis has gained increasing attention since the publications of Jenkins in 1936 and Harris in 1951. Later Harrington proposed open reduction with instrumentation. The technique of Scaglietti et al. of closed reduction and casting by traction and hyperextension allows the abnormal anatomy to accommodate the changes during 4 months before fusion is performed. The danger of producing a neurologic deficit is ever present, and thus we agree with Wiltse that reduction of a spondylolisthesis must accomplish two objectives to justify the added danger and effort: (1) extension of the flat buttocks to improve cosmesis and (2) lengthening of the torso. Most patients will do well with an in situ fusion.

In spondylolysis symptoms are often absent, and the defects are then discovered only incidentally on roentgenograms made for other purposes. In spondylolisthesis injury may aggravate any symptoms, but rarely does a single injury cause symptoms in a patient who previously had none. Usually symptoms begin insidiously during the second or third decade as an intermittent dull ache in the lower back, present with increasing frequency during walking and standing. Later, pain may develop in the but-

tocks and thighs, and still later unilateral sciatica may develop. Unilateral sciatica accompanied by sensory or motor disturbances may be caused by protrusion of an intervertebral disc, most often the one between L4 and L5. In explorations of the lumbar spine in 45 patients with spondylolisthesis, Laurent found a protruded disc in only 2 (about 4%). Henderson, however, in a review of 216 patients operated on for spondylolisthesis, reported that of 157 in whom the nerve roots were explored, a definitely abnormal intervertebral disc was found in 46 (about 29%). According to Gill, Manning, and White, the L5 and S1 nerve roots are compressed by or attached by adhesions to the fibrocartilaginous mass at the defects in the pars interarticulares, and consequently movement of the loose laminae may irritate them.

Lumbosacral spondylolisthesis associated with scoliosis presents special problems. When it is associated with a major thoracic curve, there are two treatments with separate indications: the spondylolisthesis should be fused on the basis of symptom severity, and the thoracic curve should be treated as required by its severity. When the spondylolisthesis is associated with a thoracolumbar or lumbar curve, the lumbosacral joint must be fused in a corrected position.

Treatment

Surgery is not always necessary in spondylolisthesis. Often restriction of the patient's activities, spinal and abdominal muscular rehabilitation, and other conservative measures, including the intermittent use of a rigid back brace, are sufficient. In general the younger the patient with painful spondylolisthesis, the more definite is the indication for surgery and the more likely is surgery to be successful. Persistent pain in the lower back, buttocks, and thighs without sciatica is often sufficient to incapacitate a laborer for heavy work or a homemaker for chores and thus to be an indication for surgery. For sedentary workers, on the other hand, sciatica is more often the reason for surgery because any less severe pain in the lower back and buttocks may not be disabling. For adolescents severe

hamstring tightness is often an indication for fusion; for them progression of displacement is another indication for surgery. In general about 20% of patients with symptomatic spondylolisthesis require surgery.

FUSION

Opinions vary as to the proper operation in spondylolisthesis. Fixation of the unstable spine by posterolateral fusion is the treatment that most surgeons prefer. A successful fusion in situ usually relieves symptoms enough to

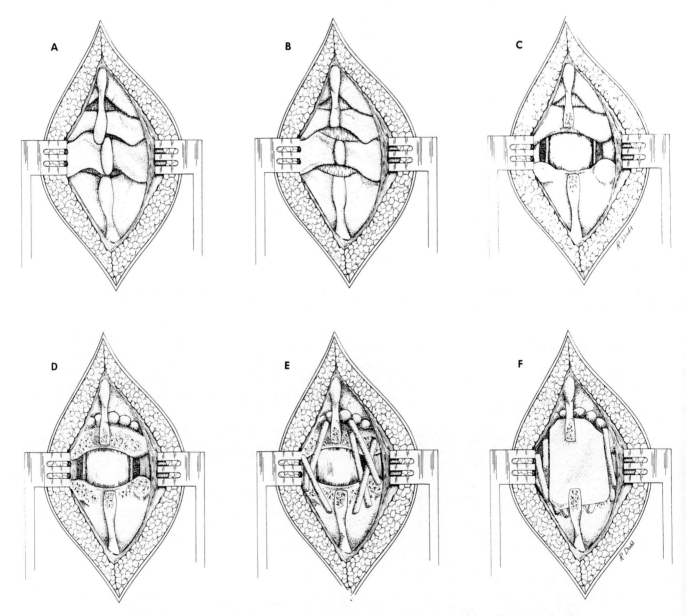

Fig. 72-10. Bosworth posterior fusion for spondylolisthesis using H graft after excision of loose neural arch. **A,** Spinous processes and laminae have been exposed. Note that deviated loose neural arch of L5 underlies and supports spinous process of L4 and maintains stability. **B,** Spinous processes of L4 and S1 have been squared to form abutments for graft. **C,** Loose neural arch has been excised. **D,** Laminae of L4 and S1 and stubs of pedicles of L4 have been roughened. **E,** Cancellous strip and chip grafts have been placed on roughened laminae and pedicles. **F,** With lumbar spine flexed, H graft has been inserted and locked in place. (From Bosworth, D.M.: In American Academy of Orthopaedic Surgeons: Instructional course lectures, vol. 9, Ann Arbor, 1952, J.W. Edwards.)

allow the patient to work. Posterior rather than anterior fusion is preferred by most because its technique is more flexible; it permits exploration of the defects, nerve roots, and intervertebral discs. In addition it is relatively safe. Spinal fusion should not be undertaken lightly, however, because it is more difficult to perform in spondylolisthesis than in other conditions. The fusion mass should extend as far proximally and distally as necessary to stabilize the affected vertebrae and interspaces. In the absence of sciatica and with an absolutely normal L4 disc and joint, fusion between L5 and S1 is sufficient but is rarely done. However, when the neural arch of L5 has been excised or when both the fourth and fifth interspaces have been explored to relieve sciatica, the fusion should extend from L4 to S1. In most instances it should extend over this longer area, that is, from L4 to S1. Details of technique vary with the preference of the surgeon. Several techniques for spinal fusion are described in this chapter and in Chapter 70. When symptoms of pressure on nerve roots are present, the fifth lumbar and first sacral roots should be inspected, and any protruding intervertebral discs and all fibrocartilaginous tissue about them should be excised before posterior fusion is performed, for otherwise radiating pain may persist even after the fusion becomes solid. The pedicle may require excision if the nerve root angulates acutely around it. When symptoms of nerve root compression are absent, posterior fusion with or without excising the loose neural arch of L5 is reasonable.

Bosworth successfully used posterior fusion with an H graft and with resection of the loose neural arch (Fig 72-10). Fusion rate was 85% initially and 90% after pseudarthrosis repair.

Several surgeons have reported successful interbody fusion through either an anterior or a posterior approach in spondylolisthesis. The anterior technique of Freebody et al. has been highly successful in their hands, but we have had no experience with it (Fig. 70-18, *B*). When the fifth lumbar vertebra is so severely displaced on the sacrum that the fifth interspace cannot be exposed and curetted, Kellogg Speed's technique of anterior fusion (p. 3249), in which a graft is inserted through the fifth lumbar vertebra and into the sacrum, has been recommended. Recently modifications of this technique in combination with posterior arthrodesis, instrumentation, or both have been used by spine surgeons such as DeWald et al., Bradford et al. and others.

Posterolateral fusion using the technique of Watkins (p. 3158) or a modification of it, with or without excision of the loose neural arch of L5, is now often used in spondylolisthesis. Rombold reported successful fusion in 96% of 73 patients treated by posterolateral fusion and resection of the arch. A high rate of successful fusion by the posterolateral technique has also been reported by Watkins, Wiltse, and others. Macnab and Dall in their study of the blood supply of the lumbar spine as applied to intertransverse fusion showed a lower pseudarthrosis rate than with other methods in a group with degenerative disc disease. They think that the intertransverse technique has special value in the treatment of spondylolisthesis, since it is easily limited to one segment and that it is the technique of choice for stabilization after extensive posterior decompression and foraminotomy. According to them, there are three reasons for a lower incidence of pseudarthrosis: (1) the graft bed includes the lateral aspects of the superior articular facets, the pars interarticularis, and the transverse process as a continuous raw bony surface (Fig. 72-11); (2) the zygoapophyseal joints are included in the fusion mass; and (3) because the graft extends to the transverse process of the most superior vertebra, this vertebral segment is more firmly incorporated in the fusion mass than with the standard posterior technique, in which the graft extends only to the spinous process and laminae of the most superior vertebra (Fig. 72-12). Kiviluoto et al. in Helsinki reported solid fusion in 78 of 80 adolescents and adults after posterolateral arthrodesis; Dawson, Lotysch, and Urist in Los Angeles reported 92% successful fusion, and Bocca-

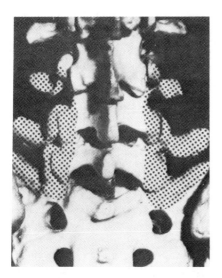

Fig. 72-11. Intertransverse fusion for spondylolisthesis. *Stippled area* indicates bed prepared for grafting. (From Macnab, I., and Dall, D.: J. Bone Joint Surg. **53-B:**628, 1971.)

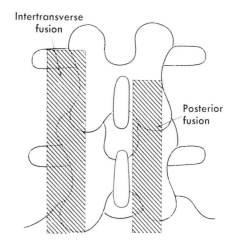

Fig. 72-12. Comparison of beds prepared for intertransverse and posterior fusions. (From Macnab, I., and Dall, D.: J. Bone Joint Surg. **53-B:**628, 1971.)

nera et al. in Bologna found that posterolateral fusion produced a high percentage of success with low risk.

In 1955, Gill, Manning, and White recommended that both the loose neural arch and the dense fibrocartilaginous tissue at the defects in the pars interarticulares be excised to free the fifth lumbar and first sacral nerve roots and to thus relieve pain without spinal fusion. They pointed out that on motion of the spine, especially extension, the proximal border of the loose neural arch might tilt anteriorly and press on the fifth lumbar roots or by this tilting stretch the first sacral roots. In 14 patients who before surgery had back pain, radiating pain, and positive neurologic signs and who had been followed after surgery from 16 to 56 months, only three had occasional mild back pain. The neurologic findings had completely disappeared in all but two, and all patients had been able to return to their former occupations. This treatment was supported in 1957 by the experience of King, Baker, and McHolick; they reported that of 29 patients in whom only the loose neural arch had been excised, the nerve roots had been explored, and fusion had not been performed, only three had any significant recurrence of pain. In 1962 Gill and White reported further results of the operation they had recommended in 1955; they followed 43 patients aged 14 to 57 years for 4 months to about 12 years (average about 5 years). Although some increase in anterior displacement occurred in 19, they rated the result as excellent (the patient asymptomatic) in 18, good in 12, and fair in 7; or to put it another way, in a total of 37 or 86.1% they considered the result satisfactory and in 13.9% a failure. They state that any increase in displacement after surgery is self-limiting, does not necessarily cause symptoms, and in their experience is not related to excision of the loose neural arch. A Gill procedure without fusion should not be performed in children with spondylolisthesis. Further slipping following the procedure has been observed by us and other investigators.

Wiltse and Hutchinson have outlined the following reasonable policy for the surgical treatment of spondylolisthesis:

1. For most patients with backache and little if any leg pain, a bilateral posterolateral fusion from L4 to S1 is performed; only when there are signs of nerve root compression is the loose neural arch of L5 excised.
2. For young adults with little if any leg pain, with minimal displacement of L5, and with large transverse processes of L5, a bilateral posterolateral fusion from L5 to S1 is performed through two incisions (p. 3158).
3. For young adults with signs of nerve root compression, with minimal anterior displacement of L5, and with large transverse processes of L5, the loose neural arch is excised and a bilateral posterolateral fusion from L5 to the sacrum is performed through a midline incision.
4. For patients with failure of previous posterior fusion, an anterior fusion through a left extraperitoneal approach is performed.
5. For patients over 60 years of age with good stability of the L5 vertebral body but with signs and symptoms of nerve root compression, the loose neural

arch is excised, care being taken to avoid traumatizing the nerve roots; fusion is omitted.

Thus opinions differ as to whether spinal fusion is necessary or whether simply excising the loose neural arch and any protruded intervertebral discs and freeing of the nerve roots are sufficient. Although we have treated a few patients surgically without arthrodesing the spine, we still believe that spinal fusion is indicated after any exploration of the nerve roots in spondylolisthesis.

According to Newman, degenerative spondylolisthesis produces the symptoms of stenosis of either the canal or the lateral recesses. Surgical management involves decompression of the appropriate roots by laminectomy. Foraminotomy may also be necessary, but extensive excision of the neural arch may result in further spinal instability, in which case the addition of a spinal fusion would be advisable. Cauchoix et al. reported immediate postoperative relief in 25 of 26 patients after this technique. Follow-up (average 3¼ years) showed 22 still leading a normal life. Four patients developed a secondary slip.

CHILDREN AND ADOLESCENTS

Posterolateral and posterior fusion in situ for spondylolisthesis in children and adolescents is recommended by many surgeons including Sherman, Rosenthal, and Hall, and Stanton, Meehan, and Lovell. Pain, other symptoms, and slipping of 50% or greater are consistent indicators for surgical treatment. Stanton et al. recommend bed rest and a pantaloon cast to prevent further slipping postoperatively, but they are in the minority; in contrast, Sherman et al. stated that additional slipping was not related to postoperative ambulation.

Verbiest of the Netherlands described an extensive anterior fusion including a strut-graft after a posterior laminectomy and foraminotomy without reduction in adolescents with 100% slips. As in all reports of in situ fusion, neurologic complications are rare, and this is stressed.

Sevastikoglou, Spangfort, and Aaro from Stockholm reported 9 patients on whom an extraperitoneal anterior interbody fusion was done also without reduction. Solid fusion and relief of symptoms were obtained in all.

Reduction of 75% to over 100% slips have been reported in relatively small numbers by several surgeons using both skeletal traction and several types of posterior instrumentation. Most techniques include an anterior interbody fusion and frequently also a posterolateral fusion. Bradford has used halo-femoral traction in bed for reduction followed by a first-stage Gill procedure and decompression with posterolateral fusion (Fig. 72-13, *A*). Through an anterior transperitoneal approach an interbody fusion with a strut graft or with iliac wedge grafts is performed as a second stage (Fig. 72-13, *B*). Because of the neurologic risk, Bradford recommends that posterior decompression be done first and the spine extended only after full length has been obtained. McPhee and O'Brien of England reported success with basically the same approach.

Reduction of spondylolisthesis has been attempted by numerous modifications of Harrington posterior distraction instrumentation. Keneda et al. of Japan used short distraction rods with posterior decompresson and posterolateral fusion. They reported no neurologic deficits from instrumentation, which is unusual, but most of their patients had less than 50% slips with an average of 26%. DeWald et al. for 50% to over 100% slips perform a posterolateral fusion and Harrington distraction reduction. A second stage consists of an anterior interbody lumbosacral fusion with two wedge-shaped iliac crest grafts.

Ohki et al. of Japan and Balderston and Bradford of Minneapolis have used posterior traction wires through the spinous processes to attach to tightening devices (on a cast or a halo-pelvic traction apparatus) to pull the lower lumbar vertebrae into place before fusion.

Sijbrandij of the Netherlands has reduced five severe slips with posterior devices using screws inserted into the lumbar vertebrae to pull them into a reduced position.

Attempts at reduction of severe slips carry a risk of neurologic deficit whether employing traction or instrumentation. Only skillful and experienced spinal surgeons should attempt procedures of this magnitude in medical centers equipped for maximum support.

POSTERIOR LUMBAR INTERBODY FUSION

A posterior lumbar interbody fusion method was devised by Cloward in 1943 and has been used extensively by him and others for treatment of spondylolisthesis. It is best suited for displacements of grades I and II and generally unsuited for displacements of grade III or higher unless reduction is accomplished by posterior Harrington or similar instrumentation as advocated by Vidal et al. in France. Bohlman and Cook of Cleveland and Takeda of Japan combine the posterior interbody fusion with other posterior fusion techniques: Bohlman and Cook, a posterolateral fusion, and Takeda, a Bosworth H-graft fusion. Retraction of nerve roots and the dural sac is necessary to insert the grafts, and cauda equina deficits are reported (Cloward reported 4% incidence of foot drop), although they usually are not permanent.

ANTERIOR LUMBAR INTERBODY FUSION

TECHNIQUE (KELLOGG SPEED). Make a midline incision from the umbilicis to the pubis and fully expose the sacral promontory. Then raise the foot of the table and pack the intestines out of the way. Palpate the relations of the fifth lumbar vertera with the sacrum and confirm the roentgenographic findings. If the bifurcation of the aorta is low, retract it with the left common iliac vein. Just to the right of the midline and avoiding the midsacral nerve and artery and the sympathetic ganglia, incise the peritoneum from the fourth lumbar interspace to the sacrum. Then determine the proper angle and depth for a drill to be inserted to pass obliquely through the body of the fifth lumbar vertebra and into the sacrum; with the patient supine the direction is almost perpendicular to the floor. Then pass a large drill through the fifth lumbar vertebra and into the sacrum; as the drill passes from the body of the fifth lumbar vertebra and into the intervertebral space, advancing the drill is easier until the body of the sacrum is reached,

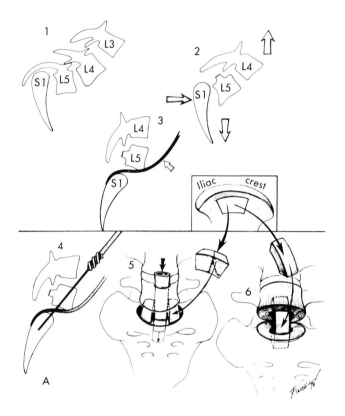

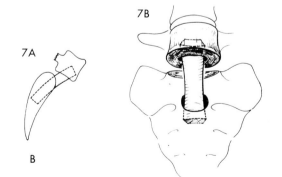

Fig. 72–13. Steps in technique of reduction of spondylolisthesis by combined posterior and anterior approach. (From Bradford, D.S.: Spine **4:**423, 1979.)

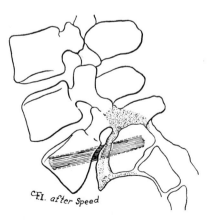

Fig. 72-14. Kellogg Speed anterior fusion for spondylolisthesis. (Redrawn from Speed, K.: Arch. Surg. **37:**715, 1938.)

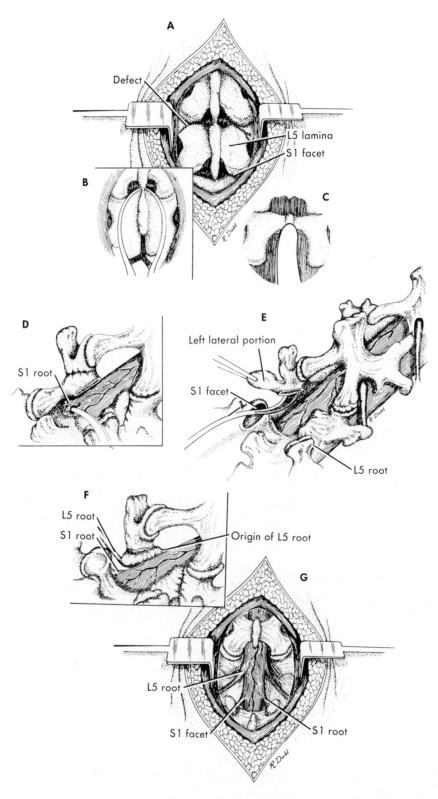

Fig. 72-15. Operation of Gill, Manning, and White for spondylolisthesis (see text). (From Gill, G.G., Manning, J.G., and White, H.L.: J. Bone Joint Surg. **37-A**:493, 1955.)

when it becomes more difficult. Then from the tibia take a cortical graft and insert it into the hole, transfixing the fifth lumbar vertebra to the sacrum (Fig. 72-14).

AFTERTREATMENT. The patient is placed on a moderately firm bed that permits nursing care without flexing the spine. At 8 weeks a rigid back brace is fitted, and the patient is allowed up.

GILL PROCEDURE

TECHNIQUE (GILL ET AL). Place the patient prone on the operating table and through a midline incision expose subperiosteally the spinous processes of the fourth and fifth lumbar and the first sacral vertebrae (Fig. 72-15, *A*). Demonstrate the mobility of the fifth lumbar neural arch and with a rongeur resect the spinous processes of all three vertebrae (Fig. 72-15, *B*). Now also with a rongeur resect the middle part of the loose fifth lumbar neural arch (Fig. 72-15, *C*). Then bite away the inferior aspect of the laminae of the fourth lumbar vertebra until the ligamentum flavum has been freed. By sharp dissection excise the ligamentum flavum from between the fourth and fifth vertebrae. Then again by sharp dissection excise on one side the lateral part of the loose fifth lumbar arch, freeing it from its articulation with the sacrum and from the tissues in the defect in the pars interarticularis (Fig. 72-15, *E*); dissect close to bone to avoid damaging the fifth lumbar nerve root. Next retract this root superiorly and medially. Carefully dissect it from the fibrocartilaginous tissue and free it laterally until it passes through the intervertebral foramen (Fig. 72-15, *F* and *G*). Resect bone from the pedicle as necessary to free the root. Then examine the exposed fourth and fifth lumbar discs and if indicated excise one or both. Now carry out the same procedure on the opposite side.

AFTERTREATMENT. No support is necessary at any time after surgery. The patient is encourged to move about in bed as desired and to sit as soon as he is able. At 3 days walking is allowed and straight leg raising exercises are begun. If by the fifth day straight leg raising is restricted to less than 75 degrees, a solution of 0.2% procaine or 0.2% lidocaine is injected extradurally through the caudal foramen. The exercises are then continued.

REFERENCES
Kyphosis

Bjekreim, I., Magnaes, B., and Semb, G.: Surgical treatment of severe angular kyphosis, Acta Orthop. Scand. **53:**913, 1982.

Bradford, D.S.: Anterior vascular pedicle bone grafting for the treatment of kyposis, Spine **5:**318, 1980.

Bradford, D.S., Ahmed, K.B., Moe, J.H., Winter, R.B., and Lonstein, J.E.: The surgical management of patients with Scheuermann's disease: a review of twenty-four cases managed by combined anterior and posterior spine fusion, J. Bone Joint Surg. **62-A:**705, 1980.

Bradford, D.S., et al.: Anterior strut-grafting for the treatment of kyphosis: review of experience with forty-eight patients, J. Bone Joint Surg. **64-A:**680, 1982.

Bradford, D.S., Moe, J.H., Montalvo, F.J., and Winter, R.B.: Scheuermann's kyphosis and roundback deformity: results of Milwaukee brace treatment, J. Bone Joint Surg. **56-A:**740, 1974.

Bradford, D.S., and Moe, J.H.: Scheuermann's juvenile kyphosis: a histologic study, Clin. Orthop. **110:**45, 1975.

Bradford D.S., Moe, J.H., Montalvo, F.J., and Winter, R.B.: Scheuermann's kyphosis: results of surgical treatment by posterior spine arthrodesis in 22 patients, J. Bone Joint Surg. **57-A:**439, 1975.

Cloward, R.B.: Treatment of ruptured intervertebral discs by vertebral body fusion: indications, operative technique and aftercare, J. Neurosurg. **10:**154, 1953.

DeWald, R.L., et al.: Severe lumbosacral spondylolisthesis in adolescents and children: reduction and staged circumferential fusion, J. Bone Joint Surg. **63-A:**619, 1981.

Fountain, S.S., Hsu, L.C.S., Yau, A.C.M.C., and Hodgson, A.R.: Progressive kyphosis following solid anterior spine fusion in children with tuberculosis of the spine: a long-term study, J. Bone Joint Surg. **57-A:**1104, 1975.

Freebody, D., Bendall, R., and Taylor, R.D.: Anterior transperitoneal lumbar fusion, J. Bone Joint Surg. **53-B:**617, 1971.

Herndon, W.A., Emans, J.B., Micheli, L.J., and Hall, J.E.: Combined anterior and posterior fusion for Scheuermann's kyphosis, Spine **6:**125, 1981.

Lonstein, J.E., et al.: Neurologic deficits secondary to spinal deformity: a review of the literature and report of 43 cases, Spine **5:**331, 1980

Moe, J.H.: Treatment of adolescent kyphosis by nonoperative and operative methods, Manitoba Med. Rev. **45:**481, 1965.

Moe, J.H., Winter, R.B., Bradford, D.S., and Lonstein, J.E.: Scoliosis and other spinal deformities, Philadelphia, 1978, W.B. Saunders Co.

Montgomery, S.P., and Hall, J.E.: Congenital kyphosis, Spine **7:**360, 1982.

Ohtani, K., Nakai, S., Fujimura, Y., Manzoku, S., and Shibasaki, K.: Anterior surgical decompresson of thoracic myelopathy as a result of ossification of the posterior longitudinal ligament, Clin. Orthop. **166:**82, 1982.

Ryan, M.D., and Taylor, T.K.F.: Acute spinal cord compression in Scheuermann's disease, J. Bone Joint Surg. **64-B:**409, 1982.

Scheuerman, H.: Kyphosis dorsalis juvenile, Ztschr. Orthop. Chir. **41:**305, 1921.

Sorenson, K.H.: Scheuermann's juvenile kyphosis, Copenhagen, 1964, Munksgaard.

Swischuk, L.E.: The beaked, notched, or hooked vertebra: its significance in infants and young children, Radiology **95:**661, 1970.

Taylor, T.C., Wenger, D.R., Stephen, J., Gillespie, R., and Bobechko, W.P.: Surgical management of thoracic kyphosis in adolescents, J. Bone Joint Surg. **61-A:**496, 1979.

Winter, R.B., Lovell, W.W., and Moe, J.H.: Excessive thoracic lordosis and loss of pulmonary function in patients with idiopathic scoliosis, J. Bone Joint Surg. **57-A:**972, 1975.

Winter, R.B., Moe, J.H., and Lonstein, J.E.: The surgical treatment of congenital kyphosis: a review of 94 patients age 5 years or older with 2 years or more follow-up in 77 patients, Spine **10:**224, 1985.

Winter, R.B., Moe, J.H., and Wang, J.F.: Congenital kyphosis: its natural history and treatment as observed in a study of one hundred and thirty patients, J. Bone Joint Surg. **55-A:**223, 1973.

Winter, R.B., and Swayze, C.: Severe neurofibromatosis kyphoscoliosis in a Jehovah's Witness: anterior and posterior spine fusion without blood transfusion, Spine **8:**39, 1983.

Spondylolisthesis

Balderston, R.A., and Bradford, D.S.: Technique for achievement and maintenance of reduction for severe spondylolisthesis using spinous process traction wiring and external fixaton of the pelvis, Spine **10:**376, 1985.

Barash, H.L., Galante, J.O., Lambert, C.N., and Ray, R.D.: Spondylolisthesis and tight hamstrings, J. Bone Joint Surg. **52-A:**1319, 1970.

Barr, J.S.: Spondylolisthesis (editorial), J. Bone Joint Surg. **37-A:**878, 1955.

Beeler, J.W.: Further evidence on the acquired nature of spondylolysis and spondylolisthesis, Am. J. Roentgenol Radium Ther. Nucl. Med. **108:**796, 1970.

Blackburne, J.S., and Velikas, E.P.: Spondylolisthesis in children and adolescents, J. Bone Joint Surg. **59-B:**490, 1977.

Boccanera, L.: Pellicioni, S., Laus, M., and Lelli, A.: Surgical treatment of isthmic spondylolisthesis in adults (review of 44 cases with long term control), Ital. J. Orthop. Traumatol. **8:**271, 1982.

Bohlman, H.H., and Cook, S.S.: One-stage decompression and posterolateral and interbody fusion for lumbosacral spondyloptosis through a posterior approach: report of two cases, J. Bone Joint Surg. **64-A:**415, 1982.

Bosworth, D.M.: Technique of spinal fusion in the lumbosacral region by the double clothespin graft (distraction graft; H graft) and results. In American Academy of Orthopaedic Surgeons: Instructional course lectures, vol. 9, Ann Arbor, 1952, J.W. Edwards.

Bosworth, D.M., Fielding J.W., Demarest, L., and Bonaquist, M.: Spondylolisthesis: a critical review of a consecutive series of cases treated by arthrodesis, J. Bone Joint Surg. **37-A**:767, 1955.

Boxall, D., Bradford, D.S., Winter, R.B., and Moe, J.H.: Management of severe spondylolisthesis in children and adolescents, J. Bone Joint Surg. **61-A**:479, 1979.

Bradford, D.S.: Treatment of severe spondylolisthesis: a combined approach for reduction and stabilization, Spine **4**:423, 1979.

Burns, B.H.: Two cases of spondylolisthesis, Proc. R. Soc. Med. **25**:571, 1932.

Capener, N.: Spondylolisthesis, Br. J. Surg. **19**:374, 1932.

Cauchoix, J., Benoist, M., and Chassaing, V.: Degenerative spondylolisthesis, Clin. Orthop. **115**:122, 1976.

Chandler, F.A.: Lesions of the "isthmus" (pars interarticularis) of the laminae of the lower lumbar vertebrae and their relation to spondylolisthesis, Surg. Gynecol. Obstet. **53**:273, 1931.

Cloward, R.B.: Spondylolisthesis: treatment by laminectomy and posterior interbody fusion: review of 100 cases, Clin. Orthop. **154**:74, 1981.

Davis, I.S., and Bailey, R.W.: Spondylolisthesis: long term follow-up study of treatment with total laminectomy, Clin. Orthop. **88**:46 1972.

Davis, I.S., and Bailey, R.W.: Spondylolisthesis: indications for lumbar nerve root decompression and operative technique, Clin. Orthop. **117**:129, 1976.

Dawson, E.G., Lotysch, M., III, and Urist, M.R.: Intertransverse process lumbar arthrodesis with autogenous bone graft, Clin. Orthop. **154**:90, 1981.

DeWald, R.L., Faut, M.M., Taddonio, R.F., and Neuwirth, M.G.: Severe lumbosacral spondylolisthesis in adolescents and children: reduction and staged circumferential fusion, J. Bone Joint Surg. **63-A**:619, 1981.

Farfan, H.F., Osteria, V., and Lamy, C.: The mechanical etiology of spondylolysis and spondylolisthesis, Clin. Orthop. **117**:40, 1976.

Fitzgerald, J.A.W., and Newman, P.H.: Degenerative spondylolisthesis, J. Bone Joint Surg. **58-B**:184, 1976.

Gill, G.G.: Treatment of spondylolisthesis and spina bifida, Exhibit, American Academy of Orthopaedic Surgeons Meeting, Chicago, January 1952.

Gill, G.G., Manning, J.G., and White, H.L.: Surgical treatment of spondylolisthesis without spine fusion, J. Bone Joint Surg. **37-A**:493, 1955.

Gill, G.G., and White, H.L.: Surgical treatment of spondylolisthesis without spine fusion: a long term follow-up of operated cases, presented at the Western Orthopaedic Association, San Francisco, November 1962.

Goldstein, L.A., et al.: Guidelines for the management of lumbosacral spondylolisthesis associated with scolosis, Clin. Orthop. **117**:135, 1976.

Hammond, G., Wise, R.E., and Haggart, G.E.: Review of seventy-three cases of spondylolisthesis treated by arthrodesis, JAMA **163**:175, 1957.

Harrington, P.R., and Dickson, J.H.: Spinal instrumentation in the treatment of severe progressive spondylolisthesis. Clin. Orthop. **117**:157, 1976.

Harrington, P.R., and Tullos, H.S.: Spondylolisthesis in children: observations and surgical treatment, Clin. Orthop. **79**:75, 1971.

Harris, R.I.: Spondylolisthesis. In Essays in surgery (presented to Dr. W.E. Gallie), Toronto, 1950, University of Toronto Press.

Harris, R.I.: Spondylolisthesis, Ann. R. Coll. Surg. Engl. **8**:259, 1951.

Henderson, E.D.: Results of the surgical treatment of spondylolisthesis, J. Bone Joint Surg. **48-A**:619, 1966.

Howorth, B.: Low backache and sciatica: results of surgical treatment: Part III. Surgical treatment of spondylolisthesis, J. Bone Joint Surg. **46-A**:1515, 1964.

Jenkins, J.A.: Spondylolisthesis, Br. J. Surg. **24**:80, 1936.

Johnson, J.R., and Kirwan, E.O'G.: The long-term results of fusion in situ for severe spondylolisthesis, J. Bone Joint Surg. **65-B**:43, 1983.

Kaneda, K., Satoh, S., Nohara, Y., and Oguma, T.: Distraction rod instrumentation with posterolateral fusion in isthmic spondylolisthesis: 53 cases followed for 18-89 months, Spine **10**:383, 1985.

King, A.B., Baker, D.R., and McHolick, W.J.: Another approach to the treatment of spondylolisthesis and spondyloschisis, Clin. Orthop. **10**:257, 1957.

Kiviluoto, O., Santavirta, S., Salenius, P., Morri, P., and Pylkkanen, P.: Postero-lateral spine fusion. a 1-4 year follow-up of 80 consecutive patients, Acta Orthop. Scand. **56**:152, 1985.

Laurent, L.E.: Spondylolisthesis: a study of 53 cases treated by spine fusion and 32 cases treated by laminectomy, Acta Orthop. Scand. **35**: Suppl., 1958.

Laurent, L.E., and Einola, S.: Spondylolisthesis in children and adolescents, Acta Orthop. Scand. **31**:45, 1961.

Laurent, L.E., and Österman, K.: Operative treatment of spondylolisthesis in young patients, Clin. Orthop. **117**:85, 1976.

Lowe, R.W., et al.: Standing roentgenograms in spondylolisthesis, Clin. Orthop. **117**:80, 1976.

Macnab, I., and Dall, D.: The blood supply of the lumbar spine and its application to the technique of intertransverse lumbar fusion, J. Bone Joint Surg. **53-B**:628, 1971.

Marmor, L., and Bechtol, C.O.: Spondylolisthesis: complete slip following the Gill procedure: a case report, J. Bone Joint Surg. **43-A**:1068, 1961.

McPhee, I.B., and O'Brien, J.P.: Reduction of severe spondylolisthesis: a preliminary report, Spine **4**:430, 1979.

Mercer, W.: Spondylolisthesis: with a description of a new method of operative treatment and notes of ten cases, Edinburgh Med. J. **43**:545, 1936.

Meyerding, H.W.: Low backache and sciatic pain associated with spondylolisthesis and protruded intervertebral disc: incidence, significance and treatment (symposium), J. Bone Joint Surg. **23**:461, 1941.

Nachemson, A.: Repair of the spondylolisthetic defect and intertransverse fusion for young patients, Clin. Orthop. **117**:101, 1976.

Newman, P.H.: Stenosis of the lumbar spine in spondylolisthesis, Clin. Orthop. **115**:116, 1976.

Newman, P.H.: Surgical treatment for spondylolisthesis in the adult, Clin. Orthop. **117**:106, 1976.

Newman, P.H., and Stone, K.H.:The etiology of spondylolisthesis, J. Bone Joint Surg. **45-A**:39, 1963.

Ohki, I., Inoue, S., Murata, T., Mikanagi, K., and Shibuya, K.: Reduction and fusion of severe spondylolisthesis using halo-pelvic traction with a wire reduction device, Inter. Orthop. (SICOT) **4**:107, 1980.

Österman, K., Lindholm, T.S., and Laurent, L.E.: Late results of removal of the loose posterior element (Gill's operation) in the treatment of lytic lumbar spondylolisthesis, Clin. Orthop. **117**:121, 1976.

Phalen, G.S., and Dickson, J.A.: Spondylolisthesis and tight hamstrings, J. Bone Joint Surg. **43-A**:505, 1961.

Rombold, C.: Treatment of spondylolisthesis by posterolateral fusion, resection of the pars interarticularis, and prompt mobilization of the patient: an end-result study of seventy-three patients, J. Bone Joint Surg. **48-A**:1282, 1966.

Scaglietti, O., Frontino, G., and Bartolozzi, P.: Technique of anatomical reduction of lumbar spondylolisthesis and its surgical stabilization, Clin. Orthop. **117**:164, 1976.

Sevastikoglou, J.A., Spangfort, E., and Aaro, S.: Operative treatment of spondylolisthesis in children and adolescents with tight hamstrings syndrome, Clin. Orthop. **147**:192, 1980.

Sherman, F.C., Rosenthal, R.K., and Hall, J.E.: Spine fusion for spondylolysis and spondylolisthesis in children, Spine **4**:59, 1979.

Sijbrandij, S.: A new technique for the reduction and stabilisation of severe spondylolisthesis: a report of two cases, J. Bone Joint Surg. **63-B**:266, 1981.

Sijbrandij, S.: Reduction and stabilisatin of severe spondylolisthesis: a report of three cases, J. Bone Joint Surg. **65-B**:40, 1983.

Speed, K.: Spondylolisthesis: treatment by anterior bone graft, Arch. Surg. **37**:175, 1938.

Stanton, R.P., Meehan, P., and Lovell, W.W.: Surgical fusion in childhood spondylolisthesis, J. Pediatr. Orthop. **5**:411, 1985.

Taillard, W.F.: Etiology of spondylolisthesis, Clin. Orthop. **117**:30, 1976.

Takeda, M.: A newly devised "three-one" method for the surgical treatment of spondylolysis and spondylolisthesis, Clin. Orthop. **147**:228, 1980.

Todd, E.M., Jr., and Gardner, W.J.: Simple excision of the unattached lamina for spondylolysis, Surg. Gynecol. Obstet. **106**:724, 1958.

Turner, R.H., and Bianco, A.J., Jr.: Spondylolysis and spondylolisthesis in children and teen-agers, J. Bone Joint Surg. **53-A**:1298, 1971.

Velikas, E.P., and Blackburne, J.S.: Surgical treatment of spondylolisthesis in children and adolescents, J. Bone Joint Surg. **63-B**:67, 1981.

Verbiest, H.: The treatment of spondyloptosis or impending lumbar spondyloptosis accompanied by neurologic deficit and/or neurogenic intermittent claudication, Spine **4:**68, 1979.

Vidal, J., Fassio, B., Fuscayret, Ch., and Allieu, Y.: Surgical reduction of spondylolisthesis using a posterior approach, Clin. Orthop. **154:**156, 1981.

Watkins, M.B.: Posterolateral fusion in pseudarthrosis and posterior element defects of the lumbosacral spine, Clin. Orthop. **35:**80, 1964.

Wiltse, L.L.: Spondylolisthesis in children, Clin. Orthop. **21:**156, 1961.

Wiltse, L.L., Bateman, J.G., Hutchinson, R.H., and Nelson, W. E.: The paraspinal sacrospinalis-splitting approach to the lumbar spine, J. Bone Joint Surg. **50-A:**919, 1968.

Wiltse, L.L., and Hutchinson, R.H.: Surgical treatment of spondylolisthesis, Clin. Orthop. **35:**116, 1964.

Wiltse, L.L., and Jackson, D.W.: Treatment of spondylolisthesis and spondylolysis in children, Clin. Orthop. **117:**92, 1976.

Wiltse, L.L., Newman, P.H., and Macnab, I.: Classification of spondylolisis and spondylolisthesis, Clin. Orthop. **117:**23, 1976.

Wiltse, L.L., Widell, E.H., Jr., and Jackson, D.W.: Fatigue fracture: the basic lesion in isthmic spondylolisthesis, J. Bone Joint Surg. **57-A:**17, 1975.

Wiltse, L.L., and Winter, R.B.: Terminology and measurement of spondylolisthesis, J. Bone Joint Surg. **65-A:**768, 1983.

Woolsey, R.D.: The mechanism of neurological symptoms and signs in spondylolisthesis at the fifth lumbar, first sacral level, J. Neurosurg. **11:**67, 1954.

CHAPTER 73

Lower back pain and disorders of intervertebral disc

George W. Wood

Humans have been plagued by back and leg pain since the beginning of recorded history. Primitive cultures attributed it to the work of demons. The early Greeks recognized the symptoms as a disease. They prescribed rest and massage for the ailment. In the eighteenth century Cotugno (Cotunnius) attributed the pain to the sciatic nerve. Gradually, as medicine advanced as a science, the number of specific diagnoses capable of causing back and leg pain increased dramatically.

A number of physical maneuvers were devised to isolate the true problem in each patient. The most notable of these is the Lasègue sign, or straight-leg raising test, described by Forst in 1881 but attributed to Lasègue, his teacher. This test was devised to distinguish hip disease from sciatica. Although sciatica was widespread as an ailment, little was known about it because only rarely did it result in

death, allowing examination at autopsy. Virchow (1857), Kocher (1896), and Middleton and Teacher (1911) described acute traumatic ruptures of the intervertebral disc that resulted in death. The correlation between the disc rupture and sciatica was not appreciated by these examiners. Goldthwait in 1911 attributed back pain to posterior displacement of the disc. Dandy in 1929 and Alajonanine in the same year reported removal of a ''disc tumor'' or chondroma from patients suffering from sciatica.

Oil contrast myelography was serendipitously introduced when iodized poppy seed oil, injected to treat sciatica in 1922, was inadvertently injected intradurally and was noted to flow freely. Finally in 1932 Barr attributed the source of sciatica to the herniated lumbar disc. Mixter and Barr in their classic paper published in 1934 again attributed sciatica to lumbar disc herniation. They suggested surgical treatment. The acceptance of myelography for confirmation of disc disease was resisted because of toxicity of the agents used in the years that followed.

As more people were treated for herniated lumbar discs, it became obvious that surgery was not universally successful. In an attempt to identify other causes of back pain Mooney popularized facet injections, thus resurrecting an idea proposed originally in 1911 by Goldthwait. Lymon Smith in 1963 approached the problem by suggesting a radical departure in treatment—enzymatic dissolution of the disc. Finally through the anatomic dissections and clinical observations of Kirkaldy-Willis and associates, spinal aging and the development of pathologic processes associated with or complicating the process of aging have evolved as a primary theory in disc disease.

EPIDEMIOLOGY

Back pain, the ancient curse, is now appearing as a modern, international epidemic. Hult estimates that up to 80% of the population is affected by this symptom at some time in life. Impairments of the back and spine are ranked as the most frequent cause of limitation of activity in people younger than 45 years by the National Center for Health Statistics.

Although back pain as a presenting complaint may account for only 2% of the patients seen by a general practitioner, Dillane reported that in 79% of men and 89% of women the specific cause was unknown. The cost to society and the patient in the form of lost work time, compensation, and treatment is staggering. Of the billions of dollars spent annually in the United States because of back complaints, it is estimated that only about one third is spent for medical treatment; the remaining costs are for disability payments. This does not include the losses from absenteeism. Although absenteeism because of back pain varies with the type of work, it rivals the common cold in total work days lost.

Multiple factors affect the development of back pain. Frymoyer et al. note that risk factors associated with severe lower back pain include jobs requiring heavy and repetitive lifting, the use of jackhammers and machine tools, and the operation of motor vehicles. They also note that patients with severe pain were more likely to be cigarette smokers and had a greater tobacco consumption. In an earlier study Frymoyer et al. noted that patients complaining of back pain reported more episodes of anxiety and depression. They also had more stressful occupations. Women with back pain had a greater number of pregnancies than those who did not. Jackson et al. noted that adult patients with scoliosis are more likely to have back pain and that the pain persists and progresses. Finally, Svensson and Anderson have associated low back pain with cardiovascular risk factors, including calf pain on exertion, high physical activity at work, smoking, and frequent worry and tension. In another report they also associated low back pain with monotonous work and less overtime work.

GENERAL DISC AND SPINE ANATOMY

The development of the spine begins in the third week of gestation and continues until the third decade of life. Formation of the primitive streak marks the beginning of spinal development, which is followed by the formation of the notochordal process. This process induces neurectodermal, ectodermal, and mesodermal differentiation.

Somites form in the mesodermal tissue adjacent to the neural tube (neurectoderm) and notochord. They number 42 to 44 in humans. The somites begin to migrate in preparation for the formation of skeletal structures. At the same time, the portion of the somites around the notochord separate into a sclerotome with loosely packed cells cephalad and densely packed cells caudally. Each sclerotome then separates at the junction of the loose and densely packed cells. The caudal dense cells migrate to the cephalad loose cells of the next more caudal sclerotome.

The space where the sclerotome separates eventually forms the intervertebral disc. Vessels that originally were positioned between the somites are now overlying the middle of the vertebral body. As the vertebral bodies form, the notochord that is in the center degenerates. The only remaining notochordal remnant forms the nucleus pulposus. Notochordal remnants usually are not distinguishable in the adult nucleus pulposus (Fig. 73-1).

In the adult the intervertebral disc is composed of the anulus fibrosus and the nucleus pulposus. The anulus fibrosus is composed of numerous concentric rings of fibrocartilaginous tissue. Fibers in each ring cross radially, and the rings attach to each other with additional diagonal fibers. The rings are thicker anteriorly (ventrally) than posteriorly (dorsally). The nucleus pulposus, a gelatinous material, forms the center of the disc. Because of the structural imbalance of the anulus, the nucleus is slightly posterior (dorsal) in relation to the disc as a whole. The discs vary in size and shape with their position in the spine.

The nucleus pulposus is composed of a loose, nonoriented, collagen fibril framework supporting a network of cells resembling fibrocytes and chondrocytes. This entire structure is embedded in a gelatinous matrix of various glucosaminoglycans, water, and salts. This material is usually under considerable pressure and is restrained by the crucible-like anulus. Inoue demonstrated that the cartilage end plate contains no fibrillar connection with the collagen of the subchondral bone of the vertebra. This lack of interconnection between the end plate and the vertebra may render the disc biomechanically weak against horizontal shearing forces. Inoue also demonstrated that the collagen fibrils in the outer two thirds of the anulus fibrosus are firmly anchored into the vertebral bodies (Fig. 73-2).

The intervertebral disc in the adult is avascular. The cells within it are sustained by diffusion of nutrients into the disc through the porous central concavity of the vertebral end plate. Histologic studies have shown regions where the marrow spaces are in direct contact with the cartilage and that the central portion of the end plate is permeable to dye. Motion and weight bearing are believed to be helpful in maintaining this diffusion. The metabolic turnover of the disc is relatively high when its avascularity is considered but slow compared with other tissues. The glycosaminoglycan turnover in the disc is quite slow, requiring 500 days. Inoue has postulated that the degeneration of the disc may be prompted by decreased permeability of the cartilage end plate, which is normally dense.

Recent studies by Bogduk and others have demonstrated

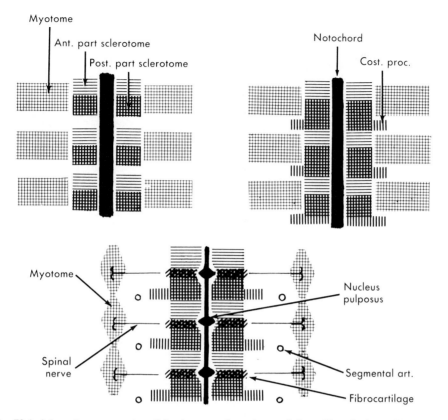

Fig. 73-1. Schematic representation of development of vertebrae and discs. (From Rothman, R.H., and Simeone, F.A.: The spine, vol. 1, Philadelphia, 1982, W.B. Saunders.)

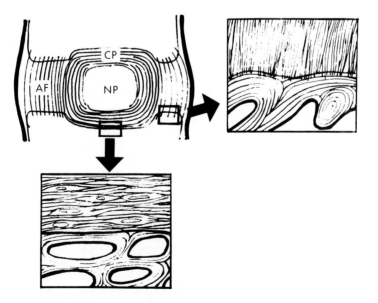

Fig. 73-2. Schematic representation of orientation of fibers in disc and end plate. *AF,* anulus fibrosus; *NP,* nucleus pulposus; *CP,* cartilaginous plate. (From Inoue, H.: Spine **6:**139, 1981.)

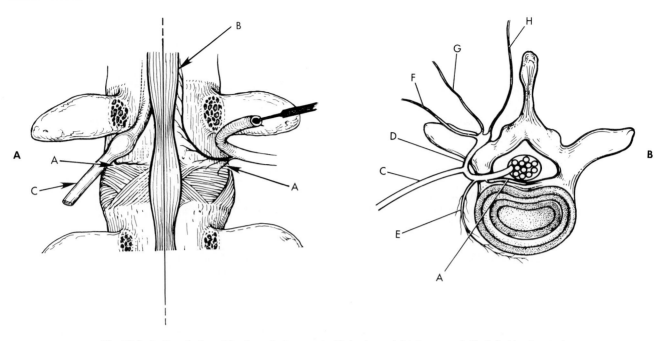

Fig. 73-3. A, Dorsal view of lumbar spinal segment with lamina and facets removed. On left side, dura and root exiting at that level remain. On right side, dura has been resected and root is elevated. Sinu-vertebral nerve, *A,* with its course and innervation of posterior longitudinal ligament, *B,* is usually obscured by nerve root, *C,* and dura. **B,** Cross sectional view of spine at level of end-plate and disc. Note that sinu-vertebral nerve, *A,* innervates dorsal surface of disc and posterior longitudinal ligament. Additional nerve branches from ventral ramus, *E,* innervate more ventral surface of disc and anterior longitudinal ligament. Dorsal ramus, *D,* arises from root immediately on leaving foramen. This ramus divides into lateral, *F,* intermediate, *G,* and medial, *H,* branches. Medial branch supplies primary innervation to facet joints dorsally.

neural fibers in the outer rings of the anulus. These fibers are branches of the sinu vertebral nerve dorsally. Ventral branches arise from the sympathetic chain that courses anterolaterally over the vertebral bodies.

Neural elements

The relational anatomy specifically with respect to the neural elements is extremely important in surgical exposure. In the *lumbar* spine each nerve root exits just below the pedicle and above the disc. This root is numbered for the vertebral body at which it exits. Each root crosses the disc above (cephalad) the vertebral body but not below (caudal) the vertebral body.

At the level of the intervertebral foramen is the dorsal root ganglion. The ganglion lies within the bony confines of the canal but near the outer confines of the foramen. Distal to the ganglion three distinct branches arise; the most prominent and important is the ventral ramus that supplies all structures ventral to the neural canal. The second branch, the sinu vertebral nerve, is a small filamentous nerve that originates from the ventral ramus and progresses medially over the posterior aspect of the disc and vertebral bodies, innervating these structures and the posterior longitudinal ligament. The third branch is the dorsal ramus. This branch courses dorsally, piercing the intertransverse ligament near the pars interarticularis. Three branches from the dorsal ramus innervate the structures dorsal to the neural canal. The lateral and intermediate branches provide

innervation to the posterior musculature and skin. The medial branch separates into three branches to innervate the facet joint at that level and the adjacent levels above and below (Fig. 73-3).

NATURAL HISTORY OF DISC DISEASE

The natural process of spinal aging has been studied by Kirkaldy-Willis and others through observation of clinical and anatomic data. A theory of spinal degeneration has been postulated that assumes that all spines degenerate and that our present methods of treatment are for symptomatic relief, not a cure.

The degenerative process has been divided into three separate stages with relatively distinct findings. The first stage is dysfunction. This stage is found in the age group between 15 and 45 years. It is characterized by circumferential and radial tears in the disc anulus and localized synovitis of the facet joints. The next stage is instability. This stage, found in 35- to 70-year-old patients, is characterized by internal disruption of the disc, progressive disc resorption, degeneration of the facet joints with capsular laxity, subluxation, and joint erosion. The final stage, present in patients older than 60 years, is stabilization. In this stage the progressive development of hypertrophic bone about the disc and facet joints leads to segmental stiffening or frank ankylosis (Table 73-1).

Each spinal segment degenerates at a different rate. As one level is in the dysfunction stage, another may be en-

Table 73-1. Spectrum of pathologic changes in facet joints and disc and the interaction of these changes

Phases of spinal degeneration	Facet joints		Pathologic result		Intervertebral disc
Dysfunction	Synovitis	→	Dysfunction	←	Circumferential tears
	Hypermobility		↓	←	
	Continuing degeneration	↗	Herniation	←	Radial tears
Instability	Capsular laxity	→	Instability	←	Internal disruption
	Subluxation	→	Lateral nerve entrapment	←	Disc resorption
Stabilization	Enlargement of articular processes	→	One level stenosis	←	Osteophytes
		↘	Multilevel spondylosis and stenosis	↙	

Modified from Kirkaldy-Willis, W.H., editor: Managing low back pain, New York, 1983, Churchill Livingstone.

tering the stabilization stage. Disc herniation in this scheme is considered a complication of disc degeneration in the dysfunction and instability stages. Spinal stenosis from degenerative arthritis in this scheme is a complication of bony overgrowth compromising neural tissue in the late instability and early stabilization stages.

Excellent long-term studies by Hakelius in 1970 and Weber in 1983 compared disc herniations on which operations were performed with those on which no surgery was done. The prognosis in disc herniation was found to be good regardless of the treatment. These studies found that patients operated on for proven disc herniations improved more rapidly during the first year than patients who had no surgery, but within 4 to 5 years the statistical difference between the groups was negligible. Neurologic recovery was noted in both the operated and unoperated patients who had neurologic deficit at the beginning of the study. Weber correlated good results with physical activity and a slightly younger age. No other variables were of statistical significance. In both studies some patients had such disabling symptoms that surgery was elected regardless of the predetermined treatment group. Acute sciatica in these studies ran a relatively short course (1 to 2 years) and was associated in most instances with neurologic recovery. Surgery provided symptomatic relief during this short course, but the long-term results were essentially the same regardless of treatment.

DIAGNOSTIC STUDIES
Roentgenograms

The simplest and most readily available diagnostic tests for back or neck pain are the anteroposterior and lateral roentgenograms of the involved spinal segment. These simple roentgenograms show a relatively high incidence of abnormal findings. Ford and Goodman reported only 7.3% normal spine roentgenograms in a group of 1614 patients evaluated for back pain. Scavone et al. reported a 46% incidence of normal or incidental findings in lumbar spine films taken over 1 year in a university hospital. Unfortunately, when these roentgenographic abnormalities are critically evaluated with respect to the patients' complaints and physical findings, the correlation is very low.

There is insignificant correlation between back pain and the roentgenographic findings of lumbar lordosis, transitional vertebra, disc space narrowing, disc vacuum sign, and claw spurs. Additionally, the entity of disc space narrowing is extremely hard to quantitate in all but the operated backs or in obviously abnormal circumstances. Frymoyer et al. in a study of 321 patients found that only when traction spurs and obvious disc space narrowing or both were present, did the incidence of severe back and leg pain, leg weakness, and numbness increase. These positive findings had no relationship to heavy lifting, vehicular exposure, or exposure to vibrating equipment. Other studies have shown some relationship between back pain and the findings of spondylolysis, spondylolisthesis, and adult scoliosis, but these findings can also be observed in the spine roentgenograms of asymptomatic patients.

Special roentgenographic views may be helpful in further defining or disproving the initial clinical roentgenographic impression. Oblique views are useful in further defining spondylolisthesis and spondylolysis but are of limited use in facet syndrome and hypertrophic arthritis of the lumbar spine. Conversely, in the cervical spine hypertrophic changes about the foramina are easily outlined. Lateral flexion and extension roentgenograms may reveal segmental instability. Unfortunately, the interpretation of these views is dependent on patient cooperation, patient positioning, and reproducible technique. Knütsen, Farfan, Kirkaldy-Willis, Stokes et al., and Macnab are excellent references on this topic. The Ferguson view (20-degree caudocephalic anteroposterior roentgenogram) has been shown by Wiltse et al. to be of value in the diagnosis of the "far out syndrome," that is, fifth root compression produced by a large transverse process of the fifth lumbar vertebra against the ala of the sacrum. Abel et al. note that angled caudal views localized to areas of concern may show evidence of facet or laminar pathology.

Myelography

Myelography of the lumbar spine and especially of the cervical spine should not be taken lightly. The recent development and popularity of computed tomography of the spine has made myelography optional or unnecessary in many instances. The value of this procedure is the ability to check all disc levels for abnormality and to define intraspinal lesions. It may be unnecessary when the clinical and computed tomographic findings are in complete agreement. The primary indications for the procedure are suspicion of an intraspinal lesion or questionable diagnosis

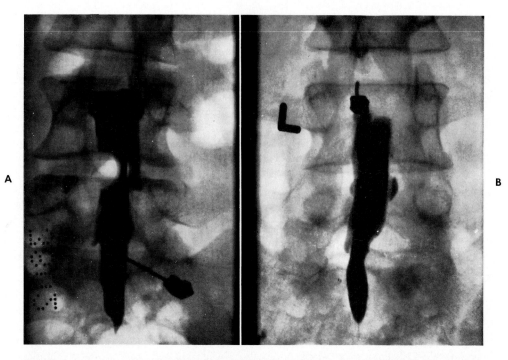

Fig. 73-4. **A,** Anteroposterior roentgenogram of iophendylate (Pantopaque) myelogram showing L-disc herniation. **B,** Oblique roentgenogram showing large L4-5 disc herniation.

resulting from conflicting clinical findings and other studies. Additionally, myelography is of value in the previously operated spine and in spinal stenosis, especially when used in conjunction with reformatted computed tomographic scans done shortly after the myelography.

Several contrast agents have been used for myelography: air, oil contrast, and water soluble (absorbable) contrast. Metrizamide (Amipaque) is now the most popular contrast agent. This is an absorbable agent that is mixed to the proper concentration for the patient and procedure just before injection. Since this agent is absorbable, the discomfort of removing it and the severity of the postmyelographic headache have been minimized.

Iophendylate (Pantopaque) was the contrast agent of choice from 1944 until the late 1970s (Fig. 73-4). This agent has a relatively low toxicity and provides excellent contrast. Unlike metrizamide, it should be removed after injection, and it does not require mixing. Because it is a more viscous material, the nerve roots are not as easily defined and its flow is more easily obstructed than is the flow of metrizamide. Iophendylate is a meningeal irritant that can cause an inflammatory response. Usually this response is mild and limited to an increase in cerebrospinal fluid white cell count but may be more severe. The usual response is headache, backache, generalized aching, and neck pain. Rarely the response is severe with transient paralysis, cauda equina syndrome, and focal neurologic defects.

Arachnoiditis is a severe complication that has been attributed on occasion to the combination of iophendylate and blood in the cerebrospinal fluid. Unfortunately, this diagnosis is usually confirmed only by repeat myelography. Attempts at surgical neurolysis have resulted in only

short-term relief and a return of symptoms in 6 to 12 months after the procedure. Fortunately, time may decrease the effects of this serious problem in some patients, but progressive paralysis has been reported in rare instances. Arachnoiditis may also be caused by tuberculosis and other types of meningitis.

Metrizamide is a water-soluble contrast medium that is rapidly becoming the standard agent for myelography (Fig. 73-5). Its advantages include absorption by the body, enhanced definition of structures, tolerance, absorption from other soft tissues, and the ability to vary the dosage for different contrasts. Like iophendylate it is a meningeal irritant, but it has not been associated with arachnoiditis. The complications of this agent include nausea, vomiting, confusion, and seizures. Rare complications include stroke, paralysis, and death. The more common complications appear to be related to patient hydration, phenothiazines, tricyclics, and migration of contrast into the cranial vault. Many of the reported complications can be prevented or minimized by using the lowest possible dose to achieve the desired degree of contrast. Adequate hydration and discontinuation of phenothiazines and tricyclic drugs before, during, and after the procedure should also minimize the incidence of the more common reactions. Likewise, maintenance of at least a 30-degree elevation of the patient's head until the contrast is absorbed should also help prevent reactions.

Iohexol (Omnipaque) is the newest nonionic contrast medium to be approved for thoracic and lumbar myelography (not cervical). The incidence of reactions to this medium is low. The most common reactions are headache (less than 20%), pain (8%), nausea (6%), and vomiting (3%). Serious reactions are very rare and include mental

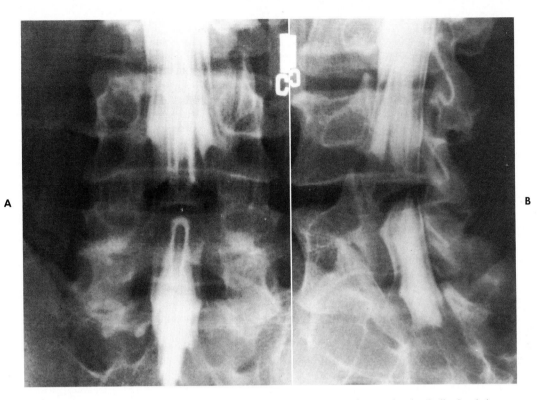

Fig. 73-5. A, Anteroposterior roentgenogram of metrizamide lumbar myelogram showing L-disc herniation. **B,** Oblique roentgenogram showing a large L4-5 disc herniation.

disturbances and aseptic meningitis (0.01%). Good hydration is essential to minimize the common reactions. The use of phenothiazine antinauseants is contraindicated when this medium is employed. Management before and after the procedure is the same as for metrizamide.

Air contrast is rarely used and should probably only be used in situations in which myelography is mandatory and the patient is extremely allergic to iodized materials. The resolution from such a procedure is poor. Recently air epidurography in conjunction with computed tomography has been suggested in patients in whom further definition between postoperative scar and recurrent disc material is required.

Myelographic technique begins with a careful explanation of the procedure to the patient before its initiation. Hydration of the patient before the procedure may minimize the postmyelographic complaints. Heavy sedation is rarely needed. Proper equipment, including a fluoroscopic unit with a spot film device, image intensification, tiltable table, and television monitoring, is useful.

TECHNIQUE. Place the patient on the fluoroscopic table in the prone position. Use of an abdominal pillow is optional. Prepare the back in the usual surgical fashion. Determine needle placement by the suspected level of pathology. Placement of the needle cephalad to L2-3 is extremely dangerous because of the chance of damage to the conus medullaris.

Infiltrate the selected area of injection with a local anesthetic. Use an 18-gauge needle for iophendylate injections and a smaller one for metrizamide injections. Midline

needle placement usually minimizes lateral nerve root irritation and epidural injection. Advance the needle with the bevel parallel to the long axis of the body. Subarachnoid placement may be enhanced by tilting the patient up to increase the intraspinal pressure and minimize the epidural space.

When the dura and arachnoid have been punctured, turn the bevel of the needle cephalad. A clear continuous flow of cerebrospinal fluid should continue with the patient in the prone position. Manometric studies may be performed at this time if desired or indicated. Remove 3 to 5 ml of cerebrospinal fluid for laboratory evaluation as indicated by the clinical suspicions. In most patients a cell count, differential white cell count, and protein analysis are performed.

Inject a test dose of the contrast material under fluoroscopic control to confirm a subarachnoid injection. If a mixed subdural-subarachnoid injection is suspected, change the needle depth; occasionally a lateral roentgenogram may be required to be sure of the proper depth. If there is good flow, inject the contrast material slowly.

Be certain of continued flow by occasionally drawing back on the syringe while injecting. If iophendylate is used, 3 to 6 ml are usually injected. The usual dose of metrizamide for lumbar myelography in an adult is 10 to 15 ml with a concentration of 170 to 190 mg/ml. Higher concentrations of water-soluble contrast are required if higher areas of the spine are to be demonstrated. Consult the package insert of the contrast used. The needle may be removed if a water-soluble contrast (metrizamide) is used.

The needle must remain in place and be covered with a sterile towel, if iophendylate is used.

Allow the contrast material to flow caudally for the best views of the lumbar roots and distal sac. Make spot films in the anteroposterior, lateral, and oblique projections. A full examination should include thoracic evaluation to about the level of T7 because lesions at the thoracic level may mimic lumbar disc disease. Take additional spot films as the contrast proceeds cranially.

If a total or cervical myelogram is desired, allow the contrast to proceed cranially. Extend the neck and head maximally to prevent or minimize intracranial migration of the contrast medium.

If iophendylate was used, then remove the contrast medium by extracting through the original needle or a multiholed stylet inserted through the original needle or by inserting another needle if extraction through the first needle is difficult. Occasionally a small amount of medium is retained, but remove as much as is physically possible.

If blood is encountered in the initial tap, abandon the procedure. It may be attempted again in several days if the patient has no symptoms related to the first tap and is well hydrated. If the proper needle position is confirmed in the anteroposterior and lateral views and cerebrospinal fluid flow is minimal or absent, suspect a neoplastic process. Then place the needle at a higher or lower level as indicated by the circumstances. If failure to obtain cerebrospinal fluid continues abandon the procedure and reevaluate the clinical picture.

The most common technical complications of myelography are significant retention of contrast medium, persistent headache from a dural leak, and epidural injection. These problems are usually minor. Persistent dural leaks are usually responsive to a blood patch. With the use of a water-soluble contrast medium, the persistent abnormalities caused by retained medium and epidural injection are eliminated.

Computed tomography

Computed tomography has revolutionized the diagnosis of spinal disease (Fig. 73-6). As with any new and revolutionary technique, the levels of technical capability vary greatly. This variation has resulted in conflicting reports as to the efficacy of computed tomographic scans in the diagnosis of disc herniations when compared with myelography and other techniques. Most clinicians now agree that computed tomography is an extremely useful diagnostic tool in the evaluation of spinal disease.

The most recent advancements in technology and computer software have resulted in the ability to reformat the standard axial cuts in almost any direction and magnify the images so that exact measurements of various structures can be made. Software is even available to evaluate the density of a selected vertebra and compare it with vertebrae of the normal population to give a numerical reproducible estimate of vertebral density to quantitate osteopenia.

Numerous types of computed tomographic studies for the spine are available. These studies vary from institution to institution and even within institutions. One must be careful in ordering the study to be certain that the areas of clinical concern are included.

Several basic routines are used in most institutions. The most common routine for lumbar disc disease is to take serial cuts through the last three lumbar intervertebral discs. If the equipment has a tilting gantry, an attempt is made to keep the axis of the cuts parallel with the disc. The problem with this is that frequently the gantry cannot tilt enough to allow a parallel beam through the lowest disc space. This technique does not allow demonstration of the canal at the pedicles. Another method is to make cuts through the discs without tilting the gantry. Once again, the entire canal is not demonstrated, and the lower cuts frequently have the lower and upper end plates of adjacent vertebrae superimposed in the same view.

The final and most complex method is to make multiple parallel cuts at equal intervals. This method allows the computer to reconstruct the images in different planes—usually sagittal and coronal. These reformatted views allow an almost three-dimensional view of the spine and most of its structures. The greatest benefit of this technique is the ability to see beyond the limits of the dural sac and root sleeves. Thus the diagnosis of foraminal encroachment by bone or disc material can now be made in the face of a normal myelogram. The proper procedure can be chosen that fits all of the pathology involved.

Optimum reformatted computed tomography should include enlarged axial and sagittal views with clear notation as to laterality and sequence of cuts. Several sections of the axial cuts should include the local soft tissue and contiguous abdominal contents. Finally, darker cuts are necessary to show bony detail with reference to the facet joints. Naturally this study should be centered on the level of greatest clinical concern. The study can be further enhanced when it is done following metrizamide myelography or with intravenous contrast medium. Enhancement techniques are especially useful when the spine being evaluated has been operated on previously.

This noninvasive, painless, outpatient procedure can supply more information about spinal disease than was previously available with a battery of invasive and noninvasive tests usually requiring hospitalization. Unfortunately, computed tomography neither demonstrates intraspinal tumors and arachnoiditis nor differentiates scar from new disc herniation. Recently Weiss et al. and Teplick et al. in separate reports have suggested that the use of intravenous contrast medium (Fig. 73-6, *E*) followed by computed tomography can improve the definition between scar and new disc herniation. Myelography is still required to demonstrate intraspinal tumors and to "run" the spine to detect occult or unsuspected lesions. New developments with low-dose metrizamide or iohexol myelography with reformatted computed tomography done as an outpatient procedure may allow a maximum of information to be obtained with a minimum of time, risk, discomfort, and cost.

Magnetic resonance imaging

Magnetic resonance imaging is the newest technologic advance in spinal imaging. This technique uses the interaction of nuclei of a selected atom with an external oscil-

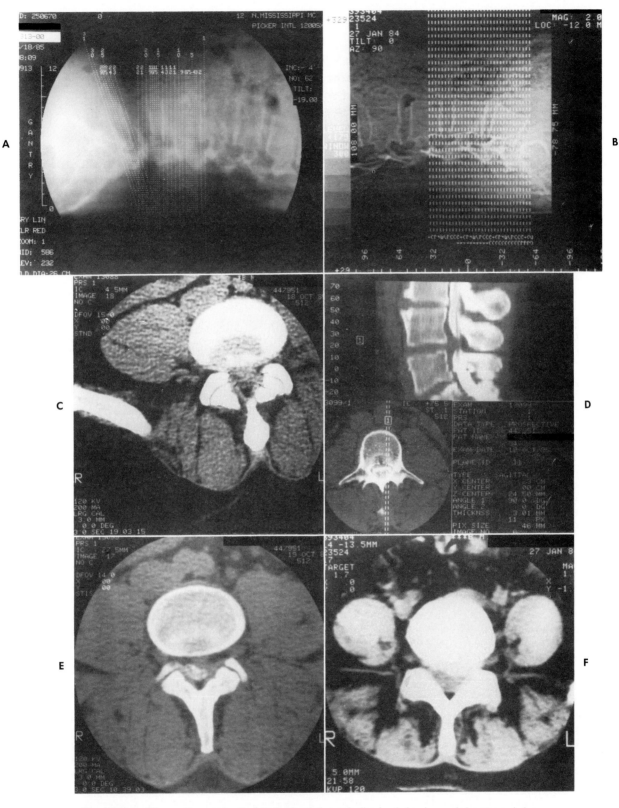

Fig. 73-6. A, CT scan "scout view" of L-disc herniation at L-disc level showing angled gantry technique. **B,** CT scan "scout view" of straight gantry technique. **C,** CT scan of L-disc herniation at L4-5 disc level showing cross sectional anatomy with gantry straight. **D,** CT scan of L4-5 disc herniation at L-disc level showing cross sectional, sagittal, and coronal anatomy using computerized reformatted technique. **E,** CT scan of L4-5 disc herniation at L-disc level showing cross sectional anatomy 2 hours after metrizamide myelography. **F,** CT scan of L-disc herniation at L4-5 disc level showing cross-sectional anatomy after intravenous injection for greater soft tissue contrast.

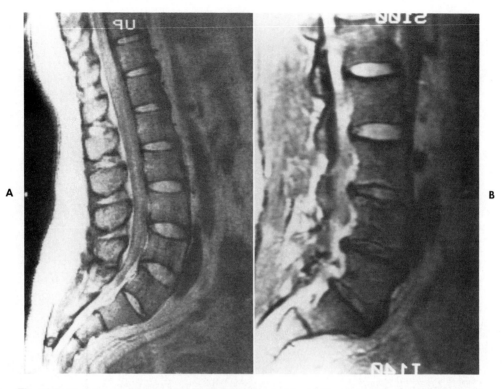

Fig. 73-7. Magnetic resonance imaging of lumbar spine. **A,** Normal T_2 weighted image. **B,** T_2 weighted image showing degenerative bulging and/or herniated discs at L3-4, L4-5, and L5-S1.

lating electromagnetic field that is changing as a function of time at a particular frequency. Energy is absorbed and subsequently released by selected nuclei at particular frequencies after irradiation with radiofrequency electromagnetic energy. This reaction is recorded and formatted by computer in a pattern similar to computed tomography. Present magnetic resonance imaging techniques concentrate on imaging the proton (hydrogen) distribution. The advantages of this technique include the ability to demonstrate intraspinal tumors, examine the entire spine, and identify degenerative discs. Unfortunately, the equipment required for this procedure is costly and requires specially constructed facilities. Currently this equipment is available in selected institutions (Fig. 73-7).

Positron emission tomography

Positron emission tomography and single-photon emission computed tomography are other similar techniques that may offer additional diagnostic information in the near future. Collier et al. and others have recently reported that single-photon emission computed tomography is more sensitive in the identification of symptomatic sites in spondylolisthesis than planar bone scintigraphy.

No test is perfect. Our present technical ability may exceed our clinical ability to identify the source of the pain. Roentgenography, computed tomography, myelography, and their combinations all may frequently show numerous areas of pathology. The question is which if any is responsible for the patient's symptoms? The incidence of lumbar disc herniation in asymptomatic patients undergoing my-

elography for other reasons is near 30%. The incidence of asymptomatic pathology in patients being studied with computed tomography is presently unknown but probably is even higher. The answer lies in a meticulous clinical evaluation and comparison with studies that one hopes will be confirmatory.

Other diagnostic tests

Numerous diagnostic tests have been used in the diagnosis of intervertebral disc disease in addition to roentgenography, myelography, and computed tomography. The primary advantage of these tests is to rule out diseases other than primary disc herniation, spinal stenosis, and spinal arthritis.

Electromyography is the most notable of these tests. One advantage of electromyography is in the identification of peripheral neuropathy and diffuse neurologic involvement indicative of higher or lower lesions. Macnab et al. report that denervation of the paraspinal muscles is found in 97% of previously operated spines as a result of the surgery.

Somatosensory evoked potentials (SSEP) are another diagnostic modality that may identify the level of root involvement. Unlike electromyography this test can only indicate a problem between the cerebral cortex and the end organs. The test cannot pinpoint the level of the lesion. This procedure is of benefit during surgery to avoid neurologic damage. Both electromyography and SSEP are dependent on the skill of the technician and interpreter.

Bone scans are another procedure in which positive

Table 73-2. Pain scale and diary

	0	No pain
	1	Mild pain that you are aware of but not bothered by
	2	Moderate pain that you can tolerate without medication
	3	Moderate pain that is discomforting and requires medication
	4-5	More severe and you begin to feel antisocial
	6	Severe pain
	7-9	Intensely severe pain
	10	Most severe pain; you might contemplate suicide over it

Activity	Comments	Location of pain	Time	Severity of pain (0 to 10)

From White, A.H.: Back school and other conservative approaches to low back pain, St. Louis, 1983, The C.V. Mosby Co.

findings usually are not indicative of intervertebral disc disease but can confirm neoplastic, traumatic, and arthritic problems in the spine. Various laboratory tests such as a complete blood count, differential white cell count, biochemical profile, urinalysis, and sedimentation rate are extremely good screening procedures for other causes of pain in the spine. Rheumatoid screening studies such as RA latex, antinuclear antibody, LE prep, and HLA-B27 are also useful when indicated by the clinical picture.

Some tests that were developed to enhance the diagnosis of intervertebral disc disease have been surpassed by the more advanced technology of reformatted computed tomography. Lumbar venography and sonographic measurement of the intervertebral canal are two examples of such technology.

INJECTION STUDIES

Whenever the diagnosis is in doubt and the complaints appear real or the pathology is diffuse, the problem is identifying the source of pain. The use of local anesthetics or contrast media in various specific anatomic areas may be useful. These techniques are relatively simple, safe, and minimally painful to the patient. Contrast media such as diatrizoate meglumine, iothalamate meglumine (Hypaque, Conray, respectively), and metrizamide have been used for discography and blocks with no reported ill effects. Recent reports of neurologic complications with contrast media used for discography and subsequent chymopapain injection are well documented. The best choice of a contrast medium for demonstrating structures outside the subarachnoid space is an absorbable medium with low reactivity if it is inadvertently injected into the subarachnoid space. Local anesthetics such as lidocaine, tetracaine, and bupivacaine (Xylocaine, Pontocaine, and Marcaine, respectively) are used frequently both epidurally and intradurally. The use of bupivacaine should be limited to low concen-

trations and low volumes because of recent reports of death following epidural anesthesia using concentrations of 0.75% or higher. Steroids prepared for intramuscular injection have also been used frequently in the epidural space with few and usually transient complications. The effect of long-acting cortisone in the intrathecal space is questionable at this time. Isotonic saline is the only other injectable medium used frequently about the spine with no reported adverse reactions.

When injection techniques are used, grading the degree of the patient's pain is helpful. This can be done by asking the patient to grade the degree of pain experienced at that moment on a 0 to 10 scale (Table 73-2). This can also be incorporated into a pain diary that is continued after the injection.

Differential spinal

The graded spinal anesthetic or differential spinal is the simplest of general screening tests for chronic, long-standing, and *constant* lower back and leg pain. The primary value of this test is to separate patients into specific clinical groups on the basis of placebo, physiologic, and nonphysiologic responses. This test appears to cover areas not touched by psychologic testing. The correlation between the abnormal responses and abnormal results on the Minnesota Multiphasic Personality Inventory is only 50%.

Our results indicate that patients who are not relieved of their pain with a full spinal anesthetic (nonphysiologic response) have not been and are not likely to be helped by spinal surgery. These patients are frequently using large doses of narcotic analgesics without relief of pain. Presently these patients are given counseling, taken off all narcotics, and encouraged to return to their previous occupations.

Patients who are relieved with a spinal anesthetic are subjected to further studies to determine the source of the pain. Patients who exhibit the placebo response are assumed to have some source for their pain, but more conservative, noninvasive treatments are used. Unfortunately, this test cannot detect the patient who is feigning pain. Such a patient may be normal in all aspects of evaluation.

The use of the differential spinal should be limited to patients with *constant,* unremitting lower back or leg pain unrelieved by usual means and with equivocal clinical and roentgenographic findings. The patient is informed that a test will be performed to see if his pain can be relieved. All narcotic pain medication, and if possible all other medication, is withdrawn for 12 hours before the procedure. No preoperative medication is given. Since this is a spinal anesthetic, we prefer that it be performed by an anesthesiologist familiar with the technique. It is suggested that the treating physician be present during the procedure to monitor the results. The patient is asked to grade his pain on a 0 to 10 scale with 0 being no pain and 10 a pain so intense that if it were to continue, suicide would be contemplated (Table 73-2). The painful areas are also delineated by the patient. An examination of the lower extremities, including straight leg raising, motor strength, deep tendon reflexes, light touch, and pin prick sensibility is performed repeatedly during the procedure.

TECHNIQUE. Position the patient with the painful side against the table (this may vary with the anesthesiologist's choice of anesthetic agent). Surgically prepare the back as for a spinal tap. Infiltrate the skin with a local anesthetic at the chosen level of entry (usually L4-5). Advance a 22-gauge spinal needle into the subarachnoid space. A good flow of cerebrospinal fluid is mandatory, and a sample should be taken for laboratory evaluation. Then ask the patient to grade his pain. Inject anesthetic agents at 10- to 15-minute intervals. Repeat patient questioning and examination before each injection. When the patient is completely relieved of his pain and the examination does not exacerbate the pain, terminate the procedure. The initial description of this procedure by Ahlgren et al. used procain hydrochloride. The reader is referred to the works of Ahlgren and others for further details of the procedure and anesthetic concentrations. We prefer to use lidocaine at concentrations of 0.5%, 1.0%, and 1.5%. The maximum dosage of lidocaine that we use is 100 mg.

Root infiltration or block

The individual areas of the spine that can produce back pain are bone, joints, nerve roots, and the outer edge of the anulus. Injection of local anesthetics into these areas for exacerbating pain has been used for some time. These procedures are invasive, mildly uncomfortable, and require some patient preparation and cooperation to get the maximum information. The simplest technique involves the instillation of 1% lidocaine into a compressed vertebral body at the time of needle biopsy. It is only slightly more complex to inject nerve roots just distal to their exit from the intervertebral foramen, individual facet joints, and the intervertebral disc.

Nerve root block or selective nerve root infiltration has been described by Macnab as a method to identify nerve root compression at the level of the intervertebral foramen.

The technique has been expanded by Tajima et al. and Krempen and Smith. The primary indications are radicular complaints or findings with inconclusive or confusing studies. This test is not of benefit in identifying patients with functional overlay. It is primarily a preoperative test to identify and confirm the area of primary pain. The test is most useful when the nerve root is entrapped laterally as in foraminal stenosis. Complete pain relief may not be obtained in simple disc herniations because more than one root may be affected.

CERVICAL NERVE ROOT INJECTION

Cervical root injection as described by Kikuchi, Macnab, and Moreau is another technique that may identify the level of symptomatic pathology. As with lumbar root injection, the nerve root is identified with the injection of contrast material, and a local anesthetic is then injected. If the patient's symptomatic pain is abolished by the injection, then that root or level is presumed to be the site of the offending pathology. Unlike the lumbar spine, cervical roots emerge from the intervertebral foramen above the level of the segment (Fig. 73-8). The roots lie anterolaterally in the costotransverse canal after they emerge from the intervertebral foramen.

The roots are covered by an epiradicular sheath peripherally. This sheath is a continuation of the epidural membrane that surrounds the dura centrally. Proper identification of the epiradicular sheath is mandatory for successful cervical root injection.

TECHNIQUE (KIKUCHI, MACNAB, MOREAU)

Anterior approach. Position the patient supine with the neck extended and rotated to the opposite side (as in cervical discography). Pull the carotid sheath laterally by the fingers, which are placed into the sulcus between the sheath and midline structures. Insert the needle, directed under image intensification control, as far as the tip of the transverse process immediately lateral to the vertebral artery. Inject a small amount of water-soluble radiopaque dye to ensure that the needle is in the epiradicular sheath. If the needle is properly positioned, the root will be outlined by the contrast material. Then inject a small amount of local anesthetic. After a short time, question the patient to determine his pain symptoms.

Lateral approach. Place the patient in the supine position with the chin pointing upwards and identify the transverse process using the fingers. Insert the needle 0.5 cm anterior to the line joining the tip of the mastoid process and the tubercle of Chassaignac, directed under image intensification control to strike the transverse process at one level above the suspected root. Then withdraw the needle and direct it caudally and medially. This avoids the inadvertent insertion of the needle into the intervertebral foramen. Inject contrast medium and anesthetic as in the anterior approach.

Posterior approach. Place the patient on his side with the affected extremity uppermost. To inject the C3, C4, C5, and C6 nerve roots insert the needle, directed under image intensification control at an angle of 45 degrees, 5 cm from the midline and advance it until it touches the transverse process. Injection of the C7 and C8 roots by this approach

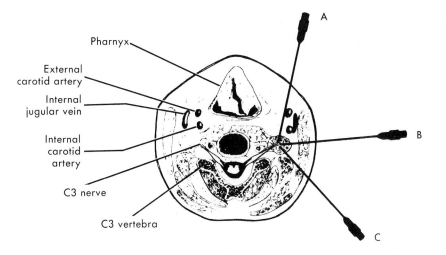

Fig. 73-8. Cross-sectional diagram of cervical spine indicating, *A,* anterior, *B,* lateral, and, *C,* posterior approaches for cervical root infiltration. (From Kikuchi, S., Macnab, I., and Moreau, P.: J. Bone Joint Surg. **63-B:**272, 1981.)

is difficult because of the thickness of the tissues at the puncture site and the size of the transverse process.

COMPLICATIONS

Potential complications of cervical root injection include puncture of a major blood vessel, penetration of the apex of the lung with resultant pneumothorax, penetration of the dura and spinal cord injury, and injury to the root with a large cutting needle. It is not uncommon to precipitate a vagal reaction with injection. The use of atropine may minimize this reaction. Kikuchi, Macnab, and Moreau used the anterior approach in all of their 75 patients. They noted no complications from this procedure. When cervical discography reproduced the symptoms of pain in this group, the symptoms were abolished by cervical root injection.

Although this series included patients with and without obvious symptomatic levels, this technique is most helpful in the identification of a painful segment in patients with refractory cervicobrachial pain with normal or equivocal studies. We have limited experience with this technique. The use of a small-bore, blunted, 45-degree needle similar to that used with cervical discography is suggested. Metrizamide and lidocaine have been the only contrast medium and anesthetic agent reported injected with this technique.

LUMBAR NERVE ROOT INFILTRATION

TECHNIQUE. The procedure is carried out with the aid of an image intensifier. Equipment with the ability to take lateral roentgenograms also is desirable. Prepare the patient by explaining the technique and asking him to gauge the level of his pain on the 0 to 10 scale with 0 being no pain and 10 being a pain so intense that its persistence might result in the contemplation of suicide. Atropine may be given before the procedure to prevent a vasovagal reaction, but no other medication is given at that time.

Place the patient on the image intensification table in the prone position. Prepare the back in the standard surgical fashion. Identify the proper level of injection by placing a needle or other metallic object at about the level of the transverse process of the involved vertebra. When the proper position is identified, anesthetize the skin with a local anesthetic agent about 3 to 4 cm from the midline or spinous process. A selection of spinal needles ranging from 10.2 to 20.3 cm (4 to 8 inches) in length in sizes from 18- to 22-gauge should be available.

Advance the needle almost perpendicularly so that it skirts the inferior edge of the transverse process near the outline of the lateral border of the vertebral body (Fig. 73-9). Slight resistance will be encountered when the needle passes through the intertransverse ligament. When the nerve is pierced, the patient will usually complain of an exacerbation or appearance of radicular pain. At this point take a lateral roentgenogram to be certain that the needle point is at the level of the intervertebral foramen.

When certain that the needle point is at the proper level, inject contrast medium if desired. Only 0.2 ml of contrast medium is needed. The nerve root sleeve should be easily outlined. If only a ball of contrast medium is seen, the needle is not in the sleeve and should be redirected. Inject 2 ml of 1% lidocaine and question the patient as to the degree of pain relief using the 0 to 10 scale. An optional method is to use a larger bolus of lidocaine and omit the contrast medium. If an 18-gauge needle is used, then a longer 22-gauge needle should be placed in it just before traversing the intertransverse ligament to avoid damage to the nerve root. We prefer to use a 22-gauge spinal needle for this technique to prevent nerve root damage.

To inject the first sacral root, place the needle through the first dorsal foramen of the sacrum on the involved side. The needle is usually placed 2 to 3 cm distal and medial to the transverse process of the fifth lumbar vertebra. The angle can vary from 90 degrees (perpendicular) to 45 degrees directed cephalad (Fig. 73-10).

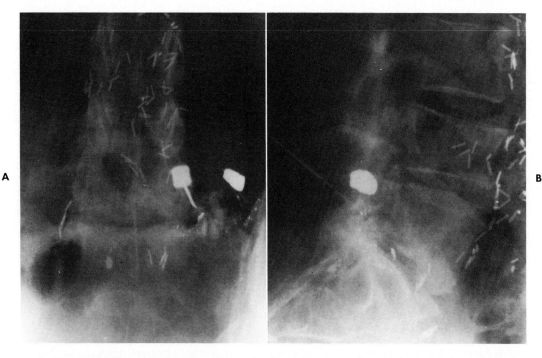

Fig. 73-9. A, Proper placement of needle about two fingerbreadths lateral to midline and inserted to level of foramen. **B,** Anteroposterior roentgenogram of L5 root injection showing metrizamide outlining root.

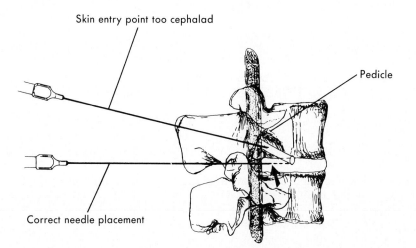

Fig. 73-10. Diagram contrasts correct needle placement with needle that entered from a point too high. (From Chung, B.U.: In Brown, J.E., and Smith, L.: Chemonucleolysis, Thorofare, N.J., 1985, Slack.)

LUMBAR FACET INJECTION

Lumbar facet injection is another simple technique that may establish a source of back and buttock pain. The term "facet syndrome" was coined in 1933 by Ghormley. Mooney reported extensively on the syndrome and added a technique for local injection of the joint as a therapeutic and diagnostic procedure. Others, most notably Shealy and Rees, have advocated operative denervation of the facet joints. Facet injection is best limited to the patient with primary lower back, buttock, or thigh pain with local point tenderness lateral to the midline and pain that is exacerbated by maneuvers that increase lumbar extension. Patients with radiculopathy should be excluded because they may have more pain after this procedure. Like any steroid injection into a joint, the degree and length of relief is variable. Most patients should be completely relieved of pain with the injection of an anesthetic, but the prolonged relief may vary from several days to months. The return of pain is usually associated with increased activity. In many patients the use of nonsteroidal antiinflammatory

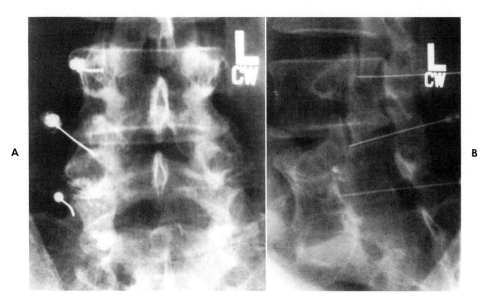

Fig. 73-11. Approximate needle position on anteroposterior, **A,** and lateral, **B,** roentgenograms of facet block. Roentgenograms also show normal facet arthrogram.

medication, a lumbar corset or brace to limit lumbar motion, and education in proper back care may be used before and after such injections to decrease the intensity of the symptoms.

Lumbar facet injection is a simple technique that can be done as an outpatient procedure. Image intensification equipment is quite helpful, but the ability to get lateral views is unnecessary. The procedure is explained to the patient, and he is asked to rate his pain on the 0 to 10 scale before initiation of the procedure. Medication before the procedure is unnecessary unless atropine is desired to prevent a vasovagal reaction.

TECHNIQUE. Place the patient prone on a radiolucent table and prepare the back in the usual sterile fashion after first determining the levels of point tenderness. Anesthetize the skin about 2 cm lateral to the midline in a linear fashion centered about the area of point tenderness. In many patients needle placement at the point of maximal tenderness will be at the level of the facet joint. It is preferable to place the needle at the inferior corner of the joint. Advance the standard 20-gauge spinal needle until the tip strikes bone.

Once proper placement in the anteroposterior plane is achieved, ask the patient to turn toward the opposite side. When the proper oblique angle to delineate the facet joint is noted by fluoroscopy, ask the patient to hold that position. Position the needle so that it appears to enter the joint (Fig. 73-11). Frequently, the patient will complain of an exacerbation of his symptoms when the capsule of the joint is entered. Occasionally in markedly arthritic joints thick, yellow synovial fluid can be aspirated. At this point inject a small amount of contrast material (0.5 ml) to verify intraarticular needle placement. Frequently two or three contiguous joints must be injected to relieve the pain. Take spot roentgenograms in the anteroposterior and oblique projections to document placement of the needles. A local anesthetic and a long-acting intramuscular steroid prepa-

ration can then be injected into and about the joint. At the completion of the procedure ask the patient to grade his pain from 0 to 10. If the patient is injected with a steroid preparation, tell him to expect some increased back soreness for the first few days. Immediate return to heavy activity is not recommended if a prolonged therapeutic response is desired.

Most patients should notice significant relief of back and buttock pain after this procedure as a result of the local anesthetic. If a patient notes increased pain after injection, primary root compression or functional overlay should be considered.

Discography

Discography has been used since the late 1940s for the experimental and clinical evaluation of disc disease in both the cervical and lumbar regions of the spine. Lindblom first described discography in 1948. Since that time, it has been used for experimental and clinical evaluation of the intervertebral disc in the cervical and lumbar spine. Discography has been and still is a technique of great controversy regarding the clinical usefulness of the data obtained.

Advocates claim that it allows the proper choice of symptomatic disc level for intervertebral fusion. Critics note the high incidence of degenerative discs in asymptomatic patients and question the reliability of pain reproduction with the technique.

It is still the most exact way to determine disc degeneration. Unfortunately, asymptomatic disc degeneration is common, and the correlation with various painful conditions about the back is hard to substantiate. In addition, the technique is not superior to myelography in the detection of disc rupture.

The application of the technique should be limited to those patients in whom conservative treatment has failed and other evaluation studies are normal or conflicting. We have found the technique of more use in identifying normal discs than pathologic ones. Kikuchi, Macnab, and Moreau warn that needle placement is critical to the accurate reproduction of pain. Needle placement in the endplate may result in pain. Therefore needle placement in the nucleus is critical before injection. Interpretation of the results on the roentgenographic finding of disc degeneration alone is not recommended. The patient response to injection is critical.

LUMBAR DISCOGRAPHY

With the advent of chemonucleolysis, lumbar discography has reemerged as a technique to confirm needle placement. The original technique described a transdural approach to the lumbar disc. This approach is *not* recommended because of the potential risk of intradural leak of neurotoxic contrast medium and other agents. We have limited the indications for this technique to those rare patients in whom the needle placement in a chemonucleolysis procedure is in doubt and to those in whom all other procedures have failed to localize the source of pain or pathology. The fear of disc degeneration initiated by this procedure has not been proven or disproven. Recently, Kahanovitz et al. found no evidence of gross histologic change in canine discs examined up to 10 weeks after injection with metrizamide, hypaque, and saline.

Lumbar discography is a simple procedure that can be done as an outpatient procedure if additional injections are not performed. The procedure is explained to the patient before its initiation. Medication is not required unless atropine is desired to prevent a vasovagal reaction. Image intensification equipment with the ability to produce anteroposterior and lateral views of the spine is necessary. A selection of spinal needles ranging from 4 to 9 inches (10 to 22.9 cm) long and 18- to 22-gauge should be available.

TECHNIQUE (FIG. 73-12). Place the patient on the image intensification table in the left lateral decubitus position with the hips and knees flexed at 45 degrees with needle placement on the right side. If the injection is to be at the L5-S1 disc, place a roll or inflatable balloon under the left iliac crest. Confirm exact anteroposterior and lateral positioning of the patient by image intensification. Prepare and drape the back in the standard surgical fashion.

Using a long radiopaque object such as a steel ruler, identify the disc levels of interest. Use a marking pen to draw a line on the back parallel with and at the level of each disc to be injected. Then make marks about 8.5 cm lateral (or a distance determined by triangulation) to the midline or spinous process bisecting the disc lines. If a plastic adhesive drape is used to cover the skin it may be advisable to remove the drape over the points of needle insertion to avoid carrying bits of drape into the disc. Infiltrate the skin with a local anesthetic at each level. Make a small stab wound with a No. 11 blade. Direct a spinal needle of at least 18-gauge and 4 inches (10 cm) long par-

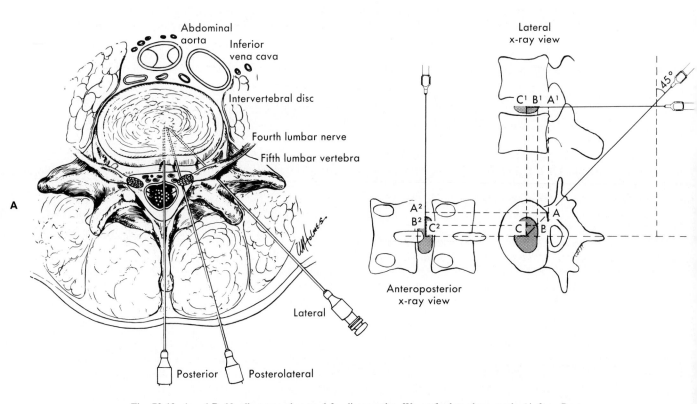

Fig. 73-12. A and **B,** Needle approaches used for discography. We prefer lateral approach. (**A** from Brown, J.E.: Lateral approach for lumbar discography and chemonucleolysis and **B** from Chung, B.U.: Bent-tip single needle technique. In Brown, J.E., Nordby, E.J., and Smith, L.: Chemonucleolysis, Thorofare, N.J., 1985, Slack.)

allel with the disc line at about 45 degrees to the back angling toward the spine. Inject additional anesthetic as the needle is advanced.

Monitor proper alignment in both anteroposterior and lateral projections as the needle is advanced. When the level of the lamina is reached, the needle should be near the outer border of the vertebral bodies and disc in the anteroposterior view and at the lamina in the lateral view. A double-needle technique is recommended. If the larger needle (usually 18 gauge) is blunted, advance the needle as far as the disc in both anteroposterior and lateral planes. Then insert the smaller needle (usually 22 gauge and at least 2 inches longer) into the larger needle and advance it into the disc.

When the needle enters the disc, a distinct change in resistance and a gritty sensation is noted. The only pain that occurs with this maneuver is the result of nerve root irritation or penetration by the needle just lateral to the disc. Aspiration of the needle should be performed if there is any question of dural penetration by the needle. If the dura is penetrated, it is probably best to abandon the procedure (this may depend on the purpose of the procedure and the contrast medium). Proper needle placement should put the needle slightly posterior in the lateral view and *dead center* over the spinous process in the anteroposterior view. Then inject 1 to 2 ml of contrast medium and take roentgenograms in the anteroposterior and lateral views for documentation (Fig. 73-13).

Usually more than one disc is injected when the procedure is done for diagnostic purposes. If the L5-S1 disc is

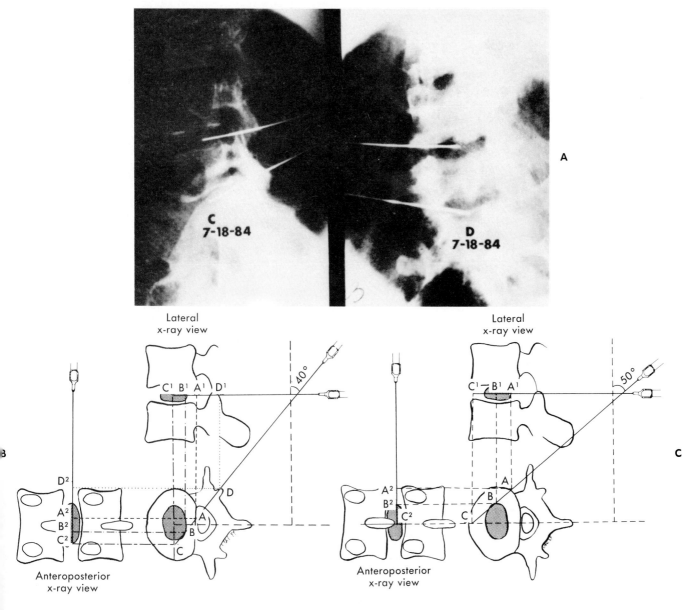

Fig. 73-13. Examples of proper and improper needle placement. **A,** Proper needle placement at center of nucleus. **B,** Needle placed too far medially. **C,** Needle placed too far laterally. *Continued.*

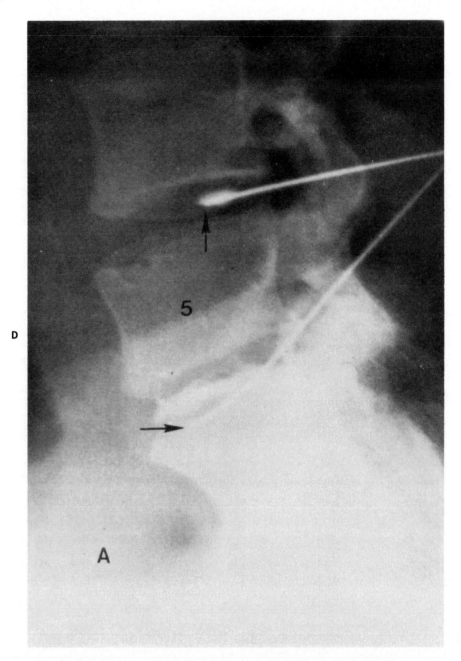

Fig. 73-13, cont'd. D and **E,** Upper needles show medial needle placement while lower needles show lateral placement. (From Chung, B.U.: Bent-tip single needle technique. In Brown, J.E., Nordby, E.J., and Smith, L.: Chemonucleolysis, Thorofare, N.J., 1985, Slack.)

to be injected, place the needle near the entrance for the L4-5 needle and advance it about 45 degrees to the plane of the back and 35 to 40 degrees caudally. Difficulty may be encountered in entering the disc at this angle. The use of the double-needle technique or putting a slight bend in the tip of the insertion needle may help "skive" the needle off the end-plate of S1. It is common to encounter the L5 root when entering this disc. In some patients with a high iliac crest it is impossible to place a needle in this disc. If a blunt 18-gauge needle and a prebent 22-gauge needle are used, the 18-gauge needle must touch the disc. Failure to do this may result in damage to neural structures when the

prebent needle is inserted. Cadaver practice with the prebent needles is suggested before attempting to use this equipment.

CERVICAL DISCOGRAPHY

The technique of cervical discography is considerably different from lumbar discography. This procedure is primarily indicated for the patient with persistent neck or arm pain without evidence of functional overlay but with normal myelography and computed tomography in whom all conservative therapy has failed. This procedure is usually done as a preoperative test for anterior intervertebral fu-

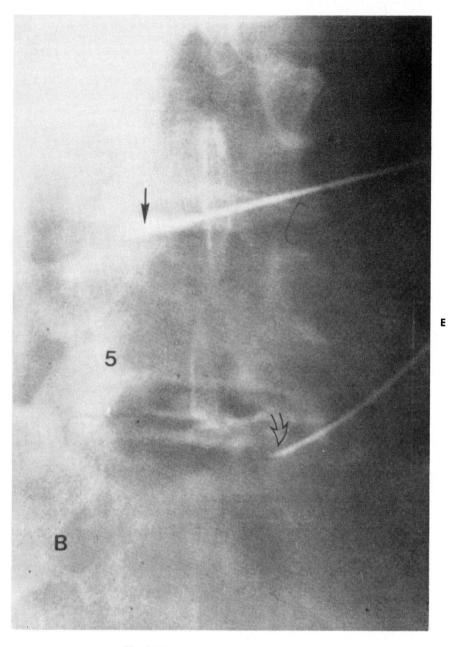

Fig. 73-13, E. For legend see opposite page.

sion. Image intensification equipment capable of both anteroposterior and lateral exposure is required. Standard 1-inch (2.5 cm), 21-gauge needles and 3- to 4-inch (7.5 to 10 cm), 25-gauge needles are also required. Minimal patient premedication is necessary. Atropine may minimize any vasovagal reaction.

TECHNIQUE. Place the patient on the image intensification table in the supine position with the head extended. Prepare and drape the neck in the standard surgical fashion. Ask the patient to grade the degree of neck and arm pain on the 0 to 10 scale. Mark the levels of disc insertion using a thin metal object such as a ruler placed parallel with the disc. Mark the skin laterally at that point using a skin marker.

Infiltrate the skin laterally near the neurovascular bundle. Use the fingers of the left hand to palpate and pull this bundle laterally. Insert the short, blunt-beveled needle, avoiding the neurovascular bundle. Direct the second needle through the first needle at an angle of about 35 degrees from the sagittal plane toward the disc. Once again, central placement of the needle confirmed by anteroposterior and lateral roentgenograms is mandatory.

Slowly inject the contrast medium. Excessive pressure must be avoided to prevent extrusion of any disc fragments. The patient's response to the injection is critical. The proper evaluation of this response usually requires the injection of multiple discs and a comparison of the responses. Ask the patient to grade the degree of his pain from 0 to 10 and localize the pain at the time of injection. Usually only one disc is painful on injection, and that disc should also be abnormal. Take great care to determine if the patient's pain pattern is recreated by the injection. The presence of a degenerative disc alone is *not* an indication for surgery. Pain at all levels of injection or a variable pain pattern should be interpreted as a negative response.

TRIANGULATION TECHNIQUE OF PERCUTANEOUS NEEDLE PLACEMENT (FORD)

Lateral needle placement for discography, needle biopsy, or chemonucleolysis is mandatory to prevent intrathecal injection or dural injury. Because of differences in body size and iliac crest height a standard starting point for needle insertion is only a rough suggestion. Considerable difficulty may occasionally be encountered with needle placement. Recently Ford has proposed a simple technique to preoperatively determine the lateral insertion distance and needle angle for lumbar chemonucleolysis and discography. This technique requires good lateral and anteroposterior roentgenograms with the skin edge visible posteriorly in the lateral.

TECHNIQUE (FORD). Mark the center of the disc spaces to be injected on both anteroposterior and lateral roentgenograms. Measure the distance in centimeters from the body surface to the apophyseal (facet) joint (*A* in Fig. 73-14 and 73-15). This is the point at which the needle should first touch the bone of, and then skid by, the apophyseal joint in its lateral approach to the anulus fibrosis and the nucleus pulposus. Then measure the distance from the apophyseal joint to the center of the disc space (*B* in Fig. 73-14 and 73-15). On the anteroposterior view of the disc space to be injected, measure the distance from the lateral edge of the apophyseal joint to the center of the nucleus pulposus (*C* in 73-15) (see also Fig. 73-16). Transfer line segments *a, b,* and *c* in centimeters, to a piece of paper, arranging them in a triangular form, as though creating a large computed tomographic scan at that vertebral level. Draw a line indicating the proper course of the needle from the skin surface and along the apophyseal joint to the center of the disc. Extend a line perpendicular to *A* at its skin-surface endpoint. The point at which the line intersects the pathway of the needle designates the approximate distance from the midline for the ideal start of the needle approach (*D* in Fig. 73-14).

If more discs are to be injected, slight modifications can be made depending on the position of the first needle. When the needle tip appears to the right of the midline and central in the lateral view, it is wise to begin needle insertion at the second disc slightly more lateral to the midline than the starting point actually derived. On the other hand, if the needle tip appears to be to the left of the midline in the first space and central in the lateral view, start the approach to the second space a little closer to the midline than indicated by triangulation.

MODIFIED TRIANGULATION TECHNIQUE. This technique uses a CT scan of the axial technique at the level to be injected with the skin edge or a sizable portion of the spinous process visible, a goniometer, ruler (metal if used for direct measurement), pencil, and paper.

Draw a line from the center of the disc or vertebral body through the spinous process to the skin line on the CT scan. Center a goniometer at the previously chosen disc center and plot a second line past the facet joint laterally. Measure the angle *x* between line *a* and line *b*. Measure the back skin to disc center as noted in Fig. 73-16, *A,* or measure the depth directly under image intensification. Using paper and pencil, draw a line equal to the length of line *ab* and construct a second line *d* at the previously calculated angle *x*. Draw a third line *e* perpendicular from the skin end of line *ab* intersecting line *d*. The distance from line *ab* to *d* along line *e* should approximate the distance the needle should be placed from the midline of the back. The angle *y* also approximates the angle of needle placement relative to the skin line *d*. Note that the curvature of the back (line *s*) may require extending the line up above the back and placing the needle at the calculated angle of insertion *z*. When the needle touches the skin, this should reasonably approximate the proper point of entry for that patient and disc level.

The lumbosacral disc always requires the most lateral starting position for injection. Midlumbar or upper lumbar discs always require a more medial starting position, sometimes even as close as 5 cm to the midline. Needle placement in patients with lateral lumbar fusions is extremely difficult.

PSYCHOLOGIC TESTING

Psychologic testing has been demonstrated to be a reasonable predictor of surgical and conservative treatment results regardless of the spinal pathology. The Minnesota Multiphasic Personality Inventory (MMPI) is the most reliable and well-documented test used for this purpose. Wiltse and Rocchio demonstrated that elevations of the

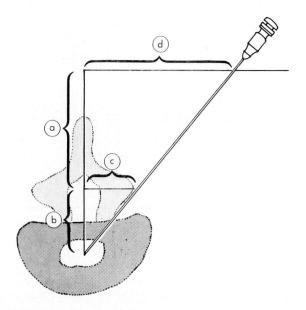

Fig. 73-14. Triangulation technique. Distances *a* and *b* are measured in centimeters from lateral view, and *c* is measured from anteroposterior view. Needle course then is sketched to produce *d*, approximate lateral distance from midline. (From Ford, L.T.: Chemonucleolysis procedure manual No. 1. Needle placement—a triangulation approach for chemonucleolysis, Smith Laboratories, 1984.)

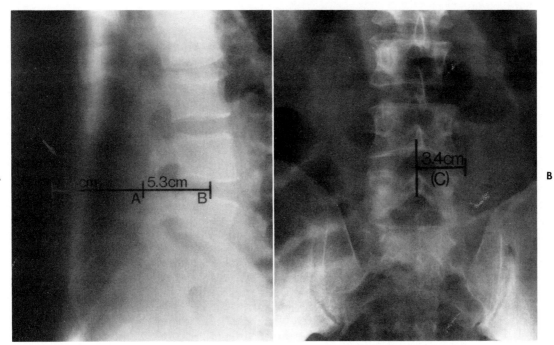

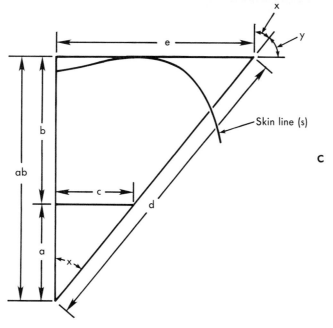

Fig. 73-15. A, Lateral roentgenogram of lumbar spine with metallic marker at highest point on skin of back. This point marks skin level. Draw line parallel with disc space or spaces to be injected. Measure length of lines from center of disc to skin line (*a* + *b*). Divide lines by selecting point that best approximates widest portion of facet joints. Line nearest disc center is line *a* and other is line *b*. (This point is usually ventral surface of facet as seen in lateral view.) **B,** Anteroposterior roentgenogram of lumbar spine with line drawn parallel to disc space or spaces to be injected. Line is measured from center of disc to lateralmost aspect of facet joint *(c)*. **C,** Line drawing showing transposition of lines *a, b,* and *c* extrapolated from above roentgenograms. Draw line *d* from center point of line *a* intersecting lateral edge of line *c* and extending beyond to level of other end of line *b*. Draw line *e* perpendicular from outer end of line *b* intersecting line *d*. Measure length of line *e*. Length of line *e* should reasonably approximate space that needle should be placed from midline of back. Note that curvature of back (line *s*) may require extending line up above back and placing needle at calculated angle of insertion *y*. When needle touches skin that should reasonably approximate proper point of entry for that patient and disc level.

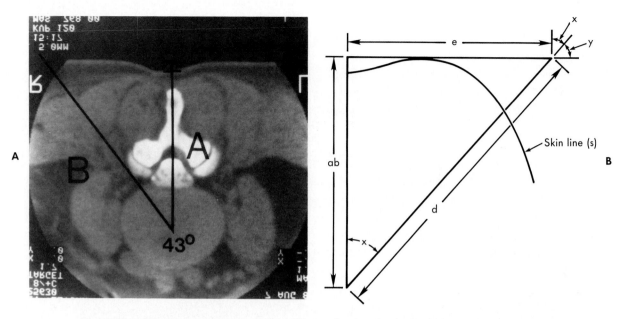

Fig. 73-16. A, Modified triangulation technique. CT scan of patient showing level of disc to be injected and skin level(s). Draw line from center of disc or vertebral body through spinous process to skin line. Center goniometer at previously chosen disc center and plot second line past facet joint laterally. Measure angle *x* between line *a* and line *b*. Measure back skin to disc center as previously noted in Fig. 73-15, *A,* or measure depth directly under image intensification. **B,** Draw line equal to length of line *ab* and construct second line *d* at previously calculated angle *x*. Draw third line *e* perpendicular from skin end of line *ab* intersecting line *d*. Distance from line *ab* to *d* along line *e* should approximate distance needle should be placed from midline of back. Angle *y* also approximates angle of needle placement relative to skin line *d*. Note that curvature of back (line *s*) may require extending line up above back and placing needle at calculated angle of insertion *z*. When needle touches skin, this should reasonably approximate proper point of entry for patient and disc level.

hysteria (Hs) and hypochondriasis (Hy) T scores above 75 are indicative of a poor postoperative response (16% good results). Their study evaluated patients treated with chymopapain and their clinical results (Tables 73-3 and 73-4).

Table 73-3 indicated the rate of good to excellent results using the MMPI test Hs and Hy scores alone in the study by Wiltse and Rocchio. Table 73-4 illustrates the lack of statistical significance between the MMPI scores and the presence of objective findings listed below.

1. Reflex changes
2. Motor weakness
3. Sensory deficits
4. Positive myelogram
5. Positive electromyogram
6. Elevated cerebrospinal fluid protein

Similar studies of surgically and conservatively treated patients have resulted in similar findings. Written reports are helpful, but the raw T score read on the far right or left side of the standard test result sheet is the simplest guide with regard to postoperative outcome. If surgery is necessary in a patient with an elevated Hs or Hy score, then psychiatric or psychologic assistance before and after the procedure may be helpful. Wiltse recommends restraint and conservative treatment in these patients.

Additional material on this test may be obtained in the excellent articles by Dennis, Wiltse, and Southwick and White. Numerous other tests are available, but none have

Table 73-3. Result expectancy related to Hs and Hy T scores on the MMPI test

Hs and Hy T scores	No. of patients	Chances of good or excellent functional recovery (percent)
85 and above	10	10
75 to 84	32	16
65 to 74	31	39
55 to 64	36	72
54 and below	21	90
Prediction from base rate	63	48

From Wiltse, L.L., and Rocchio, P.D.: J. Bone Joint Surg. **57-A**:478, 1975.

been shown to be as predictive of surgical outcome as the Hs and Hy scores on the MMPI. The main problem with the MMPI is that it requires the ability to read and comprehend the material.

A simple test that is a good screening aid is the pain drawing. The pain drawing correlates well with the Hs and Hy scores. This test also requires some ability to follow simple directions. Additional information may be obtained in the articles by Rainsford et al. and Dennis et al. (Fig. 73-17).

Table 73-4. Hs and Hy T scores of patients with good or excellent results versus number of preexisting objective deficits

Hs and Hy T scores	No. of patients	Percent good or excellent results	Per cent with the no. of preinjection objective deficits indicated*				
			1+	2+	3+	4+	5+
75 and over	42	25	95.0	57.5	30.0	7.5	2.5
64 and below	57	87	95.2	64.4	32.6	8.7	2.2

*$X^2 = <0.001$.

From Wiltse, L.L., and Rocchio, P.D.: J. Bone Joint Surg. **57-A:**478, 1975.

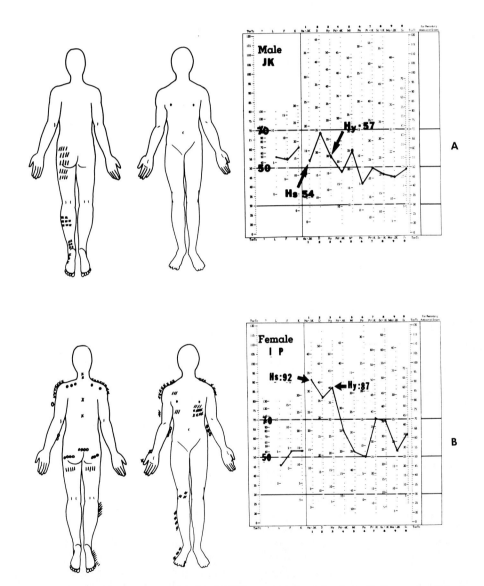

Fig. 73-17. A, Pain drawing and corresponding MMPI raw score sheet of patient with ''conversion V'' who was unrelieved of pain after disc surgery. **B,** Pain drawing and corresponding MMPI raw score sheet of patient with normal findings who was relieved of pain after disc surgery.

CERVICAL DISC DISEASE

Herniation of the cervical intervertebral disc with spinal cord compression has been identified since Key detailed the pathologic findings of two cases of cord compression by "intervertebral substance" in 1838. During the late 1800s and early 1900s there were many reports of chondromas of the cervical spine. Stokely described the clinical findings and anatomic location of cervical disc herniation in 1928 but attributed the lesion to a cervical chondroma. Finally, Mixtner and Barr reported on lumbar disc herniation in 1934 including four cervical disc protrusions.

The classic approach to discs in this region has been posteriorly with laminectomy. This approach had been used as a standard exposure for extradural tumors. In 1943 Semmes and Murphey reported four patients in whom cervical disc rupture simulated coronary disease and introduced the concept that cervical disc disease usually manifested in root symptoms and not cord compression symptoms. Bailey and Badgley, Cloward, and Robinson and Smith in the 1950s popularized the anterior approach coupled with interbody fusion. Robertson in 1972, after the initial report by Hirsch in 1960, popularized anterior cervical discectomy without fusion. He showed that simple anterior disc excision without fusion can give results similar to anterior cervical disc excision with anterior interbody fusion.

Kelsey et al. in the epidemiologic study of acute cervical disc prolapse indicated that cervical disc rupture was more common in men by a ratio of 1.4 to 1. Factors associated with the injury were frequent heavy lifting on the job, cigarette smoking, and frequent diving from a board. The use of vibrating equipment and time spent in motor vehicles were not positively associated with this problem. Participation in sports other than diving, frequent wearing of shoes with high heels, frequent twisting of the neck on the job, time spent sitting on the job, and smoking of cigars and pipes were not associated with cervical intervertebral disc collapse. Harrell reported that 40% of the population in Sweden were sometimes affected by neck pain during their lives.

The pathophysiology of cervical disc disease is the same as degenerative disc disease in other areas of the spine. Disc swelling is followed by progressive anular degeneration. Frank extrusion of nuclear material can occur as a complication of this normal degenerative process. Cramer postulated that hydraulic pressure on the disc rather than excessive motion produced traumatic disc herniation. As the disc degeneration proceeds, hypermobility of the segment can result in instability or degenerative arthritic changes or both. Unlike the lumbar spine, these hypertrophic changes are predominantly at the uncovertebral joint (uncinate process) (Fig. 73-18). Eventually hypertrophic changes develop about the facet joints and vertebral bodies. As with lumbar disease, progressive stiffening of the cervical spine and loss of motion are the usual result in the end stages. Occasionally hypertrophic spurring anteriorly can result in dysphagia.

Signs and symptoms

The signs and symptoms of intervertebral disc disease are best separated into symptoms related to the spine itself,

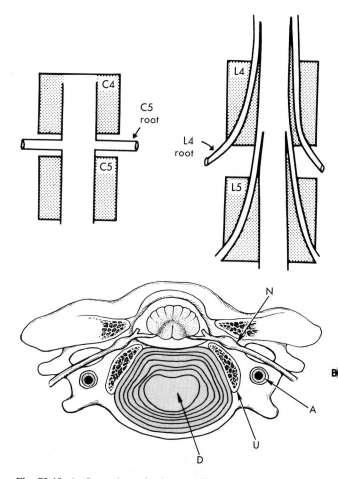

Fig. 73-18. A, Comparison of points at which nerve roots emerge from cervical and lumbar spine. **B,** Cross-sectional view of cervical spine at level of disc. Uncinate process forms ventral wall of foramen. Root exits dorsal to vertebral artery. (**A,** from Kikuchi, S., MacNab, I., and Moreau, P.: J. Bone Joint Surg. **63-B:**272, 1981.)

symptoms related to nerve root compression, and symptoms of myelopathy. Several authors have reported that when the disc is punctured anteriorly for the purpose of discography, pain is noted in the neck and shoulder. Complaints of neck pain, medial scapular pain, and shoulder pain are therefore probably related to primary pain about the disc and spine. Anatomic studies have indicated cervical disc and ligamentous innervations. This has been inferred to be similar in the cervical spine to that of the lumbar spine with its sinovertebral nerve.

Symptoms of root compression are usually associated with pain radiating into the arm or chest with numbness in the fingers and motor weakness. Cervical disc disease can also mimic cardiac disease with chest and arm pain. Usually the radicular symptoms are intermittent and combined with the more frequent neck and shoulder pain.

The signs of midline cervical compression (myelopathy) are unique and varied. The pain is poorly localized and aching in nature. Occasional sharp pain or generalized tingling may be described with neck extension. This is not unlike Lhermitte's sign in multiple sclerosis. The pain may be in both the shoulder and pelvic girdles. It is occasion-

C5 nerve root compression

(indicative of C4-5 disc rupture or other pathology at that level)

Sensory deficit
    Upper lateral arm and elbow
Motor weakness
    Deltoid
    Biceps (variable)
Reflex change
    Biceps (variable)

C6 nerve root compression

(indicative of C5-6 disc herniation or other local pathology)

Sensory deficit
    Lateral forearm, thumb, and index finger
Motor weakness
    Biceps
    Extensor carpi radialis longus and brevis
Reflex change
    Biceps
    Brachioradialis

C7 nerve root compression

(indicative of C6-7 disc rupture or other pathology at that level)

Sensory deficit
    Middle finger (variable because of overlap)
Motor weakness
    Triceps
    Wrist flexors (flexor carpi radialis)
    Finger flexors (variable)
Reflex change
    Triceps

C8 nerve root compression

(indicative of C7-T1 disc rupture or other pathology at that level)

Sensory deficit
    Ring finger, little finger, and ulnar border of palm
Motor weakness
    Interossei
    Finger flexors (variable)
    Flexor carpi ulnaris (variable)
Reflex change
    None

T1 nerve root compression

(indicative of T1-T2 disc rupture or other pathology at that level)

Sensory deficit
    Medial aspect of elbow
Motor weakness
    Interossei
Reflex change
    None

ally associated with a generalized feeling of weakness in the lower extremities and a feeling of instability.

In patients with predominant cervical spondylosis symptoms of vertebral artery compression may also be found. These symptoms consist of dizziness, tinnitus, intermittent blurring of vision, and occasional episodes of retroocular pain.

The signs of lateral root pressure from a disc or osteophytes are predominantly neurologic. By evaluating multiple motor groups, multiple levels of deep tendon reflexes and sensory abnormalities, the level of the lesion can be localized as accurately as any other lesion in the nervous system. The multiple innervation of muscles can sometimes lead to confusion in determining the exact root involved. For this reason, myelography or other studies done for roentgenographic verification of the clinical impression are usually helpful.

Rupture of the C4-5 disc with compression of the C5 nerve root should result in weakness in the deltoid and biceps muscles. The deltoid is almost entirely innervated by C5, but the biceps is poorly innervated. The biceps reflex may be diminished with injury to this nerve root, although it also has a C6 component, and this may be considered. Sensory testing should show a patch on the lateral aspect of the arm to be diminished (Fig. 73-19).

Rupture of the C5-6 disc with compression of the C6 root may be confused with other root levels because of dual innervation of structures. Weakness may be noted in the biceps and extensor carpi radialis longus and brevis. As mentioned above, the biceps is dually innervated by C5 and C6, whereas the long extensors are dually innervated by C6 and C7. The brachioradialis and biceps reflexes may also be diminished at this level. Sensory testing usually indicates a decreased sensibility over the lateral forearm, thumb, and index finger.

Rupture of the C6-7 disc with compression of the C7 root frequently results in weakness of the triceps. Weakness of the wrist flexors, especially the flexor carpi radialis, is also more indicative of C7 root problems. Weakness of the flexor carpi ulnaris is usually more affected by C8 lesions. As mentioned above, finger extensors may also be weakened in that they have both C7 and C8 innervation. The triceps reflex may be diminished. Sensation is lost in the middle finger. C7 sensibility is variable because it is so narrow and overlap is prominent. Strong sensibility change may be hard to document.

Rupture between C7 and T1 with compression of the C8 nerve root results in no reflex changes. Weakness may be noted in the finger flexors and in the interossei of the hand. Sensibility is lost on the ulnar border of the palm, including the ring and little fingers. Compression of T1 shows weakness of the interosseus muscles, decreased sensibility about the medial aspect of the elbow, and no reflex changes.

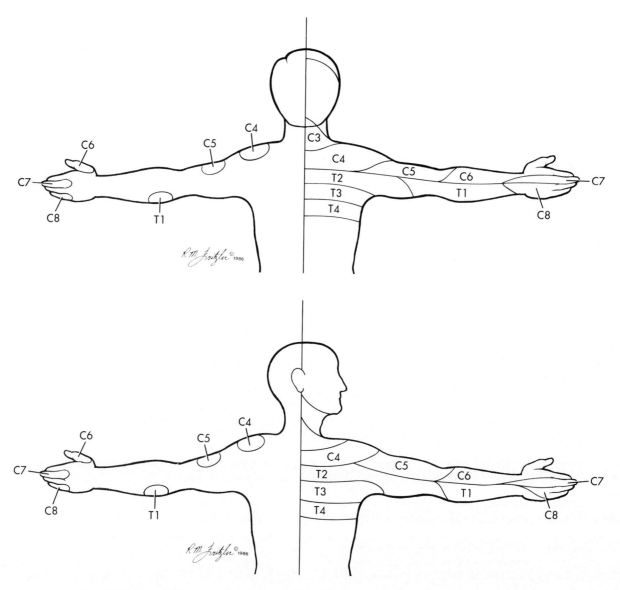

Fig. 73-19. C5 neurologic level. (After Hoppenfeld, S.: Physical examination of the spine and extremities, Norwalk, Conn., 1976, Appleton-Century-Crofts.)

The clinical series of Odom et al. noted considerable variability in the level of compression and the neurologic findings. Change in the triceps reflex was the predominant reflex change with compression of the sixth cervical root (56%). It was also the predominant reflex change in seventh root compression (64%). Similarly the index finger was the predominant digit with sensory change, with evidence of hypalgesia in both sixth (68%) and seventh (70%) cervical root compression.

Care should be taken in the examination of the extremity when radicular problems are encountered to rule out more distal compression syndromes in the upper extremities such as thoracic outlet syndrome, carpal tunnel syndrome, and cubital tunnel syndrome. Patients should also be examined in the lower extremity with special attention to long track signs indicative of myelopathy.

There are no tests for the upper extremity that correspond with straight leg raising tests in the lower extremity. Recently Davidson et al. described a shoulder test that may be helpful in the diagnosis of cervical root compression syndromes. The test consists of shoulder abduction and elbow flexion with placement of the hand on the top of the head. This should relieve the arm pain caused by radicular compression. It is interesting to note that if this position is allowed to persist for a minute or two and pain is increased, then more distal compressive neuropathies such as a tardy ulnar nerve syndrome (cubital tunnel syndrome) or primary shoulder pathologic conditions are often the cause.

Cervical paraspinal spasm and limitation of neck motion are frequent findings of cervical spine disease but are not indicative of a specific pathologic process. Special maneuvers involving neck motion may be helpful in the choice of conservative treatment and identification of pathologic processes. The distraction test, which involves placing the hands on the occiput and jaw and distracting the cervical spine in the neutral position, may relieve root compression pain but may increase pain caused by ligamentous injury. Neck extension and flexion with or without traction may be helpful in selecting conservative therapies.

Patients relieved of pain with the neck extended, with or without traction, usually have hyperextension syndromes with ligamentous injury posteriorly, whereas patients relieved of pain with distraction and neck flexion are more likely to have nerve root compression caused by either a soft ruptured disc or most likely hypertrophic spurs in the neural foramina. Pain is usually increased in any condition with compression. One must be careful before applying compression or distraction to be sure no cervical instability or fracture is present. One must also be careful in interpreting the distraction test to be certain the temporomandibular joint is not diseased or injured because distraction will also increase the pain in this area.

The signs of midline disc herniation are those of spinal cord compression. If the lesion is high in the cervical region, parasthesias, weakness, atrophy, and occasionally fasciculations may occur in the hands. Most commonly, however, the first and most prominent symptoms are those of involvement of the corticospinal tract; less commonly the posterior columns are affected. The primary signs are clonus, hyperactive reflexes, and the Babinski reflex. Lesser findings are varying degrees of spasticity, weakness in the legs, and impairment of proprioception. Equilibrium may be grossly disturbed, but sense of pain and temperature sense are rarely lost and are usually of little localizing value.

Differential diagnosis

The differential diagnosis of cervical disc disease is best separated into extrinsic and intrinsic factors. Extrinsic factors basically deal with those disease processes extrinsic to the neck resulting in symptoms similar to primary neck problems. Included in this group are tumors of the chest, nerve compression syndromes distal to the neck, degenerative processes such as shoulder and upper extremity arthritis, temporomandibular joint syndrome, and lesions about the shoulder such as acute and chronic rotator cuff tears and impingement syndromes. Intrinsic problems deal primarily with lesions directly associated with the cervical spine, the most common, of course, being cervical disc degeneration with a concomitant complication of disc herniation and later development of hypertrophic arthritis. Congenital factors such as spinal stenosis in the cervical region may also produce symptoms. Primary and secondary tumors of the cervical spine and fractures of the cervical vertebrae should also be considered as intrinsic lesions.

Cervical disc disease has been categorized by Odom et al. into four groups: (1) unilateral soft disc protrusion with nerve root compression; (2) foraminal spur, or hard disc, with nerve root compression; (3) medial soft disc protrusion with spinal cord compression; and (4) transverse ridge or cervical spondylosis with spinal cord compression. Soft disc herniations usually affect one level,

whereas hard discs can be multiple. Central lesions usually result in cord compression symptoms, and lateral lesions usually result in radicular symptoms.

Odom et al. report that most of the soft disc herniations in their series occurred at the sixth cervical interspace (70%) and fifth cervical interspace (24%). Only 6% occurred at the seventh interspace. Foraminal spurs were also found predominantly at the sixth interspace (48%). The fifth interspace (39%) and seventh interspace (13%) accounted for the remaining levels where foraminal spurs were found. They also noted the incidence of medial soft disc protrusion with myelopathy to be rare (14 of 246 patients).

Disc material is sometimes extruded into the midline of the spinal canal anteriorly, with compression of the spinal cord and without nerve root involvement. Occasionally this is the result of a violent injury to the cervical spine, with or without fracture-dislocation, and at times associated with immediate quadriplegia. In some instances, however, the symptoms are progressive and may be suggestive of spinal cord tumor or degenerative diseases of the spinal cord, such as amyotrophic lateral sclerosis, posterolateral sclerosis, and multiple sclerosis. In most of these ailments no block of the spinal canal has been reported, and for many years the mechanism whereby the cervical cord compression was produced was not understood. However, in the rare patients whom we have observed, spinal fluid block could be produced by hyperextending the neck, although with the neck in the neutral or flexed position the canal was completely open. This finding has been previously reported. It has since been observed that during operation on such patients when the neck is hyperextended, the superior edge of the lamina compresses the cord against the herniated disc, and it is therefore probable that repeated hyperextension of the neck over a period of weeks, months, or years could gradually damage the spinal cord.

The patient with a midline herniation rarely complains of pain or stiffness of the neck. The first symptom may occasionally be a shocklike sensation in the trunk and extremities as a result of flexing or hyperextending the neck, somewhat but not exactly similar to Lhermitte's sign in multiple sclerosis. If the lesion is high in the cervical region, paresthesias, weakness, atrophy, and occasionally fasciculations may occur in the hands. Most commonly, however, the first and most prominent symptoms are those of involvement of the corticospinal tract and less commonly the posterior columns with varying degrees of spasticity, weakness in the legs, and impairment of proprioception. Equilibrium may be grossly disturbed, but sense of pain and temperature sense are rarely lost and are usually of little localizing value.

In view of the disturbances of the spinal fluid dynamics just mentioned, jugular compression should be carried out during lumbar puncture with the neck in the flexed, neutral, and hyperextended positions. Roentgenographically there is more often than not little or no alteration in the cervical curve.

We are in complete agreement with Bucy, Heimburger, and Oberhill that every patient suspected of having degenerative spinal cord disease should have a spinal puncture.

All of these patients should also have a myelogram unless cranial nerve involvement is present. Neither evidence of mild cranial nerve involvement such as hypalgesia in the fifth cranial nerve distribution nor lower motor neuron abnormality in the upper or lower extremity should deter one from carrying out this procedure. However, further experience with spinal fluid dynamics with the neck in various positions may alter our opinion about the necessity of myelography in patients who do not have a block on hyperextension.

MYELOGRAPHY

Myelography is performed in the same way as for ruptured lumbar discs except that considerable attention must be paid to the flow of the column of contrast medium with the neck in hyperextended, neutral, and flexed positions. One cannot conclude that spinal cord compression is not present until one is certain that the cephalad flow of the medium is not obstructed with the neck acutely hyperextended. The neck should be hyperextended carefully because of the danger of further damage to the spinal cord.

Confirmatory testing

Roentgenographic evaluation of the cervical spine frequently shows loss of the normal cervical lordosis. Disc space narrowing and hypertrophic changes are frequently increased with age but are not indicative of cervical disc rupture. Usually roentgenograms are most helpful to rule out other problems. Oblique roentgenograms of the cervical spine may reveal foraminal encroachment.

Cervical myelography is indicated when the clinical findings fail to localize the lesion or there is a question of the level involved. Limiting the exploration and disc excision to one disc space is highly desirable because exploration of more than one root may result in increased neurologic deficit. Cervical myelography is usually more exact than lumbar myelography regardless of the contrast medium used. Iophendylate (Pantopaque) is still the contrast media of choice at this time for cervical myelography. This is primarily because cervical myelography involves more danger if the contrast medium metrizamide is allowed to proceed intracranially. The dose of metrizamide is also higher for good cervical myelography, thus increasing the side effects of nausea, vomiting, and headache, as well as the complications of seizures and mental changes. From a technical standpoint metrizamide does provide a greater degree of nerve root definition than does iophendylate. The use of low-dose water soluble myelography followed by a standard or reformatted computed tomographic scan may provide more information with less risk of illness.

Computed tomographic scans of the cervical spine are also helpful, but not as much as in the lumbar spine. In addition, reformatted tomographic scans in the cervical spine usually result in a much less distinct picture than in the lumbar spine.

Cervical discography is a highly controversial technique with limited benefits. It is not indicated in frank disc rupture, spondylosis, or spinal stenosis. The primary use is in patients with persistent neck pain without localized neurologic findings in whom standard myelographic and tomographic scan studies are negative. Some investigators believe that isolated painful discs can be identified in some patients by discography. Certainly a degenerative disc without pain on injection is not the source of the patient's complaint. The technique of cervical discography requires considerable care and caution. It should be considered a preoperative test in those patients in whom an anterior disc excision and interbody fusion are considered for primary neck and shoulder pain. Great care is required both in the technique and interpretation if reproducible results are desired. Cervical root blocks have also been suggested for the localization and confirmation of symptomatic root compression when used in conjunction with cervical discography.

Conservative therapy

Many conservative treatment modalities for neck pain are used for multiple diagnoses. The primary purpose of the cervical spine and associated musculature is to support and mobilize the head while providing a conduit for the nervous system. The forces on the cervical spine are therefore much smaller than on the lower spinal levels. The cervical spine is vulnerable to muscular tension forces, postural fatigue, and excessive motion. Most nonoperative treatments focus on one or more of these factors. The best primary treatment is rest, massage, ice, and aspirin. The position of the neck for comfort is essential for relief of pain. The position of greatest relief may suggest the offending pathologic process or mechanism of injury. Patients with hyperflexion injuries are usually more comfortable with the neck in extension over a small roll under the neck. No specific position is indicative of lateral disc herniation although most tolerate the neutral position best. Patients with spondylosis (hard disc) are most comfortable with the neck in flexion.

Cervical traction may be helpful in selected patients. Care must be exercised in instructing the patient in the proper use of the traction. It should be applied to the head in the position of maximum pain relief. Traction should never be continued if it increases pain. The weights should rarely exceed 10 pounds (weight of the head). The proper head halter and duration of traction sessions should be chosen to prevent irritation of the temporomandibular joint. Traction should also allow general relaxation of the patient.

The postural aspects of neck pain may be treated with more frequent changes in position and changes in the work area to prevent fatigue and encourage good posture. Techniques to minimize or relieve tension are also helpful.

Cervical braces usually limit excessive motion. Like traction, they should be tailored to the most comfortable neck position. They may be most helpful in situations where the patient is quite active.

Neck and shoulder exercises are most beneficial as the acute pain subsides. Isometric exercises are helpful in the acute phase. Occasionally shoulder problems such as adhesive capsulitis may be found concomitantly with cervical spondylosis. Therefore complete immobilization of the painful extremity should be avoided.

Surgery

The primary indications for surgical treatment of cervical disc disease are (1) failure of conservative therapy, (2) increasing neurologic deficit, and (3) cervical myelopathy that is progressive. In most patients the persistence of pain is the primary indication. The choice of approach should be determined by the position and type of lesion. Soft lateral discs are easily removed from the posterior approach, whereas soft central or hard discs (central or lateral) are probably best treated with an anterior approach. The decision to fuse the spine at the time of anterior discectomy is controversial. Osteophytes that were not removed at surgery have been shown to frequently be absorbed at the level of fusion. The use of a graft also prevents the collapse of the disc space and possible foraminal narrowing.

REMOVAL OF POSTEROLATERAL HERNIATIONS BY POSTERIOR APPROACH

TECHNIQUE. With the patient under general endotracheal anesthesia in the prone position and the face in a cerebellar headrest that fits comfortably, and the neck is flexed to obliterate the cervical lordosis as much as possible. The upright position for surgery decreases the venous bleeding, but concern regarding the possibility of air embolism and cerebral hypoxia in the event of a significant drop in blood pressure makes us reluctant to recommend its use. The shoulders are retracted inferiorly with tape if roentgenograms of the lower cervical levels are contemplated.

Appropriately prepare and drape the operative field. Make a midline incision 2.5 cm lower than the interspace to be explored (Fig. 73-20). Retract the edges of this incision and the skin will withdraw in a cephalad direction so that the wound becomes properly placed. Divide the ligamentum nuchae longitudinally to expose the tips of the spinous processes above and below the designated area. The correct position is reasonably well assured by palpation of the last bifid spine, which is usually the sixth cervical vertebra. However, it should be verified preoperatively by a marker on the lateral cervical spine roentgenogram. If still uncertain as to the proper level, count downward from the second cervical spinous process. Dissect subperiosteally the paravertebral muscles from the laminae on the side of the lesion and retract them with a self-retaining retractor such as the Hoen or with the help of an assistant using a Hibbs retractor. Mark the spine with an Oschner clamp or towel clip in the spinous processes and have a lateral roentgenogram made to confirm the level of dissection if there is any question.

With a small Hudson burr, rongeur, or power drill, grind away the medial edge of the facet along with the dorsal surface of the adjacent laminae. Remove a minimal portion of the trailing edge of the lamina above and the superior edge of the lamina below with a standard rongeur and with an angulated Kerrison rongeur. Sharply excise the ligamentum flavum and identify the nerve root, which is commonly displaced posteriorly and flattened by pressure from the underlying disc fragments. Removal of additional bone along the dorsal aspect of the foramen and immediately above and below the nerve root is often beneficial at this point.

The herniated nucleus pulposus most often lies slightly below the center of the nerve root but occasionally is above it. Gently retract the nerve root superiorly to expose the extruded nuclear fragments or a distended posterior longitudinal ligament. To control troublesome venous ooz-ing at this point, place tiny pledgets of cotton above and below the nerve root. Take care not to pack the pledgets tightly around the nerve. The nerve root can then be retracted slightly to enable incision of the posterior longitudinal ligament over the herniated nucleus pulposus in a cruciate manner to permit the removal of the disc fragments.

After removal of all visible loose fragments, it is imperative to make a thorough search for additional fragments, both laterally and medially. It is equally important to be sure that the nerve root is thoroughly decompressed by inserting a probe in the intervertebral foramen. If the nerve root still seems to be tight, remove more bone from the articular facets until the nerve root is completely free. Since recurrence is so rare, do not curet the intervertebral space. Remove the cotton pledgets and control bleeding with bits of Gelfoam dipped in thrombin. Hemostasis must be complete, for postoperative hemorrhage can produce cord compression and quadriplegia. Close the wound by suturing the fascia to the supraspinous ligament with interrupted sutures and then suturing the subcutaneous layers and skin.

AFTERTREATMENT. The patient is given enough opiates to control the pain and is observed closely for evidence of spinal cord compression. Motor power and sensation in the legs are checked at hourly intervals for 24 hours. The patient is allowed out of bed the next day and is usually discharged from the hospital by the seventh day. Recovery of power is usually dramatic and prompt, although hypesthesia may persist for weeks or months. The patient is allowed to return to clerical work when comfortable and to manual labor after 2 months. As a rule neither support nor physical therapy is necessary, and the patient's future activity is not restricted. Isometric neck exercises, upper extremity range of motion exercises, and posterior shoulder girdle exercises may be useful for patients in whom atrophy or inactivity has been considerable.

RESULTS

In no operation in neurosurgery are the results better than after the removal of a lateral herniated cervical disc. In the series of 250 operations reported by Simmons there were no deaths or major complications involving the brain or spinal cord. Three patients had reflex sympathetic dystrophy after operation. Two of these have completely recovered and one almost so. Two patients continued to have arm pain after operation and were reexplored during the initial hospital stay; in each, several more fragments of disc were found and removed. It is assumed that these fragments were overlooked at the initial operation. One patient had a recurrent extrusion at the same level. Two other patients have had soft extrusions on the opposite side at another level, also requiring a second operation.

Murphe and Simmons analyzed the results in a series of 150 patients who returned questionnaires concerning the success or failure of the operation. They were asked to state the percentage of benefit they derived from the procedure, whether they were performing the same work as they had done preoperatively, and if not, whether the change of work had resulted from neck trouble. The answers are given in Table 73-5. Approximately 90% had extremely good results, and there were none who were not

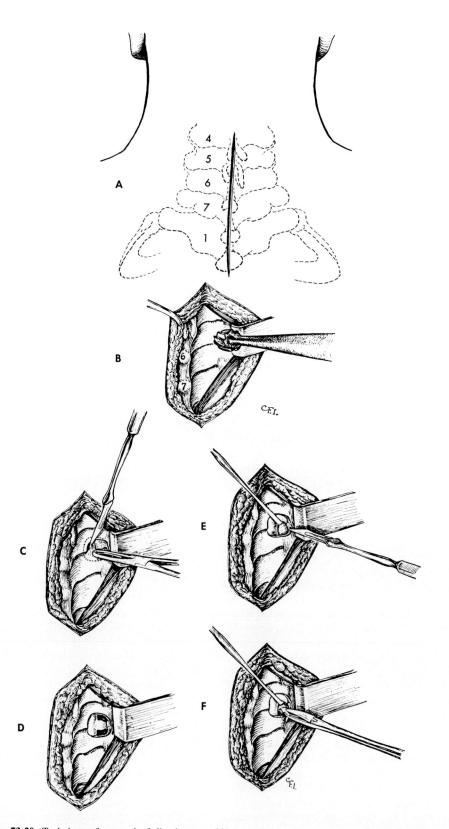

Fig. 73-20. Technique of removal of disc between fifth and sixth cervical vertebrae. **A,** Midline incision extending from spinous process of fourth cervical vertebra to that of first thoracic vertebra. **B,** Paraspinal muscles have been dissected from laminae and retracted laterally. Hole is to be drilled with Hudson burr (see text). **C,** Ligamentum flavum is being dissected. **D,** Defect measuring about 1.3 × 1.3 cm has been made (see text) to expose nerve root and lateral aspect of dura. **E,** Nerve root has been separated from nucleus and retracted superiorly to expose herniated disc. **F,** Longitudinal ligament has been incised, and loose fragment of nucleus is being removed.

Table 73-5 Results of removal of lateral herniated discs in cervical region (patient's estimate of percent improvement)

% relief	% patients improved	No. patients
95-100	65.3	98
90-94	23.3	35
75-89	8.0	12
50-74	3.3	5
TOTAL	100.0	150

significantly improved, as the data concerning work done confirm. Only 7 (6%) of the 125 patients who answered this part of the questionnaire found a change of work necessary because of neck trouble.

ANTERIOR APPROACH TO CERVICAL DISC

Smith and Robinson in 1955 were the first to recommend an anterior approach to the cervical spine in the treatment of cervical disc disease. They described an anterolateral discectomy with interbody fusion (Fig. 73-21).

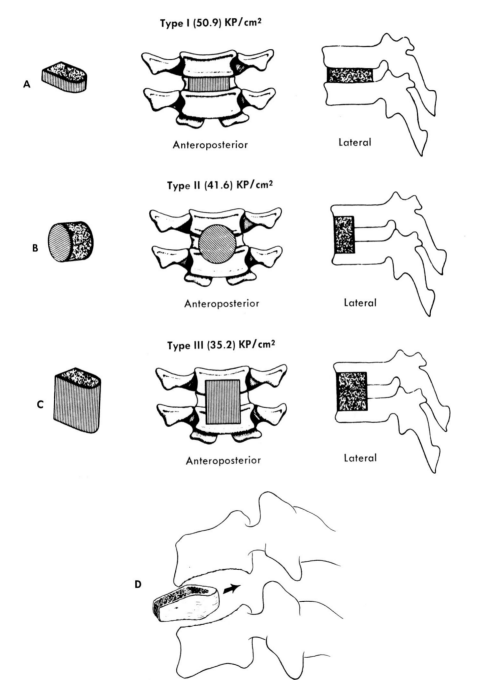

Type I (50.9) KP/cm²

Anteroposterior   Lateral

Type II (41.6) KP/cm²

Anteroposterior   Lateral

Type III (35.2) KP/cm²

Anteroposterior   Lateral

Fig. 73-21. Types of anterior cervical fusion. **A,** Smith-Robinson fusion. **B,** Cloward fusion. **C,** Bailey-Badgley fusion. **D,** Bloom-Raney modification of Smith-Robinson fusion. (**A** to **C,** From White, A.A., III, et al.: Clin. Orthop. **91:**21, 1973. **D,** From Bloom, M.H., and Raney, F.L.: J. Bone Joint Surg. **63-A:**842, 1981.)

This procedure attained widespread acceptance and application after Cloward in 1958 modified the procedure and introduced new instrumentation.

There are three basic techniques for anterior cervical disc excision and fusion. The Cloward technique involves making a round hole centered at the disc space. A slightly larger, round iliac crest plug is then inserted into the disc space hole. The Smith and Robinson technique involves inserting a tricortical plug of iliac crest into the disc space after removing the disc and cartilaginous end plate. The graft is inserted with the cancellous side facing the cord (posterior). Recently Bloom and Raney have suggested a modification of this technique by fashioning the tricortical graft to be thicker in its midportion and then inserting the graft with the cancellous portion facing anteriorly. The Bailey and Badgley technique involves the creation of a slot in the superior and inferior vertebral bodies. This technique is most applicable to reconstruction when one or more vertebral bodies are excised for tumor, stenosis, or other extensive pathology. Simmons and Bhalla have modifed this technique by using a keystone graft that increases the surface area of the graft by 30% and allows more complete locking of the graft. Biomechanically, the Smith and Robinson technique provides the greatest stability and least risk of extrusion.

White et al. reported relief of pain in 90% of 65 patients undergoing anterior cervical spine fusion for spondylosis with the technique of Smith and Robinson. Analysis of 90 patients with anterior cervical discectomies and fusion for cervical spondylosis with radiculopathy using the Cloward technique showed good to excellent results in 82% in the study by Jacobs et al. These investigators did not use discography. Others have also found that discography does not statistically improve the results.

Anterior cervical discectomy without interbody fusion was first described by Hirsch in 1960. Good relief of symptoms was first reported by Boldrey with discectomy alone. In 1971 Robertson reported a comparison of a series of patients treated by the Cloward technique with a group treated by anterior discectomy without fusion. The results were superior in those treated by discectomy alone. The procedure includes wide excision of the anterior anulus and extensive removal of the disc material. The operating microscope is used when remaining disc material is removed, and anular defects are viewed to assist in locating and removing extruded fragments. All cartilaginous plate material is curetted from the interspace, and the posterior anulus is excised. Osseous spurs or transverse bars are also removed. Murphy and Gado reported excellent results with a similar technique, and 72% of these patients obtained solid fusion at the operated level. Good clinical results and good stability occurred even in those who did not obtain fusion. Similar experiences were reported by others. Prospective studies comparing the results of anterior discectomy with and without fusion have revealed that early pain relief and return to work are faster with simple discectomy alone.

Complete discectomy, including removal of cartilaginous plates with resection of the posterior anulus and adequate bony decompression of the nerve roots and cord without bone graft, is the procedure used most commonly for soft disc disease. Hard disc disease with marked narrowing of the disc space and with an extensive posterior osteophytic spurring or ridging may be more suitable for anterior interbody fusion, for the extensive bone removed gives a better view of the posterior bony overgrowth and decompression is made easier.

The choice of right- or left-sided approach to the cervical spine is somewhat controversial. The right side of the neck is preferred by some right-handed surgeons because of the ease of dissection. The reported increased risk of recurrent laryngeal nerve trauma when operating on the right is not judged by those who use it to be a significant deterrent to choosing this exposure. Exposure from the left is more inconvenient to the right-handed surgeon but decreases the risk of recurrent laryngeal nerve injury. This nerve on the left consistently descends with the carotid sheath and exits from the carotid sheath and vagus nerve intrathoracically. The nerve then courses under the arch of the aorta and ascends in the neck beside the trachea and esophagus. The course of the nerve on the right is not as consistent. The nerve usually descends with the carotid sheath, then loops around the subclavian artery and ascends between the trachea and esophagus. Occasionally the right recurrent laryngeal nerve may exit the carotid sheath early and cross anteriorly behind the thyroid.

TECHNIQUE. Place the patient supine on the operating table with endotracheal anesthesia administered through a noncollapsible tube. Position the head turned to the right 10 to 20 degrees. The insertion of a small nasogastric tube may facilitate the positive identification of the esophagus. Place a small roll between the scapulas; and the shoulders may be pulled down with tape to allow easy roentgen exposure. Slightly extend the neck over a small roll placed beneath it. Then place a head halter on the mandible and occiput and apply several pounds of traction. Prepare and drape the area from the mandible to the upper chest. It may be necessary to suture the initial drapes in place.

A transverse incision may be used for exposure of one or two levels from C4-5 to C7-T1. Make a transverse incision following the skin folds about two finger-breadths above the clavicle. Extend it from the midline to a point just across the anterior border of the sternocleidomastoid muscle. Undermine the subcutaneous tissue both above and below and divide the platysma muscle longitudinally in the direction of its fibers. This platysmal incision reduces the postoperative scarring that is objectionable if its fibers are sectioned transversely. Open the cervical fascia along the anteromedial border of the sternocleidomastoid muscle. Develop a plane between the sternocleidomastoid laterally and the omohyoid and sternohyoid medially. The carotid artery is palpated in this plane and gently retracted laterally with a finger. With combined blunt and sharp dissection develop a relatively avascular plane between the carotid sheath laterally and the thyroid, trachea, and esophagus medially. Insert hand-held retractors initially. Identify the esophagus by palpation of the nasogastric tube. Dissect free the filmy connective tissue in the posterolateral aspect of the esophagus along the entire exposed wound to prevent ballooning of the esophagus above and below the retractor. Expose the prevertebral fascia, open it in the midline, and expose at least the anterior aspect of two full vertebral bodies and the disc in question. Insert a hypodermic needle into this disc (or in the superior exposed disc in the event more than one level is exposed) and obtain a lateral roentgenogram.

After roentgenographic localization is completed, strip the longus colli muscles laterally from the anterior surface of the vertebral bodies. Now insert a self-retaining retractor. The anterior longitudinal ligament ideally is retracted laterally along with the longus colli muscles. Excise the anterior anulus of the disc to be removed over the entire anterior aspect of its surface. With the pituitary forceps remove as much disc material as can be seen. After a portion of the disc material has been removed, insert the interspace spreader for a better view to allow more complete removal of nuclear material down to the level of the anulus posteriorly. Loupe or microscopic magnification greatly enhances the deep disc excision.

If the Cloward procedure is to be used, introduce a drill with its drill guard in a vertical position and drill the hole down as far as the posterior longitudinal ligament. It is advisable to stop several times and check the depth of the hole. Remove the drill and drill guard. Then remove free lateral cartilaginous fragments, and undercut and remove the transverse bar superiorly and inferiorly or identify the defect in the anulus. Remove anular material at this level and any lateral nuclear fragments or osteophytic spurs to achieve a good view and decompression of the nerve root on one or both sides. Obtain graft material from the ilium.

Using the Cloward technique, make a vertical incision approximately 2 cm behind the anterosuperior iliac spine down to the fascia lata, which is then opened with a T-shaped incision. Make the transverse portion of this incision approximately 2 cm below the iliac crest. Separate the muscle fibers and subperiosteally expose the cortical surface of the ilium. Using a dowel-cutting instrument, obtain one or more grafts depending on the number of interspaces to be entered. Muscle attachments to the iliac crest are not dissected free, and consequently postoperative discomfort is significantly less with this procedure. Close the periosteum, muscle, and fascia along with the subcutaneous tissue and skin. Securing hemostasis is emphasized, and a drain is not used. Determine the depth of the space and insert the graft, which must be approximately 4 mm shorter than the depth of the hole with the interspace spreader inserted. Countersink the graft 2 to 3 mm when the interspace spreader is removed. Close the anterior longitudinal ligament and longus colli muscles over the anterior aspect of the graft.

If the Smith-Robinson fusion technique or discectomy without interbody grafting is to be used, bring the microscope into position after the bulk of the nuclear material has been removed. Carefully remove all remaining nuclear and cartilaginous plate material with pituitary forceps and small angulated curets. If a soft lateral fragment is anticipated, look for the defect in the posterior anulus. Remove the anulus and identify and remove the soft extruded lateral fragment. Look carefully for additional soft nuclear fragments. If associated spurring and bar formation are encountered remove these structures adequately. With the interspace spreader in position, use a drill, curets, Kerrison

rongeur, or standard rongeurs to carefully undercut and remove the ridges and spurs. The posterior longitudinal ligament may or may not be removed; removing it allows a good view of the dural sac and nerve root on one or both sides. If interbody grafting is omitted, close the longus colli and anterior longitudinal ligament anatomically.

If the Smith-Robinson technique of fusion is used, expose the iliac crest through a linear incision made just below the crest and carried down to the periosteum. Subperiosteally free the muscles from the inner and outer tables of the iliac crest. Obtain a tricortical bone graft of the appropriate size from the crest. Before harvesting the graft, measure the width and depth of the disc space. Fashion the graft so that it is 3 to 4 mm shorter and slightly wider than the disc space. Before inserting the graft, ask the anesthesiologist to add weight to the cervical traction to allow distraction of the disc space without a spreader. Prepare the end plates by curetting off all of the cartilage. Drill several holes into the end plates if desired. Do not remove the subchondral bone, or the graft will collapse into the bodies of the vertebrae. Insert the graft with appropriate measuring of the depth and reshaping of the graft so that it is countersunk. A properly prepared graft will require some tamping to pass the anterior lip of the vertebra. But excessive force must be avoided. Release the traction and test the graft for stability. Then remove the retractors and allow the tissues to fall into place. Close the subcutaneous tissue and skin. Drain the wound if there is any question of whether hemostasis has been achieved.

AFTERTREATMENT. The patient is placed in a Philadelphia collar if a fusion is performed to protect early soft tissue and bony healing and to avoid hyperextension of the neck that may dislodge the graft. Immobilization is not necessary after simple anterior disc excision. The patient should be monitored closely for any hypoxia. If reintubation is required, perform a blind nasal intubation or tracheostomy rather than risk extrusion of the graft by hyperextending the neck for a standard intubation. The patient is allowed out of bed following surgery if he desires. When the patient begins eating, it is suggested that the physician can be present. Liquids should be started first. If the patient has no dysphagia and is able to swallow without problems, he may be slowly advanced to solid foods, but it may be several days before eating solid food is allowed. If the patient complains of any dysphagia, eating should be discontinued to prevent aspiration and respiratory problems.

MIDLINE HERNIATIONS OF CERVICAL DISCS INTO SPINAL CANAL

Once the diagnosis of midline herniation into the spinal canal is established, early operation is indicated to prevent further damage to the spinal cord. In large extrusions with immediate complete paraplegia and with block of the spinal canal, it is unlikely that any treatment will restore function, but the herniated fragments should be removed immediately. If a posterior approach is preferred, a full laminectomy should be performed, and the fragments are removed transdurally. Commonly a midline or paracentral soft disc protrusion is difficult to differentiate from a neoplasm, and approaching the lesion posteriorly through the dura is mandatory. When the lesion is unquestionably a midline or paracentral disc protrusion, however, the anterior approach may be preferred to allow complete disc removal.

Generally the results of this operation have been disappointing because irreparable damage to the cord has occurred before operation. Should the diagnosis be made early and prompt treatment instituted, however, the results should be comparable to removal of any other mass from within the spinal canal.

THORACIC DISC DISEASE

Thoracic intervertebral disc rupture is extremely rare. Most studies place the incidence between 0.25% to 0.5% of all intervertebral disc ruptures. Arseni and Nash in 1963 were able to collect only 95 cases from the literature. The first diagnosis of a ruptured thoracic disc was probably made by Antoni in 1931. Several ruptures thereafter were misinterpreted as enchondrosis. In the late 1950s sporadic case reports and small series of thoracic intervertebral disc excisions appeared. Because of the small numbers of patients affected with this problem, the exact etiology and contributing factors have not been isolated. Trauma has been indicated in some patients, although in most the onset is somewhat insidious and intermittent as is true in disc disease in other areas of the spine. There is no clear-cut preponderance of males over females. The average age appears to be about 45 years in a collection of 102 cases from the world literature in 1965. Arseni and Nash noted that the discs between T10 and T12 are the most common areas for herniation, although herniation has been recorded at all thoracic levels.

Signs and symptoms

The duration of symptoms appears to be relatively long, averaging approximately 2 years. This is believed to be attributable to the somewhat vague and misleading symptoms. Patients may complain of bowel or bladder incontinence. Pain is predominantly in the thoracic region, although the lower back is the next most frequent site of pain. Pain occasionally is found in the abdominal or leg region. Complaints of unilateral and bilateral numbness, unilateral or bilateral weakness, both unilateral and bilateral hyperesthesias, and unsteadiness of gait have also been recorded. Physical examination has shown occasional spinal deformity. Localized dorsal kyphosis is extremely rare. Weakness may be demonstrated in the lower abdominal muscles in addition to leg weakness, which is frequently bilateral. Proximal and distal muscle groups are usually comparably weak, but some patients may have symptoms similar to a more distal lumbar disc herniation. Occasionally the initial presentation may be a complete paraplegia or sudden onset of Brown-Séquard syndrome (unilateral paralysis with contralateral loss of sensibility). Sensory loss is common and is usually bilateral. Deep tendon reflexes are usually hyperreflexic. Plantar responses are frequently extensor, and clonus may be demonstrated.

Confirmatory testing

Since the level of herniation cannot be determined clinically, myelography is mandatory. With present technology, computed tomography that is performed after myelography at the area of pathology may provide additional information as to the extent and location of the herniation. Magnetic resonance imaging offers the ability to identify intradural and extradural tumors, disc degenerations, nerve root impingements, and disc herniations. This procedure may also present further evidence as to the nature of the lesion because an extradural tumor can also result in findings similar to a herniated thoracic disc. In mild ruptures in which minimal findings can be identified, cystometrograms may indicate bladder dysfunction. Somatosensory testing may also be abnormal.

Treatment results

There is no evidence to indicate the value of conservative therapy in this problem because of its low incidence of clinical detection. All patients reported in the literature have been treated surgically. The initial procedure recommended for this lesion was posterior thoracic laminectomy and disc excision. At least half of the lesions have been identified as being central, making the excision from this approach extremely difficult, and the results were somewhat disheartening. Most series reported less than half of the patients improving with some becoming worse after posterior laminectomy and discectomy. Most recent studies suggest that lateral rachiotomy (modified costotransversectomy) or an anterior transthoracic approach for discectomy produces considerably better results with no evidence of worsening after the procedure.

Costotransversectomy

Costotransversectomy is probably best suited for thoacic disc herniations that are predominantly lateral or herniations that are suspected to be extruded or sequestered. Central disc herniations are probably best approached transthoracically. Some surgeons have recommended subsequent fusion after disc removal anteriorly or laterally.

TECHNIQUE. The operation is usually done with the patient under general anesthesia with a cuffed endotracheal tube or a Carlen tube to allow lung deflation on the side of approach. Place the patient in the prone position and make a long midline incision or a curved incision concave to the midline centered over the level of involvement. Expose the spine in the usual manner out to the ribs. Remove a section of rib 5 to 7.5 cm long at the level of involvement, taking care to avoid damage to the intercostal nerve and artery. Carry the resection into the lateral side of the disc, exposing it for removal. Additional exposure can be made by laminectomy and excision of the pedicle and facet joint. Fusion is unnecessary unless more than one facet joint is removed. Close the wound in layers.

AFTERTREATMENT. The aftertreatment is similar to that for lumbar disc excision without fusion (p. 3297).

Anterior approach for thoracic disc excision

Because of the relative age of patients with thoracic disc ruptures, special care must be taken to identify those with pulmonary problems. In these patients, the anterior approach may be detrimental medically, making a posterolateral approach safer. Patients with midline protrusions are probably best treated with the transthoracic approach to ensure complete disc removal. A Carlen tube may be beneficial in allowing deflation of the lung on the side of the operation.

TECHNIQUE. The operation is performed with the patient under general anesthesia, using a cuffed endotracheal tube or Carlen tube for lung deflation on the side of the approach. Place the patient in a lateral recumbent position. A left-sided anterior approach is usually preferred, making the operative procedure easier. Make a skin incision along the line of the rib that corresponds to the second thoracic vertebra *above* the involved intervertebral disc except for approaches to the upper five thoracic segments where the approach is through the third rib. Choose the skin incision by inspection of the anteroposterior roentgenogram. Cut the rib subperiosteally at its posterior and anterior ends then insert a rib retractor. Save the rib for grafting later in the procedure. One may then decide on an extrapleural or transpleural approach depending on familiarity and ease. Exposure of the thoracic vertebrae should give adequate access to the front and opposite side. Dissect the great vessels free of the spine. Ligate the intersegmental vessels near the great vessels and not near the foramen. One should be able to insert a finger tip against the opposite side of the disc when the vascular mobilization is complete. Exposure of the intervertebral disc without disturbing more than three segmental vessels is preferable to avoid ischemic problems in the spinal cord. In the thoracolumbar region strip the diaphragm from the eleventh and twelfth ribs. The anterior longitudinal ligament is usually sectioned to allow spreading of the intervertebral disc space. Remove the disc as completely as possible. The use of the operating microscope or loupe magnification eases the removal of the disc near the posterior longitudinal ligament. Remove the disc up to the posterior longitudinal ligament using nibbling instruments. Then place a finger on the opposite side of the disc to avoid penetration when removing disc material on the more distant side. Carefully inspect the posterior longitudinal ligament for tears and extruded fragments. Remove the posterior longitudinal ligament only if necessary. Significant bleeding may occur if the venous plexus near the dura is torn. After removal of the disc, strip the end plates of their cartilage. Make a slot in one vertebral body and a hole in the body on the opposite side of the disc space to accept the graft material. Make the hole large enough to accept several sections of rib, but make the slot only large enough to accept one rib graft at a time. Then insert iliac, tibial, or rib grafts into the disc space. Tie the grafts together with heavy suture material when the maximum number of grafts have been inserted. Close the wound in the usual manner and employ standard chest drainage.

The transthoracic approach removing a rib two levels above the level of the lesion may be used up to T5. The transthoracic approach from T2 to T5 is best made by excision of the third or fourth rib and elevation of the scapula by sectioning of attachments of the serratus anterior and trapezius from the scapula. The approach to T1-2 disc is best made from the neck with a sternal splitting incision.

AFTERTREATMENT. Postoperative care is the same as for a thoracotomy. The patient is allowed to walk after the chest tubes are removed. Extension in any position is prohibited. A brace or body cast that limits extension should be used if the stability of the graft is questionable. The graft is usually stable without support if only one disc space is removed. Postoperative care is the same as for the anterior corpectomy and fusion if more than one disc level is removed.

LUMBAR DISC DISEASE
Symptoms

Although back pain is common from the second decade of life on, intervertebral disc disease and disc herniation are most prominent in otherwise healthy people in the third and fourth decades of life. Most people relate their back and leg pain to a traumatic incident, but close questioning frequently reveals that the patient has had intermittent episodes of back pain for many months or even years before the onset of severe leg pain. In many instances, the back pain is relatively fleeting in nature and is relieved by rest. This pain is often brought on by heavy exertion, repetitive bending, twisting, or heavy lifting. In other instances, an exacerbating incident cannot be elicited. The pain usually begins in the lower back, radiating to the sacroiliac region and buttocks. The pain can radiate down the posterior thigh. Back and posterior thigh pain of this type can be elicited from many areas of the spine, including the facet joints, longitudinal ligaments, and the periosteum of the vertebra. Radicular pain, on the other hand, usually extends below the knee and follows the dermatome of the involved nerve root.

The usual history of lumbar disc herniation is of repetitive, lower back and buttock pain, relieved by rest after a short period of time. This pain is then suddenly exacerbated by a flexion episode, with the sudden appearance of leg pain much greater than back pain. Most radicular pain from nerve root compression caused by a herniated nucleus pulposus is evidenced by leg pain equal to, or in many cases much greater than, the degree of back pain. Whenever leg pain is minimal and back pain is predominant, great care should be taken before making the diagnosis of a herniated intervertebral disc. The pain from disc herniation is usually intermittent in nature, increasing with activity, especially sitting. The pain may be relieved by rest, especially in the semi-Fowler position, and may be exacerbated by straining, sneezing, or coughing. Whenever the pattern of pain is bizarre or the pain itself is constant, a diagnosis of herniated disc should be viewed with some skepticism.

Other symptoms of disc herniation include weakness and paresthesias. In most patients the weakness is intermittent, variable with activity, and localized to the neurologic level of involvement. Paresthesias are also variable and limited to the dermatome of the involved nerve root. Whenever these complaints are generalized, the diagnosis of a simple unilateral disc herniation should be questioned.

Numbness and weakness in the involved leg and occasionally pain in the groin or testicle can be associated with a high or midline lumbar disc herniation. If a fragment is large or the herniation is high, symptoms of pressure on the entire cauda equina can be elicited. These include numbness and weakness in both legs, rectal pain, numbness in the perineum, and paralysis of the sphincters. This diagnosis should be the primary consideration in patients who complain of sudden loss of bowel or bladder control. Whenever the diagnosis of a cauda equina syndrome or acute midline herniation is suspected, evaluation and treatment should be aggressive.

Physical findings

The physical findings in back pain with disc disease are variable because of the time intervals involved. Usually patients with acute pain show evidence of marked paraspinal spasm that is sustained during walking or motion. A scoliosis or a list in the lumbar spine may be present, and in many patients the normal lumbar lordosis is lost. As the acute episode subsides, the degree of spasm diminishes remarkably, and the loss of normal lumbar lordosis may be the only telltale sign. Point tenderness may be present over the spinous process at the level of the disc involved and in some patients pain may extend laterally.

If there is nerve root irritation, it centers over the length of the sciatic nerve, both in the sciatic notch and more distally in the popliteal space. In addition, stretch of the sciatic nerve at the knee should reproduce buttock anbd leg pain. A Lasègue sign is usually positive on the involved

---

L4 root compression

(indicative of L3-4 disc herniation or pathology localized to the L-4 foramen)

Sensory deficit
  Posterolateral thigh, anterior knee and medial leg
Motor weakness
  Quadriceps (variable)
  Hip adductors (variable)
Reflex changes
  Patellar tendon
  Tibialis anterior tendon (variable)

L5 root compression

(indicative of L4-5 disc herniation or pathology localized to the L-5 foramen)

Sensory deficit
  Anterolateral leg, dorsum of the foot and great toe
Motor weakness
  Extensor hallucis longus
  Gluteus medius
  Extensor digitorum longus and brevis
Reflex changes
  Usually none
  Tibialis posterior (difficult to elicit)

S1 root compression

(indicative of an L5-S1 disc herniation or pathology localized to the S1 foramen)

Sensory deficit
  Lateral malleolus, lateral foot, heel, and web of fourth and fifth toes
Motor weakness
  Peroneus longus and brevis
  Gastrocnemius-soleus complex
  Gluteus maximus
Reflex changes
  Tendo calcaneus (gastrocnemius-soleus complex)

Ruptured disc between L-3 and L-4

with compression of the fourth nerve root

Pain
  Sacroiliac joint and hip
  Posterolateral aspect of thigh
  Anterior aspect of leg
Numbness
  Anteromedial aspect of leg
Weakness
  Extension of knee
Reflexes
  Decreased or absent knee jerk

Ruptured disc between L-4 and L-5

with compression of the fifth nerve root

Pain
  Sacroiliac joint and hip
  Posterolateral aspect of thigh and leg
Numbness
  Lateral aspect of leg or dorsum of foot, including great toe
Weakness
  Dorsiflexion of great toe and occasionally of foot
Reflexes
  No change

Ruptured disc between L-5 and sacrum

with compression of the first sacral nerve root

Pain
  Over sacroiliac joint and hip
  Posterolateral aspect of thigh, leg, and heel
Numbness
  Lateral aspect of leg and foot, including three lateral toes
Weakness
  Unusual; plantar flexion of foot and great toe
Reflexes
  Reduced or absent ankle jerk

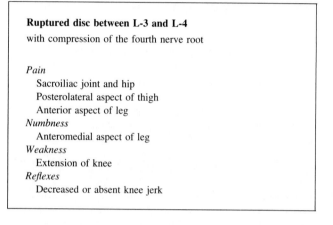

side. A positive Lasègue sign or straight leg raising should elicit buttock or leg pain or both on the side tested. Occasionally if leg pain is significant the patient will move back from a sitting position and assume the tripod stance to relieve the pain. Contralateral leg pain produced by straight leg raising should be regarded as pathognomonic of a herniated intervertebral disc. The absence of a positive Lasègue sign should make one skeptical of the diagnosis. Likewise, inappropriate findings and inconsistencies in the examination are usually nonorganic in origin. If the leg pain has persisted for any length of time, atrophy of the involved limb may be present as demonstrated by asymmetric girth of the thigh or calf. The neurologic examination will vary as determined by the level of root involvement.

Unilateral disc herniation between L3 and L4 usually compresses the fourth lumbar root as it crosses the disc before exiting at the L4 intervertebral foramen. Pain may be localized around the medial side of the leg. Numbness may be present over the anteromedial aspect of the leg. The quadriceps and hip adductor group, both innervated from L2, L3, and L4, may be weak, and in extended ruptures atrophic. Reflex testing may reveal a diminished or absent patellar tendon reflex (L2, L3, and L4) or tibialis anterior tendon reflex (L4). Sensory testing may show diminished sensibility over the L4 dermatome, the isolated portion of which is the medial leg (Fig. 73-22) and the autonomous zone is at the level of the medial malleolus.

Unilateral disc herniation between L4 and L5 results in compression of the fifth lumbar root. Fifth lumbar root radiculopathy should produce pain in the dermatomal pattern. Numbness, when present, follows the L5 dermatome along the anterolateral aspect of the leg and the dorsum of the foot, including the great toe. The autonomous zone for

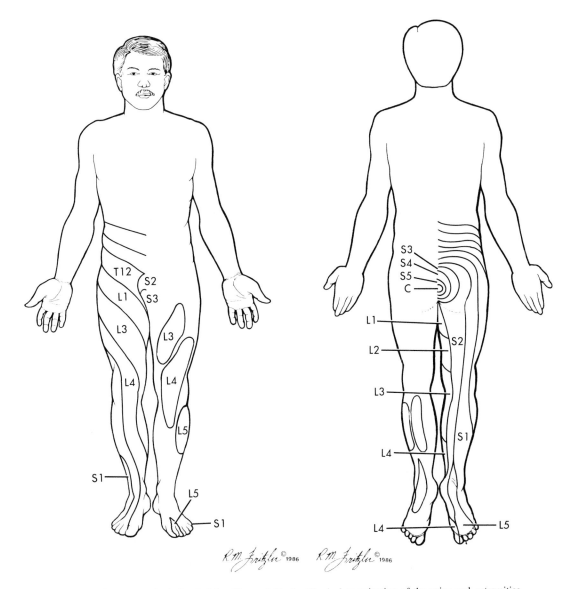

Fig. 73-22. L4 neurologic level (After Hoppenfeld, S.: Physical examination of the spine and extremities, Norwalk, Conn., 1976, Appleton-Century-Crofts.)

this nerve is the first web of the foot and the dorsum of the third toe. Weakness may involve the extensor hallucis longus (L5), gluteus medius (L5), or extensor digitorum longus and brevis (L5). Reflex change is usually not found. A diminished tibialis posterior reflex is possible but hard to elicit.

In a unilateral ruptured disc between L5 and S1 the findings of an S1 radiculopathy are noted. Pain and numbness involve the dermatome of S1. The S1 dermatome includes the lateral malleolus and the lateral and plantar surface of the foot, occasionally including the heel. There is numbness over the lateral aspect of the leg and more importantly over the lateral aspect of the foot, including the lateral three toes. The autonomous zone for this root is the dorsum of the fifth toe. Weakness may be demonstrated in the peroneus longus and brevis (S1), gastrocnemius-soleus (S1) or the gluteus maximus (S1). In general, weakness is not a usual finding in S1 radiculopathy. Occasionally mild weakness may be demonstrated by asymmetric fatigue with exercise of these motor groups. The ankle jerk is usually reduced or absent.

Massive extrusion of a disc involving the entire diameter of the lumbar canal or a large midline extrusion may produce pain in the back, legs, and occasionally the perineum. Both legs may be paralyzed, the sphincters may be incontinent, and the ankle jerks may be absent. Tay and Chacha in 1979 reported that the combination of saddle anesthesia, bilateral ankle areflexia, and bladder symptoms were the most consistent symptoms of cauda equina syndrome caused by massive intervertebral disc extrusion at any lumbar level. In these instances a cystometrogram may show bladder denervation.

More than 95% of the ruptures of the lumbar intervertebral discs occur at L4 and L5. Ruptures at higher levels in many patients are not associated with a positive straight leg raising test. In these instances, a positive femoral stretch test may be helpful. This test is carried out by placing the patient in the prone position and acutely flexing the leg while placing the hand in the popliteal fossa. When this procedure results in anterior thigh pain, the result is positive and a high lesion should be suspected. In addition, these lesions may occur with a more diffuse neurologic complaint without significant localizing neurologic signs.

Many times, the neurologic signs associated with disc disease vary over time. If the patient has been up and walking for a period of time, the neurologic findings may be much more pronounced than if he has been at bedrest for several days, thus decreasing the pressure on the nerve root and allowing the nerve to resume its normal function. Additionally, various conservative treatments may change the physical signs of disc disease. Comparative examination of a patient with back and leg pain is essential in finding a clear-cut pattern of signs and symptoms. It is not uncommon for the evaluation to change. Adverse changes in the examination may warrant more aggressive therapy, whereas improvement of the symptoms or signs should signal a resolution of the problem. Early symptoms or signs suggestive of cauda equina syndrome or severe or progressive neurologic deficit should be treated aggressively from the onset. McLaren and Bailey warn that the cauda equina syndrome is more frequent when disc excision is performed in the presence of an untreated spinal stenosis at the same level.

Differential diagnosis

The differential diagnosis of back and leg pain is extremely lengthy and complex. It includes diseases intrinsic to the spine and those involving adjacent organs but causing pain referred to the back or leg. For simplicity, lesions can be categorized as being extrinsic or intrinsic to the spine. Extrinsic lesions include diseases of the urogenital system, gastrointestinal system, vascular system, endocrine system, nervous system not localized to the spine, and the extrinsic musculoskeletal system. These lesions may include infections, tumors, metabolic disturbances, congenital abnormalities, or the associated diseases of aging. Intrinsic lesions involve those diseases that arise primarily in the spine. They include diseases of the spinal musculoskeletal system, the local hematopoietic system, and the local neurologic system. These conditions include trauma, tumors, infections, diseases of aging, and immune diseases affecting the spine or spinal nerves.

Although the predominant cause of back and leg pain in healthy people is usually caused by lumbar disc disease, one must be extremely cautious to avoid a misdiagnosis. Therefore a full physical examination must be performed before making a presumptive diagnosis of herniated disc disease. Common diseases that can mimic disc disease include ankylosing spondylitis, multiple myeloma, vascular insufficiency, arthritis of the hip, osteoporosis with stress fractures, extradural tumors, peripheral neuropathy, and herpes zoster.

Conservative therapy

The number and variety of nonoperative therapies for back and leg pain are overwhelming. Treatments range from simple rest to expensive traction apparatus. All of these therapies are reported with glowing accounts of miraculous "cures." Unfortunately, few have been evaluated scientifically. In addition, the natural history of disc disease is characterized by exacerbations and remissions with improvement eventually regardless of treatment. Finally, several distinct symptom complexes appear to be associated with disc disease. Few if any studies have isolated the response to specific and anatomically distinct diagnoses.

The simplest treatment for acute back pain is rest. Biomechanical studies indicate that lying in a semi-Fowler position or on the side with the hips and knees flexed with a pillow between the legs should relieve most pressure on the disc and nerve roots. Muscle spasm can be controlled by the application of ice, preferably in a massage over the muscles in spasm. Pain relief and antiinflammatory effect can be achieved with aspirin. Most acute exacerbations of back pain respond quickly to this therapy. As the pain diminishes, the patient should be encouraged to begin isometric abdominal and lower extremity exercises. Walking within the limits of comfort is also encouraged. Sitting, especially riding in a car, is discouraged.

Education in proper posture and body mechanics is helpful in returning the patient to his usual level of activity after the acute exacerbation is eased or relieved. This education can take many forms from individual instruction to group instruction. Back education of this type is now usually referred to as "Back School." Although the concept is excellent, the quality and quantity of information provided may vary widely. The work of Bergquist-Ullman and Larsson and others indicates that patient education of this type is extremely beneficial in decreasing the amount of time lost from work initially but does little to decrease the incidence of recurrence of symptoms or length of time from work lost during recurrences. Certainly the combination of back education and combined physical therapy is superior to placebo treatment.

Numerous medications have been used with varied results in back and leg pain syndromes. The present trend appears to be away from the use of strong narcotics and muscle relaxants in the outpatient treatment of these syndromes. This is especially true in the instances of chronic back and leg pain where drug habituation and increased depression are frequent. Oral steroids used briefly may also be beneficial as a strong antinflammatory agent. The numerous types of nonsteroidal antiinflammatory medications are also helpful when aspirin is not tolerated or is of little help. When depression is prominent, mood elevators such as amitriptyline may be beneficial in reducing sleep disturbance and anxiety without increasing depression. In addition, the use of amitriptyline also decreases the need for narcotic medication.

Physical therapy should be used judiciously. The exercises should be fitted to the symptoms and not forced as an absolute group of activities. Patients with acute back and thigh pain eased by passive extension of the spine in the prone position may be helped by extension exercises rather than flexion exercises. Improvement in symptoms with extension is indicative of a good prognosis with conservative care. On the other hand, patients whose pain is increased by passive extension may be improved by flexion exercises. These exercises should not be forced in the face of increased pain. This may avoid further disc extrusion. Any exercise that increases pain should be discontinued. Lower extremity exercises may increase strength and relieve stress on the back, but they may also exacerbate lower extremity arthritis. The true benefit of such treatments may be in the promotion of good posture and body mechanics rather than of strength.

Numerous treatment modalities have been and will be advanced for the treatment of back pain. Some patients respond to the use of transcutaneous electrical nerve stimulation (TENS). Others do well with traction varying from skin traction in bed with 5 to 8 pounds to body inversion with forces of over 100 pounds. Back braces or corsets may be helpful to other patients. Ultrasound and diathermy are other treatments used in back pain. The scientific efficacy of many of these treatments has not been proven. In addition, all therapy for disc disease is only symptomatic.

Epidural steroids

The epidural injection of a combination of a long-acting steroid with an epidural anesthetic is an excellent method of symptomatic treatment of back and leg pain from discogenic disease and other sources. Most studies show a 60% to 85% short-term success rate that falls to a 30% to 40% long-term (6-month) good result rate. The local effect of the steroids has been shown to last at least 3 weeks at a therapeutic level. In a well-controlled study Berman et al. found that the best results were obtained in patients with subacute or chronic leg pain with no prior surgery. They also found that the worst results were in patients with motor or reflex abnormalities (12% to 14% good results). A negative myelogram was also associated with a better result. Cuckler et al. in a double-blind randomized study of epidural steroid treatment of disc herniation and spinal stenosis found no difference in the results at 6 months between placebo and a single epidural injection. Our experience parallels that of Berman et al. We agree that epidural steroids are not a "cure for disc disease," but they do offer relatively prolonged pain relief without excessive narcotic intake if conservative care is elected.

In experienced hands the complication rate from this procedure should be small. White et al. have shown that the most common problem is a 25% rate of failure to place the material in the epidural space. Another technique-related problem is intrathecal injection with inadvertent spinal anesthesia. Other reported complications include transient hypotension, difficulty in voiding, severe paresthesias, cardiac angina, headache, and transient hypercorticoidism. The most serious complication reported was a bacterial meningitis. The total complication rate in most series is about 5%, and the complications are almost always transient.

This procedure is contraindicated in the presence of infection, neurologic disease (such as multiple sclerosis), hemorrhagic or bleeding diathesis, cauda equina syndrome, and a rapidly progressive neural deficit. Rapid injections of large volumes or the use of large doses of steroid may also increase the complication rate. The exact effects of intrathecal injection of steroids are not known. This technique must only be used in the low lumbar region. We prefer to abort the procedure if a bloody tap is obtained or if cerebral spinal fluid is encountered.

We prefer to perform the procedure in a room equipped for resuscitation and with the capability to monitor the patient. Experienced anesthesiologists usually perform the procedure in our institution. This procedure lends itself well to outpatient use, but the patient must be prepared to spend several hours to recover from the block. Methylprednisolone (Depo-medrol) is the usual steroid injected. The dosage may vary from 80 to 120 mg. The anesthetics used may include lidocaine, bupivacaine, or procaine. Our present protocol is to inject the patient three times. These injections are made at 48- to 72-hour intervals. This assures at least one good epidural injection and decreases the volume of material injected at each procedure.

TECHNIQUE (BROWN). The equipment needed includes material for an appropriate skin preparation, sterile rubber gloves, a 3½-inch, 20-gauge or 22-gauge disposable spinal needle (45-degree blunt- or curve-tipped epidural needles are preferred), several disposable syringes, bacteriostatic 1% lidocaine, and methylprednisolone acetate 40 mg/ml. The injection may be performed with the patient in the sitting or lateral decubitus position. Anesthetize the skin near the midline. Advance the needle until the resistance of the ligamentum flavum is encountered. Then attach a syringe and slowly advance the needle while applying light pressure on the syringe. When the epidural space is encountered, the resistance is suddenly lost and the epidural space will accommodate the air. Remove the syringe and inspect the needle opening for blood or spinal fluid. If there is no flow out of the needle, then inject 3 ml of 1% lidocaine or other appropriate anesthetic. This may be preceded or followed by the chosen dosage of methylprednisolone.

Several variations may also be used. Some physicians use a sterile balloon to indicate the proper space. Others use the ''disappearing drop'' technique which involves placing a drop of sterile saline over the hub of the needle. When the epidural space is entered, the drop will disappear. Caudal injection is also used, but this may require larger volumes to wash the steroid up to the involved level. This method is safer but less reliable than an injection at L4-5.

Surgery

When conservative treatment for lumbar disc disease fails, the next thought is surgical treatment. Before this step is taken, the surgeon must be sure of the diagnosis. The patient must be certain that the degree of pain and impairment warrants such a drastic step. Both the surgeon and the patient must realize that disc surgery is not a cure but may provide symptomatic relief. It neither stops the pathologic processes that allowed the herniation to occur nor restores the back to its previous state. The patient must still practice good posture and body mechanics after surgery. Activities involving repetitive bending, twisting, and lifting with the spine in flexion may have to be curtailed or eliminated. If prolonged relief is to be expected, then some permanent modification in the patient's lifestyle may be necessary.

The key to good results in disc surgery is appropriate patient selection. The optimum patient is one with predominant, if not only, unilateral leg pain extending below the knee that has been present for at least 6 weeks. The pain should have been decreased by rest, antiinflammatory medication, or even epidural steroids but recurred to the initial levels after a minimum of 6 to 8 weeks of conservative care. Physical examination should reveal signs of sciatic irritation and possibly objective evidence of localizing neurologic impairment. Computed tomography or myelography should confirm the level of involvement consistent with the patient's examination. Finally, psychologic testing should show a hysteria or hypochondriasis T score of 75 or less. Regardless of the technique or surgeon, one can easily predict a better than 90% chance of improvement or relief of the leg pain in this situation.

Surgical disc removal is only mandatory and urgent in cauda equina syndrome with significant neurologic deficit, especially bowel or bladder disturbance. All other disc excisions should be considered elective. This should allow a thorough evaluation to confirm the diagnosis, level of involvement, and the physical and psychologic status of the patient. Frequently when there is a rush to the operating room to relieve pain without proper investigation both the patient and physician later regret the decision.

Regardless of the method chosen to surgically treat a disc rupture, the patient should be aware that the procedure is for the symptomatic relief of leg pain. Patients with predominant back pain may not be relieved of their major complaint—back pain. Spangfort in reviewing 2504 lumbar disc excisions found that about 30% of the patients complained of back pain after disc surgery. Failure to relieve sciatica was proportional to the degree of herniation. The best results of 90% complete relief and 0.5% no relief (99.5% complete or partial pain relief) were obtained when the disc was free in the canal or sequestered. Incomplete herniation or extrusion of disc material into the canal resulted in complete relief for 82% of patients . Excision of the bulging or protruding disc that had not ruptured through the anulus resulted in complete relief in 63%, and removal of the normal or minimally bulging disc resulted in complete relief in 38% (this is near the stated level for the placebo response). Likewise the incidence of persistent back pain after surgery was inversely proportional to the degree of herniation. In patients with complete extrusions the incidence was about 25%, but with minimal bulges or negative explorations the incidence rose to over 55% (Figs. 73-23 and 73-24).

GENERAL PRINCIPLES FOR OPEN DISC SURGERY

Most disc surgery is performed with the patient under general endotracheal anesthesia, though local anesthesia has been used with minimal complications. Patient positioning varies with the operative technique and surgeon. To position the patient in a modified kneeling position, a specialized frame, or custom frame modified from the design of Hastings is gaining popularity. Positioning the patient in this manner allows the abdomen to hang free, minimizing epidural venous dilatation and bleeding (Fig. 73-25). A head lamp allows the surgeon to direct light into the lateral recesses where a large proportion of the surgery may be required. The addition of loupe magnification also greatly enhances the identification and exposure of various structures. Some surgeons also use the operative microscope to further enhance visibility. Roentgenographic confirmation of the proper level may be necessary if the exposure is small or if there is question as to the anatomic level during the dissection. Care should be taken to protect neural structures. Epidural bleeding should be controlled with bipolar electrocautery. Any sponge, pack, or cottonoid patty placed in the wound should extend to the outside. Pituitary rongeurs should be marked at a point equal to the maximum allowable disc depth to prevent accidental biopsy of viscera or aorta. Considerable research has gone into techniques to prevent epidural fibrosis. The placement of a large chunk of autogenous fat appears to be a reasonable although not foolproof or complication-free technique of minimizing postoperative epidural fibrosis.

RUPTURED LUMBAR DISC EXCISION

TECHNIQUE. After thoroughly preparing the back, identify the spinous processes of L3, L4, L5, and S1. Make a midline incision 5 to 10 cm long, in most instances from the spinous process of the fourth lumbar vertebra to the first sacral spinous process; if exploration of the third disc is contemplated, make the incision to the third lumbar spinous process. Incise the supraspinous ligament from the

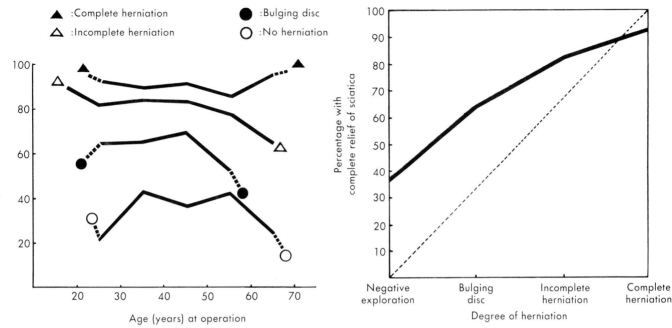

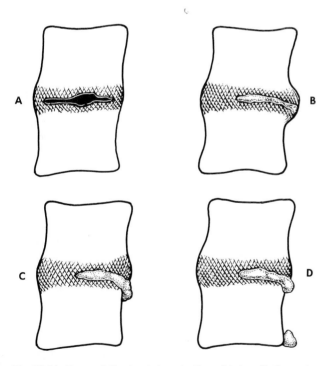

Fig. 73-23. Percent relief of sciatica with type of disc herniation. (From Spangfort, E.: Acta Orthop. Scand. Suppl. **142**:1, 1972.)

Fig. 73-24. Types of disc herniation. **A,** Normal bulge. **B,** Protrusion. **C,** Extrusion. **D,** Sequestration.

fourth lumbar to the first sacral spinous process. Then by subperiosteal dissection strip the muscles from the spines and laminae of these vertebrae on the side of the lesion. Retract the muscles either with a self-retaining retractor or with the help of an assistant and expose one interspace at a time. Verify the position of the sacrum by palpation and direct vision so that no mistake is made regarding the in-

terspaces being explored. Secure hemostasis with electrocautery, bone wax, and packs. Leave a portion of each pack completely outside the wound for ready identification.

Denude the laminae and ligamentum flavum with a curet (Fig. 73-26). Commonly the lumbosacral interspace is large enough to permit exposure and removal of a herniated nucleus pulposus without removal of any bone. If not, remove a small part of the inferior margin of the fifth lumbar lamina. Exposure of the disc at higher levels usually requires removal of a portion of the inferior lamina. Grasp the ligamentum flavum with an Allis or Kocher clamp and incise it with a bayonet-pointed knife where it fuses with the interspinous ligament. During dissection of the ligament keep the point of the knife in view so that the dura will not be nicked. Remove the flap of ligamentum flavum by sharp dissection. With an angulated Kerrison rongeur carefully remove the small shelving portion of ligamentum flavum left laterally. Next, retract the dura medially and identify the nerve root. If the root is compressed by a large extruded fragment, it will commonly be displaced posteriorly. Retract the nerve root, once identified, medially so that the underlying extruded fragment or bulging posterior longitudinal ligament can be seen. Occasionally the nerve root adheres to the fragment or to the underlying ligamentous structures and will require sharp dissection from these structures. If there is any question as to the position of the root, remove the lamina until the pedicle is visible. This will allow the identification of the upper and lower roots. Use cottonoid patties to tamponade the epidural veins both caudad and cephalad once the nerve root has been identified and retracted. Take care to minimize packing about the nerve root. Retract the root or dura, identify any bleeding vein and cauterize it with a bipolar cautery. Earlier insertion of cottonoid patties may

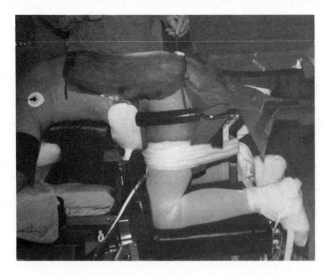

Fig. 73-25. Kneeling position for lumbar disc excision allows abdomen to be completely free of external pressure.

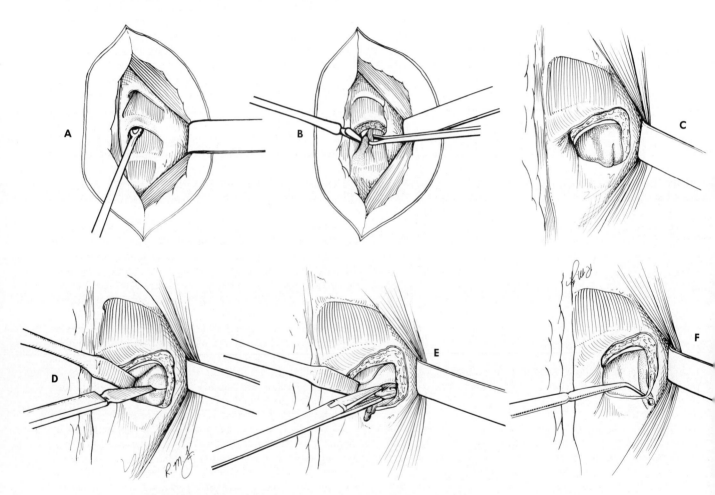

Fig. 73-26. Technique of lumbar disc excision. **A,** With lamina and ligamentum flavum exposed, use curet to remove the ligamentum flavum from inferior surface of lamina. Kerrison rongeur is used to remove bone. **B,** Ligamentum flavum is elevated at upper corner and carefully dissected back to expose dura and epidural fat below. Patties should be used to protect dura during this procedure. **C,** Dura and root are exposed. Additional bone should be removed if there is any question about adequacy of exposure. **D,** Nerve root and dural sac are retracted to expose disc. Inspect capsule for rent and extruded nuclear material. If obvious ligamentous defect is not visible, then carefully incise capsule of disc. If disc material does not bulge out, press on disc to try to dislodge herniated fragment. **E,** Carefully remove disc fragments. It is safest to not open pituitary rongeur until it is inserted into disc space. **F,** After removing disc, carefully explore foramen, subligamentous region, and beneath dura for additional fragments of disc. Obtain meticulous hemostasis using bipolar cauterization.

well displace fragments from view. The underlying disc should be clearly visible at this time.

Hold the nerve by a Love root retractor or a blunt dissector, thus exposing the herniated fragment or posterior longitudinal ligament and anulus. If an extruded fragment is not seen, carefully palpate the posterior longitudinal ligament and seek a defect or hole in the ligamentous structures. If no obvious abnormality is detected, follow the root around the pedicle or even outside the canal in search of fragments that may have migrated far laterally. Additional searching in the root axilla helps ensure that fragments that have migrated inferiorly are not missed.

If the herniated fragment is especially large, it is much better to sacrifice the facet to obtain a more lateral exposure than to risk injury to the root or cauda equina by excessive medial retraction. With such a lateral exposure the nerve root can usually be elevated, and the herniated fragment can be teased from beneath the nerve root and cauda equina, even when the fragment is large enough to block the entire canal. If the disc cannot be teased from under the root, make a cruciate incision in the disc laterally. Gently remove disc fragments until the bulge has been decompressed to allow gentle retraction of the root over the defect.

If the herniation is upward or downward, further removal of bone from the lamina and facet edges may be required. The herniated nucleus pulposus may be covered by a layer of posterior longitudinal ligament or may have ruptured through this structure. In the latter event carefully lift the loose fragments out by suction, blunt hook, or pituitary forceps. If the ligament is intact, incise it in a cruciate fashion and remove the loose fragments. The tear or hole in the anulus should then be identifiable in most instances. The cavity of the disc may be entered through this hole, or occasionally the hole may need enlargement to allow insertion of the pituitary forceps. Remember that the anterior part of the anulus is adjacent to the aorta, vena cava, or iliac arteries and that one of these structures may be injured if one proceeds too deeply. Remove other loose fragments of nucleus pulposus with the pituitary forceps and curet loose and remove the additional nuclear material along with the central portion of the cartilaginous plates, both above and below.

Early in the dissection of the disc space measure or palpate the level of the anterior anulus and take care throughout this portion of the procedure not to exceed the distance to the anterior anulus. Then carry out a complete search for additional fragments of nucleus pulposus, both inside and outside the disc space. Additional fragments commonly migrate medially beneath the posterior longitudinal ligament but outside the anulus and may easily be missed. Then remove all cotton pledgets and control residual bleeding with Gelfoam or bits of muscle or fat; remove the Gelfoam or muscle after bleeding has been controlled with bipolar cautery. Close the wound routinely with absorbable sutures in the supraspinous ligament and subcutaneous tissue. Various nonabsorbable sutures or skin staples are most commonly used in routine skin closure.

AFTERTREATMENT. The patient is allowed to turn in bed at will and to select a position of comfort such as a semi-Fowler position. Opiates are used for pain control. Bladder stimulants may be used to assist voiding. The patient is allowed to stand with assistance on the evening after surgery to go to the bathroom. The patient is encouraged to walk on the first postoperative day. Isometric abdominal and lower extremity exercises are reinstituted. Sitting is minimized, but walking is progressively increased. When the patient is walking comfortably and pain medication intake is minimal, the patient is discharged. He is instructed to minimize sitting and riding in a vehicle. Increased walking on a daily basis is recommended. Lifting, bending, and stooping are prohibited for the first several weeks. The sutures are removed in 10 to 14 days. As the patient's strength increases, gentle isotonic leg exercises are started.

Between the fourth and sixth postoperative week Back School instruction is resumed or started provided pain is minimal. Lifting, bending, and stooping are gradually restarted after the sixth week. Increased sitting is allowed after the fourth week, but long trips are to be avoided for at least 3 months. Lower extremity strength is increased from the eighth to twelfth postoperative weeks. Patients with jobs requiring much walking without lifting are allowed to return to work within 4 weeks. Patients with jobs requiring prolonged sitting are usually returned to work within 6 to 8 weeks provided minimal lifting is required. Patients with jobs requiring heavy labor or long periods of driving are not returned to work until the twelfth week and then to a modified duty. Some patients with jobs requiring exceptionally heavy manual labor may have to permanently modify their occupation or seek a lighter occupation. Note that keeping the patient out of work beyond 3 months rarely improves recovery or pain relief.

MICROLUMBAR DISC EXCISION

Microlumbar discectomy requires an operating microscope with a 400 mm lens; special retractors; a 1 mm, 45-degree Kerrison rongeur; a micropituitary rongeur; and a combination suction nerve root retractor. The procedure is performed with the patient in the prone position. A vacuum pack is molded around the patient, and an inflatable pillow is positioned under the abdomen and is removed after evacuation of the vacuum pack. The microscope is used from skin incision to closure. If the proper level is in question, a lateral roentgenogram is taken to confirm placement.

TECHNIQUE (WILLIAMS). Make the incision from the spinous process of the upper vertebra to the spinous process of the lower vertebra at the involved level. This usually results in a 1-inch (2.5 cm) skin incision (Fig. 73-27). Maintain meticulous hemostasis with electrocautery as the dissection is carried to the fascia. Incise the fascia at the midline using electrocautery. Then insert a periosteal elevator in the midline incision. Using gentle lateral movements separate the deep fascia and muscle subperiosteally from the spinous processes and lamina. Meticulously cauterize all bleeding points. Then insert a finger to palpate the interlaminar space. Insert the microlumbar retractor into the wound and adjust the microscope. Identify the ligamentum flavum and lamina. Using a No. 15 blade with the microscope set at a 25× magnification, carefully incise the ligamentum flavum superficially. Then use a Penfield No. 4 dissector to perforate the ligamentum. Minimal force should be used

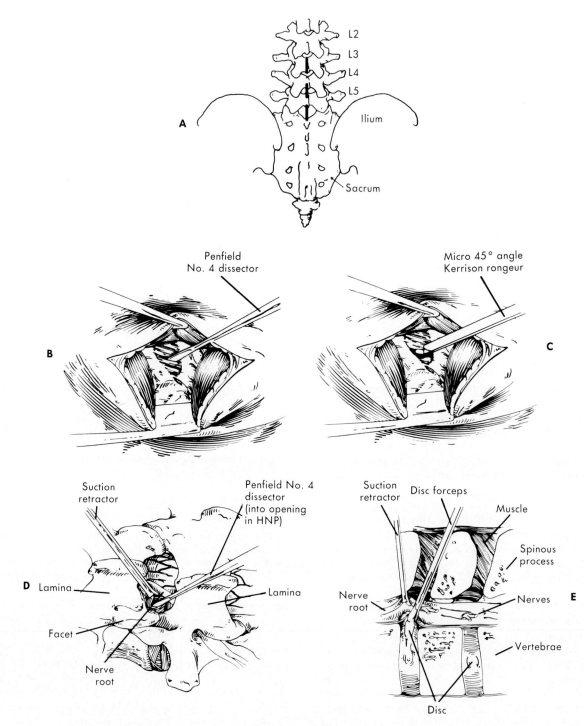

Fig. 73-27. Microlumbar disc excision. **A,** Position of skin incision for microlumbar disc excision. **B,** Entrance of epidural space by penetration of ligamentum flavum. **C,** Removal of ligamentum flavum with Kerrison rongeur. **D,** Dilation of anular defect before removal of disc fragment. **E,** Decompression of disc hernia by repeated small evacuations with discectomy forceps. (From Cauthen, J.C.: Lumbar spine surgery, Baltimore, 1983, Williams & Wilkins.)

in this maneuver to prevent penetration of the dura. Once the ligamentum is open, use a 45-degree Kerrison rongeur with a 1 mm cup to remove the ligamentum flavum toward the surgeon. The lamina, facet, and facet capsule should remain intact. Then make the extradural exploration using a blunt 90-degree hook. Gentle manipulation with the nerve hook will assist in identification of the nerve root.

In large herniations the nerve root will appear as a large, white, glistening structure and can easily be mistaken for a ruptured disc. If an epidural vein ruptures, proceed with the dissection and remove the disc.

Do not attempt to use pressure techniques or electrocautery in the limited space because severe nerve root injury may result. Epidural fat is not removed in this procedure.

Table 73-6. Results of lumbar disc excision by various methods

| Technique | Year | Number performed | Results (percentage) | | | | | | Persistent back pain |
			Excellent	Partial/good	None	Worse	Complications	Reoperation	
Open disc									
Semmes	1955	1440	53.6	43.3	1.7	1.4	NA	6.3	
Spangfort	1972	2503	76.9	17.0	5.0	0.5	8.0		31.5
Weir	1979	100	73.0	22.0	3.0	1.0	NA	NA	
Rish	1984	57	74.0	17.0	9.0		4.0	18.0	
Microdiscectomy									
Williams and Hudgins	1983	200	88.0		8.0	4.0	1.5	5.0	
Anterior lumbar interverbral fusion									
Harmon	1963	220	84.5		12.7	1.4		1.4	
Posterior lumbar intervertebral fusion									
Rish	1984	13	62.0	20.0	18.0				

NA, not available.

Insert the nerve root retractor, suction with its tip turned medially under the nerve root, and hold the manifold between the thumb and index finger. With the nerve root retracted the disc will now be visible as a white, fibrous, avascular structure. Small tears may be visible in the anulus under the magnification. Now enlarge the anular tear with a Penfield No. 4 dissector and remove the disc material with the microdisc forceps. Do not insert the instrument into the disc space beyond the angle of the jaws. Remove only exposed disc material. Do not curet the disc space. Inspect the root and adjacent dura for disc fragments. Close the fascia and skin in the usual fashion.

AFTERTREATMENT. Postoperative care is similar to that after standard open disc surgery. Those who perform this surgery indicate that a 3-day postoperative hospitalization is usual. We have no experience with this technique.

RESULTS OF OPEN SURGERY FOR DISC HERNIATION

Numerous retrospective and some prospective reviews of open disc surgery are available. The results of these series vary greatly with respect to patient selection, treatment method, evaluation method, length of follow-up, and conclusions. Good results range from 46% to 97%. Complications range from none to over 10%. The reoperation rate ranges from 4% to over 20%. The detailed studies of Spangfort, Weir, and Rush are suggested for more detailed analysis. A comparison between techniques also reveals similar reports. Few reports concerning microlumbar discectomy have appeared (Table 73-6).

Several points do stand out in the analysis of the results of lumbar disc surgery. Patient selection appears to be extremely important. The works of Wiltse and Rocchio, and Gentry indicate that valid results of the Minnesota Multiphasic Personality Inventory (hysteria and hypochondriasis T scores) are an extremely good indicator of surgical outcome regardless of the degree of pathology. The extremely detailed work of Weir suggests that the duration of the present episode, the age of the patient, the presence or

Table 73-7. Complications of lumbar disc surgery

Complication	Incidence (percentage)
1. Cauda equina syndrome	0.2
2. Thrombophlebitis	1.0
3. Pulmonary embolism	0.4
4. Wound infection	2.2
5. Pyogenic spondylitis	0.07
6. Postoperative discitis	2.0 (1,122 patients)
7. Dural tears	1.6
8. Nerve root injury	0.5
9. Cerebrospinal fluid fistula	*
10. Laceration of abdominal vessels	*
11. Injury to abdominal viscera	*

*Rare occurrence (10 and 11 not identified in Spangfort study but reported elsewhere).

Modified from Spangfort, E.V.: The lumbar disc herniation: a computer-aided analysis of 2,504 operations, Acta Orthop. Scand. Suppl. **142**:65, 1972.

absence of predominant back pain, the number of previous hospitalizations, and the presence or absence of compensation for a work injury are factors with regard to the final outcome. Spangfort's work also indicates that the softer the findings for disc herniation clinically and at the time of surgery, the lower the chance for a good result.

COMPLICATIONS OF OPEN DISC EXCISION

The complications associated with standard disc excision and microlumbar disc excision are similar. Spangfort's series (Table 73-7) of 2504 open disc excisions lists a postoperative mortality of 0.1%, thromboembolism of 1.0%, postoperative infection of 3.2%, and a deep disc space infection rate of 1.1%. Postoperative cauda equina lesions developed in 5 patients. Laceration of the aorta or iliac artery has also been described as a rare complication of this operation. Rish, in a more recent report with a 5-year follow-up, noted a total complication rate of 4% in a series of 205 patients. The major complication in his series involved a worsening neuropathy postoperatively. There were one disc space infection and one wound infection. Dural tears with cerebrospinal fluid leaks, pseudomeningocele formation, cerebrospinal fluid fistula formation, and meningitis are also possible but are more likely after reoperation. Two series of microlumbar disc excisions do not note postoperative complications.

Dural repair. The presence of a dural tear or leak results in the potentially serious problems of pseudomeningocele, cerebrospinal fluid leak, and meningitis. Eismont et al. have suggested five basic principles in the repair of these leaks (Fig. 73-28).

1. The operative field must be unobstructed, dry, and well exposed.

2. Dural suture of a 6-0 or 7-0 gauge with a tapered or reverse cutting needle is used in either a simple or running

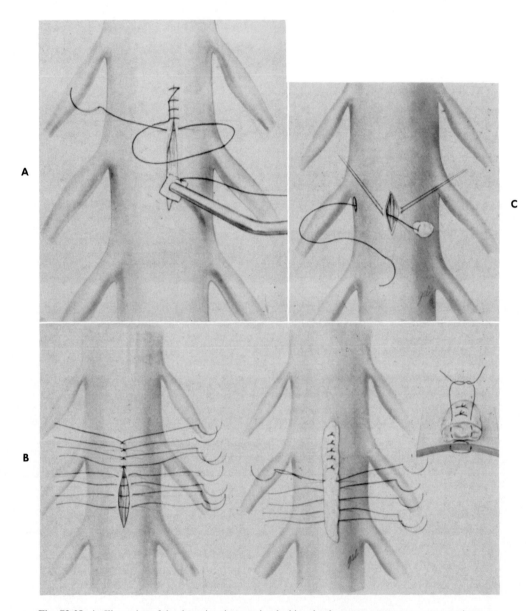

Fig. 73-28. A, Illustration of dural repair using running-locking dural suture on taper or reverse-cutting, one-half-circle needle. A smaller-size suture should be used. Use of suction with sucker and small cotton pledgets is essential to protect nerve roots while operative field is kept dry of cerebrospinal fluid. **B,** Single dural stitches may be used to achieve closure, each suture-end being left long. Second needle then is attached to free suture-end and ends of suture are passed through piece of muscle or fat, which is tied down over repaired tear to help to achieve watertight closure. Whenever dural material is inadequate to allow closure without placing excessive pressure on underlying neural tissues, a free graft fascia or fascia lata, or freeze-dried dural graft, should be secured to margins of dural tear using simple sutures of appropriate size. **C,** For small dural defects in relatively inaccessible areas, transdural approach can be used to pull small piece of muscle or fat into defect from inside out, thereby sealing cerebrospinal fluid leak. Central durotomy should be large enough to expose defect from dural sac. Durotomy is then closed in standard watertight fashion. (From Eismont, F.J., Wiesel, S.W., and Rothman, R.H.: J. Bone Joint Surg. **63-A**:1132, 1981.)

locking stitch. If the leak is large or inaccessable, a free fat graft or fascial graft may be sutured to the dura.

3. All repairs should be tested by using the reverse Trendelenburg position and Valsalva maneuvers.

4. Paraspinous muscles and overlying fascia should be closed in two layers with nonabsorbable suture used in a water-tight fashion. Drains should not be used.

5. Bed rest in the supine position should be maintained for 4 to 7 days after the repair of lumbar dural defects.

The development of headaches on standing and a stormy postoperative period should alert one to the possibility of an undetected cerebrospinal fluid leak. This can be confirmed by myelography or radioiodinated serum albumin scans. The presence of glucose in drainage fluid is not a reliable diagnostic test. On rare occasions a pseudomeningocele has been implicated as a cause of persistent pain from pressure on a nerve root by the cystic mass.

ADDITIONAL EXPOSURE TECHNIQUES

The presence of a large disc herniation or other pathology such as lateral recess stenosis or foraminal stenosis may dictate a greater exposure of the nerve root. Usually the additional pathology can be identified before surgery. If the extent of the lesion is known before surgery, the proper approach can be planned. Additional exposure includes hemilaminectomy, total laminectomy, and facetectomy. Hemilaminectomy is usually required when identifying the root is a problem. This may occur with a conjoined root. Total laminectomy is usually reserved for patients with spinal stenosis that are central in nature. Facetectomy is usually reserved for foraminal stenosis or severe lateral recess stenosis. If more than one facet is removed, then a fusion should be considered in addition. This is especially true in the removal of both facets and the disc at the same interspace in a young, active person with a normal disc height at that level.

On rare occasions disc herniation has been reported to be intradural. An extremely large disc that cannot be dissected from the dura or the persistence of a intradural mass after dissection of the disc should alert one to this potential problem. Excision of an intradural disc requires a transdural approach. This approach increases the risk of complications from cerebrospinal fluid leak and intradural scarring.

FREE FAT GRAFTING

Fat grafting for the prevention of postoperative epidural scarring has been suggested by Kiviluoto, Jacobs et al., and Bryant et al. The study by Jacobs et al. indicated that free fat grafts were superior to gelatin foam in the prevention of postoperative scarring. The present rationale for free fat grafting appears to be the possibility of making any reoperation easier. Unfortunately, the benefit of reduced scarring and its relationship to the prevention of postoperative pain has not been established; neither has the increased ease of reoperation in patients in whom fat grafting was performed. Fat grafts are also useful in the prevention of cerebrospinal fluid leaks.

The technique of free fat grafting is straightforward. At the end of the procedure, just before closing, take a large chunk of subcutaneous fat and insert it over the laminectomy defect. If the patient is thin, a separate incision over the buttock may be required to get sufficient fat to fill the defect.

Lumbar root anomalies

Lumbar nerve root anomalies (Figs. 73-29 to 73-32) are more common than may be expected, and they are rarely

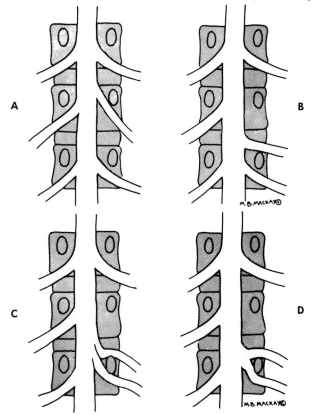

Fig. 73-30. Type II: anomalous origin of nerve roots. **A,** Cranial origin. **B,** Caudal origin. **C,** Closely adjacent nerve roots. **D,** Conjoined nerve roots. (From Kadish, L.J., and Simmons, E.H.: J. Bone Joint Surg. **66-B:**411, 1984.)

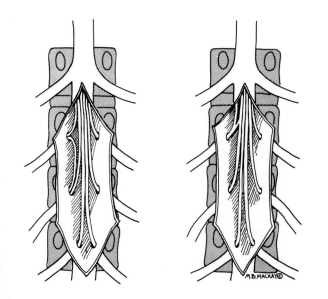

Fig. 73-29. Type I: intradural anastamosis. (From Kadish, L.J., and Simmons, E.H.: J. Bone Joint Surg. **66-B:**411, 1984.)

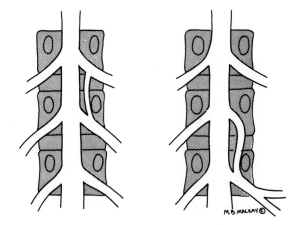

Fig. 73-31. Type III: extradural anastamosis. (From Kadish, L.J., and Simmons, E.H.: J. Bone Joint Surg. **66-B:**411, 1984.)

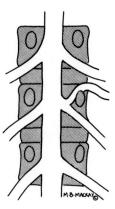

Fig. 73-32. Type IV: extradural division. (From Kadish, L.J., and Simmons, E.H.: J. Bone Joint Surg. **66-B:**411, 1984.)

correctly identified with myelography. Kadish and Simmons identified lumbar nerve root anomalies in 14% of 100 cadaver examinations. They noted nerve root anomalies in only 4% of 100 consecutive metrizamide myelograms. They identified four types of anomalies. Type I is an intradural anastomosis between rootlets at different levels. Type II is an anomalous origin of the nerve roots. They separated this into four subtypes: (1) cranial origin, (2) caudal origin, (3) combination of cranial and caudal origin, and (4) conjoined nerve roots. Type III is an extradural anastomosis between roots. Type IV is the extradural division of the nerve root. The surgeon must be aware of the possibility of anomalous roots hindering the disc excision. This may require a wider exposure. Sectioning of these roots results in irreversible neurologic damage. Traction on anomalous nerve roots has been suggested as a cause of sciatic symptoms without disc herniation.

Chemonucleolysis

Chemonucleolysis has been used experimentally in the United States for almost 30 years. The enzyme was released for general use by the FDA in December of 1982. Before its release in the United States it was used extensively in Europe and Canada. A wealth of experimental and clinical information exists concerning the technique and the enzyme. Specific guidelines have been suggested by the FDA regarding the use of the enzyme in the United States.

Because of the recent disclosure of the late development of transverse myelitis and other neurologic sequelae, the original guidelines issued in January of 1983 have been radically changed. The information presented regarding this technique reflects the most recent suggestions effective in January of 1985. Unlike other surgical procedures, this procedure requires certification of proficiency before the drug will be released to the treating physician. Those interested in performing the technique are requested to contact the pharmaceutical companies producing the drug for information regarding training and certification in the technique. Treating physicians are also encouraged to frequently check the package insert accompanying the drug and the information bulletins sent out by the FDA and the

pharmaceutical companies regarding any new changes in protocol or usage of the enzyme.

The indications for the use of chemonucleolysis are the same as for open surgery for disc herniation. Fraser reported the results of 60 patients treated for lumbar disc herniation in a 2-year double-blind study of chemonucleolysis. At 2 years 77% of the patients treated with chymopapain were improved, whereas only 47% of the saline injection group were improved. At 2 years from injection 57% of the chymopapain group were pain free compared with 23% of the placebo group. Numerous other studies of the efficacy of the drug place the good to excellent results between 50% and 85% which is comparable to the clinical reports for open surgery (Table 73-8). As with open disc surgery, this technique is not applicable in all lumbar disc herniations. The use of the drug is limited to the lumbar spine. The patient optimally has predominantly unilateral leg pain and localizing neurologic findings consistent with confirmatory testing with computed tomography or myelography. Patients with moderate lateral recess or foraminal stenosis may worsen after the procedure because of collapse of the disc space and narrowing of the foraminal opening. Large disc herniations may not shrink sufficiently to result in relief of symptoms, and sequestered discs may be untouched by the enzyme.

Chymopapain injection is specifically contraindicated in patients with a known sensitivy to papaya, papaya derivatives, or food containing papaya such as meat tenderizer. Other contraindications include severe spondylolisthesis; severe, progressive neurologic deficit or paralysis; and evidence of spinal cord tumor or a cauda equina lesion. The enzyme cannot be injected in a patient who has been previously injected, regardless of the level injected. Use of chymopapain is limited to the lumbar intervertebral discs. Relative contraindications include allergy to iodine or iodine contrast material; use of the enzyme in a previously operated disc; patients with elevated allergy studies such a RAST, ChymoFast, and skin testing with the drug; and patients with a severe allergic history, especially with a previous anaphylactic attack. Recent clinical reports indicate that patients taking beta-blockers should not be considered for the procedure or should at least be taken off

Table 73-8. Results and complications of chemonucleolysis and open disc excision

Technique	Year	Number performed	Results (percentage)				Complications	Reoperation	Persistent back pain
			Excellent	Partial/good	None	Worse			
Open disc									
Semmes	1955	1440	53.6	43.3	1.7	1.4	NA	6.3	
Spangfort	1972	2503	76.9	17.0	5.0	0.5	8.0		31.5
Weir	1979	100	73.0	22.0	3.0	1.0	NA	NA	
Rish	1984	57	74.0	17.0	9.0		4.0	18.0	
Chemonucleolysis									
Illinois trial	1982	273	90.0		10.0		1.1		
Javid	1983	40	82.0		18.0				
Nordby	1983	641	55.0	25.0	20.0		NA	NA	

NA, not available.

the drug for a time because these drugs may adversely affect epinephrine in the event of an anaphylactic reaction. It has also been suggested that the enzyme be injected without concomitant preinjection discography because of the intensification of neural damage if the enzyme is inadvertently injected intrathecally. All efforts should be made to prevent intrathecal leak or injection of the enzyme. At least 1 week should elapse between any intradural injection such as myelography and chymopapain injection. Injection should be further delayed if the patient is still experiencing a spinal headache. If spinal fluid is encountered in the process of needle placement, the procedure should be abandoned.

TECHNIQUE. The technique of chemonucleolysis (Figs. 73-33 and 73-34) begins with thorough patient preparation. This includes an explanation of the technique, possible adverse reactions, and usual postoperative occurrences and procedure. Testing for allergy or sensitivity to the enzyme is performed with adequate time to evaluate the results before the injection. The patient is started on cimetidine (Tagamet) 300 mg and diphenhydramine (Benadryl) 50 mg by mouth or intravenously every 6 hours for at least 24 hours before the procedure. Preoperative hydration is also suggested as an aid in the event of an anaphylactic reaction.

The procedure is done with the patient under local anesthesia with an anesthesiologist or an anesthetist in attendance administering oxygen and mild sedation as indicated. The injection of strong opiates is not recommended during the injection of the test dose and final injection because this may cause a drop in blood pressure, mimicking anaphylaxis. Constant monitoring of the blood pressure is essential. Insert a large-bore intravenous needle just before the initiation of the procedure. If there is any increased risk of anaphylaxis, insert an arterial line with the patient under local anesthesia. All materials for resuscitation in the event of anaphylaxis must be present in the room and available for immediate use. We presently use 1% lidocaine and 0.25% bupivacaine as the local anesthetic.

The technique requires image intensification capable of providing both anteroposterior and lateral projections. An operating platform capable of allowing the transmission of radiation is also required. The ability to provide roentgen-

ographic documentation of needle placement is also suggested. Additional materials include 4-, 6-, and 8-inch (10, 15.2, and 20.3 cm) spinal needles in 18, 20, and 22 gauges, a large metric ruler, several 5 or 10 ml syringes and two 1 ml syringes for each level injected. The draping technique is variable and possibly dictated by the image intensification equipment. We presently use a large, clear-plastic drape with an adhesive center that is also used in hip nailing procedures. Additional draping is not necessary with this method because a sterile barrier is maintained between the image intensifier and the operative field.

The anesthetist or anesthesiologist, having prepared the patient with a large-bore intravenous line and automatic blood pressure monitor or arterial line, instructs the patient to turn on the left side with the hips and knees flexed at 45 degrees. The procedure is performed on a table capable of allowing roentgen transmission and mobility of an image intensifier C-arm. The left iliac crest is elevated with a roll of towels or an inflatable bladder. This allows leveling the spine or opening the L5-S1 disc space if this level is to be injected. Absolute anteroposterior and lateral positioning of the patient is determined by image intensification. The patient is held in this position with tape if desired.

Prepare and drape the back in the standard surgical fashion. Using a long radiopaque object such as a steel ruler, identify the disc level of interest. Use a marking pen to draw a line on the back parallel with and at the level of each disc to be injected. Then make a mark about 8.5 cm lateral to the midline or spinous process bisecting the disc lines. Remove the drape from the area to be injected. Infiltrate the skin with a local anesthetic agent at each level. Make a small stab wound with a No. 11 blade. Direct a spinal needle of at least 18-gauge and 4 to 6 inches (10 to 15.2 cm) in length parallel with the disc line drawn on the skin at about 45 to 55 degrees to the back angling toward the spine. Inject additional anesthetic agent as the needle is advanced. Monitor proper alignment in both anteroposterior and lateral projections as you advance the needle.

When the disc level is reached, the needle should be at the outer border of the vertebral bodies and disc in the anteroposterior view and at the posterior edge of the bodies

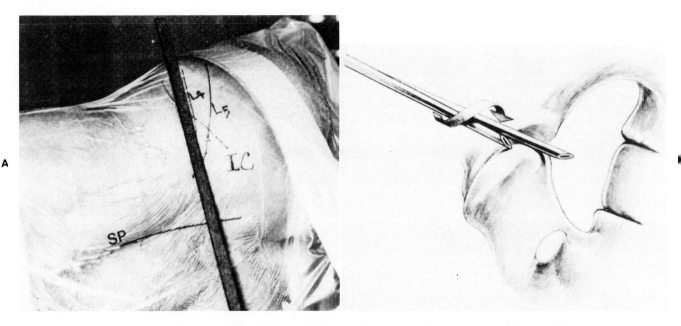

A

Fig. 73-33. A, Lines are drawn on skin parallel to disc space with metal bar or long ruler placed parallel to disc under image intensification. Lines are marked for L4-5 and L5-S1 discs. IC is the iliac crest. The smaller lines just below the iliac crest that transect the disc lines are the needle insertion points. Note the closeness of the L4-5 point to the L5-S1 point. **B,** Needle can be advanced over the facet by rotating the needle 180 degrees. Note that bevel of needle is pointing down in relation to position of insertion. (**A** From Chung, B.U.: Bent tip single needle technique. In Brown, J.E., et al.: Chemonucleolysis, Thorofare, N.J., 1985, Slack; **B** from Thomas, J.C., and Wiltse, L.L.: The double needle technique using local anesthesia. In Brown, J.E., et al.: Chemonucleolysis, Thorofare, N.J., 1985, Slack.)

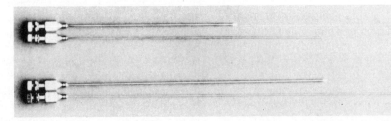

Fig. 73-34. Two sets of needles that are used in double-needle technique. Upper pair are 4-inch, 18-gauge needle and 6-inch, 22-gauge needle. Lower pair are 6-inch, 18-gauge needle and 8-inch, 22-gauge needle. The 22-gauge needle must be two inches longer than the 18-gauge needle. (From Thomas, J.C., and Wiltse, L.L.: The double needle technique using local anesthesia. In Brown, J.E., et al.: Chemonucleolysis, Thorofare, N.J., 1985, Slack.)

in the lateral view. If a double-needle technique is used, advance the larger needle (usually 18-gauge) only as far as the intertransverse ligament or lamina. Then insert the smaller needle (usually 22 gauge and at least 2 inches [10 cm] longer) into the larger needle and advance it into the disc. When the needle enters the disc, a distinct change in resistance and a "gritty" sensation are noted. The only pain that occurs during this maneuver is the result of nerve root irritation or penetration by the needle just lateral to the disc. Aspirate the needle if there is any question of dural penetration by the needle. *If the dura is penetrated, abandon the procedure.* Proper needle placement should put the needle in the center in the lateral view and dead center over the spinous process in the anteroposterior

view. If there is any question regarding the needle position, perform a saline acceptance test using about 1 ml of sterile saline from a new container. The saline should enter easily. Check the level of injection and position of the needle with standard anterioposterior and lateral roentgenograms.

If resistance to the saline acceptance test is extreme, then the needle tip is in the anulus or the disc is normal. If the needle position is satisfactory, then carry out discography using metrizamide to be sure that the disc is normal. At this point if the injection is anular or the disc is normal, redirect the needle into the proper disc or direction. If the contrast leaks into the epidural space, it may be safer to abandon the procedure to avoid the potential of mixing contrast and chymopapain intradurally. When a nerve root is encountered repeatedly injecting metrizamide into the root sleeve may be beneficial to demonstrate the nerve so as to position the needle to avoid it. Intradural injection demands termination of the procedure.

The most difficult needle placement is at L5-S1 (Fig. 73-33). The usual entry point is about ¼-inch (6 mm) caudal to the L4-5 interspace. This needle is directed 45 to 60 degrees to the sagittal plane of the back and 30 degrees caudally. It must traverse the small opening formed by the iliac crest laterally, the ala of the sacrum caudally, and the transverse process of L5 cranially. Determine accurate placement by checking the anteroposterior view when the needle reaches the level of the lamina in the lateral view. At this point, the needle should be in the center of the triangle formed by the transverse process of L5, the ala of the sacrum, and the iliac crest as viewed in the anteroposterior view. The use of the double-needle technique with a small 22-gauge needle is of value here because it may be necessary to traverse the L5 root before entering the disc space. If a large needle is used, the nerve may be permanently damaged.

The recent availability of noncutting 18-gauge needles and prebent 22-gauge needles may diminish the risk of permanent nerve damage. If a prebent needle is used, the first needle must be advanced to the edge of the anulus. Furthermore a prebent needle will begin to turn immediately on exiting the first needle and there is little control. Therefore the surgeon is urged to practice with these needles before their use to master the eccentricities of the needle turning on exit from the first needle (Fig. 73-34). Before initiating this procedure, check the lateral roentgenogram for a high iliac crest. This may indicate that entrance into the L5-S1 disc space will be difficult, and prebent needles may be necessary. Occasionally it is impossible to enter this space with a needle.

Pure oxygen is administered by the anesthesiologist for 3 minutes before injection, continuing to the end of the procedure. Inject a test dose of 0.2 ml of enzyme. Allow 15 to 20 minutes to elapse. Then inject the final dose of enzyme. The total dose injected should not exceed 1.5 ml or 4000 μl per disc or 8000 μl per patient. We suggest that only the one, symptomatic level be injected.

In the absence of any adverse reaction, the patient is transferred to the recovery room for 2 hours of constant monitoring before returning to his room. Narcotics and sedatives may be administered for the relief of back pain as indicated.

AFTERTREATMENT. Back pain and spasm are the most common occurrences after chemonucleolysis. When they occur, the patient should be placed in a position of rest such as the semi-Fowler or lateral decubitus position. Ice massage may be used for muscle spasm. Opiates and sedatives are provided as necessary. If the pain is mild, the patient is encouraged to walk wearing a lumbar corset. The patient is also instructed in the proper way to get out of bed without excessive spinal movement. The patient is discharged when the pain is easily controlled with mild pain medication and walking is comfortable. As after open disc surgery, the patient is to refrain from sitting, riding in vehicles, lifting, bending, and stooping. In uncomplicated

Table 73-9. Reported severe complications of chemonucleolysis in 57,341 patients from Smith Laboratories postmarketing survey as of February 1, 1985

Complication	No. of patients	Percentage
1. Mortality*	20	0.022
Anaphylaxis	5	
Cerebral hemorrhage	6	
Cardiorespiratory	4	
Infection	2	
Other	1	
2. Anaphylaxis	306	0.5
Male	106	0.3
Female	200	0.9
3. Neurologic complications	49	0.086
Cerebral hemorrhage	14	
Subarachnoid hemorrhage	1	
Paralysis	27	
Quadriplegia	1	
Hemiparesis	1	
Guillain-Barré	1	
Seizures	4	

*Includes all reported deaths in 90,000 injections (0.022%).
From pp. 23-25, Chemonucleolysis Resource Center Teaching Program, 1985, Smith Laboratories.

injections discharge is within 1 to 2 days. The remaining postoperative care is similar to that for open disc surgery with the exception that patients with walking and sitting jobs involving minimal lifting may return to work sooner if they are pain free. Heavy laborers are usually returned to work at 3 months.

COMPLICATIONS

The complications of chemonucleolysis (Table 73-9) have been well publicized, but similar complications of open disc surgery and myelography have received much less attention. Serious complications of chemonucleolysis are anaphylaxis (2.5% to 0.4% with five deaths in 50,000 injections), cerebral hemorrhage (eight patients in about 48,000 injections), paraplegia or paraparesis (20 patients in 48,000 injections), and disc space infection (two patients). Many of these complications can be prevented or minimized. Anaphylaxis must be considered and anticipated in all injections. Patients who could not tolerate any episode of hypotension should not be treated with this technique. Preoperative testing for sensitivity should pinpoint patients at risk. Testing with ChymoFast is 99.6% accurate with only a 0.4% false negative rate. The exact rates for the RAST test and skin testing are not known at this time. The evaluation of neurologic complications has implicated the use of a general anesthetic, dural puncture, injection of more than one level, and the concomitant use of radiopaque roentgenographic dyes as common denominators. Avoidance of these methods and meticulous attention to detail in the insertion of the needles should minimize the risk of neurologic complications. Infection can be minimized by using new sterile vials of saline for the saline acceptance test and the diluent enclosed with the drug.

Treatment of anaphylaxis. The most serious and life-threatening complication of chymopapain injection is anaphylaxis. The onset of anaphylaxis is within the first 20 minutes in 98% of the patients experiencing the complication. The risk of such a reaction is quite low 2 hours after injection. In the awake patient the first sign may be a generalized itch, a mild erythema over the trunk, respiratory difficulty or a sinking, "dying" sensation. If an arterial line is in place there may be a sudden drop in pressure of 20 to 40 torr.

Immediate response is mandatory (see protocol below); intravenous fluids are opened fully, needles and drapes are removed, and the patient is moved to the supine position. Epinephrine is injected intravenously. The initial dosage is usually 0.5 to 1 ml of a 1/10,000 solution given every 1 to 5 minutes up to a total of 2 mg per hour. The patient should be intubated. Bicarbonate, diphenhydramine, cimetidine, and steroids are also given with large volumes of fluid. Cardiopulmonary resuscitation is instituted if necessary. Vigorous and prompt reaction to this complication is mandatory if death is to be prevented. Patients with severe systemic disease who could not tolerate the insult of hypotension, epinephrine injection, and massive volume expansion should not be considered candidates for the procedure.

The recommended treatment protocol for anaphylaxis follows*:

First Priority
- Stop administration of antigen
- Administer 100% oxygen
- Stop administration of anesthetic
- Expand volume
- Intravenous infusion of 0.5 to 1.0 ml of 1:10,000 epinephrine solution not to exceed 0.5 mg over 10 minutes or intravenous bolus of 0.5 to 5 ml 1:10,000 epinephrine solution (up to 2 mg/hr)
- Obtain blood gases as soon as possible and treat acidosis appropriately or administer one 50 mEq ampule of bicarbonate prophylactically every 5 minutes for severe hypotension

Second Priority
- Initial bolus of 1 g hydrocortisone IV
- Catecholamine if slow response in peripheral blood pressure
- Loading dose of 5 to 9 mg/kg aminophylline over 20 to 30 minutes for bronchospasm
- 50 mg diphenhydramine and 300 mg cimetidine (70 kg patient) IV

After Termination of Reaction
- Check airway for laryngeal edema before extubation

SPINAL INSTABILITY FROM DEGENERATIVE DISC DISEASE

Farfan defines spinal instability (caused by degenerative disc disease) as a clinically symptomatic condition without new injury, in which a physiologic load induces abnormally large deformations at the intervertebral joint. Biomechanical studies have revealed abnormal motion at vertebral segments with degenerative discs and the transmission of the load to the facet joints. Numerous attempts at roentgenographic definition of spinal instability

with disc disease have resulted in more controversy than agreement as to a standard method of measurement. The method described by Knutsson is simple and relatively efficient in determining anterior-posterior motion. There is little controversy as to the surgical treatment of lumbar spinal instability—spinal fusion of the unstable segments. The type of fusion performed and the indications for fusion are other areas of controversy.

The major problem in spinal instability is the correlation of the patient's symptoms of giving way, catching, and predominant back pain to the roentgenographic identification of instability. Other factors such as concomitant spinal stenosis, disc herniation, and psychologic problems only complicate any evaluation of spinal instability. Presently the decision for surgery for clinically significant lumbar spine instability caused by degenerative disc disease should be decided on an individual patient basis with all the factors and risks weighed carefully.

Disc excision and fusion

The necessity of lumbar fusion at the same time as disc excision was first suggested by Mixter and Barr. In the first 20 years after their discovery the combination of disc excision and lumbar fusion was common. More recent data comparing disc excision alone with the combination of disc excision and fusion by Frymoyer et al. and others indicate that there is little if any advantage to the addition of a spinal fusion to the treatment of simple disc herniation. These studies do indicate that spinal fusion does increase the complication rate and lengthen recovery. The indications for lumbar fusion should be independent of the indications for disc excision for sciatica.

Lumbar vertebral interbody fusion

Anterior lumbar intervertebral fusion (ALIF) and posterior lumbar intervertebral fusion (PLIF) have been suggested as definitive procedures for lumbar disc disease. Biomechanically the lumbar interbody fusion offers the greatest stability. It also eliminates the disc segment as a further source of pain. The primary problems are the more involved and potentially dangerous dissection, the risk of graft extrusion, and pseudarthrosis.

Most series of these fusions include a significant number of salvage procedures and complex pathology thus making direct comparison with primary disc surgery difficult. The routine use of such procedures for simple lumbar disc herniation with sciatica is not justified.

ANTERIOR LUMBAR INTERBODY FUSION

TECHNIQUE. Place the patient in the supine position on an operating table capable of holding roentgenographic cassettes. Support the lumbar spine with a rolled sheet or inflatable bag. Prepare and drape the patient's abdomen from upper chest to groin, leaving the iliac crests exposed for obtaining bone grafts. Expose the lumbar spine through a transabdominal or retroperitoneal approach as desired. Mobilize the great vessels over the segment to be excised. Ligate the median artery and vein at the bifurcation of the aorta to prevent tearing this structure when exposing the disc at L4-5 or L5-S1.

Identify and inspect all major structures before and after

---

*Modified from Whisler, W.W.: Orthopedics **6:**1628, 1983.

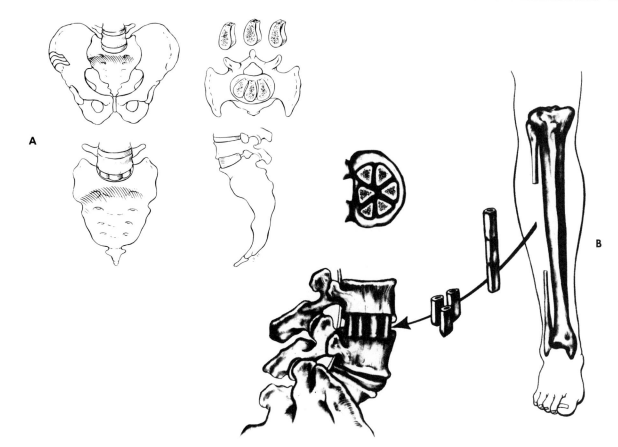

Fig. 73-35. Anterior lumbar intervertebral fusion (ALIF) can be performed using tricortical iliac crest graft, **A,** or fibular grafts, **B.** (**A** From Ruge, D., and Wiltse, L.L.: Spinal disorders: diagnosis and treatment, Lea and Febiger, Philadelphia, 1977; **B** from Wiltse, L.L.: American Academy of Orthopaedic Surgeons: Instructional course lectures, vol. 28, 1979. The C.V. Mosby Co.)

disc excision and fusion. Obtain an anteroposterior roentgenogram to confirm the proper disc level. Then incise the anterior longitudinal ligament superiorly or inferiorly over the edge of the vertebral body. Elevate the ligament as a flap if possible. Next remove the anular and nuclear material of the disc. The use of magnification may be beneficial as the dissection nears the posterior longitudinal ligament. Remove all nuclear material from the posterior longitudinal ligament.

Techniques for fusion vary. Some prefer to use dowel grafts to fill the space. Others prefer to use tricortical iliac grafts (Fig. 73-35). Obtain the grafts from the iliac crest as described for anterior cervical fusions (p. 3288). Prepare the graft area for the desired grafting technique. We prefer tricortical grafts for this fusion. Good results using fibular grafts and banked bone have also been reported. Prepare the vertebrae by curetting the end plates to cancellous bone posteriorly. Then carefully make a slot in the vertebra to accommodate the grafts; use an osteotome slightly larger than the width of the disc space for this purpose and direct the cut toward the inferior vertebral body. Try to leave the upper and lower lips of the vertebral bodies intact. Remove enough tricortical iliac bone to allow insertion of at least three individual grafts. Fashion the grafts to fit snugly in the space with a laminar spreader in place. Insert the grafts so that the cancellous portions face

the decorticated end plates. The grafts should be 3 to 4 mm shorter than the anteroposterior diameter of the vertebral body. Impact the grafts and seat them behind the anterior rim of the vertebral bodies. Usually three such grafts can be inserted. Add additional cancellous chips around the grafts. Suture the anterior longitudinal ligament. Close the retroperitoneum and abdomen in the usual manner.

AFTERTREATMENT. The patient is allowed to sit as soon as possible. Extension of the lumbar spine is prohibited for at least 6 weeks. Bracing or casting is left to the discretion of the surgeon after considering the stability of the grafts and reliability of the patient.

POSTERIOR LUMBAR INTERBODY FUSION

TECHNIQUE (CLOWARD). Position the patient in the prone or kneeling position as desired. Expose the spine through a midline incision centered over the level of pathology. Strip the muscle subperiostially from the lamina bilaterally. Insert the laminar spreader between the spinous processes at the level of pathology. Open and remove the ligamentum flavum from the midline laterally. Enlarge the opening laterally by removing the lower one third of the inferior facet and the medial two thirds of the superior facet (Fig. 73-36, *A*). The upper lamina may also be thinned by undercutting to increase the anteroposterior diameter of the canal. Retract the lower nerve root and dura to the midline

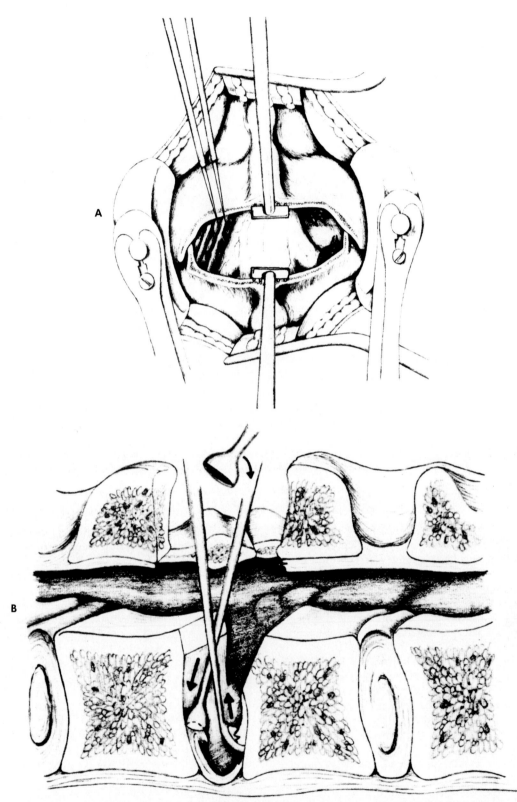

Fig. 73-36. Posterior lumbar interbody fusion technique. **A,** Bilateral laminotomy with preservation of facets. Control of epidural hemorrhage. Dipolar or insulated coagulation forceps are used on *left side*. On *right side*, epidural hemorrhage is controlled by impacted Surgicel tampons. Impacted Surgicel tampons also push nerve root medially and expose disc space without need of nerve root retractor. **B,** After intervertebral rims are removed, cleavage of disc attachment to cortical plate is identified. Curved upbite curet is used to remove concave centrum of lower cartilaginous plate. Then detached large chunks of disc material are removed with ronguer.

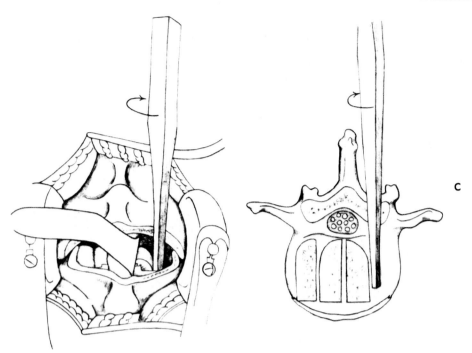

Fig. 73-36, cont'd. C, Medial graft advancement with single chisel. (From Cauthen, J.C.: Lumbar spine surgery, Baltimore, 1983, Williams & Wilkins.)

and protect it with the self-retaining nerve root retractor. Cauterize the epidural vessels with bipolar cautery. Cut out the disc and vessels over the anulus laterally. Remove as much disc material as possible (Fig. 73-36, *B*). Remove a thin layer of the end plates posteriorly. Repeat this process on the opposite side. Remove the remaining anterior edges of the end plates to the anterior longitudinal ligament. This must be done under direct vision to avoid injury to the great vessels. Prepare a surface of bleeding cancellous bone on both vertebral bodies. Obtain tricortical iliac crest grafts as previously noted from the posterior iliac crest. (Cloward uses frozen human cadaver bone grafts.) Shape the grafts to be slightly shorter and the same height or slightly higher than the disc shape. Tamp the first graft in place and lever it medially to allow insertion of the remaining grafts. Repeat the procedure on the opposite side (Fig. 73-36, *C*). Remove the laminar spreader and check the graft for stability. Close the wound in the usual fashion.

AFTERTREATMENT. Aftertreatment is the same as for lumbar discectomy (p. 3297). Early walking is encouraged.

FAILED SPINE SURGERY

One of the greatest problems in orthopaedic surgery and neurosurgery is the treatment of failed spine surgery. Numerous reasons for the failures have been advanced. The best results from repeat surgery for disc problems appears to be related to the discovery of a new problem or identification of a previously undiagnosed or untreated problem. Waddell et al. suggested that the best results from repeat surgery are when the patient had experienced 6 months or more of complete pain relief after the first procedure, when

leg pain exceeded back pain, and when a definitie recurrent disc could be identified. They identified adverse factors as scarring, previous infection, repair of pseudarthrosis, and adverse psychologic factors. Similar factors were identified by Lehmann and LaRocca and Finnegan et al. Satisfactory results from reoperation have been reported to be from 40% to 80%. Patients should expect improvement in the severity of symptoms rather than complete relief of pain. As the frequency of number of repeat back surgeries increases, the chance of a satisfactory result drops precipitously.

The recurrence or intensification of pain after disc surgery should be treated with the usual conservative methods initially. If these methods fail to relieve the pain, a complete reevaluation should be performed. Frequently a repeat history and physical examination will give some indication of the problem. Additional testing should include psychologic testing, myelography, and magnetic resonance imaging to check for tumors or a higher disc herniation, and reformatted computed tomographic scans to check for areas of foraminal stenosis or far lateral herniation. The use of the differential spinal, root blocks, facet blocks, and discograms may also help identify the source of pain. The presence of abnormal psychologic test results or an abnormal differential spinal should serve as a modifier to any suggested treatment indicated by the other testing. Satisfactory nonoperative treatment of this problem should be attempted before additional surgery is performed, provided this surgery is elective. A distinct, surgically correctable, anatomic problem should be identified before surgery is contemplated. The surgery should be specifically tailored to the anatomic problem or problems identified.

The technique of repeat lumbar disc surgery at the same level and side as the previous procedure is nearly the same as for initial surgery. The procedure will be longer and will involve more meticulous dissection.

TECHNIQUE. Approach the spine using the method described previously. Identify normal tissue first. Use a curet to carefully remove scar from the edges of the lamina. Then remove additional bone as necessary to expose normal dura. Identify the pedicles superiorly and inferiorly if there is any question of position and status of the root. Carry the dissection from the pedicles to identify each root. This will allow the development of a normal plane between the dura and scar. Maintain meticulous hemostasis with bipolar cautery. Then remove disc material as indicated by the preoperative evaluation. Meticulously check the roots, dura, and posterior longitudinal ligament after removal of the offending disc herniation. Spinal fusion is not performed unless an unstable spine is created by the dissection or was identified preoperatively as a correctable and symptomatic problem. Aftercare is the same as for disc excision (p. 3297).

REFERENCES
Epidemiology

Aird, R.: Charles Lasègue. In Haymaker, W., and Sobiller, F., editors: Founders of neurology, ed. 2, Springfield, 1970, Charles C Thomas.

Alajouanine, T.H.: From the presidential address for Professor Jean Cauchoix before the Annual Meeting of the International Society for the Study of the Lumbar Spine, San Francisco, June 1978.

Andersson, G.B.J.: Epidemiologic aspects of low-back pain in industry, Spine 6:53, 1981.

Andersson, G.B.J., Svensson, H.O., and Oden, A.: The intensity of work recovery in low back pain, Spine 8:880, 1983.

Barr, J.S.: Low-back and sciatic pain: results of treatment, J. Bone Joint Surg. 33-A:633, 1951.

Barr, J.S.: Lumbar disc lesions in retrospect and prospect, Clin. Orthop. 129:4, 1977.

Barr, J.S., Hampton, A.O., and Mixter, W.J.: Pain low in the back and "sciatica" due to lesions of the intervertebral discs, JAMA 109:1265, 1937.

Berquist-Ullman, M., and Larsson, U.: Acute low back pain in industry: a controlled perspective study with special reference to therapy and confounding factors, Acta Orthop. Scand. (Suppl.) Copenhagen, 1977, Munskgaard.

Biering-Sorensen, F., and Hilden, J.: Reproducibility of the history of low-back trouble, Spine 9:280, 1984.

Buckle, P.W., Kember, P.A., Wood, A.D., and Wood, S.N.: Factors influencing occupational back pain in Bedfordshire, Spine 5:254, 1980.

Chaffin, D.B.: Human strength capability and low-back pain, JOM 16:248, 1974.

Cotugnio, D.: Treatise on the nervous sciatica or nervous hip gout, London, 1775, J. Wilkie.

Damkot, D.K., Pope, M.H., Lord, J., and Frymoyer, J.W.: The relationship between work history, work environment and low-back pain in men, Spine 9:395, 1984.

Dandy, W.E.: Loose cartilage from the intervertebral disc simulating tumor of the spinal cord, Orthop. Surg. 19:1660, 1929.

Dandy, W.E.: Concealed ruptured intervertebral disks: a plea for the elimination of contrast mediums in diagnosis, JAMA 117:821, 1941.

Dillane, J.B., Fry, J., and Kalton, G.: Acute back syndrome: a study from general practice, Br. Med. J. 2:82, 1966.

Dimitrigevic, D.T.: Historical note: Lasègue sign, Neurology 2:453, 1952.

Dyck, P.: Lumbar nerve root: the enigmatic eponyms, Spine 9:3, 1984.

Elsberg, C.A.: Experiences in spinal surgery: observations upon 60 laminectomies for spinal disease, Surg. Gynecol. Obstet. 16:117, 1913.

Farfan, H.F., and Sullivan, J.D.: The relation of facet orientation to intervertebral disc failure, Can. J. Surg. 10:179, 1967.

Forst, J.J.: Contribution a l'etude clinique de la sciatique, thesis, Lyon, France, 1881

Frymoyer, J.W., et al.: Spine radiographs in patients with low-back pain: an epidemiological study in men, J. Bone Joint Surg. 66-A:1048, 1984.

Frymoyer, J.W., et al.: Risk factors in low-back pain. An epidemiological survey, J. Bone Joint Surg. 65-A:213, 1983.

Frymoyer, J.W., et al.: Epidemiologic studies of low-back pain, Spine 5:419, 1980.

Gardner, R.C.: The lumbar intervertebral disc: a clinicopathological correlation based on over 100 laminectomies, Arch. Surg. 100:101, 1970.

Goldthwait, J.E.: The lumbosacral articulations: an explanation of many cases of "lumbago," "sciatica" and paraplegia, Bost. Med. Surg. J. 164:365, 1911.

Goldthwait, J.E.: Backache, N. Engl. J. Med. 209:722, 1933.

Goldthwait, J.E.: Low-back lesions, J. Bone Joint Surg. 19:810, 1937.

Grabias, S.: Current concepts revue: the treatment of spinal stenosis, J. Bone Joint Surg. 62-A:308, 1980.

Hall, G.W.: Neurologic signs and their discoverers, JAMA 95:703, 1930.

Hult, L.: The Munkfors investigation, Acta Orthop. Scand. Suppl.16:1, 1954.

Jackson, R.P., Simmons, E.H., and Stripinis, D.: Incidence and severity of back pain in adult idiopathic scoliosis, Spine 8:749, 1983.

Johnsson, K., Willner, S., and Pettersson, H.: Analysis of operated cases with lumbar renal stenosis, Acta Orthop. Scand. 52:427, 1981.

Kelsey, J.L., et al.: An epidemiologic study of lifting and twisting on the job and risk for acute prolapsed lumbar intervertebral disc, J. Orthop. Res. 2:61, 1984.

Kelsey, J.L., and White, A.A., III: Epidemiology and impact of low-back pain, Spine 5:133, 1980.

Kelsey, J.L., White, A.A., III, Pastides, H., and Bisbee, G.E., Jr.: The impact of musculoskeletal disorders on the population of the United States, J. Bone Joint Surg. 61-A:959, 1979.

Kocher, T.: Die Verlitzungen der Wirbelsaule Zurleich Als Beitrag zur Physiologic des Menschichen Ruchenmarks, Mitt. Grenzgeb. Med. Chir. 1:415, 1896.

Kostuik, J.P., and Bentivoglio, J.: The incidence of low-back pain in adult scoliosis, Spine 6:268, 1981.

Knutsson, F.: The instability associated with disk degeneration in the lumbar spine, Acta Radiol. 25:593, 1944.

Lasègue, C.: Considerations sur la sciatique, Arch. Gen. Med. 2:558, 1864.

Magora, A.: Investigation of the relation between low back pain and occupation: psychological aspects, Scand. J. Rehab. Med. 5:191, 1973.

Magora, A.: Investigation of the relation between low back pain and occupation: neurologic and orthopedic conditions, Scand. J. Rehab. Med. 7:146, 1975.

Manning, D.P., and Shannon, H.S.: Slipping accidents causing low-back pain in a gearbox factory, Spine 6:70, 1981.

Middleton, G.S., and Teacher, J.H.: Injury of the spinal cord due to rupture of an intervertebral disc during muscular effort, Glasgow Med. J. 76:1, 1911.

Mixter, W.J.: Rupture of the lumbar intervertebral disk: an etiologic factor for so-called "sciatic" pain, Ann. Surg. 106:777, 1937.

Mixter, W.J., and Barr, J.S.: Rupture of the intervertebral disc with involvement of the spinal canal, N. Engl. J. Med. 211:210, 1934.

Mooney, V., and Robertson, J.: The facet syndrome, Clin. Orthop. 115:149, 1976.

Nachemson, A.L.: The lumbar spine: an orthopaedic challenge, Spine 1:59, 1976.

Nachemson, A.L.: Prevention of chronic back pain: the orthopaedic challenge for the 80's, Bull. Hosp. J. Dis. Orthop. Inst. 44:1, 1984.

Nafziger, H.C., Inman, V., and Saunders, J.B.: Lesions of the intervertebral disc and ligamenta flava, J. Surg. Gynecol. Obstet. 66:288, 1938.

Ortengren, R., Anderson, G., Broman, H., et al.: Vocational electromyography: studies of localized muscle fatigue and the assembly line, Ergonomics 18:157, 1975.

Poulsen, E.: Studies of back load, tolerance limits during lifting of burdens, Scand. J. Rehabil. Med. Suppl. 6:169, 1978.

Robinson, J.S.: Sciatica and the lumbar disk syndrome: a historic perspective, South, Med. J. 76:232, 1983.

Sandover, J.: Dynamic loading as a possible source of low-back disorders, Spine **8**:652, 1983.

Schmorl, G., and Junghanns, H.: Archiv. und Atlas der normalen und pathogischen Anatomie in typischen Röntgenbildern, Leipzig, 1932, Georg Thieme.

Semmes, R.E.: Diagnosis of ruptured intervertebral discs without contrast myelography and comment upon recent experience with modified hemilaminectomy for their removal, Yale J. Biol. Med. **11**:433, 1939.

de Sèze, S.: Sciatique "banale" et disques lombo-sacrés, Presse Med. **51-52**:570, 1940.

de Sèze, S.: Histoire de la sciatique, Rev. Neurol. **138**:1019, 1982.

Sitken, A.P., and Bradford, C.H.: End results of ruptured intervertebral discs in industry, Am. J. Surg. **73**:365, 1947.

Sjöqvist, O.: The mechanism of origin of Lasègue's sign, Acta Psych. Neurol. **46**(Suppl):290, 1947.

Smith, L., Garvin, P.J., Gesler, R.M., et al.: Enzyme dissolution of the nucleus pulposus, Nature **198**:1131, 1963.

Stolley, P.D., and Kuller, L.H.: The need for epidemiologists and surgeons to cooperate in the evaluation of surgical therapies, Surgery **78**:123, 1975.

Sugar, O.: Charles Lasègue and his "Considerations on Sciatica," JAMA **253**:1767, 1985.

Svensson, H.O., and Andersson, G.B.J.: Low back pain in 40- to 47-year-old men: work history and work environment factors, Spine **8**:272, 1983.

Svensson, H.O., Vedin, A., Wilhelmsson, C., and Andersson, G.B.J.: Low-back pain in relation to other diseases and cardiovascular risk factors, Spine **8**:277, 1983.

Troup, J.D.G., Martin, J.W., and Lloyd, D.C.E.F.: Back pain in industry: a prospective survey, Spine **6**:61, 1981.

Virchow, R.: Untersuchunger uber die Enwickelung die Schadeigrunder, Berlin, 1857, G. Reimer.

Waddell, G., Main, C.J., Morris, E.W., DiPaola, M., and Gray, I.C.M.: Chronic low-back pain, psychologic distress, and illness behavior, Spine **9**:209, 1984.

Wartenberg, R.: Lasègue sign and Kernig sign: historical notes, Arch. Neurol. Psych. **66**:58, 1951.

Wartenberg, R.: On neurologic terminology, eponyms and the Lasègue sign, Neurology **6**:853, 1956.

Weisz, G.M.: Lumbar spinal canal stenosis in Paget's disease, Spine **8**:192, 1983.

White, A.W.M.: Low back pain in men receiving workmen's compensation: a follow-up study, Can. Med. Assoc. J. **101**:61, 1969.

Wilder, D.G., Woodworth, B.B., Frymoyer, J.W., and Pope, M.H.: Vibration and the human spine, Spine **7**:1982

Wilkins, R.H., and Brody, I.A.: Lasègue's sign, Arch. Neurol. **21**:219, 1969.

General disc and spine anatomy

Adams, M.A., and Hutton, W.C.: The mechanical function of the lumbar apophyseal joints, Spine **8**:327, 1983.

Bogduk, N.: The clinical anatomy of the cervical dorsal rami, Spine **7**:319, 1982.

Bogduk, N.: The innervation of the lumbar spine, Spine **8**:286, 1983.

Bogduk, N., and Engel, R.: The menisci of the lumbar zygapophyseal joints: a review of their anatomy and clinical significance, Spine **9**:454, 1984.

Bogduk, N., and Macintosh, J.E.: The applied anatomy of the thoracolumbar fascia, Spine **9**:164, 1984.

Bose, K., and Balasubramaniam, P.: Nerve root canals of the lumbar spine, Spine **9**:16, 1984.

Bradford, F.K., and Spurling, R.G.: The intervertebral disk, ed. 2, Springfield, 1945, Charles C Thomas, Publisher.

Crock, H.V.: Normal and pathological anatomy of the lumbar spinal nerve root canals, J. Bone Joint Surg. **63**:487, 1981.

Cyriax, J.: Dural pain: mechanisms of symptoms, Lancet **1**:919, 1978.

D'Avella, D., and Mingrino, S.: Microsurgical anatomy of lumbosacral spinal roots, J. Neurosurg. **51**:819, 1979.

Edgar, M.A., and Ghadially, J.A.: Innervation of the lumbar spine, Clin. Orthop. **115**:35, 1976.

Hasue, M., and Fujiwara, M.: Epidemiologic and clinical studies of long-term prognosis of low-back pain and sciatica, Spine **4**:150, 1979.

Hasue, M., Kikuchi, S., Sakuyama, Y., and Ito, T.: Anatomic study of the interrelation between lumbosacral nerve roots and their surrounding tissues, Spine **8**:50, 1983.

Hollinshead, W.H.: Anatomy of the spine: points of interest to orthopaedic surgeons, J. Bone Joint Surg. **47-A**:209, 1965.

Inman, V.T., and Saunders, J.B., deC.M.: Referred pain from skeletal structures, J. Neurol. Ment. Dis. **99**:660, 1944.

Inoue, H.: Three-dimensional architecture of lumbar intervertebral discs, Spine **6**:139, 1981.

Jayson, M.I.V.: Compression stresses in the posterior elements and pathologic consequences, Spine **8**:338, 1983.

Jorgensen, K.: Back muscle strength and body weight as limiting factors for work in the standing slightly-stooped position, Scand. J. Rehab. Med. **2**:149, 1970.

Keegan, J.J.: Dermatome hypalgesia associated with herniation of intervertebral disc, Arch. Neurol. Psych. **50**:67, 1943.

Keyes, D.C., and Compere, E.L.: The normal and pathological physiology of the nucleus pulposus of the intervertebral disc: an anatomical, clinical, and experimental study, J. Bone Joint Surg. **14**:897, 1932.

Kikuchi, S., Hasue, M., Nishiyama, K., and Ito, T.: Anatomic and clinical studies of radicular symptoms, Spine **9**:23, 1982.

Kirkaldy-Willis, W.H.: The relationship of structural pathology to the nerve root, Spine **9**:49, 1984.

King, A.G.: Functional anatomy of the lumbar spine, Orthopedics **6**:1588, 1983.

Klausen, K.: The form and function of the loaded human spine, Acta Physiol. Scand. **65**:176, 1965.

Knutsson, F.: The instability associated with disc degeneration in the lumbar spine, Acta Radiol. **25**:593, 1944.

Macrae, I.F., and Wright, V.: Measurement of back movement, Ann. Rheum. Dis. **28**:584, 1969.

Magora, A.: Investigation of the relation between low back pain and occupation, Scand, J. Rehab. Med. **5**:191, 1973.

Miller, J.A.A., Haderspeck, K.A., and Schultz, A.B.: Posterior element loads in lumbar motion segments, Spine **8**:331, 1983.

Moll, J.M.H., and Wright, V.: Normal range of spinal mobility: an objective clinical study, Ann. Rheum. Dis. **30**:381, 1971.

Nachemson, A.: The lumbar spine and orthopaedic challenge, Spine **1**:59, 1976.

Nachemson, A., Lewin, T., Maroudas, A., et al.: In vitro diffusion of dye through the end plates and the anulus fibrosus of human intervertebral discs, Acta Orthop. Scand. **4**:589, 1970.

Postacchini, F., Urso, S., and Ferro, L.: Lumbosacral nerve-root anomalies, J. Bone Joint Surg. **64-A**:721, 1982.

Roofe, P.G.: Innervation of annulus fibrosus and posterior longitudinal ligament, fourth and fifth lumbar level, Arch. Neurol. Psychiatr. **44**:100, 1940.

Rowe, M.L.: Low back pain in industry, JOM **11**:161, 1969.

Rydevik, B., Brown, M.D., and Lundborg, G.: Pathoanatomy and pathophysiology of nerve root compression, Spine **9**:7, 1984.

Spencer, D.L., Irwin, G.S., and Miller, J.A.A.: Anatomy and significance of fixation of the lumbosacral nerve roots in sciatica, Spine **8**:672, 1983.

Wilder, D.G., Pope, M.H., and Frymoyer, J.W.: The functional topography of the sacroiliac joint, Spine **5**:575, 1980.

Willis, T.A.: Lumbosacral anomalies, J. Bone Joint Surg. **41-A**:935, 1959.

Young, A., et al.: Variations in the pattern of muscle innervation by the L5 and S1 nerve roots, Spine **8**:616, 1983.

Natural history of disc disease

Biering-Sorensen, F., and Hilden, J.: Reproducibility of the history of low-back trouble, Spine **9**:280, 1984.

Cramer, F., and McGowan, T.J.: Role of nucleus pulposus in pathogenesis of so-called "recoil" injuries of the spinal cord, Surg. Gynecol. Obstet. **79**:516, 1944.

Cyriax, J.: Dural pain: mechanisms of symptoms, Lancet **1**:919, 1978.

Dandy, W.E.: Concealed ruptured intervertebral disks: plea for elimination of contract medium in diagnosis, JAMA **117**:821, 1941.

Farfan, H.F.: The pathological anatomy of degenerative spondylolisthesis: a cadaver study, Spine **5**:412, 1980.

Farfan, H.F., and Sullivan, J.D.: The relation of facet orientation to intervertebral disc failure, Can. J. Surg. **10**:179, 1967.

Foley, R.K., and Kirkaldy-Willis, W.H.: Chronic venous hypertension in the tail of the Wistar rat, Spine **4**:251, 1979.

Frymoyer, J.W., Pope, M.H., Constanza, M.C., et al.: Epidemiological studies of low-back pain, Spine **5**:419, 1980.

Gardner, R.C.: The lumbar intervertebral disc: a correlation based on over 100 laminectomies, Arch. Surg. **100:**101, 1970.

Goldthwait, E.: Low-back lesions, J. Bone Joint Surg. **19:**810, 1937.

Hakelius, A.: Prognosis in sciatica, Acta Orthop. Scand. Suppl. **129:**1, 1970.

Jackson, R.P., Simmons, E.H., and Stripinis, D.: Incidence and severity of back pain in adult idiopathic scoliosis, Spine **8:**:749, 1983.

Jayson, M.I.V.: Compression stresses in the posterior elements and pathologic consequences, Spine **8:**338, 1983.

Kelsey, J.L., et al.: An epidemiologic study of lifting and twisting on the job and risk for acute prolapsed lumbar intervertebral disc, J. Orthop. Res. **2:**61, 1984.

Kirkaldy-Willis, W.H., and Hill, R.J.: A more precise diagnosis for low-back pain, Spine **4:**102, 1979.

Magora, A.: Investigation of the relation between low back pain and occupation: psychological aspects, Scand. J. Rehab. Med. **5:**191, 1973.

Nachemson, A.: The lumbar spine and orthopaedic challenge, Spine **1:**59, 1976.

Naylor, A.: Intervertebral disc prolapse and degeneration, Spine **1:**108, 1976.

Roland, M., and Morris, R.: A study of the natural history of back pain. Part I. Development of a reliable and sensitive measure of disability in low-back pain, Spine **8:**141, 1983.

Rydevik, B., Brown, M.D., and Lundborg, G.: Pathoanatomy and pathophysiology of nerve root compression, Spine **9:**7, 1984.

Sandover, J.: Dynamic loading as a possible source of low-back disorders, Spine **8:**652, 1983.

Scott, J.C.: Stress factor in the disc syndrome, J. Bone Joint Surg. **37-B:**107, 1955.

Weber, H.: Lumbar disc herniation: a controlled, prospective study with ten years of observation, Spine **8:**131, 1983.

Diagnostic studies

Abel, M.S., Smith, G.R., and Allen, T.N.K.: Refinements of the anteroposterior angled caudad view of the lumbar spine, Skel. Radiol. **7:**113, 1981.

Alemohammad, S., and Bouzarth, W.F.: Intracranial subdural hematoma following lumbar myelography: case report, J. Neurosurg. **52:**256, 1980.

Amundsen, P.: Cervical myelography with Amipaque: seven years experience, Radiologe **21:**282, 1981.

Andersson, G., Ortengren, R., and Nachemson, A.: Quantitive studies of the load on the back in different working-postures, Scand. J. Rehabil. Med. Suppl. **6:**173, 1978.

Andersson, G.B., and Schultz, A.B.: Effects of fluid injection on mechanical properties of intervertebral discs, J. Biomech. **12:**453, 1979.

Angiari, P., Crisi, G., and Merli, G.A.: Aphasia and right hemiplegia after cervical myelography with metrizamide: a case report, Neuroradiology **26:**61, 1984.

Asztely, M., Kadziolka, R., and Nachemson, A.: A comparison of sonography and myelography in clinically suspected spinal stenosis, Spine **8:**885, 1983.

Barrow, D.L., Wood, J.H., and Hoffman, J.C., Jr.: Clinical indications for computer-assisted myelography, Neurosurgery **12:**47, 1983.

Bladé, J., Gaston, F., Montserrat, E., et al.: Spinal subarachnoid hematoma after lumbar puncture causing reversible paraplegia in acute leukemia: case report, J. Neurosurg. **58:**438, 1983.

Bohutova, J., Vojir,R., Kolar, J., and Grepl, J.: Some unusual complications of myelography and lumbosacral radiculography, Diag. Imag. **48:**320, 1979.

Brady, L.P., Parker, L.B., and Vaughen, J.: An evaluation of the electromyogram in the diagnosis of the lumbar disc lesion, J. Bone Joint Surg. **51-A:**539, 1969.

Brem, S.S., Hafler, D.A., Van Uitert, R.L., Ruff, R.L., and Reichert, W.H.: Spinal subarachnoid hematoma: a hazard of lumbar puncture resulting in reversible paraplegia, N. Engl. J. Med. **304:**1020, 1981.

Burton, C.V.: Computed tomography scanning and the lumbar spine. Part I. Economic and historic review, Spine **4:**353, 1979.

Charles, M.F., Byrd, S.E., Cohn, M.L., and Huntington, C.T.: Metrizamide computer tomography of the postoperative lumbar spine, Orthop. Rev. **11**(10):49, 1982.

Coin, C.G.: Cervical disk degeneration and herniation: diagnosis by computerized tomography, South.Med. J. **77:**979, 1984.

Collier, B.D., Johnson, R.P., Carrera, G.F., et al.: Painful spondylolysis or spondylolisthesis studied by radiography and single-photon emission computed tomography, Radiology **154:**207, 1985.

Cook, P.L., and Wise, K.: A correlation of the surgical and radiculographic findings in lumbar disc herniation, Clin. Radiol. **30:**671, 1979.

Deburge, A., Benoist, M., and Boyer, D.: The diagnosis of disc sequestration, Spine **9:**496, 1984.

Dujovny, M., Barrionuevo, P.J., Kossovsky, N., Laha, R.K., and Rosenbaum, A.E.: Effects of contrast media on the canine subarachnoid space, Spine **3:**31, 1978.

Dvonch, V., Scarff, T., Bunch, W.H., et al.: Dermatomal somatosensory evoked potentials: their use in lumbar radiculopathy, Spine **9:**291, 1984.

Edelstein, W.A., Schenck, J.F., Hart, H.R., et al.: Surface coil magnetic resonance imaging, JAMA **253:**828, 1985.

Eisen, A., and Hoirch, M.: The electrodiagnostic evaluation of spinal root lesions, Spine **8:**98, 1983.

Eldevik, O.P.: Side effects and complications of myelography with water soluble contrast agents, J. Oslo City Hosp. **32:**121, 1982.

Fager, C.A.: Evaluation of cervical spine surgery by postoperative myelography, Neurosurgery **12:**416, 1983.

Firooznia, H., Benjamin, V., Kricheff, I.I., Rafii, M., and Golimbu, C.: CT of lumbar spine disc herniation: correlation with surgical findings, AJR **142:**587, 1984.

Fitzgerald, R.H., Reines, H.D., and Wise, J.: Diagnostic radiation exposure in trauma patients, South. Med. J. **76:**1511, 1983.

Ford, L.T., and Goodman, F.G.: X-ray studies of the lumbosacral spine, South. Med. J. **10:**1123, 1966.

Frymoyer, J.W., Hanley, E.N., and Howe, J.: A comparison of radiographic findings in fusion and nonfusion patients ten or more years following lumbar disc surgery, Spine **5:**435, 1979.

Gershater, R., and Holgate, R.C.: Lumbar epidural venography in the diagnosis of disc herniations, AJR **126:**992, 1976.

Greenberg, R.P., and Ducker, T.B.: Evoked potentials in the clinical neurosciences, J. Neurosurg. **56:**1, 1982.

Glasauer, F.E., and Alker, G.: Metrizamide enhanced computed tomography: an adjunct to myelography in lumbar disc herniation, Comput. Radiol. **7:**305, 1983.

Gulati, A.N., Guadognoli, D.A., and Quigley, J.M.: Relationship of side effects to patient position during and after metrizamide lumbar myelography, Radiology **141:**113, 1981.

Haldeman, S.: The electrodiagnosis evaluation of nerve root function, Spine **9:**42, 1984.

Harrington, H., Tyler, H.R., and Welch, K.: Surgical treatment of post-lumbar puncture dural CSF leak causing chronic headache: case report, J. Neurosurg. **57:**703, 1982.

Haughton, V.M., Eldevik, O.P., Magnaes, B., and Amundsen, P.: A prospective comparison of computed tomography and myelography in the diagnosis of herniated lumbar disks, Radiology **142:**103, 1982.

Hemminghytt, S., Daniels, D.L., Williams, A.L., and Haughton, V.M.: Intraspinal synovial cysts: natural history and diagnosis by CT, Radiology **145:**375, 1982.

Herkowitz, H.N., Romeyn, R.L., and Rothman, R.H.: The indications for metrizamide myelography: relationship with complications after myelography, J. Bone Joint Surg. **65-A:**1144, 1983.

Herkowitz, H.N., Wiesel, S.W., Booth, R.E., Jr., and Rothman, R.H.: Metrizamide myelography and epidural venography: their role in the diagnosis of lumbar disc herniation and spinal stenosis, Spine **7:**55, 1982.

Hirschy, J.C., Leue, W.M., Berninger, W.H., Hamilton, R.H., and Abbott, G.F.: CT of the lumbosacral spine: importance of tomographic planes parallel to vertebral end plate, AJR **136:**47, 1981.

Hitselberger, W.E., and Witten, R.M.: Abnormal myelograms in asymptomatic patients, J. Neurosurg. **28:**204, 1968.

Howie, D.W., Chatterton, B.E., and Hone, M.R.: Failure of ultrasound in the investigation of sciatica, J. Bone Joint Surg. **65-B:**144, 1983.

Hudgins, W.R.: Computer-aided diagnosis of lumbar disc herniation, Spine **8:**604, 1983.

James, A.E., Jr., Partain, C.L., Patton, J.A., et al.: Current status of magnetic resonance imaging, South. Med. J. **78:**580, 1985.

Jajic, I.: The role of HLA-B27 in the diagnosis of low back pain, Acta Orthop. Scand. **50:**411, 1979.

Jepson, K., Nada, A., and Rymaszewski, L.: The role of radiculography in the management of lesions of the lumbar disc, J. Bone Joint Surg. **64-B:**405, 1982.

Johansen, J.P., Fossgreen, J., and Hansen, H.H.: Bone scanning in lumbar disc herniation, Acta. Orthop. Scand. **51:**617, 1980.

Kapoor, W., Hemmer, K., Herbert, D., and Karpf, M.: Abdominal computed tomography: comparison of the usefulness of goal-directed vs non-goal-directed studies, Arch. Intern. Med. **143:**249, 1983.

Keller, R.H.: Traumatic displacement of the cartilaginous vertebral rim: a sign of intervertebral disc prolapse, Radiology **110:**21, 1974.

Kelsey, J.L., Githens, P.B., Walter, S.D., et al.: An epidemiological study of acute prolapsed cervical intervertebral disc, J. Bone Joint Surg. **66-A:**907, 1984.

Kieffer,S.A., Cacyorin, E.D., and Sherry, R.G.: The radiological diagnosis of herniated lumbar intervertebral disk: a current controversy, JAMA **251:**1192, 1984.

Kieffer, S.A., Sherry, R.G., Wellenstein, D.E., and King, R.B.: Bulging lumbar intervertebral disk: myelographic differentiation from herniated disk with nerve root compression, AJR **138:**709, 1982.

Kikuchi, S., Macnab, I., and Moreau, P.: Localisation of the level of symptomatic cervical disc degeneration, J. Bone Joint Surg. **63-B:**272, 1981.

Killebrew, K., Whaley, R.A., Hayward, J.N., and Scatliff, J.H.: Complications of metrizamide myelography, Arch. Neurol. **40:**78, 1983.

MacGibbon, B., and Farfan, H.F.: A radiologic survey of various configurations of the lumbar spine, Spine **4:**258, 1979.

Macnab, I.: The traction spur: an indicator of segmental instability, J. Bone Joint Surg. **53-A:**663, 1971.

Macnab, I., Cuthbert, H., and Godfrey, C.M.: The incidence of denervation of the sacrospinales muscles following spinal surgery, Spine **2:**294, 1977.

Macnab, I., St. Louis, E.L., Grabias, S.L., and Jacob, R.: Selective ascending lumbosacral venography in the assessment of lumbar disc herniation, J. Bone Joint Surg. **58-A:**1093, 1976.

Macon, J.B., and Poletti, C.E.: Conducted somatosensory evoked potentials during spinal surgery, Part 1. Control conduction velocity measurements, J. Neurosurg. **57:**349, 1982.

Macon, J.B., Poletti, C.E., Sweet, W.H., Ojemann, R.G., and Zervas, N.T.: Conducted somatosensory evoked potentials during spinal surgery. Part 2. Clinical applications, J. Neurosurg. **57:**354, 1982.

MacPherson, P., Teasdale, E., and MacPherson, P.Y.: Radiculography: is routine bed rest really necessary? Clin. Radiol. **34:**325, 1983.

McNeill, T.W., et al.: A new advance in water-soluble myelography, Spine **1:**72, 1976.

Meador, K., Hamilton, W.J., El Gammal, T.A.M., Demetropoulos, K.C., and Nichols, F.T., III: Irreversible neurologic complications of metrizamide myelography, Neurology **34:**817, 1984.

Moufarrij, N.A., Hardy, R.W., Jr., and Weinstein, M.A.: Computed tomographic, myelographic, and operative findings in patients with suspected herniated lumbar discs, Neurosurgery **12:**184, 1983.

Murphey, F., Pascucci, L.M., Meade, W.H., and Van Zwaluwenburg, B.R.: Myelography in patients with ruptured cervical intervertebral discs, Am. J. Roentgenol. Radium Ther. **56:**27, 1946.

Nelson, M.A., Allen, P., Clamp, S.E., et al.: Reliability and reproducibility of clinical findings in low-back pain, Spine **4:**97, 1979.

Paleari, G.L., Ballarati, P., Gambrioli, P.L., and Paleari, M.: Recent progress in vertebral body section roentgenography in the study of the pathology of the lumbar vertebrae, Ital. J. Orthop. Traumatol. **8:**109, 1982.

Peters, N.D., and Ehni, G.: Xeorradiography in evaluation of cervical spine injuries, J. Neurosurg. **49:**620, 1978.

Pope, M.H., Hanley, E.N., Matteri, R.E., Wilder, D.G., and Frymoyer, J.W.: Measurement of intervertebral disc space height, Spine **2:**282, 1977.

Post, M.J.D., Brown, M.D., and Gargano, F.P.: The technique and interpretation of lumbar myelograms, Spine **2:**214, 1977.

Rab, G.T., and Chao, E.Y.: Verification of roentgenographic landmarks in the lumbar spine, Spine **2:**287, 1977.

Raskin, S.P., and Keating, J.W.: Recognition of lumber disk disease: comparison of myelography and computed tomography, AJR **139:**349, 1982.

Risius, B., Modic, M.T., Hardy, R.W., Jr., Duchesneau, P.M., and Weinstein, M.A.: Sector computed tomographic spine scanning in the diagnosis of lumbar nerve root entrapment, Radiology **143:**109, 1982.

Scavone, J.G., Latshaw, R.F., and Rohrer, G.V.: Use of lumbar spine films: statistical evaluation of a university teaching hospital, JAMA **246:**1105, 1981.

Schelkun, S.R., Wagner, K.F., Blanks, J.A., and Reinert, C.M.: Bacterial meningitis following pantopaque myelography: a case report and literature review, Orthopedics **8**(1):74, 1985.

Schutte, H.E., and Park, W.M.: The diagnostic value of bone scintigraphy in patients with low back pain, Skel. Rad. **10:**1, 1983.

Sheldon, J.J., Russin, L.A., and Gargano, F.P.: Lumbar spinal stenosis: radiographic diagnosis with special reference to transverse axial tomography, Clin. Orthop. **115:**53, 1976.

Shima, F., Mihara, K., and Hachisuga, S.: Angioma in the paraspinal muscles complicated by spinal epidural hematoma: case report, J. Neurosurg. **57:**274, 1982.

Siddiqi, T.S., and Buchheit, W.A.: Herniated nerve root as a complication of spinal tap: case report, J. Neurosurg. **56:**565, 1982.

Siqueira, E.B., Kranzler, L.I., and Schaffer, L.: Intraoperative myelography: technical note, J. Neurosurg. **58:**786, 1983.

Splithoff, C.A.: Lumbosacral junction: roentgenographic comparison of patients with and without backaches, JAMA **152:**1610, 1953.

Steiner, R.E.: Nuclear magnetic resonance: its clinical application, J. Bone Joint Surg. **65-B:**533, 1983.

Stokes, I.A.F., Wilder, D.G., Frymoyer, J.W., and Pope, M.H.: Assessment of patients with low-back pain by biplanar radiographic measurement of intervertebral motion, Spine **6:**233, 1981.

Tchang, S.P.K., Howie, J.L., Kirkaldy-Willis, W.H., Paine, K.W.E., and Moola, D.: Computed tomography versus myelography in diagnosis of lumbar disc herniation, J. Canadian Assoc. Radiol. **33:**15, 1982.

Teplick, J.G., and Haskin, M.E.: Intravenous contrast-enhanced CT of the postoperative lumbar spine: improved identification of recurrent disk herniation, scar, arachnoiditis, and diskitis, AJR **143:**845, 1984.

Torgerson, W.R., and Dotter, W.E.: Comparative roentgenographic study of the asymptomatic and symptomatic lumbar spine, J. Bone Joint Surg. **58-A:**850, 1976.

Waddell, G., et al.: Nonorganic physical signs in low-back pain, Spine **5:**117, 1980.

Weiss, T., Treisch, J., Kazner, E., Claussen, C., Schörner, W., and Feigler, W.: Intervenöse Kontrastmittelgabe bei der Computertomographie (CT) der operierten Lendenwirbelsäule, Fortschr. Röntgenstr. **141:**30, 1984.

Weiss, T., et al.: CT of the postoperative lumbar spine: the value of intravenous contrast, Neuroradiology **28:**241, 1986.

Whelan, M.A., and Gold, R.P.: Computed tomography of the sacrum. Part 1. Normal anatomy, AJR **139:**1183, 1982.

Whelan, M.A., Hilal, S.K., Gold, R.P., Luken, M.G., and Michelson, W.J.: Computed tomography of the sacrum. Part 2. pathology, AJR **139:**1191, 1982.

Whiteleather, J.E., Semmes, R.E., and Murphey, F.: The roentgenographic signs of herniation of the cervical intervertebral disk, Radiology **46:**213, 1946.

Wilberger, J.E., Jr., and Pang, D.: Syndrome of the incidental herniated lumbar disc, J. Neurosurg. **59:**137, 1983.

Williams, P.C.: Reduced lumbosacral joint space: Its relation to sciatic irritation, JAMA **99:**1677,1932.

Williams, A.L., Haughton, V.M., Daniels, D.L., and Thornton, R.S.: CT recognition of lateral lumbar disc herniation, AJR **139:**345, 1982.

Wiltse, L.L.: The effect of the common anomalies of the lumbar spine upon disc degeneration and low back pain, Orthop. Clin. North Am. **2:**569, 1971.

Wiltse, L.L., Guyer, R.D., Spencer, C.W., Glenn, W.V., and Porter, I.S.: Alar transverse process impingement of the L5 spinal nerve: the far-out syndrome, Spine **9:**31, 1984.

Winston, K., Rumbaugh, C., and Colucci, V.: The vertebral canals in lumbar disc disease, Spine **9:**414, 1984.

Witt, I., Vestergaard, A., and Rosenklint, A.: A comparative analysis of x-ray findings of the lumbar spine in patients with and without lumbar pain, Spine **9:**298, 1984.

Injection studies

Ahlgren, E.W., Stephen, R., Lloyd, E.A.C., and McCollum, D.E.: Diagnosis of pain with a graduated spinal block technique, JAMA **195:**125, 1966.

Angtuaco, E.J.C., Holder, J.C., Boop, W.C., and Binet, E.F.: Computed tomographic discography in the evaluation of extreme lateral disc herniation, Neurosurgery **14:**350, 1984.

Benner, B., and Ehni, G.: Spinal arachnoiditis: the postoperative variety in particular, Spine **3:**40, 1978.

Benoist, M., Ficat, C., Baraf, P., and Cauchoix, J.: Postoperative lumbar epiduro-arachnoiditis: diagnostic and therapeutic aspects, Spine **5**:432, 1980.

Berman, A.T., Garbarino, J.L., Jr., Fisher, S.M., and Bosacco, S.J.: The effects of epidural injection of local anesthetics and corticosteroids on patients with lumbosciatic pain, Clin. Orthop. **188**:144, 1984.

Bogduk, N., and Long, D.M.: The anatomy of the so-called "articular nerves" and their relationship to facet denervation in the treatment of low-back pain, J. Neurosurg. **51**:172, 1979.

Brodsky, A.E.: Cauda equina arachnoiditis: a correlative clinical and roentgenologic study, Spine **3**:51, 1978.

Brodsky, A.E., and Binder, W.F.: Lumbar discography: its value in diagnosis and treatment of lumbar disc lesions, Spine **4**:110, 1979.

Bromley, J.W., et al.: Double-blind evaluation of collagenase injections for herniated lumbar discs, Spine **9**:486, 1984.

Brooks, S., Dent, A.R., and Thompson, A.G.: Anterior rupture of the lumbosacral disc: report of a case, J. Bone Joint Surg. **65-A**:1186, 1983.

Brothers, M.A., and Finlayson, D.C.: Evaluation of low back pain by differential spinal block, Can. Anaes. Soc. J. **15**:478, 1968.

Brown, F.W.: Management of discogenic pain using epidural and intrathecal steroids, Clin. Orthop. **129**:72, 1977.

Burton, C.V.: Lumbosacral Arachnoiditis, Spine **3**:24, 1978.

Butt, W.P.: Lumbar discography, J. Can. Assoc. Radiol. **14**:172, 1963.

Cloward, R.B., and Buzaid, L.L.: Discography: technique, indications and evaluation of the normal and abnormal intervertebral disc, Am. J. Roentgenol. **68**:552, 1952.

Collins, H.R.: An evaluation of cervical and lumbar discography, Clin. Orthop. **107**:133, 1975.

Cuckler, J.M., Bernini, P.A., Wiesel, S.W., et al.: The use of epidural steroids in the treatment of lumbar radicular pain: a prospective, randomized, double-blind study, J. Bone Joint Surg. **67-A**:63, 1985.

Dandy, W.E.: Concealed ruptured intervertebral disks: a plea for the elimination of contrast mediums in diagnosis, JAMA **117**:821, 1941.

De La Porte, C., and Siegfried, J.: Lumbosacral spinal fibrosis (spinal arachnoiditis): its diagnosis and treatment by spinal cord stimulation, Spine **8**:593, 1983.

Deburge, A., Benoist, M., and Rocolle, J.: La chirurgie dans les echecs de la nucleolyse des hernies discales lombaires, Rev. Chir. Orthop. **70**:637, 1984.

Destouet, J.M., Bilula, L.A., Murphy, W.A., and Monsees, B.: Lumbar facet joint injection: indicaton, technique, clinical correlation, and preliminary results, Radiology **145**:321, 1982.

Dory, M.A.: Arthrography of the lumbar facet joints, Radiology **140**:23, 1981.

Eng, R.H.K., and Seligman, S.J.: Lumbar puncture-induced meningitis, JAMA **245**:1456, 1981.

Feffer, H.L.: Regional use of steroids in the management of lumbar intervertebral disc disease, Orthop. Clin. North Am. **6**:249, 1975.

Ford, L.: Personal communication, 1984.

Fox, A.J.: Lumbar discography: a dissenting opinion letter, J. Can. Assoc. Radiol. **34**:88, 1983.

Gentry, W.D., Newman, M.C., Goldner, J.L., and von Baeyer, C.: Relation between graduated spinal block technique and MMPI for diagnosis and prognosis of chronic low-back pain, Spine **2**:210,1977.

Ghia, J.N., Duncan, G.H., and Teeple, E.: Differential spinal block for diagnosis of chronic pain, Compr. Ther. **8**:55, 1982.

Ghia, J.N., Duncan, G., Toomey, T.C., Mao, W., and Gregg, J.M.: The pharmacologic approach in differential diagnosis of chronic pain, Spine **4**:447, 1979.

Ghia, J.N., Mao, W., Toomey, T.C., and Gregg, J.M.: Acupuncture and chronic pain mechanisms, Pain **2**:285, 1976.

Ghormley, R.K.: Low back pain with special reference to the articular facets with presentation of an operative procedure, JAMA **101**:1773, 1933.

Goldthwait, E.: Low-back lesions, J. Bone Joint Surg. **19**:810, 1937.

Green, P.W.B., Burke, A.J., Weiss, C.A., and Langan, P.: The role of epidural cortisone injection in the treatment of diskogenic low back pain, Clin. Orthop. **153**:121, 1980.

Hauelsen, D.C., Smith, B.S., Myers, S.R., and Pryce, R.L.: The diagnostic accuracy of spinal nerve injection studies, Clin. Orthop. **198**:179, 1985.

Haughton, V.M., Eldevik, O.P., Ho, K.C., Larson, S.J., and Unger, G.F.: Arachnoiditis from experimental myelography with aqueous contrast media, Spine **3**:65, 1978.

Hoffman, G.S., Ellsworth, C.A., Wells, E.E., Franck, W.A., and Mackie, R.W.: Spinal arachnoiditis. What is the clinical spectrum? Part II. Arachnoiditis induced by pantopaque/autologous blood in dogs, a possible model for human disease, Spine **8**:541, 1983.

Hudgins, W.R.: Diagnostic accuracy of lumbar discography, Spine **2**:305, 1977.

Johnston, J.D.H., and Matheny, J.B.: Microscopic lysis of lumbar adhesive arachnoiditis, Spine **3**:36, 1978.

Kahanovitz, N., Arnoczky, S.P., Sissons, H.A., Steiner, G.C., and Schwarez, P.: The effect of discography on the canine intervertebral disc, Spine **11**:26, 1986.

Kikuchi, S., Macnab, I., and Moreau, P.: Localisation of the level of symptomatic cervical disc degeneration, J. Bone Joint Surg. **63-B**:272, 1981.

Krempen, J.F., and Smith, B.S.: Nerve-root injection: a method for evaluating the etiology of sciatica, J. Bone Joint Surg. **56-A**:1435, 1974.

Krempen, J.F., Silver, R.A., and Hadley, J.: An analysis of differential epidural spinal anesthesia and penthothal pain study in the differential diagnosis of back pain: aids in avoiding unncessary back surgery, Spine **4**:452, 1979.

Laun, A., Lorenz, R., and Agnoli, A.L.: Complications of cervical discography, J. Neurosurg. Sci. **25**:17, 1981.

Legré, J., Louis, R., Serrano, R., and Debaene, A.: Anatomo-radiological considerations about lumbar discography: an experimental study, Neuroradiology **17**:77, 1979.

Lindblom, K.: Diagnostic puncture of intervertebral discs in sciatica, Acta Orthop. Scand. **17**:231, 1948.

Macnab, I.: Negative disc exploration: an analysis of the causes of nerve-root involvement in sixty-eight patients, J. Bone Joint Surg. **53-A**:891, 1971.

Macnab, I., Grabias, S.L., and Jacob, R.: Selective ascending lumbosacral venography in the assessment of lumbar-disc herniation: an anatomical study and clinical experience, J. Bone Joint Surg. **58-A**:1093, 1976.

McCall, I.W., Park, W.M., and O'Brien, J.P.: Induced pain referral from posterior lumbar elements in normal subjects, Spine **4**:441, 1979.

McLaughlin, R.E., Miller, W.R., and Miller, C.W.: Quadriparesis after needle aspiration of the cervical spine: report of a case, J. Bone Joint Surg. **58-A**:1167, 1976.

Merriam, W.F., and Stockdale, H.R.: Is cervical discography of any value? Europ. J. Radiol. **3**:138, 1983.

Milette, P.C., and Melanson, D.: A reappraisal of lumbar discography, J. Can. Assoc. Radiol. **33**:176, 1982.

Mooney, V.: Alternative approaches for the patient beyond the help of surgery, Orthop. Clin. North Am. **6**:331, 1975.

Mooney, V., and Robertson, J.: The facet syndrome, Clin. Orthop. **115**:149, 1976.

Nelson, M.A., Allen, P., Clamp, S.E., et al.: Reliability and reproducibility of clinical findings in low-back pain, Spine **4**:97, 1979.

Oudenhoven, R.C.: The role of laminectomy, facet rhizotomy, and epidural steroids, Spine **4**:145, 1979.

Park, W.M., McCall, I.W., O'Brien, J.P., and Webb, J.K.: Fissuring of the posterior annulus fibrosus in the lumbar spine, Br. J. Radiol. **53**:382, 1979.

Quiles, M., Marchisello, P.J., and Tsairis, P.: Lumbar adhesive arachnoiditis: etiologic and pathologic aspects, Spine **3**:45, 1978.

Quinnell, R.C., and Stockdale, H.R.: The significance of osteophytes on lumbar vertebral bodies in relation to discographic findings, Clin. Radiol. **33**:197, 1982.

Quinell, R.C., and Stockdale, H.R.: Flexion and extension radiography of the lumbar spine: a comparison with lumbar discography, Clin. Radiol. **34**:405, 1983.

Quinell, R.C., Stockdale, H.R., and Harmon, B.: Pressure standardized lumbar discography, Br. J. Radiol. **53**:1031, 1980.

Shealy, C.N.: Facet denervation in the management of back and sciatic pain, Clin. Orthop. **115**:157, 1976.

Simmons, E.H., and Segil, C.M.: An evaluation of discography in the localization of symptomatic levels in discogenic disease of the spine, Clin. Orthop. **108**:57, 1975.

Skalpe, I.O.: Adhesive arachnoiditis following lumbar myelography, Spine **3**:61, 1978.

Sneider, S.E., Winslow, O.P., Jr., and Pryor, T.H.: Cervical diskography: is it relevant, JAMA **185**:163, 1963.

Stambough, J.L., Booth, R.E., Jr., and Rothman, R.H.: Transient hypercorticism after epidural steroid injection: a case report, J. Bone Joint Surg. **66-A:**1115, 1984.

Steindler, A., and Luck, J.V.: Differential diagnosis of pain low in the back: allocation of the source of pain by the procaine hydrochloride method, JAMA **110:**106, 1938.

Sussman, B.J., Bromley, J.W., and Gomez, J.C.: Injection of collagenase for herniated lumbar disk: initial clinical report, JAMA **245:**730, 1981.

Tajima, T., Furukawa, K., and Kuramochi, E.: Selective lumbosacral radiculography and block, Spine **5:**68, 1980.

Teeple, E., Scott, D.L., and Ghia, J.N.: Intrathecal normal saline without preservative does not have a local anesthetic effect, Pain **14:**3, 1982.

Weinberg, J.A.: The surgical excision of psoas abscesses resulting from spinal tuberculosis, J. Bone Joint Surg. **39-A:**17, 1957.

White, A.H., Derby, R., and Wynne, G.: Epidural injections for the diagnosis and treatment of low-back pain, Spine **5:**78, 1980.

Wilkinson, H.A.: Field block anesthesia for lumbar puncture (letter), JAMA **249:**2177, 1983.

Psychological testing

Caldwell, A.B., and Chase, C.: Diagnosis and treatment of personality factors in chronic low back pain, Clin. Orthop. **129:**141, 1977.

Carron, H., DeGood, D.E., and Tait, R.: A comparison of low back pain patients in the United States and New Zealand: psychosocial and economic facturs affecting severity of disability, Pain **21:**77, 1985.

Cohen, C.A., Foster, H.M., and Peck, E.A., III: MMPI evaluation of patients with chronic pain, South Med. J. **76:**316, 1983.

Colligan, R.C., Osborne, D., Swenson, W.M., and Offord, K.P.: The aging MMPI: development of contemporary norms, Mayo Clin. Proc. **59:**377, 1984.

Dennis, M.D., Greene, R.L., Farr, S.P., and Hartman, J.T.: The Minnesota Multiphasic Personality Inventory: general guidelines to its use and interpretation of orthopedics, Clin. Orthop. **150:**125, 1980.

Dennis, M.D., Rocchio, P.O., and Wiltse, L.L.: The topographical pain representation and its correlation with MMPI scores, Orthopaedics **5:**433, 1981.

Deyo, R.A., and Diehl, A.K.: Measuring physical and psychosocial function in patients with low-back pain, Spine **8:**635, 1983.

Evanski, P.M., Carver, D., Nehemkis, A., and Waugh, T.R.: The Burns' test in low back pain: correlation with the hysterical personality, Clin. Orthop. **140:**42, 1979.

Gentry, W.D.: Chronic back pain: does elective surgery benefit patients with evidence of psychologic disturbance? South. Med. J. **75:**1169, 1982.

Gentry, W.D., Shows, W.D., and Thomas, M.: Chronic low back pain: a psychological profile, Psychosomatics **15:**174, 1974.

Herron, L.D., and Pheasant, H.C.: Changes in MMPI profiles after low-back surgery, Spine **7:**591, 1982.

Leavitt, F., Garron, D.C., McNeill, T.W., and Whisler, W.W.: Organic status, psychological disturbance, and pain report characteristics in low-back-pain patients on compensation, Spine **7:**398, 1982.

Long, C.J., Brown, D.A., and Engelberg, J.: Intervertebral disc surgery: strategies for patient selection to improve surgical outcome, J. Neurosurg. **52:**818, 1980.

Luck, J.: Psychomatic problems in military orthopaedic surgery, J. Bone Joint Surg. **28:**213, 1946.

Nehemkis, A.M., Carver, D.W., and Evanski, P.M.: The predictive utility of the orthopaedic examination in identifying the low back pain patient with hysterical personality features, Clin. Orthop. **145:**158, 1979.

Pheasant, H.C., Gilbert, D., Goldfarb, J., and Herron, L.: The MMPI as a predictor of outcome in low-back surgery, Spine **4:**78, 1979.

Rainsford, A.O., Cairns, D., and Mooney, V.: The pain drawing as an aid to the psychologic evaluation of patients with low-back pain, Spine **1:**127, 1976.

Rockwood, C.A., and Eilert, R.E.: Camptocormia, J. Bone Joint Surg. **51-A:**533, 1969.

Southwick, S.M., and White, A.A.: The use of psychological tests in the evaluation of low-back pain, J. Bone Joint Surg. **65-A:**560, 1983.

Sternback, R.A.: Psychological aspects of chronic pain, Clin. Orthop. **129:**150, 1977.

Waddell, G., McCullouch, J.A., Kummel, E., et al.: Nonorganic physical signs in low-back pain, Spine **5:**117, 1980.

Westrin, C., Hirsch, C., and Lindegard, B.: The personality of the back patient, Clin. Orthop. **87:**209, 1972.

Wilfling, B.A., Klonoff, H., and Kokan, P.: Psychological, demographic and orthopaedic factors associated with prediction of outcome of spinal fusion, Clin. Orthop. **90:**153, 1973.

Wiltse, L.L., and Rocchio, P.: Preoperative psychological tests as predictors of success of chemonucleolysis in the treatment of the low-back syndrome, J. Bone Joint Surg. **57-A:**478, 1975.

Cervical disc

Bailey, R.W., and Badgley, C.E.: Stabilization of the cervical spine by anterior fusion, J. Bone Joint Surg. **42-A:**565, 1960.

Bloom, M.H., and Raney, F.L.: Anterior intervertebral fusion of the cervica spine: a technical note, J. Bone Joint Surg. **63-A:**842, 1981.

Boldrey, E.B.: Anterior cervical decompression (without fusion). Presented to the 25th annual meeting of the American Academy of Neurological Surgery, Key Biscayne, Florida, November 12, 1964.

Braun, I.R., Pinto, R.S., De Fillip, G.J., et al.: Brain stem infarction due to chiropractic manipulation of the cervical spine, South. Med. J. **76:**1507, 1983.

Bucy, P.C., Heimburger, R.F., and Oberhill, H.R.: Compression of the cervical spinal cord by herniated intervertebral discs, J. Neurosurg. **5:**471, 1948.

Bull, J.W.D.: Rupture of the interverteral disk in the cervical region, Proc. R. Soc. Med. **41:**513, 1948.

Cloward, R.B.: The treatment of ruptured lumbar intervertebral discs by vertebral body fusion: I. Indications, operative technique, after care, J. Neurosurg. **10:**154, 1953.

Cloward, R.B.: The anterior approach for removal of ruptured cervical discs, J. Neurosurg. **15:**602, 1958.

Coventry, M.B., Ghormley, R.K., and Kernohan, J.W.: The intervertebral disc: its microscopic anatomy and pathology. Part II. Changes in the intervertebral disc concomitant with age, J. Bone Joint Surg. **27:**233, 1945.

Coventry, M.B., Ghormley, R.K., and Kernohan, J.W.: the intervertebral disc: its microscopic anatomy and pathology. Part III. Pathological changes in the intervertebral disc. J. Bone Joint Surg. **27:**460, 1945.

Davidson, R.I., Dunn, E.J., and Metzmaker, J.N.: The shoulder abduction test in the diagnosis of radicular pain in cervical extradural compressive monoradiculopathies, Spine **6:**441, 1981.

De Palma, A.F., and Cooke, A.J.: Results of anterior interbody fusion of the cervical spine, Clin. Orthop. **60:**169, 1966.

Dunsker, S.B.: Anterior cervical discectomy with and without fusion, Clin. Neurosurg. **24:**516, 1976.

Evans, D.K.: Anterior cervical subluxation, J. Bone Joint Surg. **58-B:**318, 1976.

Garcia, A.: Cervical traction, an ancient modality, Orthop. Rev. **13:**429, 1984.

Harris, R.I., and Macnab, I.: Structural changes in the lumbar intervertebral disc: their relationship to low back pain and sciatica, J. Bone Joint Surg. **36-B:**304, 1954.

Hartman, J.T., Palumob, F., and Hill, B.J.: Cineradiography of the braced normal cervical spine: a comparative study of five commonly used cervical orthoses, Clin. Orthop. **109:**97, 1975.

Hirsch, D.: Cervical disc rupture; diagnosis and therapy, Acta Orthop. Scand. **30;**172, 1960.

Horal, J.: The clinical appearance of low back disorders in the city of Gothenburg, Sweden: comparisons of incapacitated probands with matched controls, Acta Orthop. Scand. Suppl. **116:**1, 1969.

Jacobs, B., Krueger, E.G., and Leivy, D.M.: Cervical spondylosis with radiculopathy: results of anterior diskectomy and interbody fusion, JAMA **211:**2135, 1970.

Josey, A.I., and Murphey, F.: Ruptured intervertebral disk simulating angina pectoria, JAMA **131:**581, 1946.

Keegan, J.J.: Dermatome hypalgesia associated with herniation or intervertebral disc, Arch Neurol. Psychiatr. **50:**67, 1943.

Kelsey, J.L., et al.: An epidemiological study of acute prolapsed cervical intervertebral disc, J. Bone Joint Surg. **66-A:**907, 1984.

Key, C.A.: On paraplegia depending on the ligaments of the spine, Guy's Hosp. Rep. **7:**1737, 1838.

Kikuchi, S., et al.: Anatomic and clinical studies of radicular symptoms, Spine **9:**23, 1984.

Kikuchi, S., Macnab, I., and Moreau, P.: Localisation of the level of symptomatic cervical disc degeneration, J. Bone Joint Surg. **63-B:**272, 1981.

Koop, S.E., Winter, R.B., and Lonstein, J.E.: The surgical treatment of instability of the upper part of the cervical spine in children and adolescents, J. Bone Joint Surg. **66-A:**403, 1984.

Lourie, H., Shende, M.C., and Stewart, D.H.: The syndrome of central cervical soft disk herniation, JAMA **226:**302, 1973.

Lunsford, L.D., Bissonette, D.J., Jannetta, P.J., Sheptak, P.E., and Zorub, D.S.: Anterior surgery for cervical disc disease. Part 1. Treatment of lateral cervical disc herniation in 253 cases, J. Neurosurg. **53:**1, 1980.

Murphey, M.G., and Gado, M.: Anterior cervical discectomy without interbody bone graft, J. Neurosurg. **37:**71, 1972.

Murphey, F., Simmons, J.C.H., and Brunson, B.: Surgical treatment of laterally ruptured cervical discs: a review of 648 cases, 1939 to 1972, J. Neurosurg. **38:**679, 1973.

Odom, G.L., Finney, W., and Woodhall, B.: Cervical disk lesion, JAMA **166:**23, 1958.

O'Laoire, S.A., and Thomas, D.G.T.: Spinal cord compression due to prolapse of cervical intervertebral disc (herniation of nucleus pulposes), J. Neurosurg. **59:**847, 1983.

Pennecot, G.F., Gouraud, D., Hardy, J.R., and Pouliquen, J.C.: Roentgenographical study of the stability of the cervical spine in children, J. Pediatr. Orthop. **4:**346, 1984.

Rainer, J.K.: Cervical disc surgery: a historical review, J. Tenn. Med. Assoc. **77:**12, 1984.

Rath, W.W.: Cervical traction: a clinical perspective, Orthop. Rev. **13:**430, 1984.

Robertson, J.T.: Anterior removal of cervical disc without fusion, Clin. Neurosurg. **20:**259, 1973.

Robertson, J.T., and Johnson, S.D.: Anterior cervical discectomy without fusion: long-term results, Clin. Neurosurg. **27:**440, 1980.

Robinson, J.S.: Sciatica and the lumbar disc syndrome: a historic perspective, South. Med. J. **76:**232, 1983.

Robinson, R.A., and Southwick, W.O.: Surgical approaches to the cervical spine. In AAOS: Instructional course lectures, volume 17, St. Louis, 1960, The C.V. Mosby Co.

Roda, J.M., et al.: Intradural herniated cervical disc: case report, J. Neurosurg. **57:**278, 1982.

Rosenorn, J., Hansen, E.B., and Rosenorn, M.A.: Anterior cervical discectomy with and without fusion, J. Neurosurg. **59:**252, 1983.

Rothman, R.H., and Marvel, J.P., Jr.: The acute cervical disk, Clin. Orthop. **109:**59, 1975.

Scoville, W.B.: Types of cervical disk lesions and their surgical approaches, JAMA **196:**105, 1966.

Scoville, W.B., Whitcomb, B.B., and McLaurin, R.: The cervical ruptured disk: report of 115 operative cases, Trans. Am. Neurol. Assoc. 76th Ann. Meet., 222, 1951.

Semmes, R.E., and Murphey, F.: The syndrome of unilateral rupture of the sixth cervical intervertebral disk, with compression of the seventh nerve root: a report of four cases with symptoms simulating coronary disease, JAMA **121:**1209, 1943.

Seddon, H.J., and Alexander, G.L.: Discussion on spinal caries with paraplegia, Proc. R. Soc. Med. **39:**723, 1946.

Sherk, H.H., Watters, W.C., III, and Zeiger, L.: Evaluation and treatment of neck pain, Orthop. Clin. North Am. **13:**439, 1982.

Simmons, E.H., and Bhalla, S.K.: Anterior cervical discectomy and fusion: a clinical and biomechanical study with eight-year follow-up, with a note on discography: technique and interpretation of results by W.P. Butt, J. Bone Joint Surg. **51-B:**225, 1969.

Simmons, J.C.H.: Rupture of cervical intervertebral discs. In Edmonson, A.S., and Crenshaw, A.H., editors: Campbell's Operative Orthopaedics, 6th ed., St. Louis, 1980, The C.V. Mosby Co.

Smith, G.W., and Robinson, R.A.: Anterior lateral cervical disc removal and interbody fusion for cervical disc syndrome, Bull. Johns Hopkins Hosp. **96:**223, 1955.

Spurling, R.G., and Scoville, W.B.: Lateral rupture of the cervical intervertebral discs: a common cause of shoulder and arm pain, Surg. Gynecol. Obstet. **78:**350, 1944.

Spurling, R.G., and Segerberg, L.H.: Lateral intervertebral disk lesions in the lower cervical region, JAMA **151:**354, 1953.

Stookey, B.: Cervical chondroma, Arch. Neurol. Psych. **20:**275, 1928.

White, A.A., Jupiter, J., Southwick, W.O., and Panjabi, M.M.: An experimental study of the immediate load bearing capacity of three surgical constructions for anterior spine fusions, Clin. Orthop. **91:**21, 1973.

White, A.A., et al.: Relief of pain by anterior cervical spine fusion for spondylosis: a report of sixty-five cases, J. Bone Joint Surg. **55-A:**525, 1973.

Whitecloud, T.S.: Management of radiculopathy and myelopathy by the anterior approach: the cervical spine, The Cervical Spine Research Society, Philadelphia, 1983, J.B. Lippincott Co.

Thoracic disc

Albrand, O.W., and Corkill, G.: Thoracic disc herniation: treatment and prognosis, Spine **4:**41, 1979.

Antoni, N.: Fall av kronisk rotkompression med ovanlig orsak, hernia nuclei pulposi disci intervertebralis, Sv. Lakartidn. **28:**436, 1931.

Arseni, C., and Nash, F.: Protrusion of thoracic intervertebral discs, Acta Neurochir. **11:**1, 1963.

Benson, M.K.D., and Byrnes, D.P.: The clinical syndromes and surgical treatment of thoracic intervertebral disc prolapse, J. Bone Joint Surg. **57-B:**471, 1975.

Hochman, M.S., Pena, C., and Ramirez, R.: Calcified herniated thoracic disc diagnosed by computerized tomography: case report, J. Neurosurg. **52:**722, 1980.

Hulme, A.: The surgical approach to thoracic intervertebral disc protrusions, J. Neurol. Neurosurg. Psychiat. **23:**133, 1960.

Logue, V.: Thoracic intervertebral disc prolapse with spinal cord compression, J. Neurol. Neurosurg. Psychiat. **15:**227, 1952.

Love, J.G., and Kiefer, E.J.: Root pain and paraplegia due to protrusions of thoracic intervertebral disks, J. Neurosurg. **15:**62, 1950.

Maiman, D.J., Larson, S.J., Luck, E., and El-Ghatit, A.: Lateral extracavity approach to the spine for thoracic disc herniation: report of 23 cases, Neurosurgery **14:**178, 1984.

Martucci, E., Mele, C., and Martella, P.: Thoracic intervertebral disc protrusion, Ital. J. Orthop. Traumatol. **10:**333, 1984.

Marzluff, J.M., Hungerford, G.D., Kempe, L.G., Rawe, S.E., Trevor, R., and Perot, P.L., Jr.: Thoracic myelopathy caused by osteophytes of the articular process, J. Neurosurg. **50:**779, 1979.

Muller, R.: Protrusion of thoracic intervertebral disks with compression of the spinal cord, Acta Med. Scand. **139:**99, 1951.

O'Leary, P.F., Camins, M.B., Polifroni, N.V., and Floman, Y.: Thoracic disc disease: clinical manifestations and surgical treatment, Bull. Hosp. Jt. Dis. Orthop. Inst. **44:**27, 1984.

Omojola, M.F., Cardoso, E.R., Fox, A.J., Drake, C.G., and Durward, Q.J.: Thoracic myelopathy secondary to ossified ligamentum flavum: case report, J. Neurosurg. **56:**448, 1982.

Otani, K., Manzoku, S., Shibasaki, K., and Nomachi, S.: The surgical treatment of thoracic and thoracolumbar disc lesions using the anterior approach: report of six cases, Spine **2:**266, 1977.

Panjabi, M.M., Krag, M.H., Dimnet, J.C., Walter, S.D., and Brand, R.A.: Thoracic spine centers of rotation in the sagittal plane, J. Orthop. Res. **1:**387, 1984.

Perot, P.L., Jr., and Munro, D.D.: Transthoracic removal of midline thoracic disc protrusions causing spinal cord compression, J. Neurosurg. **31:**452, 1969.

Seddon, H.J.: Pott's paraplegia. In Platt, H., editor: Modern trends in orthopaedics (second series), London, 1956, Butterworth & Co., Ltd.

Sekhar, L.N., and Jannetta, P.J.: Thoracic disc herniation: operative approaches and results, Neurosurgery **12:**303, 1983.

Tovi, D., and Strang, R.R.: Thoracic intervertebral disk protrusions, Acta Chir. Scand. **267,** 1960.

Lumbar disc

Agre, K., Wilson, R.R., Brim, M., and McDermott, D.J.: Chymodiactin postmarketing surveillance: demographic and adverse experience data in 29,075 patients, Spine **9:**479, 1984.

Aho, A.J., Auranen, A., and Pesonen, K.: Analysis of cauda equina symptoms in patients with lumbar disc prolapse, Acta Chir. Scand. **135:**413, 1969.

Aitken, A.P., and Bradford, C.H.: End results of ruptured intervertebral discs in industry, Am. J. Surg. **73:**365, 1947.

Anderson, B.J.G., Ortengren, R., Nachemson, A., and Elfstrom, G.: Lumbar disc pressure and myoelectric back muscle activity during sitting. Part 1. Scand. J. Rehab. Med. **6:**104, 1974.

Anderson, B.J.G., and Ortengren, R.: Lumbar disc pressure and myo-electric back muscle activity during sitting. Part 2, Scand. J. Rehab. Med. **6**:115, 1974.

Andrews, E.T.: A unique frame for back surgery, Orthopedics **2**:130, 1979.

Apfelbach, H.W.: Technique for chemonucleolysis, Orthopedics **6**:1613, 1983.

Arnoldi, C.C., et al.: Lumbar spinal stenosis and nerve root entrapment syndromes: definition and classification, Clin. Orthop. **115**:4, 1976.

Barach, E.M., Nowak, R.M., Lee, T.G., and Tomlanovich, M.C.: Epinephrine for treatment of anaphylactic shock, JAMA **251**:2118, 1984.

Barr, J.S.: Low-back and sciatic pain: results of treatment, J. Bone Joint Surg. **33-A**:633, 1951.

Barr, J.S., et al.: Evaluation of end results in treatment of ruptured lumbar intervertebral discs with protrusion of nucleus pulposus, J. Surg. **123**:250, 1967.

Battit, G.E.: Anaphylaxis associated with chymopapain injections, JAMA **253**:977, 1985.

Bell, G.R., and Rothman, R.H.: The conservative treatment of siatica, Spine **9**:54, 1984.

Benezech, et al.: Microsurgery of common discal sciatica: technics and results, Neurochirurgie **29**:371, 1983.

Benner, B., and Ehni, G.: Degenerative lumbar scoliosis, Spine **4**:548, 1979.

Benoist, M., et al.: Treatment of lumbar disc herniation by chymopapain chemonucleolysis: a report on 120 patients, Spine **7**:613, 1982.

Benoist, M., Ficat, C., Baraf, P., and Cauchoix, J.: Postoperative lumbar epiduro-arachnoiditis: diagnostic and therapeutic aspects, Spine **5**:432, 1980.

Bergquist-Ullman, M., and Larsson, U.: Acute low back pain in industry: a controlled prospective study with special reference to therapy and confounding factors, Acta Orthop. Scand. Suppl. **170**, 1977.

Berman, A.T., Garbarino, J.L., Fisher, S.T., and Bosacco, S.J.: The effects of epidural injection of local anesthetics and corticosteroids on patients with lumbosciatic pain, Clin. Orthop. **188**:144, 1984.

Bernstein, I.L.: Adverse effects of chemonucleolysis, JAMA **250**:1167, 1983.

Blower, P.W.: Neurologic patterns in unilateral sciatica: a prospective study of 100 new cases, Spine **6**:175, 1981.

Borgesen, S.E., and Vang, P.S.: Herniation of the lumbar intervertebral disk in children and adolescents, Acta Orthop. Scand. **45**:540, 1974.

Bradford, D.S., and Garcia, A.: Lumbar intervertebral disk herniations in children and adolescents, Orthop. Clin. North Am. **2**:583, 1971.

Bradford, D.S., Cooper, K.M., and Oegema, T.R., Jr.: Chymopapain, chemonucleolysis, and nucleus pulposus regeneration, J. Bone Joint Surg. **65-A**:1220, 1983.

Breig, A., and Troup, J.D.G.: Biomechanical considerations in the straight-leg-raising test, Spine **4**:242, 1979.

Brown, F.W.: Management of diskogenic pain using epidural and intrathecal steroids, Clin. Orthop. **129**:72, 1977.

Brown, M.D.: Diagnosis of pain syndromes of the spine, Orthop. Clin. North Am. **6**:233, 1975.

Bryant, M.S., Bremer, A.M., and Nguyen, T.Q.: Autogeneic fat transplants in the epidural space in routine lumbar spine surgery, Neurosurgery **13**:367, 1983.

Capanna, A.H., et al.: Lumbar discectomy-percentage of disc removal and detection of anterior anulus perforation, Spine **6**:610, 1981.

Carruthers, C.C., and Kousaie, K.N.: Surgical treatment after chemonucleolysis failure, Clin. Orthop. **165**:172, 1982.

Castellvi, A.E., Goldstein, L.A., and Chan, D.P.K.: Lumbosacral transitional vertebrae and their relationship with lumbar extradural defects, Spine **9**:493, 1984.

Cauchoix, J., Ficat, C., and Girard, B.: Repeat surgery after disc excision, Spine **3**:256, 1978.

Cauthen, C.: Lumbar spine surgery, Baltimore, 1983, Williams & Wilkins.

Charnley, J.: Orthopaedic signs in the diagnosis of disc protrusion, Lancet, **1**:186, 1951.

Choudhury, A.R., and Taylor, J.C.: Cauda equina syndrome in lumbar disc disease, Acta Orthop. Scand. **51**:493, 1980.

Choudhury, A.R., Taylor, J.C., Worthington, B.S., and Whitaker, R.: Lumbar radiculopathy contralateral to upper lumbar disc herniation: report of three cases, Br. J. Surg. **65**:842, 1978.

Chow, S.P., Leong, J.C.Y., and Yau, A.C.M.C.: Anterior spinal fusion for deranged lumbar intervertebral disc: a review of 97 cases, Spine **5**:452, 1980.

Clark, K.: Significance of the small lumbar spinal canal: cauda equina compression syndromes due to sponylosis. Part 2. Clinical and surgical significance. J. Neurosurg. **31**:495, 1969.

Clarke, H.A., and Fleming, I.D.: Disk disease and occult malignancies, South. Med. J. **66**:449, 1973.

Clarke, N.M.P., and Cleak, D.K.: Intervertebral lumbar disc prolapse in children and adolescents, J. Pediatr. Orthop. **3**:202, 1983.

Compere, E.L.: Spinal fusion following removal of intervertebral disk, South. Med. J. **39**:301, 1946.

Cook, P.L., and Wise, K.: A correlation of the surgical and radiculographic findings in lumbar disc herniation, Clin. Radiol. **30**:671, 1979.

Coyer, A.B., and Curwen, I.H.M.: Low back pain treated by manipulation, Br. Med. J. 705, March 19, 1955.

Crawshaw, C., Frazer, A.M., Merriam, W.F., Mulholland, R.C., and Webb, J.K.: A comparison of surgery and chemonucleolysis in the treatment of sciatica: a prospective randomized trial, Spine **9**:195, 1984.

Crock, H.V.: Normal and pathological anatomy of the lumbar spinal nerve roots, J. Bone Joint Surg. **63-B**:487, 1981.

Cuckler, J.M., et al.: The use of epidural steroids in the treatment of lumbar radicular pain, J. Bone Joint Surg. **67-A**:63, 1985.

Cyriax, J.: Dural pain: mechanisms of symptoms, Lancet **1**:919, 1978.

Di Lauro, L., Poli, R., Bortoluzzi, M., and Marini, G.: Paresthesias after lumbar disc removal and their relationship to epidural hematoma, J. Neurosurg. **57**:135, 1982.

Dimitrigevic, D.T.: Historical note: Laseègue sign, Neurology **2**:453, 1952.

Dujovny, M., Barrionuevo, P.J., Kossovsky, N., Laha, R.K., and Rosenbaum, A.E.: Effects of contrast media on the canine subarachnoid space, Spine **3**:31, 1978.

Dvonch, V., et al.: Dermtomal somatosensory evoked potentials: their use in lumbar radiculopathy, Spine **9**:291, 1984.

Dyck, P.: The stoop-test in lumbar entrapment radiculopathy, Spine **4**:89, 1979.

Edgar, M.A., and Park, W.M.: Induced pain patterns on passive straight-leg raising in lower lumbar disc protrusion: a prospective clinical, myelographic and operative study in fifty patients, J. Bone Joint Surg. **56-B**:658, 1974.

Eguro, H.: Transverse myelitis following chemonucleolysis: report of a case, J. Bone Joint Surg. **65-A**:1328, 1983.

Eie, N., Solgaard, T., and Kleppe, H.: The knee-elbow position in lumbar disc surgery: a review of complications, Spine **8**:897, 1983.

Eismont, F.J., Wiesel, S.W., and Rothman, R.H.: The treatment of dural tears associated with spinal surgery, J. Bone Joint Surg. **63-A**:1132, 1981.

El-Gindi, S., Aref, S., Salama, M., and Andrew, J.: Infection of the intervertebral discs after surgery, J. Bone Joint Surg. **58-B**:114, 1976.

Epstein, B.S., Epstein, J.A., and Lavine, L.: The effect of anatomic variations in the lumbar vertebrae and spinal canal on cauda equina and nerve root syndromes, Am. J. Roentgenol. Radium Ther. Nucl. Med. **91**:105, 1964.

Epstein, J.A., Carras, R., Ferrar, J., Hyman, R.A., and Khan, A.: Conjoined lumbosacral nerve roots, J. Neurosurg. **55**:585, 1981.

Epstein, J.A., Epstein, B.S., and Jones, M.D.: Symptomatic lumbar scoliosis with degenerative changes in the elderly, Spine **4**:542, 1979.

Estridge, M.N., Rouhe, S.A., and Johnson, N.G.: The femoral stretching test: a valuable sign in diagnosing upper lumbar disc herniations, J. Neurosurg. **57**:813, 1982.

Evanski, P.M., Carver, D., Nehemkis, A. and Waugh, T.R.: The Burns' test in low back pain: correlation with the hysterical personality, Clin. Orthop. **140**:42, 1979.

Fairbank, J.C.T., and O'Brien, J.P.: The iliac crest syndrome: a treatable cause of low-back pain, Spine **8**:220, 1983.

Farfan, H.F.: The torsional injury of the lumbar spine, Spine **9**:53, 1984.

Finneson, B.E., and Cooper, V.R.: A lumbar disc surgery predictive score card: a retrospective evaluation, Spine **4**:141, 1979.

Fisher, R.G., and Saunders, R.L.: Lumbar disc protrusion in children, J. Neurosurg. **54**:480, 1981.

Floman, Y., Wiesel, S.W., and Rothman, R.H.: Cauda equina syndrome presenting as a herniated lumbar disc, Clin. Orthop. **147**:234, 1980.

Flynn, J.C., and Price, C.T.: Sexual complications of anterior fusion of the lumbar spine, Spine **9**:489, 1984.

Fraser, R.D.: Chymopapain for the treatment of intervertebral disc herniation: a preliminary report of a double-blind study, Spine **7**:608, 1982.

Fraser, R.D.: Chymopapain for the treatment of intervertebral disc herniation: the final report of a double-blind study, Spine **9:**815, 1984.

Friberg, O.: Clinical symptoms and biomechanics of lumbar spine and hip joint in leg length inequality, Spine **8:**643, 1983.

Frymoyer, J.W., Hanaley, E.N., and Howe, J.: A comparison of radiographic findings in fusion and nonfusion patients ten or more years following lumbar disc surgery, Spine **5:**435, 1979.

Gardner, R.C.: The lumbar intervertebral disk: a clinicopathological correlation based on over 100 laminectomies, Arch. Surg. **100:**101, 1970.

Garrido, E., and Rosenwasser, R.H.: Painless footdrop secondary to lumbar disc herniation: report of two cases, Neurosurgery **8:**484, 1981.

Getty, C.J.M., Johnson, J.R., Kirwan, E., and Sullivan, M.F.: Partial undercutting facetectomy for bony entrapment of the lumbar nerve root, J. Bone Joint Surg. **63-B:**330, 1981.

Giles, L.G.F., and Taylor, J.R.: Low back pain associated with leg length inequality, Spine **6:**510, 1981.

Goald, H.J.: Microlumbar discectomy: followup of 147 patients, Spine **3:**183, 1978.

Gokalp, H.Z., and Ozkai, E.: Intradural tuberculomas of the spinal cord: report of two cases, J. Neurosurg. **55:**289, 1981.

Grammer, L.C., Ricketti, A.J., Schafer, M.F., and Patterson, R.: Chymopapain allergy: case reports and identification of patients at risk for chymopapain anaphylaxis, Clin. Orthop. **188:**139, 1984.

Grant, F.C.: Operative results in intervertebral discs, Ann. Surg. **124:**1066, 1946.

Greenberg, R.P., and Ducker, T.B.: Evoked potentials in the clinical neurosciences, J. Neurosurg. **56:**1, 1982.

Grobler, L.J., Simmons, E.H., and Barrington, T.W.: Intervertebral disc herniation in the adolescent, Spine **4:**267, 1979.

Gurdjian, E.S., and Webster, J.E.: Lumbar herniations of the nucleus pulposus: an analysis of 196 operated cases, Am. J. Surg. **76:**235, 1948.

Hakelius, A.: Prognosis in sciatica, Acta Orthop. Scand. Suppl. **129:**6, 1970.

Hall, B.B., and McCulloch, J.A.: Anaphylactic reactions following the intradiscal injection of chymopapain under local anesthesia, J. Bone Joint Surg. **65-A:**1215, 1983.

Hall, G.W.: Neurologic signs and their discoverers, JAMA **95:**703, 1930.

Hanman, B.: The evaluation of physical ability, N. Engl. J. Med. **258:**986, 1958.

Harbison, S.P.: Major vascular complications of intervertebral disc surgery, Ann. Surg. **140:**342, 1954.

Hastings, D.E.: A simple frame of operations of the lumbar spine, Can. J. Surg. **12:**251, 1969.

Healy, K.M.: Does preoperative instruction make a difference?, Am. J. Nurs. **68:**62, 1968.

Herron, L.D., and Pheasant, H.C.: Prone knee-flexion provocative testing for lumbar disc protrusion, Spine **5:**65, 1980.

Hirsch, C.: Reflections on the use of surgery in lumbar disc disease, Orthop. Clin. **2:**493, 1971.

Hirsh, L.F., and Finneson, B.E.: Intradural sacral nerve root metastasis mimicking herniated disc: case report, J. Neurosurg. **49:**764, 1978.

Hitselberger, W.E., and Witten, R.M.: Abnormal myelograms in asymptomatic patients, J. Neurosurg. **28:**204, 1968.

Hodge, C.J., Binet, E.F., and Kieffer, S.A.: Intradural herniation of lumbar intervertebral discs, Spine **3:**346, 1978.

Hollinshead, W.H.: Anatomy of the spine: points of interest to orthopaedic surgeons, J. Bone Joint Surg. **47-A:**209, 1965.

Holmes, H.E., and Rothman, R.H.: The Pennsylvania plan: an algorithm for the management of lumbar degenerative disc disease, Spine **4:**156, 1979.

Holscsher, E.C.: Vascular complication of disc surgery, J. Bone Joint Surg. **30-A:**968, 1948.

Jacobs, R.R., McClain, O., and Neff, J.: Control of postlaminectomy scar formation: an experimental and clinical study, Spine **5:**223, 1980.

Javid, M.J., et al.: Safety and efficacy of chymopapain (chymodiactin) in herniated nucleus pulposus with sciatica: results of a randomized, double-blind study, JAMA **249:**2489, 1983.

Kadish, L., and Simmons, E.H.: Anomalies of the lumbosacral nerve roots and anatomical investigation and myelographic study, J. Bone Joint Surg. **66-B:**411, 1984.

Kane, R.L., Olsen, D., and Leymaster, C., et al.: Manipulating the patient, Lancet **1:**1333, 1974.

Keegan, J.J.: Dermatome hypalgesia associated with herniation of intervertebral disc, Arch. Neurol. Psych. **50:**67, 1943.

Keller, J.T., et al.: The fat of autogenous grafts to the spinal dura, J. Neurosurg. **49:**412, 1978.

Kelley, J.H., Voris, D.C., Svien, H.J., and Ghormley, R.K.: Multiple operations for protruded lumbar intervertebral disk, Mayo Clin. Proc **29:**546, 1954.

Key, J.A.: Intervertebral-disk lesions in children and adolescents, J. Bone Joint Surg. **32-A:**97, 1950.

Kieffer, S.A., Sherry, R.G., Wellenstein, D.E., and King, R.B.: Bulging lumbar intervertebral disk: myelographic differentiation from herniated disk with nerve root compression, AJR **138:**709,1982.

Kikuchi, S., Hasue, M., Nishiyama, K., et al.: Anatomic and clinical studies of radicular symptoms, Spine **9:**23, 1984.

Kirkaldy-Willis, W.H., and Hill, R.J.: A more precise diagnosis for low-back pain, Spine **4:**102, 1979.

Kiviluoto, O.: Use of free fat transplants to prevent epidural scar formation: an experimental study, Acta Orthop. Scand. Suppl **164:**1, 1976.

Klier, I., and Santo, M.: Low back pain as presenting symptoms of chronic granulocytic leukemia, Orthop. Rev. **11:**111, 1982.

Kostuik, J.P., and Bentivoglio, J.: The incidence of low-back pain in adult scoliosis, Spine **6:**268, 1981.

Kostuik, J.P., et al.: Cauda equina syndrome and lumbar disc hernia, J. Bone Joint Surg. **68-A:**386, 1986.

LaRocca, H., and Macnab, I.: The laminectomy membrane: studies in its evolution, characteristics, effects and prophylaxis in dogs, J. Bone Joint Surg. **56-B:**545, 1974.

Leavitt, F., Garron, D.C., Whisler, W.W., and D'Angelo, C.M.: A comparison of patients treated by chymopapain and laminectomy for low back pain using a multidimensional pain scale, Clin. Orthop. **146:**136, 1980.

Leong, J.C.Y., et al.: Long-term results of lumbar intervertebral disc prolapse, Spine **8:**793, 1983.

Lidstrom, A., and Zachrisson, M.: Physical therapy on low back pain and sciatica, Scand. J. Rehab. Med. **2:**37, 1970.

Lindholm, T.S., and Pylkkanen, P.: Discitis following removal of intervertebral disc, Spine **7:**618, 1982.

Macnab, I.: Management of low back pain, In Ahstrom, J.P., Jr., editor: Current practice in orthopaedic surgery, St. Louis, 1973, The C.V. Mosby Co.

Macnab, I., Cuthbert, H., and Godfrey, C.M.: The incidence of denervation of the sacrospinales muscles following spinal surgery, Spine **2:**294, 1977.

Macon, J.B., and Poletti, C.E.: Conducted somatosensory evoked potentials during spinal surgery. Part 1: Control, conduction velocity measurements, J. Neurosurg. **57:**349, 1982.

Macon, J.B., Poletti, C.E., Sweet, W.H., Ojemann, R.G., and Zervas, N.T.: Conducted somatosensory evoked potentials during spinal surgery. Part 2: Clinical applications, J. Neurosurg. **57:**354, 1982.

Martins, A.N., Ramirez, A., Johnston, J., and Schwetschenau, P.R.: Double-blind evaluation of chemonucleolysis for herniated lumbar discs: late results, J. Neurosurg. **49:**816, 1978.

May, A.R.L., Brewster, D.C., and Darling, R.C., et al.: Arteriovenous fistula following lumbar disc surgery, Br. J. Surg. **68:**41, 1981.

McCulloch, J.A.: Chemonucleolysis: experience with 2000 cases, Clin. Orthop. **146:**128, 1980.

McCulloch, J.A.: Outpatient discolysis with chymopapain, Orthopedics **6:**1624, 1983.

McCulloch, J.A., and Ferguson, J.M.: Outpatient chemonucleolysis, Spine **6:**606, 1981.

McLaren, A.C., and Bailey, S.I.: Cauda equina syndrome: a complication of lumbar discectomy, Clin. Orthop. **204:**143, 1986.

Moll, J.M.H., and Wright, V.: Normal range of spinal mobility: an objective clinical study, Ann. Rheum. Dis. **30:**381, 1971.

Mullen, J.B., and Cook, W.A., Jr.: Reduction of postoperative lumbar hemilaminectomy pain with marcaine, J. Neurosurg. **51:**126, 1975.

Nachemson, A.: Physiotherapy for low back pain patients: a critical look, Scand. J. Rehab. Med. **1:**85, 1969.

Nachemson, A.L.: The lumbar spine: an orthopaedic challenge, Spine **1:**59, 1976.

Nachemson, A.: Adult scoliosis and back pain, Spine **4:**513, 1979.

Nachemson, A.L.: Prevention of chronic back pain: the orthopaedic challenge for the 80's, Bull. Hosp. J. Dis. Orthop. Inst. **44:**1, 1984.

Nachemson, A., and Lindh, M.: Measurement of abdominal and back muscle strength with and without low back pain, Scand. J. Rehab. Med. **1**:60, 1969.

Nachlas, I.W.: End-result study of the treatment of herniated nucleus pulposus by excision with fusion and without fusion, J. Bone Joint Surg. **34-A**:981, 1952.

Nafziger, H.C., Inman, V., and Saunders, J.B.: Lesions of the intervertebral disc and ligamenta flava, J. Surg. Gyn. Obstet. **66**:288, 1938.

Nakano, N., and Tomita, T.: Results of surgical treatment of low back pain: a comparative study of the anterior and posterior approach, Inter. Orthop. (SICOT) **4**:101, 1980.

Naylor, A., Earland, C., and Robinson, J.: The effect of diagnostic radiopaque fluids used in discography on chymopapain activity, Spine **8**:875, 1983.

Neidre, A., and Macnab, I.: Anomalies of the lumbosacral nerve roots, Spine **8**:294, 1983.

Nelson, M.A., Allen, P., and Clamp, S.E., et al.: Reliability and reproducibility of clinical findings in low-back pain, Spine **4**:97, 1979.

Nielsen, B., deNully, M., Schmidt, K., and Hansen, R.I.: A urodynamic study of cauda equina syndrome due to lumbar disc herniation, Urol. Int. **35**:167, 1980.

Nordby, E.J.: Current concepts review: chymopapain in intradiscal therapy, J. Bone Joint Surg. **65-A**:1350, 1983.

Nordby, E.J., and Lucas, G.L.: A comparative analysis of lumbar disk disease treated by laminectomy or chemonucleolysis, Clin. Orthop. **90**:119, 1973.

O'Brien, J.P.: Anterior spinal tenderness in low-back pain syndromes, Spine **4**:85, 1979.

Offierski, C.M., and Macnab, I.: Hip-spine syndrome, Spine **8**:316, 1983.

Oudenhoven, R.C.: The role of laminectomy, facet rhizotomy, and epidural steroids, Spine **4**:145, 1979.

Parkinson, D.: Late results of treatment of intervertebral disc disease with chymopapain, J. Neurosurg. **59**:990, 1983.

Pásztor, E., and Szarvas, I.: Herniation of the upper lumbar discs, Neurosurg. Rev. **4**:151, 1981.

Pau, A., Viale, E.S., Turtas, S., and Zirattu, G.: Redundant nerve roots of the cauda equina, Ital. J. Orthop. Traumatol. **4**:95, 1984.

Pheasant, H.C.: Sources of failure in laminectomies, Orthop. Clin. North Am. **6**:319, 1975.

Pheasant, H., Bursk, A., Goldfarb, J., et al.: Amitriptyline and chronic low-back pain: a randomized double-blind crossover study, Spine **8**:552, 1983.

Posner, I., White, A.A., III, Edwards, W.T., and Hayes, W.C.: A biomechanical analysis of the clinical stability of the lumbar and lumbosacral spine, Spine **7**:374, 1982.

Postacchini, F., and Monttanaro, A.: Extreme lateral hernations of lumbar disks, Clin. Orthop. **138**:222, 1979.

Postacchini, F., Urso, S., and Ferro, L.: Lumbosacral nerve-root anomalies. J. Bone Joint Surg. **64-A**:721, 1982.

Postacchini, F., Urso, S., and Tovaglia, V.: Lumbosacral intradural tumours simulating disc disease, Inter. Orthop. (SICOT) **5**:283, 1981.

Postacchini, F., et al.: Computerised tomography in lumbar stenosis: a preliminary report, J. Bone Joint Surg. **62-B**:78, 1980.

Puranen, J., Makela, J., and Lahde, S.: Postoperative intervertebral discitis, Acta Orthop. Scand. **55**:461, 1984.

Quinet, R.J., and Hadler, N.M.: Diagnosis and treatment of backache, Semin. Arthritis Rheum. **8**:261, 1979.

Ramamurthi, B.: Absence of limitation of straight leg raising in proved lumbar disc lesion: case report, J. Neurosurg. **52**:852, 1980.

Rechtine, G.R., Reinert, C.M., and Bohlman, H.H.: The use of epidural morphine to decrease postoperative pain in patients undergoing lumbar laminectomy, J. Bone Joint Surg. **66-A**:1, 1984.

Rish, B.L.: A critique of the surgical management of lumbar disc disease in a private neurosurgical practice, Spine **9**:500, 1984.

Robinson, J.S.: Sciatica and the lumbar disk syndrome: a historic perspective, South. Med. J. **76**:232, 1983.

Rockwood, C.A., and Eilert, R.E.: Camptocormia, J. Bone Joint Surg. **51-A**:533, 1969.

Rosen, J.: Lumbar intervertebral disc surgery: review of 300 cases, Can. Med. Ass. J. **101**:317, 1969.

Rothman, R.H.: The clinical syndrome of lumbar disc disease, Orthop. Clin. North Am. **2**:463, 1971.

Salander, J.M., Youkey, J.R., and Rich, N.M., et al.: Vascular injury related to lumbar disc surgery, J. Trauma **24**:628, 1984.

Sandover, J.: Dynamic loading as a possible source of low-back disorders, Spine **8**:652, 1983.

Schoendinger, G.R., III, and Ford, L.T., Jr.: The use of chymopapain in ruptured lumbar discs, South. Med. J. **64**:333, 1971.

Seeley, S.F., Hughes, C.W., and Jahnke, E.J.: Major vessel damage in lumbar disc operation, Surgery **35**:421, 1954.

Semmes, R.E.: Diagnosis of ruptured intervertebral discs without contrast myelography and comment upon recent experience with modified hemilaminectomy for their removal, Yale J. Biol. Med. **11**:433, 1939.

de Sèze, S.: Sciatique "banale" et disques lombo-sacrés, La Presse Medicale 51-52:570, 1940.

de Sèze, S.: Histoire de la sciatique, Rev. Neurol. **138**:1019, 1982.

Shaw, E.D., Scarborough, J.T., and Beals, R.K.: Bowel injury as a complication of lumbar discectomy: a case report and review of the literature, J. Bone Joint Surg. **63-A**:478, 1981.

Shinners, B.M., and Hamby, W.B.: The results of surgical removal of protruded laminar intervertebral discs, J. Neurosurg. **1**:117, 1944.

Simeone, F.A.: The neurosurgical approach to lumbar disc disease, Orthop. Clin. **2**:499, 1971.

Simmons, J.W., Dennis, M.D., and Rath, D.: The back school: a total back management program, Orthopedics **7**(9):1453, 1984.

Simmons, J.W., Stavinoha, W.B., and Knodel, L.C.: Update and review of chemonucleolysis, Clin. Orthop. **183**:51, 1984.

Sitken, A.P., and Bradford, C.H.: End results of ruptured intervertebral discs in industry, Am. J. Surg. **73**:365, 1947.

Sjöqvist, O.: The mechanism of origin of Lasègue's sign, Acta Psych. Neurol. **46**(Suppl.):290, 1947.

Smith, R.V.: Intradural disc rupture: report of two cases, J. Neurosurg. **55**:117, 1981.

Solgaard, T., and Kleppe, H.: Long-term results of lumbar intervertebral disc prolapse, Spine **8**:793, 1983.

Solheim, L.F., Siewers, P., and Paus, B.: The piriformis muscle syndrome: sciatic nerve entrapment treated with section of the piriformis muscle, Acta Orthop. Scand. **52**:73, 1981.

Spangfort, E.V.: The lumbar disc hernation: a computer-aided analysis of 2,504 operations, Acta Orthop. Scand. **142**(suppl.):1, 1972.

Spencer, D.L., Irwin, G.S., and Miller, J.A.: Anatomy and significance of fixation of the lumbosacral nerve roots in sciatica, Spine **8**:672, 1983.

Spengler, D.M.: Lumbar discectomy: results with limited disc excision and selective foraminotomy, Spine **7**:604, 1982.

Spengler, D.M., and Freeman, C.W.: Patient selection for lumbar discectomy: an objective approach, Spine **4**:129, 1979.

Spurling, R.G.: Lesions of the lumbar intervertebral disk, ed. 1, Springfield, Ill., 1953, Charles C Thomas, Publisher.

Spurling, R.G., and Grantham, E.G.: The end-results of surgery for ruptured lumbar intervertebral disks, J. Neurosurg. **6**:57, 1949.

Steindler, A., and Luck, J.V.: Differential diagnosis of pain low in the back: allocation of the source of pain by the procaine hydrochloride method, JAMA **110**(2):106, 1938.

Tay, E.C.K., and Chacha, P.B.: Midline prolapse of a lumbar intervertebral disc with compression of the cauda equina, J. Bone Joint Surg. **61-B**:43, 1979.

Techakapuch, S., and Bangkok, T.: Rupture of the lumbar cartilage plate into the spinal canal in an adolescent, J. Bone Joint Surg. **63-A**:481, 1981.

Tonelli, L., Falasca, A., Argentieri, C., Andreoli, M., and Merli, G.A.: Influence of psychic distress on short-term outcome of lumbar disc surgery, J. Neurosurg. Sci. **27**:237, 1983.

Troup, J.D.G.: Straight-leg raising (SLR) and the qualifying tests for increased root tension: their predictive value after back and sciatic pain, Spine **6**:526, 1981.

Tsay, Y.-G., et al.: A preoperative chymopapain sensitivity test for chemonucleolysis candidates, Spine **9**:764, 1984.

Verta, M.J., Jr., Vitello, J., and Fuller, J.: Adductor canal compression syndrome, Arch. Surg. **119**:345, 1984.

Waddell, G., Main, C.J., Morris, E.W., DiPaola, M., and Gray, I.C.M.: Chronic low-back pain, psychologic distress, and illness behavior, Spine **9**:209, 1984.

Waddell, G., McCulloch, J.A., Kummel, E., et al.: Nonorganic physical signs of low-back pain, Spine **5**:117, 1980.

Wakano, K., Kasman, R., Chao, E.Y., Bradford, D.S., and Oegema, T.R.: Biomechanical analysis of canine intervertebral discs after chymopapain injection: a preliminary report, Spine **8**:59, 1983.

Wartenberg, R.: Lasègue sign and Kernig sign: historical notes, Arch. Neurol. Psych. **66**:58, 1951.

Wartenberg, R.: On neurologic terminology, eponyms and the Lasègue sign, Neurology **6**:853, 1956.

Wayne, S.J.: A modification of the tuck position for lumbar spine surgery: a 15-year follow-up study, Clin. Orthop. **184**:212, 1984.

Weber, H.: Lumber disc herniation: a controlled, prospective study with ten years of observation, Spine **8**:131, 1983.

Weinstein, J., Spratt, K.F., Lehmann, T., McNeill, T., and Hejna,W.: Lumbar disc hernation: a comparison of the results of chemonucleolysis and open discectomy after ten years, J. Bone Joint Surg. **68-A**:43, 1986.

Weinstein, J.N., Scafuri, R.L., and McNeill, T.W.: The Rush-Presbyterian-St. Luke's lumbar spine analysis form: a prospective study of patients with "spinal stenosis," Spine **8**:891, 1983.

Weir, B.K.A.: Prospective study of 100 lumbosacral discectomies, J. Neurosurg. **50**:283, 1979.

Weise, M.D., Garfin, S.R., Gelberman, R.H., Katz, M.M., and Thorne, R.P.: Lower-extremity sensibility testing in patients with herniated lumbar intervertebral discs, J. Bone Joint Surg. **67-A**:1219, 1985.

Weitz, E.M.: The lateral bending sign, Spine **6**:388, 1981.

Weitz, E.M.: Paraplegia following chymopapain injection: a case report, J. Bone Joint Surg. **66-A**:1131, 1984.

Whisler, W.W.: Anaphylaxis secondary to chymopapain, Orthopedics **6**:1628, 1983.

White, A.A., III, and Gordon, S.L.: Synopsis: workshop on idiopathic low-back pain, Spine **7**:141, 1982.

White, A.H., Derby, R., and Wynne, G.: Epidural injections for the diagnosis and treatment of low-back pain, Spine **5**:78, 1980.

White, A.H., Taylor, L.W., Wynne, G., and Welch, R.B.: Appendix: a diagnostic classification of low-back pain, Spine **5**(1):83, 1980.

Wilberger, J.E., Jr., and Pang, D.: Syndrome of the incidental herniated lumbar disc, J. Neurosurg. **59**:137, 1983.

Wilkins, R.H., and Brody, I.A.: Lasègue's sign, Arch. Neurol. **21**:219, 1969.

Wilkinson, H.A., Baker, S., and Rosenfeld, S.: Gelfoam paste in experimental laminectomy and cranial trephination: hemostasis and bone healing, J. Neurosurg. **54**:664, 1981.

Williams, R.W.: Microlumbar discectomy: a conservative surgical approach to the virgin herniated lumbar disc, Spine **3**:175, 1978.

Williams, R.W.: Microcervical foraminotomy: a surgical alternative for intractable radicular pain, Spine **8**:708, 1983.

Willis, J. (ed.): Chymopapain administration procedures modified, FDA Drug Bull. **14**:14, 1984.

Willis, T.A.: Lumbosacral anomalies, J. Bone Joint Surg. **41-A**:935, 1959.

Wiltberger, B.R.: Surgical treatment of degenerative disease of the back, J. Bone Joint Surg. **45-A**:1509, 1963.

Wiltse, L.L., Widell, E.H., and Yuan, H.A.: Chymopapain chemonucleolysis in lumbar disk disease, JAMA **231**:474, 1975.

Yong-Hing, K., Reilly, J., de Korompay, V., and Kirkaldy-Willis, W.H.: Prevention of nerve root adhesions after laminectomy, Spine **5**(1):59, 1980.

Young, A., et al.: Variations in the pattern of muscle innervation by the L5 S1 nerve roots, Spine **8**:616, 1983.

Zaleske, D.J., Bode, H.H., Benz, R., and Kirshnamoorthy, K.S.: Association of sciatica-like pain and Addison's disease: a case report, J. Bone Joint Surg. **66-A**:297, 1984.

Zamani, M.H., and MacEwen, G.D.: Herniation of the lumbar disc in children and adolescents, J. Pediatr. Orthop. **2**:528, 1982.

Spinal instability

Bailey, R.W., and Badgley, C.E.: Stabilization of the cervical spine by anterior fusion, J. Bone Joint Surg. **42-A**:565, 1960.

Benton, B.F., and Calandruccio, R.A.: Surgical technic of anterior lumbar fusion, Am. Surg. **32**:134, 1966

Bloom, M.H., and Raney, F.L., Jr.: Anterior intervertebral fusion of the cervical spine: a technical note, J. Bone Joint Surg. **63-A**:842, 1981.

Cauthen, C.: Lumbar spine surgery, Baltimore, 1983, Williams & Wilkins Co.

Chow, S.P., Leong, J.C.Y., and Ma, A., et al.: Anterior spinal fusion for deranged lumbar intervertebral disc: a review of 97 cases, Spine **5**:452, 1980.

Cloward, R.B.: Vertebral body fusion for ruptured cervical discs: description of instruments and operative technic, Am. J. Surg. **98**:722, 1959.

Cohen, C.A., Young, H.F., Howell, J.R., Griffith, E.R., and Becker, D.P.: Chronic neck and back pain: a reassessment of usual surgical treatment, South. Med. J. **73**:40, 1980.

Cyron, B M., and Hutton, W.C.: Articular tropism and stability of the lumbar spine, Spine **5**:168, 1980.

Farfan, H.F., and Gracovetsky, S.: The nature of instability, Spine **9**:714, 1984.

Farfan, H.F., and Sullivan, J.D.: The relation of facet orientation to intervertebral disc failure, Can. J. Surg. **10**:179, 1967.

Flynn, T.B.: Neurologic complications of anterior cervical interbody fusion, Spine **7**:536, 1982.

Freebody, D., Bendall, R., and Taylor, R.D.: Anterior transperitoneal lumbar fusion, J. Bone Joint Surg. **53-B**:617, 1971.

Frymoyer, J.W., Hanley, E.N., Jr., Howe, J., Kuhlmann, D., and Matteri, R.E.: A comparison of radiographic findings in fusion and nonfusion patients ten or more years following lumbar disc surgery, Spine **4**:435, 1979.

Gentry, W.D.: Chronic back pain: does elective surgery benefit patients with evidence of psychologic disturbance?, South. Med. J. **75**:1169, 1982.

Giles, L.G.F.: Lumbosacral facetal 'joint angles' associated with leg length inequality, Rheum. Rehabil. **20**:233, 1981.

Goldner, J.L., Urbaniak, J.R., and McCollum, D.E.: Anterior disc excision and interbody spinal fusion for chronic low back pain, Orthop. Clin. North Am. **2**(2):543, 1971.

Harmon, P.H.: Subtotal anterior lumbar disc excision and vertebral body fusion. III. Application to complicated and recurrent multilevel degeneration, Am. J. Surg. **97**:649, 1959.

Harmon, P.H.: Anterior disc excision and fusion of the lumbar vertebral bodies: a review of diagnostic level testing, with operative results in more than seven hundred cases, J. Int. Coll. Surg. **40**:572, 1963.

Harmon, P.H.: Anterior excision and vertebral body fusion operation for intervertebral disk syndromes of the lower lumbar spine: three- to five-year results in 244 cases, Clin. Orthop. **26**:107, 1963.

Hazlett, J.W., and Kinnard, P.: Lumbar apophyseal process excision and spinal instability, Spine **7**:171, 1982.

Herron, L.D., and Pheasant, H.C.: Bilateral laminotomy and discectomy for segmental lumbar disc disease: decompression with stability, Spine **8**:86, 1983.

Hodgson, A.R., and Wong, S.K.: A description of a technic and evaluation of results in anterior spinal fusion for deranged intervertebral disk and spondylolisthesis, Clin. Orthop. **56**:133, 1968.

Humphries, A.W., Hawk, W.A., and Berndt, A.L.: Anterior interbody fusion of lumbar vertebrae: a surgical technique, Surg. Clin. North Am. **41**:1685, 1961.

Kirkaldy-Willis, W.H., and Farfan, H.F.: Instability of the lumbar spine, Clin. Orthop. **165**:110, 1982.

Koop, S.E., Winter, R.B., and Lonstein, J.E.: The surgical treatment of instability of the upper part of the cervical spine in children and adolescents, J. Bone Joint Surg. **66-A**:403, 1984.

Knutsson, F.: The instability associated with disk degeneration in the lumbar spine, Acta Radiol. **25**:593, 1944.

Lane, J.D., Jr., and Moore, E.S., Jr.: Transperitoneal approach to the intervertebral disc in the lumbar area. Ann. Surg. **127**:537, 1948.

Lee, C.K.: Lumbar spinal instability (olisthesis) after extensive posterior spinal decompression, Spine **8**:429, 1983.

Macnab, I.: The traction spur: an indicator of segmental instability, J. Bone Joint Surg. **53-A**:663, 1971.

McCarroll, H.R., and Odell, R.: Use of barrel stave grafts in spinal fusion, Arch. Surg. **58**:42, 1949.

Mensor, M.C., and Duvall, G.: Absence of motion at the fourth and fifth lumbar interspaces in patients with and without low-back pain, J. Bone Joint Surg. **41-A**:1047, 1959.

Nachlas, I.: End-results of the treatment of herniated nucleus pulposus by excision with fusion and without fusion, J. Bone Joint Surg. **34-A**:981, 1952.

Nakano, N., and Tomita, T.: Results of surgical treatment of low back pain: a comparative study of the anterior and posterior approach, Int. Orthop. **4**:101, 1980.

Naylor, A.: Intervertebral disc prolapse and degeneration, Spine **1**:108, 1976.

Pennecot, G.F., Gouraud, D., Hardy, J.R., and Pouliquen, J.C.: Roentgenographical study of the stability of the cervical spine in children, J. Pediatr. Orthop. **4**:346, 1984.

Robinson, R.A., and Smith, G.W.: Anterolateral cervical disk: removal and interbody fusion for cervical disk syndrome, Bull. Johns Hopkins Hosp. **96:**223, 1955.

Robinson, R.A., Walker, E., Ferlic, D.C., and Wieckling, D.K.: The results of anterior interbody fusion of the cervical spine, J. Bone Joint Surg. **44-A:**1569, 1962.

Sacks, S.: Anterior interbody fusion of the lumbar spine, J. Bone Joint Surg. **47-B:**211, 1965.

Saunders, E.A., and Jacobs, R.R.: The multiply operated back: fusion of the posterolateral spine with and without nerve root compression, South. Med. J. **69:**868, 1976.

Shenkin, H.A., and Hash, C.J.: Spondylolisthesis after multiple bilateral laminectomies and facetectomies for lumbar spondylosis, J. Neurosurg. **50:**45, 1979.

Stauffer, R.N., and Coventry, M.B.: Anterior interbody lumbar spine fusion: analysis of Mayo Clinic series, J. Bone Joint Surg. **54-A:**756, 1972.

Straight, T.A., and Hunter, S.E.: Intraspinal extradural sensory rhizotomy in patients with failure of lumbar disc surgery, J. Neurosurg. **54:**193, 1981.

Tanz, S.S.: Motion of the lumbar spine: a roentgenologic study, Amer. J. Roentgenol. **69:**399, 1953.

Wenger, D.R., Bobechko, W.P., and Gilday, D.L.: The spectrum of intervertebral disc-space infection in children, J. Bone Joint Surg. **60-A:**100, 1978.

Wilder, D.G., Seligson, D., Frymoyer, J.W., and Pope, M.H.: Objective measurement of L4-5 instability: a case report, Spine **5:**56, 1980.

Wiltberger, B.R.: Surgical treatment of degenerative disease of the back, J. Bone Joint Surg. **45-A:**1509, 1963.

Failed spine

Burton, C.V., Kirkaldy-Willis, W.H., Yong-Hong, K., and Heithoff, K.B.: Causes of failure of surgery on the lumbar spine, Clin. Orthop. **157:**191, 1981.

Cauchoix, J., Ficat, C., and Girard, B.: Repeat surgery after disc excision, Spine **3:**256, 1978.

Cohen, C.A., Young, H.F., Howell, J.R., Griffith, E.R., and Becker, D.P.: Chronic neck and back pain: a reassessment of usual surgical treatment, South. Med. J. **73:**40, 1980.

Crock, H.V.: Observations on the management of failed spinal operations, J. Bone Joint Surg. **58-B:**193, 1976.

Egbert, L.D., Battit, G.E., Welch, C.E., and Bartlett, M.K.: Reduction of postoperative pain by encouragement and instruction of patients: a study of doctor-patient rapport, N. Engl. J. Med. **270:**825, 1964.

Fager, C.A., and Friedberg, S.R.: Analysis of failures and poor results of lumbar spine surgery, Spine **5:**87, 1980.

Finnegan, W.J., Fenlin, J.M., Marvel, J.P., Nardini, R.J., and Rothman, R.H.: Results of surgical intervention in the symptomatic multiply-operated back patient: analysis of sixty-seven cases followed for three to seven years, J. Bone Joint Surg. **61-A:**1077, 1979.

Finneson, B.E., and Cooper, V.R.: A lumbar disc surgery predictive score card: a retrospective evaluation, Spine **4:**141, 1979.

Frymoyer, J.W., Hanley, E., Howe, J., Kuhlmann, D., and Matteri, R.: Disc excision and spine fusion in the management of lumbar disc disease, Spine **3:**1, 1978.

Frymoyer, J.W., Matteri, R.E., Hanley, E.N., Kuhlmann, D., and Howe, J.: Failed lumbar disc surgery requiring second operation: a long-term follow-up study, Spine **3:**7, 1978.

Gentry, W.D.: Chronic back pain: does elective surgery benefit patients with evidence of psychologic disturbance? South. Med. J. **75:**1169, 1982.

Hasue, M., and Fujiwara, M.: Epidemiologic and clinical studies of long-term prognosis of low-back pain and sciatica, Spine **4:**150, 1979.

Holmes, H.E., and Rothman, R.H.: The Pennsylvania plan: an algorithm for the management of lumbar degenerative disc disease, Spine **4:**156, 1979.

Hurme, M., Alaranta, H., Torma, T., and Einola, S.: Operated lumbar disc herniation: epidemiological aspects, Ann. Chir. Gynaecol. **72**(1):33, 1983.

Lehmann, T.R., and LaRocca, H.S.: Repeat lumbar surgery: a review of patients with failure from previous lumbar surgery treated by spinal canal exploration and lumbar spinal fusion, Spine **6:**615, 1981.

Macnab, I.: Negative disc exploration: an analysis of the causes of nerve-root involvement in sixty-eight patients, J. Bone Joint Surg. **53-A:**891, 1971.

Mooney, V., and Cairns, D.: Management in the patient with chronic low back pain, Orthop. Clin. North Am. **9**(2):543, 1978.

Pheasant, H.C., and Dyck, P.: Failed lumbar disc surgery: cause, assessment, treatment, Clin. Orthop. **164:**93, 1982.

Rothman, R.H., and Bernini, P.M.: Algorithm for salvage surgery of the lumbar spine, Clin. Orthop. **154:**14, 1981.

Rothman, R.H., and Tarlov, E.: Failed back surgery syndrome, JAMA **251:**657, 1984.

Saunders, E.A., and Jacobs, R.R.: The multiply operated back: fusion of the posterolateral spine with and without nerve root compression, South. Med. J. **69:**868, 1976.

Spengler, D.M., and Freeman, C.W.: Patient selection for lumbar discectomy: an objective approach, Spine **4:**129, 1979.

Strait, T.A., and Hunter, S.E.: Intraspinal extradural sensory rhizotomy in patients with failure of lumbar disc surgery, J. Neurosurg. **54:**193, 1981.

Waddell, G., et al.: Failed lumbar disc surgery and repeat surgery following industrial injuries, J. Bone Joint Surg. **61-A:**201, 1979.

Wilberger, J.E., Jr., and Pang, D.: Syndrome of the incidental herniated lumbar disc, J. Neurosurg. **59:**137, 1983.

CHAPTER 74

Infections of spine

George W. Wood

Before the use of antibiotics, mortality in infections of the spine and contiguous tissues was 40% to 70%. Advances in chemotherapy over the past 40 years have also dramatically altered the natural history of these serious diseases. Today spinal infections are relatively rare, accounting for only 2% to 4% of all osteomyelitis. Present mortality is estimated at 1% to 20% and is steadily declining. The rate of paralysis is reported to be up to 50% depending on the patient population reviewed. The major problems today are the delay in diagnosis (estimated to average 3 months) and the long recovery period (averaging 12 months or more).

Major infections of the spine are often referred to as disc space infections, which is frequently inaccurate. Coventry et al. have demonstrated that the intervertebral disc has a blood supply until age 30. The subsequent studies of Wiley and Trueta, Hassler, and most recently Crock and Yoshizawa confirm the absence of a blood supply to the intervertebral disc in the adult, but a good blood supply at the periphery of the disc and in all other areas of the spine.

The venous plexus has been shown by Crock and Yoshizawa to mimic the arterial supply (Fig. 74-1). The drainage system of the pelvis through the venous plexus of Batson has been postulated to be the primary reason for the high percentage of lumbar vertebral infections originating from urinary tract infections. Whalen et al. have recently reported that even the developing vertebrate intervertebral discs are avascular. They note that the blood supply ends in the vertebral end plate adjacent to the disc.

Spinal infection has most commonly been identified in the vertebral bodies. It has also been reported in the posterior elements of the spine, the epidural space, the intervertebral disc, and the perispinal soft tissues. The mechanisms of infection are bloodborne metastasis, direct implantations and indirect local extension. The most common source of infection is by hematogenous spread from more distant infections, most frequently from the urinary tract and respiratory system. Usually two vertebrae and an intervening disc are affected. Occasionally only one vertebra or multiple vertebrae at the same or different sites are affected. Stauffer emphasizes the importance of distinguishing vertebral osteomyelitis from true disc space infection. In the former the disc space is involved *secondarily as a result of hematogenous seeding in the subchondral bone of the vertebral body*. This follows a bacteremia. *Disc space infection,* on the other hand, most commonly occurs following surgical excision of the disc.

Staphylococcus aureus is the most common bacterial organism identified in spinal infections. The incidence of isolation of this organism varies from 40% to 90%. (Recently, the incidence of infection with this organism has been declining, but over half of the isolates of the organism were resistant to penicillin and over one third of that group were resistant to methicillin.) The present trend is a decrease in the frequency of *Staphylococcus aureus* infections but an increase in the resistant strains of the organism.

Other types of bacteria have been reported but at a much lower incidence. Several reports of *Brucella* infection of the spine have noted the chronic nature of this infection and the similarity to tuberculous spinal infection. Morrey et al. reported a patient with *Streptococcus viridans* spinal osteomyelitis associated with bacterial endocarditis from the same organism. They also noted that 24% of patients with bacterial endocarditis complained of back pain but few progressed to detectable spinal osteomyelitis.

Fungal infections of the spine are rare. These infections frequently resemble tuberculous infections in their insidious development and tendency to produce abscesses and paralysis. Spinal infections by *Actinomyces, Aspergillus, Arachnia, Cryptococcus,* and most frequently by *Coccidioides* have been reported. Santos et al. noted a 50% spinal involvement in disseminated coccidioidomycosis infections that affect bone. This organism is endemic to the south-

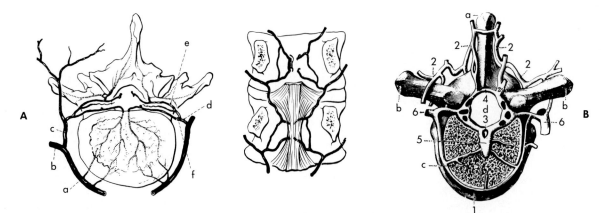

Fig. 74-1. A, Blood supply to vertebra as seen from below and behind with laminae removed: *a,* segmental artery; *b,* ventral continuation; *c,* dorsal branch; *d,* spinal branch; *e* and *f,* spinal branch's dorsal and ventral twigs to tissue of epidural space and vertebral column. In middle figure, only branches to vertebral bodies are seen. **B,** Venous drainage of vertebra: *a* and *b,* spinous and transverse processes; *c,* body of vertebra; *1, 2, 3,* and *4,* vertebral venous plexuses; *5,* chief vein of vertebral bodies; *6,* segmental veins and tributaries. (From Hollinshead, W.H.: Anatomy for surgeons, vol. 3. The back and limbs, ed. 3, Harper & Row, 1982.)

western regions of the United States and the arid regions of Central America and South America. Winter et al. reported that no fungal agent is capable of eradicating this infection.

Mycobacterium tuberculosis is now an infrequent cause of spinal infection in the United States because of advancements in chemotherapy and preventive medicine. Other countries are not as fortunate. Most of the studies of the efficacy of various methods of treatment now originate in Asia and Africa.

The lumbar spine is the area most often affected by spinal osteomyelitis. The thoracic and cervical areas are affected to lesser degrees in that order. The incidence of paralysis is greatest for cervical infections, less for thoracic, and least for lumbar infections. The age distribution for spinal infections is bimodal. The first peak is in children (age 1 to 15 years) and the second is in older adults (age 50 to 80 years). Paralysis is more frequent in the older population.

Paralysis from spinal infection may occur early or late. Early onset of paralysis frequently suggests epidural extension of an abscess. Late paralysis can occur from the development of significant kyphosis, vertebral collapse with retropulsion of bone and debris, or late abscess formation in more indolent infections. Eismont et al. identified four factors that indicate an increased predisposition to paralysis in pyogenic and fungal vertebral osteomyelitis. They noted that the incidence of paralysis increased with (1) age, (2) a higher vertebral level of infection (cervical), (3) the presence of debilitating disease such as diabetes mellitus, rheumatoid arthritis, or chronic steroid usage, and (4) *Staphylococcus aureus* infections. Paralysis from tuberculosis is not related to those factors.

CLINICAL FINDINGS AND DIAGNOSIS

Pain is the most frequent complaint in vertebral infection. The location of the pain varies from the region of spinal infection to the extremities. Early symptoms may not suggest an infection of the spine, and consequently the

correct diagnosis may not be made for several weeks. In fact, symptoms may be so bizarre as to be thought functional. Constitutional symptoms include anorexia, weight loss, and intermittent fever. Puig-Guri described four clinical syndromes that may be caused by the disease:

1. Hip joint syndrome, with acute pain in the hip, flexion contracture, and limited motion
2. Abdominal syndrome, with symptoms and signs that may suggest acute appendicitis
3. Meningeal syndrome, with symptoms and signs that suggest acute suppurative or tuberculous meningitis
4. Back pain syndrome, in which the onset of pain may be acute or insidious; pain may be so severe that jarring the bed is agonizing, or it may be mild

Severe muscle spasm is the most frequent sign of spinal infection. Temperature elevations if present are usually minor. Additional signs noted in less than 50% of patients include loss of hip joint motion and the hip assuming a flexed attitude, localized tenderness, positive Kenrig's sign, hamstring spasm, and generalized weakness. Occasionally, a fluctuant mass can be palpated. Such masses are most readily detectable in the cervical and thoracic spine in thin people, in the groin below Poupart's ligament, and in the adductor region of the thigh. Abscesses are usually associated with tuberculous and fungal infections. The presence of neurologic signs should alert the examiner to the possible development of epidural extension of the infection or vertebral collapse with spinal cord compression.

The erythrocyte sedimentation rate is the laboratory test most frequently abnormal; it is elevated from the low 20s to over 100 mm per hour. Leukocytosis is infrequent. Roentgenographic changes are slow to develop. Digby and Kersley noted a characteristic sequence of roentgenographic changes in nontuberculous spinal infection. At 2 weeks only disc space narrowing may be seen. Rarefaction of adjacent vertebral bodies is noted at 6 weeks. Reactive sclerosis is noted at about 8 weeks, and new bone formation is present at 12 weeks. Intervertebral fusion usually signifies a resolution of the process. This can occur between 6 months and 2 years. Technetium bone scans are rarely positive in the early stages of the infection. Gallium bone scans have been reported to be positive within 48 hours in experimentally produced disc space infection. Computed tomographic scans are helpful in delineating the extent of the infection and the presence of a paravertebral abscess. Magnetic resonance imaging (MRI) should provide even greater information. Unfortunately, the computed tomographic scan is not helpful in the early stages of the infection.

Bacteriologic diagnosis should be sought primarily by blood cultures of percutaneous needle biopsy. Needle biopsy should be performed through the posterolateral approach in the thoracic and lumbar spines. A Craig needle is helpful in obtaining a subcortical biopsy, but its use should be limited to the thoracic and lumbar spines. Much smaller needles are necessary for biopsy of the cervical spine and the L5 vertebra, and cortical bone penetration is difficult with small needles. The techniques for this procedure are the same as for lateral discography p. 3270. Infections of the upper cervical spine and the sacrum are not readily or safely accessible to needle aspiration.

TREATMENT OF PYOGENIC AND FUNGAL VERTEBRAL OSTEOMYELITIS

The primary treatment of pyogenic osteomyelitis is rest. Some infections heal spontaneously with recumbency or immobilization alone. We prefer to withhold antibiotics until an adequate biopsy of the infected area is obtained. The initial antibiotic choice is determined by the clinical history and physical examination, supplemented by a gram stain of the specimen if possible. The final antibiotic choice is determined by the culture report. Usually vertebral osteomyelitis requires antibiotics for a considerable period of time. Intravenous antibiotics are usually administered initially and are followed by oral antibiotics (if available). The timing of antibiotic usage is determined by the patient's progress and the return of his erythrocyte sedimentation rate to normal. The gallium scan can be used to follow the resolution of the infection. Cast immobilization is also useful in selected patients.

Conservative treatment should be abandoned if the clinical condition deteriorates despite adequate antibiotic therapy. The development of neurologic deficits is a serious complication that demands aggressive evaluation and treatment. The surgical options available include open biopsy; incision, drainage, and debridement of necrotic tissue; and radical debridement of necrotic tissue and bone grafting. Laminectomy for neurologic deficits is beneficial only in the drainage and debridement of posterior element infections and localized epidural abscesses. Eismont et al. noted significant improvement in patients with paralysis from cervical or thoracic infections after debridement and grafting using an anterior approach. Patients treated by laminectomy alone rarely improved.

Clinically, spine infections can be subdivided into several groups. The major division is between infections in children and in adults. Infections in children are usually hematogenous in origin and pyogenic, viral, or tuberculous. Infections in adults are usually hematogenous or postoperative in origin, and infection is usually pyogenic

or tuberculous. The treatment of these infections is generally similar, but there are several exceptions with regard to spinal infections in children, postoperative disc space infections, and tuberculous infections in children and adults.

Pyogenic vertebral osteomyelitis in children

Infected lesions of the spine should always be suspected in the child who is irritable and has back or hip pain or a change in walking pattern. Clinically this is combined with limited spine motion, muscle spasm, and an increased erythrocyte sedimentation rate. *Staphylococcus aureus* is the primary offending bacterium. Primary treatment consists of rigid immobilization of the spinal column in a plaster jacket or spica cast and is generally adequate. As recommended by Boston et al., antibiotics are not generally used but are reserved for atypical infections that do not respond to immobilization and in patients with persistent pain and spasm and a high erythrocyte sedimentation rate. Disc space aspiration is not necessary unless improvement does not occur. Immobilization results in improvement in 6 to 12 weeks. On the other hand, Wenger, Bobechko, and Gilday believe that infected disc disease in children is a vertebral osteomyelitis with disc involvement. This view is based on the studies by Wiley and Trueta showing by injection studies that the vertebral end plate in children contains vascular channels that allow nutrition of the intervertebral disc and that could be a site of entry for septic emboli. This has been supported by bone scanning that suggests that the process originates in the vertebral body rather than in the disc itself. The preferred treatment of Wenger, Bobechko, and Gilday consists of rest and antibiotics continued for an arbitrary 3 weeks. Prolonged immobilization after discharge from the hospital is required only for those with protracted symptoms.

Saenger and others have described a lesion of an intervertebral disc in children that causes narrowing of the disc space and mild erosion of the adjacent vertebrae; these changes occur slowly during 1 to 2 months. The disc space is usually restored, especially in young children; calcium may be deposited in the disc only to disappear eventually. Epiphysitis of the spine, brucellosis, or viral infection must be considered in the differential diagnosis.

POSTOPERATIVE DISC SPACE INFECTIONS

Postoperative disc space infections are a rare but serious and debilitating complication of intervertebral disc surgery. The onset of this complication is usually slow with the appearance of severe back pain, muscle spasm, and an elevated erythrocyte sedimentation rate 2 to 6 weeks after surgery. It is rarely associated with a frank wound infection and wound drainage. The usual infecting organism is *Staphylococcus aureus*, but other bacterial and fungal organisms have also been reported. A needle biopsy of the disc space for culture or cultures of the blood, or both will result in a positive diagnosis in over 50% of patients when these are done before the administration of antibiotics. Specific or empiric antibiotics have been suggested in most reports of postoperative disc space infection. Antibiotics should be continued until the erythrocyte sedimentation rate returns to normal. Immobilization in a body cast is frequently helpful in relieving pain. The pain from this infection usually lasts for 8 to 24 months. Spontaneous intervertebral fusion usually resolves the problem. Occasionally spontaneous fusion does not occur. The indications for surgery are the same as for vertebral osteomyelitis, p. 3325.

TUBERCULOSIS WITHOUT PARAPLEGIA

During the past few decades the trend in the treatment of tuberculosis of the spine has been toward more radical surgery. Some such as Campos, Allen and Stevenson, Bosworth, and Smith have adhered to the principles of Albee, Hibbs, and others, advocating early arthrodesis and usually allowing paraspinal abscesses to regress spontaneously. Smith reports that this treatment is satisfactory for the average patient seen in the United States in whom vertebral destruction is not severe. On the other hand, paraspinal abscesses have been drained by Karlén and others, effecting cures in some children, as shown by spontaneous bony fusion of the affected vertebrae.

Tuli and Kumar, in a study of 100 patients in India on triple drug therapy for spinal tuberculosis, showed favorable results without surgery. They state that in economically underdeveloped countries (when certain circumstances prevail) this regimen is the treatment of choice. (See Chapter 29 for the medical treatment of tuberculosis.) Operative treatment is reserved for those patients not responding favorably to drug therapy after 6 months and for those with neural complications or with recrudescence of the disease. Operative treatment is combined with 6 to 12 months of bed rest and 18 to 24 months of spinal bracing thereafter.

Tuli et al. and Friedman have reported cures in some adults treated by antibacterial therapy and drainage of some paraspinal abscesses. Surprisingly, Konstam and Blesovsky as well as Dickson reported cures in many patients, both children and adults, using the same treatment but allowing most of the patients to walk and be out of the hospital. Others such as Wilkinson, Felländer, Kondo and Yamada, Roaf et al., and Hodgson et al. have applied to the spine the principle of debridement that has been effective in other regions. Some of these and others, including Shaw and Thomas, Kohli, and Kirkaldy-Willis and Thomas have inserted bone grafts directly into the defects after debridement. Arct reported 119 elderly patients with tuberculosis of the spine without paraplegia. Those treated by debridement and the insertion of bone grafts did much better and required much briefer hospitalization than those treated without such surgery. In a report by Neville and Davis, 27 patients with spinal tuberculosis were reviewed at the Medical College of Virginia. Thirteen were treated by surgical fusion and 14 by surgical drainage of the abscess only. Spontaneous fusion occurred in 50% of the nonfusion group in an average 15.2 months. Three patients in this group had poor results. Surgical fusion occurred in 92% of the fusion group in an average time of 7.3 months, and there were no poor results.

Kemp et al. believe that in the adult, stable bony fusion with the least risk of collapse into kyphos is obtained by a radical anterior clearance of diseased tissue and an autogenous iliac crest inlay graft. They reserved posterior fusion for use only if there were destruction of two or more vertebral bodies or instability from destruction of posterior elements. In these instances we prefer the use of a corticocancellous fibular anterior graft combined with rib grafts. Collapse is prevented by ensuring that the fibular graft reaches from the superior end plate of the vertebra above the area of resection to the inferior end plate of the vertebra below. Any placement of the graft short of this may allow collapse of the graft into the cancellous area until it finds its stability at the respective end plates with resultant kyphotic deformity. On the other hand, in a review of 241 consecutive anterior spinal fusions for tuberculosis to detect late progression of a kyphotic deformity, Hodgson found 3 of 31 patients with kyphosis had an increase in deformity, which may have resulted from growth retardation of the anterior ring epiphyses and posterior element overgrowth. Such patients therefore require careful follow-up, and if the kyphos progresses, supplemental posterior fusion will arrest the progression. Martin also stresses that correction of angulation and stabilization are indispensable when extensive diseased tissue is excised.

Reports of the Medical Research Council Working Party from two centers in Korea and one in Rhodesia were compared with a study made in Hong Kong. Patients in the former study received as outpatients isoniazid plus para-aminosalicylic acid (PAS) for 18 months and daily streptomycin for 3 months, whereas in Hong Kong resection of the tuberculous focus and repair of the resulting gap by bone grafting was added to the treatment by Hodgson and Stock. After 5 years all groups had a favorable response. However, in the radical operation series of Hong Kong a significantly higher percentage of the patients achieved healing with bony fusion with less vertebral body loss. Fusion was achieved in 93%, compared with 68% for those with debridement only. Thus at 5 years the radical operation in expert hands gave better results in terms of healing by bony fusion, less vertebral loss and deformity, and more rapid resolution of mediastinal abscess shadows.

Wilkinson selected for debridement *mostly* patients whose prognosis without surgery seemed doubtful or poor. Felländer performed radical surgery on all patients unless complications were severe or the disease was mild or inactive. Hodgson et al. have gone even further, doing debridement and anterior arthrodesis in *all* patients as soon as possible after the diagnosis is established. If exploration shows that the disease has healed, they arthrodese for stability. Chu in 1967 reported satisfactory healing in 71 of 74 consecutive patients treated by the method of Hodgson. One hundred consecutive children, age 18 months to 10 years, as reported by Bailey, Gabriel, Hodgson, and Shin, treated between December, 1955, and June, 1959, were reviewed. Forty-three of the 100 children had paraplegia. In this group 37 made a complete recovery and 6 a partial recovery. In 74 patients solid fusion and healing of the tuberculous lesion occurred; in 16 there was a stable nonunion with apparent healing of the disease; the remaining 10 were classified as having unstable nonunions requiring further treatment. On the basis of this study they reached the following conclusions:

1. The anterior approach gives direct wide access to the diseased area in the treatment of Pott's disease in

children. It is through this approach that it is possible to remove all pathologic foci and make an accurate diagnosis.

2. In children with thoracic lesions early decompression of the abscess is recommended to avoid further destruction that may result in severe kyphosis, paraplegia, or impairment of cardiopulmonary function.

3. With penetration of the lung the anterior approach to the spine is the only method of dealing with both lesions simultaneously.

4. Only surgical exposure permits a definite and accurate diagnosis of the cause of paraplegia.

5. The prognosis for recovery from a pressure type of paraplegia is remarkably good if the cause of the pressure is removed soon after the onset of symptoms.

6. In Pott's paraplegia the prognosis for recovery is far better in children than in adults.

7. An anterior interbody fusion can be made more stable if needed by an additional posterior fusion over the same segments, especially at the cervicothoracic and thoracolumbar junctions.

8. In the treatment of tuberculosis of the spine in children, evacuation of the contents of the abscess combined with removal of all avascular bone and anterior fusion with strut grafts has given results superior to those obtained by other methods.

In the absence of excellent facilities and trained assistants, Roaf et al. recommend surgical treatment in two stages: (1) evacuation of an abscess, if present, and (2) arthrodesis posteriorly at a later date.

Tuberculous abscesses of spine

Abscesses associated with tuberculosis of the spine may be palpable externally, depending on their size, on the vertebrae involved, and the distribution of the adjacent fascial planes and musculature, or they may present no outward manifestations until sufficiently large to cause pressure symptoms on various organs such as the pharynx or spinal cord.

In 1960 Hodgson et al. reported a series of 412 patients treated by radical removal of the diseased area and anterior spinal arthrodesis. Their technique entails a more extensive excision of bone than that of Roaf et al., but their mortality was only 2.9%, and no deaths occurred in patients with disease of limited extent or of short duration and who had no pulmonary involvement. No patient developed paraplegia after operation. They advise the operation for all patients with early tuberculosis of the spine and believe that it should supplant conservative treatment in most instances. They have operated on all patients, even those in whom the disease was far advanced, and of the first 100 patients followed from 2 to 4 years, 93 had solid arthrodesis consisting of an uninterrupted bridge of mature bone and healing of the tuberculous focus.

TUBERCULOSIS WITH PARAPLEGIA

Paraplegia, the result of interference with the conductivity of the spinal cord, is most often associated with tuberculosis of the dorsal spine. The chief reasons for this are that (1) tuberculosis is more prevalent in the dorsal spine, (2) the spinal cord terminates below the level of the first lumbar vertebra, and (3) the spinal canal is smallest in the dorsal portion. Seddon noted that the normal curve of the dorsal spine encourages marked kyphos after destruction of the vertebrae and a squeezing of tuberculous products toward the cord. Furthermore, the anterior ligament in the dorsal region loosely confines the abscess; in contrast, abscesses in the lumbar region can escape into the psoas muscle.

Clonus is the most prominent early sign of Pott's paraplegia, and the diagnosis of the disease is not difficult. The paralysis may pass with varying rapidity through the following stages: muscle weakness, spasticity, and incoordination, progressing to paraplegia in extension and later to paraplegia in flexion. In paraplegia in extension the cord is not completely involved and some nerve tracts continue to function, whereas in paraplegia in flexion the whole thickness of the cord is affected. Urinary and rectal incontinence occur. In the severe forms all spasticity disappears, and paralysis becomes flaccid.

Lumbar puncture may be valuable in assessing Pott's paraplegia. It is true that a negative Queckenstedt test and a low spinal fluid protein level are not diagnostic because irreparable damage to the spinal cord may take place without a complete block within the spinal canal. However, Hodgson et al. recommend lumbar puncture in those patients in whom involvement of the spinal cord by the infection is suspected. The Queckenstedt test should indicate the severity of any block. Furthermore, in patients with tuberculous meningomyelitis, they usually have found an increase in the white cell count and protein in the spinal fluid.

Types of Pott's paraplegia

According to Seddon, Sorrel-Dejerine in 1925 described two main types of Pott's paraplegia. Butler and Seddon, after working independently, agreed with her in 1935, dividing the disease into two types: (1) paraplegia of early onset, coming on during the florid phase of the spinal disease usually within the first 2 years, and (2) paraplegia of late onset, appearing even many years after the disease has become quiescent and sometimes without evidence of reactivation.

Pathology of Pott's paraplegia

Seddon gives the following causes of Pott's paraplegia secondary to changes in the vertebral column:

A. Early onset
   1. Inflammatory
      a. Swelling because of an abscess, inflammatory tissue, or a caseating mass; may spontaneously shrink to a varying degree, but last of these is least likely to
      b. Circumscribed tuberculous focus, arising usually from the posterior aspect of the vertebral body, producing a clinical picture resembling that of an intraspinal tumor; hence the name *spinal tumor syndrome;* this type is rare, and only type in which neurologic signs precede

roentgenographic picture of spinal tuberculosis
  c. Posterior spinal disease, wherein primary
  bone lesion is in neural arch
  d. Infective thrombosis of cord; extremely rare;
  only one fully documented case recorded
  2. Mechanical
    a. Pathologic dislocation, ridge of living bone
    pressing cord and embarrassing its circulation
    b. Compression by sequestra, loose fragments of
    dead bone or disc being squeezed posteriorly
    against the cord; rarely, concertina collapse
    may occur without angulation, squeezing
    granulation tissue and debris against cord
  B. Late onset
    1. Cord almost always shrunken longitudinally and
    tight against the anterior wall of spinal canal;
    therefore peculiarly susceptible to compression
      a. Inflammatory: continued activity or reactiva-
      tion of disease, producing pressure on cord by
      abscess or inflammatory tissue
      b. Mechanical: cord more and more tightly
      stretched over debris or bone in spinal canal
      until its circulation at this level insufficient;
      stretching aggravated by increasing angulation
      of spine in absence of arthrodesis

Intrinsic cord lesions without compression may be responsible. In the past these lesions have not been understood and were thought probably to result from edema
from vascular stasis or local toxicity.

Seddon stated that although these several mechanisms
have been described as acting separately to produce a paraplegia, more than one cause may be found in a single
patient, and which is prominent is often difficult if not
impossible to tell.

Hodgson et al. have pointed out that it was Michaud in
1871 who first suggested that tuberculous infection in
Pott's disease may pass through the dura to involve the
cord and produce an irreversible paraplegia. Through the
years histologic evidence of such involvement has been
presented by others. As late as 1950 Garceau and Brady,
from postmortem studies and from observations in patients
explored surgically, showed that the dura can be invaded
by tuberculous granulation tissue. Hodgson et al. treated
two patients who did not improve after anterior debridement and fusion. Additional surgery was carried out in
each; in one adhesions and other evidence of inflammation
were found about the cord, and in the other granulation
tissue had invaded the dura, and two small abscesses were
found within the cord itself. The paraplegia changed little,
if at all, in either patient. After these experiences they
biopsied the dura in nine consecutive paraplegics. All
specimens except one showed granulomatous inflammation
with typical epithelioid tubercle formation or with caseous
necrosis on the outer surface. Some showed varying degrees of more severe involvement. Two showed typical
tuberculous, granulomatous inflammation on the outer surface, extending into and through the dura, and spreading
onto the inner surface. The pattern of inflammation suggested direct spread through the dura, presumably from the
outer to the inner surface. They were disturbed to note that

in four of the nine patients the duration of paraplegia had
been less than 6 months, and in one patient less than 1
month. Thus it appeared to them that tuberculous inflammatory change within the dura is the rule in this disease.
Accordingly they proposed that causes of Pott's paraplegia
be classified as follows:
  Extrinsic causes
  1. In active disease
    a. Abscess (fluid or caseous)
    b. Granulation tissue
    c. Sequestrated bone and disc
    d. Pathologic subluxation
    e. Dislocation of vertebrae
  2. In healed disease
    a. Transverse ridge of bone anterior to spinal cord
    b. Fibrosis of the dura
  Intrinsic causes
  1. Passage of tuberculous inflammation through the
  dura to involve the meninges and eventually the
  spinal cord
  Rare causes
  1. Infective thrombosis of the cord
  2. Spinal tumor syndrome

Treatment of Pott's paraplegia

At least three schools of thought exist on the treatment
of Pott's paraplegia. According to Bosworth, Campos, and
others, the most reliable treatment is immobilization and
early posterior arthrodesis. Bosworth stated that 80% of
the patients in whom this complication is recognized early
will recover after successful arthrodesis. In his opinion,
anterior decompression is indicated only for those few patients who do not recover after such treatment. Hodgson et
al. treat all patients by radical anterior decompression and
arthrodesis (p. 3333). Similarly Kohli, Ahn, Guirguis, and
others treat all patients by anterior or anterolateral decompression with or without arthrodesis. But according to
Roaf et al., Griffiths, James, and others, the usual treatment is immobilization. If this treatment *within specified
limits* does not produce improvement and recovery, they
decompress the cord. They usually arthrodese the spine
only after recovery is progressing or is complete. Seddon
estimated that despite nonoperative treatment paraplegia of
early onset will persist or increase in one fourth of the
patients and of late onset in one half.

Indications for surgery. The following summary of the in-
dications for surgery is adapted from Griffiths and from
Seddon.
  A. Absolute indications
    1. Paraplegia with onset during usual conservative
    treatment; operation not performed for pyramidal
    tract signs, but delayed until important motor
    weakness occurs
    2. Paraplegia getting worse or remaining stationary
    despite sufficient conservative treatment
    3. Complete loss of motor power for 1 month de-
    spite sufficient conservative treatment
    4. Paraplegia accompanied by uncontrollable spas-
    ticity of such severity that reasonable rest and
    immobilization are impossible or there is risk of
    pressure necrosis of skin

5. Severe paraplegia of rapid onset; may indicate unusually severe pressure from mechanical accident or abscess; may also result from vascular thrombosis, but this cannot be diagnosed

6. Any severe paraplegia; flaccid paraplegia, paraplegia in flexion, complete sensory loss, or complete loss of motor power for more than 6 months—all indications for immediate surgery without trial of conservative treatment

B. Relative indications

1. Recurrent paraplegia even with paralysis that would cause no concern in first attack

2. Paraplegia with onset in old age; indications for surgery stronger because of hazards of immobilization.

3. Painful paraplegia, pain resulting from spasm or root compression

4. Complications such as urinary tract infections and stones

C. Rare indications

1. Posterior spinal disease

2. Spinal tumor syndrome

3. Severe paralysis secondary to cervical disease

4. Severe cauda equina paralysis

Pott's paraplegia itself is always an indication for surgery according to Hodgson et al., Ahn, Goel, Kohli, and others. They recommend early operation consisting of evacuation of the diseased material, and some insert bone grafts at the same time. Hodgson et al. believe that immediate operation results in the most cures in the shortest possible time. To them operation is urgent because of their observations that tuberculous infection can penetrate the dura and infect the cord and that when this occurs, the paraplegia is likely to be permanent.

Selection of proper operation. According to Roaf et al., Griffiths, James, and Seddon the surgical procedures for Pott's paraplegia are (1) costotransversectomy, (2) anterolateral decompression, and (3) laminectomy. Arthrodesis of the spine is usually necessary as an adjunct to these operations, but is of secondary importance.

When a tense paravertebral abscess is suspected, costotransversectomy is indicated. According to James, if this procedure yields pus under pressure, one is justified in proceeding no further and should wait up to 6 weeks for improvement. If no improvement occurs during this time, anterolateral decompression should be done without further delay. If pus under pressure is not found during costotransversectomy, the procedure should be continued as an anterolateral decompression. Anterolateral decompression is the procedure of choice for Pott's paraplegia not accompanied by a tense abscess, except in those instances listed in the preceding outline as rare indications. Spinal tumor syndrome and paraplegia from posterior spinal disease require laminectomy. Paralysis secondary to cervical disease is treated by either laminectomy and posterior arthrodesis or debridement and anterior arthrodesis, and severe cauda equina paralysis is treated by lumbar transversectomy.

According to Hodgson et al., except in spinal tumor syndrome and paraplegia resulting from posterior spinal disease, early radical anterior decompression and arthrodesis (p. 3333) are indicated in all patients; Kohli, Guirguis, Ahn, Goel, and others prefer a less radical anterior or anterolateral decompression and some omit the arthrodesis.

ABSCESS DRAINAGE BY ANATOMIC LEVEL

Any abscess cavity about the spine can be drained by the following techniques.

Cervical spine

If the cervical spine is involved, the abscess may be present retropharyngeally in the posterior triangle of the neck or supraclavicular area, or the tuberculous detritus may gravitate downward under the prevertebral fascia to form a mediastinal abscess.

DRAINAGE OF RETROPHARYNGEAL ABSCESS

Drainage of a retropharyngeal abscess through an incision in the posterior wall of the pharynx is warranted only in an emergency, as indicated by cyanosis and respiratory

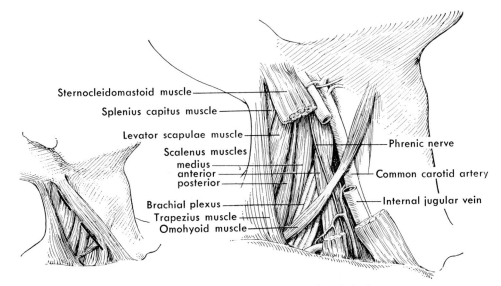

Fig. 74-2. Drainage of tuberculous abscess of cervical spine.

difficulty. Usually drainage should be through an extraoral approach (Fig. 74-2).

TECHNIQUE. Make a 7.5 cm incision along the posterior border of the sternocleidomastoid muscle at the junction of its middle and upper thirds. Incise the superficial layer of cervical fascia and protect the spinal accessory nerve that pierces the sternocleidomastoid muscle and runs obliquely across the posterior triangle. Retract the sternocleidomastoid muscle medially or divide it transversely. Using blunt dissection, expose the levator scapulae and splenius muscles, displace the internal jugular vein anteriorly, and palpate the abscess in front of the transverse processes and bodies of the vertebrae. Puncture the abscess wall with a hemostat, enlarge the opening, and gently but thoroughly evacuate the abscess. If the abscess is unusually large and symptoms are severe, do not close the wound; if not, close the wound in layers. A tracheostomy set should be available should the patient develop respiratory difficulty from edema of the larynx or should the abscess rupture into the pharynx.

DRAINAGE OF ABSCESS OF POSTERIOR TRIANGLE OF NECK

TECHNIQUE. Incise obliquely the skin and superficial fascia for 6.3 cm along the posterior border of the sternocleidomastoid muscle. Retract this muscle medially, but carefully protect the superficial nerves and external jugular vein. Identify the scaleni muscles without injuring the phrenic nerve. Locate and divide the line of cleavage between the scalenus anterior and longus colli muscles by blunt dissection obliquely inward to the abscess beneath the paravertebral fascia. Evacuate the cavity and close the wound.

Dorsal spine

Most abscesses caused by disease of the dorsal spine may be evacuated by costotransversectomy (Fig. 74-3). This procedure, originally performed by Haidenhaim, was described by Ménard in 1894.

TECHNIQUE. Make a midline incision over three spinous processes. Reflect the periosteum and soft tissues laterally from the spinous processes and laminae on the side containing the abscess. Expose fully the middle transverse process and resect it at its base. After reflecting the periosteum from the contiguous rib, resect its medial end by division 5 cm from the tip of the transverse process. Bevel the end of the rib, taking care to avoid puncture of the pleura. Open the abscess by blunt dissection close to the vertebral body. The opening should be large enough to permit thorough exploration of the cavity and removal of all debris. If resection of more than one rib is necessary, enlarge the initial incision accordingly. After resecting the ribs, doubly ligate and divide the intervening neurovascular bundle. Close the wound in layers.

TECHNIQUE (SEDDON). Begin a semicircular skin incision in the midline about 10 cm proximal to the apex of the kyphos, curve distally and laterally to a point 10 cm from the midline at this apex, and continue distally and medially to the midline at a point 10 cm distal to the apex (Fig. 74-4). If the infection is pyogenic without a kyphosis, a midline incision can be used. Elevate the skin flap and retract it medially. Cut the superficial muscles and turn them in whatever direction is appropriate for the particular level. Divide the erector spinae muscles transversely opposite the apex of the deformity. Using diathermy dissection, expose

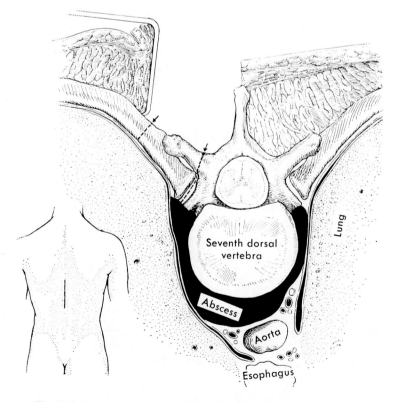

Fig. 74-3. Costotransversectomy to drain tuberculous abscess of dorsal spine.

the medial 8.3 cm of not less than three ribs, the corresponding transverse processes, and the lateral third of the laminae (Fig. 74-5).

Resect the rib that roentgenograms show to be level with the widest bulge of the abscess as follows. After dividing the costotransverse ligaments, remove the transverse process in one piece with large bone-cutting forceps. Using subperiosteal dissection, expose the rib, being careful not to perforate the pleura. If such a perforation occurs, place a small swab over it and try to close it as soon as the rib has been removed. The use of a Carlen tube will allow deflation of the lung. Transect the rib at a point not less than 6.8 cm (in the adult) lateral to the costotransverse joint. Use a curved gouge to free the medial end of the rib, pushing the gouge gently anteriorly and medially until it strikes the head of the rib or the vertebral column. Gently rotate the medial end of the rib and use the gouge to divide any remaining attachment. If the operation is successful, pus will pour out of the hole; remove it immediately with a sucker. Explore the abscess with a finger, reaching the vertebral bodies, opening small cavities, and dislodging necrotic material. If the abscess is unusually large, remove a second transverse process and rib for more exposure. Remove the tuberculous material from the abscess cavity and superficial tissues. After dusting the wound and the cavity with streptomycin powder, close the muscles and skin without a drain.

Lumbar and pelvic drainage
DRAINAGE OF PARAVERTEBRAL ABSCESS

TECHNIQUE. Make a 7.5 to 10 cm longitudinal incision 5.0 to 7.5 lateral to the midline parallel to the spinous processes. Divide the lumbodorsal fascia in line with the incision and pass a hemostat bluntly around the lateral and anterior borders of the erector spinae muscles to the transverse processes (Fig. 74-6). Usually the abscess is encountered immediately; if not, puncture the layer of lumbodorsal fascia that separates the quadratus lumborum muscle from the erector spinae group and force the hemostat along the anterior border of the transverse processes. After thorough evacuation of the abscess, close the incision in layers.

DRAINAGE OF PSOAS ABSCESS

Psoas abscesses are entirely extraperitoneal and follow the course of the iliopsoas muscle. Drainage may be accomplished posteriorly through Petit's triangle, by a lateral

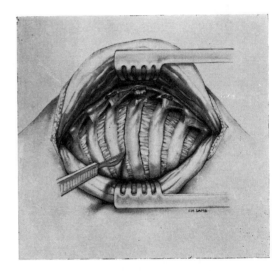

Fig. 74-5. Exposure of ribs and resection of transverse processes. (From Seddon, H.J.: In Platt, H., editor: Modern trends in orthopedics, second series, London, 1956, Butterworth & Co., Ltd.)

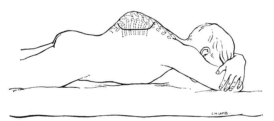

Fig. 74-4. Incision for costotransversectomy or anterolateral decompression. (From Seddon, H.J.: In Platt, H., editor: Modern trends in orthopedics, second series, London, 1956, Butterworth & Co., Ltd.)

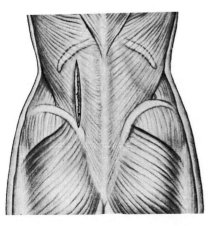

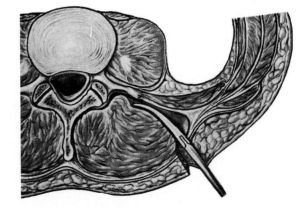

Fig. 74-6. Drainage of paravertebral abscess.

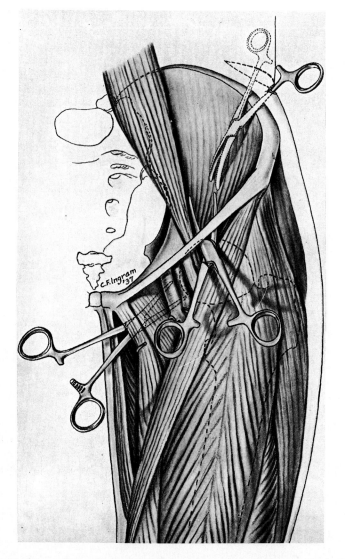

Fig. 74-7. Drainage of psoas abscess. Hemostat in adductor region is pointed toward inferior edge of acetabulum; abscess is usually located nearer junction of femoral head and neck. (Adapted from Freiberg, J.A., and Perlman, R.: J. Bone Joint Surg. **18:**417, 1936.)

incision along the crest of the ilium, or anteriorly under Poupart's ligament, depending on the size of the abscess and the area in which it appears. Occasionally an abscess burrows beneath Poupart's ligament and is seen subcutaneously in the proximal third of the thigh in the adductor region (Fig. 74-7).

DRAINAGE THROUGH PETIT'S TRIANGLE

The sides of this triangle are formed by the lateral margin of the latissimus dorsi muscle and the medial border of the obliquus externus abdominis muscle and its base by the crest of the ilium. The floor of the triangle is the obliquus internus abdominis muscle.

TECHNIQUE. Make a 7.5 cm incision 2.5 cm proximal to and parallel with the posterior crest of the ilium, beginning lateral to the erector spinae group of muscles (Fig. 74-8). After exposure of Petit's triangle, bluntly dissect through the obliquus internus abdominis muscle directly into the

abscess. After thorough evacuation of the abscess close the incision in layers.

AFTERTREATMENT. Since flexion contracture of the hip usually accompanies a psoas abscess, Buck's extension should be employed to correct the deformity and relax the spastic muscles until the hip is fully extended.

DRAINAGE BY LATERAL INCISION

TECHNIQUE. Make a 10 cm incision along the middle third of the crest of the ilium and free the attachments of the internal and external obliquus abdominis muscles. Puncture with a hemostat the abscess, which may be palpated as a fluctuant extraperitoneal mass on the inner surface of the wing of the ilium. Avoid rupture of the peritoneum.

DRAINAGE BY ANTERIOR INCISION

TECHNIQUE. Begin a longitudinal skin incision at the anterosuperior spine and continue it distally for 5 to 7.5 cm

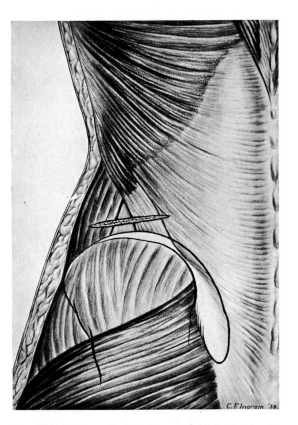

Fig. 74-8. Drainage of pelvic abscess through Petit's triangle.

on the anterior aspect of the thigh. Identify the sartorius muscle and carry the dissection deep to its medial border to the level of the anteroinferior spine. Protect the femoral nerve, which lies just medial to this area. Now insert a long hemostat along the medial surface of the wing of the ilium under Poupart's ligament and puncture the abscess. Separate the blades of the hemostat to enlarge the opening and permit complete evacuation. Close the incision in layers.

DRAINAGE BY LUDLOFF INCISION

When a psoas abscess points subcutaneously in the adductor region of the thigh, drainage is accomplished by a Ludloff incision, as described on p. 72.

Weinberg has described a method of excising a psoas abscess when simpler treatment has failed or is likely to fail because of the size of the abscess, its chronicity, or involvement with mixed bacterial infection. He removes the abscess and also any bony or cartilaginous sequestra lodged in the tract or in the diseased vertebrae. The reader is referred to his work for details of technique and aftertreatment.

DRAINAGE OF PELVIC ABSCESS

Lougheed and White have noted that when tuberculosis involves the lower lumbar and lumbosacral areas, soft tissue abscesses may gravitate into the pelvis, forming a large abscess anterior to the sacrum. These may point to the skin on the anterior surface of the thigh or above the iliac crest, but drainage at these sites alone is insufficient,

resulting only in a chronically draining sinus despite antibacterial therapy. The pelvic abscess usually can be demonstrated roentgenographically by retrograde injection of an opaque medium. They have devised a method of establishing dependent drainage posteriorly by coccygectomy. Their results in treatment of 10 patients by this method have been uniformly good. The wound usually healed within 6 to 8 weeks, and the spinal lesions all became inactive.

TECHNIQUE (LOUGHEED AND WHITE). Make a 15 cm elliptical incision over the coccyx, removing a strip of skin. After freeing the coccyx from soft tissues, disarticulate it from the sacrum. With careful hemostasis carry the dissection upward, staying close to the sacrum until the resulting pyramidal tunnel communicates with the abscess cavity. After evacuating the purulent matter, insert an irrigating catheter to the top of the cavity and pack the wound with iodoform gauze.

AFTERTREATMENT. For 2 to 3 weeks the wound is irrigated through the catheter several times daily with a solution of streptomycin. The packing is changed at intervals until the wound has healed by granulation tissue from within.

RADICAL DEBRIDEMENT AND ARTHRODESIS FOR TUBERCULOSIS OF SPINE

TECHNIQUE (HODGSON ET AL.). Approach the *upper cervical* area (C1 and C2) through either the transoral or transthyrohyoid approach. In either approach perform a tracheostomy before operation. Have the anesthesia given through the tracheostomy opening, thus leaving the pharynx free of endotracheal tubing that would obstruct the view.

In the transoral approach, place the head in hyperextension and pack the hypopharynx. Turn back the soft palate upon itself and anchor it with stay sutures exposing the nasopharynx. Next in the posterior pharyngeal wall make a midline incision 5 cm long with its center 1 fingerbreadth inferior to the anterior tubercle of the atlas that is palpable (Fig. 74-9, *A*). Carry the incision down to bone. Now strip the posterior pharyngeal wall subperiosteally as far laterally as the lateral margin of the lateral masses of the atlas and the axis. Retract the raised soft tissue flaps with long stay sutures (Fig. 74-9, *B*) and control any oozing of blood by packing. The anterior arch of the atlas, the body of the axis, and the atlantoaxial joints on either side now are exposed.

For the transthyrohyoid approach, make a collar incision along the uppermost crease of the neck between the hyoid bone and the thyroid cartilage extending as far laterally as the carotid sheaths (Fig. 74-10, *A*). Divide the sternohyoid and thyrohyoid muscles exposing the thyrohyoid membrane. Detach this membrane as near to the hyoid bone as possible to avoid damaging the internal laryngeal nerve and the superior laryngeal vessels that pierce it from the side nearer to its inferior attachment (Fig. 74-10, *B*). Next enter the hypopharynx by cutting into the exposed mucous membrane from the side to avoid damaging the epiglottis. Expose the posterior pharyngeal wall by retracting the hyoid bone and the epiglottis; make a midline incision in it down to bone (Fig. 74-10, *C*). Raise subperiosteally soft tissue flaps on either side and retract them to expose the bodies of C2, C3, and C4 (Fig. 74-10, *D*).

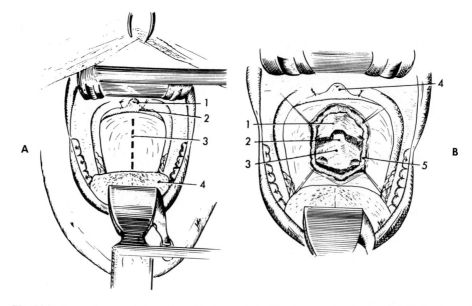

Fig. 74-9. Transoral approach to upper cervical area. **A,** Incision in posterior pharyngeal wall. *1,* Uvula; *2,* soft palate; *3,* incision in posterior pharyngeal wall; *4,* tongue. **B,** Atlas and axis exposed. *1,* Atlas; *2,* odontoid process; *3,* axis; *4,* uvula; *5,* edge of posterior pharyngeal wall retracted. (From Fang, H.S.Y., and Ong, G.B.: J. Bone Joint Surg. **44-A:**1588, 1962.)

Approach the *lower cervical* vertebrae (C3 through C7) through a collar incision or one along the anterior or posterior border of the sternocleidomastoid muscle p. 3094). Incise the abscess longitudinally, exposing the spine.

Approach the *lower cervical and upper dorsal* vertebrae (C7 through D3) on the side with the larger abscess through a periscapular incision similar to that used for a first-stage thoracoplasty. Elevate the scapula with a mechanical retractor and resect the third rib. The pleura is usually opened, but if it is adherent, or if for other reasons it is necessary, make an extrapleural approach. Divide the superior intercostal artery at its origin, along with the accompanying vein.

Approach the *middorsal* vertebrae (D4 through D11) usually from the left side. Select the rib that in the midaxillary line lies opposite the maximum convexity of the kyphos. It is usually two ribs superior to the center of the vertebral focus. Make an incision along this rib, resect it, and do a standard thoracotomy. The abscess is usually seen immediately, or there may be adhesions between it and the adjacent lung. Mobilize the lung and push it anteriorly. Now make a longitudinal incision in the pleura close to the aorta in the groove between the aorta and the abscess. Displace the aorta anteriorly and medially, revealing the intercostal vessels; secure and divide these for the entire length of the abscess cavity. Divide also elements of the splanchnic nerves. Now displace the aorta anteriorly away from the spine and palpate the abscess across the anterior aspects of the vertebrae. Make a T-shaped incision through the abscess wall: the first incision is transverse and opposite the center of the disease process, and the second is longitudinal and medial to the distally placed ligatures on the intercostal vessels. Now raise the two triangular flaps, revealing the diseased area including the inside of the abscess cavity (Fig. 74-11).

Approach the *dorsolumbar area* (D12 through L2) through an incision along the left eleventh rib. Keep the dissection extrapleural and retroperitoneal and separate the diaphragm from the spine. Divide the psoas muscle transversely and turn it distally. Ligate the lumbar arteries and veins, as just described for the intercostals, and proceed with the approach as for the middorsal area.

Expose the *lower lumbar* vertebrae (L3 through L4) through a renal approach, using a left twelfth rib incision. The psoas muscle is usually divided transversely at a more distal level, often going through an ill-defined abscess between the muscle fibers. Avoid the trunks of the lumbar plexus posterior to the muscle.

Expose the *fifth lumbar and first sacral* vertebrae through an extraperitoneal approach. Start the incision in the midline midway between the symphysis pubis and the umbilicus and carry it to the left in a lazy-S fashion to a point midway between the iliac crest and the lowest rib in the flank (Fig. 74-12, *A*). Divide the skin, superficial fascia, and deep fascia in line with the incision. Divide the obliquus internus abdominis muscle in the same line but across its fibers. Divide also the transversus abdominis muscle and fascia in the same line. Then expose and dissect the peritoneum from the lateral wall of the abdomen, the left psoas muscle, and the lower lumbar spine. If the bifurcation of the aorta is high, the easiest approach to the lumbosacral region is between the common iliac vessels. The only vessels encountered are the middle sacral artery and vein; cauterize and divide these (Fig. 74-12, *B*). Retract or divide any fibers of the presacral plexus as necessary. If the bifurcation of the aorta is low, make the approach lateral to the aorta, the vena cava, and the common iliac vessels. Ligate and divide the iliolumbar and ascending lumbar veins to mobilize adequately the left common iliac vein (Fig. 74-12, *C*). If necessary ligate and divide

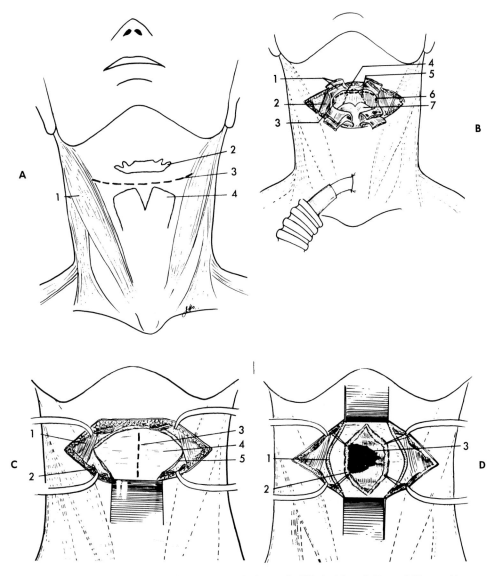

Fig. 74-10. Transthyrohyoid approach to upper cervical area. **A,** Skin incision. *1,* Sternocleidomastoid muscle; *2,* hyoid bone, *3,* skin incision; *4,* thyroid cartilage. **B,** Incision in thyrohyoid membrane. *1,* Cut ends of sternohyoid and thyrohyoid muscles; *2,* omohyoid muscle; *3,* thyrohyoid membrane; *4,* incision in thryohyoid membrane; *5,* epiglottis; *6,* internal laryngeal nerve and superior laryngeal artery;; *7,* thyroid cartilage. **C,** Incision in posterior pharyngeal wall. *1,* Omohyoid muscle; *2,* cut ends of sternohyoid and thyrohyoid muscles; *3,* incision; *4,* posterior pharyngeal wall; *5,* cut edges of thyrohyoid membrane and hypopharyngeal mucosa. **D,** Vertebral bodies exposed. *1,* Cut edges of thyrohyoid membrane and hypopharyngeal mucosa; *2,* retracted edge of posterior pharyngeal wall; *3,* bodies of C2, C3, and C4 are exposed. (From Fang, H.S.Y., Ong, G.B., and Hodgson, A.R.: Clin. Orthop. **35:**16, 1964.)

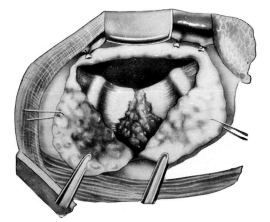

Fig. 74-11. Abscess opened with T-shaped incision through its wall. (From Hodgson, A.R., and Stock, F.E.: In Rob, C., and Smith, R., editors: Operative surgery service, vol. 9, London, 1960, Butterworth & Co., Ltd.)

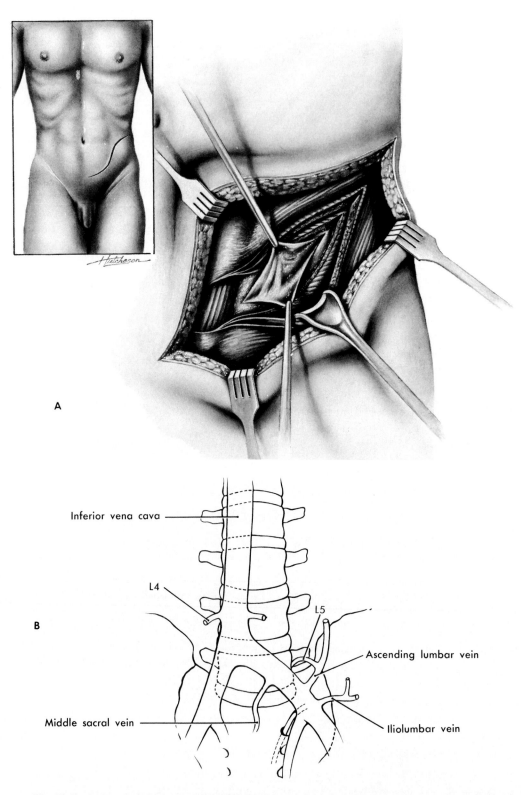

Fig. 74-12. A, Extraperitoneal approach to fifth lumbar and first sacral vertebrae (see text). *Inset,* Skin incision. **B,** In high bifurcation of aorta, middle sacral artery and vein are cauterized and divided. In low bifurcation of aorta, iliolumbar and ascending lumbar vein.

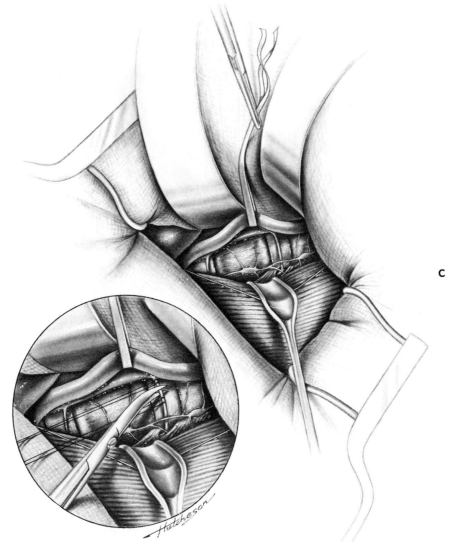

Fig. 74-12, cont'd. C, Exposed vertebrae are crossed by ascending lumbar vein. *Inset,* Ascending lumbar vein is ligated and divided. (From Hoover, N.W.: J. Bone Joint Surg. **50-A:**194, 1968.)

the fifth lumbar artery and vein and, if a higher approach is required, the fourth lumbar artery and vein as well. Then displace the large vessels to the right side and protect them with retractors.

The technique of excision of the diseased tissue and of anterior arthrodesis is about the same at all levels of the spine. Remove debris, pus, and sequestrated bone or disc by suction or with a pituitary rongeur. If possible, pass the sucker across anterior to or between diseased vertebrae into the abscess cavity on the opposite side, and evacuate all material. Remove with an osteotome, rongeur, or chisel all diseased bone, both soft and sclerotic, exposing the spinal canal for the whole length of the disease. Also remove with a knife or rongeur the posterior common ligament and tuberculous granulation and fibrous tissue, exposing the dura. Excise the entire vertebral body affected by the disease, since collections of pus or sequestrated bone or disc material are often found in the spinal canal

posterior to apparently normal posterior parts of diseased bodies. If there is a definite indication, open the dura for inspection of the cord.

Now remove the disc at each end of the cavity, exposing normal bleeding bone (Fig. 74-13). Partially correct the kyphosis by direct pressure posteriorly on the spine. After cutting a mortise in the vertebrae at each end, insert one or more strut grafts of the correct length, keeping the vertebrae sprung apart (Fig. 74-14). For the dorsal area, fashion the grafts from the rib removed during thoracotomy (Fig. 74-15); bank grafts may be added. For the cervical area obtain the grafts from the bank or from the iliac crest. For the lumbar area take a massive graft from the iliac crest (Figs. 74-16 and 74-17).

Put streptomycin and isoniazid into the cavity before closure. After thoracotomy close the chest in the usual way and maintain suction drainage of the pleural space for 2 or 3 days.

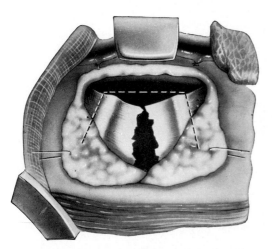

Fig. 74-13. Excision of diseased bone. (From Hodgson, A.R., and Stock, F.E.: In Rob, C., and Smith, R., editors: Operative surgery service, vol. 9, London, 1960, Butterworth & Co., Ltd.)

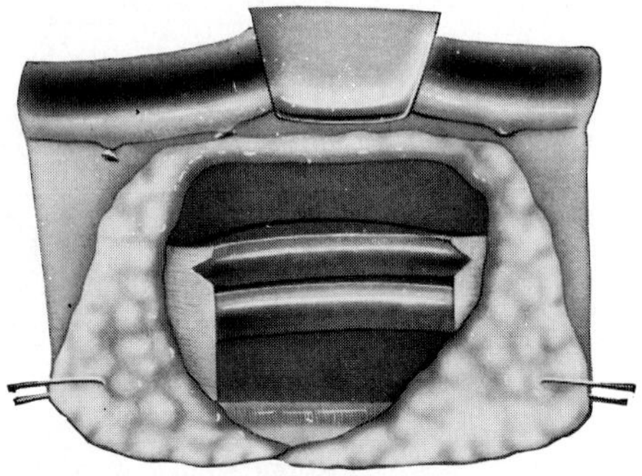

Fig. 74-14. Grafts inserted keeping vertebrae sprung apart. (From Hodgson, A.R., and Stock, F.E.: In Rob, C., and Smith, R., editors: Operative surgery service, vol. 9, London, 1960, Butterworth & Co., Ltd.)

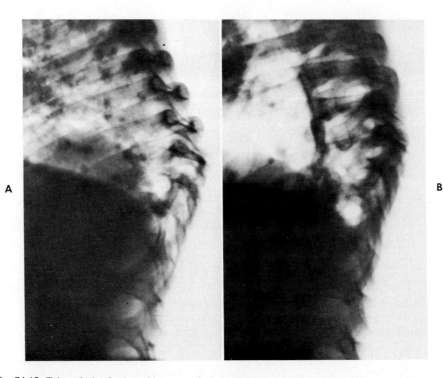

Fig. 74-15. Tuberculosis of spine without paraplegia in girl 4 years old. **A,** Destruction of vertebral bodies before surgery. **B,** Six months after a thoracotomy approach, excision of diseased bone, and anterior fusion from D6 to D11 using resected ribs for grafts; 4½ years later, pain and evidence of activity are absent.

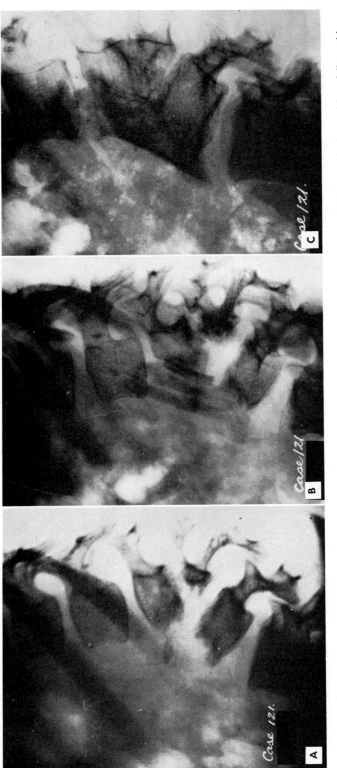
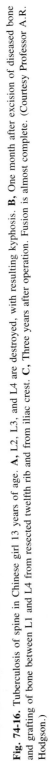

Fig. 74-16. Tuberculosis of spine in Chinese girl 13 years of age. **A,** L2, L3, and L4 are destroyed, with resulting kyphosis. **B,** One month after excision of diseased bone and grafting of bone between L1 and L4 from resected twelfth rib and from iliac crest. **C,** Three years after operation. Fusion is almost complete. (Courtesy Professor A.R. Hodgson.)

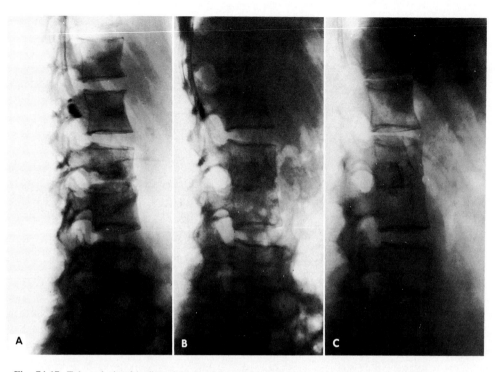

Fig. 74-17. Tuberculosis of bodies of L2 and L3 without paraplegia in woman 23 years of age. **A,** Before surgery. **B,** Six months after debridement and anterior arthrodesis through left extraperitoneal approach; grafts were from ilium. **C,** Four years after surgery; fusion is complete.

AFTERTREATMENT. The patient is placed in a plaster bed consisting of anterior and posterior shells and remains there until the spine is judged to have united clinically. The time of immobilization after surgery averages about 3½ months. Mobilization is then gradually started and is continued for 6 to 8 weeks, the patient being carefully watched for increasing kyphosis or other signs of activity of the disease.

ROAF TECHNIQUE WITH DORSOLATERAL APPROACH TO DORSAL SPINE. Expose the dorsal spine through a dorsolateral approach. Maintain careful hemostasis throughout. Select the side with the larger abscess shadow, or in the absence of an abscess use the left side, and make a curved incision. Begin posteriorly 3.8 cm from the midline, 7.5 cm proximal to the center of the lesion, and curve distally and laterally to a point 12.5 cm from the midline at the center of the lesion; continue medially and distally, ending 3.8 cm from the midline 7.5 cm distal to the center of the lesion (Fig. 74-18). Divide the superficial and deep fascia and the underlying muscles down to the ribs in the line of the incision. Retract the flap of the skin and muscle medially. Now locate the rib opposite the center of the focus and remove 7.5 to 10 cm of this rib and the one proximal and distal in the following manner. Free the ribs with a periosteal elevator and divide them with rib shears 7.5 to 10 cm from the tips of the transverse processes. Now resect each at the tip of the transverse process. Divide under direct vision the ligaments and muscles attached to the rib heads and transverse processes and resect these bony parts. Identify two and preferably three intercostal nerves and trace them medially to the intervertebral foramina. These nerves, as they pass into the foramina, indicate the level of the cord in the spinal canal. Expose the intercostal vessels near the spinal column and cut them between clamps. Divide the intercostal muscles near the vertebral column. Separate the pleura from the spinal column by blunt dissection, exposing the lateral and anterolateral aspects of the vertebral bodies. Take care to avoid perforating the pleura, as it is often adherent and thickened; if a perforation should occur, suture it at once. Locate the center of the lesion by passing a finger into the wound anterior to the vertebral bodies. Remove all pus, granulation tissue, and necrotic matter. Occasionally one or more vertebral bodies may be sequestrated and lying free in the abscess cavity. Usually two or three small bony sequestra and pieces of necrotic disc material are found. If the paravertebral shadow, thought to be an abscess, is found to be mainly fibrous tissue, it is more difficult to find the lesion. Under these circumstances using roentgenographic control, explore the bone with a fine gouge, burr, and rongeur. After thorough debridement decide whether bone grafts are advisable. The simplest method of grafting is to pack the cavity with bone chips. Or a more extensive procedure may be undertaken: with a chisel or gouge roughen the lateral and anterolateral aspects of the diseased vertebral bodies and if possible of one healthy vertebra above and below and cut a groove in them, passing from healthy bone above to healthy bone below. Wedge a full-thickness rib graft into the groove and sink it deeply within the vertebral bodies. Place cancellous bone chips obtained from the remaining portion of the resected ribs in the groove and laterally along the roughened surface of the vertebral bodies. If the pleura has been accidentally opened, drain the pleural cavity with a chest tube inserted through a small stab incision in the eighth intercostal space in the midaxillary line and connected to an underwater seal for 48 hours after surgery.

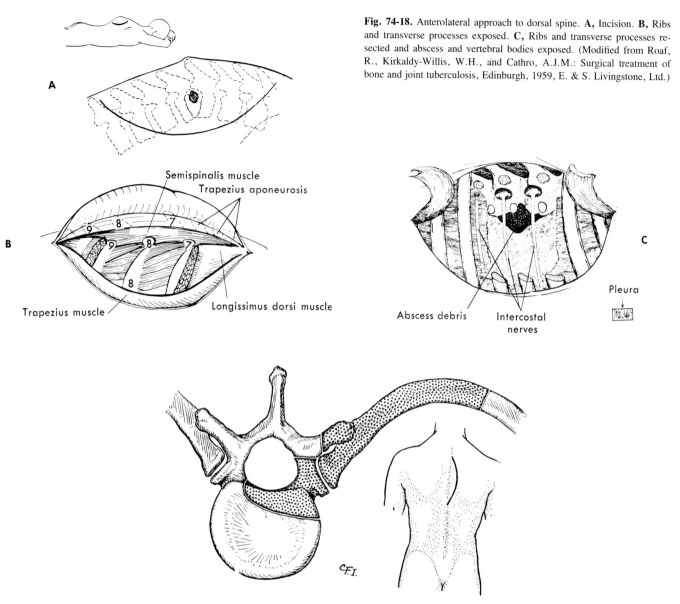

Fig. 74-18. Anterolateral approach to dorsal spine. **A,** Incision. **B,** Ribs and transverse processes exposed. **C,** Ribs and transverse processes resected and abscess and vertebral bodies exposed. (Modified from Roaf, R., Kirkaldy-Willis, W.H., and Cathro, A.J.M.: Surgical treatment of bone and joint tuberculosis, Edinburgh, 1959, E. & S. Livingstone, Ltd.)

Semispinalis muscle
Trapezius aponeurosis
Trapezius muscle
Longissimus dorsi muscle

Abscess debris   Intercostal nerves   Pleura

Fig. 74-19. Capener anterolateral decompression for tuberculous abscess of dorsal spine. *Stippled areas,* extent of bone resection. *Inset,* Skin incision.

COSTOTRANSVERSECTOMY

Costotransversectomy is discussed on p. 3330.

ANTEROLATERAL DECOMPRESSION (LATERAL RHACHOTOMY)

In 1933 Capener originated a procedure that he called lateral rhachotomy and that is now popularly known as anterolateral decompression, in which the spine is opened from its lateral side. This affords access to the front and side of the cord, permitting decompression by the removal of bony spurs, granulation tissue, and sequestra or the evacuation of abscesses. Since the procedure entails resection of one or more pedicles, it is contraindicated if the spine is unstable. The operation, at best difficult, is easiest when there is a sharp kyphos.

TECHNIQUE (CAPENER). If the disease is in the middorsal region, begin the incision in the midline at a point 10 cm proximal to the lesion, gently curve it laterally a distance of 7.5 cm, and return to the midline at a point 10 cm distal to the lesion (Fig. 74-19). Reflect the skin and superficial and deep fasciae as a thick flap. Now incise and retract laterally the origin of the trapezius muscle; divide the erector spinae muscles transversely over the rib leading to the affected intervertebral space and retract them proximally and distally. After exposing the rib subperiosteally, resect it from its angle to the transverse process; if necessary, resect the rib proximal and distal in the same manner. Now separate the intercostal nerve from its accompanying vessels and divide it, using the proximal end as a guide to further dissection and later for traction on the cord. Carefully retract the pleura along with the intercostal vessels and remove the medial end of the rib and the transverse process and pedicle of the vertebra with a rongeur; a

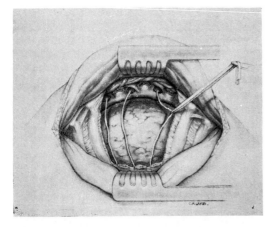

Fig. 74-20. Intercostal nerves isolated and pedicles exposed. (From Seddon, H.J.: In Platt, H., editor: Modern trends in orthopedics, second series, London, 1956, Butterworth & Co., Ltd.)

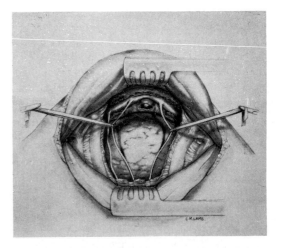

Fig. 74-21. Exposure of spinal cord after resection of three pedicles. Material anterior to cord may now be removed. Sequestrum is shown within abscess. (From Seddon, H.J.: In Platt, H., editor: Modern trends in orthopedics, second series, London, 1956, Butterworth & Co., Ltd.)

sphenoid punch and a motor-driven burr are of assistance at this stage. The dura and the posterolateral aspect of the vertebral body are seen after anterior depression of the pleura and the intercostal vessels and traction on the intercostal nerve. Now work from the more normal tissues in the vertebral canal toward the site of compression. Gently remove diseased bone with a curet; also remove all impinging and encroaching tissues so carefully that the dura is not even momentarily dented. Thoroughly evacuate a paravertebral abscess if present. Close the wound in layers.

AFTERTREATMENT. Anterior and posterior plaster shells, prepared before surgery, are applied; when the lesion is in the cervical or upper dorsal region, skeletal traction should be employed.

Alexander has recommended that three or more ribs be widely resected to provide better exposure; currently, Griffiths, Seddon, and Roaf also endorse the more extensive approach.

TECHNIQUE (SEDDON). The approach and the method of rib resection are as described for costotransversectomy on p. 3330. Resect not less than three and not more than four ribs. Isolate the intercostal nerves and trace them medially to the intervertebral foramina; now cut away the intervening intercostal muscles (Fig. 74-20). Gently push the pleura anteriorly with the fingers and determine by palpation the position of the two or three pedicles to be resected. To increase exposure, cut away small parts of the overhanging neural arches. Remove as little bone as possible dorsal to the pedicles, since anything in the least approaching hemilaminectomy is likely to be followed by a lateral subluxation of the spine. Now resect the pedicles by nibbling away from their lateral surfaces with a rongeur (Fig. 74-21). Use utmost care to avoid tearing the dura, which may be adherent to the inner surface of the pedicles. If a rent occurs, suture it as soon as possible.

Remove the offending material such as a caseous mass, granulation tissue, a necrotic disc, or a nest of sequestra.

This may be accomplished easily, but the removal of a ridge of living bone is difficult. Do not retract the cord, but leave it untouched and attack the bony ridge from the side or from beneath. Drill the ridge in several places with a slowly rotating hand drill and then nibble away from the side and below with a small rongeur. The mass may be further broken up with an osteotome. The cord now rests on a shell of bone; gently push this bone anteriorly with a blunt instrument. Be sure to leave no offending ridges. Now pass a probe along the anterior surface of the cord both proximally and distally to locate any second cause of compression inside the spinal canal, such as an encapsulated caseous mass. Wash the wound with saline solution and dust it with streptomycin. Suture the muscles and skin without drainage.

AFTERTREATMENT. Aftertreatment is the same as for the Capener technique (see above).

REFERENCES
Infection of spine

Ahn, B.H.: Treatment of Pott's paraplegia, Acta Orthop. Scand. **39:**145, 1968.

Albee, F.H.: Orthopedic and reconstruction surgery, Philadelphia, 1919, W.B. Saunders Co.

Albee, F.H., Powers, E.J., and McDowell, H.C.: Surgery of the spinal column, Philadelphia, 1945, F.A. Davis Co.

Alexander, G.L.: Neurological complications of spinal tuberculosis, Proc. R. Soc. Med. **39:**730, 1945-1946.

Allen, A.R., and Stevenson, A.W.: The results of combined drug therapy and early fusion in bone tuberculosis, J. Bone Joint Surg. **39-A:**32, 1957.

Allen, A.R., and Stevenson, A.W.: A ten-year follow-up of combined drug therapy and early fusion in bone tuberculosis, J. Bone Joint Surg. **49-A:**1001, 1967.

Altemeier, W.A., and Largen, T.: Antibiotic and chemotherapeutic agents in infections of the skeletal system, JAMA **150:**1462, 1952.

Ambrose, G.B., Alpert, M., and Neer, C.S.: Vertebral osteomyelitis: a diagnostic problem, JAMA **197:**619, 1966.

Arct, W.: Operative treatment of tuberculosis of the spine in old people, J. Bone Joint Surg. **50-A:**255, 1968.

Avila, L., Jr.: Primary pyogenic infections of the sacro-iliac articulation: a new approach to the joint, J. Bone Joint Surg. **23:**922, 1941.

Badgley, C.E.: Osteomyelitis of the ilium, Arch. Surg. **28**:83, 1934.

Bailey, H.L., Gabriel, M., Hodgson, A.R., and Shin, J.A.: Tuberculosis of the spine in children: operative findings and results in one hundred consecutive patients treated by removal of the lesion and anterior grafting, J. Bone Joint Surg. **54-A**:1633, 1972.

Bakalim, G.: Tuberculosis spondylitis: a clinical study with special reference to the significance of spinal fusion and chemotherapy, Acta Orthop. Scand., Suppl. 47, 1960.

Bakalim, G.: Results of radical evacuation and arthrodesis in sacro-iliac tuberculosis, Acta Orthop. Scand. **37**:375, 1966.

Batson, O.V.: The vertebral vein system as a mechanism for the spread of metastases, Am. J. Roentgenol. Radium Ther. **48**:715, 1942.

Bickel, W.H.: Tuberculosis of bones and joints, Mayo Clin. Proc. **28**:370, 1953.

Bickham, W.S.: Operative surgery, vol. 2, Philadelphia, 1924, W.B. Saunders Co.

Blanche, D.W.: Osteomyelitis in infants, J. Bone Joint Surg. **34-A**:71, 1952.

Bonfiglio, M., Lange, T.A., and Kim, Y.M.: Pyogenic vertebral osteomyelitis: disk space infections, Clin. Orthop. **96**:234, 1973.

Boston, H.C., Jr., Bianco, A.J., Jr., and Rhodes, K.H.: Disk space infections in children, Orthop. Clin. North Am. **6**:953, 1975.

Bosworth, D.: Tuberculosis of the osseous system: Part 4. Operative methods, Quart. Bull. Sea View Hosp. **5**:441, 1940.

Bosworth, D.M.: The treatment of tuberculous lesions of bones and joints with ipronazid (Marsilid), NY State J. Med. **56**:1281, 1956.

Bosworth, D.M.: Surgery of the spine. In American Academy of Orthopaedic Surgeons: Instructional course lectures, vol. 14, Ann Arbor, 1957, J.W. Edwards.

Bosworth, D.M.: Treatment of bone and joint tuberculosis in children, J. Bone Joint Surg. **41-A**:1255, 1959.

Bosworth, D.M.: Treatment of tuberculosis of bone and joint, Bull. NY Acad. Med. **35**:167, 1959.

Bosworth, D.M., Della Pietra, A., and Rahilly, G.: Paraplegia resulting from tuberculosis of the spine, J. Bone Joint Surg. **35-A**:735, 1953.

Bosworth, D.M., and Wright, H.A.: Streptomycin in bone and joint tuberculosis, J. Bone Joint Surg. **34-A**:255, 1952.

Bosworth, D.M., Wright, H.A., Fielding, J.W., and Wilson, H.J., Jr.: The use of ipronazid in the treatment of bone and joint tuberculosis, J. Bone Joint Surg. **35-A**:577, 1953.

Brant-Zawadzki, M., Burke, V.D., and Jeffrey R.B.: CT in the evaluation of spine infection, Spine **8**:358, 1983.

Brashear, H.R., Jr., and Rendleman, D.A.: Pott's paraplegia, South. Med. J. **71**:1379, 1978.

Butler, R.W.: Paraplegia in Pott's disease with special reference to the pathology and etiology, Br. J. Surg. **22**:738, 1934-1935.

Campos, O.P.: Bone and joint tuberculosis and its treatment, J. Bone Joint Surg. **37-A**:937, 1955.

Capener, N.: Personal communication to Girdlestone, G.R., 1934. Cited in Platt, H., editor: Modern trends in orthopaedics, New York, 1950, Paul B. Hoeber, Inc.

Capener, N.: The evolution of lateral rhachotomy, J. Bone Joint Surg. **36-B**:173, 1954.

Chu, C.-B.: Treatment of spinal tuberculosis in Korea, using focal debridement and interbody fusion, Clin. Orthop. **50**:235, 1967.

Conrad, S.E., Breivis, J., and Fried, M.A.: Vertebral osteomyelitis, caused by *Arachni propionica* and resembling actinomycosis, J. Bone Joint Surg. **60-A**:549, 1978.

Coventry, M.B., Ghormley, R.K., and Kernohan, J.W.: The intervertebral disc: its microscopic anatomy and pathology. Part 1. Anatomy, development, and physiology, J. Bone Joint Surg. **27-A**:105, 1945.

Crock, H.V., and Yoshizawa, H.: The blood supply of the lumbar vertebral column, Clin. Orthop. **115**:6, 1976.

Davies, P.D.O., et al.: Bone and joint tuberculosis: a survey of notifications in England and Wales, J. Bone Joint Surg. **66-B**:326, 1984.

Dickson, J.A.: Spinal tuberculosis in Nigerian children: a review of ambulant treatment, J. Bone Joint Surg. **49-B**:682, 1967.

Digby, J.M., and Kersley, J.B.: Pyogenic non-tuberculous spinal infection, J. Bone Joint Surg. **61-B**:47, 1979.

Dott, N.M.: Skeletal traction and anterior decompression in the management of Pott's paraplegia, Edinburgh Med. J. **54**:620, 1947.

Dove, J., Hsu, L.C.S., and Yau, A.C.M.C.: The cervical spine after halo-pelvic traction: an analysis of the complications in 83 patients, J. Bone Joint Surg. **62-B**:158, 1980.

Editorial: Chemotherapy in orthopaedic tuberculosis, Lancet **1**:1227, 1954.

Eismont, F.J., Bohlman, H.H., Soni, P.L., Goldberg, V.M., and Freehafer, A.A.: Pyogenic and fungal vertebral osteomyelitis with paralysis, J. Bone Joint Surg. **65-A**:19, 1983.

El-Gindi, S., Aref, S., Salama, M., and Andrew, J.: Infection of intervertebral discs after operation, J. Bone Joint Surg. **58-B**:114, 1976.

Erlacher, P.J.: The radical operative treatment of bone and joint tuberculosis, J. Bone Joint Surg. **17**:536, 1935.

Evans, E.T.: Tuberculosis of the bones and joints, J. Bone Joint Surg. **34-A**:267, 1952.

Fang, H.S.Y., Ong, G.B., and Hodgson, A.R.: Anterior spinal fusion, the operative approaches, Clin. Orthop. **35**:16, 1964.

Felländer, M.: Radical operation in tuberculosis of the spine, Acta Orthop. Scand., Suppl. 19, 1955.

Fifth report of the Medical Research Council Working Party on Tuberculosis of the Spine, Brompton Hospital, London, England: A five-year assessment of controlled trials of in-patient and out-patient treatment and of plaster-of-Paris jackets for tuberculosis of the spine in children on standard chemotherapy: studies in Masan and Pusan, Korea, J. Bone Joint Surg. **58-B**:399, 1976.

First report of the Medical Research Council Working Party on Tuberculosis of the Spine: A controlled trial of ambulant out-patient treatment and in-patient rest in bed in management of tuberculosis of the spine in young Korean patients on standard chemotherapy: a study in Masan, Korea, J. Bone Joint Surg. **55-B**:678, 1973.

Ford, L.T.: Postoperative infection of lumbar intervertebral disk space, South. Med. J. **69**:1477, 1977.

Fountain, S.S., Hsu, L.C.S., Yau, A.C.M.C., and Hodgson, A.R.: Progressive kyphosis following solid anterior spine fusion in children with tuberculosis of the spine: a long term study, J. Bone Joint Surg. **57-A**:1104, 1975.

Fourth report of the Medical Research Council Working Party on Tuberculosis of the Spine: A controlled trial of anterior spinal fusion and debridement in the surgical management of tuberculosis of the spine in patients on standard chemotherapy: a study in Hong Kong, Br. J. Surg. **61**:853, 1974.

Freehafer, A.A., Heiser, D.P., and Saunders, A.P.: Infection of the lower lumbar spine with Neisseria meningitidis, J. Bone Joint Surg. **60-A**:1001, 1978.

Friedman, B.: Chemotherapy of tuberculosis of the spine, J. Bone Joint Surg. **48-A**:451, 1966.

Friedman, B., and Kapur, V.N.: Newer knowledge of chemotherapy in the treatment of tuberculosis of bones and joints, Clin. Othop. **97**:5, 1973.

Garceau, G.J., and Brady, T.A.: Pott's paraplegia, J. Bone Joint Surg. **32-A**:87, 1950.

Garcia, A., Jr., and Grantham, S.A.: Hematogenous pyogenic vertebral osteomyelitis, J. Bone Joint Surg. **42-A**:429, 1960.

Ghormley, R.K., Bickel, W.H., and Dickson, D.D.: A study of acute infectious lesions of the intervertebral disks, South. Med. J. **33**:347, 1940.

Girdlestone, G.R.: The operative treatment of Pott's paraplegia, Br. J. Surg. **19**:121, 1931.

Girdlestone, G.R.: Tuberculosis of bones and joints. In Platt, H., editor: Modern trends in orthopaedics, New York, 1950, Paul B. Hoeber, Inc.

Girdlestone, G.R., and Somerville, E.W.: Tuberculosis of bone and joint, ed. 2, New York, 1952, Oxford University Press.

Goel, M.K.: Treatment of Pott's paraplegia by operation, J. Bone Joint Surg. **49-B**:674, 1967.

Golimbu, C., Firooznia, H., and Rafii, M.: CT of osteomyelitis of the spine, AJR **142**:159, 1984.

Griffiths, D.L.: Pott's paraplegia and its operative treatment, J. Bone Joint Surg. **35-B**:487, 1953.

Griffiths, H.E.D., and Jones, D.M.: Pyogenic infection of the spine: a review of twenty-eight cases, J. Bone Joint Surg. **53-B**:383, 1971.

Guirguis, A.R.: Pott's paraplegia, J. Bone Joint Surg. **49-B**:658, 1967.

Hale, J.E., and Aichroth, P.: Vertebral osteomyelitis: a complication of urological surgery, Br. J. Surg. **61**:867, 1974.

Hallock, H., and Jones, J.B.: Tuberculosis of the spine, J. Bone Joint Surg. **36-A**:219, 1954.

Halpern, A.A., Rinsky, L.A., Fountain, S., and Nagel, D.A.: Coccidioidomycosis of the spine: unusual roentgenographic presentation, Clin. Orthop. **140**:78, 1979.

Harris, R.I., Coulthard, H.S., and Dewar, F.P.: Streptomycin in the treatment of bone and joint tuberculosis, J. Bone Joint Surg. **34-A:**279, 1952.

Harris, H.N., and Kirkaldy-Willis, W.H.: Primary subacute pyogenic osteomyelitis, J. Bone Joint Surg. **47-B:**526, 1965.

Hartman, J.T., and Phalen, G.S.: Needle biopsy of bone: report of three representative cases, JAMA **200:**201, 1967.

Hassler, O.: The human intervertebral disc: a microangiographical study on its vascular supply at various ages, Acta Orthop. Scand. **40:**765, 1969.

Hazlett, J.W.: Pyogenic osteomyelitis of the spine, Can. J. Surg. **1:**243, 1958.

Henson, S.W., Jr., and Coventry, M.B.: Osteomyelitis of the vertebrae as the result of infection of the urinary tract, Surg. Gynecol. Obstet. **102:**207, 1956.

Hodgson, A.R., Skinsnes, O.K., and Leong, C.Y.: The pathogenesis of Pott's paraplegia, J. Bone Joint Surg. **49-A:**1147, 1967.

Hodgson, A.R., and Stock, F.E.: Anterior spinal fusion: a preliminary communication on the radical treatment of Pott's disease and Pott's paraplegia, Br. J. Surg. **44:**266, 1956.

Hodgson, A.R., and Stock, F.E.: Anterior fusion. In Rob, C., and Smith, R., editors: Operative surgery service, vol. 9, London, 1960, Butterworth & Co., Ltd.

Hodgson, A.R., and Stock, F.E.: Anterior spine fusion for the treatment of tuberculosis of the spine: the operative findings and results of treatment of the first one hundred cases, J. Bone Joint Surg. **42-A:**295, 1960.

Hodgson, A.R., Stock, F.E., Fang, H.S.Y., and Ong, G.B.: Anterior spinal fusion: the operative approach and pathological findings in 412 patients with Pott's disease of the spine, Br. J. Surg. **48:**172, 1960.

Hodgson, A.R., Yau, A., Kwon, J.S., and Kim, D.: A clinical study of 100 consecutive cases of Pott's paraplegia, Clin. Orthop. **36:**128, 1964.

Hoover, M.J., Jr.: The treatment of the tuberculous psoas abscess, South. Surg. **16:**729, 1950.

Hoover, N.W.: Methods of lumbar fusion, J. Bone Joint Surg. **50-A:**194, 1968.

Hsieh, C.K., Miltner, L.J., and Chang, C.P.: Tuberculosis of the shaft of the large bones of the extremities, J. Bone Joint Surg. **16:**545, 1934.

James, J.I.P.: Pott's paraplegia, Med. Pregl. **13:**9, 1960.

Janeway, T., and Moseberg, W.H., Jr.: Tuberculous paraplegia with lateral vertebral dislocation: a case report, J. Bone Joint Surg. **59-A:**554, 1977.

Jenkins, D.H.R., et al.: Stabilization of the spine in the surgical treatment of severe spinal tuberculosis in children, Clin. Orthop. **110:**69, 1975.

Johnson, R.W., Jr., Hillman, J.W., and Southwick, W.O.: The importance of direct surgical attack upon lesions of the vertebral bodies, particularly in Pott's disease, J. Bone Joint Surg. **35-A:**17, 1953.

Jones, A.R.: The influence of Hugh Owen Thomas on the evolution of treatment of skeletal tuberculosis, J. Bone Joint Surg. **35-B:**309, 1958.

Jones, B.S.: Pott's paraplegia in the Nigerian, J. Bone Joint Surg. **40-B:**16, 1958.

Kaplan, C.J.: Conservative therapy in skeletal tuberculosis: an appraisal based on experience in South Africa, Tubercle **40:**355, 1959.

Karlén, A.: Early drainage of paraspinal tuberculous abscesses in children: a preliminary report, J. Bone Joint Surg. **41-B:**491, 1959.

Kattapuram, S.V., Phillips, W.C., and Boyd, R.: Computed tomography in pyogenic osteomyelitis of the spine, AJR **140:**1199, 1983.

Kemp, H.B.S., Jackson, J.W., Jeremiah, J.D., and Cook, J.: Anterior fusion of the spine for infective lesions in adults, J. Bone Joint Surg. **55-B:**715, 1973.

Kemp, H.B.S., Jackson, J.W., Jeremiah, J.D., and Hall, A.J.: Pyogenic infections occurring primarily in intervertebral discs, J. Bone Joint Surg. **55-B:**698, 1973.

Kemp, H.B.S., Jackson, J.W., and Shaw, N.C.: Laminectomy in paraplegia due to infective spondylosis, Br. J. Surg. **61:**66, 1974.

King, D.M., and Mayo, K.M.: Infective lesions of the vertebral column, Clin. Orthop. **96:**248, 1973.

Kirkaldy-Willis, W.H., and Thomas, T.G.: Anterior approaches in the diagnosis and treatment of infections of the vertebral bodies, J. Bone Joint Surg. **47-A:**87, 1965.

Kite, J.H.: Tuberculosis of the spine with paraplegia, South. Med. J. **29:**883, 1936.

Kocher, T.: Textbook of operative surgery, London, 1911, A. & C. Black, Ltd.

Kohli, S.B.: Radical surgical approach to spinal tuberculosis, J. Bone Joint Surg. **49-B:**668, 1967.

Kondo, E., and Yamada, K.: End results of focal débridement in bone and joint tuberculosis and its indications, J. Bone Joint Surg. **39-A:**27, 1957.

Konstam, P.G., and Blesovsky, A.: The ambulant treatment of spinal tuberculosis, Br. J. Surg. **50:**26, 1962-1963.

Lame, E.L.: Vertebral osteomyelitis following operation on the urinary tract or sigmoid: the third lesion of an uncommon syndrome, Am. J. Roentgenol. Radium Ther. Nucl. Med. **75:**938, 1956.

Langenskiöld, A., and Riska, E.B.: Pott's paraplegia treated by anterolateral decompression in the thoracic and lumbar spine: a report of twenty-seven cases, Acta Orthop. Scand. **38:**181, 1967.

Lindholm, T.S., and Pylkkänen, P.: Discitis following removal of intervertebral disc, Spine **7:**618, 1982.

Ling, C.M.: Pyogenic osteomyelitis of the spine, Orthop. Rev. **4:**23, September 1975.

Lougheed, J.C., and White, W.G.: Anterior dependent drainage for tuberculous lumbosacral spinal lesions: coccygectomy and dependent drainage in treatment of tuberculous lesions of the lower spine with associated soft-tissue abscesses, Arch. Surg. **81:**961, 1960.

Malawski, S.K.: Pyogenic infection of the spine, Inter. Orthop. **1:**125, 1977.

Martin, N.S.: Tuberculosis of the spine: a study of the results of treatment during the last twenty-five years, J. Bone Joint Surg. **52-B:**613, 1970.

Martin, N.S.: Pott's paraplegia: a report of 120 cases, J. Bone Joint Surg. **53-B:**596, 1971.

Matsushita, T., and Suzuki, K.: Spastic paraparesis due to cryptococcal osteomyelitis: a case report, Clin. Orthop. **196:**279, 1985.

Mawk, J.R., Erickson, D.L., Chou, S.N., and Seljeskog, E.L.: *Aspergillus* infections of the lumbar disc spaces: report of three cases, J. Neurosurg. **58:**270, 1983.

Mazet, R., Jr.: Skeletal lesions of coccidioidomycosis, Arch. Surg. **70:**633, 1955.

Medical Resource Council Working Party on Tuberculosis of the Spine: Five-year assessments of controlled trials of ambulatory treatment, debridement and anterior spinal fusion in the management of tuberculosis of the spine: studies in Bulawayo (Rhodesia) and in Hong Kong, J. Bone Joint Surg. **60-B:**163, 1978.

Menelaus, M.B.: Discitis: an inflammation affecting the intervertebral discs in children, J. Bone Joint Surg. **46-B:**16, 1964.

Ménard, V.: Étude pratique sur le mal du Pott, Paris, 1900, Masson et Cie.

Morrey, B.F., Kelly, P.J., and Nichols, D.R.: Viridans streptococcal osteomyelitis of the spine, J. Bone Joint Surg. **62-A:**1009, 1980.

Nagel, D.A., Albright, J.A., Keggi, K.J., and Southwick, W.O.: Closer look at spinal lesions: open biopsy of vertebral lesions, JAMA **191:**975, 1965.

Naim-Ur-Rahman: Atypical forms of spinal tuberculosis, J. Bone Joint Surg. **62-B:**162, 1980.

Neville, C.H., Jr., and Davis, W.L.: Is surgical fusion still desirable in spinal tuberculosis? Clin. Orthop. **75:**179, 1971.

Norris, S.H., Ehrlich, M.G., McKusick, K., and Provine, H.: The radioisotopic study of an experimental model of disc space, J. Bone Joint Surg. **60-B:**281, 1978.

O'Connor, B.T.: Steel, W.M., and Sanders, R.: Disseminated bone tuberculosis, J. Bone Joint Surg. **57-A:**537, 1970.

Puig-Guri, J.: Pyogenic osteomyelitis of the spine: differential diagnosis through clinical and roentgenographic observations, J. Bone Joint Surg. **28:**29, 1946.

Puranen, J., Mäkelä, J., and Lähde, S.: Postoperative intervertebral discitis, Acta Orthop. Scand. **55:**461, 1984.

Ray, M.J., and Bassett, R.L.: Pyogenic vertebral osteomyelitis, Orthopedics **8:**506, 1985.

Risko, T., and Novoszel, T.: Experiences with radical operations in tuberculosis of the spine, J. Bone Joint Surg. **45-A:**53, 1963.

Roaf, R.: Tuberculosis of the spine (editorial), J. Bone Joint Surg. **40-B:**3, 1958.

Roaf, R., Kirkaldy-Willis, W.H., and Cathro, A.J.M.: Surgical treatment of bone and joint tuberculosis, Edinburgh, 1959, E. & S. Livingstone, Ltd.

Robertson, R.C., and Ball, R.P.: Destructive spine lesions: diagnosis by needle biopsy, J. Bone Joint Surg. **17**:749, 1935.

Ross, P.M., and Fleming, J.L.: Vertebral body osteomyelitis: spectrum and natural history: a retrospective analysis of 37 cases, Clin. Orthop. **118**:190, 1976.

Ryan, L.M., Carrera, G.F., Lightfoot, R.W., Jr., Hoffman, R.G., and Kozen, F.: The radiographic diagnosis of sacroiliitis: a comparison of different views with computed tomograms of the sacroiliac joint, Arthritis Rheum. **26**:760, 1983.

Saenger, E.L.: Spondylarthritis in children, Am. J. Roentgenol. Radium Ther. **64**:20, 1950.

Scoles, P.V., and Quinn, T.P.: Intervertebral discitis in children and adolescents, Clin. Orthop. **162**:31, 1982.

Seddon, H.J.: Pott's paraplegia, Br. J. Surg. **22**:769, 1935.

Seddon, H.J.: The pathology of Pott's paraplegia, Proc. R. Soc. Med. **39**:723, 1945-1946.

Seddon, H.J.: Antero-lateral decompression of Pott's paraplegia, J. Bone Joint Surg. **33-B**:461, 1951.

Seddon, H.J.: Treatment of Pott's paraplegia by anterolateral decompression, Mém. Acad. Chir. **79**:281, 1952.

Seddon, H.J.: Pott's paraplegia and its operative treatment, J. Bone Joint Surg. **35-B**:487, 1953.

Seddon, H.J.: Pott's paraplegia. In Platt, H., editor: Modern trends in orthopaedics (second series), London, 1956, Butterworth & Co., Ltd.

Seddon, H.J. and Alexander, G.L.: Discussion of spinal caries with paraplegia, Proc. R. Soc. Med. **39**:723, 1946.

Shaw, N.E., and Thomas, T.G.: Surgical treatment of chronic infective lesions of the spine, Br. Med. J. **1**:162, 1963.

Sherman, M., and Schneider, G.T.: Vertebral osteomyelitis complicating postabortal and postpartum infection, South. Med. J. **48**:333, 1955.

Siebert, W.T., Moreland, N., and Williams, T.W., Jr.: Methicillin-resistant Staphylococcus epidermidis, South. Med. J. **7**:1353, 1978.

Smith, A.D.: The treatment of bone and joint tuberculosis, J. Bone Joint Surg. **37-A**:1214, 1955.

Smith, A.D.: Tuberculosis of the spine: results in 70 cases treated at the New York Orthopaedic Hospital from 1945 to 1960, Clin. Orthop. **58**:171, 1968.

Speed, J.S., and Boyd, H.B.: Bone syphilis, South. Med. J. **29**:371, 1936.

Spiegel, P.G., Kengla, K.W., Isaacson, A.S., and Wilson, J.C., Jr.: Intervertebral disc-space inflammation in children, J. Bone Joint Surg. **54-A**:284, 1972.

Stauffer, R.N.: Pyogenic vertebral osteomyelitis, Orthop. Clin. North Am. **6**:1015, 1975.

Steindler, A.: Posterior mediastinal abscess in tuberculosis of the dorsal spine, Illinois Med. J. **50**:201, 1926.

Steindler, A.: Posterior mediastinal abscess in tuberculosis of the dorsal spine (Abstract). In Osgood, R.B., et al.; editors: Thirty-third report of progress in orthopaedic surgery.

Steindler, A.: Diseases and deformities of the spine and thorax, St. Louis, 1929, The C.V. Mosby Co.

Steindler, A.: On paraplegia in Pott's disease, Lancet **54**:281, 1934.

Stern, W.E., and Balch, R.E.: Surgical aspects of nonspecific inflammatory and suppurative disease of the vertebral column, Am. J. Surg. **122**:314, 1966.

Stevenson, F.H.: The chemotherapy of orthopaedic tuberculosis, J. Bone Joint Surg. **36-B**:5, 1954.

Surgarman, B.: Osteomyelitis in spinal cord injury, Arch. Phys. Med. Rehabil. **65**:132, 1984.

Torres-Rojas, J., Taddonio, R.F., and Sanders, C.V.: Spondylitis caused by *Brucella abortus,* South Med. J. **72**:1166, 1979.

Tuli, S.M.: Tuberculosis of the craniovertebral region, Clin. Orthop. **104**:209, 1974.

Tuli, S.M.: Results of treatment of spinal tuberculosis by ''middle-path'' regime, J. Bone Joint Surg. **57-B**:13, 1975.

Tuli, S.M., and Kumar, S.: Early results of treatment of spinal tuberculosis of triple drug therapy, Clin. Orthop. **81**:56, 1971.

Tuli, S.M., Sprivastava, T.P., Varma, B.P., and Sinha, G.P.: Tuberculosis of spine, Acta Orthop. Scand. **38**:445, 1967.

Waldvogel, F.A., Medoff, G., and Swartz, M.N.: Osteomyelitis: a review of clinical features, therapeutic considerations and unusual aspects (first of three parts), N. Engl. J. Med. **282**:198, 1976.

Wedge, J.H., Oryschak, A.F., Robertson, D.E., and Kirkaldy-Willis, W.H.: Atypical manifestations of spinal infections. Clin. Orthop. **123**:155, 1977.

Weinberg, J.A.: The surgical excision of psoas abscesses resulting from spinal tuberculosis, J. Bone Joint Surg. **39-A**:17, 1957.

Wenger, D.R., Bobechko, W.P., and Gilday, D.L.: The spectrum of intervertebral disc-space infection in children, J. Bone Joint Surg. **60-A**:100, 1978.

Whalen, J.L., Parke, W.W., Mazur, J.M., and Stauffer, E.S.: The intrinsic vasculature of developing vertebral end plates and its nutritive significance to the intervertebral discs, J. Ped. Ortho. **5**:403, 1985.

Wiley, A.M., and Trueta, J.: The vascular anatomy of the spine and its relationship to pyogenic vertebral osteomyelitis, J. Bone Joint Surg. **41-B**:796, 1959.

Wilkinson, M.C.: The treatment of tuberculosis of the spine by evacuation of the paravertebral abscess and curettage of the vertebral bodies, J. Bone Joint Surg. **37-B**:382, 1955.

Wiltberger, B.R.: Resection of the vertebral bodies and bone-grafting for chronic osteomyelitis of the spine, J. Bone Joint Surg. **34-A**:215, 1952.

Winter, W.G., Jr., Larson, R.K., Zettas, J.P., and Libke, R.: Coccidioidal spondylitis, J. Bone Joint Surg. **60-A**:240, 1978.

Yau, A.C.M.C., and Hodgson, A.R.: Penetration of the lung by the paravertebral abscess in tuberculosis of the spine, J. Bone Joint Surg. **50-A**:243, 1968.

Yau, A.C.M.C., Hsu, L.C.S., O'Brien, J.P., and Hodgson, A.R.: Tuberculous kyphosis: correction with spinal osteotomy, halo-pelvic distraction, and anterior and posterior fusion, J. Bone Joint Surg. **56-A**:1419, 1974.

CHAPTER 75

Other disorders of spine

George W. Wood

In this chapter are discussed spinal stenosis, congenital anomalies of the spine, rheumatoid arthritis of the spine, tumors of the spine, and spinal deformity after late treatment.

SPINAL STENOSIS

The initial description of lumbar spinal stenosis relieved by two-level laminectomy was that of Sachs and Fraenkel. Bailey and Casamajor in 1911 and Elsberg in 1913 wrote similar adequate descriptions of the symptoms, pathologic findings, and relief following surgery. The syndrome was not widely diagnosed, however, until Verbiest in 1954 described the rather classic findings of middle-aged and older adults with back and lower extremity pain precipitated by standing and walking and aggravated by hyperextension. He delineated congenital narrowing of the spinal canal as a contributing factor in many and the secondary develop-

ment of degenerative changes to further narrow the lumbar canal and precipitate symptoms. Myelographic block in the midlumbar region with the characteristic degenerative hypertrophic changes about the discs, facets, and ligamentous structures was described in detail. A subsequent article by Verbiest on lumbar spondylosis documented detailed measurements of the spinal canal obtained during surgery with an appropriate instrument for obtaining these operative measurements. Since that time the syndrome has been well recognized and numerous well-documented series have been reported. An excellent four-part review of the entire topic was published by Ehni, Clark, Wilson, and Alexander in 1969.

Classification

Spinal stenosis can be categorized according to the anatomic area of the spine affected, the local area of each vertebral segment affected, and by the specific pathologic entity involved. Stenosis can be generalized or localized to specific areas of the cervical, thoracic, or lumbar spine. It is most common in the lumbar region, but cervical stenosis is just now being recognized. It has been rarely reported in the thoracic spine. Spinal stenosis can be localized, affecting only one segment or a portion of one segment. The most recent terminology for localized stenosis is central, lateral recess, foraminal, and far-out. This terminology deals primarily with the area of root compression. It is most frequently used to describe lumbar spinal stenosis but it can be applied to all areas of the spine. Finally, spinal stenosis can be categorized by the pathologic process. Arnoldi et al. proposed a classification scheme for the lumbar spine. This classification separates spinal stenosis into congenital stenosis and acquired stenosis. Although this classification was developed for the lumbar spine, it can be applied to all other areas of the spine as well. The anatomic and pathologic classification of spinal stenosis is helpful in the proper selection of both treatment modality and prognosis.

The most common type of spinal stenosis is caused by degenerative arthritis of the spine. Congenital forms caused by such disorders as achondroplasia and congenital spondylolisthesis are much less frequent. Finally, other processes such as Paget's disease, fluorosis, kyphosis, scoliosis, and fracture with canal narrowing have been reported to result in spinal stenosis. Hypertrophy and ossification of the posterior longitudinal ligament in the cervical spine (diffuse idiopathic skeletal hyperostosis [DISH] syndrome) is another example of a disease that may result in

3347

an acquired form of spinal stenosis. This disease is usually confined to the cervical spine.

The radiographic identification and confirmation of lumbar spinal stenosis has improved with the development of new imaging techniques. Initially only central spinal stenosis was recognized. Canal narrowing to 10 mm was considered diagnostic. This could be measured using roentgenograms or preferably myelography. In 1985 Bolender et al. reported a comparison of the identification of central spinal stenosis with anteroposterior canal measurement by computed tomography to the measurement of the dural sac with myelography in patients undergoing surgery for spinal stenosis. They found no correlation between the transverse area of the bony canal in normal patients and patients with spinal stenosis. A dural sac transverse area of 100 square mm or less did correlate with symptomatic spinal stenosis.

REGIONAL CLASSIFICATION

Ciric et al. and others have used computed tomography to further define lateral recess stenosis and foraminal stenosis. These types of stenosis are rarely identified with myelography. The lateral recess is anatomically the area bordered laterally by the pedicle, posteriorly by the superior articular facet, and anteriorly by the posterolateral surface of the vertebral body and the adjacent intervertebral disc. The superior and rostral border of the corresponding pedicle is the narrowest portion of the lateral recess. Measurement of the recess in this area using the tomographic cross section is usually 5 mm or greater in normal patients but in symptomatic patients the diagnosis is confirmed if the height is 2 mm or less (Fig. 75-1). The foramen is the area of the spine bordered by the inferior edge of the pedicle cephalad, the pars interarticularis with the associated inferior articular facet and the superior articular facet from the lower segment dorsally, the superior edge of the pedicle of the next lower vertebra caudally, and the vertebral body and disc ventrally. This area can rarely be seen with myelography. Standard computed tomography in the cross-sectional mode can suggest narrowing. This is suggested when the foraminal space immediately after the pedicle cut is only present for one or two more cuts (provided the cuts are close together). The best way to appreciate foraminal narrowing is to reformat the lumbar scan. This technique can create sagittal views through the pedicles and structures situated laterally.

Wiltse et al. have described a far-out compression of the root seen predominantly in spondylolisthesis when the root is compressed by a large L5 transverse process subluxed below the root and pressing the root against the ala of the sacrum. This diagnosis is best confirmed with a reformatted computed tomography scan with coronal cuts (Fig. 75-2).

PATHOLOGIC CLASSIFICATION

Differentiation between the pathologic processes causing spinal stenosis is relatively simple. Congenital spinal stenosis is usually central. In achondroplasia the canal is narrowed in both the anteroposterior measurement (pedicle height) and lateral width (distance between the pedicles) in addition to showing other stigmata of achondroplasia. Id-

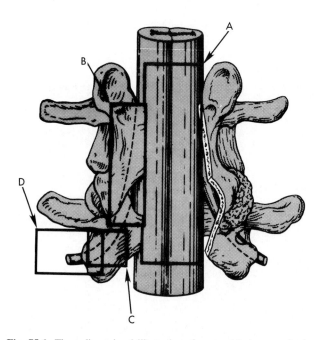

Fig. 75-1. Three dimensional illustration of segmental stenoses. **A,** Anatomic. **B,** Segmental. **C,** Pathologic. (Redrawn from Ciric, I., et al.: J. Neurosurg. **53:**433, 1980.)

iopathic congenital narrowing usually involves one dimension of canal measurement, and the patient is otherwise normal.

Acquired forms of spinal stenosis are caused by degenerative arthritis, spondylolisthesis, posttraumatic deformity, and other disease processes. Degenerative forms of stenosis are usually localized to the facet joints with additional evidence of roentgenographically visible changes in the joints. Frequently, these abnormalities are symmetric. The L4-5 level is the most commonly involved followed by L5-S1 and L3-4. Disc herniation and spondylolisthesis may further increase the narrowing. Spondylolisthesis and spondylolysis rarely cause spinal stenosis in the young. The combination of degenerative change, aging, and spondylolisthesis or spondylolysis in patients 50 years old or older frequently results in stenosis of the lateral recess or foraminal variety. Paget's disease and fluorosis have been reported to result in central or lateral spinal stenosis. Paget's disease causes one form of spinal stenosis that responds well to treatment with calcitonin.

Etiology of degenerative stenosis

Dunlop et al. have experimentally identified the presence of a significant increase in pressure on the facet joints with disc space narrowing and increasing angles of extension. Degenerative spinal stenosis has been attributed to simple hypertrophic overgrowth of the superior articular facets that is the result of a progressive degeneration of the disc with resultant instability or hypermobility in the facet joints. As joint destruction progresses, the hypertrophic process finally results in local anklyosis. Calcification and hypertrophy of the ligamentum flavum and venous hypertension resulting in generalized bone overgrowth may also

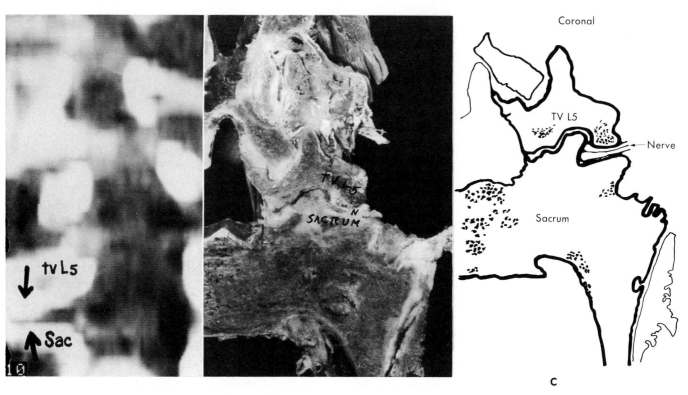

Fig. 75-2. A, Coronal view of computed tomography scan showing impingement of transverse process of L5 on sacrum. **B,** Coronal section showing right transverse process. **C,** Line drawing of coronal section. (From Wiltse, L.L., et al.: Spine **9:**31, 1984.)

be factors in this disease. Mild trauma and occupational activity do not appear to significantly affect the development of this disease but they may exacerbate a preexisting condition.

Natural history and clinical symptoms

The natural course of patients with all forms of spinal stenosis is the insidious development of symptoms occasionally exacerbated by trauma or heavy activity. Many patients have significant roentgenographic findings with minimal complaints and physical findings. Porter et al. note that most patients can be treated conservatively for many years. The physical complaints of lumbar spinal stenosis vary. Most patients complain of back pain relieved by rest and increased by activity. Radicular symptoms do occur but they are infrequent. Most pain may be centered in the buttocks and thigh, making differentiation from hip disease mandatory. The pain is eased with sitting or recumbancy and increased with standing and walking. Staying in any position for any length of time may be uncomfortable. About one third of the patients complain of increasing leg pain with walking. Neurogenic claudication of this type usually begins very rapidly, intensifies with walking and is not relieved by standing. Vascular claudication on the other hand usually begins after walking some distance and is relieved by standing. Claudication is more frequent in central or advanced stenosis and rare in fora-

minal stenosis. Moderate lateral recess stenosis and foraminal stenosis may mimic osteoarthritis of the hip.

Physical findings

The physical findings with all forms of spinal stenosis are vague. Distal pulses should be strong and internal and external rotation of the hips in extension should be full and painless. Straight leg raising and sciatic tension tests are usually normal. The neurologic examination is usually normal but some abnormality may be detected if the patient is allowed to walk to the limit of pain and is then reexamined. The gait and posture after walking may reveal a positive "stoop test." This test is performed by asking the patient to walk briskly. As the pain intensifies, the patient may complain of sensory symptoms followed by motor symptoms. If the patient is asked to continue to walk he may assume a stooped posture and the symptoms may be eased or if he sits in a chair bent forward the same resolution of symptoms will occur.

Conservative treatment

The conservative treatment of symptomatic spinal stenosis is similar to disc disease. Rest, nonsteroidal antiinflammatory medication (usually aspirin) and decreased activity may be all that is necessary for the initial attack. A back support that decreases lumbar motion and increases lumbar flexion may also help. Strong narcotics and seda-

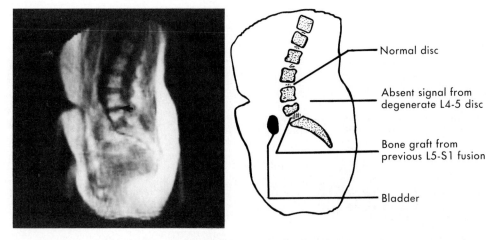

Fig. 75-3. Sagittal section showing normal discs above L4-5 with abnormal disc at this level (reduced signal). Fusion site is also demonstrated. (From Crawshaw, C., et al.: J. Bone Joint Surg. **66-B:**711, 1984.)

tives are rarely necessary. Epidural steroids may also produce significant symptomatic relief if combined with decreased activity. As in disc disease the Back School is essential to teach good posture and body mechanics. When spinal stenosis is present with coexistent degenerative arthritis in the hips or knees some permanent limitation in activity may be necessary regardless of the treatment.

Confirmation of diagnosis

The best method of confirming the diagnosis is with metrizamide thoracic and lumbar myelography and a reformatted computed tomography scan of the suspected lumbar segments. In the near future magnetic resonance imaging may surpass these techniques in the identification of localized areas of spinal stenosis. Crewshaw et al. reported 21 patients with lateral canal entrapment identified by magnetic resonance imaging (MRI). They identified the entrapment by a reduction of epidural fat around the nerve root in the foraminal sagittal reconstructions. This abnormality was identified by myelography in only 7 of the patients (Fig. 75-3).

Frequently, multiple areas are affected with stenosis as indicated by imaging techniques, but usually the symptoms are unilateral. The use of a lumbar root block with or without contrast may indicate the symptomatic root if all pain is relieved with one block. As with disc disease psychologic testing is of benefit as a predictor of outcome.

Indications for surgery

The primary indication for surgery in spinal stenosis is increasing pain resistant to conservative measures. Since the primary complaint is back and some leg pain the relief after surgery may only be in degrees. The results of most series show about a 70% rate of improvement, and most patients still have some minor complaints usually referable to the preexisting degenerative arthritis of the spine. When neurologic findings are present, they rarely decrease after surgery. Roentgenographic findings alone are never an indication for surgery. The best results in most reported series are with localized lesions without general involvement.

Lumbar spinal stenosis

PRINCIPLES OF SPINAL STENOSIS SURGERY

Whenever possible the source of pain should be localized preoperatively using root blocks. At surgery specific attention should be directed to that area. If radical decompression of only one root is necessary then additional stabilization is not needed. The removal of two or more facet joints usually requires some additional stabilization unless the patient is elderly or has a narrow disc at that level. It is advisable to prepare the patient for a fusion in case the findings at surgery require a more radical approach then anticipated. Positioning the patient in the kneeling position minimizes bleeding. As in disc surgery, the use of magnifying loupes and a head lamp is helpful. When proceeding with the decompression, care should be taken to watch for adhesions that may result in dural tears. Frequently the narrowing in the lateral recess and foramen is so great that the use of a Kerrison rongeur may be impossible without damaging the root. Dissection in the lateral recess and foramen usually requires a small sharp osteotome. Unlike disc surgery the lateral gutter is best seen from the opposite side of the table. The operating surgeon may find it necessary to switch sides during the operation to better view the pathology and nerve root. When the lamina is extremely thick, the use of a high-speed drill with a diamond burr may decrease the thickness of the lamina to afford easier removal with a Kerrison rongeur or chisel. Blunt probes with increasing diameters are also useful to determine adequate foraminal enlargement. Bailey and McLoren reviewed six patients with postoperative cauda equina syndrome. In five of these a disc was removed from a stenotic spine without adequate decompression of the stenosis. Spinal stenosis should be treated at the same time as the disc herniation.

MIDLINE DECOMPRESSION (NEURAL ARCH RESECTION)

TECHNIQUE. Perform the procedure with the patient under general endotrachial anesthesia. Position the patient kneeling using the frame of choice. Make the incision in the midline centered over the level of stenosis. Localizing roentgenograms should be taken if the level of dissection is in question. Carry the incision vertically to the fascia. Strip the fascia and muscle subperiosteally from the spinous processes and laminae to the facet joints. Take care to avoid damaging facet joints that are not involved in the bony dissection. Identify and remove the spinous processes of the levels to be decompressed. Then clear the soft tissue with a sharp curet. Dissect the lower edge of ligmentum flavum from the lamina with a curet and remove the lamina with a Kerrison rongeur. If the lamina is extremely thick, a high-speed drill with a diamond burr may be used to thin the outer cortex to allow easier removal of the inner portion with a Kerrison rongeur. Take special care in removal of the lamina and ligamentum flavum. The neural structures will be found compressed, and the usual space for instrument insertion may not be available. Remove the lamina until the pedicles can be seen. Using the pedicle as a guide, identify the nerve root and trace it out to the foramen. Carefully with a chisel remove the medial portion of the superior facet that forms the upper portion of the lateral recess. Check the foramen for patency with a Murphy ball elevator or graduated probes. If there is further restriction, carry the dissection laterally and open the foramen. Inspect the disc and remove gross herniations. Usually the disc is bulging, and the anulus is firm. Remove the anulus and bony ridge ventrally if it is kinking the nerve. This procedure involves some risk of nerve injury and requires a bloodless field. If safety is in question, then a more radical removal of the facet may be better. Complete the dissection at all symptomatic levels. Carefully advance a red rubber catheter caudally and cranially to check for central obstructions. If no obstructions are noted and all areas have been adequately decompressed, close the wound, or if desired, take a large fat graft from the wound or buttock and place it over the laminectomy defect and then close the wound.

SELECTIVE DECOMPRESSION (GETTY ET AL.)

TECHNIQUE. Expose the spine as described above. Localize the dissection to the level of compression unilaterally near the foramen previously identified as the source of painful constriction. Confirm the level of resection with roentgenograms if in doubt. Remove the lamina in the standard fashion and identify the pedicle. Place an osteotome (or preferably a chisel) over the medial portion of the inferior articular facet. Advance the bone cut in an oblique direction as noted. Identify the nerve root proximally. Make the initial cut in the direction of the nerve root. This line is roughly parallel to the longitudinal axis of the spinal canal where the root passes under the facet joint before turning outward below the pedicle. Possible damage to the nerve root is minimized with such a cut. If possible, interpose a Penfield elevator between root and facet to provide additional safety. Advance the osteotome or chisel with the percussion effect of rapid blows to reduce further the risk of sudden uncontrolled advance. Make the initial osteotomy through the inferior articular process of the facet. When the articular process of the superior facet is reached, twist the osteotome to free the osteotomized fragment and then ease it out with a rongeur. Advance the osteotome into the superior articular facet in the same direction. Remove this fragment in the same careful manner. Perform a complete facetectomy if further restriction is present. Check the disc and canal for herniations and obstructions. If no obstructions are found, apply a fat graft over the laminar defect if desired. Close the wound in layers.

AFTERTREATMENT. Special considerations are not necessary after a simple decompression. The patient should be examined carefully for the first few days for new neurologic changes which may indicate the formation of an epidural hematoma. The patient is encouraged to walk on the first day. Sutures are removed at 14 days. The same limitations as after disc surgery (p. 3297) apply to decompressions. Patients engaged in heavy manual labor may require a permanent job change. Return to work is also similar to disc surgery.

SURGICAL RESULTS

The results of decompression for spinal stenosis vary with the extent of disease and the primary diagnosis. Patients with extensive disease, central stenosis, and degenerative joint disease do not improve as much as patients with localized, segmental, central, and lateral stenosis. Figures are not available regarding the inclusion of a lateral spinal fusion or anterior interbody spinal fusion with this procedure. In many instances the age of the patient, an already decreased activity level, disc space narrowing at the operated level, and an absence of motion at this level preoperatively make fusion unnecessary.

The complete removal of one facet does not result in instability. When two facets are removed at the same level or at contiguous areas, instability may result. Shenkin and Hash noted a 6% incidence of postoperative spondylolisthesis in patients with bilateral facetectomy and a 15% incidence when three or more facets were removed. If the patient is young and active, then a unilateral lateral fusion of the opposite side or bilateral lateral fusion (see Chapter 70) may be necessary when multiple facetectomies are performed on the opposite side. When the facetectomies are bilateral at the same level, the addition of a lateral fusion may be difficult and the bone graft may impinge on the exposed neural elements. In this instance an anterior interbody fusion may be necessary at a later date if symptoms of instability are noted. Some surgeons suggest performing this procedure two weeks after an extensive destabilizing decompressive procedure.

The complications of this procedure are similar to those of disc surgery. However, the risk of nerve root damage and dural laceration is greater. The rate of infection, thrombophelibitis, and pulmonary embolism is also slightly greater. When a facet has been narrowed, later facet or pars fracture may account for any recurrence of symptoms. However, Getty et al. found that the most important reason for failure to relieve symptoms in their series was inadequate decompression.

• • •

Spinal stenosis in spondylolisthesis may be treated in the same manner as degenerative spinal stenosis with respect to the central, lateral, or foraminal stenosis found. Children and young patients with spondylolisthesis rarely if ever require decompression. Such patients respond well to bilateral lateral fusion alone. In older but active patients with degenerative changes and spondylolisthesis decompression with fusion of the asymptomatic side is preferred. Wiltse et al. reported 90% good to excellent results when decompression of the compressed nerve root was combined with spinal fusion to treat symptomatic spondylolisthesis in adults. Sedentary patients without motion at the segment involved may be decompressed without fusion, but Wiltse notes only a 50% good result rate after this procedure. Patients with severe slips (50% or greater) may be fused with greater ease and less additional level involvement through the anterior approach.

Cervical spinal stenosis

Cervical spinal stenosis is frequently referred to by its neurologic presentation of cervical myelopathy. Hypertrophic arthritis both segmental and more generalized is the most common cause of acquired spinal stenosis. Ossification of the posterior longitudinal ligament, a manifestation of diffuse idiopathic skeletal hyperostosis (DISH) syndrome, is another infrequent cause of diffuse cervical spinal stenosis.

The treatment of diffuse cervical spinal stenosis is extremely difficult. Treatments have varied from radical anterior decompression of multiple vertebral bodies with fibular strut or iliac crest grafting to expansive cervical laminoplasty posteriorly. Extensive cervical laminectomies lead to late deformity or instability or both in young people. A long-term study by Crandall and Gregorius revealed late worsening of symptoms in patients treated by multiple level laminectomy. They noted only 31% improvement after this method compared with 71% improvement after anterior disc excision and fusion at multiple levels. The greatest improvement occurred in patients who were symptomatic for less than 12 months. Boni et al. reported 39

patients with spondylotic myelopathy treated by multiple subtotal somatectomy with 51% good and 47% moderate improvement. Kimura et al. reported 24 patients treated with expansive laminaplasty. They noted 16% excellent and 75% good results.

Many patients with cervical spinal stenosis become symptomatic after trauma or minor repeated trauma. The presenting symptoms may be multiple and varied, including pain, weakness, and spasticity. Some patients may complain of sharp, tingling sensations on neck extension similar to Lhermitte's sign of multiple sclerosis. Physical findings may include signs of root compression, clonus, Babinski's sign, hyperactive reflexes, muscle wasting, and generalized sensory loss.

Myelography to rule out an intradural lesion is mandatory in the evaluation of this problem. In the future magnetic resonance imaging (MRI) may replace myelography for this purpose. Cervical spinal canal measurement in the lateral dimension on standard roentgenograms is helpful in the identification of this disorder. The normal lateral cervical spine canal measures about 17 mm in the adult. The spinal cord at this level measures about 10 mm. When the canal is narrowed to 10 mm, significant symptoms of myelopathy are usually present. Edwards and LaRocca observed that narrowing of 13 mm or more on the lateral cervical spine view was predictive of myelopathy or a premyelopathic state.

Subtotal somatectomy

TECHNIQUE. Position and prepare the patient in the supine position as for an anterior cervical disc excision. Approach the spine from the left. Because of the extent of the exposure, a longitudinal incision is recommended. Continue the approach as described for anterior cervical disc excision (p. 3287). Elevate or excise the anterior longitudinal

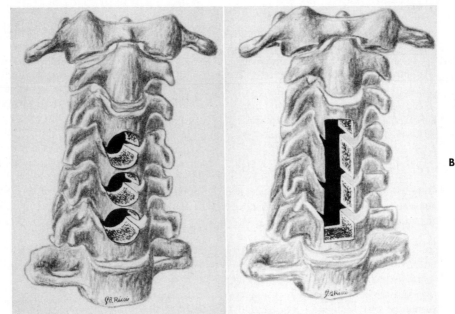

Fig. 75-4. Multiple subtotal somateotomy. Excision of multiple anterior cervical vertebral bodies using Cloward instrumentation. **A,** Initial excision of discs at symptomatic levels. **B,** Final trough. (From Boni, M., et al.: Spine **9:**358, 1984.)

ligament over the segments involved. Remove the central portion of the vertebral bodies. Boni et al. use the Cloward drill to remove the bone and disc at each level indicated (Fig. 75-4, *A*). The remaining areas of bone are then removed leaving a trough down to the posterior longitudinal ligament (Fig. 75-4, *B*). Another method is to create a trough in the involved vertebral bodies using a high-speed burr. Depending on the length of the trough, use a tricortical iliac crest graft or a fibular strut graft. Prepare the ends of the caudal and cranial end plates by drilling down to cancellous bone centrally. Then trim the graft to allow insertion into the holes in the end plates. We prefer to shape the graft to resemble a keystone. Boni et al. describe making a notch in the graft so the cortical edge of the vertebral bodies has a place to rest in the notch.

AFTERTREATMENT. The patient is placed in a Philadelphia collar with a chest extension initially. Boni et al. recommend the use of a minerva cast followed by a SOMI brace. A halo vest or cast may be substituted for the minerva cast. Bracing should be continued until early evidence of union is noted.

EXPANSIVE LAMINAPLASTY

TECHNIQUE (TSUJI). Position the patient prone with the head in a cervical rest. Retract the shoulders with tape to allow satisfactory roentgenographic exposure. Then prepare and drape the patient in the usual manner. Expose the cervical (or thoracic) spine in the usual manner bilaterally. Remove the spinous processes at the involved vertebral levels. Clear the remaining soft tissue from the laminae to the lateral edge of the facet joints. Make a longitudinal groove bilaterally at the point of intersection of the lamina and the facet (Fig. 75-5, *B*). Use a power drill with a diamond burr to make the grooves. Lengthen the grooves to include all involved segments. Deepen them until the ligamentum flavum is identified. Then on both sides widely expose the ligamentum flavum at the caudal and cranial ends of the dissection (usually C3 and C7). Carefully open the ligamentum flavum caudally, cranially, and on one side laterally. Mobilize the laminae by gently rolling them up and peeling them off the dura (Fig. 75-5, *A* and *C*). The flap resulting should float and pulsate with the dura at this point. Suture the flap slightly open with nonabsorbable sutures from the ligamentum flavum to the muscle and fascia on the side of the ligamentous hinge. Then close the wound in the usual fashion.

AFTERTREATMENT. The patient is kept supine with the neck in the neutral position for 2 to 3 weeks. A Philadelphia collar or SOMI brace is then worn for 6 to 12 weeks as indicated by symptoms.

CONGENITAL ANOMALIES OF SPINE

Segmentation of the mesoderm about the neural tube occurs early in the third week of gestation and comes to lie

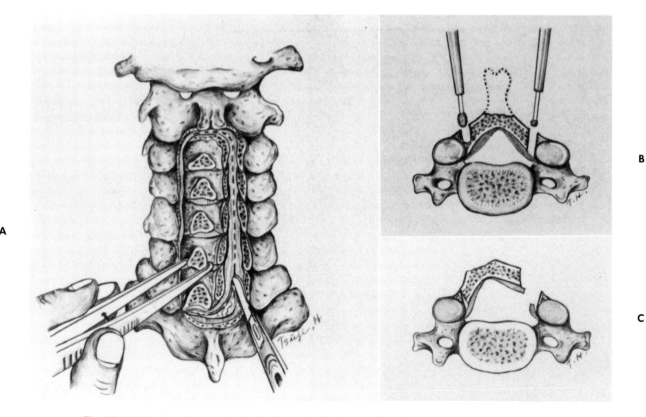

Fig. 75-5. Technique of expansive laminaplasty. **A,** Laminotomy from C3 to C7 with cutting of yellow ligaments with gentle rolling-reelevation maneuver of floated lamina. Knife should be used as shown. **B,** Position and direction of air drills. Long steel burr can only be used until internal cortex is exposed. Internal cortex is to be chiseled with a small-tipped diamond burr in perforator fashion. **C,** Horizontal view of completion of widening of spinal canal. Note opposite cut surfaces of laminae contact each other in one side of groove at which site bony union can easily be obtained. (From Tsuji, H.: Spine 7:28, 1982.)

dorsal and lateral to the notochord. At 4 to 5 weeks of gestation, fusion of the mesenchymal tissue occurs in the cephalocaudal direction. Hemivertebrae are formed and fuse to form the vertebral bodies at 6 weeks. Other mesenchymal cells migrate dorsolaterally to form two ossification centers, giving rise to the laminae and pedicles. At birth there are three primary ossification centers—one in the body and one in each half of the neural arch—that unite during the first year of life. This process starts in the lumbar region and progresses cephalad.

Zimbler and Belkin studied this development and the many problems that may result. Among them are the following nine anomalies:

1. *Basilar impression.* This is characterized by a cephalad displacement of the cervical spine on the skull and an occipital indentation of the posterior foramen magnum. Symptoms usually begin in the second decade because of pressure on vital structures such as the brainstem, cerebellar tonsils, and vertebral arteries. These symptoms include ataxia, nystagmus, headache, neck pain, spasticity, hyperreflexia, weakness, syncope, seizures, difficulty with speech and deglutition, and intellectual impairment. There is an association with Morquio's syndrome, Klippel-Feil syndrome, and cleidocranial dysostosis.

The diagnosis of basilar impression is based on the

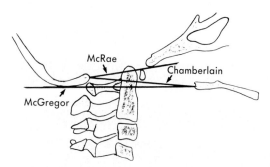
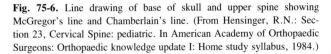

Fig. 75-6. Line drawing of base of skull and upper spine showing McGregor's line and Chamberlain's line. (From Hensinger, R.N.: Section 23, Cervical Spine: pediatric. In American Academy of Orthopaedic Surgeons: Orthopaedic knowledge update I: Home study syllabus, 1984.)

roentgenographic evaluation of the dens with respect to Chamberlain's line. Chamberlain's line is drawn from the hard palate to the inner aspect of the posterior rim of the foramen magnum. McGregor's line is similar to Chamberlain's line except that it is drawn to the outer cortex of the posterior rim of the foramen magnum. Whenever the dens protrudes above Chamberlain's line, some degree of basilar impression is present (Fig. 75-6). Symptomatic basilar impression usually requires significant dens protrusion. Menezes et al. suggest the addition of air contrast myelography and lateral tomography to identify indention of the brain stem. They also suggest measurement of the clivus-canal angle which is the angle formed by a line bisecting the clivus and the cervical vertebral bodies. This angle should be greater than 130 degrees. Basilar impression should not be confused with platybasia. Platybasia is a benign flattening of the base of the skull.

The symptoms and signs of basilar impression are many and varied. They include signs and symptoms of cord compression, cranial nerve palsies, sudden syncope, and visual and vestibular dysfunction.

Menezes et al. have outlined a logical approach to the treatment of craniocervical abnormalities based on stability, reducibility, and area of compression (Fig. 75-7). They suggest posterior occipitocervical fusion for lesions that become reduced in tong traction. Nonreducible lesions are decompressed at the area of encroachment. Ventral encroachment is decompressed through a transoral approach with removal of the anterior rim of the foramen magnum, the ring of C1, and the odontoid. Posterior encroachment is decompressed through a posterior approach with removal of the ring of C1 and the posterior edge of the foramen magnum. If instability is demonstrated after the decompression, a posterior occiput to C3 fusion is performed.

2. *Congenital atlantoaxial instability.* Because of ligamentous laxity of the transverse ligament of the atlas or bony anomolies of the odontoid, C1-2 instability results as in Down syndrome. Roentgenographic diagnosis includes a measurement from the anterior ring of the atlas to the

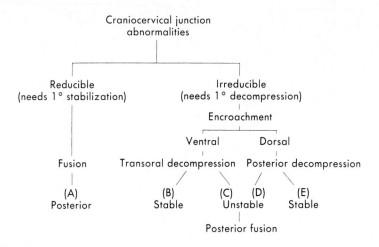

Fig. 75-7. Approach to abnormalities of the cervicobasilar junction. (From Menezes, A., et al.: J. Neurosurg. **3:**444, 1980.)

odontoid. This space is greater than 4 mm in children and 3 mm in adults. The distance from the posterior aspect of the odontoid to the anterior edge of the arch of the atlas is abnormal if it is less than 14 mm. This space is also called the space available for the spinal cord (SAC) (Fig. 75-8).

Treatment in these patients consists of reduction of the atlantoaxial displacement by traction and cervical fusion.

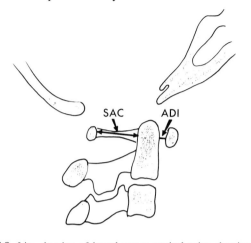

Fig. 75-8. Line drawing of lateral upper cervical spine showing space available for the cord (SAC) and atlanto-dens interval (ADI). (From Hensinger, R.N.: Section 23, Cervical Spine: pediatric. In American Academy of Orthopaedic Surgeons: Orthopaedic knowledge update I: Home study syllabus, 1984.)

Irreducible situations demand decompression of the spinal cord and brainstem at that level, using the rationale of Menezes et al.

3. *Atlantooccipital fusion.* In this anomaly partial or complete synostosis is present between the ring of the atlas and the occiput, resulting in a short-neck appearance with a low hairline. These individuals have a 20% incidence of associated anomalies. Treatment of this condition, if symptomatic, may require decompression and suboccipital craniectomy combined with fusion of the occiput to C2 or C3 if unstable.

4. *Congenital anomalies of odontoid.* Aplasia or hyperplasia of the odontoid or os odontoideum may produce atlantoaxial instability. The separate ossification centers of the odontoid should be fused by the age of 5 years. The diagnostic problem persists in differentiating the os odontoideum from a posttraumatic nonunion of a fracture of the odontoid. (Fig. 75-9). Patients with congenital odontoid dysplasia may have normal atlantoaxial stability. However, in those with generalized ligamentous laxity atlantoaxial instability may lead to a chronic compressive myelopathy of the cervical spinal cord (Fig. 75-10). In a study by Perovic, Kopits, and Thompson, gas myelography revealed loss of the subarachnoid space mainly on the ventral aspect; this was caused by a thick mass of soft tissue posterior to the dysplastic odontoid at a point where the posterior longitudinal ligament blended with the transverse atlantal ligament. They thought that this structure underwent hypertrophy resulting from the abnormal motion be-

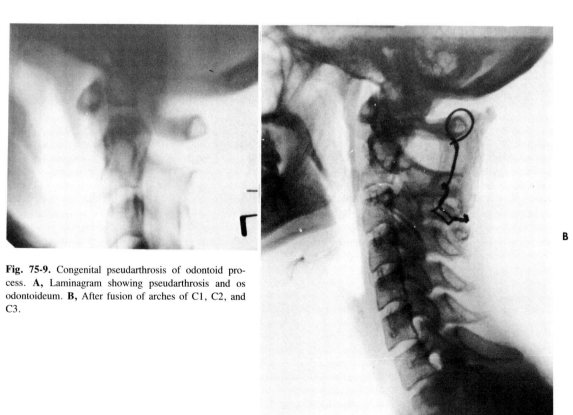

Fig. 75-9. Congenital pseudarthrosis of odontoid process. **A,** Laminagram showing pseudarthrosis and os odontoideum. **B,** After fusion of arches of C1, C2, and C3.

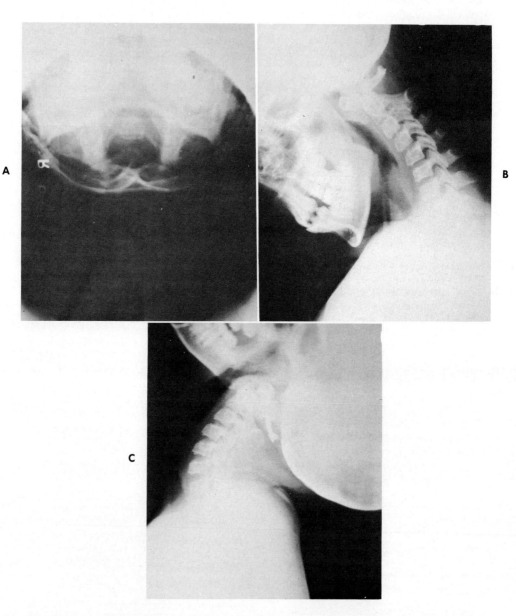

Fig. 75-10. Congenital pseudarthrosis of odontoid. **A,** This basal view of skull demonstrates os odontoideum better than routine open mouth view because occiput is not superimposed. **B** and **C,** Roentgenograms in flexion and extension demonstrate marked subluxation of atlas on axis. (Courtesy Dr. C.H. Herndon; from Garber, J.N.: J. Bone Joint Surg. **46-A:**1782, 1964.)

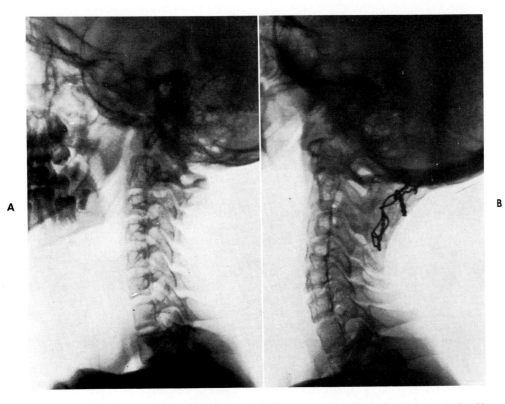

Fig. 75-11. Congenital pseudarthrosis of odontoid. **A,** Before surgery. **B,** After fusion of occiput to C1, C2, C3, and C4.

cause an atlantoaxial fusion, suppressing the motion, resulted in atrophy of this tissue and an increase in the space provided for the spinal canal. It was also noted that this mass of tissue produced a flattening in the sagittal dimension and displaced it laterally, thus explaining the predominance of lateralizing neurologic signs. An atlantoaxial fusion is indicated when motion is painful or transitory neurologic signs are present. If the neural arch of C1 is intact and not malformed, arthrodesis of C1 and C2 is sufficient. With a deficient neural arch of C1, an occipitocervical arthrodesis is done (Fig. 75-11).

Aplasia of the odontoid (Fig. 75-12) has been studied in 21 patients by the Piedmont Orthopaedic Society. A neurologic deficit was present in nine; its onset was sudden in three and gradual in six. The remaining 12 patients had no neurologic abnormality, but symptoms after an injury were sufficient to justify roentgenographic evaluation. Associated congenital defects at the base of the skull were found in four. Six patients were treated by fusions of the cervical spine, three from the occiput to C3, and three between C1 and C2. Those from the occiput to C3 were all successful; those between C1 and C2 failed, but sufficiently strong fibrous union developed to stabilize the spine. It was concluded that fusion is indicated when any patient with aplasia of the odontoid develops neurologic signs or symptoms, either transient or permanent.

Care should be taken in the choice of C1-2 fusion technique to avoid fusion in a hyperextended position.

5. *Congenital laxity of the transverse atlantal ligament.* There is a reported 20% incidence of this abnormality in Down's syndrome. Instability shown on flexion-extension roentgenograms in the symptomatic patient requires fusion from the occiput to C2 or C3.

6. *Klippel-Feil syndrome.* Congenital cervical synostosis was first described by Klippel and Feil in 1912 and consisted of a short neck, low hairline, and decreased range of motion of the cervical spine. Webbing of the neck and torticollis may also be seen. If symptoms ensue, they usually occur in young adulthood. This is often associated with Sprengel's deformity (30%), deafness (30%), urinary tract abnormality (30%), or scoliosis or kyphosis. Congenital heart disease and synkinesia are common. Roentgenographic studies show fusion of two or more cervical vertebrae and a decreased number of vertebral bodies. Treatment is directed toward investigation of any neurologic abnormality and management of the associated spinal deformities of kyphosis or scoliosis.

7. *Diastematomyelia.* Diastematomyelia is discussed in Chapter 66.

8. *Lumbar and sacral agenesis.* This is a rare anomaly; about 18% occur with diabetic mothers. There is motion between the last lumbar vertebra and the pelvis. Motor loss corresponds to the last vertebra present, and the anus is usually patulous and horizontal. The lower extremities may have flexed and abducted hips, flexed knees, and equinovarus feet. There is a 35% incidence of association

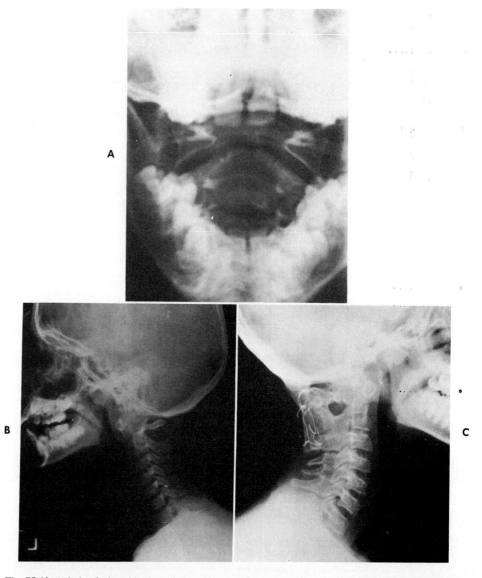

Fig. 75-12. Aplasia of odontoid process in boy 10 years of age. **A,** Open mouth roentgenogram shows absence of odontoid process. **B,** Lateral roentgenogram shows anterior displacement of atlas on axis. **C,** Lateral roentgenogram made 4 years after fusion of C1, C2, and C3; spontaneous fusion occurred between atlas and occiput. (From Garber, J.N.: J. Bone Joint Surg. **46-A:**1782, 1964.)

with visceral anomalies. Renshaw studied 23 patients with sacral agenesis and provided a working classification:

Type I—Either total or partial unilateral sacral agenesis (Fig. 75-13, *A*)

Type II—Partial sacral agenesis with partial but bilaterally symmetrical defect in the stable articulation between the ilia and a normal or hypoplastic first sacral vertebra (Fig. 75-13, *B*)

Type III—Variable lumbar and total sacral agenesis with the ilia articulating with the sides of the lowest vertebra present (Fig. 75-13, *C*)

Type IV—Variable lumbar and total sacral agenesis with caudal end plate of the lowest vertebra resting above either fused ilia or an iliac amphiarthrosis (Fig. 75-13, *D*)

The type II defect is the most common and type I the least common: type IV is the most severe. Types I and II defects usually have a stable vertebropelvic articulation, whereas types III and IV show instability and possibly a progressive kyphosis. The clinical picture ranges from one of severe deformities of the pelvis and lower extremities to those with no deformity or weakness whatsoever.

Scoliosis is the most common associated spinal abnormality. Progressive scoliosis or kyphosis necessitates surgical stabilization as indicated, and occasionally stabilization is required for spinopelvic instability. Additionally, lower extremity abnormalities will require treatment.

9. *Congenital kyphosis and scoliosis.* See Chapters 72 and 71.

Other congenital abnormalities of the spine involving

Text continued on p. 3363

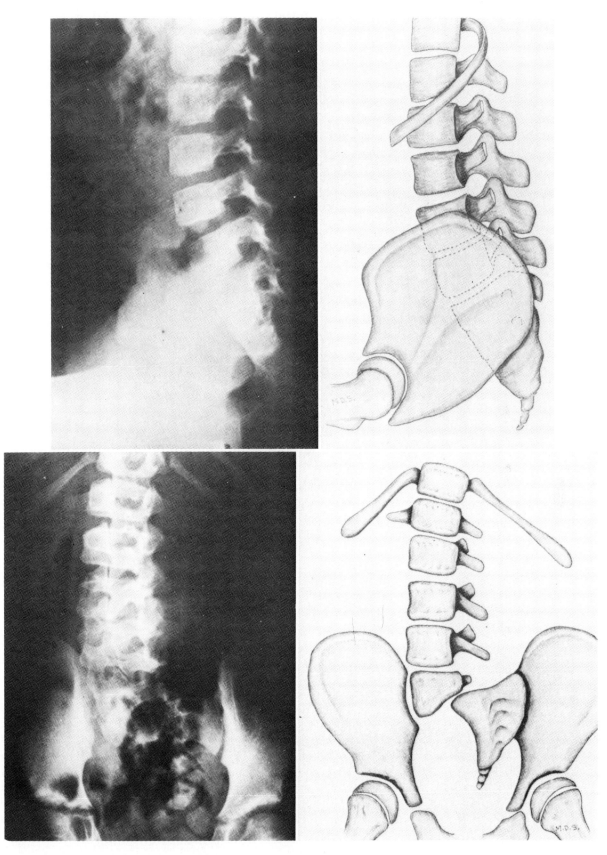

Fig. 75-13. Types of sacral agenesis (see text). **A,** Type 1.
Continued.

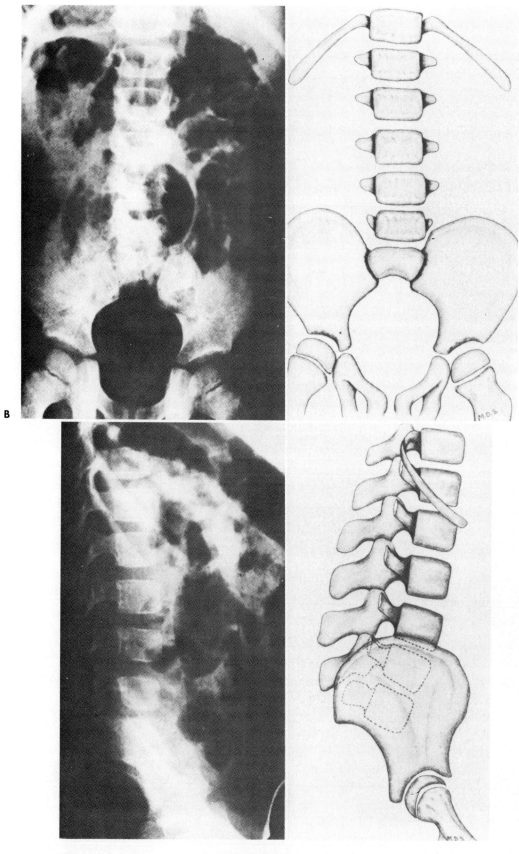

Fig. 75-13, cont'd. B, Type II.

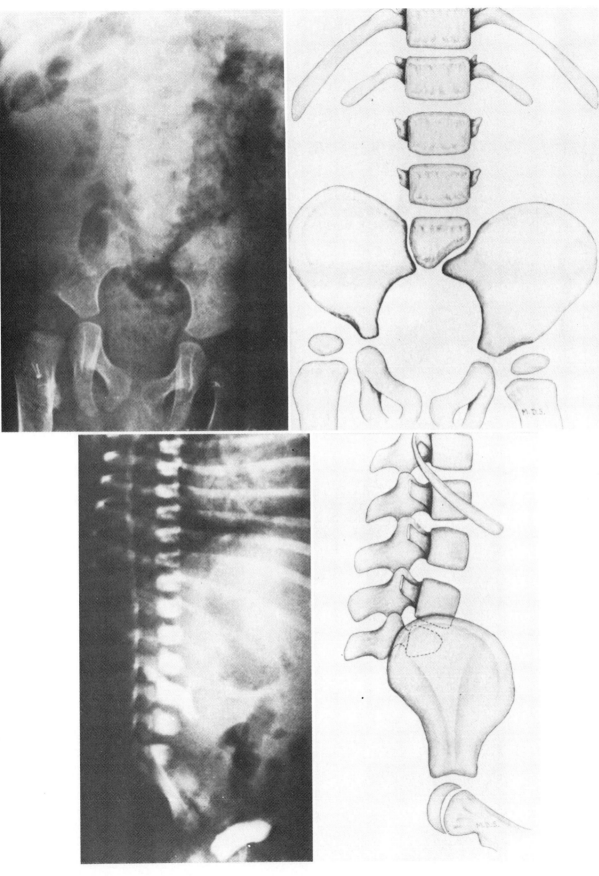

Fig. 75-13, cont'd. C, Type III.

Continued.

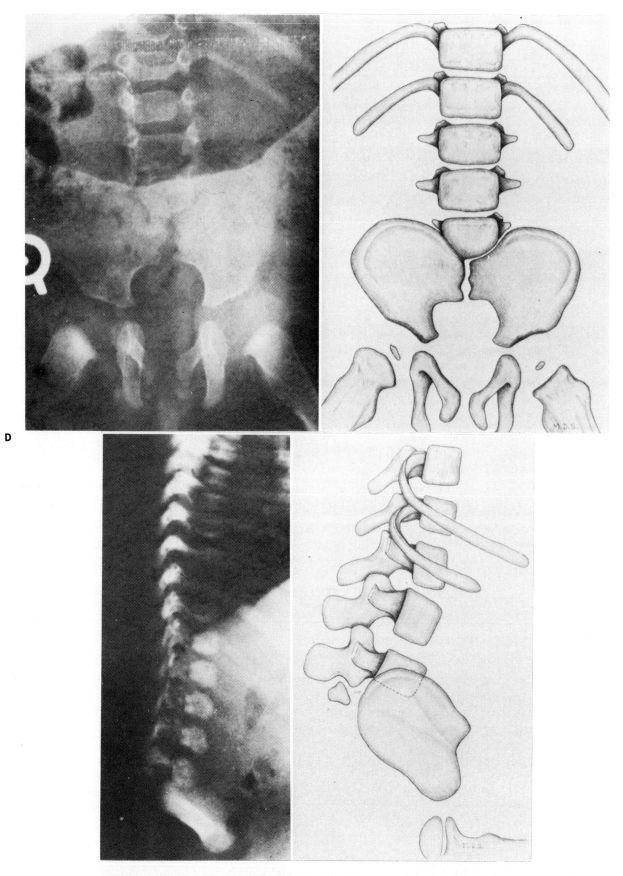

Fig. 75-13, cont'd. D, Type IV. (From Renshaw, T.S.: J. Bone Joint Surg: **60-A:**373, 1978.)

segmentation are usually asymptomatic. These include absence of pedicles or of the posterior arch. The significance of these abnormalities is their association with more serious congenital abnormalities. Absence of a pedicle in children is usually congenital. This abnormality has been reported in all areas of the spine. In the lumbar spine it is associated with urologic defects. Absence of the arch or portions of the arch is not associated with instability of the spine or other significant abnormalities.

RHEUMATOID ARTHRITIS OF THE SPINE

Cervical instability is the most serious and potentially lethal manifestation of rheumatoid arthritis. Three basic types of cervical instability occur in this disease: (1) basilar impression or atlantoaxial impaction, (2) atlantoaxial instability, and (3) subaxial subluxation. Lipson notes that the incidence of all types of cervical instability in rheumatoid arthritis is 43% to 86%. The incidence of neck pain is 40% to 88%, and the incidence of neurologic findings is from 7% to 34%. Lipson also notes that the incidence of sudden death from the combination of basilar impression and atlantoaxial instability is about 10%.

Basilar impression or atlantoaxial impaction is the settling of the skull onto the atlas and the atlas onto the axis from erosive arthritis and bone loss. This settling can result in vertebral artery thrombosis. As in congenital basilar impression, atlantoaxial impaction is measured using McGregor's line. Atlantoaxial impaction is considered present in men when the tip of the odontoid is 8 mm above the line and in women when 9.7 mm above. Menezes et al. suggest the use of air myelography with lateral tomography to confirm the medullary compression. This also allows the determination of the point of primary compression.

Atlantoaxial subluxation can be anterior, posterior, or lateral. Anterior atlantoaxial subluxation is the most common instability. It is usually determined by measuring the distance between the posterior edge of the ring of C1 and the anterior edge of the odontoid. This distance is called the atlantodens interval (ADI) and normally it should not be greater than 3.5 mm in the adult. Subluxation greater than 10 to 12 mm is clinically significant and indicative of complete ligamentous disruption. Posterior subluxation is best determined by acute angulation of the cord and upper cervical spine as identified by sagittal reformatted computed tomography or lateral air contrast tomography. Magnetic resonance imaging may replace these techniques in the future. Lateral subluxation implies some rotation of the atlas. It is present when the lateral masses of C1 lie 2 mm or more laterally on those of C2. Menezes et al. suggest the use of air myelography and lateral tomography to confirm the cord and medullary compression from these instabilities.

Subaxial subluxations are more subtle and frequently multiple. They may result in root compression from foraminal narrowing. Myelography may show root cut off and partial or complete block. Absolute subluxation distances of clinical significance are not available for this problem.

The signs and symptoms of these instability patterns include findings of pyramidal tract involvement, vertebrobasilar insufficiency, root findings, and symptoms similar to Lhermitte's sign in multiple sclerosis. Menezes et al. suggest air or metrizamide myelography to confirm med-

ullary or cord compression. The availability of magnetic resonance imaging may eliminate the need for this uncomfortable and dangerous confirmatory testing.

The indication for surgery in these problems is the development of neurologic impairment and to a lesser degree severe pain. Menezes et al. suggest fusion for instabilities that are reducible, and decompression anteriorly or posteriorly combined with fusion if instability is present. In atlantoaxial impression a trial of halo or tong traction for reduction is suggested. If reduction is accomplished, then a posterior occipitocervical fusion is performed. If reduction is not possible posterior fusion is performed after anterior transoral decompression or posterior decompression. Atlantoaxial subluxation is best treated by posterior C1 and C2 fusion. Lipson suggests halo traction followed by occipitocervical fusion reinforced with metal mesh, wire, and polymethylmethacrylate to treat posterior subluxation at C1 and C2. Symptomatic subaxial subluxation is probably best treated by posterior fusion. The results of anterior cervical decompression and fusion for this problem reported by Ranawat et al. were not satisfactory. Decompression is occasionally necessary when reduction is not possible and clinically significant narrowing of the space available for the cord is present. Four of five patients treated this way in their series did not improve. Stabilization may be increased by the use of polymethylmethacrylate placed around the wires. A bone graft is placed laterally to provide long-term stability. The mortality associated with surgery for these problems is 8% to 20%. The complication rate is also high, including a nonunion rate of 20% to 33%.

Kudo et al. identified extradural granulation tissue as a cause of myelopathy in five patients with rheumatoid arthritis and mild subaxial subluxations of the cervical spine. They suggested longitudinal division of the dura and a fascial patch graft; three of the five patients improved after this treatment. Similar compressive myelopathies have been reported with synovial swelling caused by gout.

Osteotomy of lumbar spine

Smith-Petersen, Larson, and Aufranc in 1945 described an osteotomy of the spine to correct the flexion deformity that develops often in Marie-Strümpell arthritis and sometimes in rheumatoid arthritis. Since then, La Chapelle, Herbert, Wilson, Law, Simmons, and others have reported similar procedures. The technique described by Smith-Petersen et al. is carried out in one stage. Others have described methods in two stages, one consisting of division of the anterior longitudinal ligament under direct vision instead of allowing it to rupture when the deformity is corrected by gentle manipulation as in the method of Smith-Petersen et al.

When the flexion deformity is severe, the patient's field of vision is limited to a small area near his feet, and walking is extremely difficult. Respiration becomes almost completely diaphragmatic, and gastrointestinal symptoms resulting from pressure of the costal margin on the contents of the upper abdomen are common. Needless to say, in addition to improvement in function, the improvement in appearance made by correcting the deformity is of great importance to the patient. When extreme, the deformity should be corrected in two or more stages because of contracture of soft tissues and the danger of damaging the aorta, the inferior vena cava, and the major nerves to the lower extremities. Lichtblau and Wilson reported one instance of transverse rupture of the aorta caused by manipulating the spine for Marie-Strümpell arthritis with severe flexion deformity. The patient had previously received 2000 units of roentgen therapy. These authors think that the roentgen therapy once used for this type of arthritis, not the arthritis itself, causes the aorta to adhere to the anterior longitudinal ligament and makes it subject to rupture during manipulation or osteotomy. They advocate a procedure in two stages in which the aorta is freed from the anterior longitudinal ligament in the first and the osteotomy is made in the second. They point out that in all of their patients, regardless of the number of levels at which osteotomies were made, all correction took place at only one level. Law reported a series of 114 patients and Herbert one of 50 in which the patients were treated by osteotomy; in each series the mortality was about 10%, but in each most of the deaths occurred early in the series, and both surgeons believed that the rate in the future should be lower. In fact, Goel has since reported a series of 15 patients in whom no deaths or serious complications occurred. According to Law, 25 to 45 degrees of correction can usually be obtained, resulting in marked improvement both functionally and cosmetically.

Adams suggests that the operation be carried out with the patient lying on the side. This lateral position has several advantages: the grossly deformed patient is easier to place on the table, danger of injuring the ankylosed cervical spine by pressure of the forehead against the table is eliminated, the anesthesia is easier to manage because maintaining a clear airway and free respiratory exchange is less difficult, and the operation is easier because any blood will flow out from the depth of the wound rather than into it. He hyperextends the spine with an ingenious three-point pressure apparatus.

Osteotomy is usually made at the upper lumbar level because the spinal canal here is large, and the osteotomy is distal to the end of the cord. A lumbar lordosis is created to compensate for the thoracic kyphosis; motion of the spine is not increased.

Simmons performs surgery with the patient under local anesthesia on his side. When the osteotomy is complete the patient is turned prone, carefully fracturing the anterior longitudinal ligament with the patient briefly under nitrous oxide and fentanyl anesthesia.

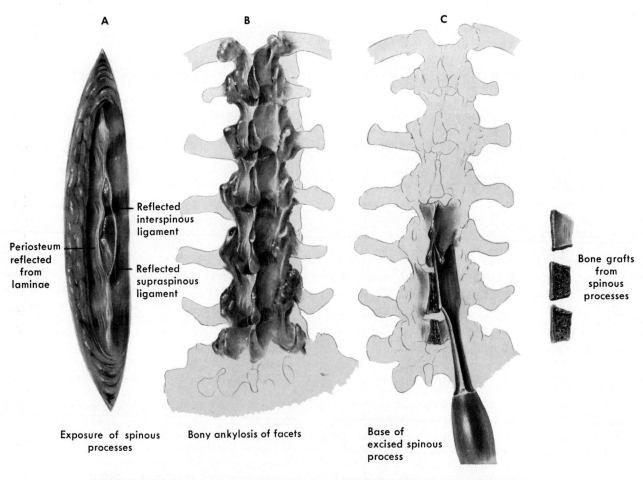

Fig. 75-14. Smith-Petersen osteotomy of spine for correction of flexion deformity in rheumatoid arthritis. **A,** Incision, exposure, and reflection of supraspinous and interspinous ligaments. Subperiosteal reflection of muscles from spinous processes and laminae. **B,** Bony ankylosis of facets. **C,** Osteotomy of spinous processes.

TECHNIQUE (SMITH-PETERSEN ET AL.). Place the patient prone on the operating table. Expose the spinous processes and laminae of three or more vertebrae subperiosteally through a midline incision (Fig. 75-14); the extent of exposure will depend on whether the osteotomy is to be made at one, two, or three levels. Carefully maintain hemostasis throughout the operation. Resect the spinous processes and cut them into small strips for grafting later. At the level of osteotomy detach the ligamentum flavum from the inferior margin of the lamina and the inferior articular facet with a small periosteal elevator. Carefully insert the elevator beneath the lamina and inferior articular facet and bring it out through the intervertebral foramen laterally. The elevator now serves as a guide for the osteotomy through the superior articular facet of the vertebra below and the inferior facet of the vertebra above. Make the osteotomy oblique, its angle approximately 45 degrees with the coronal plane. Widen the osteotomy with small osteotomes, gouges, and rongeurs to at least 6.2 to 9.4 mm. When the ligaments are ossified, take great care to avoid injuring the dura and nerves. Now repeat the procedure on the opposite side. The osteotomy may be made at two or three levels if necessary. Simmons emphasizes preplanning the amount of wedge to be removed so that proper coaptation of the osteotomy results and the patient achieves an optimum functional upright position.

After completing the osteotomy (or osteotomies), extend the spine by raising the head and foot of the operating table very slowly. The obliquity of the osteotomy ensures locking of the vertebrae and prevents serious displacement. Raise flaps of bone from the laminae adjacent to the osteotomy and bridge the defect with the bone grafts obtained from the spinous processes. Now carefully close the wound with interrupted sutures and apply a plaster shell to maintain the corrected position.

AFTERTREATMENT. The plaster is removed at 4 to 6 weeks, and a plaster jacket or back brace for walking is fitted. A back support is worn continuously for at least a year. To prevent recurrence of the deformity, the patient must wear the brace part of the time for 2 or 3 years more. Postural and deep breathing exercises are carried out regularly.

Goel uses no bone grafts or internal fixation and reports that abundant callus may be seen on the roentgenograms made as early as 3 weeks after surgery. He discards the final plaster jacket at 6 months and uses no external support thereafter.

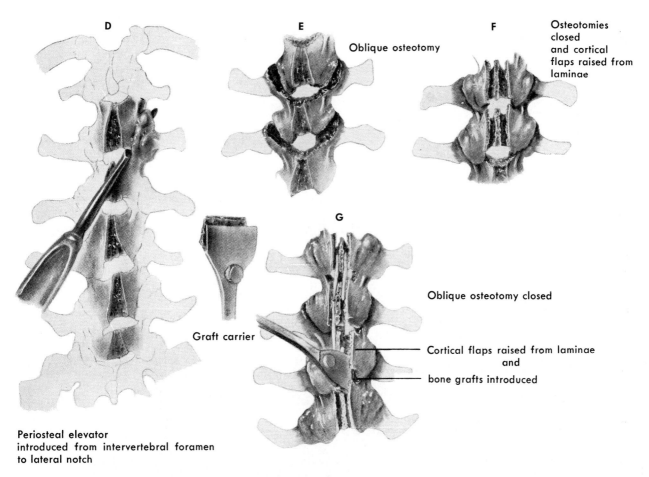

Fig. 75-14, cont'd. D, Periosteal elevator has been introduced deep to lamina and articular process, and its tip is visible at intervertebral foramen. **E,** Oblique osteotomies have been completed at two levels (see text). **F,** Spine has been extended, and spaces created by osteotomies have been closed. Flaps of cortical bone have been raised from laminae. **G,** Bone grafts obtained from spinous processes are being inserted beneath cortical flaps. (From Smith-Petersen, M.N., Larson, C.B., and Aufranc, O.E.: J. Bone Joint Surg. **27:**1, 1945.)

Osteotomy of cervical spine

In patients with severe cervicodorsal kyphosis in rheumatoid arthritis, often the mandible is so near the sternum that opening the mouth and chewing properly are difficult. Law reported a series of 14 patients treated by osteotomy of the cervical spine for this deformity. He points out that cervicodorsal kyphosis can usually be treated satisfactorily by lumbar osteotomy, which provides a compensatory lumbar lordosis and results in an erect posture. But according to him cervical osteotomy may be indicated (1) to elevate the chin from the sternum, thus improving the appearance, the ability to eat, and the ability to see ahead; (2) to prevent atlantoaxial and cervical subluxations and dislocations, which result from the weight of the head being carried forward by gravity; (3) to relieve tracheal and esophageal distortion, which causes dyspnea and dysphasia; and (4) to prevent irritation of the spinal cord tracts or excessive traction on the nerve roots, which cause neurologic disturbances. The appropriate level for osteotomy is determined by the deformity and the degree of ossification of the anterior longitudinal ligament. Law has successfully performed osteotomies at the levels of C3 and C4, C5 and C6, and C6 and C7. He prefers to fix the spine internally with the plates devised by Wilson and Straub for use in lumbosacral arthrodesis. However, wiring of the spinal processes as described by Rogers (p. 3126) should also be effective. Correcting the deformity too much must be avoided because otherwise the trachea and esophagus could be overstretched and become obstructed. Law usually obtained correction of 20 to 30 degrees. After surgery he supports the neck either by skeletal traction with Crutchfield tongs, a Minerva plaster jacket, or a halo attached to a plaster jacket. There were two deaths among his 14 patients, one at 3 weeks after surgery and one at 2 months.

Freeman reported treating by skeletal traction a patient with severe cervicodorsal kyphosis who could not actively lift his chin from the sternum but in whom minimal passive motion of the cervical spine was demonstrated by skeletal traction. The traction reduced a subluxation of C4 on C5 but failed to restore acceptable alignment. The Crutchfield tongs were then removed and a plaster jacket with an attached halo was applied. The neck was gradually extended until some of the cervical lordosis had been restored. Then with the halo still in place and the patient under a local anesthesia an arthrodesis from the occiput to T3 was carried out successfully.

TECHNIQUE (SIMMONS). Simmons applies a plaster body jacket incorporating halo supports 2 to 3 days preoperatively. The operation is carried out with the patient sitting in a dental chair and inclined forward with the arms resting on an operating table.

Apply a halo to the skull with local anesthesia and support the skull by 9 pounds (4 kg) of traction along the axis of neck deformity. Carry out the exposure with local anesthesia and identify the bifid spinous process of C6. Remove the spinous process and laminae of C7 together with the inferior portion of C6 and the upper portion of D1. Remove bone laterally through the fused posterior joints, exposing the eighth nerve root. Remove approximately 1.25 to 1.5 cm of bone bilaterally to thoroughly decom-press the eighth nerve root, leaving beveled edges to oppose later. After decompression is complete, the patient is given nitrous oxide and halothane (Fluothane) and the spine is fractured. As the gap closes posteriorly, the dura will buckle as the lateral masses come together. Verify the absence of root compression and close the wound routinely over a suction drain. Then stabilize the head by connection of the halo to the previously applied cast. Being fully conscious, the patient is checked for neurologic function in all extremities and can be assisted in ambulation to the CircOlectric bed.

AFTERTREATMENT. The patient is allowed to walk and move about but remains immobilized in the halo and cast until healing is complete at approximately 4 months after operation.

TUMORS

Osteoid osteoma of spine

The osteoid osteoma, first described by Jaffe in 1935, may be seen in the spine and involves males more commonly than females and is most common in the second decade. The lumbar spine is the most common location, the cervical next, and the thoracic last, and the lesion is almost invariably located in the posterior elements.

Pain is usually the patient's complaint, is worse at night, and often is relieved by aspirin. A painful scoliosis may result, with the concavity of the curve on the side of the lesion. Various curve types may result and usually demonstrate poor flexibility on side bending.

Diagnosis may be difficult since early roentgenograms may look normal. Later the usual configuration of a central nidus with surrounding sclerosis may be found, but in only half the patients will it be typical in appearance. Oblique roentgenograms may be helpful when the pedicle, facet, and pars interarticularis are studied. A radioisotopic bone scan will be most helpful in accurate localization.

Treatment should consist of surgical excision of the lesion. If the spine is considered unstable by virtue of facet or pedicle removal, we prefer to perform a one-level fusion at the same time. Complete excision should result in improvement in the angular degree of the scoliosis. Brace management may be necessary in the immature patient, and regular follow-up is advised.

Vertebral body tumors

BENIGN TUMORS

Lesions such as aneurysmal bone cyst, giant cell tumor, and others were once considered inaccessible surgically when found in the vertebrae. The older literature recommended irradiation or chemotherapy. Although this treatment still may apply in special circumstances such as in highly radiosensitive malignant tumors, angular deformity with potential paraplegia may result because of subsequent spinal instability. Benign tumors are best treated without irradiation to avoid secondary sarcomatous change. With other tumors, however, optimum treatment may be anterior resection of the tumor to effect a cure or for tumor debulking.

Significant advances in anterior spinal surgery have made possible the resection of vertebral bodies with minimal morbidity. A clearer understanding of the meaning of spinal instability has led to improvements in results. As reported by Stener and Johnsen, we have resected up to three thoracic vertebral bodies but have emphasized the achievement of spinal stability to avoid the late angulatory deformity they described. Our experience has included giant cell tumors, aneurysmal bone cysts, and lymphomas. One giant cell tumor recurred after initial resection of one vertebral body along with the tumor. The fibular graft was eroded by the recurrent tumor that then involved the adjacent cephalad and caudad vertebral bodies. At reoperation three bodies were resected and replaced using a construction of two rib grafts and one fibular strut graft.

Ultimate spinal stability to allow ambulation has been our goal. This we have achieved by first-stage tumor resection and fibular strut grafting followed in 10 to 14 days by posterior Harrington instrumentation and fusion (Fig. 75-15) in thoracic and lumbar lesions.

The symptoms of vertebral body tumors may include paraparesis that has been treated by a neurosurgeon with a laminectomy. The combination of anterior instability from tumor destruction of the body and that resulting from the laminectomy produces a most unstable situation. The surgeon must be prepared to properly decompress such a spine via the anterior route and stabilize the spine with a strut graft while preserving the only stability the patient has remaining, that is, the posterior arch and ligament complex. This approach will achieve complete removal of the tumor, decompression of the spinal cord, and stabilization of the spine. Since there are exceptions, each case must be considered on its own merits and involve oncologists, radiotherapists, and other interested specialists.

METASTATIC TUMORS

Recent advances in chemotherapy, radiation therapy, and other cancer therapies have resulted in a significant improvement in survival for many types of cancer. With the improved survival, previously silent spinal metastases are becoming clinically apparent and significantly impairing the quality of life. The standard methods of treatment for benign tumors involving excision and grafting are usually insufficient for the early mobilization of the patient. Siegal et al. estimate that 5% of patients with metastatic cancer will develop spinal cord compression. Kawabata et al. noted that 2% of 3880 patients autopsied with the diagnosis of metastatic cancer had previous clinical evidence of spinal metastasis but at autopsy the rate of metastasis varied from 21% to 48%. Schaberg and Gainor analyzed 322 patients with metastatic cancer. The rate of spinal metastases varied from 2.2% to 31%. Breast, lung, and prostate tumors were the most frequent. Of patients with spinal metastases, 36% did not have back pain. Spinal cord compression was noted in 20% of the patients. Prostatic tumors were the most common cause of epidural impingement. Hypernephroma was the most common malignancy to present with neurologic impairment as the first sign of malignancy.

Dewald et al. suggested a classification of patients with spinal metastases. Class I is destruction without collapse but with pain. This class is further divided into (a) less than 50% destruction, (b) greater than 50% destruction, and (c) pedicle destruction. In this class they considered surgery only in *b* and *c*. Class II is the addition of moderate deformity and collapse with immune competence. This class is considered a good risk for surgery. Class III is the addition of immune incompetence. This class carries greater risk for surgery. Class IV adds paralysis with immune competence. This class is considered a relative surgical emergency. Class V adds immune incompetence with paralysis. This class is not considered a good surgical risk.

Scoville et al. in 1967 were the first to use polymethylmethacrylate to fill defects in the vertebral bodies. Keggi et al. reported the use of polymethylmethacrylate as an adjunct to internal fixation in situations where bone fixation is questionable. There have been numerous reports on the efficacy of this material as an adjunct to internal fixation and bone grafting. Fear of neural injury from this technique has been a frequent concern. Wang et al. have shown that although the temperature of the curing cement may reach 176° to 194° F the temperature measured beneath an intact lamina and under gelfoam covering the dura at a laminar defect were significantly less (45° F). Later examination of the spinal cord in test animals did not show evidence of neural injury. Clinically, we have noted a fall in amplitude of somatosensory evoked potentials during the curing phase that returns to normal within 20 to 30 minutes of insertion of polymethylmethacrylate. Injury after the use of the material near the spinal cord has not been reported.

Numerous methods have been devised to provide additional stability with polymethylmethacrylate. Wang et al. tested 11 different methods of anterior and posterior fixation in the cervical spine. They concluded that anterior fixation with chain, screws, and cement provided the greatest rigidity in extension. The addition of a posterior wiring with cement further improved the degree of rigidity. Clark et al. have recommended the use of polymethylmethacrylate incorporating the wires in a posterior fusion, leaving the lateral edges of the spine, the lateral two thirds of the bone graft, and the tops of the spinous processes for revascularization and fusion. Anteriorly, they suggest the use of a wire mesh against the dura or posterior longitudinal ligament and threaded Steinmann pins drilled into the vertebral bodies as additional fixation with the cement. This popular anterior construction was not included in the group tested by Wang et al.

Panjabi et al. in a postmortem biomechanical evaluation concluded that the initial rigidity decreased with time. The spontaneous fusion that occurred in their patient enhanced the long-term stability. Whitehill et al. compared posterior cervical fusions in dogs with and without polymethylmethacrylate. Fusions with the cement showed loosening by the second month while fusions with bone grafting were mechanically equal to or stronger than controls at the same time.

Excellent results with significant neurologic improvement have been reported in numerous patients. This technique allows immediate walking of debilitated patients with minimal or no external spinal support. Additionally, significant pain relief is obtained in almost all patients. Further pain relief can be obtained with additional radiation or chemotherapy. This method of treatment is rapidly replacing simple laminectomy in patients with neural involvement from metastatic cancer.

The indications for the use of the technique are varied and will probably expand as further experience is acquired. The primary indications are (1) the development of a neural deficit and (2) intractable pain. Before surgery is performed the patient should be evaluated for (1) additional areas of metastasis, (2) general medical condition, (3) efficacy or use of nonoperative methods, (4) location and extent of the metastatic lesion, and (5) estimation of the expected life span (Clark et al. suggested a minimum of 4 to 6 weeks) considering current therapy, tumor type, and aggressiveness. Each patient should be considered on his own merits in relation to this evaluation. A careful preoperative evaluation is mandatory since multiple spinal lesions with skip areas are common.

Lesions situated in the vertebral bodies are best approached from anteriorly. Frequently, the excision of one

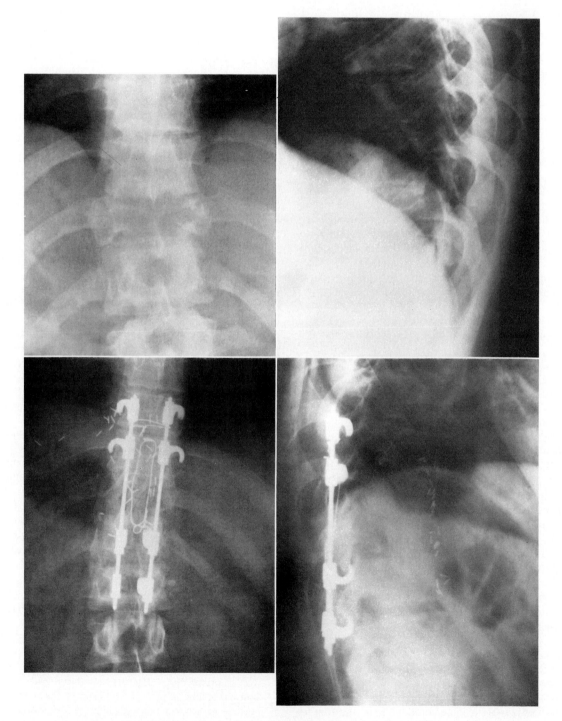

Fig. 75-15. Example of polymethylmethacrylate for cervical spine stability.

or more vertebral bodies is involved. One should be prepared to extend the dissection in the event of the discovery of additional metastatic disease. If the predominant lesion is posterior, then the posterior approach for that region of the spine should be used. Cement-augmented internal fixation should be considered if the spine is unstable (Fig. 75-15). Autogenous bone grafting is performed only if considerable longevity is assumed. Some case reports and clinical series have used the posterior approach exclusively to prevent or reduce anterior collapse, dislocation, or both. This may be a consideration in the severely debilitated patient with a short anticipated life span. Clark et al. suggest a combined anterior and posterior resection with polymethylmethacrylate and metal fixation. They suggest posterior decompression and cement fusion first to prevent anterior implant displacement or turning postoperatively.

TECHNIQUE (ANTERIOR). Approach the spinal segment using the standard anterior approach for that spinal segment but choose an approach that allows for more radical or extensive exposure if necessary. Identify normal bone cranially and caudally. Then excise the tumor mass. Remove all disc and central end plate material in the normal caudal and cranial vertebral bodies. Prepare the normal cancellous bone in these vertebral bodies as desired for the method of fixation desired. (We presently use threaded Steinmann pins.) Cover the exposed dura or anterior longitudinal ligament or both with gelfoam. Insert the polymethylmethacrylate in a semiliquid or doughy state. (We presently use a small amount of cement to line the floor of the cavity before inserting the threaded Steinmann pins superiorly and inferiorly.) Remove excess cement. (This is especially important in the cervical spine where a large mass of cement may cause dysphagia.) Take care to avoid pushing the cement against the dura and spinal cord. As soon as the cement has been trimmed begin continuous irrigation of the wound with normal saline. (We presently prefer the irrigation solution used for arthroscopy which comes in 3-liter bags.) Continue the irrigation for at least 20 minutes. Test the construction for stability before closing. Remove and replace the cement and metal fixation if it is loose. Close the wound in the standard fashion.

TECHNIQUE (POSTERIOR). Approach the spine using the standard posterior approach for the spinal segment involved. Allow for extension of the exposure if indicated. Then perform laminectomies as indicated by the pathology. Clean the remaining normal lamina and spinous processes of all soft tissue for at *least* two segments above and below the pathology. Pass wires through the remaining spinous processes. Clark et al. suggest wiring 2 spinous processes above and below large laminar defects. Cover the exposed dura with gelfoam. Then insert other internal fixation as indicated by the spinal level. (We usually add Harrington compression rods in the thoracic region and Harrington distraction rods at the thoracolumbar junction or lower. Others have used the Luque instrumentation.) Apply the cement in a semiliquid or doughy consistency. Allow the tips of the spinous processes to be exposed. If autogenous bone grafting is performed place the grafts laterally and allow the cement to cover only their inner one third or add the grafts laterally after application of the cement. Close the wound in the standard fashion.

AFTERTREATMENT. Rigid immobilization is not necessary if the surgical construction is deemed solid. Clark et al. suggest only soft collar immobilization of the cervical spine until soft tissue healing is complete. In the thoracic and lumbar spine we have allowed immediate sitting and early walking in a long Thomas back brace. The use of radiation or chemotherapy after the procedure is left to the judgment of the oncologist.

• • •

The use of polymethylmethacrylate as an adjunct to spinal fusion is also applicable in other pathologic conditions in which the rate of successful fusion is low or the patient is unable to tolerate prolonged immobilization. Such conditions include fusions for cervical instability in rheumatoid arthritis, instability in renal osteodystrophy, and selected fractures or spondylosis in elderly and debilitated patients.

LATE DEFORMITY AFTER TREATMENT
Intraspinal tumors in childhood

Although fortunately rare, spinal tumors in children may lead to significant spinal deformity, instability, or paraplegia. The orthopaedic surgeon may be presented with this problem, both early and for long-term management, and must be aware of its symptoms and management.

The diagnosis of intraspinal tumors should be considered whenever an otherwise healthy, active child has symptoms of back pain, especially at night. Pain radiating to an extremity, a limp with demonstrated atrophy or weakness but no local cause, and sphincter disturbance are other symptoms. Fraser et al., reporting on 40 children, recorded 67% presenting with weakness of a limb, 60% with back or radiating extremity pain, and 22% with sphincter disturbance.

Presenting clinical signs may include painful scoliosis, muscle weakness, sensory loss, or pathologic reflexes. Definite paravertebral muscle spasm may also be seen. Fraser et al. reported that 30% of their patients were first seen with paraparesis or paraplegia.

The initial diagnosis is often missed and the symptoms and signs are minimized. Diagnoses such as back strain, discitis, osteomyelitis, and others may be made. Again it must be emphasized that since back pain in children is so rare, special attention must be paid to those having the above complaints and a thorough investigation must be made.

Plain roentgenograms should be taken and carefully scrutinized for erosion of the neural arch or vertebral body, erosions, widened interpedicular distances, and paraspinal masses of calcifications. Myelography is then indicated with laboratory investigation of the cerebrospinal fluid. An elevated protein determination in the cerebrospinal fluid is the most significant finding in support of intraspinal tumors. A wide variety of tumors is possible, and specific information should be sought in articles dealing with this subject.

Neurosurgeons will primarily care for these children, but the orthopaedic surgeon will be presented with the long-term problems inherent with the necessary laminectomy. Fraser et al. emphasize that the higher the laminectomy is in the spine, the more likely is instability or deformity. Yasuoka et al. reviewed 58 patients who had extensive laminectomies before the age of 25. Spinal deformity developed in 46% of the patients age 12 to 24 years. The incidence of cervical deformity in this group was 100% and the incidence of thoracic deformity was 36%. There was no deformity after lumbar laminectomy. Swan-neck deformity occurs in the cervical area and scoliosis and kyphosis in the thoracic area, whereas the lumbar area is relatively free of deformity.

Treatment of any resulting deformity must follow the guidelines for paralytic or nonparalytic spinal deformity discussed elsewhere. It must be remembered, as pointed out by Ingraham and Matson in 1954, that a childhood laminectomy might result in spinal deformity. Anterior or posterior fusion and appropriate bracing are necessary depending on the specific deformity.

Spinal irradiation in childhood

Despite studies of the effect of irradiation on the growing spine, little is really known regarding growth retardation. Probert et al. are presently using a prospective protocol at Stanford University to further delineate this problem. Their previous studies suggest periods of accelerated growth under 6 years of age and at puberty and an increased sensitivity to irradiation. Neuhauser et al. suggest a dose and age relationship with the ultimate effect on the vertebral bodies. Studies continue to lower the irradiation dose for protection of growth and still remain effective on the primary tumor pathology.

Probert et al. and Riseborough et al. reported vertebral body abnormalities following irradiation consisting of subcortical osteoporosis in the mildest type to complete cessation of growth in the most severe. Growth arrest lines, end plate irregularity, altered trabecular pattern, decreased vertebral body height, contour abnormalities, and asymmetric or symmetric body maldevelopment were listed by Riseborough et al. in their study of 81 patients. They also showed a 70% incidence of scoliosis, 26% of kyphosis, and 27% with no abnormality in axial alignment.

Riseborough et al. found a statistically significant correlation between the amount of irradiation, the severity of the spinal changes, the age of the patient, and the type of deformity. Those patients receiving more than 3070 rads had a higher rate of scoliosis, those receiving less than 3070 rads had a lower than expected rate of scoliosis. If irradiation occurred before the age of 5 years, more than 2600 rads resulted in deformity. Their data also showed that the younger the patient, the greater the deformity.

The deformities progress rapidly during the adolescent growth period. The curves are rigid and frequently are associated with kyphosis; hence bracing is of little value. Surgical stabilization is necessary and is best accomplished by a two-stage anterior and posterior fusion as in other kyphoscoliotic deformities.

Spinal deformity in acquired spinal cord injury

Mayfield et al. report that spinal cord injury before the adolescent growth spurt is associated with a 100% rate of deformity of which 96% is progressive. Conservative bracing is difficult. They recommend bracing with a bivalved underarm polypropylene body jacket for curves of 20 to 30 degrees until the age of 10 to 12 years. Surgery is then performed using a staged anterior and posterior fusion. They suggest fusion from the upper thoracic spine to the sacrum.

REFERENCES
Spinal stenosis

Arnoldi, C.C., et al.: Lumbar spinal stenosis and nerve root entrapment syndromes: definition and classification, Clin. Orthop. **115:**4, 1976.

Bailey, P., and Casamajor, L.: Osteoarthritis of spine compressing cord, J. Nerv. Ment. Dis. **38:**588, 1911.

Bell, G.R., and Rothman, R.H.: The conservative treatment of sciatica, Spine **9:**54, 1984.

Bohl, W.R., and Steffee, A.D.: Lumbar spinal stenosis: a cause of continued pain and disability after total hip arthroplasty, Spine **4:**168, 1979.

Ciric, I., Mikhael, M.A., Tarkington, J.A., and Vick, N.A.: The lateral recess syndrome: a variant of spinal stenosis, J. Neurosurg. **53:**433, 1980.

Claussen, C.D., Lohkamp, F.W., and v. Bazan, U.B.: The diagnosis of congenital spinal disorders in computed tomography (CT), Neuropadiatrie **8:**405, 1977.

Cranston, P.E., Patel, R.B., and Harrison, R.B.: Computed tomography for metastatic lesions of the osseous pelvis, South. Med. J. **76:**1503, 1983.

Crawshaw, C., et al.: The use of nuclear magnetic resonance in the diagnosis of lateral canal entrapment, J. Bone Joint Surg. **66-B:**711, 1984.

Dunlop, R.B., Adams, M.A., and Hutton, W.C.: Disc space narrowing and the lumbar facet joints, J. Bone Joint Surg. **66-B:**706, 1984.

Dyck, P.: The stoop-test in lumbar entrapment radiculopathy, Spine **4:**89, 1979.

Ehni, G., Clark, K., Wilson, C.B., and Alexander, E., Jr.: Significance of the small lumbar spinal canal cauda equina compression syndromes due to spondylosis (parts 1 to 4), J. Neurosurg. **31:**490, 1969.

Elsberg, C.A.: Experiences in spinal surgery, Surg. Gynecol. Obstet. **16:**117, 1913.

Farfan, H.F.: The pathological anatomy of degenerative spondylolisthesis: a cadaver study, Spine **5:**412, 1980.

Foley, R.K., and Kirkaldy-Willis, W.H.: Chronic venous hypertension in the tail of the wistar rat, Spine **4:**251, 1979.

Getty, C.J.M.: Lumbar spinal stenosis: the clinical spectrum and the results of operation, J. Bone Joint Surg. **62-B:**481, 1980.

Getty, C.J.M., Johnson, J.R., Kirwan, E., and Sullivan, M.F.: Partial undercutting facetectomy for bony entrapment of the lumbar nerve root, J. Bone Joint Surg. **63-B:**330, 1981.

Gokalp, H.Z., and Ozkai, E.: Intradural tuberculomas of the spinal cord: report of two cases, J. Neurosurg **55:**289, 1981.

Grabias, S.: The treatment of spinal stenosis: current concepts review, J. Bone Joint Surg. **62-A:**308, 1980.

Herron, L.D., and Pheasant, H.C.: Bilateral laminotomy and discectomy for segmental lumbar disc disease: decompression with stability, Spine **8:**86, 1983.

Hirsh, L.F., and Finneson, B.E.: Intradural sacral nerve root metastasis mimicking herniated disc; case report, J. Neurosurg. **49:**764, 1978.

Johnsson, K., Willner, S., and Pettersson, H.: Analysis of operated cases with lumbar spinal stenosis, Acta Orthop. Scand. **52:**427, 1981.

Karayannacos, P.E., Yashon, D., and Vasko, J.S.: Narrow lumbar spinal canal with "vascular" syndromes, Arch. Surg. **111:**803, 1976.

Kimura, I., Oh-Hama, M., and Shingu, H.: Cervical myelopathy treated by canal-expansive laminaplasty: computed tomographic and myelographic findings, J. Bone Joint Surg. **66-A:**914, 1984.

Kirkaldy-Willis, W.H.: The relationship of structural pathology to the nerve root, Spine **9:**49, 1984.

Kirkaldy-Willis, W.H., Paine, K.W.E., Cauchoix, J., and McIvor, G.: Lumbar spinal stenosis, Clin. Orthop. **99:**30, 1974.

Kirkaldy-Willis, W.H., Wedge, J.H., Yong-Hing, K., and Reilly, J.: Pathology and pathogenesis of lumbar spondylosis and stenosis, Spine **4:**319, 1978.

Kirkaldy-Willis, W.H., et al.: Lumbar spinal nerve lateral entrapment, Clin. Orthop. **169:**171, 1982.

Macnab, I.: Cervical spondylosis, Clin. Orthop. **109:**69, 1975.

Messersmith, R.N., Cronan, J., and Esparza, A.R.: Computed tomography-guided percutaneous biopsy: combined approach to the retroperitoneum, Neurosurgery **14:**218, 1984.

Paine, K.W.E.: Clinical features of lumbar spinal stenosis, Clin. Orthop. **115:**77, 1976.

Porter, R.W., Hibbert, C., and Evans, C.: The natural history of root entrapment syndrome, Spine **9:**418, 1984.

Porter, R.W., Hibbert, C., and Wellman, P.: Backache and the lumbar spinal canal, Spine **5:**99, 1980.

Posner, I., White, A.A., III, Edwards, W.T., and Hayes, W.C.: A biomechanical analysis of the clinical stability of the lumbar and lumbosacral spine, Spine **7:**374, 1982.

Postacchini, F., et al.: Computerized tomography in lumbar stenosis: a preliminary report, J. Bone Joint Surg. **62-B:**78, 1980.

Raskin, S.P.: Degenerative changes of the lumbar spine: assessment by computed tomography, Orthopedics **4:**186, 1981.

Rinaldi, I., Mullins, W.J., Delandy, W.F., Fitzer, P.M., and Tornberg, D.M.: Computerized tomographic demonstration of rotational atlanto-axial fixation: case report, J. Neurosurg. **50:**115, 1979.

Rydevik, B., Brown, M.D., and Lundborg, G.: Pathoanatomy and pathophysiology of nerve root compression, Spine **9:**7, 1984.

San Martino, A., D'Andria, F.M., and San Martino, C.: The surgical treatment of nerve root compression caused by scoliosis of the lumbar spine, Spine **8:**261, 1983.

Schonstrom, N.S.R., Bolender, N., Spengler D.M.: The pathomorphology of spinal stenosis as seen on CT scans of the lumbar spine, Spine **10:**806, 1985.

Shenkin, H.A., and Hash, C.J.: Spondylolisthesis after multiple bilateral laminectomies and facetectomies for lumbar spondylosis, J. Neurosurg. **50:**45, 1979.

Surin, V., Hedelin, E., and Smith, L.: Degenerative lumbar spinal stenosis: results of operative treatment, Acta Orthop. Scand. **53:**79, 1982.

Tile, M.: The role of surgery in nerve root compression, Spine **9:**57, 1984.

Tile, M., et al.: Spinal stenosis: results of treatment, Clin. Orthop. **115:**104, 1976.

Tile, M., et al.: Lumbar spinal stenosis and nerve root entrapment syndromes: definition and classification, Clin. Orthop. **115:**4, 1976.

Verbiest, H.: Pathological influence of developmental narrowness of bony lumbar vertebral canal, J. Bone Joint Surg. **37-B:**576, 1954.

Verbiest, H.: Results of surgical treatment of idiopathic developmental stenosis of the lumbar vertebral canal: a review of twenty-seven years' experience, J. Bone Joint Surg. **59-B:**181, 1977.

Verbiest, H.: The significance and principles of computerized axial tomography in idiopathic developmental stenosis of the bony lumbar vertebral canal, Spine **4:**369, 1979.

Walpin, L.A., and Singer, F.R.: Paget's disease: reversal of severe paraparesis using calcitonin, Spine **4:**213, 1979.

Weinstein, J.M., Scafuri, R.L., and McNeill, T.W.: The Rush-Presbyterian-St. Luke's lumbar spine analysis form: a prospective study of patients with "spinal stenosis", Spine **8:**891, 1983.

Wiesz, G.M.: Stenosis of the lumbar spinal canal in Forestier's disease, Int. Orthop. **7:**61, 1983.

Weisz, M.: Lumbar spinal canal stenosis in Paget's disease, Spine **8:**192, 1983.

Wiltse, L.L., et al.: Alar transverse process impingement of the L5 spinal nerve: the far-out syndrome, Spine **9:**31, 1984.

Wiltse, L.L., Kirkaldy-Willis, W.H., and McIvor, G.W.D.: The treatment of spinal stenosis, Clin. Orthop. **115:**83, 1976.

C1-2 instability

Dawson, E.G., and Smith, L.: Atlanto-axial subluxation in children due to vertebral anomalies, J. Bone Joint Surg. **61-A:**582, 1979.

Fielding, J.W., Hawkins, R.J., and Ratzen, S.A.: Spine fusion for atlanto-axial instability, J. Bone Joint Surg. **58-A:**400, 1976.

Fielding, J.W., Hensinger, R.N., and Hawkins, R.J.: Os odontoideum, J. Bone Joint Surg. **62-A:**376, 1980.

Hawkins, R.J., Fielding, J.W., and Thompson, W.J.: Os odontoideum: congenital or acquired—a case report, J. Bone Joint Surg. **58-A:**413, 1976.

Hukuda, S., Ota, H., Okabe, N., and Tazima, K.: Traumatic atlantoaxial dislocation causing os odontoideum in infants, Spine **5:**207, 1980.

Lee, P.C., Chun, S.Y., and Leong, J.C.Y.: Experience of posterior surgery in atlanto-axial instability, Spine **9:**231, 1984.

Nordt, J.C., and Stauffer, E.S.: Sequelae of atlantoaxial stabilization in two patients with Down's syndrome, Spine **6:**437, 1981.

Perovic, M.N., Kopits, S.E., and Thompson, R.C.: Radiological evaluation of the spinal cord in congenital atlanto-axial dislocation, Radiology **109:**713, 1973.

Pueschel, S.M., et al.: Symptomatic atlantoaxial subluxation in persons with Down syndrome, J. Pediatr. Orthop. **4:**682, 1984.

Ricciardi, J.E., Kaufer, H., and Louis, D.S.: Acquired os odontoideum following acute ligament injury: report of a case, J. Bone Joint Surg. **58-A:**410, 1976.

Roach, J.W., Duncan, D., Wenger, D.R., Maravilla, A., and Maravilla, K.: Atlanto-axial instability and spinal cord compression in children: diagnosis by computerized tomography, J. Bone Joint Surg. **66-A:**708, 1984.

Sherk, H.H., and Dawoud, S.: Congenital os odontoideum with Klippel-Feil anomaly and fatal atlanto-axial instability: report of a case, Spine **6:**42, 1981.

Spierings, E.L.H., and Braakman, R.: The management of os odontoideum: analysis of 37 cases, J. Bone Joint Surg. **64-B:**422, 1982.

Wollin, D.G.: The os odontoideum: separate odontoid process, J. Bone Joint Surg. **45-A:**1459, 1963.

Occiput-C1 problems

Menezes, A.H., VanGilder, J.C., Graf, C.J., and McDonnell, D.E.: Craniocervical abnormalities: a comprehensive surgical approach, J. Neurosurg. **53:**444, 1980.

Wolf, J.W., Jr., and Kahler, S.G.: Atlanto-axial rotary fixation associated with the 18q-syndrome, J. Bone Joint Surg. **62-A:**295, 1980.

Sacral agenesis

Abraham, E.: Sacral agenesis with associated anomalies (caudal regression syndrome): autopsy case report, Clin. Orthop. **145:**168, 1979.

Abraham, E.: Lumbosacral coccygeal agenesis: autopsy case report, J. Bone Joint Surg. **58-A:**1169, 1976.

Andrish, J., Kalamchi, A., and MacEwen, G.D.: Sacral agenesis: a clinical evaluation of its management, heredity, and associated anomalies, Clin. Orthop. **139:**52, 1979.

Denton, J.R.: The association of congenital spinal anomalies with imperforate anus, Clin. Orthop. **162:**91, 1982.

Ezaki, M., and Herring, J.A.: Congenital hyperextension of the lumbar spine: a case report, J. Bone Joint Surg. **63-A;**1177, 1981.

Renshaw, T.S.: Sacral agenesis: a classification and review of twenty-three cases, J. Bone Joint Surg. **60-A:**373, 1978.

Stanley, J.K., Owen, R., and Koff, S.: Congenital sacral anomalies, J. Bone Joint Surg. **61-B;**401, 1979.

Congenital anomalies of spine

Bassett, F.H., III: Aplasia of the odontoid process (Piedmont Orthopaedic Society), personal communication, 1969.

Cattell, J.S., and Filtzer, D.L.: Pseudosubluxation and other normal variations in the cervical spine in children, J. Bone Joint Surg. **47-A:**1295, 1965.

Coventry, M.B., and Harris, L.E.: Congenital muscular torticollis in infancy, some observations regarding treatment, J. Bone Joint Surg. **41-A:**815, 1959.

Dalinka, M.K., Rosenbaum, A.E., and Van Houten, F.: Congenital absence of the posterior arch of the atlas, Radiology **103:**581, 1972.

Guthkelch, A.N.: Diastematomyelia with median septum, Brain **97:**729, 1974.

Herring, J.A.: Rapidly progressive scoliosis in multiple epiphyseal dysplasia: a case report, J. Bone Joint Surg. **58-A:**703, 1976.

Hilal, S.K., Marton, D., and Pollack, E.: Diastematomyelia in children: radiographic study of 34 cases, Radiology **112:**609, 1974.

Huick, V.C., Hopkins, C.E., and Savara, B.S.: Sagittal diameter of the cervical spinal canal in children, Radiology **79:**971, 1962.

James, C.C.M., and Lassman, L.P.: Spinal dysraphism: the diagnosis and treatment of progressive lesions in spina bifida occulta, J. Bone Joint Surg. **44-B:**828, 1962.

Klippel, M., and Feil, A.: Un cas d'absence des vertebres cervicales, Bull. et Mems. Soc. Anat. de Paris **87:**185, 1912.

Ling, C.M., and Low, H.S.: Sternomastoid tumor and muscular torticollis, Clin. Orthop. **86:**144, 1972.

Micheli, L.J., Hall, J.E., and Watts, H.G.: Spinal instability in Larsen's syndrome: report of three cases, J. Bone Joint Surg. **58-A;**562, 1976.

Mongeau, M., and Leclaire, R.: Complete agenesis of the lumbosacral spine: a case report, J. Bone Joint Surg. **54-A:**161, 1972.

Perovic, M.N., Kopits, S.E., and Thompson, R.C.: Radiological evaluation of the spinal cord in congenital atlanto-axial dislocation, Radiology **109:**713, 1973.

Perry, J., Bonnett, C.A., and Hoffer, M.M.: Vertebral pelvic fusions in the rehabilitation of patients with sacral agenesis, J. Bone Joint Surg. **52-A:**288, 1970.

Polga, J.P., and Cramer, G.G.: Cleft anterior arch of atlas simulating odontoid fracture, Radiology **113:**341, 1974.

Renshaw, T.S.: Sacral agenesis: a classification and review of twenty-three cases, J. Bone Joint Surg. **60-A:**373, 1978.

Richardson, E.G., Boone, S.C., and Reid, R.L.: Intermittent quadriparesis associated with a congenital anomaly of the posterior arch of the atlas: case report, J. Bone Joint Surg. **57-A:**853, 1975.

Scatliff, J.H., Till, K., and Hoare, R.D.: Incomplete, false, and true diastematomyelia: radiological evaluation by air myelography and tomography, Radiology **116:**349, 1975.

Winter, R.B., Moe, J.H., and Eikers, V.E.: Congenital scoliosis: a study of 234 patients treated and untreated, J. Bone Joint Surg. **50-A:**1, 1968.

Winter, R.B., Moe, J.H., and Lagaard, S.M.: Diastematomyelia and congenital spine deformities, J. Bone Joint Surg. **56-A:**27, 1974.

Zimbler, S., and Belkin, S.: Birth defects involving the spine, Orthop. Clin. North Am. **7:**303, 1976.

Rheumatoid arthritis

Adams, J.C.: Technic, dangers and safeguards in osteotomy of the spine, J. Bone Joint Surg. **34-B:**226. 1952.

Calabro, J.J., and Maltz, B.A.: Current concepts: ankylosing spondylitis, N. Engl. J. Med. **282:**606, 1970.

Conlon, P.W., Isdale, I.C., and Rose, B.S.: Rheumatoid arthritis of the cervical spine: an analysis of 333 cases, Ann. Rheum. Dis. **25:**120, 1966.

Detenbeck, L.C.: Rheumatoid arthritis of the spinal column: pathologic aspects and treatment, Orthop. Clin. North Am. **2:**679, 1971.

Fam, A.G., and Cruickshank, B.: Subaxial cervical subluxation and cord compression in psoriatic spondylitis, Arthritis Rheum. **25:**101, 1982.

Freeman, G.E., Jr.: Correction of severe deformity of the cervical spine in ankylosing spondylitis with the halo device, J. Bone Joint Surg. **43-A:**547, 1961.

Goel, M.K.: Vertebral osteotomy for correction of fixed flexion deformity of the spine, J. Bone Joint Surg. **50-A:**287, 1968.

Harta, S., Thono, S., and Kawagishi: Osteoarthritis of the atlanto-axial joint, Int. Orthop. **5:**277, 1981.

Helfet, A.J.: Spinal osteotomy, S. Afr. Med. J. **26:**773, 1952.

Herbert, J.J.: Vertebral osteotomy, technique, indications, and results, J. Bone Joint Surg. **30-A:**680, 1948.

Herbert, J.J.: Vertebral osteotomy for kyphosis, especially in Marie-Strümpell arthritis: a report on fifty cases, J. Bone Joint Surg. **41-A:**291, 1959.

Kudo, H., Iwano, K., and Yoshizawa, H.: Cervical cord compression due to extradural granulation tissue in rheumatoid arthritis, J. Bone Joint Surg. **66-B:**426, 1984.

LaChapelle, E.H.: Osteotomy of the lumbar spine for correction of kyphosis in a case of ankylosing spondylarthritis, J. Bone Joint Surg. **28:**851, 1946.

Law, W.A.: Osteotomy of the spine and the treatment of severe dorsal kyphosis: four cases, Proc. R. Soc. Med. **42:**594, 1949.

Law, W.A.: Arthritis: surgical treatment of chronic arthritis. In Carling, E.R., and Ross, J.P., editors: British surgical practice, surgical progress, London, 1952, Butterworth & Co., Ltd.

Law, W.A.: Surgical treatment of the rheumatic diseases, J. Bone Joint Surg. **34-B:**215, 1952.

Law, W.A.: Lumbar spinal osteotomy, J. Bone Joint Surg. **41-B:**270, 1959.

Law, W.A.: Osteotomy of the spine, J. Bone Joint Surg. **44-A:**1199, 1962.

Law, W.A.: The spine in rheumatoid spondylitis, Clin. Orthop. **36:**35, 1964.

Lichtblau, P.O., and Wilson, P.D.: Possible mechanism of aortic rupture in orthopaedic correction of rheumatoid spondylitis, J. Bone Joint Surg. **38-A:**123, 1956.

Lipson, S.J.: Rheumatoid arthritis of the cervical spine, Clin. Orthop. **182:**143, 1984.

Lourie, H. and Stewart, W.A.: Spontaneous atlantoaxial dislocation: a complication of rheumatoid disease, N. Engl. J. Med. **265:**677, 1961.

Martel, W., and Page, J.W.: Cervical vertebral erosions and subluxations in rheumatoid arthritis and ankylosing spondylitis, Arthritis Rheum. **3:**546, 1960.

Matthews, J.A.: Atlanto-axial subluxation in rheumatoid arthritis: a five-year follow-up study, Ann. Rheum. Dis. **33:**526, 1974.

McMaster, P.E.: Osteotomy of the spine for fixed flexion deformity, J. Bone Joint Surg. **44-A:**1207, 1962.

Ranawat, C.S., et al.: Cervical spine fusion in rheumatoid arthritis, J. Bone Joint Surg. **61-A:**1003, 1979.

Rombouts, J.J., and Rombouts-Lindemans C.: Scoliosis in juvenile rheumatoid arthritis, J. Bone Joint Surg. **56-B:**478, 1974.

Sachs, B., and Fraenkel, J.: Progressive ankylotic rigidity of the spine (spondylose rhizomelique), J. Nerv. Mental Dis., **27:**1, 1900.

Sharp, J., and Purser, D.W.: Spontaneous atlanto-axial dislocation in ankylosing spondylitis and rheumatoid arthritis, Ann. Rheum. Dis. **20:**47, 1961.

Simmons, E.H.: Surgery of the spine in rheumatoid arthritis and ankylosing spondylitis. In Cruess, R.L., and Mitchell, N.S., editors: Surgery of rheumatoid arthritis, Philadelphia, 1971, J.B. Lippincott Co.

Simmons, E.H.: The surgical correction of flexion deformity of the cervical spine in ankylosing spondylitis, Clin. Orthop. **86:**132, 1972.

Smith, H.P., Challa, V.R., and Alexander, E., Jr.: Odontoid compression of the brain stem in a patient with rheumatoid arthritis: case report, J. Neurosurg. **53:**841, 1980.

Smith-Petersen, M.N., Larson, C.B., and Aufranc, O.E.: Osteotomy of the spine for correction of flexion deformity in rheumatoid spondylitis, J. Bone Joint Surg. **27:**1, 1945.

Stern, W.E., and Balch, R.E.: Surgical aspects of nonspecific inflammatory and suppurative disease of the vertebral column, Am. J. Surg. **112:**314, 1966.

Thomas, W.H.: Surgical management of the rheumatoid cervical spine, Orthop. Clin. North Am. **6:**793, 1975.

Weinstein, P.R., Karpman, R.R., Gall, E.P., and Pitt, M.: Spinal cord injury, spinal fracture, and spinal stenosis in ankylosing spondylitis, J. Neurosurg. **57:**609, 1982.

Wilson, M.J., and Turkell, J.H.: Multiple spinal wedge osteotomy: its use in a case of Marie-Strumpell spondylitis, Am. J. Surg. **77:**777, 1949.

Wilson, P.D.: Surgical reconstruction of the arthritic cripple, Med. Clin. N. Am. **21:**1623, 1937.

Wilson, P.D., and Osgood, R.B.: Reconstructive surgery in chronic arthritis, N. Engl. J. Med. **209:**117, 1933.

Winfield, J., Cooke, D., Brook, A.S., and Corbett, M.: A prospective study of the radiological changes in the cervical spine in early rheumatoid disease, Ann. Rheum. Dis. **40:**109, 1981.

Young, H.H., and Regan, J.M.: Total excision of the patella for arthritis of the knee, Minn. Med. **28:**909, 1945.

Cervical myelopathy

Abe, H., Tsuru, M., Ito, T., Iwasaki, Y., and Koiwa, M.: Anterior decompression for ossification of the posterior longitudinal ligament of the cervical spine, J. Neurosurg. **55:**108, 1981.

Alenghat, J.P., and Hallett, M., and Kido, D.K.: Spinal cord compression in diffuse idiopathic skeletal hyperostosis, Radiology **142:**119, 1982.

Boni, M., Cherubino, P., Denaro, V., and Benazzo, F.: Multiple subtotal somatectomy: technique and evaluation of a series of 39 cases, Spine **9:**358, 1984.

Crandall, P.H., and Gregorius, F.K.: Long-term followup of surgical treatment of cervical spondylotic myelopathy, Spine **2:**139, 1977.

Edwards, W.C., and LaRocca, H.: The developmental segmental sagittal diameter of the cervical spinal canal in patients with cervical spondylosis, Spine **8:**20, 1983.

Epstein, J.A., Carras, R., Hyman, R.A., and Costa, S.: Cervical myelopathy caused by developmental stenosis of the spinal canal, J. Neurosurg. **51:**362, 1979.

Govoni, A.F.: Developmental stenosis of a thoracic vertebra resulting in narrowing of the spinal canal, Am. J. Roentgenol. Radium Ther. Nucl. Med. **112:**401, 1971.

Gui, L., Merlini, L., Savini, R., and Davidovits, P.: Cervical myelopathy due to ossification of the posterior longitudinal ligament, Ital. J. Orthop. Traumatol. **9:**269, 1983.

Hirabayashi, K., et al.: Expansive open-door laminoplasty for cervical spinal stenotic myelopathy, Spine 8:693, 1983.

Hoff, J., et al.: The role of ischemia in the pathogenesis of cervical spondylotic myelopathy: a review and new microangiographic evidence, Spine 2:100, 1977.

Hukuda, S., Mochizuki, T., Ogata, M., and Shichikawa, K.: The pattern of spinal and extraspinal hyperostosis in patients with ossification of the posterior longitudinal ligament and the ligamentum flavum causing myelopathy, Skel. Rad. 10:79, 1983.

Jacobs, B., Krueger, E.G., and Leivy, D.M.: Cervical spondylosis with radiculopathy, JAMA 211:2135, 1970.

Kimura, I., Oh-hama, M., Shingu, H., and Shingu, H.: Cervical myelopathy treated by canal-expansive laminaplasty, J. Bone Joint Surg. 66-A:914, 1984.

Kubota, M., Baba, I., and Sumida, T.: Myelopathy due to ossification of the ligamentum flavum of the cervical spine: a report of two cases, Spine 6:553, 1981.

Lunsford, L.D., Bissonette, D.J., and Zorub, D.S.: Anterior surgery for cervical disc disease. Part 2. Treatment of cervical spondylotic myelopathy in 32 cases, J. Neurosurg. 53:12, 1980.

Mayfield, F.H.: Cervical spondylosis: a comparison of the anterior and posterior approaches, Clin. Neurosurg. 13:181, 1966.

Ono, K., Ota, H., Tada, K., and Yamamoto, T.: Cervical myelopathy secondary to multiple spondylotic protrusions: a clinicopathologic study, Spine 2:109, 1977.

Robinson, R.A., Afeiche, N., Dunn, E.J., and Northrup, B.E.: Cervical spondylotic myelopathy: etiology and treatment concepts, Spine 2:89, 1977.

Tsuji, H.: Laminoplasty for patients with compressive myelopathy due to so-called spinal canal stenosis in cervical and thoracic regions, Spine 7:28, 1982.

Veidlinger, O.F., Colwill, J.C., Smyth, H.S., and Turner, D.: Cervical myelopathy and its relationship to cervical stenosis, Spine 6:550, 1981.

Zanasi, R., Fioretta, G., Rotolo, F., and Zanasi, L.: "Open door" operation to raise the vertebral arch in myelopathy due to cervical spondylosis, Ital. J. Orthop. Traumatol. 10:21, 1984.

Zhang, Z., et al.: Anterior intervertebral disc excision and bone grafting in cervical spondylotic myelopathy, Spine 8:16, 1983.

Tumors

Aarabi, B., Pasternak, G., Hurko, O., and Long, D.M.: Familial intradural arachnoid cysts: report of two cases, J. Neurosurg. 50:826, 1979.

Archer, C.R., and Smith, K.R., Jr.: Extradural lipomatosis simulating an acute herniated nucleus pulposus: case report, J. Neurosurg. 57:559, 1982.

Asnis, S.E., Lesniewski, P., and Dowling, T., Jr.: Anterior decompression and stabilization with methylmethacrylate and a bone bolt for treatment of pathologic fractures of the cervical spine: a report of two cases, Clin. Orthop. 187:139, 1984.

Boruta, P.M., and LaBan, M.M.: Electromyographic findings in patients with low back pain due to unsuspected primary and metastatic spinal or paraspinal muscle disease, Clin. Orthop. 161:235, 1981.

Breuer, A.C., Kneisley, L.W., and Fischer, E.G.: Treatable extramedullary cord compression: meningioma as a cause of the Brown-Sequard syndrome, Spine 5:19, 1980.

Broderick, T.W., Resnick, D., Goergen, T.G., and Alazraki, N.: Enostosis of the spine, Spine 3:167, 1978.

Calderoni, P., Gusella, A., and Martucci, E.: Multiple osteoid osteoma in the 7th dorsal vertebra, Ital. J. Orthop. Traumatol. 10:257, 1984.

Cantore, G., Ciappetta, P., Delfini, R., Vagnozzi, R., and Nolletti, A.: Intramedullary spinal neurinomas: report of two cases, J. Neurosurg. 57:143, 1982.

Capanna, R., et al.: Aneurysmal bone cyst of the spine, J. Bone Joint Surg. 67-A:527, 1985.

Cattell, H.S., and Clark, G.L.: Cervical kyphosis and instability following multiple laminectomies in children, J. Bone Joint Surg. 49-A:713, 1967.

Chadduck, W.M., and Boop, W.C., Jr.: Acrylic stabilization of the cervical spine for neoplastic disease: evolution of a technique for vertebral body replacement, Neurosurgery 13:23, 1983.

Clark, C.R., Keggi, K.J., and Panjabi, M.M.: Methylmethacrylate stabilization of the cervical spine, J. Bone Joint Surg. 66-A:40, 1984.

Clarke, H.A., and Fleming, I.D.: Disk disease and occult malignancies, South. Med. J. 66:449, 1973.

Conley, R.K., Britt, R.H., Hanbery, J.W., and Silverberg, G.D.: Anterior fibular strut graft in neoplastic disease of the cervical spine, J. Neurosurg. 51:677, 1979.

Constans, J.P., et al.: Spinal metastases with neurological manifestations: review of 600 cases, J. Neurosurg. 59:111, 1983.

Cross, G.O., White, H.L., and White, L.P.: Acrylic prosthesis of the fifth cervical vertebra in multiple myeloma: technical note, J. Neurosurg. 35:112, 1971.

Cusick, J.F., Larson, S.J., Walsh, P.R., and Steiner, R.E.: Distraction rod stabilization in the treatment of metastatic carcinoma, J. Neurosurg. 59:861, 1983.

Dawson, W.B.: Growth impairment following irradiation in childhood, Clin. Radiol. 19:241, 1968.

Decker, R.E., Augustin, W.S., and Epstein, J.A.: Spinal epidural venous angioma causing foraminal enlargement and erosion of a vertebral body, J. Neurosurg. 49:605, 1978.

DeSousa, A.L., Kalsbeck, J.E., Mealey, J., Jr., Campbell, R.L., and Hockey, A.: Intraspinal tumors in children: a review of 81 cases, J. Neurosurg. 51:437, 1979.

DeWald, R.L., et al.: Reconstructive spinal surgery as palliation for metastatic malignancies of the spine, Spine 10:21, 1985.

Dunn, E.J.: The role of methyl methacrylate in the stabilization and replacement of tumors of the cervical spine, Spine 2:15, 1977.

Evans, J.A., and Lougheed, W.L.M.: Intradural cysts of the cervical spine: report of three cases, J. Bone Joint Surg. 60-A:123, 1978.

Ferris, R.A., et al.: Eosinophilic granuloma of the spine: an unusual radiographic presentation, Clin. Orthop. 99:57, 1974.

Fett, H.C., and Russo, V.P.: Osteoid osteoma of a cervical vertebra: report of a case, J. Bone Joint Surg. 41-A:948, 1959.

Fidler, M.W.: Pathological fractures of the cervical spine: palliative surgical treatment, J. Bone Joint Surg. 67-B:352, 1985.

Fielding, J.W., Fietti, V.G., Hughes, J.E.O., and Gabrielian, J.Z.: Primary osteogenic sarcoma of the cervical spine: a case report, J. Bone Joint Surg. 58-A:892, 1976.

Flatley, T.J., Anderson, M.H., and Anast, G.T.: Spinal instability due to malignant disease: treatment by segmental spinal stabilization, J. Bone Joint Surg. 66-A:47, 1984.

Fornasier, V.L., and Czitrom, A.A.: Collapsed vertebrae: a review of 659 autopsies, Clin. Orthop. 131:261, 1978.

Fountain, S.S.: A single-stage combined surgical approach for vertebral resections, J. Bone Joint Surg. 61-A:1011, 1979.

Fraser, R.D., Paterson, D.C., and Simpson, D.A.: Orthopaedic aspects of spinal tumours in children, J. Bone Joint Surg. 59-B:143, 1977.

Gelberman, R.H., and Olson, C.O.: Benign osteoblastoma of the atlas: a case report, J. Bone Joint Surg. 56-A:808, 1974.

Glenn, J.N., Reckling, F.W., and Mantz, F.A.: Malignant hemangioendothelioma in a lumbar vertebra: a rare tumor in an unusual location, J. Bone Joint Surg. 56-A:1279, 1974.

Goldberg, M.J., Belsky, R., Brader, I., and Prager, H.J.: Solitary osteochondroma of the cervical spine, Orthopedics 3:759, 1980.

Gore, D.R., and Mueller, H.A.: Osteoid-osteoma of the spine with localization aided by 99 mTc-polyphosphate bone scan: case report, Clin. Orthop. 113:132, 1975.

Griffin, J.B.: Benign osteoblastoma of the thoracic spine: case report with fifteen-year follow-up, J. Bone Joint Surg. 60-A:833, 1978.

Guarnaschelli, J.J., Wehry, S.M., Serratoni, F.T., and Dzenitis, A.J.: Atypical fibrous histiocytoma of the thoracic spine: case report, J. Neurosurg. 51:415, 1979.

Guegan, Y., Fardoun, R., Launois, B., and Pecker, J.: Spinal cord compression by extradural fat after prolonged corticosteroid therapy: case report, J. Neurosurg. 56:267, 1982.

Haft, H., Ransohoff, J., and Carter, S.: Spinal cord tumors in children, Pediatrics 23:1152, 1959.

Hamby, W.B., and Glaser, H.T.: Replacement of spinal intervertebral discs with locally polymerizing methyl methacrylate: experimental study of effects upon tissues and report of a small clinical series, J. Neurosurg. 16:311, 1959.

Hansebout, R.R., and Blomquist, G.A., Jr.: Acrylic spinal fusion: a 20-year clinical series and technical note, J. Neurosurg. 53:606, 1980.

Hejgaard, N., and Larsen, E.: Value of early attention to spinal compression syndromes, Acta Orthop. Scand. 55:234, 1984.

Ingraham, F.D., and Matson, D.D.: Neurosurgery of infancy and childhood, Springfield, Ill., 1954, Charles C Thomas, Publisher.

Jaffe, H.L.: "Osteoidosteoma." Benign osteoblastic tumour composed of osteoid and atypical bone, Arch. Surg. **31:**709, 1935.

Kagan, A.R.: Diagnostic oncology case study: lytic spine lesion and cold bone scan, AJR **136:**129, 1981.

Katzman, H., Waugh, T., and Berdon, W.: Skeletal changes following irradiation of childhood tumors, J. Bone Joint Surg. **51-A:**825, 1969.

Kawabata, M., Sugiyama, M., Suzuki, T., and Kumano, K.: The role of metal and bone cement fixation in the management of malignant lesions of the vertebral column, Int. Orthop. **4:**177, 1980.

Keggi, K.J., Southwick, W.O., and Keller, D.J.: Stabilization of the spine using methylmethacrylate (abstract), J. Bone Joint Surg. **58-A:**738, 1976.

Ker, N.B., and Jones, C.B.: Tumours of the cauda equina: the problem of differential diagnosis, J. Bone Joint Surg. **67-B:**358, 1985.

Kirwan, E.O.G., Hutton, P.A.N., Pozo, J.L., and Ransford, A.O.: Osteoid osteoma and benign osteoblastoma of the spine: clinical presentation and treatment, J. Bone Joint Surg. **66-B:**21, 1984.

Kleinman, G.M., Dagi, F., and Poletti, C.E.: Villonodular synovitis in the spinal canal: case report, J. Neurosurg. **52:**846, 1980.

Kwok, D.M.F., and Jeffreys, R.V.: Intramedullary enterogenous cyst of the spinal cord: case report, J. Neurosurg. **56:**270, 1982.

Leaney, B.J., and Calvert, J.M.: Tophaceous gout producing spinal cord compression: case report, J. Neurosurg. **58:**580, 1983.

Lindholm, T.S., Snellman, O., and Osterman, K.: Scoliosis caused by benign osteoblastoma of the lumbar spine: a report of three patients, Spine **2:**276, 1977.

Maresca, L., Meland, N.B., Maresca, C., and Field, E.M.: Ganglion cyst of the spinal canal: case report, J. Neurosurg. **57:**140, 1982.

McCarthy, E.F., and Dorfman, H.D.: Idiopathic segmental sclerosis of vertebral bodies, Skel. Radiol. **9:**88, 1982.

McCrum, C., and Williams, B.: Spinal extradural arachnoid pouches: report of two cases, J. Neurosurg. **57:**849, 1982.

Nagashima, C., Iwasaki, T., Okada, K., and Sakaguchi, A.: Reconstruction of the atlas and axis with wire and acrylic after metastatic destruction: case report, J. Neurosurg. **50:**668, 1979.

Neuhauser, E.B.D., et al.: Irradiation effects of roentgen therapy on the growing spine: Radiology **59:**637, 1952.

Palmer, F.J., and Blum, P.W.: Osteochondroma with spinal cord compression: report of three cases, J. Neurosurg. **52:**842, 1980.

Panjabi, M.M., et al.: Biomechanical study of cervical spine stabilization with methylmethacrylate, Spine **10:**198, 1985.

Postacchini, F., Urso, S., and Tovaglia, V.: Lumbosacral intradural tumours simulating disc disease, Int. Orthop. **5:**283, 1981.

Probert, J.C., Parker, B.R., and Kaplan, H.S.: Growth retardation in children after megavoltage irradiation of the spine, Cancer **32:**634, 1973.

Ransford, A.O., Pozo, J.L., Hutton, P.A.N., and Kirwan, E.O.G.: The behaviour pattern of the scoliosis associated with osteoid osteoma or osteoblastoma of the spine, J. Bone Joint Surg. **66-B:**16, 1984.

Raycroft, J.F., Hockman, R.P., Albright, J.A., and Southwick, W.O.: Surgery of malignant tumors of the cervical spine, J. Bone Joint Surg. **54-A:**1794, 1972.

Raycroft, J.F., Hockman, R.P., and Southwick, W.O.: Metastatic tumors involving the cervical vertebrae: surgical palliation, J. Bone Joint Surg. **60-A:**763, 1978.

Resnick, D.: The sclerotic vertebral body, JAMA **249:**1761, 1983.

Riseborough, E.J., Grabias, S.L., Burton, R.I., and Jaffe, N.: Skeletal alterations following irradiation for Wilms' tumor, with particular reference to scoliosis and kyphosis, J. Bone Joint Surg. **58-A:**526, 1976.

Schaberg, J., and Gainor, B.J.: A profile of metastatic carcinoma of the spine, Spine **10:**19, 1985.

Scoville, W.B., Palmer, A.H., Samra, K., and Chong, G.: The use of acrylic plastic for vertebral replacement or fixation in metastatic disease of the spine, J. Neurosurg. **27:**274, 1967.

Siegal, T., Tiqva, P., and Siegal, T.: Vertebral body resection for epidural compression by malignant tumors: results of forty-seven consecutive operative procedures, J. Bone Joint Surg. **67-A:**375, 1985.

Silverberg, I.J., and Jacobs, E.M.: Treatment of spinal cord compression in Hodgkin's disease, Cancer **27:**308, 1971.

Simmons, E.H., and Grobler, L.J.: Acute spinal epidural hematoma: a case report, J. Bone Joint Surg. **60-A:**395, 1978.

Stener, B.: Total spondylectomy in chondrosarcoma arising from the seventh thoracic vertebra, J. Bone Joint Surg. **53-B:**288, 1971.

Stener, B., and Gunterberg, B.: High amputation of the sacrum for extirpation of tumors: principles and technique, Spine **3:**351, 1978.

Stener, B., and Johnsen, O.E.: Complete removal of three vertebrae for giant-cell tumour, J. Bone Joint Surg. **53-B:**278, 1971.

Stevens, W.W., and Weaver, E.N.: Giant cell tumors and aneurysmal bone cysts of the spine: report of four cases, South. Med. J. **63:**218, 1970.

Stillwell, W.T., and Fielding, J.W.: Aneurysmal bone cyst of the cervicodorsal spine, Clin. Orthop. **187:**144, 1984.

Suit, H.D., et al.: Definitive radiation therapy for chordoma and chondrosarcoma of base of skull and cervical spine, J. Neurosurg. **56:**377, 1982.

Sundaresan, N., Galicich, J.H., Lane, J.M., and Greenberg, H.S.: Treatment of odontoid fractures in cancer patients, J. Neurosurg. **54:**187, 1981.

Symeonides, P.P.: Osteoid osteoma of the lumbar spine, South. Med. J. **63:**975, 1970.

Tachdjian, M.O., and Matson, D.D.: Orthopaedic aspects of intraspinal tumors in infants and children, J. Bone Joint Surg. **47-A:**223, 1965.

Turner, M.L., Mulhern, C.B., and Dalinka, M.K.: Lesions of the sacrum: differential diagnosis and radiological evaluation, JAMA **245:**275, 1981.

Wald, S.L., McLennan, J.E., Carroll, R.M., and Segal, H.: Extradural spinal involvement by gout: case report, J. Neurosurg. **50:**236, 1979.

Wang, G., et al.: Comparative strengths of various anterior cement fixations of the cervical spine, Spine **8:**717, 1983.

Wang, G., Reger, S.I., McLaughlin, R.E., Stamp, W.G., and Albin, D.: The safety of cement fixation in the cervical spine: studies of a rabbit model, Clin. Orthop. **139:**276, 1979.

Wang, G., et al.: Safety of anterior cement fixation in the cervical spine: in vivo study of dog spine, South. Med. J. **77:**178, 1984.

White, W.A., Patterson, R.H., Jr., and Bergland, R.M.: Role of surgery in the treatment of spinal cord compression by metastatic neoplasm, Cancer **27:**558, 1971.

Whitehill, R., et al.: Use of methylmethacrylate cement as an instantaneous fusion mass in posterior cervical fusions: a canine in vivo experimental model, Spine **9:**246, 1984.

Wilkinson, R.H., and Hall, J.E.: The sclerotic pedicle: tumor or pseudotumor? Radiology **111:**683, 1974.

Young, R.F., Post, E.M., and King, G.A.: Treatment of spinal epidural metastases: randomized prospective comparison of laminectomy and radiotherapy, J. Neurosurg. **53:**741, 1980.

Growth problems

Dawson, W.B.: Growth impairment following radiotherapy in childhood, Clin. Radiol. **19:**241, 1968.

Mayfield, J.K., Erkkila, J.C., and Winter, R.B.: Spine deformity subsequent to acquired childhood spinal cord injury, J. Bone Joint Surg. **63-A:**1401, 1981.

Probert, J.C., Parker, B.R., and Kaplan, H.S.: Growth retardation in children after megavoltage irradiation of the spine, Cancer **32:**634, 1973.

Riseborough, E.J., Grabias, S.L., Burton, R.I., and Jaffe, N.: Skeletal alteration following irradiation for Wilms' tumor, with particular reference to scoliosis and kyphosis, J. Bone Joint Surg. **58-A:**526, 1976.

White, W.A., Patterson, R.H., Jr., and Bergland, R.M.: Role of surgery in the treatment of spinal cord compression by metastatic neoplasm, Cancer **27:**558, 1971.

Yasuoka, S., Peterson, H.A., and MacCarty, C.S.: Incidence of spinal column deformity after multilevel laminectomy in children and adults, J. Neurosurg. **57:**441, 1982.

Miscellaneous anomalies

Bernard, T.N., Jr., Burke, S.W., Johnston, C.E., III, and Roberts, J.M.: Congenital spine deformities: a review of 47 cases, Orthopedics **8:**777, 1985.

Bethem, D., et al.: Spinal disorders of dwarfism: review of the literature and report of eighty cases, J. Bone Joint Surg. **63-A:**1412, 1981.

Kahanovitz, N., Rimoin, D.L., and Sillence, D.O.: The clinical spectrum of lumbar spine disease in achondroplasia, Spine **7:**137, 1982.

Mattews, L.S., Vetter, W.L., and Tolo, V.T.: Cervical anomaly simulating hangman's fracture in a child: case report, J. Bone Joint Surg. **64-A:**299, 1982.

Author Index

Subject index

Arthritic hand—cont'd
  postoperative splint and cast immobilization
      in, 381
  progressive systemic sclerosis and, 380
  psoriatic arthritis and, 378
  Reiter's syndrome and, 378
  rheumatoid arthritis and, 378
  scleroderma and, 380
  staging of operations in, 380
  tendon rupture in, 391-392
  tenosynovitis of flexor tendon sheaths in,
      392-393
  thumb deformities in, 393-400
    carpometacarpal joint, 396-400
    infection after silastic prosthesis insertion
        and, 400
    metacarpophalangeal joint, 393-395
    synovectomy of interphalangeal joint, 400
  ulnar drift or deviation of fingers in, 385-
      391
  wrist deformities in, 401-404
    arthrodesis versus arthroplasty in, 402-403
    synovitis and, 401-402
    total wrist prosthesis in, 403-404
Arthritis
  degenerative, 1413, 1417
    spinal stenosis and, 3347
    total hip arthroplasty and, 1330, 1331,
        1332, 1333, 1364, 1368
  of elbow, 2514, 2515
  of foot, 964-978
  intrapelvic protrusion of acetabulum and,
      1361, 1363
  infectious; see Infectious arthritis
  greater trochanter fracture with, 1364, 1368
  of hand; see Arthritic hand
  Marie-Strümpell, 1342
  psoriatic, 1330
  shoulder arthroscopy and, 2609
  spinal, 3363-3366
  traumatic
    ankle, 2268
    elbow, 2514, 2515
    patellar affections and, 2477
Arthrodesis, 1091; see also Fusion
  ankle, 1091-1106, 2957
    Adams, 1099
    anterior, 1092-1099
    Barr and Record, 2961
    compression, 1093, 1094
    equinovarus deformity and, 2961
    Garceau and Brahms, 2961
    Horwitz, 1099
    intraarticular, 1106
    malunited fracture and, 2023
    posterior, 1104-1106
    revision of, 1154
    talipes equinus and, 2951
    transmalleolar techniques of, 1099-1104
  bony ankylosis and, 1091
  of calcaneocuboid joint, 2644-2645
  of calcaneonavicular coalition, triple, 913
  of calcaneus, 1624, 2018, 2967, 2968
  cervical
    Robinson and Riley, 3150-3151
    Whitecloud and Larocca, 3151

Arthrodesis—cont'd
  dorsal and lumbar spine; see Spinal
      arthrodesis, dorsal and lumbar
  of elbow, 1140-1144
  of first carpometacarpal joint, 330
  flexor digitorum sublimis function and, 156
  of foot
    calcaneocuboid joint, 2644-2645
    calcaneonavicular coalition, triple, 913
    calcaneus, 1624, 2018, 2967, 2968
    cone, hallux rigidus and, 889-890
    clubfoot and, 2640
    first metarsal-first cuneiform and first
        cuneiform-navicular joint, 892-894
    first metatarsophalangeal joint, 877-879,
        886-889, 973, 974
    Grice subtalar extraarticular, 2871, 2872-
        2873
    hallux varus and, 847
    hammertoe and, 941, 942, 944-945
    navicular, 895, 989
    pantalar, 2950-2951, 2968
    pes planus and, 892-894, 897-899
    primary triple, 1624
    spinal bifida and, 3031-3032
    subtalar, 2019-2020, 2871-2873, 2963
    talar, 2017
    talocalcaneal coalition and, 916-917
    triplane, pes planus and, 897-899
  hand and, 280-283
  hemophilia and, 1063
  of hip, 1091, 1113-1127
    cerebral palsy and, 2907
    Charcot, 1059-1060
    difficult and unusual cases in, 1125-1127
    extraarticular, 1116-1118
    Gill, nonunion of femoral neck and, 2091
    internal fixation techniques in, 1118-1121
    intraarticular, 1115-1118
    osteoarthritis and, 1047
    paralytic dislocation and, 2997
    rheumatoid arthritis and, 1014
    tuberculosis and, 705
  incision for, 119
  interphalangeal joint
    hammertoe and, 941, 942, 944-945
    poliomyelitis and, 2940
    Shriver and Johnson technique for, 848-
        851
    ulnar drift and, 388-391
  intraarticular, grafts and, 1092
  of knee, 1106-1113; see also Knee,
      arthrodesis of
  metacarpophalangeal joint, 393-395
    thumb, 330
  metatarsal, first cuneiform, and first
      cuneiform-navicular joint, 892-894
  metatarsophalangeal joint of hallux, 877-
      879, 886-889, 973, 974
  osteochondrosis of navicular and, 989
  pantalar, 2968
    talipes equinus and, 2950-2951
  pes planus and, 892-894
  of phalangeal joint, buttonhole deformity
      and, 385
  postpoliomyelitis and, 2927, 2933-2934,
      2935

Arthrodesis—cont'd
  sacroiliac joint, 1127
  of shoulder, 1016, 1131-1139
    poliomyelitis and, 3009-3010
  spinal; see Spinal arthrodesis
  subtalar, 2019-2020
  talar, 2017
  total hip arthroplasty versus, 1265
  triple
    calcaneus, 2018
    Charcot-Marie-Tooth disease and, 3083
    clubfoot and, 2640
    pes planus and, 897-899
    poliomyelitis and, 2933-2934, 2935
    Siffert, Forster, and Nachamie technique
        for talipes calcaneus, 2967
    for talipes calcaneocavus, 2968
    talocalcaneal coalition and, 916-917
  trophic joint disorders and, 1057
  upper extremity, 1131-1144
  of wrist, 105, 401, 402-403
    disadvantages of, 2930
    hand fractures, 222-225
    Millender and Nalebuff, 402
    reduplication of ulna and, 438
Arthrofibrosis, knee, 2602
Arthrography
  ankle, Gordon and Broström technique for,
      2268
  hip dislocation and
    congenital, 2727-2721
    recurrent, 2184, 2185
  knee, 2307-2308
  shoulder, pathognomonic sign in, 2508
Arthrogryposis multiplex congenita, 2926,
    3035-3042, 3227
  congenital dislocation of patella and, 2681
  deformities in, 3035, 3037
Arthrokatadysis, 1060, 1361, 1363
Arthrometer, stress-testing, 2327
Arthro-onycho-dsyplasia, 2668
Arthropathy
  cuff-tear, 2507
  hemophilic, 1148
  total knee arthroplasty and, 1158
Arthroplasty
  abrasion, arthroscopy and, 2602-2603
  ankle, 1145-1152
  Charnley, successful, 1434
  cup
    osteoarthritis of hip and, 1047
    total hip procedures for, 1375-1378, 1379
  elbow, 1524-1551; see also Elbow
    complications of, 1536-1540
    fascial, 1019, 1533-1536
    history of, 1524
    interpositional, 1533-1536
    rheumatoid arthritis and, 1019
    types of, 1529-1533
  forefoot, 968
  hallux rigidus and, 886
  hallux varus and, 847
  hand, 283-284
    Ashworth technique for, 396
    carpometacarpal joint, 393, 396-400
    Eaton carpometacarpal, 398
    implant, 393, 396-400

Myelography
cervical, 3282, 3283
computed tomography after, 3262
indications for, 3259-3260
lower back pain and, 3259-3262
technical complications of, 3262
technique of, 3261-3262
Myelolipoma, 812
Myeloma
bone, 792-797
multiple, 792, 793, 794
solitary, 792, 794-795, 796
Myeloma kidney, 796
Myelomeningocele, 3226-3227
epidemiology of, 3024
general considerations of, 3024
neurologic lesion and deformity in, 3024-3027
orthopaedic management of, 3027-3035
prevention of, 3024
Myelopathy, cervical, 1073, 3278-3279
Myoblastoma, granular cell, 818
Myocardial infarction, 1242, 1460
Myoglobin, 530
Myositis
ischemic, 2221-2225
proliferative, 809
Myositis fibrosa, progressive, 810
Myositis ossificans, 809, 821-823
Myotomy
cerebral palsy and, 2877
thumb intrinsic muscle, 374
Myotonic dystrophy, 3061, 3079-3080
Myxoid tumor well-differentiated, 812
chondrosarcoma, 819
Myxoma, 818-819

N

Nafcillin, 1446
Nahai tensor fascia lata flap, 554
Nail(ing)
Calandruccio, 1758, 1762
and congenital pseudarthrosis of fibula and tibia, 2676-2677
femoral shaft, 1683
interlocking, 1695-1704, 1746
Schneider technique for, 1690-1691
Harris condylocephalic
intertrochanteric fractures and, 1737-1741
subtrochanteric fractures and, 1746
Jewett; see Jewett nail
Küntscher; see Küntscher nail
Lottes, 1637, 1641, 1643-1646
Massie, 1758, 1766
medullary, 2074
bending of, 1706, 1707
Christenson method of, 2079-2082
contraindications to, 1683, 1687-1689
diameter of, 1580
failed insertion of, 2672, 2673
Grosse-Kempf interlocking, 1701-1704
humeral nonunions and, 2094
knee arthrodesis and, 1106
loose, in canal, 1704, 1706
miscalculation of length and diameter of, 1704

Nail(ing)—cont'd
medullary—cont'd
nonunions and, 2077, 2078
osteogenesis imperfecta and, 1069-1073
transarticular, Beall, Waebel, and Bailey technique with, 2077, 2078
prophylactic, 799, 800
Pugh, 1758
Russell-Taylor interlocking, 1746
Smith-Petersen, hip arthrodesis and, 1114
tibial shaft fracture and, 1637, 1641, 1646-1653
Zickel, 1743-1746
Nail fold removal or reduction, ingrown toenail and, 926-932
Nail guide pin, 1698
Nail plate devices
femoral neck fractures and, 1766
subtrochanteric fractures and, 1741-1746
Nail-patella syndrome, 2668
Nalebuff and Millender lateral band mobilization and skin release, 384
Narcotic analgesics, 533
Nassif parascapular flap, 562
Natatory ligament, 247
National Academy of Science Committee on Prosthetic Research and Development, 597
Navicular
accessory, 903-908
clubfoot and, 2635-2636
osteochondrosis of, 989
tuberculosis of foot and, 701
Navicular pads, 891
Navicular end first cuneiform arthrodesis, 894
Naviculocapitate fracture syndrome, 213
Neck
cervical spine fusion for, 3002
drainage of abscess of posterior triangle, 3330
exercises for, 3283
motion limitation of, 3280
pain of, 3283
paralysis of muscles of, 3000-3002
Necrosis
abdominal flap and, 145
amputation and, 605
avascular; see Avascular necrosis
irreversible, 524
skin, after replantation, 533-534
around sutures, 122, 123
Needle biopsy
of knee, 1007
tumor and, 714-716
Needle test, tendon rupture and, 2226
Needling and aspiration of calcified deposits, 2502-2503
Neer classification of shoulder displaced fractures and fracture- dislocations, 1672, 1787-1788
type III and type IV fracture in, 1889
Neer prosthesis, 1506, 1507, 1791-1794
giant cell tumor of, 767
humeral nonunions and, 2093-2094
Neer II thicker humeral component in, 1513
two neck lengths of, 1506-1508

Neer technique
for acromioplasty, 2505, 2506, 2509-2510
for hemiarthroplasty, 1505-1508
for open reduction and internal fixation of three-part greater tuberosity segment, 1798-1791
for proximal humeral prosthetic replacement, 1791-1794
for total shoulder arthroplasty, unconstrained, 1508-1518
Neibauer and Glynn transection of brachialis, 2521
Neisseria, 501
Neonate; *see* Newborn
Nerve; *see also* Nerve graft; Nerve injuries; Nerve repair
acute hand injury and, 139
age and, 2796
anatomy of, 2785, 2786
axillary, deltoid and teres paralysis of, 2810
conduction studies of, 2794
crossing of, 2803
damage to, arthroscopy and, 2543-2544
degeneration and regeneration of, 2787-2788
delay between time of injury and repair of, 2796-2798
disease of, differentiated from muscle disease, 3061-3064
effects of injury to, 2789-2792
fibers of, myelinated, 2785, 2786
hand
regeneration of, 232
technique of suture of, 231
injury to; see Nerve injuries
inspection of hand injury and, 141
limb lengthening and, 2700
median, injury to, 2792, 2793
mixed spinal, 2784
peripheral
anatomy of, 231
suture of, 231
tumors of, 817-818
peroneal, injury to, 2792
radial
injury to, 2792-2793
paralysis of elbow, wrist, fingers and, 2810
repair of; see Nerve repair
spinal, anatomy of, 2784-2787
stress-strain relationship in, 3187
subscapular, 2810
thoracodorsal, paralysis of latissimus dorsi and, 2810
tibial, injury to, 2792, 2793
transplantation and, 2802
ulnar, injury to, 2792
Nerve block
phenol, stroke and, 2914
replantation and, 533
Nerve deficit, 2799
Nerve ends
condition of, 2799
gap between; see Nerve gaps
Nerve gaps, 2796
methods of closing, 2796, 2802-2803

Steroids—cont'd
  avascular necrosis and, 1334
  epidural, 3265
    back pain and, 3293-3294
    spinal stenosis and, 3350
  osteitis pubis and, 1061
  postoperative infection and, 1444
  rheumatoid arthritis and, 1332, 1334, 1335
    foot, 968
    hand and, 377, 380, 385
  tendon rupture and, 2226
  tenosynovitis and, 462
Steward technique for acromioclavicular joint
    dislocation, 2146, 2147
Steward and Harley ankle arthrodesis, 1100-
    1102
  modifications of, 1102, 1103
Stewart technique
  for styloidectomy, 1048
  for tendo calcaneus lengthening, 2640, 2641
STH-2; see Sarmiento femoral component
Stiles-Bunnell transfer, Burkhalter modification
    of, 345, 352, 354
Still's disease, 1330
Stimulation of muscle, electric, stroke patients
    and, 2914
Stimulation therapy, sensorimotor, 2850
Stockinette, hand surgery and, 128, 129, 130
Stone staple, 12, 14
  posterolateral rotary instability
    reconstruction and, 2394
Stone hip arthrodesis, 1114-1115
Stool for surgeon, 111
Stoop test, 3349
Storen intraepiphyseal osteotomy, Siffert
    modification of, 1067-1068
Storen modification
  of Irwin osteotomy, 2979
Straight leg raising test, 3255, 3280, 3291
Straight tension band plate, 1567-1574
Straight-stemmed metal hinged elbow, 1524
Strain, definition of, 2325; see also Sprain
Straub technique for congenital absence of
    ulna, 448
Strawberry hemangioma, 813-814
Strayer technique for gastrocnemius
    lengthening, 2861-2862, 2863
Street diamond-shaped nail insertion, 1690-
    1691
Street and Stevens humeral replacement, 1547-
    1548
Streptococci
  hematogenous osteomyelitis and, 652
  human bite injury and, 501
  spinal infections and, 3323-3324
  total hip arthroplasty and, 1446, 1447
    revision of, 1462, 1486
Streptokinase, 1460
Streptomycin
  Pott's disease and, 3337
  total hip arthroplasty and, 1446
Stress
  acetabulum and distribution of, 1228, 1230
  arthrometers for testing, 2327; see also
    Stress test
  to femur, 1228; see also Stress fracture
  knee, 2548

Stress—cont'd
  in pelvis, 1228, 1230
  per unit area, ankle trauma and, 2268
Stress fracture
  femoral neck, 1768, 1907, 1908
  metatarsal, 1995
    after Keller procedure, 856-857
  Paget's disease and, 1337
Stress roentgenogram
  ankle trauma and, 2271
  proximal tibial epiphyseal fracture and,
    1964, 1965
Stress test
  ankle trauma and, 2266, 2267
  for knee, 2327-2330
Stress-strain diagram, 1231, 1232
Stress-testing arthrometers, 2327
Stretch test, cervical spine injury and, 3111
Stretching
  of clubfoot in newborn, 2638
  nerve, 6
  stroke and, 2911
Strickland tendon repair in zone II, 156, 158-
    159, 160
Stroke, lower extremity deformities and, 2910-
    2913
Struthers
  arcade of, 2821
  ligament of, 2824
Stryker dermatome, 124
Stump, amputation
  dressing of, 603-605
  as footlike end organ, 607
  painful, 305
  unsatisfactory Syme, 609
Styloidectomy, 1048
  nonunion of scaphoid hand fractures and,
    210
Subacromial bursitis, 1016-1017, 2258
Subacute osteomyelitis, 657
Subaxial subluxation, 3363
Subchondral bone
  excision of defects of, 2479
  Müller hip arthroplasty and, 1292
Subclavian steal syndrome, 2775, 2776
Subclavius, 2186
Subcondylar osteotomy, 2026
Subcutaneous fasciotomy, Dupuytren's
    contracture and, 453-455
Subcutaneous fat dissection, 144, 145
Subcutaneous fibroplasia, 451, 808
Subcutaneous tenotomy, 2759-2762
  adductor; see Adductor tenotomy
  tibialis posterior, 3071
Subdeltoid bursitis, 2258
Subepidermal nodular fibrosis, 819
Subgluteal bursa, 2257
Sublimis tendon
  repair of
    primary suture, 160-162
    zone II, 156
    zone V, 157
  rupture of, 392
  severed, 150
  tenodesis of, Curtis, 374
  transfer of
    Brand, 332, 337

Sublimis tendon—cont'd
  transfer of—cont'd
    Groves and Goldner, 333-335
    Omer, 337
    paralytic hand and, 333-335
    Riordan, 330-332
Subluxation; see also Dislocation
  atlantoaxial, 3363
  of C1 on C2, rotary, 3117-3118
  elbow, 2212
  glenohumeral, 2810
  hip
    cerebral palsy and, 2896, 2897, 2902
    congenital, 2729, 2730, 2733; see also
      Congenital dislocation of hip
    spina bifida and, 3033
  knee, 2678
    poliomyelitis and, 2985
  metacarpophalangeal joint, 387
  patellar, 1201, 2175, 2478
    cerebral palsy and, 2890-2891
  shoulder, 2187, 2250
    arthroscopy in, 2610
  subaxial, 3363
  term of, 2713
  thumb, 241; see also Thumb
  of toe, 2627
  total hip arthroplasty and, 1345-1356
    complications of, 1151, 1405-1412
  ulnar, 380, 387
Subpatellar crepitus, 2477
Subpectoral flap, 142
Subperiosteal decortication, 2079
Subscapular nerve, 2810
Subscapularis, 2497, 2498
  bursitis of, 2258-2260
  function of, 3003
  paralysis of, 2810
  reattachment of, to humerus, 2196-2198,
    2199
  tendon and muscle transfers for paralysis of,
    3007-3009
Subtalar
  arthrodesis of, 2019-2020
    Gallie, 2020-2021
    Grice, spina bifida and, 3032
    Grice and Green, 2963-2964
    pes planus and, 897-899
    primary, 1624
    talar fractures and, 1613
    talipes equinovalgus and, 2963
    triple, 2018
  biomechanics of, 1148
  dislocation of, 2123-2125
  facets of, angles of middle and posterior,
    915
  fracture treatment and, 1616
Subtotal somatectomy, 3352-3353
Subtrochanteric femoral fracture; see Femur,
    subtrochanteric fractures of
Subtrochanteric osteotomy, 1113
  coxa vara and, 2036, 2750
  hip arthrodesis and, 1121
  valgus, femoral fracture nonunion and,
    1905-1907, 1908-1910
Subungual exostosis, 758
Suction drainage
  total hip arthroplasty and, 1402

Upper extremities—cont'd
paralysis of, cerebral palsy and, 2907-2909
rheumatoid arthritis and, 1015-1020
segmental innervation of muscles of, 3036
stroke and, 2913-2914
Upper plexus injury, 2809
Urbaniak technique for hand, 561-562
in replantation, 530
in wraparound toe flap, 572-576
Urethritis, Reiter's syndrome and, 378
Uric acid, 379
Urinary diversion for incontinence, 3024
Urinary tract complications in total hip
arthroplasty and, 1402
Urine creatine, 3064
Urokinase, 1460

V

V osteotomy, 690, 861
Vac-Pac, 2611
Valgus deformity
femoral
poliomyelitis and, 2997
preoperative determination of, in fracture,
1908-1910
of foot and ankle
in cerebral palsy, 2865, 2870-2873
in rheumatoid foot, 977
triple arthrodesis for, 2935, 2936
hallux; see Hallux valgus
knee
in cerebral palsy, 2889-2890
in rheumatoid arthritis, 1012
after tibial fracture, 1967, 1968, 1969, 1970
total knee arthroplasty and, 1162
Valgus night splint, hallux, 843
Valgus osteotomies
Coventry, through lateral approach, 1023,
1024, 1025-1027
for developmental coxa vara, 2751
MacEwen and Shands technique for,
2728, 2729
femoral fracture nonunion and, 1905-1910
hip osteoarthritis and, 1031
indications for, 1031
proximal tibial osteotomy and, 1022-1025
Valgus position
elbow prosthesis and, 1525
of femoral neck, disadvantage of, 2086-
2087
of hip prosthesis, 1221-1223
Valgus stress test for knee, 2327
Valium; see Diazepam
Van Gorder technique for hip, 59-60
Vancomycin, 1446
Vanillylmandelic acid, 797
Varicose veins, 485
Varus
arthritic knee and, 1012
foot fractures in child and, 1988
Varus deformity
foot
cerebral palsy and, 2865-2870
rheumatoid arthritis and, 977
split tendon transfer for, 2867
stroke and, 2913
triple arthrodesis for, 2935, 2936

Varus deformity—cont'd
hallux
Keller procedure and, 855
modified McBride bunionectomy and,
845-851
rheumatoid foot and, 977
knee
proximal tibial osteotomy and, 1022-1025
total knee arthroplasty and, 1162
Varus osteotomies
femoral, 2729, 2730, 2733
derotational, 996-999, 2186, 2901-2905
hip
compression blade plate for, 1037-1044
congenital subluxation and, 1032
osteoarthritis and, 1031
poliomyelitis and, 2997-2999
wedges cut for, 1042, 1043
of proximal tibia through medial approach,
1023-1025
Varus position of hip prosthesis, 1221-1223
Varus stress
elbow prosthesis and, 1525
knee, 2327-2328
Vasconez tensor fascia lata flap, 554
Vascular bone tumor, 753
Vascular deficiency; see Vascular insufficiency
Vascular disease, peripheral, 598, 607
Vascular insufficiency
femoral neck nonunion and, 2084
knee dislocations with, 2126
total hip arthroplasty complications and,
1400-1401
in Volkmann's ischemia, 409
Vascular spasm
free flap transfer and, 539
microvascular anastomosis and, 512
replantation and, 531, 532-533
Vascularized fibular graft to tibia, 557-558
Vascularized patellar tendon graft, 2439-2441
Vascularized rib grafts, 560
Vasculitis, 378
Vasocystic tumor, 752
Vasomotor paralysis in autonomous zone,
2790
Vasospasm; see Vascular spasm
free flap transfer and, 539
replantation and, 532-533
Vastamäki technique for serratus anterior
paralysis, 3001, 3050-3052
Vastus intermedius contracture, 2247
Vein grafts
compression of ulnar nerve in fibrooseous
tunnel and, 461
harvesting of, 513-514, 531
interpositional, 522
microvascular, 513-514
replantation and, 522, 531
Veins
in dorsum of toes, 563, 565
grafts of; see Vein grafts
toe-to-hand transfer skin marking for, 578
total knee arthroplasty and, 1160
Veleanu, Rosianu, and Ionescu obturator
neurectomy and adductor tenotomy,
2899

Velpeau bandage, 1519-1520, 2243
Venac comitantes, 555
Venous thrombosis, 1160
Ventral spinothalamic tract, 2784
Ventriculoperitoneal shunts, 530
Verdan for osteoplastic thumb reconstruction,
309
Verebelyi-Ogston procedure for spina bifida,
3029, 3031
Verruca plantaris, 952-953
Vertebra; see Spine
Vertebral artery compression, 3279
Vertebral body
corpectomy of, 3136
excision of anterior, for burst fractures,
3138
radiation damage to, 3370
Vertebrectomy, Bohlman technique for
cervical, 3126-3127
Vertical laminar flow room, 1160, 1161, 1270-
1272
Vertical shear disruptions, pelvic fractures and,
1591
Vertical talus, congenital, 2647-2652
Vessel shifting, replantation and, 531; see also
Blood vessels
Vicryl suture in meniscus, 2321
Villonodular synovitis, pigmented, 821, 1006,
1007
Vincular accessorium, 150, 151
Vinertia, ASTM designation of, 1234
Viridans streptococci, 1446
Vitallium
acetabular cup of, femoral focal deficiency
and, 2668
ASTM designation of, 1234
in cap prosthesis for patella, 2481
elbow hinge and, Chatzidakis, 1524
humeral replacement prosthesis of, Neer's,
1791-1794
shoulder arthroplasty and, 1503
tolerance for, 2088
Vitallium-W, ASTM designation of, 1234
Vitamin D, rickets and, 1063, 1064, 1065
VMA; see Vanillylmandelic acid
Volar flap, hand surgery on, 120, 121
Volar forearm incision, 412
Volar ligament reconstruction, Eaton and
Littler, 241, 242
Volar plate
anatomy of, 160, 161
phalangeal neck fracture with interposition
of, 1843
Volar surface of finger, 142
Volar synovectomy, 402
Volar transfer, Volkmann's contracture and,
412
Volar transscaphoid perilunar dislocations, 213
Volkmann's ischemic contracture, 409-418
child and, 1864
definition of, 409
diagnosis of acute ischemia and, 411
established, 412-413
incision in, 412
tibial shaft fractures and, 1636
vascularized nerve grafts and, 584